Augoustides and Kaplan's
CARDIAC ANESTHESIA
REVIEW

Augoustides and Kaplan's
CARDIAC ANESTHESIA REVIEW

JOHN G.T. AUGOUSTIDES, MD, FASE, FAHA

Professor
Anesthesiology and Critical Care
University of Pennsylvania
Philadelphia, Pennsylvania
United States

JOEL A. KAPLAN, MD, FACC

Professor
Anesthesiology
University of California San Diego
San Diego, California;
Dean Emeritus, School of Medicine
Former Chancellor, Health Sciences
University of Louisville
Louisville, Kentucky
United States

ELSEVIER

Elsevier
1600 John F. Kennedy Blvd.
Ste 1800
Philadelphia, PA 19103-2899

AUGOUSTIDES AND KAPLAN'S CARDIAC ANESTHESIA REVIEW   ISBN: 978-0-443-11576-9

Senior Content Development Manager: Somodatta Roy Choudhury
Senior Content Strategist: Kayla Wolfe
Senior Content Development Specialist: Rishabh Gupta
Publishing Services Manager: Shereen Jameel
Project Manager: Vishnu T. Jiji
Senior Designer: Renee Duenow

Printed in India

Last digit is the print number: 9 8 7 6 5 4 3 2

Working together
to grow libraries in
developing countries

www.elsevier.com • www.bookaid.org

To our families and loved ones for their support and understanding.
Thank you to the authors of the chapters in the
7th edition of Kaplan's Cardiac Anesthesia.

John G.T. Augoustides
Joel A. Kaplan

ASSOCIATE EDITORS

Brigid Flynn, MD, FCCM
Professor
Department of Anesthesiology
University of Kansas Medical Center
Kansas City, Kansas
United States

Theresa Anne Gelzinis, MD
Professor
Department of Anesthesiology and Perioperative Medicine
University of Pittsburgh
Pittsburgh, Pennsylvania
United States

Alexander Mittnacht, MD
Professor
Department of Anesthesiology
Westchester Medical Center
Valhalla, New York
United States

Harish Ramakrishna, MD, FACC, FESC, FASE
Professor
Division of Cardiovascular and Thoracic Anesthesiology
Mayo Clinic
Rochester, Minnesota
United States

Matthew M. Townsley, MD, FASE
Professor
Department of Anesthesiology and Perioperative Medicine
University of Alabama at Birmingham
Birmingham, Alabama
United States

Matthew W. Vanneman, MD
Clinical Assistant Professor
Anesthesiology, Perioperative and Pain Medicine
Stanford University School of Medicine
Stanford, California
United States

CONTRIBUTORS

Cheen Alkhatib, MD, BA
Associate Professor
Department of Anesthesiology
University of Kansas Medical Center
Kansas City, Kansas
United States

John G.T. Augoustides, MD, FASE, FAHA
Professor
Anesthesiology and Critical Care
University of Pennsylvania
Philadelphia, Pennsylvania
United States

Daniel Bainbridge, MD, FRCPC
Professor
Department of Anesthesia and Perioperative Medicine
Western University
London, Ontario
Canada

Michael L. Boisen, MS, FASE
Associate Professor
Department of Anesthesiology and Perioperative Medicine
University of Pittsburgh
Pittsburgh, Pennsylvania
United States

Christopher Cassara, MD
Assistant Professor
Department of Anesthesiology
University of Wisconsin
Madison, Wisconsin
United States

Brigid Flynn, MD, FCCM
Professor
Department of Anesthesiology
University of Kansas Medical Center
Kansas City, Kansas
United States

Theresa Anne Gelzinis, MD
Professor
Department of Anesthesiology and Perioperative Medicine
University of Pittsburgh
Pittsburgh, Pennsylvania
United States

Jennette Hansen, MD
Assistant Professor
Department of Anesthesiology
University of Kansas Medical Center
Kansas City, Kansas
United States

Patrick Hussey, MD
Assistant Professor
Department of Anesthesiology and Perioperative Medicine
University of Alabama at Birmingham
Birmingham, Alabama
United States

Joel A. Kaplan, MD, FACC
Professor
Anesthesiology
University of California San Diego
San Diego, California;
Dean Emeritus, School of Medicine
Former Chancellor, Health Sciences
University of Louisville
Louisville, Kentucky
United States

Gerard Manecke, MD
Professor Emeritus
University of California San Diego
San Diego, California;
Staff Anesthesiologist
Veterans Affairs Medical Center
San Diego, California
United States

J. Bradley Meers, MD, FASE
Associate Professor
Anesthesiology and Perioperative Medicine
University of Alabama at Birmingham
Birmingham, Alabama
United States

Alexander Mittnacht, MD
Professor
Department of Anesthesiology
Westchester Medical Center
Valhalla, New York
United States

Steven T. Morozowich, DO, FASE, FASA
Assistant Professor
Division of Cardiovascular and Thoracic Anesthesiology
Mayo Clinic Arizona
Phoenix, Arizona
United States

Harish Ramakrishna, MD, FACC, FESC, FASE
Professor
Division of Cardiovascular and Thoracic Anesthesiology
Mayo Clinic
Rochester, Minnesota
United States

Iwan Sofjan, MD
Assistant Professor of Anesthesiology
Westchester Medical Center
Valhalla, New York
United States

Alexander D. Stoker, MD
Assistant Professor
Department of Anesthesiology
Mayo Clinic Arizona
Phoenix, Arizona
United States

Shea Stoops, MD
Assistant Professor
Department of Anesthesiology
University of Kansas Medical Center
Kansas City, Kansas
United States

Harikesh Subramanian, MBBS
Assistant Professor
Department of Anesthesiology and Perioperative Medicine
University of Pittsburgh
Pittsburgh, Pennsylvania
United States

Justin Tawil, MD, FASA
Associate Professor
Department of Anesthesiology
University of Wisconsin
Madison, Wisconsin
United States

Matthew M. Townsley, MD, FASE
Professor
Department of Anesthesiology and Perioperative Medicine
University of Alabama at Birmingham
Birmingham, Alabama
United States

Matthew W. Vanneman, MD
Clinical Assistant Professor
Anesthesiology, Perioperative and Pain Medicine
Stanford University School of Medicine
Stanford, California
United States

Soojie Yu, MD
Assistant Professor; Senior Associate Consultant
Anesthesiology and Perioperative Medicine
Associate Program Director, Anesthesiology
Mayo Clinic Arizona
Phoenix, Arizona
United States

The first edition of *Augoustides and Kaplan's Cardiac Anesthesia Review* has been written to facilitate comprehensive assessment of important knowledge in the perioperative management of patients with cardiac disease. The specialty of cardiac anesthesia has steadily evolved to include dedicated textbooks, specialty journals such as the *Journal of Cardiothoracic and Vascular Anesthesia*, accredited fellowships, examinations in perioperative echocardiography, and more recently board certification in cardiac anesthesia. The ongoing advances in perioperative cardiovascular care have also enhanced the roles of cardiac anesthesiologists in preoperative evaluation, cardiovascular monitoring, and imaging, as well as postoperative management. The 7th edition of *Kaplan's Cardiac Anesthesia* has captured the latest progress in these domains, including novel cardiovascular medications, advanced cardiopulmonary assist devices, and transcatheter interventions for structural heart disease, as well as the evolution of the multidisciplinary heart team that typically includes cardiac anesthesiologists.

As a consequence of all these advances, this first edition of *Augoustides and Kaplan's Cardiac Anesthesia Review* has been indexed to the 7th edition of *Kaplan's Cardiac Anesthesia* to encourage systematic evaluation of knowledge in the perioperative care of cardiac surgical patients. Although perioperative echocardiography and noncardiac surgery are covered in the 7th edition of *Kaplan's Cardiac Anesthesia*, these domains have largely been omitted in this review book to allow a greater focus on the rest of the specialty that is the current emphasis for the written board examination in cardiac anesthesia.

To assist the reader, each chapter has a standardized layout that begins with a summary of the key points to introduce the topic. The multiple-choice questions then follow to allow thorough self-assessment across the topic of interest. The correct answers with explanations are then presented to inform the reader's self-assessment in the covered specialty area. The references have been condensed to include the 7th edition of *Kaplan's Cardiac Anesthesia* and related journal articles to provide the detail for each question item and the corresponding answer. The content that is reviewed ranges from the basic sciences to translational medicine, including preoperative assessment and management, cardiovascular physiology and pharmacology, monitoring, cardiac surgical procedures, and extracorporeal circulation, as well as postoperative management. The emphasis throughout this first edition is to review the scientific basis of perioperative practice in cardiac anesthesia, including society guidelines where relevant.

The educational aids in each chapter go beyond the included key points at the beginning of each chapter. Where relevant, graphics and teaching boxes have been included to highlight the important take-home messages. The content of the first edition has also been enhanced with access to both a printed and an electronic format to suit the full spectrum of learning styles. Furthermore, the chapters have been carefully coordinated in an effort to maximize their utility for effective review of the material. The electronic version will also be accessible by a variety of devices to ensure enhanced learner compatibility.

In preparing this first edition, we have been tremendously assisted by the talented team of associate editors and authors who have collaborated so effectively to ensure timely production of their chapters. This first edition of over 1000 review questions will help the reader identify content gaps that require further study as well as reinforce existing knowledge in cardiac anesthesia. Although the cognitive processes of reading questions, weighing options, and considering the background information will often enhance the integration and recall of important information, this review platform is intended to complement rather than replace standard textbooks in the specialty, including the 7th edition of *Kaplan's Cardiac Anesthesia*. Along with our authors and associate editors, we trust that this book will assist our readers in enhancing their cognitive expertise in cardiac anesthesia.

John G. T. Augoustides, MD, FASE, FAHA
Editor

Joel A. Kaplan, MD, FACC
Editor

CONTENTS

CHAPTER 1

Assessment of Cardiac Risk

Soojie Yu, Steven T. Morozowich, and Harish Ramakrishna

KEY POINTS

1. Perioperative cardiac morbidity is multifactorial, and understanding the predictive risk factors helps define the risk for individual patients.
2. Assessment of myocardial injury is based on the integration of information from myocardial imaging (e.g., echocardiography), electrocardiography, and serum biomarkers, with significant variability in the diagnosis depending on the criteria selected.
3. Multivariate modeling has been used to develop risk indices that focus on preoperative variables, intraoperative variables, or both.
4. Key predictors of perioperative risk are dependent on the type of cardiac operation and the outcome of interest.
5. New risk models have become available for valvular heart surgery and for combined coronary and valvular cardiac procedures.

---

1. Coronary artery bypass graft surgery has an operative mortality rate of:
   A. 1%–2%
   B. 2%–3%
   C. 3%–4%
   D. 5%–6%

Correct Answer: D

Explanation: Coronary artery bypass graft surgery (CABG) had a mortality risk of 1% to 2% in the early 1980s. The morbidity and mortality rates have gradually increased as more urgent, emergent, and repeat sternotomy procedures became more common. Currently, as percutaneous coronary interventions treat low risk patients, the operative mortality rate has further increased to a range of 5% to 6%. The risk of mortality is high after CABG, especially in the first postoperative year due to cardiac causes. Despite significant progress, patients undergoing CABG are still at greater risk of death than the general population. Risk calculators such as the model from the Society of Thoracic Surgeons can estimate the perioperative mortality and morbidity for a given patient based on readily available clinical parameters.

References:

1. Bansal M, Fuster V, Narula J, et al. Chapter 1: Assessment of Cardiac Risk and the Cardiology Consultation. In: Kaplan JA, Augoustides JGT, Manecke GR, et al., eds. Kaplan's Cardiac Anesthesia. 7th ed. Elsevier; 2017:3-9.
2. Aittokallio J, Kauko A, Palmu J, et al. Predictors and outcomes of coronary artery bypass grafting: a systemic and untargeted analysis of more than 120,000 individuals and 1300 disease traits. J Cardiothorac Vasc Anesth, 2021; 35: 3232-3240.
3. Ferguson Jr T, Hammill B, Peterson ED, et al. A decade of change—risk profiles and outcomes for isolated coronary artery bypass grafting procedures, 1990-1999: a report from the STS National Database Committee and the Duke Clinical Research Institute. Society of Thoracic Surgeons. Ann Thorac Surg, 2002; 73: 480-489.

2. For patients who experience perioperative myocardial infarction after coronary bypass graft surgery, what percentage remain free from adverse cardiac events after 2 years?
   A. 60%
   B. 65%
   C. 51%
   D. 72%

Correct Answer: C

Explanation: Patients who experience perioperative myocardial infarction (MI) have a poorer prognosis both in the short term and beyond. Compared with the patients who did not experience perioperative MI, patients who did have about a 50% risk of ongoing adverse cardiac events after 2 years. Force et al. studied 59 patients with perioperative MI and 115 patients without perioperative MI. If patients with perioperative MI have been adequately revascularized and had a postoperative left ventricular ejection fraction greater than 40%, then this adverse outcome risk was significantly attenuated. This outcome effect explains the ongoing focus on detection and prevention of perioperative MI.

References:

1. Bansal M, Fuster V, Narula J, et al. Chapter 1: Assessment of Cardiac Risk and the Cardiology Consultation. In: Kaplan JA, Augoustides JGT, Manecke GR, et al., eds. Kaplan's Cardiac Anesthesia. 7th ed. Elsevier; 2017:3-9.
2. Force T, Hibberd P, Weeks G, et al. Perioperative myocardial infarction after coronary artery bypass surgery. Clinical significance and approach to risk stratification. Circulation, 1990; 82: 903-912.
3. Goeddel L, Hopkins AN, Fernando RJ, et al. Analysis of the 4th universal definition of myocardial infarction – key concepts and perioperative implications. J Cardiothorac Vasc Anesth, 2019; 33: 3486-3495.

3. Following prolonged myocardial ischemia, when does myocardial infarction (i.e., necrosis) start to occur?
  A. Within seconds
  B. Within minutes
  C. Within hours
  D. Within days

Correct Answer: B

Explanation: Myocardial ischemia occurs when there is a sudden insufficiency of the coronary blood supply.

Myocardial infarction (i.e., necrosis/cellular death) begins within minutes following prolonged ischemia. This process of cell death is characterized by release of cellular myocardial enzymes such as cardiac troponins. Cardiac troponins are protein components of the contractile apparatus of myocardial cells and are expressed almost exclusively in the heart. Based on this understanding, the clinical definition of myocardial infarction requires (1) the presence of abnormal/elevated troponin values; and (2) evidence of myocardial ischemia such as symptoms of ischemia, new ischemic electrocardiographic changes, imaging evidence of ischemia, and/or coronary thrombus by angiography.

References:

1. Bansal M, Fuster V, Narula J, et al. Chapter 1: Assessment of Cardiac Risk and the Cardiology Consultation. In: Kaplan JA, Augoustides JGT, Manecke GR, et al., eds. Kaplan's Cardiac Anesthesia. 7th ed. Elsevier; 2017:3-9.
2. Thygesen K, Alpert JS, Jaffe AS, et al. Fourth universal definition of myocardial infarction. Circulation, 2018; 138: e618-e651.

3. Goeddel L, Hopkins AN, Fernando RJ, et al. Analysis of the 4th universal definition of myocardial infarction – key concepts and perioperative implications. J Cardiothorac Vasc Anesth, 2019; 33: 3486-3495.

4. The most frequent complication after cardiac surgery and the most important cause of hospital complications and death is which of the following?
  A. Myocardial injury
  B. Atrial fibrillation
  C. Ventilator associated pneumonia
  D. Heart block

Correct Answer: A

Explanation: Myocardial injury can present as transient cardiac dysfunction such as stunning, acute myocardial infarction, or both. With regard to myocardial infarction, the incidence of postoperative myocardial infarction found in studies is dependent on the definition and ranges between approximately 2% and 10%.

References:

1. Bansal M, Fuster V, Narula J, et al. Chapter 1: Assessment of Cardiac Risk and the Cardiology Consultation. In: Kaplan JA, Augoustides JGT, Manecke GR, et al., eds. Kaplan's Cardiac Anesthesia. 7th ed. Elsevier; 2017:3-9.
2. Nicolas J, Soriano K, Salter B, et al. Myocardial infarction after cardiac surgery: When to intervene? J Thorac Cardiovasc Surg, 2021; 21: 01279-4.

5. The most influential determinants of postoperative outcome in cardiac surgery include which of the following?
  A. Duration of surgery and duration of anesthesia
  B. Duration of aortic cross clamp and lowest mean arterial pressure
  C. Duration of aortic cross clamp and duration of cardiopulmonary bypass
  D. Duration of cardiopulmonary bypass and lowest mean arterial pressure

Correct Answer: C

Explanation: As myocardial necrosis occurs due to the interruption of blood flow, the duration of aortic cross clamp affects the extent of myocardial injury. As myocardial injury is an important cause of hospital complications and mortality, the duration of cross clamp is often a significant factor in postoperative outcome. Prolonged aortic cross clamp time was found to be an independent risk factor for postoperative morbidity and mortality in both high-risk and low-risk patients. Cardiopulmonary bypass duration is also an independent predictor of outcomes after cardiac surgery due to the multiple detrimental effects that occur.

References:

1. Bansal M, Fuster V, Narula J, et al. Chapter 1: Assessment of Cardiac Risk and the Cardiology Consultation. In: Kaplan JA,

Augoustides JGT, Manecke GR, et al., eds. Kaplan's Cardiac Anesthesia. 7th ed. Elsevier; 2017:3-9.

2. Salis S, Mazzanti V, Meri G, et al. Cardiopulmonary bypass duration is an independent predictor of morbidity and mortality after cardiac surgery. J Cardiothorac Vasc Anesth, 2008; 22: 814-822.

3. Al-Sarraf N, Lukman T, Hughes A, et al. Cross-clamp time is an independent predictor of mortality and morbidity in low- and high-risk cardiac patients. Int J Surg, 2011; 9: 104-109.

6. After complex cardiac surgery with cardiopulmonary bypass, which of the following has NOT been correlated with decreased patient survival?
   A. Duration of cardiopulmonary bypass
   B. Anesthetic technique
   C. Lowest myocardial pH recorded during aortic cross-clamping
   D. Lower preoperative ejection fraction

Correct Answer: B

Explanation: Clinical trials have demonstrated a direct relationship between the lowest mean myocardial pH recorded during aortic cross clamping on cardiopulmonary bypass and postoperative mortality. As myocardial acidosis reflects an accumulation of hydrogen ions in myocardial tissue due to anaerobic metabolism, it is a surrogate marker for the duration of aortic cross clamp time and cardiopulmonary bypass, which both also are associated with patient survival. A lower preoperative ejection fraction is also a significant risk factor for low cardiac output syndrome after complex cardiac surgery due to decreased myocardial reserve combined with a prolonged period of myocardial ischemia during cardiopulmonary bypass. These considerations highlight the outcome importance of aggressive myocardial protection during cardiopulmonary bypass. Anesthetic technique has not been directly correlated with patient survival after complex surgery with cardiopulmonary bypass.

References:

1. Bansal M, Fuster V, Narula J, et al. Chapter 1: Assessment of Cardiac Risk and the Cardiology Consultation. In: Kaplan JA, Augoustides JGT, Manecke GR, et al., eds. Kaplan's Cardiac Anesthesia. 7th ed. Elsevier; 2017:3-9.

2. Khuri S. Evidence, sources, and assessment of injury during cardiac surgery. Ann Thorac Surg, 2001; 72: PS2205-PS2207.

3. Khabbaz K, Zankoul F, Warner K. Intraoperative metabolic monitoring of the heart: II. Online measurement of myocardial tissue pH. Ann Thorac Surg, 2001; 72: PS2227-PS2233.

7. Which of the following best describes the observation that, after a period of myocardial ischemia, myocardial viability can be maintained if reperfusion is instituted within a reasonable period but risks extending injury beyond the initial insult?
   A. No-reflow phenomenon
   B. Myocardial stunning
   C. Myocardial acidosis
   D. Myocardial reperfusion injury

Correct Answer: D

Explanation: Myocardial reperfusion injury occurs after a prolonged period of ischemia. Despite the restoration of tissue viability, the metabolic cascade that accompanies ischemia-reperfusion may lead to myocardial injury that can extend beyond the initial ischemic area. Myocardial reperfusion injury can cause irreversible consequences, which include microvascular obstruction and myocardial infarction. The no-reflow phenomenon refers to the failure of reperfusion despite the resolution of proximal coronary obstruction. This event may be due to damaged distal microvasculature and may be part of the overall process of ischemia-reperfusion injury. Significant acidosis occurs during myocardial ischemia, and its gradual resolution often accompanies ischemia-reperfusion injury. Myocardial stunning refers to the transient myocardial dysfunction that occurs after ischemia-reperfusion and is not accompanied by myocardial necrosis, but rather a slow process of cellular recovery.

References:

1. Bansal M, Fuster V, Narula J, et al. Chapter 1: Assessment of Cardiac Risk and the Cardiology Consultation. In: Kaplan JA, Augoustides JGT, Manecke GR, et al., eds. Kaplan's Cardiac Anesthesia. 7th ed. Elsevier; 2017:3-9.

2. Frohlich G, Meier P, White SK, et al. Myocardial reperfusion injury: looking beyond primary PCI. Eur Heart J, 2013; 34: 1714-1722.

3. Verma S, Fedak PWM, Weisel RD, et al. Fundamentals of reperfusion injury for the clinical cardiologist. Circulation, 2002; 105: 2332-2336.

8. Reperfusion should be reinitiated after myocardial ischemia before irreversible myocardial injury occurs within which of the following time frames?
   A. 10 minutes
   B. 20 minutes
   C. 45 minutes
   D. 60 minutes

Correct Answer: B

Explanation: The myocardium can usually tolerate brief periods of severe and even total myocardial ischemia without myocyte death. Although the myocardium may experience injury, it can be reversed if perfusion is reestablished within 16 to 20 minutes. After 20 minutes of ischemia, irreversible myocardial damage develops and additional myocardium is subsequently predisposed to reperfusion injury.

References:

1. Bansal M, Fuster V, Narula J, et al. Chapter 1: Assessment of Cardiac Risk and the Cardiology Consultation. In: Kaplan JA, Augoustides JGT, Manecke GR, et al., eds. Kaplan's Cardiac Anesthesia. 7th ed. Elsevier; 2017:3-9.

2. Verma S, Fedak PWM, Weisel RD, et al. Fundamentals of reperfusion injury for the clinical cardiologist. Circulation, 2002; 105: 2332-2336.

9. The phenomenon where tissue necrosis originates in the subendocardial region of the ischemic myocardium and then extends to the subepicardial region is known as which of the following?
   A. Wavefront phenomenon
   B. Reperfusion phenomenon
   C. No-reflow phenomenon
   D. Myocardial stunning phenomenon

Correct Answer: A

Explanation: The wavefront phenomenon is when tissue necrosis originates in the subendocardial region of the ischemic myocardium and then extends to the subepicardial region. If reperfusion is initiated after 20 minutes, the level of tissue necrosis that develops is directly related to the length of the ischemic event. Cardiac magnetic resonance imaging may demonstrate the areas of irreversible myocardial injury if ischemia persists beyond 20 minutes. The reperfusion phenomenon refers to the process of ischemia-reperfusion injury after termination of ischemia and restoration of tissue perfusion. The no-reflow phenomenon describes the failure of myocardial reperfusion despite the resolution of proximal coronary obstruction due to damaged distal microvasculature. Myocardial stunning describes the transient myocardial dysfunction that occurs after ischemia-reperfusion with a slow process of cellular recovery.

References:

1. Bansal M, Fuster V, Narula J, et al. Chapter 1: Assessment of Cardiac Risk and the Cardiology Consultation. In: Kaplan JA, Augoustides JGT, Manecke GR, et al., eds. Kaplan's Cardiac Anesthesia. 7th ed. Elsevier; 2017:3-9.
2. Marra M, Lima JAC, Iliceto S. MRI in acute myocardial infarction. Eur Heart J, 2011; 32: 264-293.

10. According to the universal definition, the diagnosis of myocardial infarction can be reached with evidence of myocardial ischemia on electrocardiogram or imaging, as well as a rise and fall of cardiac biomarkers, with at least one value above:
   A. The 90th percentile of the upper reference limit
   B. The 95th percentile of the upper reference limit
   C. The 99th percentile of the upper reference limit
   D. The 85th percentile of the upper reference limit

Correct Answer: C

Explanation: The definition of myocardial infarction is reasonable with acute myocardial injury with clinical evidence of acute ischemia that is accompanied by a rise and/or fall of cardiac biomarkers with at least one value above the 99th percentile. Furthermore, clinical evidence of ischemia may be evident with new ischemic electrocardiographic changes, the development of pathological Q waves, imaging evidence of new loss of viable myocardium or new regional wall motion abnormality, and identification of coronary thrombus by angiography.

References:

1. Bansal M, Fuster V, Narula J, et al. Chapter 1: Assessment of Cardiac Risk and the Cardiology Consultation. In: Kaplan JA, Augoustides JGT, Manecke GR, et al., eds. Kaplan's Cardiac Anesthesia. 7th ed. Elsevier; 2017:3-9.
2. Thygesen K, Alpert J, Jaffe AS, et al. Fourth universal definition of myocardial infarction (2018). Circulation, 2018; 138: e618-e651.

11. For the diagnosis of myocardial infarction during the immediate period after cardiac surgery, cardiac biomarkers values have to be more than:
   A. 5 times the 99th percentile of the upper reference limit
   B. 10 times the 99th percentile of the upper reference limit
   C. 2 times the 99th percentile of the upper reference limit
   D. 20 times the 99th percentile of the upper reference limit

Correct Answer: B

Explanation: Increases in cardiac biomarkers should be expected after coronary artery bypass graft surgery due to the extent of procedural myocardial injury. To help ensure consistency, the current definition of myocardial infarction in this setting is reasonable if cardiac biomarkers are 10 times the 99th percentile of the upper reference limit during the first 48 hours postoperatively. It is important that the elevated cardiac biomarkers are accompanied by electrocardiographic, angiographic, or imaging evidence of new myocardial ischemia. It is important to note, however, that ST segment and T wave changes are common in this setting due to epicardial injury rather than myocardial ischemia.

References:

1. Bansal M, Fuster V, Narula J, et al. Chapter 1: Assessment of Cardiac Risk and the Cardiology Consultation. In: Kaplan JA, Augoustides JGT, Manecke GR, et al., eds. Kaplan's Cardiac Anesthesia. 7th ed. Elsevier; 2017:3-9.
2. Thygesen K, Alpert J, Jaffe AS, et al. Fourth universal definition of myocardial infarction (2018). Circulation, 2018; 138: e618-e651.

12. Evidence of perioperative acute myocardial infarction is characterized by what changes on the postoperative electrocardiogram?
   A. New ST segment abnormalities
   B. New atrial fibrillation
   C. New T wave inversions
   D. New persistent Q waves

Correct Answer: D

Explanation: New persistent Q waves of at least 0.03 seconds in duration, broadening of existing Q waves, or new QS deflections on the postoperative electrocardiogram are considered indicators of new acute myocardial infarction. New Q waves, though, are not necessarily evidence of new acute myocardial infarction and could be unmasking of an old myocardial infarction. However, new Q waves accompanied by an elevation in cardiac biomarkers provide stronger evidence of significant myocardial ischemia. The presence of new pathological Q waves in leads V1 to V5 in the first week after cardiac surgery has been significantly associated with major cardiac events and/or mortality in the first year after surgery. Atrial fibrillation is common after cardiac surgery and is typically not accompanied by acute myocardial ischemia. New ST segment and T wave inversions after cardiac surgery may indicate ischemia but are also commonly associated with diverse etiologies that include pericarditis and electrolyte abnormalities.

References:

1. Bansal M, Fuster V, Narula J, et al. Chapter 1: Assessment of Cardiac Risk and the Cardiology Consultation. In: Kaplan JA, Augoustides JGT, Manecke GR, et al., eds. Kaplan's Cardiac Anesthesia. 7th ed. Elsevier; 2017:3-9.
2. Mauermann E, Bolliger D, Fassl J, et al. Significance of new Q waves and their location in postoperative ECGs after elective on-pump cardiac surgery: An observational cohort study. Euro J Anaesthesiol, 2017; 34: 271-279.
3. Crescenzi G, Bove T, Pappalardo F, et al. Clinical significance of a new Q wave after cardiac surgery. Euro J Cardiothorac Surg, 2004; 25: 1001-1005.

13. Serum biomarkers indicative of myocardial infarction include creatine kinase–MB subtype and troponins T and I, as well as lactate dehydrogenase. What is the most sensitive and most specific of these markers for detecting myocardial infarction?
A. Creatine kinase–MB subtype
B. Troponin I
C. Lactate dehydrogenase
D. Troponin T

Correct Answer: B

Explanation: Cardiac troponins I and T are components of the contractile apparatus of myocardial cells and are expressed almost exclusively in the heart. Based on this, either of these assays are currently recommended for routine clinical use. It is worth noting, however, that increases in troponin I values have not been reported to occur following infarction of noncardiac tissues. In contrast, skeletal muscle expresses proteins that may be detected by the troponin T assay. Because of this, troponin I is the biomarker of choice for the diagnosis of myocardial infarction. Rises in lactate dehydrogenase and creatine kinase–MB fraction may also accompany myocardial infarction, but with less sensitivity and specificity than the troponin biomarkers.

References:

1. Bansal M, Fuster V, Narula J, et al. Chapter 1: Assessment of Cardiac Risk and the Cardiology Consultation. In: Kaplan JA, Augoustides JGT, Manecke GR, et al., eds. Kaplan's Cardiac Anesthesia. 7th ed. Elsevier; 2017:3-9.
2. Thygesen K, Alpert JS, Jaffe AS, et al. Fourth universal definition of myocardial infarction (2018). Circulation, 2018; 138: e618-e651.

14. In patients undergoing coronary artery bypass graft surgery, increases in which of following cardiac biomarkers have been independently associated with late adverse outcomes?
A. Creatine kinase–MB subtype
B. Lactate dehydrogenase
C. Myoglobin
D. Troponin T

Correct Answer: A

Explanation: In patients undergoing coronary artery bypass grafting, acute postoperative elevations of the biomarker creatine kinase–MB have been significantly associated with increased risk for mortality, repeat acute myocardial infarction, and additional late adverse outcomes. This significant association highlights the outcome importance of perioperative myocardial ischemia in adult cardiac surgery and explains the ongoing focus on this important outcome variable.

References:

1. Bansal M, Fuster V, Narula J, et al. Chapter 1: Assessment of Cardiac Risk and the Cardiology Consultation. In: Kaplan JA, Augoustides JGT, Manecke GR, et al., eds. Kaplan's Cardiac Anesthesia. 7th ed. Elsevier; 2017:3-9.
2. Mahaffey K, Roe M, Kilaru R, et al. Creatinine Kinase-MB elevation after coronary artery bypass grafting surgery in patients with non-ST segment elevation acute coronary syndromes predict worse outcomes: results of four large clinical trials. Eur Heart J, 2007; 28: 425-432.

15. Which of the following biomarkers can be detected in the early stages of myocardial injury with subsequent decreases shortly after the insult?
A. Myoglobin
B. Brain natriuretic peptide
C. Lactate dehydrogenase
D. Total creatine kinase

Correct Answer: B

Explanation: Brain natriuretic peptide is a natriuretic hormone initially identified in the brain that is also released from the ventricles. It is actively synthesized and released from the ventricles in response to increases in pressure and volume, myocardial injury, and/or inflammation. This biomarker is prognostic in both heart failure and acute coronary syndromes. Furthermore, it is elevated early in myocardial injury and decreases quickly after the insult, and therefore can detect new subsequent injury. This biomarker is significantly elevated after coronary artery bypass graft surgery in patients who experience adverse outcome events including major cardiovascular events, longer hospital stays, and a decline in physical function.

References:

1. Bansal M, Fuster V, Narula J, et al. Chapter 1: Assessment of Cardiac Risk and the Cardiology Consultation. In: Kaplan JA, Augoustides JGT, Manecke GR, et al., eds. Kaplan's Cardiac Anesthesia. 7th ed. Elsevier; 2017: 3-9.
2. Nadir MA, Dow E, et al. Myocardial ischemia is associated with an elevated brain natriuretic peptide level in the presence of left ventricular systolic dysfunction. Eur J Heart Fail, 2014; 16: 56-67.
3. Fox AA, Marcantonio ER, et al. Elevated peak postoperative B-type natriuretic peptide predicts decreased longer-term physical function after primary coronary artery bypass graft surgery. Anesthesiology, 2011; 14: 807-816.

16. Which of the following studies defined the initial clinical and angiographic predictors of operative mortality in coronary artery disease?
A. Coronary artery surgery study
B. Arterial revascularization therapy study
C. Coronary calcium scoring study
D. Predictors of mortality after coronary artery bypass study

Correct Answer: A

Explanation: The landmark Coronary Artery Surgery Study looked at 780 patients with stable ischemic heart disease from 1975 to 1983. The patients were randomly assigned to receive surgical or nonsurgical treatment. The results from this landmark trial identified predictors for mortality for both surgical and medical management of coronary artery disease, including a higher severity of angina, manifestations of heart failure, and more severe coronary artery disease. The findings from this important trial also provided evidence to refine the indications for surgical management of coronary artery disease.

References:

1. Bansal M, Fuster V, Narula J, et al. Chapter 1: Assessment of Cardiac Risk and the Cardiology Consultation. In: Kaplan JA, Augoustides JGT, Manecke GR, et al., eds. Kaplan's Cardiac Anesthesia. 7th ed. Elsevier; 2017:3-9.
2. CASS Principal Investigators and their associates. Coronary Artery Surgery Study (CASS): a randomized trial of coronary artery bypass surgery survival data. Circulation, 1983; 68: 939-950.

17. The risk factors identified for the landmark simple classification of risk in cardiac surgery study from Canada include left ventricular dysfunction, congestive heart failure, unstable angina, recent myocardial infarction, age above 65 years, severe obesity, reoperation, emergency surgery, and:
A. Hypothyroidism
B. Diabetes
C. Other significant or uncontrolled comorbidities
D. Dementia

Correct Answer: C

Explanation: Paiement and associates from Canada reported this risk scoring scheme for cardiac surgery in 1983. The risk factors identified poor left ventricular function, congestive heart failure, unstable angina or recent myocardial infarction, age above 65 years, severe obesity, reoperation, emergency surgery, and other significant or uncontrolled comorbidities. Considering these eight risk factors, three classes of patients were identified: those with no risk factors, those with one risk factor, and those with more than one risk factor. The operative mortality was found to be associated with a higher number of risk factors. Significant or uncontrolled comorbidities were defined as systolic pulmonary arterial pressure greater than 50 mmHg, uncontrolled systemic arterial hypertension, renal insufficiency, chronic lung disease, poor hepatic function, cerebrovascular insufficiency, severe arrhythmias, active endocarditis, and/or cachexia.

References:

1. Bansal M, Fuster V, Narula J, et al. Chapter 1: Assessment of Cardiac Risk and the Cardiology Consultation. In: Kaplan JA, Augoustides JGT, Manecke GR, et al., eds. Kaplan's Cardiac Anesthesia. 7th ed. Elsevier; 2017:3-9.
2. Paiement B, Pelletier C, Dyrda I, et al. A simple classification of the risk in cardiac surgery. Canadian Anesth Soc J, 1983; 30: 61-68.

18. The preoperative risk factors associated with the greatest operative mortality rates based on the Society of Thoracic Surgeons database include salvage status, renal failure, emergent status, multiple reoperations, and which of the following factors?
A. Age over 65 years
B. New York Heart Association class IV status
C. Left ventricular function
D. Severe obesity

Correct Answer: B

Explanation: The national adult cardiac surgery database of the Society of Thoracic Surgeons has a large data archive for calculating risk-adjusted scores. It was created in 1989 and allows participants to benchmark their risk-adjusted results against regional and national standards. The preoperative risk factors with the highest operative mortality rates were salvage status, renal failure (with or without renal replacement therapy), emergent status, multiple reoperations, and New York Heart Association class IV status. The New York Heart Association classification of heart failure has four classes, with class IV disease characterized by symptoms of heart failure at rest.

References:

1. Bansal M, Fuster V, Narula J, et al. Chapter 1: Assessment of Cardiac Risk and the Cardiology Consultation. In: Kaplan JA, Augoustides JGT, Manecke GR, et al., eds. Kaplan's Cardiac Anesthesia. 7th ed. Elsevier; 2017:3-9.

2. LePar DJ, Filardo G, Crosby IK, et al. The challenge of achieving 1% operative mortality for coronary artery bypass grafting: A multi-institution Society of Thoracic Surgeons Database analysis. Acq Cardiovasc Dis, 2014; 148: 2686-2696.

19. The Society of Thoracic Surgeons has developed risk models for coronary artery bypass graft (CABG) surgery and heart valve surgery, as well as valve and CABG surgery. How many specific, defined procedures do these risk models account for?
   A. Five
   B. Six
   C. Seven
   D. Eight

Correct Answer: C

Explanation: There are three risk models from the Society of Thoracic Surgeons: coronary artery bypass graft (CABG) surgery; valve surgery; and valve and CABG surgery. These three risk models are comprised of seven specifically defined procedures. The CABG model is only for isolated CABG (#1). The valve model is for isolated aortic valve replacement (#2), mitral valve replacement (#3), and mitral valve repair (#4). The CABG plus valve model includes aortic valve replacement with CABG (#5), mitral valve replacement with CABG (#6), and mitral valve repair with CABG (#7).

References:

1. Bansal M, Fuster V, Narula J, et al. Chapter 1: Assessment of Cardiac Risk and the Cardiology Consultation. In: Kaplan JA, Augoustides JGT, Manecke GR, et al., eds. Kaplan's Cardiac Anesthesia. 7th ed. Elsevier; 2017:3-9.
2. O'Brien S, Feng L, He X, et al. The Society of Thoracic Surgeons 2018 Adult Cardiac Surgery Risk Models: Part 2 – statistical methods and results. Ann Thorac Surg, 2018; 105: 1419-1428.

20. All of the following risk factors have been associated with greater 30-day readmission after coronary artery bypass graft surgery EXCEPT:
   A. Male gender
   B. Advanced age
   C. Increased body surface area
   D. Infection

Correct Answer: D

Explanation: Clinical trials looking at 30-day readmission rates in patients after coronary artery bypass grafting identified the most common reasons for readmission, including postoperative infections and heart failure. Further risk factors for readmissions included older age, female sex, African-American race, greater body surface area, and previous acute myocardial infarction within 1 week.

References:

1. Bansal M, Fuster V, Narula J, et al. Chapter 1: Assessment of Cardiac Risk and the Cardiology Consultation. In: Kaplan JA, Augoustides JGT, Manecke GR, et al., eds. Kaplan's Cardiac Anesthesia. 7th ed. Elsevier; 2017:3-9.
2. Hannan EL, Racz MJ, Walford G, et al. Predictors of readmission for complications of coronary artery bypass graft surgery. JAMA, 2003; 290: 773-780.
3. Hannan EL, Zhong Y, Lahey SJ, et al. 30-day readmissions after coronary artery bypass graft surgery in New York State. JACC Cardiovasc Interv, 2011; 4: 569-576.

21. After controlling for patient risk factors, all of the following factors have been associated with a higher risk of hospital readmission after cardiac surgery EXCEPT:
   A. Low annual case volume
   B. Discharge to a nursing home
   C. Length of hospital stay less than 5 days
   D. Discharge to a rehabilitation facility

Correct Answer: C

Explanation: Factors associated with greater readmission rates after cardiac surgery include both patient and provider risk factors. After careful controlling for patient-level risk factors, provider-level risk factors included annual coronary artery bypass graft surgery volume under 100 cases per year and hospital risk-adjusted mortality rate in the highest decile. Further postoperative factors for higher risk of readmission after cardiac surgery included hospital discharge to a nursing home or a rehabilitation/acute care facility, as well as a length of hospital stay greater than 5 days.

References:

1. Bansal M, Fuster V, Narula J, et al. Chapter 1: Assessment of Cardiac Risk and the Cardiology Consultation. In: Kaplan JA, Augoustides JGT, Manecke GR, et al., eds. Kaplan's Cardiac Anesthesia. 7th ed. Elsevier; 2017:3-9.
2. Hannan EL, Racz MJ, Jones RH, et al. Predictors of mortality for patients undergoing cardiac valve replacements in New York State. Ann Thorac Surg, 2000; 70: 1212-1218.

22. All of the following major variables are consistently present in most prediction models for outcomes after cardiac surgery EXCEPT:
   A. Patient age
   B. Functional status
   C. Male gender
   D. Left ventricular function

Correct Answer: C

Explanation: There are many different factors that have been significantly associated with increased risk during cardiac surgery. These risk factors have typically been captured in the spectrum of currently available risk models, including the risk calculators from the Society of Thoracic Surgeons and the European System of Cardiac Operative Risk Evaluation (EuroSCORE). Consistent predictors of increased outcome risk in this setting across risk models include advanced age, female gender, left ventricular function, body habitus, reoperation, type of surgery, and urgency of surgery.

References:

1. Bansal M, Fuster V, Narula J, et al. Chapter 1: Assessment of Cardiac Risk and the Cardiology Consultation. In: Kaplan JA, Augoustides JGT, Manecke GR, et al., eds. Kaplan's Cardiac Anesthesia. 7th ed. Elsevier; 2017:3-9.
2. Nashef SA, Roques F, Michel P, et al. European System of Cardiac Operative Risk Evaluation (EuroSCORE). Eur J Cardiothorac Surg, 1999; 16: 9-13.
3. Pittams AP, Iddawela S, Zaidi S, et al. Scoring systems for risk stratification in patients undergoing cardiac surgery. J Cardiothorac Vasc Anesth, 2022; 36: 1148-1156.

23. In addition to renal dysfunction, which of the following comorbidities has been found to be a consistent significant risk factor for adverse outcomes after cardiac surgery?
    A. Hypothyroidism
    B. Diabetes
    C. Mild anemia
    D. Transient ischemic attack

Correct Answer: B

Explanation: Renal dysfunction and diabetes are consistent risk factors for adverse outcomes after cardiac surgery. Diabetes has been associated with adverse outcomes after cardiac surgery, including wound infections, ischemic events, renal complications, strokes, and mortality. Patients with inadequate blood glucose control are at higher risk for pulmonary, renal, and gastrointestinal complications after cardiac surgery. Although hypothyroidism, mild anemia, and transient ischemic attacks may increase outcome risk after cardiac surgery, they are much weaker risk factors than renal dysfunction and diabetes in this setting.

References:

1. Bansal M, Fuster V, Narula J, et al. Chapter 1: Assessment of Cardiac Risk and the Cardiology Consultation. In: Kaplan JA, Augoustides JGT, Manecke GR, et al., eds. Kaplan's Cardiac Anesthesia. 7th ed. Elsevier; 2017:3-9.
2. Ascione R, Rogers CA, Rajakaruna C, et al. Inadequate blood glucose control is associated with in-hospital mortality and morbidity in diabetic and nondiabetic patients undergoing cardiac surgery. Circulation, 2008; 118: 113-123.

24. In cardiac surgery, certain preoperative patient risk factors such as age, gender, prior coronary surgery, diabetes, and preoperative intra-aortic balloon pump are associated with adverse outcomes. The presence of these risk factors is most strongly associated with which of the following complications?
    A. Acute kidney injury
    B. Prolonged intubation
    C. Surgical site infection
    D. Delirium

Correct Answer: A

Explanation: Acute kidney injury is highly prevalent after cardiac surgery. Risk factors associated with this adverse outcome include older age, gender, prior coronary artery surgery, diabetes, and preoperative intra-aortic balloon pump. Further risk factors in this setting include preoperative anemia, intraoperative red blood cell transfusion, and postoperative mediastinal exploration.

References:

1. Bansal M, Fuster V, Narula J, et al. Chapter 1: Assessment of Cardiac Risk and the Cardiology Consultation. In: Kaplan JA, Augoustides JGT, Manecke GR, et al., eds. Kaplan's Cardiac Anesthesia. 7th ed. Elsevier; 2017:3-9.
2. Karkouti K, Wijeysundera DN, Yau TM, et al. Acute kidney injury after cardiac surgery: focus on modifiable risk factors. Circulation, 2009; 119: 495-502.

25. The determinants of perioperative myocardial injury after cardiac surgery include insufficient blood supply, reperfusion of ischemic myocardium, and which of the following?
    A. Hypothermia
    B. Adverse systemic effects of cardiopulmonary bypass
    C. Inotropic medication administration
    D. Hypotension

Correct Answer: B

Explanation: Myocardial injury is due to prolonged ischemia (i.e., insufficient blood supply). In cardiac surgery, this occurs during partial or complete aortic cross clamping, with ischemic changes occurring in the myocardium within minutes. When the myocardium has been exposed to prolonged periods of ischemia, reperfusion injury may occur when the blood flow is restored. In addition, during cardiopulmonary bypass, myocardial injury may occur due to the systemic effects of cardiopulmonary bypass via protease cascades, leukocyte and platelet activation, and other inflammatory mediators.

References:

1. Bansal M, Fuster V, Narula J, et al. Chapter 1: Assessment of Cardiac Risk and the Cardiology Consultation. In: Kaplan JA, Augoustides JGT, Manecke GR, et al., eds. Kaplan's Cardiac Anesthesia. 7th ed. Elsevier; 2017:3-9.
2. Khuri S. Evidence, sources, and assessment of injury during and following cardiac surgery. Ann Thorac Surg, 2001; 72: S2205-SS207.
3. Murphy GJ, Angelini GD. Side effects of cardiopulmonary bypass: What is the reality? J Card Surg, 2004; 19: 481-488.

26. Which of the following combinations resulting in myocardial injury are most associated with adverse outcomes in cardiac surgery?
    A. The combination of myocardial ischemia and reperfusion injury
    B. The combination of myocardial ischemia injury and hypotension
    C. The combination of myocardial reperfusion injury and hyperglycemia
    D. The combination of myocardial reperfusion injury and hypothermia

Correct Answer: A

Explanation: Myocardial reperfusion injury is characterized by death of myocytes that were alive at time of reperfusion. The amount of reperfusion injury is directly related to the amount of ischemic injury that occurred before reperfusion. In cardiac surgery, adequate myocardial protection during aortic cross clamping is important in preventing myocardial reperfusion injury after release of the aortic cross clamp. Even with improvements in myocardial protection, the mortality risk is still high in the first month after coronary bypass graft surgery, suggesting there is still risk of ischemic and reperfusion injury during the cross clamp period.

References:

1. Bansal M, Fuster V, Narula J, et al. Chapter 1: Assessment of Cardiac Risk and the Cardiology Consultation. In: Kaplan JA, Augoustides JGT, Manecke GR, et al., eds. Kaplan's Cardiac Anesthesia. 7th ed. Elsevier; 2017:3-9.
2. Khuri S. Evidence, sources, and assessment of injury during and following cardiac surgery. The Ann Thorac Surg, 2001; 72: S2205-S2207.
3. Ferguson Jr TB. Ischemia/reperfusion injury in coronary artery bypass grafting: Time to revisit? J Thorac Cardiovasc Surg, 2011; 141: 1-2.

27. Which of the following phenomena describes the most severe form of reperfusion injury?
    A. Reactive hyperemia phenomenon
    B. Low-flow phenomenon
    C. No-reflow phenomenon
    D. Ceased-flow phenomenon

Correct Answer: C

Explanation: The no-reflow phenomenon occurs when blood flow to ischemic tissues remains impaired following the relief of coronary occlusion or obstruction and is typically associated with the most severe form of reperfusion injury. This is due to damage to the microvasculature that prevents the restoration of normal blood flow despite relief of the proximal occlusion or obstruction. The phenomenon is more pronounced after prolonged periods of ischemia and is associated with malignant arrhythmias, lower ejection fraction, and extension of myocardial infarction.

References:

1. Bansal M, Fuster V, Narula J, et al. Chapter 1: Assessment of Cardiac Risk and the Cardiology Consultation. In: Kaplan JA, Augoustides JGT, Manecke GR, et al., eds. Kaplan's Cardiac Anesthesia. 7th ed. Elsevier; 2017:3-9.
2. Rezkalla SH, Kloner RA. No-reflow phenomenon. Circulation, 2002; 105: 656-662.

28. Which of the following is a proinflammatory protein that is a biomarker for myocardial ischemia and may contribute to the thrombotic and inflammatory complications associated with cardiopulmonary bypass?
    A. Chemokine ligand 20
    B. Cytochrome P450 2D6
    C. Natural Killer Group 2D ligands
    D. CD40 ligand

Correct Answer: D

Explanation: CD40 ligand is a signaling molecule associated with thrombosis and inflammatory responses. This biomarker is derived from platelets and contributes to the thrombotic and inflammatory complications associated with cardiopulmonary bypass. Its plasma levels increase during bypass and return to baseline approximately 8 hours after bypass. In acute coronary syndromes, patients with elevated values of this protein have an increased risk of death or nonfatal myocardial infarction at 6-month follow-up.

References:

1. Bansal M, Fuster V, Narula J, et al. Chapter 1: Assessment of Cardiac Risk and the Cardiology Consultation. In: Kaplan JA, Augoustides JGT, Manecke GR, et al., eds. Kaplan's Cardiac Anesthesia. 7th ed. Elsevier; 2017:3-9.
2. Heeschen C, Dimmeler S, Hamm CW, et al. Soluble CD40 ligand in acute coronary syndromes. N Engl J Med, 2003; 348: 1104-1111.
3. Nannizzi-Alaimo L, Rubenstein MH, Alves VL, et al. Cardiopulmonary bypass induces release of soluble CD40 ligand. Circulation, 2002; 105: 2349-2354.

29. Echocardiography is a rapid and sensitive monitor for myocardial ischemia. When monitoring with transesophageal echocardiography, how quickly can regional wall motion abnormalities be detected after the onset of myocardial ischemia?
    A. Less than 5 seconds
    B. 10 to 15 seconds
    C. 1 to 2 minutes
    D. More than 2 minutes

Correct Answer: B

Explanation: Cardiac contractile dysfunction is the most prominent feature of myocardial ischemia and may be measured with a variety of modalities including transesophageal echocardiography. With this imaging modality, regional wall motion abnormalities, indicative of myocardial ischemia, are seen within 10 to 15 seconds following the onset of ischemia. If they become irreversible, then the ischemia has likely progressed to myocardial necrosis.

References:

1. Bansal M, Fuster V, Narula J, et al. Chapter 1: Assessment of Cardiac Risk and the Cardiology Consultation. In: Kaplan JA, Augoustides JGT, Manecke GR, et al., eds. Kaplan's Cardiac Anesthesia. 7th ed. Elsevier; 2017:3-9.
2. Swaminathan M, Morris RW, De Meyts DD, et al. Deterioration of regional wall motion immediately after coronary artery bypass graft surgery is associated with long-term major adverse cardiac events. Anesthesiology, 2007; 107: 739-745.

30. Which of the following is a common cause of new postoperative regional wall motion abnormalities and decreased left ventricular systolic function that is often transient?
  A. Myocardial stunning
  B. Myocardial ischemia
  C. Myocardial infarction
  D. Myocardial reperfusion

Correct Answer: A

Explanation: Myocardial stunning describes the period of postischemic left ventricular dysfunction that occurs following reperfusion of an area of ischemia. It is a common cause of new regional wall motion abnormalities and decreased left ventricular systolic function. The myocardium eventually recovers fully but might require transient inotropic support until it does. The mechanism causing myocardial stunning is thought to be due to either oxygen free radical damage or altered calcium flux with calcium overload.

References:

1. Bansal M, Fuster V, Narula J, et al. Chapter 1: Assessment of Cardiac Risk and the Cardiology Consultation. In: Kaplan JA, Augoustides JGT, Manecke GR, et al., eds. Kaplan's Cardiac Anesthesia. 7th ed. Elsevier; 2017:3-9.
2. Kloner RA. Stunned and hibernating myocardium: where are we nearly 4 decades later? J Am Heart Assoc, 2020; 9: e015502.

CHAPTER 2

Cardiovascular Imaging

Alexander D. Stoker, Steven T. Morozowich, and Harish Ramakrishna

KEY POINTS

1. Echocardiography is the most widely used modality for cardiac imaging in almost any form of cardiac disease.
2. Echocardiography is noninvasive, safe, readily available, and portable, and it has the ability to provide vast amounts of information about cardiac structure and function. Additionally, echocardiography is the only modality available for imaging during the intraoperative period.
3. A combination of transthoracic and transesophageal imaging permits comprehensive evaluation of most cardiac pathologies. The advent of three-dimensional transesophageal echocardiography has further enhanced the utility of this modality, especially in the evaluation of mitral valve disease.
4. Stress echocardiography is helpful in the assessment of inducible myocardial ischemia, myocardial viability, and certain valve disorders.
5. Myocardial perfusion imaging can be performed using single-photon emission computed tomography or positron emission tomography and is useful in the evaluation of myocardial ischemia and viability.
6. Cardiac computed tomography and cardiac magnetic resonance are increasingly used when there are conflicting results or when further information is required in the preoperative phase of care.
7. Cardiac magnetic resonance is the gold standard for quantitative assessment of ventricular volumes, ejection fraction, and mass. It is also used to evaluate ventricular and valvular function, atherosclerosis, and plaque composition.
8. Computed tomographic aortography is the best modality for the evaluation of aortic aneurysms and dissections. Additionally, computed tomographic coronary angiography offers an alternative to invasive coronary angiography for excluding significant coronary artery disease in patients undergoing noncoronary surgery.

1. What two transthoracic echocardiography views are needed to determine left ventricular ejection fraction using the Simpson summation-of-discs method?
   A. Apical four-chamber and apical two-chamber views
   B. Apical four-chamber and apical long axis views
   C. Apical two-chamber and apical long axis views
   D. Apical five-chamber and apical long axis views

Correct Answer: A

Explanation: The Simpson method considers the left ventricular cavity as a stack of discs of equal height. Left ventricular volume is calculated by summing the volumes of all discs by manually tracing the endocardial border in the apical four- and two-chamber views, both at end-diastole and end-systole. By using the apical four- and two-chamber views, the left ventricle is assessed in two orthogonal planes and allows better estimation of ventricular volume. This method remains applicable even when the ventricle is distorted, but accuracy depends heavily on adequate visualization of the blood-endocardium interface.

References:

1. Bansal M, Fuster V, Narula J, et al. Chapter 2: Cardiovascular Imaging. In: Kaplan JA, Augoustides JGT, Manecke GR, et al., eds. Kaplan's Cardiac Anesthesia. 7th ed. Elsevier; 2017:20-45.
2. Lashin H, Olusanya O, Smith A, et al. Left ventricular ejection fraction correlation with stroke volume as estimated by Doppler echocardiography in cardiogenic shock: a retrospective observational study. J Cardiothorac Vasc Anesth, 2022; 36: 3511-3516.

2. When assessing regional left ventricular function using echocardiography, which of the follow parameters is most indicative of normal myocardial function?
   A. Preserved left ventricular ejection fraction
   B. Myocardial wall thickening
   C. Presence of endocardial motion
   D. Preserved global longitudinal strain

Correct Answer: B

Explanation: During echocardiography, left ventricular (LV) regional function assessment is performed by visual inspection of the extent of wall thickening in each myocardial segment. Depending on the extent of wall thickening, the wall motion can be classified as normal, hypokinetic, akinetic, or dyskinetic. When assessing regional wall motion, distinction must be made between actual wall thickening and endocardial motion, which is affected by tethering effects from adjacent myocardial segments and by the translational movement of the heart. The inferior and inferolateral LV segments may be classified incorrectly as hypokinetic by less experienced clinicians. Wall thickening is the gold standard for assessing regional LV function. Disease of the coronary arteries is the most common cardiac illness that affects the LV regionally, and the presence of regional LV systolic dysfunction is virtually diagnostic of underlying coronary artery disease.

References:

1. Bansal M, Fuster V, Narula J, et al. Chapter 2: Cardiovascular Imaging. In: Kaplan JA, Augoustides JGT, Manecke GR, et al., eds. Kaplan's Cardiac Anesthesia. 7th ed. Elsevier; 2017:20-45.
2. Niimi Y, Morita S, Watanabe T, et al. Effects of nitroglycerin infusion on segmental wall motion abnormalities after anesthetic induction. J Cardiothorac Vasc Anesth, 1996; 10: 734-740.

3. Which of the following parameters of right ventricular systolic function assessment is abnormal?
   A. Tricuspid annular plane systolic excursion of 23 mm
   B. Fractional area change of 33%
   C. Right ventricular free wall strain of −22%
   D. Right ventricular ejection fraction by three-dimensional echocardiogram of 47%

Correct Answer: B

Explanation: Because of the complex shape of the right ventricle (RV), it is impossible to image the entire RV from one echocardiographic window. It is possible to measure RV ejection fraction by three-dimensional echocardiography, although this can be time-consuming. A number of alternative parameters are used to assess RV function including tricuspid annular plane systolic excursion (normal value >16 mm), fractional area change (normal value ≥35%), RV free wall strain (normal value equal to or more negative than −20%), and tricuspid annular peak systolic velocity (normal value >10 cm/s). A normal RV ejection fraction as assessed by three-dimensional echocardiogram is 45% or more.

References:

1. Bansal M, Fuster V, Narula J, et al. Chapter 2: Cardiovascular Imaging. In: Kaplan JA, Augoustides JGT, Manecke GR, et al., eds. Kaplan's Cardiac Anesthesia. 7th ed. Elsevier; 2017:20-45.
2. Rudski LG, Lai WW, Afilalo J, et al. Guidelines for the echocardiographic assessment of the right heart in adults: a report from the American Society of Echocardiography endorsed by the European Association of Echocardiography, a registered branch of the European Society of Cardiology, and the Canadian Society of Echocardiography. J Am Soc Echocardiogr, 2010; 23: 685-713.

4. Which of the following parameters would be expected in a spontaneously breathing patient with an elevated central venous pressure?
   A. Right ventricular systolic pressure of 28 mmHg
   B. Inferior vena cava diameter of 12 mm
   C. Inferior vena cava collapsibility of 30% upon deep inspiration
   D. Systolic dominant hepatic vein flow pattern (S wave > D wave) as measured by pulsed wave spectral Doppler echocardiography

Correct Answer: C

Explanation: A dilated inferior vena cava (IVC) greater than 21 mm in diameter that collapses by less than 50% on inspiration indicates significantly elevated right atrial (RA) pressure (~15 mmHg with a range of 10–20 mmHg). If the IVC is normal in size and collapses by more than 50% on deep inspiration the RA pressure is considered to be normal (~3 mmHg with a range of 0–5 mmHg). When the IVC size and collapsibility are discrepant with one another the RA pressure is assumed to be in the intermediate range (~8 mmHg with a range of 5–10 mmHg). Because the IVC size and collapsibility are affected by positive pressure ventilation, this approach cannot be used for estimating RA pressure in patients who are mechanically ventilated. The right ventricular systolic pressure may be elevated in a patient with a high central venous pressure or in a patient with elevated pulmonary vascular resistance and thus cannot be used to determine RA pressure. Systolic dominant hepatic vein flow pattern is normal. Patients with a high RA pressure or severe tricuspid regurgitation would be expected to have hepatic vein systolic flow reversal.

References:

1. Bansal M, Fuster V, Narula J, et al. Chapter 2: Cardiovascular Imaging. In: Kaplan JA, Augoustides JGT, Manecke GR, et al., eds. Kaplan's Cardiac Anesthesia. 7th ed. Elsevier; 2017:20-45.
2. Rudski LG, Lai WW, Afilalo J, et al. Guidelines for the echocardiographic assessment of the right heart in adults: a report from the American Society of Echocardiography endorsed by the European Association of Echocardiography, a registered branch of the European Society of Cardiology, and the Canadian Society of Echocardiography. J Am Soc Echocardiogr, 2010; 23: 685-713.

5. Which of the following echocardiography findings would NOT be expected in a patient with rheumatic mitral stenosis?
   A. Mitral leaflet thickening with doming of the anterior mitral leaflet
   B. Flail posterior mitral leaflet
   C. Calcification of commissures
   D. Thickening, shortening, and calcification of the sub-valvular apparatus

Correct Answer: B

Explanation: Rheumatic heart disease is the most common cause of mitral stenosis even in developed nations. Mitral annular calcification, which is common in elderly persons and in those undergoing hemodialysis, can also produce mitral inflow obstruction, although mitral regurgitation is more frequent. Echocardiography typically reveals restriction of the posterior mitral leaflet, not a flail posterior mitral leaflet. These patients typically have mitral leaflet thickening with doming of the anterior mitral leaflet, variable amounts of leaflet calcification, fusion and calcification of the commissures, and thickened and calcified subvalvular apparatus.

References:

1. Bansal M, Fuster V, Narula J, et al. Chapter 2: Cardiovascular Imaging. In: Kaplan JA, Augoustides JGT, Manecke GR, et al., eds. Kaplan's Cardiac Anesthesia. 7th ed. Elsevier; 2017:20-45.
2. Reid CL, Chandraratna PA, Kawanishi DT, et al. Influence of mitral valve morphology on double-balloon catheter balloon valvuloplasty in patients with mitral stenosis. Analysis of factors predicting immediate and 3-month results. Circulation, 1989; 80: 515-524.
3. Koshy T, Tambe SP, Sinha PK, et al. Case-2 – 2008: Rheumatic mitral stenosis associated with partial anomalous venous return. J Cardiothorac Vasc Anesth, 2008; 22: 302-310.

6. Which of the follow physiologic factors would be expected to increase the mean diastolic gradient across a stenotic mitral valve?
   A. Left-to-right shunting through an atrial septal defect
   B. Decreased heart rate
   C. Increased heart rate
   D. Decreased cardiac output

Correct Answer: C

Explanation: Mitral diastolic gradient assessed by Doppler echocardiography is often utilized to assess the degree of mitral stenosis. A mean mitral valve gradient of less than 5 mmHg is consistent with mild mitral stenosis, while a mean gradient between 5 and 10 mmHg is consistent with moderate mitral stenosis, and a mean gradient above 10 mmHg is consistent with severe mitral stenosis. A number of factors can increase the mean diastolic gradient across the mitral valve, including increased heart rate and increased cardiac output. A left-to-right shunt through an atrial septal defect would result in less flow across the mitral valve and a reduced mitral valve gradient.

References:

1. Bansal M, Fuster V, Narula J, et al. Chapter 2: Cardiovascular Imaging. In: Kaplan JA, Augoustides JGT, Manecke GR, et al., eds. Kaplan's Cardiac Anesthesia. 7th ed. Elsevier; 2017:20-45.
2. Baumgartner H, Hung J, Bermejo J, et al. American Society of Echocardiography; European Association of Echocardiography. Echocardiographic assessment of valve stenosis: EAE/ASE recommendations for clinical practice. J Am Soc Echocardiogr, 2009; 22: 1-23.
3. Koshy T, Tambe SP, Sinha PK, et al. Case-2 – 2008: Rheumatic mitral stenosis associated with partial anomalous venous return. J Cardiothorac Vasc Anesth, 2008; 22: 302-310.

7. Which of the following echocardiographic parameters is consistent with severe mitral regurgitation?
   A. Vena contracta width of 0.6 cm
   B. Regurgitant volume of 55 mL/beat
   C. Regurgitant fraction of 58%
   D. Effective regurgitant orifice area of 0.35 cm^2

Correct Answer: C

Explanation: A regurgitation fraction of greater than 50% is consistent with severe mitral regurgitation (MR). A vena contracta greater to or equal to 0.7 cm, a regurgitant volume greater than or equal to 60 mL/beat, and/or an effective regurgitant orifice area greater than or equal to 0.4 cm^2 is consistent with severe MR. MR is a complex entity with a multitude of etiologies and pathogenic mechanisms, including rheumatic heart disease, degenerative disease, systemic inflammatory disease, infective endocarditis, and ischemic heart disease (resulting chordal or papillary muscle rupture), as well as congenital malformations. The mitral valve may also be normal; however, there may be poor leaflet coaptation during systole as a result of regional or global dilation and left ventricular systolic dysfunction.

References:

1. Bansal M, Fuster V, Narula J, et al. Chapter 2: Cardiovascular Imaging. In: Kaplan JA, Augoustides JGT, Manecke GR, et al., eds. Kaplan's Cardiac Anesthesia. 7th ed. Elsevier; 2017:20-45.
2. Zoghbi WA, Enriquez-Sarano M, Foster E, et al. American Society of Echocardiography. Recommendations for evaluation of the severity of native valvular regurgitation with two-dimensional and Doppler echocardiography. J Am Soc Echocardiogr, 2003; 16: 777-802.
3. Mahmood F, Sharkey A, Maslow A, et al. Echocardiographic assessment of the mitral valve for suitability of repair: an intraoperative approach from a mitral center. J Cardiothorac Vasc Anesth, 2022; 36: 2164-2176.

8. A 64-year-old male presenting with an acute myocardial infarction is found to have severe eccentric mitral regurgitation that was not present on previous echocardiographic imaging. Which Carpentier classification of mitral regurgitation would be expected in this patient?
   A. Type I
   B. Type II
   C. Type IIIa
   D. Type IIIb

Correct Answer: B

Explanation: This patient most likely is experiencing an acute papillary muscle rupture due to an acute myocardial infarction, which results in excessive mitral leaflet motion and would be classified as Carpentier type II mitral regurgitation. This typically results in an eccentric mitral regurgitant jet directed away from the leaflet involved. Carpentier type I involves normal mitral leaflet motion and may be due to dilation of the mitral annulus or a mitral leaflet perforation. Type II involves excessive mitral leaflet motion, and type III involves restricted mitral leaflet motion. Type IIIa involves restricted leaflet motion in both systole and diastole and is classically caused by rheumatic heart disease. Type IIIb involves restricted closure of mitral leaflets only in systole and may be due to functional mitral regurgitation or ischemic mitral regurgitation.

References:

1. Bansal M, Fuster V, Narula J, et al. Chapter 2: Cardiovascular Imaging. In: Kaplan JA, Augoustides JGT, Manecke GR, et al., eds. Kaplan's Cardiac Anesthesia. 7th ed. Elsevier; 2017:20-45.
2. Mahmood F, Sharkey A, Maslow A, et al. Echocardiographic assessment of the mitral valve for suitability of repair: an intraoperative approach from a mitral center. J Cardiothorac Vasc Anesth, 2022; 36: 2164-2176.

9. Which of the follow would result in a low transaortic gradient despite a stenotic aortic valve with significantly reduced aortic valve area?
   A. High cardiac output state
   B. Decreased left ventricular diastolic function
   C. Concomitant aortic regurgitation and aortic stenosis
   D. Decreased left ventricular systolic function

Correct Answer: D

Explanation: The most common causes of aortic stenosis include senile degeneration, bicuspid aortic valve disease, and rheumatic heart disease. Aortic stenosis can be classified by a number of echocardiographic parameters, including aortic jet peak velocity, aortic valve mean gradient, aortic valve area, indexed aortic valve area, and velocity ratio. A discrepancy between an inappropriately low transaortic gradient and a significantly reduced aortic valve area is commonly seen in the setting of left ventricular systolic dysfunction. Dobutamine echocardiography may help in further evaluation of these patients. Dobutamine echocardiography may also be used to differentiate pseudosevere from true severe aortic stenosis.

References:

1. Bansal M, Fuster V, Narula J, et al. Chapter 2: Cardiovascular Imaging. In: Kaplan JA, Augoustides JGT, Manecke GR, et al., eds. Kaplan's Cardiac Anesthesia. 7th ed. Elsevier; 2017:20-45.
2. Pibarot P, Dumesnil JG. Paradoxical low-flow, low-gradient aortic stenosis. J Am Coll Cardiol, 2011; 58: 413-415.
3. Baumgartner H, Hung J, Bermejo J, et al. American Society of Echocardiography; European Association of Echocardiography. Echocardiographic assessment of valve stenosis: EAE/ASE recommendations for clinical practice. J Am Soc Echocardiogr, 2009; 22: 1-23.

10. Which of the following is most likely to result in tricuspid stenosis?
    A. Placement of right ventricular transvenous pacing lead
    B. Carcinoid tumor
    C. Chronic renal failure
    D. Severe left ventricular dysfunction

Correct Answer: B

Explanation: Tricuspid stenosis is very rare and is usually congenital, associated with carcinoid tumor, or rheumatic in origin, Rheumatic disease involving the tricuspid valve almost always occurs in the setting of concomitant mitral stenosis. Right-sided cardioverter-defibrillator or pacing leads may become infected and develop associated vegetations, which can cause functional tricuspid stenosis or become adherent to components of the subvalvular apparatus leading to changes in the tricuspid valve geometry. This is less likely to result in tricuspid stenosis than carcinoid tumor, however.

References:

1. Bansal M, Fuster V, Narula J, et al. Chapter 2: Cardiovascular Imaging. In: Kaplan JA, Augoustides JGT, Manecke GR, et al., eds. Kaplan's Cardiac Anesthesia. 7th ed. Elsevier; 2017:20-45.
2. Essandoh M, Zuleta-Alarcon A, Weiss R, et al. Transesophageal echocardiographic diagnosis of severe functional tricuspid stenosis during infected implantable cardioverter-defibrillator lead extraction. J Cardiothorac Vasc Anesth, 2015; 29: 412-416.
3. Castillo J, Silvay G, Weiner M. Anesthetic management of patients with carcinoid syndrome and carcinoid heart disease: the Mount Sinai algorithm. J Cardiothorac Vasc Anesth, 2018; 32: 1023-1031.

11. Which of the following imaging modalities is considered to be the best for diagnosing infective endocarditis?
    A. Transthoracic echocardiography
    B. Transesophageal echocardiography
    C. Computed tomography
    D. Fluoroscopy

Correct Answer: B

Explanation: Infective endocarditis is a common indication for valve surgery in patients with either native or prosthetic valves. Diagnosis is usually based on visualization of vegetations by echocardiography, which is the primary modality for diagnosing infective endocarditis. In severe cases, valve perforations, paravalvular abscesses, and prosthetic heart valve dehiscence can also be seen. The sensitivity for detection of native valve endocarditis in the range of 82% to 89% for transthoracic echocardiography and 90% to 100% for transesophageal echocardiography. Computed tomography can also be used to diagnose vegetation lesions, with a lower sensitivity and limited assessment of the hemodynamic effects of valvular lesions.

References:

1. Bansal M, Fuster V, Narula J, et al. Chapter 2: Cardiovascular Imaging. In: Kaplan JA, Augoustides JGT, Manecke GR, et al., eds. Kaplan's Cardiac Anesthesia. 7th ed. Elsevier; 2017:20-45.
2. Hansalia S, Biswas M, Dutta R, et al. The value of live/real time three-dimensional transesophageal echocardiography in the assessment of valvular vegetations. Echocardiography, 2009; 26: 1264-1273.

12. Pulmonary artery systolic pressure can be estimated by measuring the peak tricuspid regurgitation jet gradient in the absence of which of the following cardiac lesions?
    A. Tricuspid stenosis

B. Pulmonary insufficiency
C. Pulmonary stenosis
D. Atrial septal defect

Correct Answer: C

Explanation: A wide range of intracardiac pressures can be derived using the simplified Bernouli equation, which states that the pressure gradient driving a blood flow jet across a given valve is equal to $4v^2$, where v is the peak jet velocity. If the pressure within the upstream or downstream chamber is known, the pressure in the other chamber can be calculated. Right ventricular systolic pressure is commonly estimated by measuring the peak tricuspid regurgitation jet velocity and adding the mean right atrial pressure (which can be determined from assessment of the inferior vena cava and/or direct measurement with a central venous catheter). If there is no right ventricular outflow tract obstruction, the right ventricular systolic pressure will be equal to the pulmonary artery systolic pressure. In the setting of pulmonic stenosis, the measured right ventricular systolic pressure will be higher than the pulmonary artery systolic pressure due to the pressure gradient across the pulmonic valve.

References:

1. Bansal M, Fuster V, Narula J, et al. Chapter 2: Cardiovascular Imaging. In: Kaplan JA, Augoustides JGT, Manecke GR, et al., eds. Kaplan's Cardiac Anesthesia. 7th ed. Elsevier; 2017:20-45.
2. Thunberg CA, Gaitan BD, Grewal A, et al. Pulmonary hypertension in patients undergoing cardiac surgery: pathophysiology, perioperative management, and outcomes. J Cardiothorac Vasc Anesth, 2013; 27: 551-572.

13. Which of the following is not needed to calculate systemic vascular resistance using echocardiography in a patient with an intraarterial catheter?
A. Stroke volume
B. Heart rate
C. Mean right atrial pressure
D. Mean pulmonary artery pressure

Correct Answer: D

Explanation: Systemic vascular resistance (SVR) can be estimated using the principle of Ohm's law, which states that the resistance across any vascular circuit is equal to the pressure gradient across the circuit divided by the flow. SVR can be calculated using the following formula: SVR = (mean aortic pressure − mean right atrial pressure) / cardiac output. Cardiac output is determined by multiplying the left ventricular outflow tract (LVOT) area by the LVOT velocity time integral by the heart rate. Right atrial pressure can be determined by echocardiographic evaluation of the inferior vena cava and/or by central venous catheter measurement. Mean arterial pressure can be measured by invasive or noninvasive means and can be used as the mean aortic pressure. Mean pulmonary artery pressure is used to calculate pulmonary vascular resistance but not SVR.

References:

1. Bansal M, Fuster V, Narula J, et al. Chapter 2: Cardiovascular Imaging. In: Kaplan JA, Augoustides JGT, Manecke GR, et al., eds. Kaplan's Cardiac Anesthesia. 7th ed. Elsevier; 2017:20-45.
2. Quiñones MA, Otto CM, Stoddard M, et al. Recommendations for quantification of Doppler echocardiography: a report from the Doppler Quantification Task Force of the Nomenclature and Standards Committee of the American Society of Echocardiography. J Am Soc Echocardiogr, 2002; 15: 167-184.

14. Which of the following factors most contributes to the development of cardiac tamponade?
A. Size of pericardial effusion
B. Rapidity of fluid collection
C. Circumferential distribution of pericardial fluid
D. Presence of clots within pericardial fluid collection

Correct Answer: B

Explanation: Pericardial effusions can occur due to a number of conditions, including immune reactions after inflammatory or infectious processes, after myocardial infarction, or due to bleeding after cardiac surgery. Pericardial fluid or blood collections can be circumferential or localized and may contain fibrinous bands, septa, or frank clots. The size of the effusion itself is not a reliable indicator of the presence of cardiac tamponade. The rapidity of fluid accumulation is a more important factor contributing to cardiac tamponade

References:

1. Bansal M, Fuster V, Narula J, et al. Chapter 2: Cardiovascular Imaging. In: Kaplan JA, Augoustides JGT, Manecke GR, et al., eds. Kaplan's Cardiac Anesthesia. 7th ed. Elsevier; 2017:20-45.
2. Tuck BC, Townsley MM. Clinical update in pericardial diseases. J Cardiothorac Vasc Anesth, 2019; 33: 184-199.

15. Which of the following echocardiographic features is NOT associated with the presence of cardiac tamponade in a spontaneously breathing patient?
A. Diastolic right atrial and right ventricular collapse
B. Dilated, noncollapsing inferior vena cava
C. Increased tricuspid valve inflow velocity during inspiration with decreased inflow during expiration
D. Increased transmitral velocity with inspiration and decreased velocity during expiration

Correct Answer: D

Explanation: When a pericardial effusion is visualized, an important question is whether there is any evidence of cardiac tamponade. Evidence of diastolic right atrial and/or right ventricular collapse, a dilated and noncollapsing inferior vena cava, and a restrictive type of mitral inflow pattern with significant respiratory variation in mitral and tricuspid inflow velocities indicates the presence of cardiac tamponade. In a spontaneously breathing patient, inspiration will decrease intrathoracic pressure and augment venous return across the tricuspid valve. Due to the increased pericardial pressure, increased filling of the right ventricle will shift the interventricular septum to the left, limit left ventricular filling, and decrease transmitral flow. This is an example of ventricular interdependence.

References:

1. Bansal M, Fuster V, Narula J, et al. Chapter 2: Cardiovascular Imaging. In: Kaplan JA, Augoustides JGT, Manecke GR, et al., eds. Kaplan's Cardiac Anesthesia. 7th ed. Elsevier; 2017:20-45.
2. Tuck BC, Townsley MM. Clinical update in pericardial diseases. J Cardiothorac Vasc Anesth, 2019; 33: 184-199.

16. A patient with echocardiographic findings of a medial e' that is larger than the lateral e', as well as a septal bounce and a dilated, noncollapsing inferior vena cava, is likely to have which of the following pathologic conditions?
   A. Mitral stenosis
   B. Constrictive pericarditis
   C. Restrictive cardiomyopathy
   D. Cardiac tamponade

Correct Answer: B

Explanation: Constrictive pericarditis is another common pericardial pathology and is itself an indication for cardiac surgery. In patients with suspected chronic constrictive pericarditis, pericardial thickening and calcification may be visualized on echocardiography. The echocardiographic findings suggestive of constriction include (1) exaggerated ventricular interdependence as evidenced by significant respiratory variation in mitral and tricuspid inflow velocities, (2) a restrictive-type mitral inflow pattern with a relatively preserved or exaggerated mitral e' (known as annulus paradoxus) or a medial mitral e' that is taller than the lateral e' (known as annulus reversus), and (3) a dilated, noncollapsing inferior vena cava. A septal bounce and annulus paradoxus would not be expected in a restrictive cardiomyopathy. Furthermore, respiratory variation in ventricular filling velocity is usually minimal in restrictive cardiomyopathy.

References:

1. Bansal M, Fuster V, Narula J, et al. Chapter 2: Cardiovascular Imaging. In: Kaplan JA, Augoustides JGT, Manecke GR, et al., eds. Kaplan's Cardiac Anesthesia. 7th ed. Elsevier; 2017:20-45.
2. Amaki M, Savino J, Ain DL, et al. Diagnostic concordance of echocardiography and cardiac magnetic resonance-based tissue tracking for differentiating constrictive pericarditis from restrictive cardiomyopathy. Circ Cardiovasc Imaging, 2014; 7: 819-827.
3. Tuck BC, Townsley MM. Clinical update in pericardial diseases. J Cardiothorac Vasc Anesth, 2019; 33: 184-199.

17. Which of the following is primarily a cause of descending aortic aneurysms rather than ascending aortic aneurysms?
   A. Hypertension
   B. Marfan syndrome
   C. Bicuspid aortic valve
   D. Atherosclerosis

Correct Answer: D

Explanation: Ascending aortic aneurysms usually occur because of cystic medial degeneration; they frequently involve the aortic root and cause aortic insufficiency. These aneurysms are more common in patients with hypertension, bicuspid aortic valve, or connective tissue disease such as in Marfan or Ehlers-Danlos syndrome. In contrast, descending aortic aneurysms are mostly caused by atherosclerosis and are associated with the same risk factors as for coronary artery disease. Abdominal aortic aneurysms are more common than descending thoracic aortic aneurysms.

References:

1. Bansal M, Fuster V, Narula J, et al. Chapter 2: Cardiovascular Imaging. In: Kaplan JA, Augoustides JGT, Manecke GR, et al., eds. Kaplan's Cardiac Anesthesia. 7th ed. Elsevier; 2017:20-45.
2. Nistri S, Sorbo MD, Marin M, et al. Aortic root dilatation in young men with normally functioning bicuspid aortic valves. Heart, 1999; 82: 19-22.

18. Which of the following is the most common location for aortic dissections to originate from?
   A. Descending aorta just distal to the subclavian artery
   B. Aortic arch
   C. Ascending aorta just above the sinuses of Valsalva
   D. Abdominal aorta

Correct Answer: C

Explanation: Ascending aortic dissections are true cardiac surgical emergencies that need to be diagnosed urgently and treated surgically. In aortic dissections, there is a tear in the intima that forms communication with the aortic true lumen. A false lumen forms as the media is exposed to blood flow, and the dissection can extend in either an anterograde or retrograde fashion, often involving branch arteries. Aortic dissections most commonly originate in one of two locations that experience the greatest stress: the ascending aorta just above the sinuses of Valsalva (65%) or the descending aorta just distal to the subclavian artery (20%). Other less common sites include the aortic arch (10%) and the abdominal aorta (5%).

References:

1. Bansal M, Fuster V, Narula J, et al. Chapter 2: Cardiovascular Imaging. In: Kaplan JA, Augoustides JGT, Manecke GR, et al., eds. Kaplan's Cardiac Anesthesia. 7th ed. Elsevier; 2017:20-45.
2. Baumgartner D, Baumgartner C, Mátyás G, et al. Diagnostic power of aortic elastic properties in young patients with Marfan syndrome. J Thorac Cardiovasc Surg, 2005; 129: 730-739.

19. Aortic insufficiency (AI) in the setting of acute ascending aortic dissection is LEAST likely to be due to which of the following mechanisms?
   A. AI related to intimal flap prolapse
   B. AI related to leaflet prolapse
   C. AI related to bicuspid aortic valve
   D. AI related to coronary cusp perforation

Correct Answer: D

Explanation: Echocardiography is an excellent modality for the initial assessment of patients with aortic dissection, particularly those with proximal aortic dissection. Transesophageal echocardiography can demonstrate intimal tears in most cases and permits recognition of true and false lumina. Both transthoracic and transesophageal echocardiography are helpful in defining the mechanism of aortic insufficiency if present, as well as recognizing pericardial extension of the dissection. Mechanisms for aortic insufficiency in patients with acute ascending aortic dissection include intimal flap prolapse, leaflet prolapse, presence of bicuspid aortic valve, or incomplete leaflet closure. Aortic insufficiency due to coronary cusp perforation is more likely to be due to infective endocarditis.

References:

1. Bansal M, Fuster V, Narula J, et al. Chapter 2: Cardiovascular Imaging. In: Kaplan JA, Augoustides JGT, Manecke GR, et al., eds. Kaplan's Cardiac Anesthesia. 7th ed. Elsevier; 2017:20-45.
2. Thorsgard ME, Morrissette GJ, et al. Impact of intraoperative transesophageal echocardiography on acute type-A aortic dissection. J Cardiothorac Vasc Anesth, 2014; 28: 1203-1207.
3. Patel PA. Bavaria JE, Ghadimi K, et al. Aortic regurgitation in acute type A dissection: a clinical classification for the perioperative echocardiographer. J Cardiothorac Vasc Anesth, 2018; 32: 586-597.

20. When using dobutamine echocardiography to assess myocardial viability, which of the following findings is most likely to indicate that the affected myocardium will benefit from revascularization?
    A. Myocardium that improves in function at low doses but worsens at peak doses
    B. Myocardium that lacks improvement in contractility at low doses
    C. Myocardium with a sustained improvement in contractility at both low and high doses
    D. Myocardium that improves in contractility only at high doses

Correct Answer: A

Explanation: Dobutamine echocardiography is the primary echocardiographic modality used for the assessment of myocardial viability in clinical practice. This involves initiating a dobutamine infusion at a low dose (typically 2.5–5 mcg/kg/min) and then doubling the dose every 3 minutes to a maximum rate of 40 mcg/kg/min. At low doses (up to 10 mcg/kg/min) dobutamine augments cardiac contractility without any appreciable increase in myocardial oxygen demand. However, when the dose is increased further, there is a progressive increase in heart rate and myocardial oxygen demand. As a result, a dysfunctional but viable segment that is underperfused (hibernating segment) will improve at low doses but worsen again at peak doses (biphasic response). This is considered an accurate predictor of function recovery after revascularization. Stunned myocardium will demonstrate a sustained improvement in contractility at both low and peak doses and is a segment that will likely improve over time without the need for revascularization. If there is no improvement with a low dose, this is considered a lack of myocardial viability and the likelihood of functional recovery is very low.

References:

1. Bansal M, Fuster V, Narula J, et al. Chapter 2: Cardiovascular Imaging. In: Kaplan JA, Augoustides JGT, Manecke GR, et al., eds. Kaplan's Cardiac Anesthesia. 7th ed. Elsevier; 2017:20-45.
2. Afridi I, Kleiman NS, Raizner AE, et al. Dobutamine echocardiography in myocardial hibernation. Optimal dose and accuracy in predicting recovery of ventricular function after coronary angioplasty. Circulation, 1995; 9: 663-670.

21. Which of the follow modalities of stress echocardiography is considered to be the most sensitive for detection of inducible ischemia?
    A. Dobutamine echocardiography
    B. Dipyridamole echocardiography
    C. Adenosine echocardiography
    D. Exercise echocardiography

Correct Answer: D

Explanation: The accuracy of stress echocardiography for detection of inducible ischemia has been examined in numerous studies. In a large meta-analysis, the average sensitivity and specificity of exercise echocardiography were found to be 83% and 84%, respectively. These values were 80% and 85%, respectively, for dobutamine echocardiography; 71% and 92%, respectively, for dipyridamole echocardiography; and 68% and 81%, respectively, for adenosine stress echocardiography. A number of factors can influence the accuracy of stress echocardiography, including the adequacy of stress, delayed imaging after stress, the extent of coronary disease, use of beta-blockers and other antianginal agents, preexisting wall motion abnormalities, previous coronary surgery, the presence of concomitant conduction abnormalities, and the acoustic quality of the grey-scale images.

References:

1. Bansal M, Fuster V, Narula J, et al. Chapter 2: Cardiovascular Imaging. In: Kaplan JA, Augoustides JGT, Manecke GR, et al., eds. Kaplan's Cardiac Anesthesia. 7th ed. Elsevier; 2017:20-45.
2. Noguchi Y, Nagata-Kobayashi S, Stahl JE, et al. A meta-analytic comparison of echocardiographic stressors. Int J Cardiovasc Imaging, 2005; 21: 189-207.

22. Which of the following findings indicate the presence of pseudosevere aortic stenosis as investigated by low-dose dobutamine echocardiography?
    A. Increase in transaortic gradient without a concomitant increase in valve area
    B. Decrease in transaortic gradient with a decrease in valve area
    C. Increase in valve area without significant increase in transaortic gradient

D. Increase in valve area with significant increase in transaortic gradient

Correct Answer: C

Explanation: A specific indication for stress echocardiography is in the evaluation of low-gradient severe aortic stenosis (AS) in the presence of left ventricular (LV) systolic dysfunction. The AS may be truly severe, and the gradients may be low due to LV systolic dysfunction. The AS may not be severe, and the reduced valve area may be a function of inadequate opening force (pseudosevere AS). Low-dose dobutamine echocardiography (max dose 10–20 mcg/kg/min) can help to differentiate these two clinical situations. In true AS an increase in LV contractility with dobutamine will significantly increase the transaortic gradient without a concomitant increase in valve area. In these patients the LV systolic dysfunction is likely related to AS and is expected to improve after aortic valve replacement. In contrast, if the valve area increases with dobutamine and improved LV contractility but the gradients do not increase much, then the patient has pseudosevere AS, and the LV systolic dysfunction is likely not related to AS. Of note, patients may have advanced LV systolic dysfunction with no contractile reserve, which precludes making the distinction between severe AS and pseudosevere AS. These patients have high associated surgical mortality rates and poor long-term outcomes, although aortic valve replacement may still improve LV function and outcome in selected individuals.

References:

1. Bansal M, Fuster V, Narula J, et al. Chapter 2: Cardiovascular Imaging. In: Kaplan JA, Augoustides JGT, Manecke GR, et al., eds. Kaplan's Cardiac Anesthesia. 7th ed. Elsevier; 2017:20-45.
2. Monin JL, Quéré JP, Monchi M, et al. Low-gradient aortic stenosis: operative risk stratification and predictors for long-term outcome: a multicenter study using dobutamine stress hemodynamics. Circulation, 2003; 108: 319-324.

23. Which of the following assessments is not able to be made by myocardial nuclear scintigraphy?
A. Myocardial viability
B. Distribution of coronary artery disease
C. Beta-receptor density
D. Valvular disease severity

Correct Answer: D

Explanation: Myocardial nuclear scintigraphy is the most widely used modality for assessment of myocardial ischemia and viability, at least in the preoperative setting. There are two main forms of myocardial nuclear imaging: single-photon emission computed tomography (SPECT) and positron emission tomography (PET). Both use the principles of radioactive decay to evaluate the myocardium and its blood supply. Technetium 99m and thallium 201 are most commonly used in SPECT, and rubidium 82, N-ammonia 13, and fluorine 18 are most commonly used in PET. Detection of myocardial ischemia is the most common indication for performing myocardial perfusion imaging. Either SPECT or PET can be used for this purpose and is based on assessments of myocardial uptake of the radioisotope at rest and after stress. Myocardial uptake is reduced after stress in myocardial regions where significant coronary artery stenosis is present. Viability assessment using SPECT imaging involves taking advantage of the long half-life of thallium. The time for uptake is short in normal myocardium, but 24 hours may be needed for hibernating myocardium. Patients are imaged 24 hours after the initial injection of thallium to assess viability and delayed metabolic activity. SPECT imaging of the myocardial uptake of an iodine 123-labeled analog of norepinephrine (metaiodobenzylguanidine) provides an assessment of the beta-receptor density and has been used in evaluation of patients with heart failure.

References:

1. Bansal M, Fuster V, Narula J, et al. Chapter 2: Cardiovascular Imaging. In: Kaplan JA, Augoustides JGT, Manecke GR, et al., eds. Kaplan's Cardiac Anesthesia. 7th ed. Elsevier; 2017:20-45.
2. Merlet P, Pouillart F, Dubois-Randé JL, et al. Sympathetic nerve alterations assessed with 123I-MIBG in the failing human heart. J Nucl Med, 1999; 40: 224-231.

24. Which of the following is considered the imaging modality of choice for evaluation of aortic pathologies such as aortic aneurysms and nonemergency dissections?
A. Transesophageal echocardiography
B. Nuclear scintigraphy
C. Computed tomography with aortography
D. Cardiovascular magnetic resonance imaging

Correct Answer: C

Explanation: Computed tomography with aortography is the imaging modality of choice for evaluation of aortic pathologies such as aortic aneurysms and nonemergency dissections. It is important to have the scan gated to the patient's electrocardiogram because the ascending aorta moves significantly during the cardiac cycle. Nongated scans have inherent motion artifacts that can be confused for a dissection. Once the images are acquired by specialized imaging workstations, the aorta is evaluated in multiple orthogonal views to measure the true short axis throughout the length of the aorta. The excellent spatial and contrast resolution of this modality makes it useful for the evaluation of aortic dissections. Entry points of dissection, intimal flap location, false lumen, extension into branch arteries, and the abdominal aortic circulation are easily identified.

References:

1. Bansal M, Fuster V, Narula J, et al. Chapter 2: Cardiovascular Imaging. In: Kaplan JA, Augoustides JGT, Manecke GR, et al., eds. Kaplan's Cardiac Anesthesia. 7th ed. Elsevier; 2017:20-45.
2. Maslow A, Atalay MK, Sodha N. Intramural hematoma. J Cardiothorac Vasc Anesth, 2018; 32: 1341-1362.

25. Which of the following imaging modalities exposes the patient to ionizing radiation?
  A. Cardiac magnetic resonance imaging
  B. Transesophageal echocardiography
  C. Transthoracic echocardiography
  D. Cardiac computed tomography

Correct Answer: D

Explanation: Cardiac computed tomography uses ionizing radiation for the production of images. Concern about excessive medical radiation exposure has been raised. Although several techniques, such as prospective gated acquisition, may be implemented to reduce the radiation dose, a risk-benefit assessment must be done for the selection of patients who have appropriate indications for cardiac computed tomography.

References:

  1. Bansal M, Fuster V, Narula J, et al. Chapter 2: Cardiovascular Imaging. In: Kaplan JA, Augoustides JGT, Manecke GR, et al., eds. Kaplan's Cardiac Anesthesia. 7th ed. Elsevier; 2017:20-45.
  2. Scheffel H, Alkadhi H, Leschka S, et al. Low-dose CT coronary angiography in the step-and-shoot mode: diagnostic performance. Heart, 2008; 94: 1132-1137.

26. Which of the following is considered the gold standard for quantitative assessment of biventricular volumes and ejection fraction?
  A. Three-dimensional transesophageal echocardiography
  B. Nuclear scintigraphy
  C. Cardiovascular magnetic resonance imaging
  D. Cardiac computed tomography

Correct Answer: C

Explanation: Cardiovascular magnetic resonance imaging (CMR) is the gold standard for the quantitative assessment of biventricular volumes, ejection fraction, and mass while also offering excellent reproducibility. CMR has good spatial and temporal resolution. In dynamic contrast-enhanced CMR, gadolinium is used to enhance the magnetization of protons in nearby water and create a stronger signal. Additionally, gadolinium contrast permeates through the intercellular space in necrotic or fibrotic myocardium, enabling myocardial scar detection on late gadolinium enhancement. CMR can also be used for perfusion imaging by evaluating the first pass of gadolinium contrast through the myocardium.

References:

  1. Bansal M, Fuster V, Narula J, et al. Chapter 2: Cardiovascular Imaging. In: Kaplan JA, Augoustides JGT, Manecke GR, et al., eds. Kaplan's Cardiac Anesthesia. 7th ed. Elsevier; 2017:20-45.
  2. Pujadas S, Reddy GP, Weber O, et al. MR imaging assessment of cardiac function. J Magn Reson Imaging, 2004; 19: 789-799.

27. Signs of pulmonary hypertension on cardiac computed tomography include all the following EXCEPT:
  A. Enlargement of peripheral pulmonary vessels
  B. Right ventricular hypertrophy
  C. Enlargement of proximal pulmonary vessels
  D. Right ventricle and right atrial enlargement

Correct Answer: A

Explanation: Computed tomography with pulmonary angiography can evaluate for signs of pulmonary hypertension, which include reduced right ventricular systolic function, right atrial and right ventricular enlargement, right ventricular hypertrophy, enlargement of proximal pulmonary vessels, and an abrupt narrowing of peripheral pulmonary vessels. Further diagnostic modalities to assess for the presence of pulmonary hypertension include transthoracic or transesophageal echocardiography and right heart catheterization.

References:

  1. Bansal M, Fuster V, Narula J, et al. Chapter 2: Cardiovascular Imaging. In: Kaplan JA, Augoustides JGT, Manecke GR, et al., eds. Kaplan's Cardiac Anesthesia. 7th ed. Elsevier; 2017:20-45.
  2. Ranka S, Mohananey D, Agarwal N, et al. Chronic thromboembolic pulmonary hypertension-management strategies and outcomes. J Cardiothorac Vasc Anesth, 2020; 34: 2513-2523.

28. Which of the following is NOT an indication for coronary angiography before a cardiac surgical procedure?
  A. Age greater than 40 years for men
  B. Postmenopausal status for women
  C. Symptoms suggestive of coronary ischemia
  D. Left ventricular diastolic dysfunction

Correct Answer: D

Explanation: Conventional coronary angiography remains the gold standard for evaluation of coronary anatomy and the anatomic extent and severity of coronary artery disease. The planning for a coronary revascularization procedure typically relies on prior invasive coronary angiography. The indications for coronary angiography before a cardiac surgical procedure include age greater than 40 years for men, postmenopausal status for women, symptoms suggestive of coronary ischemia, left ventricular systolic dysfunction, and the presence of one or more major cardiovascular risk factors. Cardiac computed tomography with angiography is an alternative in patients when the pretest probability of coronary artery disease is relatively low; however, classic coronary angiography is often preferred because of its superior accuracy, feasibility regardless of heart rate and rhythm, the need for smaller amounts of contrast agents, and noninterference from calcium present in the coronary arteries or the aortic valve.

References:

  1. Bansal M, Fuster V, Narula J, et al. Chapter 2: Cardiovascular Imaging. In: Kaplan JA, Augoustides JGT, Manecke GR, et al., eds. Kaplan's Cardiac Anesthesia. 7th ed. Elsevier; 2017:20-45.
  2. Otto CM, Nishimura RA, Bonow R, et al. 2020 ACC/AHA Guideline for the Management of Patients With Valvular Heart Disease: Executive Summary: A Report of the American

College of Cardiology/American Heart Association Joint Committee on Clinical Practice Guidelines. Circulation, 2021; 143: e35-e71.

29. Which of the following echocardiographic findings is consistent with severe mitral regurgitation?
  A. Pulmonary vein flow pattern showing systolic wave blunting
  B. Continuous wave Doppler showing a parabolic jet contour
  C. Continuous wave Doppler showing early peaking triangular jet contour
  D. Color flow jet area of 8 cm^2

Correct Answer: C

Explanation: Early peaking triangular jet contour of a continuous wave spectral Doppler profile is consistent with severe mitral regurgitation, while a parabolic jet contour is typically found in mild or moderate mitral regurgitation. Pulmonary vein flow pattern showing systolic flow reversal would be expected in severe mitral regurgitation, while systolic blunting is generally found in moderate mitral regurgitation. A color flow jet area greater than 10 cm^2 is consistent with severe mitral regurgitation, although a wall-hugging jet with a jet area less than 10 cm^2 can also be present in cases of severe mitral regurgitation due to the Coanda effect.

References:

1. Bansal M, Fuster V, Narula J, et al. Chapter 2: Cardiovascular Imaging. In: Kaplan JA, Augoustides JGT, Manecke GR, et al., eds. Kaplan's Cardiac Anesthesia. 7th ed. Elsevier; 2017:20-45.
2. Zoghbi WA, Enriquez-Sarano M, Foster E, et al. American Society of Echocardiography. Recommendations for evaluation of the severity of native valvular regurgitation with two-dimensional and Doppler echocardiography. J Am Soc Echocardiogr, 2003; 16: 777-802.
3. Otto CM, Nishimura RA, Bonow R, et al. 2020 ACC/AHA Guideline for the Management of Patients With Valvular Heart Disease: Executive Summary: A Report of the American

College of Cardiology/American Heart Association Joint Committee on Clinical Practice Guidelines. Circulation, 2021; 143: e35-e71.

30. When using vascular Doppler ultrasound to determine the severity of carotid artery stenosis, which of the following is LEAST likely to lead to an inaccurate estimation of stenosis severity?
  A. Presence of severe aortic insufficiency
  B. Presence of reduced left ventricular systolic function
  C. Presence of an upper extremity arteriovenous fistula
  D. Presence of left ventricular diastolic dysfunction

Correct Answer: D

Explanation: Stroke is a severely debilitating disease, with carotid artery stenosis being the major cause. Atherosclerotic plaques most often form in the proximal internal carotid artery; however, the common carotid artery may also be involved. Stroke often occurs as the first symptom of the disease. Several imaging modalities can be used for diagnosis, including computed tomography with angiography and vascular ultrasound. Vascular ultrasound is easily accessible, inexpensive, and excellent for the evaluation of carotid anatomy and flow dynamics. Doppler ultrasound can be used to measure velocity and pressure gradients across lesions; however, it can give false measurements in scenarios of decreased velocity of blood from the heart to the carotid arteries such as in the setting of reduced left ventricular systolic function or significant valvular disease, or through shunting in arteriovenous fistulas.

References:

1. Bansal M, Fuster V, Narula J, et al. Chapter 2: Cardiovascular Imaging. In: Kaplan JA, Augoustides JGT, Manecke GR, et al., eds. Kaplan's Cardiac Anesthesia. 7th ed. Elsevier; 2017:20-45.
2. Baron EL, Fremed DI, Tadros RO, et al. Surgical versus percutaneous therapy of carotid artery disease: an evidence-based outcomes analysis. J Cardiothorac Vasc Anesth, 2017; 31: 755-767.

CHAPTER 3

Cardiac Catheterization Laboratory

Alexander D. Stoker, Steven T. Morozowich, and Harish Ramakrishna

KEY POINTS

1. The cardiac catheterization laboratory has evolved from a purely diagnostic facility to a therapeutic one in which many facets of cardiovascular disease can be effectively modified or treated. Despite improvements in equipment, the quality of the procedure depends on well-trained and experienced physicians with proper certification, adequate procedural volume, and personnel committed to the continuous quality improvement process.

2. Guidelines for diagnostic cardiac catheterization have established indications, contraindications, and criteria to identify high-risk patients. Careful evaluation of the patient before the procedure is critical to minimize risks.

3. Interventional cardiology began in the late 1970s as balloon angioplasty, with a success rate of 80% and emergent coronary artery bypass graft (CABG) surgery rates of 3% to 5%. Although current success rates exceed 95%, with CABG rates of less than 1%, failed percutaneous coronary intervention (PCI) presents a challenge for the anesthesiologist because of hemodynamic problems, concomitant medications, and the underlying cardiac disease.

4. Since the introduction of drug-eluting stents (DESs), acute closure due to coronary dissection has diminished significantly, and restenosis rates have fallen precipitously.

5. The first-generation DESs (Cypher, Cordis, Miami Lakes, FL, and Taxus, Boston Scientific, Marlborough, MA) were extremely effective at reducing in-stent restenosis compared with bare metal stents (BMSs). However, DESs have demonstrated higher rates of late stent thrombosis (LST), especially in the setting of premature discontinuation of dual antiplatelet therapy. Second-generation DESs (Xience, Abbott Vascular, Abbott Park, IL, and Resolute, Medtronic, Minneapolis, MN) have LST rates comparable to those of BMSs and therefore are the preferred stent type.

6. As a treatment strategy for patients with acute myocardial infarction, primary PCI is preferred to the administration of thrombolytic therapy because of its higher rates of infarct artery patency and Thrombolysis In Myocardial Infarction grade 3 flow, as well as lower rates of recurrent ischemia, reinfarction, intracranial hemorrhage, and death.

7. In the United States, increasing numbers of diagnostic coronary angiograms and PCIs are performed from a transradial approach because of lower vascular complication rates and patient preference for this approach compared with the more traditional transfemoral approach.

8. In multivessel coronary artery disease, an angiographic SYNTAX score should be calculated to assist with decision making regarding percutaneous versus surgical revascularization. A multidisciplinary heart team meeting (including a cardiologist, a cardiovascular surgeon, and, occasionally, an anesthesiologist) should then convene to discuss and optimize patient care by providing an individualized treatment recommendation.

9. Extensive thrombus, heavy calcification, degenerated saphenous vein graft, and chronic total occlusion present specific challenges in PCI. Various specialty devices have been developed to address these problems and have had varying degrees of success.

10. Acute thrombotic PCI complications can usually be overcome with more aggressive antithrombotic and antiplatelet pharmacotherapy. These medications can complicate the management of an unstable patient who requires transfer for bailout CABG. Appropriate understanding of the pharmacokinetics is essential for the cardiac anesthesiologist.

11. The reach of the interventional cardiologist has extended beyond coronary vessels to include closure of congenital defects and percutaneous treatment of valvular disease. These complex procedures are more likely to require general anesthesia but also can be effectively managed with monitored anesthesia care or regional anesthesia techniques.

1. Which of the following strategies is LEAST likely to prevent contrast-induced nephropathy?
   A. Intravenous hydration with normal saline before contrast administration
   B. Avoiding high-osmolar contrast dyes
   C. Limiting the amount of contrast dye administered
   D. Maintaining an interval of 24 hours between contrast dye exposures

Correct Answer: D

Explanation: Contrast-induced nephropathy is defined as an increase in serum creatinine concentration of more than 0.5 mg/dL or 25% above baseline level within 48 hours of contrast administration. Risk factors for this type of acute kidney injury include diabetes mellitus, preexisting chronic kidney disease, and heart failure. The risk in each patient must be weighed against the potential benefit of contrast administration. In a patient with a serum creatinine level greater than 1.5 mg/dL, particularly in the presence of diabetes mellitus or a glomerular filtration rate less than 60 mL/min, the administration of contrast may need to be delayed due to the risk of contrast-induced nephropathy. This nephropathy is dependent on the amount of dye reaching the renal arteries and can be reduced by hydrating the patient before the procedure, avoiding high-osmolar contrast dyes and nephrotoxic agents, limiting the amount of dye administered, and maintaining an interval of 72 hours between contrast dye exposures if multiple studies are required.

References:

1. Gelzinis T, Kozak M, Chambers C, et al. Chapter 3: Cardiac Catheterization Laboratory: Diagnostic and Therapeutic Procedures in the Adult Patient. In: Kaplan JA, Augoustides JGT, Manecke GR, et al., eds. Kaplan's Cardiac Anesthesia. 7th ed. Elsevier; 2017:46-95.
2. Schweiger MJ, Chambers CE, Davidson CJ, et al. Prevention of contrast induced nephropathy: recommendations for the high-risk patient undergoing cardiovascular procedures. Catheter Cardiovasc Interv, 2007; 69: 135-140.

2. Which of the following conditions would NOT cause a step-up in venous oxygen saturation as detected during a right heart catheterization?
   A. Post–myocardial infarction ventricular septal defect
   B. Partial anomalous pulmonary venous return
   C. Intrapulmonary shunting
   D. Gerbode defect

Correct Answer: C

Explanation: A left-to-right shunt can be detected during right heart catheterization by the presence of a step-up in venous oxygenation. Examples of left-to-right shunts include a ventricular septal defect, which would cause a step-up in oxygen saturation in the right ventricle, a partial anomalous pulmonary venous return, which would cause a step-up in the superior vena cava or right atrium, and a Gerbode defect, which would cause a step-up in the right atrium. A Gerbode defect is a communication from the left ventricle to the right atrium and may be congenital or acquired. Acquired cases of Gerbode defect have occurred due to infective endocarditis, previous cardiac surgery, and myocardial infarction. Intrapulmonary shunting, as occurs in hepatopulmonary syndrome, causes a right-to-left shunt and may cause hypoxemia, but would not cause a step-up during right heart catheterization.

References:

1. Gelzinis T, Kozak M, Chambers C, et al. Chapter 3: Cardiac Catheterization Laboratory: Diagnostic and Therapeutic Procedures in the Adult Patient. In: Kaplan JA, Augoustides JGT, Manecke GR, et al., eds. Kaplan's Cardiac Anesthesia. 7th ed. Elsevier; 2017:46-95.
2. Ting PC, Lee KT, Chou AH, et al. Surgical repair of acquired Gerbode defect (left ventricle-to-right atrium shunt) caused by intramyocardial dissection after redo mitral valve replacement. J Cardiothorac Vasc Anesth, 2020; 34: 1573-1576.

3. Which of the following lesions is most likely to result in the clinical finding of *pulsus parvus et tardus*?
   A. Tricuspid regurgitation
   B. Aortic stenosis
   C. Hypertrophic cardiomyopathy
   D. Aortic regurgitation

Correct Answer: B

Explanation: The normal adult aortic valve area is 2.6 to 3.5 cm^2. As the valve area decreases, as in aortic stenosis, the left ventricle exhibits a more rounded appearance at its peak systolic pressure, and there is a progressive increase in left ventricular end-diastolic pressure. The left ventricle hypertrophies, and filling becomes more dependent on the contraction of the left atrium. Widening of the systolic pressure gradient from the left ventricle to the aorta, a decrease in the rate of rise of the upstroke on the aortic pressure tracing, and a delay in time to peak aortic pressure are seen. A delayed and weak peripheral pulse, which can be appreciated on physical exam in patients with aortic stenosis, is known as *pulsus parvus et tardus*.

References:

1. Gelzinis T, Kozak M, Chambers C, et al. Chapter 3: Cardiac Catheterization Laboratory: Diagnostic and Therapeutic Procedures in the Adult Patient. In: Kaplan JA, Augoustides JGT, Manecke GR, et al., eds. Kaplan's Cardiac Anesthesia. 7th ed. Elsevier; 2017:46-95.
2. Zimmerman J, Birgenheier N. Appropriate use criteria for the treatment of patients with severe aortic stenosis: a review of the 2017 American College of Cardiology Guideline for the Cardiac Anesthesiologist. J Cardiothorac Vasc Anesth, 2019; 33: 3127-3142.

4. Bland-White-Garland syndrome consists of which of the following anatomical findings?
   A. Fistula formation from the right coronary artery to the right ventricle

B. Left coronary artery arising from the pulmonary artery

C. Left coronary artery arising from right sinus of Valsalva

D. Fistula formation from the left circumflex to left atrium

Correct Answer: B

Explanation: Coronary anomalies can be encountered during coronary angiography and may or may not be of clinical significance. Anomalous coronary origins can involve the left main, circumflex, or right coronary artery. An anomalous course of a coronary artery between the aorta and pulmonary artery can cause compression of the vessel and may require surgical intervention due to the risk of myocardial ischemia and sudden death. A fistula between a coronary artery and a heart chamber is known as a coronary-cameral fistula, with most being small and of no clinical significance. Bland-White-Garland syndrome occurs when the left coronary artery arises from the pulmonary artery, with most patients presenting early in life, although adults may present with sudden cardiac death, angina, or ischemic cardiomyopathy.

References:

1. Gelzinis T, Kozak M, Chambers C, et al. Chapter 3: Cardiac Catheterization Laboratory: Diagnostic and Therapeutic Procedures in the Adult Patient. In: Kaplan JA, Augoustides JGT, Manecke GR, et al., eds. Kaplan's Cardiac Anesthesia. 7th ed. Elsevier; 2017:46-95.
2. Maddali MM, Al-delamie TY, Al-Maskari SN, et al. Unusual cause of chest pain at an unusual age. J Cardiothorac Vasc Anesth, 2011; 25: 501-504.

5. In the setting of coronary artery disease with circumferential narrowing, a 70% reduction in vessel diameter as detected on coronary angiography would result in what percent reduction in cross-sectional area of the vessel?

A. 59%

B. 91%

C. 70%

D. 85%

Correct Answer: B

Explanation: By convention, the severity of coronary vessel stenosis is quantified by percentage diameter reduction. Multiple views of each vessel are recorded in coronary angiography, and the worst narrowing is used to make a clinical decision. Diameter reduction can be used to estimate luminal cross-sectional area reductions. If the narrowing is circumferential, a 70% diameter reduction would result in a 91% cross-sectional area reduction given that area is proportional to the square of the radius. Using the reduction in diameter as a measure of lesion severity may be difficult at times, particularly in cases of diffuse coronary artery disease, which can make it difficult to define the normal coronary diameter. This scenario may be encountered in patients with insulin-dependent diabetes and in individuals with severe lipid disorders.

References:

1. Gelzinis T, Kozak M, Chambers C, et al. Chapter 3: Cardiac Catheterization Laboratory: Diagnostic and Therapeutic Procedures in the Adult Patient. In: Kaplan JA, Augoustides JGT, Manecke GR, et al., eds. Kaplan's Cardiac Anesthesia. 7th ed. Elsevier; 2017:46-95.
2. Shekhar S, Mohananey D, Villablanca P, et al. Revascularization strategies for stable left main coronary artery disease: analysis of current evidence. J Cardiothorac Vasc Anesth, 2022; 36(8 Pt B): 3370-3378.

6. Which of the following pairs of a coronary artery branch and the corresponding originating vessel is INCORRECT?

A. Septal perforator; left anterior descending artery

B. Acute marginal; right coronary artery

C. Diagonal artery; left anterior descending artery

D. Ramus intermedius; right coronary artery

Correct Answer: D

Explanation: In most patients the left main coronary artery bifurcates into the circumflex and left anterior descending artery. Occasionally, these branches arise from separate ostia, or the left main artery may trifurcate, creating a middle branch, known as the ramus intermedius, which supplies the high lateral wall of the left ventricle. Septal perforators and diagonal branch arteries arise from the left anterior descending artery. The obtuse marginal branch arteries arise from the circumflex artery. The acute marginal artery arises from the right coronary artery, as does the sinus node branch. The posterior descending artery originates from the right coronary artery in 85% to 90% of patients, and from the circumflex artery in 10% to 15% of patients.

References:

1. Gelzinis T, Kozak M, Chambers C, et al. Chapter 3: Cardiac Catheterization Laboratory: Diagnostic and Therapeutic Procedures in the Adult Patient. In: Kaplan JA, Augoustides JGT, Manecke GR, et al., eds. Kaplan's Cardiac Anesthesia. 7th ed. Elsevier; 2017:46-95.
2. Dhawan R, Prakash A, Kundu A, et al. A rare case of recurrent coronary cameral fistula: a unique surgical challenge. J Cardiothorac Vasc Anesth, 2019; 33: 1068-1072.

7. Which of the following mechanisms is currently the most significant cause of restenosis in the first 6 months after a percutaneous coronary intervention?

A. Stent fracture

B. Neointimal hyperplasia

C. Vessel recoil

D. Negative remodeling

Correct Answer: B

Explanation: Restenosis usually occurs within the first 6 months after percutaneous coronary intervention and may be caused by several mechanisms. Vessel recoil is caused by the elastic tissue in the vessel and occurs early after balloon dilation. It is no longer a significant contributor to restenosis, because metal stents are almost 100% effective in preventing recoil. Negative remodeling refers to late narrowing of the external elastic lamina and adjacent tissue, which accounted for up to 75% of lumen loss in the past. This process is prevented by metal stents and is no longer a significant contributor to restenosis. Neointimal hyperplasia is the major component of in-stent restenosis in the modern era. Neointimal hyperplasia is more pronounced in diabetic patients, who are at increased risk for restenosis. Drug-eluting stents limit neointimal hyperplasia and have dramatically reduced the frequency of in-stent thrombosis. Stent fracture is uncommon.

References:

1. Gelzinis T, Kozak M, Chambers C, et al. Chapter 3: Cardiac Catheterization Laboratory: Diagnostic and Therapeutic Procedures in the Adult Patient. In: Kaplan JA, Augoustides JGT, Manecke GR, et al., eds. Kaplan's Cardiac Anesthesia. 7th ed. Elsevier; 2017:46-95.
2. Mauermann WJ, Rehfeldt KH, Bell MR, et al. Percutaneous coronary interventions and antiplatelet therapy in the perioperative period. J Cardiothorac Vasc Anesth, 2007; 21: 436-442.

8. Which of the following is the correct mechanism of action of clopidogrel?
   A. It binds irreversibly to the P2Y12 adenosine diphosphate receptor on platelets
   B. It results in glycoprotein IIb/IIIa platelet receptor inhibition
   C. It acetylates cyclooxygenase
   D. It inhibits factor Xa

Correct Answer: A

Explanation: Thrombosis is a major component of acute coronary syndrome during percutaneous coronary intervention. The primary pathway for clot formation and acute in-stent thrombosis is platelet-mediated. Dual antiplatelet therapy is commonly used to prevent stent thrombosis and typically continued for a minimum of 6 to 12 months after placement of drug-eluting stents. Clopidogrel and aspirin are commonly combined for dual antiplatelet therapy. Clopidogrel acts by irreversibly binding to the adenosine diphosphate receptor P2Y12 on platelets. Aspirin acts by blocking platelet activation by irreversible acetylation of cyclooxygenase. Glycoprotein IIb/IIIa inhibitors include abciximab, eptifibatide, and tirofiban. Factor Xa inhibitors include apixaban and rivaroxaban.

References:

1. Gelzinis T, Kozak M, Chambers C, et al. Chapter 3: Cardiac Catheterization Laboratory: Diagnostic and Therapeutic Procedures in the Adult Patient. In: Kaplan JA, Augoustides JGT, Manecke GR, et al., eds. Kaplan's Cardiac Anesthesia. 7th ed. Elsevier; 2017:46-95.
2. Mauermann WJ, Rehfeldt KH, Bell MR, et al. Percutaneous coronary interventions and antiplatelet therapy in the perioperative period. J Cardiothorac Vasc Anesth, 2007; 21: 436-442.

9. Which of the following antiplatelet agents has a rapid onset of action and a rapid return of platelet function after cessation?
   A. Clopidogrel
   B. Prasugrel
   C. Aspirin
   D. Cangrelor

Correct Answer: D

Explanation: Cangrelor is a P2Y12 platelet receptor inhibitor that is delivered in the form of an intravenous infusion. The advantages of cangrelor include its rapid onset of action and rapid return of platelet function after cessation, which is of particular interest in the perioperative period and allows for its therapeutic application as a bridge to surgery. Cangrelor has a half-life of 3 to 6 minutes and an offset of platelet inhibition within 30 to 60 minutes. Clopidogrel and prasugrel irreversibly bind to the P2Y12 receptor on platelets. Aspirin also has an irreversible platelet inhibition effect through its mechanism of acetylation of cyclooxygenase.

References:

1. Gelzinis T, Kozak M, Chambers C, et al. Chapter 3: Cardiac Catheterization Laboratory: Diagnostic and Therapeutic Procedures in the Adult Patient. In: Kaplan JA, Augoustides JGT, Manecke GR, et al., eds. Kaplan's Cardiac Anesthesia. 7th ed. Elsevier; 2017:46-95.
2. Laehn SJ, Feih JT, Saltzberg MT, et al. Pharmacodynamic-guided cangrelor bridge therapy for orthotopic heart transplant. J Cardiothorac Vasc Anesth, 2019; 33: 1054-1058.

10. Which of the following characteristics of coronary lesions is LEAST likely to increase the complexity of percutaneous coronary intervention?
    A. Discrete lesion
    B. Total occlusion greater than 3 months old
    C. Angulated segment greater than 90 degrees
    D. Excessive tortuosity of proximal segment

Correct Answer: A

Explanation: Beginning in 1988, the American College of Cardiology/American Heart Association task force developed a lesion morphology classification of coronary artery disease in an attempt to correlate complexity of lesions with outcomes and success rates of percutaneous coronary intervention. The most complex lesions described are diffuse (>2 cm in length) rather than discrete (<10 mm), have excessive tortuosity of proximal segments, and involve angulated segments over 90 degrees. Further markers of complex coronary lesions are those with total occlusions greater than 3 months old, degenerated vein grafts with friable lesions, and those with an inability to protect major side branches.

References:

1. Gelzinis T, Kozak M, Chambers C, et al. Chapter 3: Cardiac Catheterization Laboratory: Diagnostic and Therapeutic Procedures in the Adult Patient. In: Kaplan JA, Augoustides

JGT, Manecke GR, et al., eds. Kaplan's Cardiac Anesthesia. 7th ed. Elsevier; 2017:46-95.

2. Vanneman MW. Anesthetic considerations for percutaneous coronary intervention for chronic total occlusions-a narrative review. J Cardiothorac Vasc Anesth, 2022; 36: 2132-2142.

11. At what point in the cardiac cycle should an intra-aortic balloon pump deflate?
   A. At the beginning of isovolumetric contraction
   B. At the time of aortic valve closure
   C. At the beginning of diastole
   D. At the beginning of isovolumetric relaxation

Correct Answer: **A**

Explanation: The intra-aortic balloon pump augments diastolic pressure and myocardial perfusion by inflating when the aortic valve is closed, which increases the coronary pressure gradient from the aorta to the coronary circulation. The optimal timing of balloon deflation is at the beginning of isovolumetric contraction and immediately before the onset of systole. This creates a dead space in the thoracic aorta, which reduces afterload and promotes forward flow. The net result is a reduction in left ventricular end-diastolic pressure, left ventricular volume, wall tension, myocardial work, and oxygen demand with preserved or increased stroke volume, ejection fraction, and cardiac output.

References:

1. Gelzinis T, Kozak M, Chambers C, et al. Chapter 3: Cardiac Catheterization Laboratory: Diagnostic and Therapeutic Procedures in the Adult Patient. In: Kaplan JA, Augoustides JGT, Manecke GR, et al., eds. Kaplan's Cardiac Anesthesia. 7th ed. Elsevier; 2017:46-95.

2. Loforte A, Comentale G, Botta L, et al. How would the authors treat their own temporary left ventricular failure with mechanical circulatory support? J Cardiothorac Vasc Anesth, 2022; 36: 1238-1250.

12. Contraindications for intra-aortic balloon pump counterpulsation include all the following EXCEPT:
   A. Aortic stents
   B. Aortic insufficiency
   C. Aortic dissection
   D. Coagulopathy

Correct Answer: **D**

Explanation: The disadvantages of an intra-aortic balloon pump include a limited ability to increase cardiac output (generally about 0.3 to 0.5 L/min); reliance on synchronization with the cardiac cycle and unreliable function in the setting of dysrhythmias; and reduced function with increases in aortic compliance, reduction in systemic vascular resistance, or higher heart rates. The complications of this device include balloon displacement, balloon rupture, balloon entrapment, aortic dissection or rupture, lower limb ischemia, thrombus formation, hemolysis, and bleeding at the insertion site. The contraindications for its placement include aortic

regurgitation, aortic dissections, and aortic stents. Coagulopathy is typically not considered a contraindication, and an intra-aortic balloon pump can be placed in patients systemically heparinized for cardiopulmonary bypass.

References:

1. Gelzinis T, Kozak M, Chambers C, et al. Chapter 3: Cardiac Catheterization Laboratory: Diagnostic and Therapeutic Procedures in the Adult Patient. In: Kaplan JA, Augoustides JGT, Manecke GR, et al., eds. Kaplan's Cardiac Anesthesia. 7th ed. Elsevier; 2017:46-95.

2. Loforte A, Comentale G, Botta L, et al. How would the authors treat their own temporary left ventricular failure with mechanical circulatory support? J Cardiothorac Vasc Anesth, 2022; 36: 1238-1250.

13. Which of the following is NOT considered a contraindication to Impella placement?
   A. Mechanical aortic valve
   B. Left ventricular mural thrombus
   C. Ventricular septal defect
   D. Mitral stenosis

Correct Answer: **D**

Explanation: The Impella device is an axial flow left ventricular assist device that is positioned across the aortic valve using fluoroscopic or echocardiographic guidance. The Impella can augment cardiac output up to 5.5 L/min and does not require a stable cardiac rhythm, cardiac output, or blood pressure signal for optimal function; however, it does require adequate left ventricular filling. The Impella is typically placed in the femoral artery or axillary artery, and has a higher risk of limb ischemia, hemolysis, and bleeding at the insertion site compared to an intra-aortic balloon pump. The Impella is contraindicated in patients with ventricular septal defects, mechanical aortic valves, left ventricular rupture, mural thrombus in the left ventricle, aortic dissection, or severe aortic insufficiency.

References:

1. Gelzinis T, Kozak M, Chambers C, et al. Chapter 3: Cardiac Catheterization Laboratory: Diagnostic and Therapeutic Procedures in the Adult Patient. In: Kaplan JA, Augoustides JGT, Manecke GR, et al., eds. Kaplan's Cardiac Anesthesia. 7th ed. Elsevier; 2017:46-95.

2. Crowley J, Cronin B, Essandoh M, et al. Transesophageal echocardiography for impella placement and management. J Cardiothorac Vasc Anesth, 2019; 33: 2663-2668.

14. The correct position for the inflow cannula of a TandemHeart is in which of the following locations?
   A. Left ventricle
   B. Left atrium
   C. Right atrium
   D. Superior vena cava

Correct Answer: **B**

Explanation: The TandemHeart is a centrifugal-flow left ventricular assist device in which the inflow cannula is inserted via the femoral vein into the left atrium through a trans-septal puncture. The outflow cannula is inserted in the femoral artery and positioned at the aortic bifurcation, providing flows up to 5 L/min. The TandemHeart reduces filling pressures including pulmonary artery pressure, pulmonary capillary wedge pressure, and central venous pressure, thereby decreasing myocardial workload and demand. The disadvantages include the limited availability, a requirement for expertise in transseptal puncture, hypoxemia due to shunting if the left atrial cannula slips back into the right atrium, prolonged implantation time, use of large cannulas (which increase the risk of vascular compromise), and limb ischemia.

References:

1. Gelzinis T, Kozak M, Chambers C, et al. Chapter 3: Cardiac Catheterization Laboratory: Diagnostic and Therapeutic Procedures in the Adult Patient. In: Kaplan JA, Augoustides JGT, Manecke GR, et al., eds. Kaplan's Cardiac Anesthesia. 7th ed. Elsevier; 2017:46-95.
2. Cole SP, Martinez-Acero N, Peterson A, et al. Imaging for temporary mechanical circulatory support devices. J Cardiothorac Vasc Anesth, 2022; 36: 2114-2131.

15. Which of the following types of mechanical circulatory support can increase left ventricular afterload and wall stress?
   A. Intra-aortic balloon pump
   B. Impella
   C. Veno-arterial extracorporeal membrane oxygenation
   D. TandemHeart

Correct Answer: C

Explanation: Veno-arterial extracorporeal membrane oxygenation (ECMO) is a modified cardiopulmonary bypass circuit that provides continuous nonpulsatile cardiac output and can be placed peripherally or centrally. It can oxygenate the blood, remove carbon dioxide, and support the circulation for several weeks. Unlike the Impella, intra-aortic balloon pump, or TandemHeart, veno-arterial ECMO can increase the left ventricular afterload and wall stress and can increase myocardial oxygen demand. The risks of veno-arterial ECMO include limb ischemia, arterial rupture, aortic dissection, differential hypoxia, left ventricular distention, and left ventricular thrombus.

References:

1. Gelzinis T, Kozak M, Chambers C, et al. Chapter 3: Cardiac Catheterization Laboratory: Diagnostic and Therapeutic Procedures in the Adult Patient. In: Kaplan JA, Augoustides JGT, Manecke GR, et al., eds. Kaplan's Cardiac Anesthesia. 7th ed. Elsevier; 2017:46-95.
2. Cole SP, Martinez-Acero N, Peterson A, et al. Imaging for temporary mechanical circulatory support devices. J Cardiothorac Vasc Anesth, 2022; 36: 2114-2131.

16. Which of the following patient comorbidities is most likely to contribute to coronary artery restenosis following percutaneous coronary intervention and may benefit from coronary artery bypass grafting in the setting of multivessel coronary artery disease?
   A. Obesity
   B. Hyperlipidemia
   C. Diabetes mellitus
   D. Hypertension

Correct Answer: C

Explanation: Patients with diabetes mellitus have been shown to have increased rates of restenosis following percutaneous coronary intervention, likely due to accelerated neointimal hyperplasia. Multiple trials have evaluated the roles of percutaneous coronary intervention and coronary artery bypass grafting for myocardial revascularization. In patients with diabetes and multivessel coronary artery disease, surgical revascularization has been associated with a survival advantage as compared to transcatheter options.

References:

1. Gelzinis T, Kozak M, Chambers C, et al. Chapter 3: Cardiac Catheterization Laboratory: Diagnostic and Therapeutic Procedures in the Adult Patient. In: Kaplan JA, Augoustides JGT, Manecke GR, et al., eds. Kaplan's Cardiac Anesthesia. 7th ed. Elsevier; 2017:46-95.
2. Cormican D, Jayaraman A, Sheu R, et al Coronary artery bypass grafting versus percutaneous coronary interventions: analysis of outcomes in myocardial revascularization. J Cardiothorac Vasc Anesth, 2019; 33: 2569-2588.

17. The placement of a MitraClip during transcatheter mitral valve repair is most similar to which of the following surgical techniques?
   A. Balloon valvuloplasty
   B. Annuloplasty ring
   C. Alfieri repair
   D. Park's stitch

Correct Answer: C

Explanation: The Alfieri repair was developed by Dr. Alfieri in 1991 for treatment of mitral regurgitation due to anterior mitral valve leaflet prolapse. He approximated the central segments of the anterior and posterior mitral valve leaflets, creating a double-orifice valve. Techniques in mitral valve repair include mitral annuloplasty that remodels the mitral annulus to improve the durability of the mitral repair. The MitraClip is a transcatheter technique for mitral valve repair that produces an edge-to-edge repair by the middle scallops of the mitral leaflets to simulate the Alfieri stitch. Balloon valvuloplasty is used to treat mitral stenosis, not mitral regurgitation. The Park's stitch is a central coaptation repair of the aortic valve to manage aortic insufficiency during placement of a left ventricular assist device and causes the aortic valve to become immobile in the closed position.

References:

1. Gelzinis T, Kozak M, Chambers C, et al. Chapter 3: Cardiac Catheterization Laboratory: Diagnostic and Therapeutic

Procedures in the Adult Patient. In: Kaplan JA, Augoustides JGT, Manecke GR, et al., eds. Kaplan's Cardiac Anesthesia. 7th ed. Elsevier; 2017:46-95.
2. Wu IY, Barajas MB, Hahn RT. The MitraClip procedure-a comprehensive review for the cardiac anesthesiologist. J Cardiothorac Vasc Anesth, 2018; 32: 2746-2759.

18. Which of the following is NOT included in the selection criteria for transcatheter mitral valve repair with the MitraClip device?
   A. Flail width less than 15 mm and flail gap less than 10 mm
   B. Calcification in the leaflet grasping area
   C. Mitral valve area greater or equal to 4.0 cm
   D. Coaptation length greater than 2 mm and depth less than 11 mm

Correct Answer: B

Explanation: The anatomical mechanism of mitral regurgitation must be evaluated to determine the feasibility and appropriateness of using a MitraClip to correct the mitral valve pathology. The mitral regurgitation jet should arise from the central two-thirds of the coaptation line, and there should be minimal calcification in the leaflet grasping area. Further selection criteria include a mitral valve area 4 cm^2 or more to minimize the risk of creating mitral stenosis; a coaptation length of at least 2 mm and a depth less than 11 mm; a flail width less than 15 mm; and a flail gap less than 10 mm. There should also be no leaflet cleft in the grasping area.

References:
1. Gelzinis T, Kozak M, Chambers C, et al. Chapter 3: Cardiac Catheterization Laboratory: Diagnostic and Therapeutic Procedures in the Adult Patient. In: Kaplan JA, Augoustides JGT, Manecke GR, et al., eds. Kaplan's Cardiac Anesthesia. 7th ed. Elsevier; 2017:46-95.
2. Wu IY, Barajas MB, Hahn RT. The MitraClip procedure-a comprehensive review for the cardiac anesthesiologist. J Cardiothorac Vasc Anesth, 2018; 32: 2746-2759.

19. Which of the following describes the best location for trans-septal puncture during transcatheter mitral valve repair with the MitraClip device?
   A. Posterior and superior
   B. Posterior and inferior
   C. Anterior and superior
   D. Anterior and inferior

Correct Answer: A

Explanation: A well placed trans-septal puncture is important as it allows the interventional cardiologist the necessary space to safely and effectively maneuver the MitraClip delivery system within the left atrium. The optimal puncture site typically is located midposteriorly along the interatrial septum, approximately 4.5 cm above the level of the systolic mitral leaflet position and close to the medial commissure. Transesophageal echocardiography can guide trans-septal

puncture with the following midesophageal views: the aortic valve short axis view, the bicaval view, and the four-chamber view. Furthermore, biplane imaging can provide assessment of the transseptal puncture site in two views simultaneously.

References:
1. Gelzinis T, Kozak M, Chambers C, et al. Chapter 3: Cardiac Catheterization Laboratory: Diagnostic and Therapeutic Procedures in the Adult Patient. In: Kaplan JA, Augoustides JGT, Manecke GR, et al., eds. Kaplan's Cardiac Anesthesia. 7th ed. Elsevier; 2017:46-95.
2. Wu IY, Barajas MB, Hahn RT. The MitraClip procedure-a comprehensive review for the cardiac anesthesiologist. J Cardiothorac Vasc Anesth, 2018; 32: 2746-2759.

20. Indirect annuloplasty via a percutaneous approach to correct mitral regurgitation involves placing a catheter into which of the following anatomical locations?
   A. Left atrial appendage
   B. Left atrium
   C. Coronary sinus
   D. Left ventricular outflow tract

Correct Answer: C

Explanation: Indirect annuloplasty has been developed because of the close relationship of the coronary sinus to the posterior and lateral mitral valve annulus. A device is inserted into the coronary sinus and used to shorten or reshape the annulus. The catheter is inserted via a transjugular approach. An anchoring device is placed in the distal coronary sinus with a connection that creates tension with the device anchored in the proximal coronary sinus. This tension is transmitted to the annulus and decreases its circumference and improves leaflet coaptation. This technique has been considered in high-risk patients with degenerative prolapse and ischemic mitral regurgitation. This procedure has the potential to compromise the circumflex coronary artery, and the patient should be monitored closely for signs of ischemia during the procedure.

References:
1. Gelzinis T, Kozak M, Chambers C, et al. Chapter 3: Cardiac Catheterization Laboratory: Diagnostic and Therapeutic Procedures in the Adult Patient. In: Kaplan JA, Augoustides JGT, Manecke GR, et al., eds. Kaplan's Cardiac Anesthesia. 7th ed. Elsevier; 2017:46-95.
2. Webb JG, Harnek J, Munt BI, et al. Percutaneous transvenous mitral annuloplasty: initial human experience with device implantation in the coronary sinus. Circulation, 2006; 113: 851-855.
3. Khatib D, Neuburger PJ, Pan S, et al. Transcatheter mitral valve interventions for mitral regurgitation: a review of mitral annuloplasty, valve replacement, and chordal repair devices. J Cardiothoracic Vasc Anesth, 2022; 36: 3887-3903.

21. Alcohol septal ablation may be used to treat which of the following conditions?
   A. Dilated cardiomyopathy
   B. Hypertrophic cardiomyopathy
   C. Noncompaction cardiomyopathy
   D. Tachycardia-induced cardiomyopathy

Correct Answer: B

Explanation: Hypertrophic cardiomyopathy is a genetic disorder that can manifest with sudden cardiac death or heart failure. These patients may have asymmetric septal hypertrophy that leads to dynamic outflow tract obstruction with severe symptoms. If this condition is refractory to medical therapy, more invasive therapy may be needed such as a transcatheter alcohol septal ablation, which involves injection of ethanol into a large septal perforator coronary artery. Further treatment strategies include a septal myectomy with or without concomitant mitral valve intervention. These interventions aim to reduce the left ventricular outflow tract obstruction and relieve symptoms. A potential complication of a septal myectomy is a ventricular septal defect if too much myocardium is removed. Of note, a septal myectomy may unroof sepal perforator arteries, causing flow into the left ventricle that can be detected by color flow Doppler. Septal perforator arteries can be distinguished from a ventricular septal defect by the occurrence of flow in diastole rather than systole.

References:

1. Gelzinis T, Kozak M, Chambers C, et al. Chapter 3: Cardiac Catheterization Laboratory: Diagnostic and Therapeutic Procedures in the Adult Patient. In: Kaplan JA, Augoustides JGT, Manecke GR, et al., eds. Kaplan's Cardiac Anesthesia. 7th ed. Elsevier; 2017:46-95.
2. Jain P, Patel PA, Fabbro M 2nd. Hypertrophic cardiomyopathy and left ventricular outflow tract obstruction: expecting the unexpected. J Cardiothorac Vasc Anesth, 2018; 32: 467-477.

22. Which of the following locations is the best place to cross the interatrial septum to place a left atrial appendage occlusion device?
    A. Superior and anterior
    B. Superior and posterior
    C. Inferior and anterior
    D. Inferior and posterior

Correct Answer: D

Explanation: It is important to have an optimal trans-septal puncture location to facilitate the approach of the occlusion device to the left atrial appendage for achieving the proper final position. The recommended position for the trans-septal crossing is the inferoposterior part of the septum, as imaged with tranesophageal echocardiography. In the midesophageal bicaval view, the inferior portion of the septum will be seen near the inferior vena cava. By viewing the interatrial septum in the midesophageal aortic valve short axis view, the trans-septal access sheath can be guided posteriorly away from the aortic valve. Live three-dimensional imaging with transesophageal echocardiography can also guide and confirm proper crossing of the interatrial septum.

References:

1. Gelzinis T, Kozak M, Chambers C, et al. Chapter 3: Cardiac Catheterization Laboratory: Diagnostic and Therapeutic Procedures in the Adult Patient. In: Kaplan JA, Augoustides

JGT, Manecke GR, et al., eds. Kaplan's Cardiac Anesthesia. 7th ed. Elsevier; 2017:46-95.
2. Mitrev L, Trautman N, Vadlamudi R, et al. Anesthesia and transesophageal echocardiography for WATCHMAN device implantation. J Cardiothorac Vasc Anesth, 2016; 30: 1685-1692.

23. What should be the ideal size of a WATCHMAN left atrial appendage occlusion device in relation to the widest portion of the left atrial appendage (LAA) orifice?
    A. 20% to 30% wider than the measured LAA orifice
    B. 20% to 30% narrower than the measure LAA orifice
    C. 12% to 20% wider than the measured LAA orifice
    D. 12% to 20% narrower than the measure LAA orifice

Correct Answer: C

Explanation: After deploying the WATCHMAN device into the left atrial appendage (LAA), the multiple fixation anchors engage the atrial tissue to provide stability. The occlusion device is kept in place largely by radial forces generated from the compression of the device. Because of this, it is recommended to have 12% to 20% compression of the device once it is implanted, and the device should therefore be selected to be 12% to 20% wider than the widest measurement of the LAA orifice. The device should not be smaller than the LAA orifice, as this can place the device at risk of dislodgement or embolization. Undersizing of the device also allows residual space for blood to enter the LAA, increasing the risk for thromboembolic complications.

References:

1. Gelzinis T, Kozak M, Chambers C, et al. Chapter 3: Cardiac Catheterization Laboratory: Diagnostic and Therapeutic Procedures in the Adult Patient. In: Kaplan JA, Augoustides JGT, Manecke GR, et al., eds. Kaplan's Cardiac Anesthesia. 7th ed. Elsevier; 2017:46-95.
2. Mitrev L, Trautman N, Vadlamudi R, et al. Anesthesia and transesophageal echocardiography for WATCHMAN device implantation. J Cardiothorac Vasc Anesth, 2016; 30: 1685-1692.

24. Which of the following described morphologies of the left atrial appendage is likely to be the easiest to close with a WATCHMAN left atrial appendage occlusion device?
    A. Cactus morphology
    B. Chicken-wing appearance
    C. Cauliflower morphology
    D. Windsock appearance

Correct Answer: D

Explanation: The shape of the left atrial appendage (LAA) is highly variable among the population. The described subtypes of the LAA include "cactus" (30%), "chicken-wing" (48%), "windsock" (19%), and "cauliflower" (3%). The cactus morphology has a dominant central lobe with secondary lobes extending both in the superior and inferior directions. The chicken-wing type of LAA has a bend in the proximal or middle part of the dominant lobe. The windsock morphology has a single elongated lobe as the primary structure. The cauliflower type of LAA has a limited overall length with a wide orifice and a variable number of lobes. The windsock type of LAA is easiest to occlude because it consists of one long tube-like space. The cauliflower type of LAA is typically short relative to the size of its orifice, making it hard to occlude with a WATCHMAN device. The chicken-wing morphology may have a short proximal portion, which is less optimal for occlusion.

References:

1. Gelzinis T, Kozak M, Chambers C, et al. Chapter 3: Cardiac Catheterization Laboratory: Diagnostic and Therapeutic Procedures in the Adult Patient. In: Kaplan JA, Augoustides JGT, Manecke GR, et al., eds. Kaplan's Cardiac Anesthesia. 7th ed. Elsevier; 2017:46-95.
2. Mitrev L, Trautman N, Vadlamudi R, et al. Anesthesia and transesophageal echocardiography for WATCHMAN device implantation. J Cardiothorac Vasc Anesth, 2016; 30: 1685-1692.

25. Which of the following techniques is considered the most sensitive for detecting a patent foramen ovale?
    A. Transthoracic echocardiography with saline contrast injection
    B. Transthoracic echocardiography with color flow Doppler
    C. Transesophageal echocardiography with saline contrast injection
    D. Transesophageal echocardiography with color flow Doppler

Correct Answer: C

Explanation: Transesophageal echocardiography with saline contrast injection and additional provocative maneuvers is the current gold standard for detection of patent foramen ovale (PFO), with a 100% sensitivity and a 92% specificity. Transthoracic echocardiography is the least invasive and most common diagnostic method for detecting a suspected PFO. Color flow Doppler with this echocardiographic approach only detects 5% to 10% of interatrial shunts. The prevalence of a PFO in the general population is approximately 20% to 25%. A PFO or atrial septal defect closure can be performed percutaneously in the cardiac catheterization suite and may be guided by fluoroscopy and/or transesophageal echocardiography.

References:

1. Gelzinis T, Kozak M, Chambers C, et al. Chapter 3: Cardiac Catheterization Laboratory: Diagnostic and Therapeutic Procedures in the Adult Patient. In: Kaplan JA, Augoustides JGT, Manecke GR, et al., eds. Kaplan's Cardiac Anesthesia. 7th ed. Elsevier; 2017:46-95.
2. Lai Y, Dalia AA. PFO! Should I stay, or should I go? J Cardiothorac Vasc Anesth, 2020; 34: 2069-2071.

26. Which of the following types of atrial septal defects (ASDs) is most likely to be amenable to transcatheter closure?
    A. Ostium primum ASD
    B. Ostium secundum ASD
    C. Sinus venosus ASD
    D. Coronary sinus ASD

Correct Answer: B

Explanation: Percutaneous device closure of a patent foramen ovale (PFO) or atrial septal defect (ASD) may be considered in patients to reduce the risk of recurrent stroke and is less invasive than surgical closure. A PFO is a separation between the septum primum and septum secundum and is not a true deficiency of atrial septal tissue. Among the true ASDs, ostium secundum is the most common type and also the most amenable to device closure due to its location near the center of the interatrial septum. Ostium primum ASDs are positioned more inferiorly near the tricuspid valve. The sinus venosus defect may be located at the junction of the right atrium and superior vena cava, or less commonly at the junction of the right atrium and inferior vena cava. The coronary sinus septal defect involves a defect between the coronary sinus and the left atrium.

References:

1. Gelzinis T, Kozak M, Chambers C, et al. Chapter 3: Cardiac Catheterization Laboratory: Diagnostic and Therapeutic Procedures in the Adult Patient. In: Kaplan JA, Augoustides JGT, Manecke GR, et al., eds. Kaplan's Cardiac Anesthesia. 7th ed. Elsevier; 2017:46-95.
2. McGrail D, Sehgal S, Tuttle MK, et al. The many faces of the interatrial septum: a diagnostic dilemma and considerations for defect closure device selection. J Cardiothorac Vasc Anesth, 2022; 36: 3156-3162.

27. Which of the following conditions is associated with partial anomalous pulmonary venous return?
    A. Ostium primum atrial septal defect (ASD)
    B. Ostium secundum ASD
    C. Sinus venosus ASD
    D. Coronary sinus ASD

Correct Answer: C

Explanation: Sinus venosus atrial septal defects account for about 5% to 10% of all atrial septal defects. They are located outside the confines of the true septum and occur either superiorly or inferiorly in association with the relevant vena cava. The superior type is more common than the inferior types. The majority of sinus venosus atrial septal defects are associated with partial anomalous pulmonary venous return, usually with connection of the right upper pulmonary vein to the superior vena cava.

References:

1. Gelzinis T, Kozak M, Chambers C, et al. Chapter 3: Cardiac Catheterization Laboratory: Diagnostic and Therapeutic Procedures in the Adult Patient. In: Kaplan JA, Augoustides JGT, Manecke GR, et al., eds. Kaplan's Cardiac Anesthesia. 7th ed. Elsevier; 2017:46-95.
2. Naqvi N, McCarthy KP, Ho SY. Anatomy of the atrial septum and interatrial communications. J Thorac Dis, 2018; 10: S2837-S2847.

28. Which of the following is NOT true regarding the comparison of right ventricular (RV) and pulmonary artery (PA) catheter pressure waveforms?

A. The RV and PA systolic pressures are equal in the absence of obstruction in the RV outflow tract or pulmonic stenosis

B. The diastolic pressure is lower in the RV compared to the PA

C. There is a dicrotic notch in the PA and RV waveform in systole

D. There is an upslope of the diastolic waveform in the RV and a downslope of the diastolic waveform in the PA

Correct Answer: C

Explanation: Right heart catheterization may be used in the catheterization laboratory as a diagnostic tool or in the perioperative period for monitoring and to guide clinical care. Right heart catheterization is commonly performed with a pulmonary artery catheter and may be guided to the desired location by transesophageal echocardiography direct visualization, analysis of pressure waveforms, or fluoroscopy. There are several distinct features that can be used to differentiate the pressure waveforms of the right ventricle (RV) and pulmonary artery (PA). In the absence of pulmonic stenosis or other RV outflow tract obstruction, the RV and PA peak systolic pressures should be nearly identical. The diastolic pressure in the PA should be higher than the RV in a normal, functioning RV and is known as the diastolic pressure step-up. There should be a dicrotic notch in the PA waveform and not in the RV waveform. The dicrotic notch represents a sudden increase in pressure due to pulmonic valve closure, similar to the dicrotic notch seen in a systemic arterial catheter. In the PA, there should be a diastolic run-off or down-sloping of the PA pressure waveform in diastole, whereas an RV diastolic pressure waveform is expected to be nearly flat in a fully compliant RV or upsloping due to RV filling in diastole.

References:

1. Gelzinis T, Kozak M, Chambers C, et al. Chapter 3: Cardiac Catheterization Laboratory: Diagnostic and Therapeutic Procedures in the Adult Patient. In: Kaplan JA, Augoustides JGT, Manecke GR, et al., eds. Kaplan's Cardiac Anesthesia. 7th ed. Elsevier; 2017:46-95.
2. Bootsma IT, Boerma EC, de Lange F, et al. The contemporary pulmonary artery catheter. Part 1: placement and waveform analysis. J Clin Monit Comput, 2022; 36: 5-15.

29. Which of the following conditions is LEAST likely to result in difficulty advancing a pulmonary artery catheter to the pulmonary artery?

A. Right atrial dilation

B. Tricuspid regurgitation

C. Right ventricular dilation

D. Right ventricular hypertrophy

Correct Answer: D

Explanation: Pulmonary artery catheters can be used to measure cardiac output, central venous pressure, pulmonary artery pressure, and pulmonary capillary wedge pressure and to calculate both pulmonary vascular resistance and systemic vascular resistance. There are a number of factors that may impede successful advancement of a pulmonary artery catheter into the pulmonary artery, including dilation of the right atrium or right ventricle, tricuspid regurgitation, low cardiac output state, pulmonary hypertension, or the presence of right-sided devices such as pacing wires. In addition to pressure waveform analysis, transesophageal echocardiography or fluoroscopy may be used to successfully guide pulmonary artery catheter placement.

References:

1. Gelzinis T, Kozak M, Chambers C, et al. Chapter 3: Cardiac Catheterization Laboratory: Diagnostic and Therapeutic Procedures in the Adult Patient. In: Kaplan JA, Augoustides JGT, Manecke GR, et al., eds. Kaplan's Cardiac Anesthesia. 7th ed. Elsevier; 2017:46-95.
2. Cronin B, Kolotiniuk N, Youssefzadeh K, et al. Pulmonary artery catheter placement aided by transesophageal echocardiography versus pressure waveform transduction. J Cardiothorac Vasc Anesth, 2018; 32: 2578-2582.

30. If the distance from an ionizing radiation source is doubled, how will the radiation exposure level change?

A. Decrease by 50%

B. Decrease by 25%

C. Decrease by 75%

D. Decrease by 94%

Correct Answer: C

Explanation: Radiation safety is particularly important in the cardiac catheterization laboratory. Lead-lined walls, lead-glass partitions, and mobile lead shielding with aprons and thyroid guards help to reduce radiation exposure to cardiac catheterization laboratory personnel. Several principles of radiation exposure should be considered to minimize radiation exposure. Radiation exposure can be reduced by minimizing duration of imaging (and thereby generating less radiation), decreasing x-ray scatter by placing the imaging equipment as close to the patient as possible, and increasing the distance between personnel and the radiation source. The amount of radiation exposure is inversely related to the square of the distance from the source. If the distance from the radiation source is doubled, the exposure will be decreased to one fourth of the original exposure (or a 75% decrease in exposure).

References:

1. Gelzinis T, Kozak M, Chambers C, et al. Chapter 3: Cardiac Catheterization Laboratory: Diagnostic and Therapeutic Procedures in the Adult Patient. In: Kaplan JA, Augoustides JGT, Manecke GR, et al., eds. Kaplan's Cardiac Anesthesia. 7th ed. Elsevier; 2017:46-95.
2. Fujii S, Zhou JR, Dhir A. Anesthesia for cardiac ablation. J Cardiothorac Vasc Anesth, 2018; 32: 1892-1910.

CHAPTER 4

Cardiac Electrophysiology: Diagnosis and Treatment

Steven T. Morozowich and Harish Ramakrishna

KEY POINTS

1. Cardiac arrhythmias are common and result from an ectopic focus or a reentry circuit.
2. Surgical and catheter-based ablative therapies can abolish the origins of arrhythmias by interposition of scar tissue along the reentrant pathway or by isolation of an ectopic area.
3. Supraventricular arrhythmias can be hemodynamically unstable, especially in the setting of structural heart disease. In some cases, persistent tachycardia can lead to tachycardia-induced cardiomyopathy.
4. Accessory pathways are typically interrupted using percutaneous, catheter-based techniques, producing high success rates with minimal complications.
5. Atrioventricular nodal reentrant tachycardia results from altered electrophysiologic properties of the anterior fast pathway and posterior slow pathway fibers that provide input to the atrioventricular node. Interruption of the involved pathway is curative.
6. Atrial flutter typically involves a reentrant circuit that circles the tricuspid valve and crosses the myocardial isthmus between the inferior vena cava and tricuspid valve. Catheter ablation of this region can remedy the arrhythmia.
7. Paroxysmal atrial fibrillation often results from ectopic beats originating in the pulmonary veins. Pulmonary vein isolation with catheter-based ablative energy is indicated for patients who have failed antiarrhythmic therapy and are symptomatic or have evidence of structural heart disease due to atrial fibrillation.
8. Catheter ablation for persistent or long-standing atrial fibrillation is less effective than for paroxysmal atrial fibrillation. Although pulmonary vein isolation is recommended, adjuvant ablation strategies are also employed, including abatement of complex fractionated atrial electrograms and targeting areas of ganglionated plexus.
9. Surgical treatment of atrial fibrillation (i.e., maze procedure) has been employed with good success and has been modified to avoid the sinus node in an effort to minimize occurrences of chronotropic incompetence.
10. In adults, most episodes of sudden cardiac death are the result of ventricular tachyarrhythmias due to ischemic and nonischemic cardiomyopathy. Other conditions associated with an increased risk of sudden death include infiltrative cardiac diseases (e.g., cardiac sarcoidosis, amyloidosis) and genetically based abnormalities such as hypertrophic cardiomyopathy, long QT syndrome, Brugada syndrome, catecholaminergic polymorphic ventricular tachycardia, and arrhythmogenic right ventricular dysplasia.
11. Substantial evidence supports use of an implantable cardioverter-defibrillator for primary and secondary prevention of sudden cardiac death.

1. Following initiation of the heartbeat in the sinoatrial node and depolarization of the atria and then the atrioventricular node, the action potential activates which of the following next?
   A. Purkinje fiber network
   B. Bundle of His
   C. Left bundle branch
   D. Right bundle branch

Correct Answer: B

Explanation: The human heart beats 2.5 billion times during a normal life span. The sinoatrial node (the most proximal part of the conduction system) exhibits the most automaticity due to its rate of spontaneous diastolic depolarization. Consequently, it typically functions as the dominant pacemaker to start the heartbeat in normal circumstances. Thereafter, the wave of depolarization travels to activate the atria, the atrioventricular node, the bundle of His, the left and right bundle branches, and then the Purkinje fiber network throughout the ventricles.

BOX 4.1   Anatomy of the cardiac pacemaker and conduction system

- Sinus node
- Internodal conduction
- Atrioventricular junction
- Intraventricular conduction system
  - Left bundle branch
    - Anterior fascicle
    - Posterior fascicle
- Right bundle branch
- Purkinje fibers

References:

1. Hensley N, Cheng A, Shah A, et al. Chapter 4: Cardiac Electrophysiology: Diagnosis and Treatment. In: Kaplan JA, Augoustides JGT, Manecke GR, et al., eds. Kaplan's Cardiac Anesthesia. 7th ed. Elsevier; 2017:96-117.
2. Park DS, Fishman GI. The cardiac conduction system. Circulation, 2011; 123: 904-915.

2. In the majority of patients, the blood supply to the sinoatrial node is from which of the following:
   A. Left anterior descending artery
   B. Left circumflex artery
   C. Right coronary artery
   D. Obtuse marginal artery

Correct Answer: C

Explanation: The sinoatrial node is located in the superior right atrium on the lateral aspect of the junction of the superior vena cava and the right atrium. The blood supply to the sinoatrial node via its nodal artery is provided from the right coronary artery in approximately 60% to 70% of the population. In the remainder of patients, the sinoatrial nodal artery is derived from the circumflex coronary artery or both the circumflex and right coronary arteries. The sinoatrial node exhibits the most automaticity and functions as the dominant pacemaker to start the heartbeat in normal circumstances.

References:

1. Hensley N, Cheng A, Shah A, et al. Chapter 4: Cardiac Electrophysiology: Diagnosis and Treatment. In: Kaplan JA, Augoustides JGT, Manecke GR, et al., eds. Kaplan's Cardiac Anesthesia. 7th ed. Elsevier; 2017:96-117.
2. Futami C, Tanuma K, Tanuma Y, et al. The arterial blood supply of the conducting system in normal human hearts. Surg Radiol Anat, 2003; 25: 42-49.
3. Park DS, Fishman GI. The cardiac conduction system. Circulation, 2011; 123: 904-901.

3. In approximately 80% to 85% of patients, the blood supply to the atrioventricular node is from the right coronary artery. In the remaining 15% to 20% of patients it is supplied by the:
   A. Circumflex artery
   B. Left anterior descending artery
   C. Posterior descending artery
   D. Diagonal artery

Correct Answer: A

Explanation: The compact portion of the atrioventricular node is located superficially and anterior to the ostium of the coronary sinus and above the insertion of the septal leaflet of the tricuspid valve. The longitudinal segment of the compact atrioventricular node penetrates the central fibrous body and becomes the bundle of His. In 80% to 85% of the population the blood supply to the atrioventricular node is from the right coronary artery, and the circumflex artery (and/or both the left circumflex and the right coronary artery) supplies the remainder.

References:

1. Hensley N, Cheng A, Shah A, et al. Chapter 4: Cardiac Electrophysiology: Diagnosis and Treatment. In: Kaplan JA, Augoustides JGT, Manecke GR, et al., eds. Kaplan's Cardiac Anesthesia. 7th ed. Elsevier; 2017:96-117.
2. Futami C, Tanuma K, Tanuma Y, et al. The arterial blood supply of the conducting system in normal human hearts. Surg Radiol Anat, 2003; 25: 42-49.

4. The PR segment on the electrocardiogram represents which of the following?
   A. Atrial depolarization
   B. Atrial repolarization
   C. Impulse conduction through the atrioventricular node and bundle of His
   D. Interventricular septum depolarization

Correct Answer: C

Explanation: The PR interval includes both the P wave and the PR segment. Following electrical impulse initiation in the sinoatrial node, the depolarization of the atria generates the P wave. The PR segment that follows the P wave is a period of electrical silence that represents impulse conduction through the atrioventricular node and bundle of His, which are small structures and thus do not generate any electrocardiographic activity. The PR segment is then followed by depolarization of the interventricular septum resulting in the Q wave, and subsequently, the depolarization of the remaining left and right ventricular myocardium resulting in the QRS complex. Atrial repolarization is usually not distinctly visible on the electrocardiogram because it has low magnitude and occurs during ventricular depolarization.

References:

1. Hensley N, Cheng A, Shah A, et al. Chapter 4: Cardiac Electrophysiology: Diagnosis and Treatment. In: Kaplan JA, Augoustides JGT, Manecke GR, et al., eds. Kaplan's Cardiac Anesthesia. 7th ed. Elsevier; 2017:96-117.
2. Magnani JW, Wang N, Nelson KP, et al. Electrocardiographic PR interval and adverse outcomes in older adults: the Health, Ageing and Body Composition Study. Circ Arrhythm Electrophysiol, 2013; 6: 84-90.
3. Stracina T, Ronzhina M, Redina R, et al. Golden standard or obsolete method? Review of ECG applications in clinical and experimental context. Front Physiol, 2022; 13: 867033.

5. The Q wave on the electrocardiogram represents:
   A. Atrial depolarization
   B. Impulse conduction through the atrioventricular node and bundle of His
   C. Interventricular septum depolarization
   D. Left and right ventricular depolarization

Correct Answer: C

Explanation: Following the P wave and PR interval on the electrocardiogram, depolarization of the interventricular septum produces a small Q wave, followed by depolarization of the remaining left and right ventricular myocardium that generates the QRS complex. The T wave represents ventricular repolarization, and a U wave, if present, represents repolarization of the Purkinje fiber network.

References:

1. Hensley N, Cheng A, Shah A, et al. Chapter 4: Cardiac Electrophysiology: Diagnosis and Treatment. In: Kaplan JA,

BOX 4.2   **Arrhythmia mechanisms**

- Focal mechanisms
  - Automatic
  - Triggered
- Re-entrant arrhythmias
- Normal automaticity
  - Sinoatrial node
  - Subsidiary atrial foci
  - Atrioventricular node
  - His-Purkinje system
- Triggered mechanisms occur from repetitive delayed or early afterdepolarizations.
- Re-entry
  - Unidirectional block is necessary
- Slowed conduction in the alternate pathway exceeds the refractory period of cells at the site of unidirectional block

Augoustides JGT, Manecke GR, et al., eds. Kaplan's Cardiac Anesthesia. 7th ed. Elsevier; 2017:96-117.
2. Stracina T, Ronzhina M, Redina R, et al. Golden standard or obsolete method? Review of ECG applications in clinical and experimental context. Front Physiol, 2022; 13: 867033.

6. Which of the following is typically NOT part of the initial evaluation of a cardiac arrhythmia?
   A. History and physical examination
   B. Twelve-lead electrocardiogram
   C. Electrophysiology study
   D. Transthoracic echocardiogram

Correct Answer: C

Explanation: If the initial history, for example, is consistent with the abrupt onset and abrupt termination of palpitations this may suggest a supraventricular tachycardia. Further, if palpitations are irregular this may indicate atrial fibrillation. The initial evaluation after the history and physical examination includes a 12-lead electrocardiogram that should be obtained at baseline and during symptoms if possible. A transthoracic echocardiogram is typically included to assess cardiac structural abnormalities and ventricular function. Beyond these aspects, 24-hour Holter monitoring of patient-triggered events may be useful for further diagnostic evaluation that may also in select patients require an invasive electrophysiologic study.

BOX 4.3   **Diagnostic evaluation of arrhythmias**

- History of palpitations, syncope, and constitutional symptoms
- Physical examination
- Twelve-lead electrocardiogram at baseline and during tachycardia if available
- Two-dimensional echocardiogram
- Twenty-four–hour Holter monitoring of patient-triggered events
- Invasive electrophysiologic testing

References:

1. Hensley N, Cheng A, Shah A, et al. Chapter 4: Cardiac Electrophysiology: Diagnosis and Treatment. In: Kaplan JA, Augoustides JGT, Manecke GR, et al., eds. Kaplan's Cardiac Anesthesia. 7th ed. Elsevier; 2017:96-117.
2. Nelson JA, Gue YX, Christensen JM, et al. Analysis of the ESC/EACTS 2020 Atrial Fibrillation Guidelines with perioperative implications. J Cardiothorac Vasc Anes, 2022; 36: 2177-2195.

7. The evolving management of cardiac arrhythmias is BEST characterized by:
   A. More emphasis on pharmacologic therapy
   B. Less emphasis on procedural ablation therapy
   C. Improved survival for patients with implantable cardioverter-defibrillators
   D. All of the above

Correct Answer: C

Explanation: The management of life-threatening ventricular tachyarrhythmias has shown improved survival for patients with implantable cardioverter-defibrillators versus antiarrhythmic drug therapy in prospective randomized trials. The management of cardiac arrhythmias has also shifted away from pharmacologic therapy and toward procedural ablation therapy with catheter-based and surgical approaches. The catheter-based ablations aim to render the endocardium electrically inert at specific locations through targeted cautery with radiofrequency ablation, cryoballoon ablation, and/or laser ablation.

As procedural ablation therapies continue to improve clinical outcomes, it is likely that these procedures will only increase in the future. Consequently, based on their associated complexities with respect to both the procedure and the patient population, there will be a growing demand for involvement from the cardiac anesthesiologist.

References:

1. Hensley N, Cheng A, Shah A, et al. Chapter 4: Cardiac Electrophysiology: Diagnosis and Treatment. In: Kaplan JA, Augoustides JGT, Manecke GR, et al., eds. Kaplan's Cardiac Anesthesia. 7th ed. Elsevier; 2017:96-117.
2. Zipes DP. Implantable cardioverter-defibrillator: A Volkswagen or a Rolls Royce: how much will we pay to save a life? Circulation, 2001; 103: 1372-1374.
3. Mahajan A, Chua J. Pro: a cardiovascular anesthesiologist should provide services in the catheterization and electrophysiology laboratory. J Cardiothorac Vasc Anesth, 2011; 25: 553-556.

8. An invasive electrophysiologic study is characterized by all of the following, EXCEPT:
   A. Catheters are most often introduced through the jugular vessels
   B. Systemic heparinization may be required
   C. Most complications are associated with the catheterization process
   D. Placement of external cardioverter-defibrillator pads

Correct Answer: A

Explanation: An electrophysiologic study is a collection of techniques used to analyze the mechanisms of cardiac arrhythmias and their site of origin as part of the mapping process and to provide definitive treatment via catheter-based ablation techniques when applicable. During this type of study, catheters are typically introduced through the femoral vessels under local anesthesia, not the jugular vessels.

Systemic heparinization may be required when accessing left-sided cardiac chambers. If a trans-septal puncture is performed, heparin is administered at the time of trans-septal puncture to prevent thrombus formation, which could result in systemic embolization. The target activated clotting time is typically in the range of 275 to 350 seconds.

During an electrophysiologic study, most complications are typically associated with the intravascular catheters. These complications include vascular injury, tricuspid valve damage, pulmonary embolism, hemorrhage requiring transfusion therapy, cardiac chamber perforation resulting in tamponade, sepsis from catheterization site infection, abscess, myocardial infarction, stroke, and death. The placement of external cardioversion electrodes facilitates cardioversion and/or defibrillation of persistent or hemodynamically unstable tachyarrhythmia resulting from stimulation protocols.

> **BOX 4.4 Electrophysiologic ablative treatment indications**
>
> - Drug-resistant arrhythmias
> - Drug intolerance
> - Severe symptoms
> - Avoiding lifelong treatments

References:

1. Hensley N, Cheng A, Shah A, et al. Chapter 4: Cardiac Electrophysiology: Diagnosis and Treatment. In: Kaplan JA, Augoustides JGT, Manecke GR, et al., eds. Kaplan's Cardiac Anesthesia. 7th ed. Elsevier; 2017:96-117.
2. Malladi V, Naeini PS, Razavi M, et al. Endovascular ablation of atrial fibrillation. Anesthesiology, 2014; 120: 1513-1519.
3. Siegrist KK, Robles CF, Kertai MD, et al. The electrophysiologic laboratory: anesthetic considerations and staffing models. J Cardiothorac Vasc Anesth, 2021; 35: 2775-2783.

9. During electrical mapping prior to cardiac ablation, electrophysiology catheters are positioned in all of the following structures, EXCEPT:
   A. Superior vena cava
   B. Right atrium
   C. Coronary sinus
   D. Right ventricle

Correct Answer: A

Explanation: Most ablation procedures require mapping to create an electrical map of the heart to localize lesion targets for the arrhythmia of interest. The electrical map is created by electrophysiologic catheters, which are complex, multielectrode systems that capture information on timing, position, and voltage of arrhythmias. These catheters are typically positioned in the right atrium, right ventricular apex, and coronary sinus to record and map intracardiac electrograms from the right atrium, right ventricle, and left atrium and left ventricle, respectively.

References:

1. Hensley N, Cheng A, Shah A, et al. Chapter 4: Cardiac Electrophysiology: Diagnosis and Treatment. In: Kaplan JA, Augoustides JGT, Manecke GR, et al., eds. Kaplan's Cardiac Anesthesia. 7th ed. Elsevier; 2017:96-117.
2. Fujii S, Zhou JR, Dhir A. Anesthesia for cardiac ablation. J Cardiothorac Vasc Anesth, 2018; 32:1892-1910.

10. When left-heart access is required during cardiac ablation in the electrophysiology suite it may typically be obtained by trans-septal puncture and/or which of the following approaches?
    A. Retrograde aortic approach
    B. Transaortic approach

C. Transapical approach

D. All of the above

Correct Answer: A

Explanation: Electrophysiology catheters enter the right atrium typically via femoral vein access, and left-heart access is often obtained by crossing the intra-atrial septum with a trans-septal puncture guided by fluoroscopy, intracardiac echocardiography, and/or transesophageal echocardiography. In addition, left-heart access may also be obtained by a retrograde aortic approach via percutaneous femoral artery access, where catheters are then advanced through the aortic valve. In contrast, interventional cardiovascular procedures such as transcatheter aortic valve replacement at times require alternative arterial access that includes transaortic and transapical approaches, which do not typically apply to electrophysiologic procedures. In addition, these invasive procedures require a minithoracotomy or partial sternotomy.

References:

1. Hensley N, Cheng A, Shah A, et al. Chapter 4: Cardiac Electrophysiology: Diagnosis and Treatment. In: Kaplan JA, Augoustides JGT, Manecke GR, et al., eds. Kaplan's Cardiac Anesthesia. 7th ed. Elsevier; 2017:96-117.
2. Fujii S, Zhou JR, Dhir A. Anesthesia for cardiac ablation. J Cardiothorac Vasc Anesth, 2018; 32: 1892-1910.
3. Morozowich ST, Sell-Dottin KA, Crestanello JA, et al. Trans-carotid versus transaxillary/subclavian transcatheter aortic valve replacement (TAVR): analysis of outcomes. J Cardiothorac Vasc Anesth, 2022; 36: 1771-1776.

11. What is the preferred anesthesia type for supraventricular tachycardia ablation?

A. General anesthesia

B. Regional anesthesia

C. Monitored anesthesia care

D. All of the above

Correct Answer: C

Explanation: Some of the supraventricular arrhythmias that may require ablation include atrioventricular re-entry tachycardias, atrioventricular nodal re-entry tachycardia, and atrial tachycardia. The preferred anesthesia type for these procedures is monitored anesthetic care. The procedure is typically started with either no sedation or minimal sedation to avoid arrhythmia suppression during mapping, with the transition to moderate sedation once mapping is complete. These precautions are typically made because sedation and anesthetic drugs affect the inducibility of a given supraventricular arrhythmia by prolonging cardiac repolarization and modulating the autonomic nervous system. These arrhythmias have a variety of mechanisms that are summarized in the following teaching box.

References:

1. Hensley N, Cheng A, Shah A, et al. Chapter 4: Cardiac Electrophysiology: Diagnosis and Treatment. In: Kaplan JA, Augoustides JGT, Manecke GR, et al., eds. Kaplan's Cardiac Anesthesia. 7th ed. Elsevier; 2017:96-117.

BOX 4.5 Anesthesia considerations for supraventricular arrhythmia surgery and ablation procedures

- Familiarity with electrophysiologic study results and associated treatments
- Transcutaneous cardioversion-defibrillation pads placed before induction
- Hemodynamically tolerated tachyarrhythmias treated by slowing conduction across accessory pathway rather than the atrioventricular node
- Hemodynamically significant tachyarrhythmias treated with cardioversion
- Avoidance of sympathetic stimulation

---

2. Fujii S, Zhou JR, Dhir A. Anesthesia for cardiac ablation. J Cardiothorac Vasc Anesth, 2018; 32: 1892-1910.

12. All of the following regarding atrial fibrillation are true, EXCEPT:

A. It is uncommon in the general population

B. Prevalence is associated with older age

C. It is associated with stroke

D. It is associated with mortality

Correct Answer: A

Explanation: Atrial fibrillation is the most common arrhythmia in the general population, affecting more than 2.3 million Americans. Atrial flutter may also be associated with atrial fibrillation. The prevalence of atrial fibrillation is strongly associated with age, occurring in less than 1% of those younger than 55 years old but in nearly 10% of those older than 80 years. In the perioperative period, atrial fibrillation is also very common after cardiothoracic procedures. Overall, this common atrial arrhythmia is associated with increased healthcare cost, stroke, and long-term mortality.

References:

1. Hensley N, Cheng A, Shah A, et al. Chapter 4: Cardiac Electrophysiology: Diagnosis and Treatment. In: Kaplan JA,

---

BOX 4.6 Atrial flutter

- Re-entry results from a large anatomic circuit
- Macro re-entrant pathway is amenable to catheter ablation

BOX 4.7 Atrial fibrillation features

- Associated with multiple re-entrant circuits
- May originate from automatic foci in a pulmonary vein or the vena cava
- Treatment with catheter ablation
  - Atrioventricular node ablation with pacemaker placement
  - Curative ablation to restore sinus rhythm
- Surgical therapy with the maze procedure

Augoustides JGT, Manecke GR, et al., eds. Kaplan's Cardiac Anesthesia. 7th ed. Elsevier; 2017:96-117.

2. Nelson JA, Gue YX, Christensen JM, et al. Analysis of the ESC/EACTS 2020 Atrial Fibrillation Guidelines with perioperative implications. J Cardiothorac Vasc Anesth, 2022; 36: 2177-2195.

13. Which is the most common arrhythmia seen in the perioperative setting?
- **A.** Atrial tachycardia
- **B.** Atrial flutter
- **C.** Atrial fibrillation
- **D.** Atrioventricular nodal re-entry tachycardia

Correct Answer: C

Explanation: Postoperative atrial fibrillation is the most common arrhythmia seen in the perioperative setting, with an incidence as high as 60%, but this varies widely based on type of surgery (higher with cardiothoracic and esophageal surgery). Recent meta-analysis demonstrated that new-onset postoperative atrial fibrillation was associated with increased risk of early stroke and early mortality. Its pathogenesis is multifactorial, with contributors being preexisting cardiovascular disease, chronic renal failure, obstructive sleep apnea, medications (both chronic and newly administered), and surgical stressors.

Atrial flutter occurs in many of the same situations as atrial fibrillation, but atrial fibrillation is much more common. In the intensive care unit, new-onset supraventricular arrhythmias were atrial fibrillation in 73% and atrial flutter in 4%. Further examples of supraventricular arrhythmias include focal atrial tachycardia, atrioventricular nodal re-entrant tachycardia, and atrioventricular reciprocating tachycardia.

BOX 4.8   Atrioventricular reciprocating tachycardia accessory pathway characteristics

- Concealed: accessory pathway displays retrograde conduction.
- Manifest: accessory pathway displays antegrade conduction. Pathways often exhibit retrograde conduction.
- Orthodromic: antegrade conduction from atria to ventricles occurs through the normal atrioventricular (AV) nodal conduction system and retrograde conduction through the accessory pathway.
- Antidromic: antegrade conduction from atria to ventricles occurs through the accessory pathway and retrograde conduction through the AV nodal pathway.
- Abnormal pathways are treated with percutaneous radiofrequency ablation.
- Abnormal pathways are treated surgically from the endocardium to epicardium by transection and/or cryoablation.

BOX 4.9   Atrioventricular nodal re-entrant tachycardia

- Altered electrophysiologic properties of the anterior fast and posterior slow pathways provide input to the atrioventricular node.
- Successful fast pathway ablation occurs when the PR interval is prolonged or fast-pathway conduction is eliminated.
- Successful slow pathway ablation occurs when induced atrioventricular nodal re-entrant tachycardia is eliminated.
- Surgical techniques include selective cryoablation.

BOX 4.10   Focal atrial tachycardia

- Mechanisms include abnormal automaticity, triggered activity, and micro re-entry
- Catheter-based treatment uses radiofrequency ablation
- Surgical-based treatment uses an incision and cryoablation

References:

1. Hensley N, Cheng A, Shah A, et al. Chapter 4: Cardiac Electrophysiology: Diagnosis and Treatment. In: Kaplan JA, Augoustides JGT, Manecke GR, et al., eds. Kaplan's Cardiac Anesthesia. 7th ed. Elsevier; 2017:96-117.

2. Vanneman MW, Madhok J, Weimer JM, et al. Perioperative implications of the 2020 American Heart Association Scientific Statement on Drug-Induced Arrhythmias—a focused review. J Cardiothorac Vasc Anesth, 2022; 36: 952-961.

3. Goodman S, Shirov T, Weissman C. Supraventricular arrhythmias in intensive care unit patients: short and long-term consequences. Anesth Analg, 2007; 104: 880-886.

14. All of the following characterize the atrial fibrillation ablation procedure, EXCEPT:
- **A.** The goal is to restore normal sinus rhythm
- **B.** Ablation strategies involve electrical isolation of the pulmonary veins
- **C.** Access to the left heart
- **D.** Ablation of the atrioventricular node

Correct Answer: D

Explanation: In an attempt to restore normal sinus rhythm during ablation for atrial fibrillation, ablation strategies involve electrical isolation of the pulmonary veins, not ablation of the atrioventricular node. It is thought that myocardial sleeves involving the ostium of the pulmonary veins can initiate atrial fibrillation due to their inherently different electrophysiologic properties. Thus, during this type of ablation, the pulmonary veins are electrically isolated to prevent the development of atrial fibrillation. To perform pulmonary vein isolation, the femoral vein is typically accessed, followed by trans-septal puncture to gain access to the pulmonary veins on the left side of the heart.

References:

1. Hensley N, Cheng A, Shah A, et al. Chapter 4: Cardiac Electrophysiology: Diagnosis and Treatment. In: Kaplan JA, Augoustides JGT, Manecke GR, et al., eds. Kaplan's Cardiac Anesthesia. 7th ed. Elsevier; 2017:96-117.
2. Malladi V, Naeini PS, Razavi M, et al. Endovascular ablation of atrial fibrillation. Anesthesiology, 2014; 120: 1513-1519.
3. Siegrist KK, Robles CF, Kertai MD, et al. The electrophysiologic laboratory: anesthetic considerations and staffing models. J Cardiothorac Vasc Anesth, 2021; 35: 2775-2783.

15. Anesthesia considerations for atrial fibrillation ablations include all of the following, EXCEPT:
    A. Anesthesia type is typically monitored anesthesia care
    B. Procedural complications include cardiac tamponade
    C. Monitoring is needed for acute increases in esophageal temperature
    D. Several liters of intravenous fluid administration via the ablation catheters throughout the procedure should be anticipated

Correct Answer: A

Explanation: The anesthesia type for ablation of atrial fibrillation is typically general anesthesia due to case duration of several hours and procedure-related pain (patient movement could require remapping and can affect tissue contact with the catheters), and because superior outcomes have been demonstrated compared to monitored anesthesia care. Specifically, trials have found that general anesthesia reduces the prevalence of pulmonary vein reconnection in repeat ablations compared with monitored anesthesia care.

Because trans-septal puncture is required to gain access to the left heart to perform atrial fibrillation ablations, radial arterial lines are usually placed to monitor for hemodynamic instability, which assists in the identification of procedure-related complications such as cardiac tamponade. Sudden increases in esophageal temperature are monitored to avoid esophageal burn injury during radiofrequency catheter ablation. Because several liters of intravenous fluid are typically administered via the ablation catheters throughout the procedure, minimizing further volume administration should be considered, as many patients have underlying cardiac dysfunction.

References:

1. Hensley N, Cheng A, Shah A, et al. Chapter 4: Cardiac Electrophysiology: Diagnosis and Treatment. In: Kaplan JA, Augoustides JGT, Manecke GR, et al., eds. Kaplan's Cardiac Anesthesia. 7th ed. Elsevier; 2017:96-117.
2. Malladi V, Naeini PS, Razavi M, et al. Endovascular ablation of atrial fibrillation. Anesthesiology, 2014; 120: 1513-1519.
3. Osorio J, Rajendra A, Varley A, et al. General anesthesia during atrial fibrillation ablation: Standardized protocol and experience. Pac Clin Electrophysiol, 2020; 43: 602-608.

16. When conducting general anesthesia for atrial fibrillation ablations, which of the following is INCORRECT?
    A. Case duration is typically several hours
    B. Paralysis is maintained during phrenic nerve pacing
    C. Intravenous line air filters may be present
    D. Monitoring for cardiac tamponade is performed

Correct Answer: B

Explanation: The case duration for transcatheter ablations of atrial fibrillation is typically several hours.

The absence (or reversal) of paralysis may be required for phrenic nerve pacing to observe for diaphragmatic contractions. This is done because of the proximity of the phrenic nerve to the right upper pulmonary vein and since isolation carries a significantly higher incidence of phrenic nerve palsy. Careful monitoring of the phrenic nerve pacing can mitigate this complication.

Patients undergoing trans-septal puncture may be at higher risk of systemic embolism and, to mitigate this, intravenous air filters may be placed during the preoperative preparation of the patient on the day of surgery. Radial arterial lines are typically placed during ablations for atrial fibrillation to monitor for hemodynamic instability, which assists in the identification of procedure-related complications such as cardiac tamponade.

References:

1. Hensley N, Cheng A, Shah A, et al. Chapter 4: Cardiac Electrophysiology: Diagnosis and Treatment. In: Kaplan JA, Augoustides JGT, Manecke GR, et al., eds. Kaplan's Cardiac Anesthesia. 7th ed. Elsevier; 2017:96-117.
2. Fujii S, Zhou JR, Dhir A. Anesthesia for cardiac ablation. J Cardiothorac Vasc Anesth, 2018; 32: 1892-1910.
3. Madhavan M, Yao X, Sangaralingham LR, et al. Ischemic stroke or systemic embolism after transseptal ablation of arrhythmias in patients with cardiac implantable electronic devices. J Am Heart Assoc, 2016; 5: e003163.

17. What is the approximate incidence of cardiac tamponade as a complication of transcatheter ablation for atrial fibrillation?
    A. 10%
    B. 8%
    C. 5%
    D. <2%

Correct Answer: D

Explanation: Cardiac tamponade is a rare complication of catheter-based ablation for atrial fibrillation. A high-volume center studied 1000 transcatheter ablation procedures for atrial fibrillation and found the incidence of cardiac tamponade to be approximately 1.3%. Furthermore, this complication was often managed by percutaneous drainage. Another study demonstrated that death as a complication of atrial fibrillation ablation occurs in 0.1% of cases, with cardiac tamponade being the leading cause.

References:

1. Hensley N, Cheng A, Shah A, et al. Chapter 4: Cardiac Electrophysiology: Diagnosis and Treatment. In: Kaplan JA, Augoustides JGT, Manecke GR, et al., eds. Kaplan's Cardiac Anesthesia. 7th ed. Elsevier; 2017:96-117.

2. Dagres N, Hindricks G, Kottkamp H, et al. Complications of atrial fibrillation ablation in a high-volume center in 1,000 procedures: still cause for concern? J Cardiovasc Electrophysiol, 2009; 20: 1014-1019.
3. Cappato R, Calkins H, Chen SA, et al. Prevalence and causes of fatal outcome in catheter ablation of atrial fibrillation. J Am Coll Cardiol, 2009; 53: 1798-1803.

18. Approximately what percentage of iatrogenic atrial septal defects are still present 1 year after trans-septal puncture?
  A. 100%
  B. 50%
  C. 20%
  D. 0%

Correct Answer: C

Explanation: After trans-septal ablation of atrial arrhythmias, approximately 20% of iatrogenic atrial septal defects due to these trans-septal punctures are still present at 1 year, but the clinical relevance of these is currently unknown. Regardless, these patients may remain at higher risk of systemic embolism. At times, these iatrogenic atrial septal defects may require transcatheter closure.

References:

1. Hensley N, Cheng A, Shah A, et al. Chapter 4: Cardiac Electrophysiology: Diagnosis and Treatment. In: Kaplan JA, Augoustides JGT, Manecke GR, et al., eds. Kaplan's Cardiac Anesthesia. 7th ed. Elsevier; 2017:96-117.
2. Madhavan M, Yao X, Sangaralingham LR, et al. Ischemic stroke or systemic embolism after transseptal ablation of arrhythmias in patients with cardiac implantable electronic devices. J Am Heart Assoc, 2016; 5: e003163.
3. Sieira J, Chierchia GB, Di Giovanni G, et al. One year incidence of iatrogenic atrial septal defect after cryoballoon ablation for atrial fibrillation. J Cardiovasc Electrophysiol, 2014; 25: 11-15.

19. In preparation for an atypical atrial flutter ablation with trans-septal puncture, an intravenous line air filter has been placed as a precaution. Administration of which of the following medications could clog this filter?
  A. Fentanyl
  B. Lidocaine
  C. Propofol
  D. Rocuronium

Correct Answer: C

Explanation: The anesthesia type for atypical atrial flutter ablations is typically general anesthesia as with atrial fibrillation ablations due to left-heart access and a case duration of several hours. Furthermore, procedure-related pain can thus be effectively limited to prevent patient movement with its consequent risks for electrical remapping and ineffective ablation with a risk of recurrence of the targeted arrhythmia.

When administering propofol, most anesthesiologists do not inject it through a running intravenous line if there is an air filter in place, since propofol is known to clog filters with a pore size of less than 5 microns, and many available air filters have a pore size of 0.2 microns. The published filter recommendations for propofol are that, in general, the filter pore size be should be 5 microns or more; otherwise it can restrict the flow of the emulsion or cause the emulsion to break down. To avoid these potential issues, most will induce anesthesia via a separate proximal injection port that does not have an air filter in place and will use a deaired normal saline flush syringe to complete the injection, since these ports are usually not connected to a running intravenous line.

References:

1. Hensley N, Cheng A, Shah A, et al. Chapter 4: Cardiac Electrophysiology: Diagnosis and Treatment. In: Kaplan JA, Augoustides JGT, Manecke GR, et al., eds. Kaplan's Cardiac Anesthesia. 7th ed. Elsevier; 2017:96-117.
2. Osorio J, Rajendra A, Varley A, et al. General anesthesia during atrial fibrillation ablation: Standardized protocol and experience. Pac Clin Electrophysiol, 2020; 43: 602-608.
3. Lundström S, Twycross R, Mihalyo M, et al. Propofol. J Pain Sympt Manag, 2010; 40: 466-470.

20. Esophageal temperature is monitored closely during atrial fibrillation ablation procedures to monitor for which of the following aspects?
  A. Malignant hyperthermia
  B. Esophageal temperature during cryoablation
  C. Esophageal temperature during radiofrequency ablation
  D. Patient core temperature due to the intravenous fluid administered via the ablation catheters

Correct Answer: C

Explanation: If radiofrequency ablation is planned during transcatheter ablation for atrial fibrillation, an esophageal temperature probe is inserted and positioned under fluoroscopy to position it close to the ablation catheter. This probe is monitored carefully for a sudden increase in temperature to avoid esophageal burn injury that can lead to esophageal ulceration and/or perforation with development of an atrial-esophageal fistula. Acute increases in esophageal temperature of only 0.1 degrees Celsius are communicated to the electrophysiologist so immediate cooling measures can be taken.

During radiofrequency ablation, electrical energy is converted to thermal energy by resistive heating. Overheating cardiac tissue causes irreversible coagulation necrosis and nonconducting myocardial scaring. Successful radiofrequency ablation achieves permanent transmural lesions. In contrast, cryoablation uses catheter tip cooling to freeze the endocardium to impair tissue conduction and is not associated with esophageal injury.

References:

1. Hensley N, Cheng A, Shah A, et al. Chapter 4: Cardiac Electrophysiology: Diagnosis and Treatment. In: Kaplan JA, Augoustides JGT, Manecke GR, et al., eds. Kaplan's Cardiac Anesthesia. 7th ed. Elsevier; 2017:96-117.

2. Malladi V, Naeini PS, Razavi M, et al. Endovascular ablation of atrial fibrillation. Anesthesiology, 2014; 120: 1513-1519.
3. Fujii S, Zhou JR, Dhir A. Anesthesia for cardiac ablation. J Cardiothorac Vasc Anesth, 2018; 32: 1892-1910.

21. Heparin is administered during atrial fibrillation ablations to prevent:
  A. Left atrial appendage thrombus
  B. Left ventricular thrombus
  C. Thrombus formation at the time of trans-septal puncture
  D. Deep vein thrombosis

Correct Answer: C

Explanation: Heparin is titrated at the time of trans-septal puncture to prevent thrombus formation that could result in systemic embolization and stroke with a target activated clotting time in the range of 275 to 350 seconds. Heparinization is another reason why constant vigilance is required to identify procedure-related complications such as hematomas, and cardiac tamponade.

References:

1. Hensley N, Cheng A, Shah A, et al. Chapter 4: Cardiac Electrophysiology: Diagnosis and Treatment. In: Kaplan JA, Augoustides JGT, Manecke GR, et al., eds. Kaplan's Cardiac Anesthesia. 7th ed. Elsevier; 2017:96-117.
2. Malladi V, Naeini PS, Razavi M, et al. Endovascular ablation of atrial fibrillation. Anesthesiology, 2014; 120: 1513-1519.
3. Siegrist KK, Robles CF, Kertai MD, et al. The electrophysiologic laboratory: anesthetic considerations and staffing models. J Cardiothorac Vasc Anesth, 2021; 35: 2775-2783.

22. During cardiac ablation procedures requiring general anesthesia, reducing the volatile anesthetic depth is associated with:
  A. Burst suppression with monitoring of the processed electroencephalogram
  B. Awareness in geriatric patients
  C. Prolonged recovery in the postanesthesia care unit
  D. Best practice guidelines in patients over 65 years of age

Correct Answer: D

Explanation: Reduced volatile anesthetic depth refers to volatile anesthetic minimum alveolar concentrations of 0.5 to 0.7 and/or titration of volatile anesthetic to a value of 50 (range 40–60) with bispectral index monitoring. In contrast, values below 40 correspond to a deep hypnotic state, with values below 20 typically correlating with burst suppression. Reduced volatile anesthetic depth is safe in geriatric patients and is not associated with an increased risk of awareness. Furthermore, it may shorten and improve postoperative recovery and is supported in current best practice guidelines for optimizing perioperative brain health in patients older than 65 years of age.

References:

1. Hensley N, Cheng A, Shah A, et al. Chapter 4: Cardiac Electrophysiology: Diagnosis and Treatment. In: Kaplan JA,

Augoustides JGT, Manecke GR, et al., eds. Kaplan's Cardiac Anesthesia. 7th ed. Elsevier; 2017:96-117.
2. Short TG, Campbell D, Frampton C, et al. Anesthetic depth and complications after major surgery: an international, randomised controlled trial. Lancet, 2019; 394: 1907-1914.
3. Berger M, Schenning KJ, Brown CHT, et al. Best practices for postoperative brain health: recommendations from the Fifth International Perioperative Neurotoxicity Working Group. Anesth Analg, 2018; 127: 1406-1413.

23. Regarding surgical therapy for atrial fibrillation, which of the following is INCORRECT?
  A. It may be performed concomitant with another cardiac operation or as a stand-alone procedure
  B. Maze procedure may be performed
  C. Epicardial pulmonary vein isolation may be performed
  D. Right-sided lesions are always treated

Correct Answer: D

Explanation: Surgical ablation for atrial fibrillation may be done concomitant with another cardiac operation or as a stand-alone procedure as in video-assisted thoracoscopic surgery. The conventional maze procedure operation creates a maze-like pattern of surgical incisions (and subsequent scar) to interrupt the electrophysiologic substrate for atrial fibrillation and thus restore normal sinus rhythm to optimize myocardial performance. The conventional maze procedure has since been simplified by the availability of newer energy sources to produce atrial scar, such as bipolar radiofrequency and cryoablation. This simplification of the procedural complexity has allowed the expansion of eligibility criteria.

The modified maze procedure, representing the ongoing evolution of the conventional maze procedure, involves treatment of both left-sided and right-sided lesions that contribute to atrial fibrillation. However, some surgeons omit the treatment of right-sided lesions. If atrial fibrillation or atrial flutter subsequently develops, then ablation of the right-sided tricuspid isthmus (an area between the coronary sinus, tricuspid annulus, and eustachian valve) is subsequently performed, since it is a straightforward procedure typically performed under monitored anesthesia care in the electrophysiology suite.

References:

1. Hensley N, Cheng A, Shah A, et al. Chapter 4: Cardiac Electrophysiology: Diagnosis and Treatment. In: Kaplan JA, Augoustides JGT, Manecke GR, et al., eds. Kaplan's Cardiac Anesthesia. 7th ed. Elsevier; 2017:96-117.
2. Dooley N, Lowe M, Ashley EMC. Advances in management of electrophysiology and atrial fibrillation in the cardiac catheter laboratory: implications for anesthesia. BJA Education, 2018; 18: 349-356.
3. Finnerty DT, Griffin M. Recent developments in cardiology procedures for adult congenital heart disease: the anesthesiologist's perspective. J Cardiothorac Vasc Anesth, 2021; 35: 741-751.

24. Which of the following is NOT characteristic of atrial flutter?
  A. Typical lesions involve the right heart
  B. Typical atrial flutter ablations are usually performed under general anesthesia

C. Atypical lesions involve the left heart

D. Atypical atrial flutter ablations are usually performed under general anesthesia

Correct Answer: B

Explanation: Atrial flutter may be classified as typical if originating in the right heart or as atypical if originating in the left heart. Transcatheter ablation for typical right-heart lesions are shorter procedures and may be amenable to monitored anesthesia care. In contrast, ablation procedures for atypical left-heart lesions require general anesthesia and are conducted in a similar fashion to atrial fibrillation ablations, with a transseptal puncture to gain access to the left-heart and placement of a radial arterial line to monitor for hemodynamic instability, including complications such as cardiac tamponade.

References:

1. Hensley N, Cheng A, Shah A, et al. Chapter 4: Cardiac Electrophysiology: Diagnosis and Treatment. In: Kaplan JA, Augoustides JGT, Manecke GR, et al., eds. Kaplan's Cardiac Anesthesia. 7th ed. Elsevier; 2017:96-117.
2. Dooley N, Lowe M, Ashley EMC. Advances in management of electrophysiology and atrial fibrillation in the cardiac catheter laboratory: implications for anesthesia. BJA Education, 2018; 18: 349-356.
3. Finnerty DT, Griffin M. Recent developments in cardiology procedures for adult congenital heart disease: the anesthesiologist's perspective. J Cardiothorac Vasc Anesth, 2021; 35: 741-751.

25. Perioperative considerations for atrioventricular node ablation include all of the following, EXCEPT:

A. Indications include refractory tachycardia due to atrial fibrillation

B. Anesthesia type is typically monitored anesthesia care

C. The procedure requires placement of an implantable cardioverter-defibrillator with pacing capability

D. Perioperative anticoagulation is often encountered

Correct Answer: C

Explanation: When drug therapy fails to adequately control heart rate in atrial fibrillation, atrioventricular node ablation with ventricular pacing is an alternative. In patients with atrial fibrillation the procedure does not aim to restore sinus rhythm and does not eliminate the need for anticoagulation. The procedure requires implantation of a permanent pacemaker rather than a cardioverter-defibrillator. In select patients, biventricular pacing may be indicated, compared to right ventricular pacing alone, to improve symptoms and cardiac performance. The typical objective of atrioventricular node ablation is to ablate the node, leaving a stable junctional escape rhythm. The anesthesia type is usually monitored anesthesia because the most common approach is right-sided with access via the femoral vein to permit radiofrequency ablation of the right atrium near the atrioventricular node. Anatomically, the atrioventricular node is contained within the triangle of Koch, a discrete region bounded by the tendon of Todaro, tricuspid valve annulus, and ostium of the coronary sinus. During the ablation procedure, the atrioventricular node is identified with fluoroscopic landmarks and electrogram recordings.

References:

1. Hensley N, Cheng A, Shah A, et al. Chapter 4: Cardiac Electrophysiology: Diagnosis and Treatment. In: Kaplan JA, Augoustides JGT, Manecke GR, et al., eds. Kaplan's Cardiac Anesthesia. 7th ed. Elsevier; 2017:96-117.
2. Nelson JA, Gue YX, Christensen JM, et al. Analysis of the ESC/EACTS 2020 Atrial Fibrillation Guidelines with perioperative implications. J Cardiothorac Vasc Anesth, 2022; 36: 2177-2195.
3. Vlachos K, Letsas KP, Korantzopoulos P, et al. A review on atrioventricular junction ablation and pacing for heart rate control of atrial fibrillation. J Geriatr Cardiol, 2015; 12: 547-554.

26. Anesthesia considerations for transcatheter ablation of ventricular tachycardia typically include all of the following, EXCEPT:

A. Monitored anesthesia care with minimal sedation may be indicated

B. Procedures are typically brief in duration

C. Hemodynamic instability is common

D. Percutaneous or surgical subxiphoid epicardial approaches may be indicated

Correct Answer: B

Explanation: Preoperative discussion with the electrophysiologist is recommended to plan the ablation procedure and design the anesthetic accordingly. Right-heart lesions may be amenable to monitored anesthesia care that can thus avoid arrhythmia suppression and optimize electrophysiologic mapping. Alternatively, with complex lesions with considerable ventricular scar, general endotracheal anesthesia is typically required due to anticipated long case duration as well as the possibility of percutaneous and/or surgical subxiphoid epicardial approaches. A preinduction radial arterial line is often considered for close blood pressure monitoring prior to the induction of anesthesia due to considerable patient comorbidities, including advanced coronary artery disease and severely impaired ventricular function. Furthermore, central venous access may be necessary if the administration of vasoactive drugs is anticipated based on comorbidity.

Regardless of anesthesia type, recommended additional monitors include cerebral oximetry and serial arterial blood gas sampling to monitor for end-organ hypoperfusion/metabolic acidemia, since hemodynamic instability during induction of ventricular tachycardia during these procedures is common.

References:

1. Hensley N, Cheng A, Shah A, et al. Chapter 4: Cardiac Electrophysiology: Diagnosis and Treatment. In: Kaplan JA, Augoustides JGT, Manecke GR, et al., eds. Kaplan's Cardiac Anesthesia. 7th ed. Elsevier; 2017:96-117.
2. Mittnacht AJ, Dukkipati S, Mahajan A. Ventricular tachycardia ablation: a comprehensive review for anesthesiologists. Anesth Analg, 2015; 120: 737-748.

BOX 4.11 Ventricular arrhythmias

- Most episodes of ventricular tachycardia or fibrillation result from coronary artery disease and dilated or hypertrophic cardiomyopathy.
- Implantable cardioverter-defibrillator placement is the standard of care with or without medical treatment for life-threatening ventricular arrhythmias and structural heart disease.
- Catheter ablation is adjuvant therapy for medically refractory monomorphic ventricular tachycardia.
- Surgical therapy includes endocardial resection with cryoablation.
- Anesthesia considerations focus on preoperative catheterization, echocardiography, and electrophysiologic testing.
- Monitoring of surgical patients is dictated by the underlying cardiac disease.

BOX 4.12 Implantable cardioverter-defibrillators

- ICDs can pace and provide tiered therapy for tachyarrhythmias (e.g., shocks, antitachycardia pacing).
- Insertion of modern devices typically is done with percutaneous techniques.
- ICDs are indicated for the primary or secondary prevention of sudden cardiac death.
- ICDs reduce overall mortality rates compared with standard treatment alone.
- ICDs are indicated for patients surviving sudden death without a reversible cause, those with ischemic cardiomyopathy with an ejection fraction ≤30%, and those with ischemic or nonischemic cardiomyopathy with an ejection fraction of ≤35% and NYHA class II or III heart failure symptoms.

ICD, Implantable cardioverter-defibrillator; *NYHA*, New York Heart Association.

3. Siegrist KK, Robles CF, Kertai MD, et al. The electrophysiologic laboratory: anesthetic considerations and staffing models. J Cardiothorac Vasc Anesth, 2021; 35: 2775-2783.

27. Current implantable cardioverter defibrillators are capable of all of the following, EXCEPT:
  A. Antitachycardia function
  B. Single-chamber pacing
  C. Dual-chamber pacing
  D. Asynchronous pacing with magnet application

Correct Answer: D

Explanation: Modern implantable cardioverter-defibrillators (ICDs) provide both antitachycardia function and pacing capability. Antitachycardia function includes both antitachycardia pacing and shock therapies such as cardioversion and/or defibrillation. Contemporary ICDs can typically pace as a single-chamber, dual-chamber, or biventricular system. For ICDs with pacing capability, magnet application will generally not alter the pacing mode and specifically will not create asynchronous pacing, but in many cases applying a magnet will suspend the antitachycardia function. Calling the manufacturer remains the most reliable method for determining the magnet response of a given device.

References:

1. Hensley N, Cheng A, Shah A, et al. Chapter 4: Cardiac Electrophysiology: Diagnosis and Treatment. In: Kaplan JA, Augoustides JGT, Manecke GR, et al., eds. Kaplan's Cardiac Anesthesia. 7th ed. Elsevier; 2017:96-117.
2. Cronin B, Essandoh MK. Update on cardiovascular implantable electronic devices for anesthesiologists. J Cardiothorac Vasc Anesth, 2018; 32: 1871-1884.
3. Practice Advisory for the Perioperative Management of Patients with Cardiac Implantable Electronic Devices: Pacemakers and Implantable Cardioverter–Defibrillators 2020: An Updated Report by the American Society of Anesthesiologists Task Force on Perioperative Management of Patients with Cardiac Implantable Electronic Devices. Anesthesiology, 2020; 132: 225-252.

28. The procedural conduct for implantable cardioverter defibrillator insertion is characterized by all of the following, EXCEPT:
  A. Performed in the electrophysiology suite
  B. Induction of ventricular tachycardia or ventricular fibrillation
  C. Defibrillation testing
  D. External cardioverter-defibrillator pads are not required

Correct Answer: D

Explanation: Insertion of implantable cardioverter-defibrillators is usually performed in the electrophysiologic suite and typically includes defibrillation testing to ensure an acceptable margin of safety for the device. Ventricular tachycardia and/or fibrillation is induced by the introduction of premature beats timed to the vulnerable repolarization period. External cardioverter-defibrillator pads are always placed before the procedure to provide backup shocks if the device is ineffective.

References:

1. Hensley N, Cheng A, Shah A, et al. Chapter 4: Cardiac Electrophysiology: Diagnosis and Treatment. In: Kaplan JA, Augoustides JGT, Manecke GR, et al., eds. Kaplan's Cardiac Anesthesia. 7th ed. Elsevier; 2017:96-117.
2. Fujii S, Zhou JR, Dhir A. Anesthesia for cardiac ablation. J Cardiothorac Vasc Anesth, 2018; 32: 1892-1910.

29. Which of the following is NOT an anesthesia consideration during implantable cardioverter-defibrillator implantation?
  A. Anesthesia type is usually general anesthesia
  B. The need for continuous arterial blood pressure monitoring is determined on a case-by-case basis
  C. Defibrillation testing is done
  D. Simultaneous insertion of biventricular pacing systems may be done

BOX 4.13   American College of Cardiology, American Heart Association, and Heart Rhythm Society guidelines for insertion of implantable cardioverter-defibrillators

Class I Heart Failure

- Survivors of cardiac arrest due to VF or sustained VT after excluding reversible causes
- Patients with structural heart disease and spontaneous, sustained VT, whether hemodynamically stable or unstable
- Patients with syncope of undetermined origin with clinically relevant sustained VT or VF induced at electrophysiology study
- Patients with an LVEF ≤35% due to prior MI occurring at least 40 days earlier and who have NYHA functional class II or III disease
- Patients with nonischemic dilated cardiomyopathy who have an LVEF ≤35% and NYHA functional class II or III disease
- Patients with LV dysfunction due to prior MI occurring at least 40 days earlier with an LVEF ≥30% and who have NYHA class I disease
- Patients with nonsustained VT due to prior MI with an LVEF ≤40% with inducible VF or sustained VT at electrophysiology study

Class IIa Heart Failure

- Patients with unexplained syncope, LV dysfunction, and nonischemic cardiomyopathy
- Patients with sustained VT and normal LV function
- Patients with hypertrophic cardiomyopathy and at least one risk factor for sudden cardiac death
- Patients with arrhythmogenic RV dysplasia with at least one risk factor for sudden cardiac death
- Patients with long QT syndrome with syncope and/or sustained VT while on β-blockers
- Nonhospitalized patients awaiting heart transplantation

- Patients with Brugada syndrome who have syncope or those with documented VT not resulting in cardiac arrest
- Patients with catecholaminergic polymorphic VT who have syncope and/or documented sustained VT while receiving β-blockers
- Patients with cardiac sarcoidosis, giant cell myocarditis, or Chagas disease

Class IIb Heart Failure

- Patients with nonischemic heart disease who have an LVEF ≤35% and who have NYHA class I disease
- Patients with long QT syndrome and risk factors for sudden cardiac death
- Patients with syncope and structural heart disease when evaluation has failed to define a cause
- Patients with familial cardiomyopathy associated with sudden cardiac death
- Patients with LV noncompaction

Class III Heart Failure

- ICD implantation is not indicated for patients whose reasonable life expectancy at an acceptable functional status is <1 year even if they meet other criteria

Therapeutic Indications by Functional Class

- Class I: There is evidence or general agreement that the treatment is useful and effective.
- Class IIa: Weight of the data or evidence favors benefit of the therapy.
- Class IIb: The conditions for which usefulness or efficacy of the treatment are less well established.
- Class III: Intervention is not indicated.

ICD, Implantable cardioverter-defibrillator; *LV,* left ventricular; *LVEF,* left ventricular ejection fraction; *MI,* myocardial infarction; *NYHA,* New York Heart Association; *RV,* right ventricular; *VF,* ventricular fibrillation; *VT,* ventricular tachycardia.

Correct Answer: A

Explanation: Monitored anesthesia care is typically chosen as the anesthesia type for transvenous implantation of cardioverter defibrillators. However, brief periods of general anesthesia may be necessary for defibrillation testing to ensure an acceptable margin of safety for the device. In contrast, when placing a subcutaneous implantable cardioverter-defibrillator, adequate analgesia cannot typically be achieved with monitored anesthesia care, since greater surgical dissection and tunneling is required. For these reasons, these devices are typically placed under general anesthesia and/or regional anesthesia. In addition to standard patient monitoring, continuous arterial blood pressure monitoring may be considered on a case-by-case basis to rapidly assess return of blood pressure after defibrillation testing. Simultaneous insertion of biventricular pacing systems is being performed more frequently, as this patient population often has concomitant left ventricular dysfunction.

References:

1. Hensley N, Cheng A, Shah A, et al. Chapter 4: Cardiac Electrophysiology: Diagnosis and Treatment. In: Kaplan JA, Augoustides JGT, Manecke GR, et al., eds. Kaplan's Cardiac Anesthesia. 7th ed. Elsevier; 2017:96-117.
2. Mittnacht AJC, Shariat A, Weiner MM, et al. Regional techniques for cardiac and cardiac-related procedures. J Cardiothorac Vasc Anesth, 2019; 33: 532-546.
3. Siegrist KK, Robles CF, Kertai MD, et al. The electrophysiologic laboratory: anesthetic considerations and staffing models. J Cardiothorac Vasc Anesth, 2021; 35: 2775-2783.

30. Which of the following procedural complications is LEAST likely to occur with implantable cardioverter-defibrillator implantation?

  A. Pneumothorax
  B. Cardiac perforation
  C. Myocardial injury
  D. Vascular and/or cardiac avulsion

Correct Answer: D

Explanation: Vascular and/or cardiac avulsion resulting in injuries to the great vessels and/or cardiac structures represent a set of complications associated with transvenous lead extraction due to fibrous adhesions connections that associate with indwelling venous electrophysiologic leads over time. Therefore, they are associated with acute device implantation. Known complications associated with implantation of cardioverter-defibrillators include pneumothorax, cardiac perforation, and myocardial injury due to defibrillation testing/multiple shocks. In addition, device infections may occur and are particularly difficult to manage, often requiring device and lead extraction.

References:

1. Hensley N, Cheng A, Shah A, et al. Chapter 4: Cardiac Electrophysiology: Diagnosis and Treatment. In: Kaplan JA, Augoustides JGT, Manecke GR, et al., eds. Kaplan's Cardiac Anesthesia. 7th ed. Elsevier; 2017:96-117.
2. Maus TM, Shurter J, Nguyen L, et al. Multidisciplinary approach to transvenous lead extraction: a single center's experience. J Cardiothorac Vasc Anesth, 2015; 29: 265-270.
3. Siegrist KK, Robles CF, Kertai MD, et al. The electrophysiologic laboratory: anesthetic considerations and staffing models. J Cardiothorac Vasc Anesth, 2021; 35: 2775-2783.

CHAPTER 5

Cardiovascular Implantable Electrical Devices

Steven T. Morozowich and Harish Ramakrishna

KEY POINTS

Preoperative Key Points

1. Identify the type of cardiac implantable electronic device (CIED) (e.g., transvenous implantable pacemaker, intracardiac pacemaker, transvenous implantable cardioverter-defibrillator [ICD], subcutaneous ICD) and the manufacturer of the generator.

2. Establish contact with the patient's CIED physician or clinic to obtain records and perioperative prescription (Heart Rhythm Society [HRS] expert consensus statement). Have the CIED interrogated by a competent authority shortly before the procedure (American Society of Anesthesiologists [ASA] practice advisory).

3. Obtain appropriate records from the CIED clinic (HRS expert consensus statement) or preoperative interrogation (ASA practice advisory). Ensure that the device will appropriately pace the heart.

4. Consider replacing any CIED near its elective replacement period in a patient scheduled to undergo either a major operation or surgery within 25 cm of the generator.

5. Determine the patient's underlying rate, rhythm, and pacing dependency to determine the need for asynchronous or external backup pacing support.

6. If magnet use is planned, then ensure that magnet behavior (pacing mode, rate, atrioventricular delay, shock therapy suspension) is appropriate for the patient.

7. Consider programming minute ventilation and other rate-responsiveness features off, if present.

8. Consider programming rate enhancements off, if present.

9. Consider increasing the pacing rate to optimize oxygen delivery to tissues for major operations.

10. If electromagnetic interference is likely, or if a central venous catheter guidewire will be placed into the chest, then consider asynchronous pacing for the pacing-dependent patient and suspension of antitachycardia therapy for any ICD patient. Magnet application might be effective, although magnet use has been associated with inappropriate ICD discharge. Magnet application will never create asynchronous pacing in any type of ICD.

Intraoperative Key Points

1. Monitor cardiac rhythm/peripheral pulse with pulse oximeter (plethysmography) or arterial waveform.

2. Consider disabling the "artifact filter" on the electrocardiographic monitor. If a minute ventilation sensor is active, then ensure that respiratory rate monitoring is disabled.

3. Ask the surgeon to avoid the use of the monopolar electrosurgical unit (ESU) or limit ESU bursts to <4 seconds separated by at least 2 seconds. Use the bipolar ESU if possible; if not possible, then pure cut (monopolar ESU) is better than "blend" or "coag."

4. Place the ESU dispersive electrode in such a way as to prevent electricity from crossing the generator-heart circuit, even if the electrode must be placed on the distal forearm and the wire covered with sterile drape.

5. If the ESU causes ventricular oversensing, resulting in pacing quiescence or atrial oversensing with inappropriate high-rate ventricular pacing, then limit the period(s) of asystole, relocate the dispersive electrode, or place a magnet over the pacemaker (not indicated for any ICD).

6. Temporary pacing might be needed, and consideration should be given to the possibility of CIED failure.

7. Consider avoiding sevoflurane, isoflurane, or desflurane in the patient with long QT syndrome.

Postoperative Key Points

1. Have the CIED interrogated by a competent authority postoperatively. Some rate enhancements can be reinitiated, and optimum heart rate and pacing parameters should be determined. The ICD patient must be monitored until the antitachycardia therapy is restored.

1. All of the following are typical examples of transvenous cardiovascular implantable electronic devices (CIEDs), EXCEPT:
- **A.** Permanent pacemaker
- **B.** Cardiac resynchronization therapy
- **C.** Subcutaneous implantable cardioverter-defibrillator
- **D.** Implantable cardioverter-defibrillator

Correct Answer: C

Explanation: Due to the clinical challenges and morbidity inherent in intravascular lead management with cardiovascular implantable electronic devices, new technology includes options that do not require intravascular leads. These include subcutaneous implantable cardioverter-defibrillators (S-ICDs) and leadless pacemaker systems. The S-ICD is an extrathoracic device that detects ventricular tachyarrhythmias and intervenes with antitachycardia pacing and shock therapy such as cardioversion or defibrillation. Leadless pacemakers also do not require intravascular leads, are a permanent implant placed typically via the transfemoral venous approach with fluoroscopic guidance, and are anchored within the right ventricular endocardium.

References:

1. Rozner MA. Chapter 5: Cardiac Implantable Electrical Devices. In: Kaplan JA, Augoustides JGT, Manecke GR, et al., eds. Kaplan's Cardiac Anesthesia. 7th ed. Elsevier; 2017:118-139.
2. Kusumoto FM, Schoenfeld MH, Wilkoff BL, et al. 2017 HRS expert consensus statement on cardiovascular implantable electronic device lead management and extraction. Heart Rhythm, 2017; 14: e503-e51.
3. Cody J, Graul T, Holliday S, et al. Nontransvenous cardiovascular implantable electronic device technology—a review for the anesthesiologist. J Cardiothorac Vasc Anesth, 2021; 35: 2784-2791.

2. Which of the following BEST characterizes a CardioMEMS device?
- **A.** It is a leadless pacemaker
- **B.** It is an implantable hemodynamic monitor
- **E.** It is an implantable cardioverter-defibrillator
- **C.** It is not a cardiovascular implantable electronic device

Correct Answer: B

Explanation: Cardiovascular implantable electronic devices are continually evolving to advance cardiovascular monitoring and management throughout the world. The CardioMEMS device is an implantable hemodynamic monitor. It has a wireless pressure sensor without a battery and is implanted via the femoral or internal jugular vein with anchoring in the left pulmonary artery. It is intended to prevent hospital admissions from heart failure decompensation by measuring and transmitting pulmonary artery pressure data that can then guide optimal management such as titration of medical therapy.

References:

1. Rozner MA. Chapter 5, Cardiac Implantable Electrical Devices. In: Kaplan JA, Augoustides JGT, Manecke GR, et al., eds. Kaplan's Cardiac Anesthesia. 7th ed. Elsevier; 2017: 118-139.
2. Ijaz SH, Shah SP, Majithia A. Implantable devices for heart failure monitoring. Prog Cardiovasc Dis, 2021; 69: 47-53.

3. Regarding implantable cardioverter-defibrillators (ICDs), which of the following is CORRECT?
- **A.** ICDs provide both antitachycardia function and pacing
- **B.** ICDs provide only pacing
- **C.** ICDs provide only defibrillation shock therapy
- **D.** ICDs provide only cardioversion shock therapy

Correct Answer: A

Explanation: Cardiovascular implantable electronic devices were first introduced in 1958 and continue to evolve. Contemporary implantable cardioverter-defibrillators provide both antitachycardia function and pacing capability. The antitachycardia function includes both antitachycardia pacing and shock therapies such as cardioversion and/or defibrillation.

References:

1. Rozner MA. Chapter 5, Cardiac Implantable Electrical Devices. In: Kaplan JA, Augoustides JGT, Manecke GR, et al., eds. Kaplan's Cardiac Anesthesia. 7th ed. Elsevier; 2017:118-139.
2. Cronin B, Essandoh MK. Update on cardiovascular implantable electronic devices for anesthesiologists. J Cardiothorac Vasc Anesth, 2018; 32: 1871-1884.

4. Complications associated with the implantation of transvenous cardiovascular implantable electronic devices include all of the following, EXCEPT:
- **A.** Bleeding
- **B.** Pneumothorax

C. Cardiac perforation

D. Perioperative mortality 5%

Correct Answer: D

Explanation: The continued enhancements in the technology of cardiovascular implantable electronic devices (CIEDs) will expand their clinical indications. For example, the demand for implantable cardioverter-defibrillators has accelerated based on data regarding the primary prevention of sudden cardiac death in patients with low left ventricular ejection fraction. In an analysis of over 800,000 patients who underwent initial CIED implantation between 2010 and 2014, the observed in-hospital mortality rate was less than 1% (0.9%). The complications associated with transvenous CIED lead implantation include bleeding, pneumothorax, air embolism, cardiac perforation, infection, lead dislodgement, and thrombosis of the implant vein.

References:

1. Rozner MA. Chapter 5, Cardiac Implantable Electrical Devices. In: Kaplan JA, Augoustides JGT, Manecke GR, et al., eds. Kaplan's Cardiac Anesthesia. 7th ed. Elsevier; 2017:118-139.
2. Pasupula DK, Rajaratnam A, Rattan R, et al. Trends in hospital admissions for and readmissions after cardiac implantable electronic device procedures in the United States: an analysis from 2010 to 2014 using the national readmission database. Mayo Clin Proc, 2019; 94: 588-598.

5. Which of the following BEST characterizes transvenous lead extraction?

    A. Removal of lead implanted less than 1 year ago

    B. Removal of lead performed with manual traction

    C. Removal of lead performed with telescoping laser sheaths

    D. Considered low-risk

Correct Answer: C

Explanation: With the aging population and increasing indications for the implantation of cardiovascular implantable electronic devices (CIEDs), lead removal will become increasingly common as well. Transvenous lead removal is the general term used when the benefits of lead removal exceed the potential risks of the procedure. It implies a percutaneous approach, but open approaches can be used if the patient failed prior percutaneous removal, if the patient needs other cardiac surgery, and/or if large vegetations are present. The term lead extraction (also known as transvenous lead extraction) specifically refers to leads implanted more than 1 year ago, with removal performed typically with telescoping laser sheaths. Lead extraction procedures are generally considered high-risk because fibrous connections to adjacent veins and/or endocardial surfaces develop over time, and thus extraction may result in catastrophic vascular/cardiac avulsion requiring superior vena cava occlusion balloon deployment and/or rapid surgical rescue with sternotomy. In contrast, the term lead explantation (also known as lead revision) specifically refers to leads implanted less than 1 year ago, with removal performed with manual traction via the implant vein, with relatively low risk.

References:

1. Rozner MA. Chapter 5, Cardiac Implantable Electrical Devices. In: Kaplan JA, Augoustides JGT, Manecke GR, et al., eds. Kaplan's Cardiac Anesthesia. 7th ed. Elsevier; 2017:118-139.
2. Kusumoto FM, Schoenfeld MH, Wilkoff BL, et al. 2017 HRS expert consensus statement on cardiovascular implantable electronic device lead management and extraction. Heart Rhythm, 2017; 14: e503-e551.

6. Which of the following is an indication for transvenous lead removal?

    A. Lead malfunction

    B. Infection including endocarditis and/or pocket infection

    C. Venous occlusion including superior vena cava syndrome

    D. All of the above

Correct Answer: D

Explanation: Lead removal for cardiovascular implantable electronic device lead removal is no longer an uncommon procedure. All the given options in this question are indications for transvenous lead removal and illustrate the complications associated with transvenous leads, including malfunction, infection, and thrombosis. The indications for transvenous lead removal have been categorized as follows: lead management in approximately 53% of cases, infection in 37%, and venous thrombosis in the remaining approximately 10% of cases.

References:

1. Rozner MA. Chapter 5, Cardiac Implantable Electrical Devices. In: Kaplan JA, Augoustides JGT, Manecke GR, et al., eds. Kaplan's Cardiac Anesthesia. 7th ed. Elsevier; 2017:118-139.
2. Maus TM, Shurter J, Nguyen L, et al. Multidisciplinary approach to transvenous lead extraction: a single center's experience. J Cardiothorac Vasc Anesth, 2015; 29: 265-270.

7. Which of the following factors determine patient risk during transvenous lead removal?

    A. Preprocedural evaluation by the heart team

    B. Presence of implantable cardioverter-defibrillator leads that are higher risk compared to permanent pacemaker leads

    C. Risk factors such as multiple or long-standing leads, as well the geriatric or pediatric age groups

    D. All of the above

Correct Answer: D

Explanation: All of the above factors are used to determine patient risk for transvenous lead removal. Lead extraction is a difficult procedure and is prone to severe complications due to adherence of the leads to vascular structures, and thus the perioperative engagement of the full heart team is required.

The preprocedural evaluation by the heart team includes review of the patient clinical presentation and related special studies. Chest imaging including computerized tomography will permit identification of calcification, high-risk areas of adhesion such as the superior vena cava, and impending complications such as subclinical cardiac perforation. A detailed review of echocardiographic data will characterize baseline ventricular function and the degree of tricuspid regurgitation. Further important aspects include identifying prior cardiac surgery, determining pacemaker-dependency, excluding the presence of inferior vena cava filter, planning for reversal of anticoagulation, and arranging blood availability.

Lead type is another consideration when determining patient risk. Implantable cardioverter-defibrillator as compared to permanent pacemaker leads are associated with more substantial adhesions to endovascular structures since they are larger and provide a greater surface area for adherence. Further risk factors in this setting include multiple or long-standing leads, the geriatric or pediatric age group, and female gender.

References:

1. Rozner MA. Chapter 5, Cardiac Implantable Electrical Devices. In: Kaplan JA, Augoustides JGT, Manecke GR, et al., eds. Kaplan's Cardiac Anesthesia. 7th ed. Elsevier; 2017: 118-139.
2. Kusumoto FM, Schoenfeld MH, Wilkoff BL, et al. 2017 HRS expert consensus statement on cardiovascular implantable electronic device lead management and extraction. Heart Rhythm, 2017; 14: e503-e551.
3. Epstein LM, Love CJ, Wilkoff BL, et al. Superior vena cava defibrillator coils make transvenous lead extraction more challenging and riskier. J Am Coll Cardiol, 2013; 61: 987-989.

8. What is the approximate rate of major complications associated with transvenous lead removal?
  A. Less than 5%
  B. 5% to 10%
  C. 10% to 20%
  D. More than 20%

Correct Answer: A

Explanation: The main concern with transvenous lead removal is injury of adjacent veins and/or endocardial surfaces (also referred to as vascular/cardiac avulsion) due to dense fibrous adhesions associated with indwelling venous leads over time. During transvenous lead extraction, transesophageal echocardiography can detect major complications. These complications occur at a rate of less than 5% (1%–4%) and include right ventricular perforation, right atrial tears, and great vein injuries that collectively can lead to life-threatening bleeding as well as pericardial tamponade and/or hemothorax. Further, the mortality rate (directly related to the procedure) has been shown to be less than 1% (0.28%). Additional complications include traumatic tricuspid regurgitation and pulmonary embolism.

References:

1. Rozner MA. Chapter 5, Cardiac Implantable Electrical Devices. In: Kaplan JA, Augoustides JGT, Manecke GR, et al., eds. Kaplan's Cardiac Anesthesia. 7th ed. Elsevier; 2017:118-139.
2. Maus TM, Shurter J, Nguyen L, et al. Multidisciplinary approach to transvenous lead extraction: a single center's experience. J Cardiothorac Vasc Anesth, 2015; 29: 265-270.
3. Wazni O, Epstein LM, Carrillo RG, et al. Lead extraction in the contemporary setting: the LExICon study: an observational retrospective study of consecutive laser lead extractions. J Am Coll Cardiol, 2010; 55: 579-586.

9. Compared to a transvenous implantable cardioverter-defibrillator, a subcutaneous implantable cardioverter-defibrillator is characterized by which of the following?
  A. Higher defibrillation thresholds
  B. Smaller device size
  C. Similar anesthetic requirements for device placement
  D. The use of intravascular leads

Correct Answer: A

Explanation: Subcutaneous implantable cardioverters-defibrillators (S-ICDs) are larger devices compared to their transvenous counterparts and generally have higher defibrillation thresholds. Due to the greater surgical dissection and tunneling required for S-ICD placement, general and/or regional anesthesia is/are selected for placement. The main advantage of nontransvenous devices such as S-ICDs is the absence of intravascular leads and consequent freedom from their related complications.

References:

1. Rozner MA. Chapter 5, Cardiac Implantable Electrical Devices. In: Kaplan JA, Augoustides JGT, Manecke GR, et al., eds. Kaplan's Cardiac Anesthesia. 7th ed. Elsevier; 2017:118-139.
2. Mittnacht AJC, Shariat A, Weiner MM, et al. Regional techniques for cardiac and cardiac-related procedures. J Cardiothorac Vasc Anesth, 2019; 33: 532-546.
3. Cody J, Graul T, Holliday S, Streckenbach S, et al. Nontransvenous cardiovascular implantable electronic device technology—a review for the anesthesiologist. J Cardiothorac Vasc Anesth, 2021; 35: 2784-2791.

10. Indications for the placement of subcutaneous implantable cardioverter-defibrillator include all of the following, EXCEPT:
  A. Patients who require both antitachycardia function and pacing
  B. Young patients
  C. Patients with infectious risks
  D. Patients with difficult vascular access

Correct Answer: A

Explanation: Cardiovascular implantable electronic devices that do not require intravascular leads include leadless pacemakers and subcutaneous implantable cardioverter-defibrillators (S-ICDs). These devices can only provide single therapy: either antitachycardia function (S-ICDs) or pacing (leadless pacemakers). Thus, S-ICDs differ in this regard from their conventional counterparts that can provide both antitachycardia function and pacing. The main advantage of S-ICDs is that the absence of transvenous leads avoids complications such as infection, endocarditis, vascular occlusion, and lead fracture or displacement, as well as lead-related tricuspid valve complications. For these reasons, S-ICDs are typically indicated for younger patients, those at higher risk for infection, and/or those with difficult vascular access.

References:

1. Rozner MA. Chapter 5, Cardiac Implantable Electrical Devices. In: Kaplan JA, Augoustides JGT, Manecke GR, et al., eds. Kaplan's Cardiac Anesthesia. 7th ed. Elsevier; 2017:118-139.
2. Cody J, Graul T, Holliday S, et al. Nontransvenous cardiovascular implantable electronic device technology—a review for the anesthesiologist. J Cardiothorac Vasc Anesth, 2021; 35: 2784-2791.
3. Kusumoto FM, Schoenfeld MH, Wilkoff BL, et al. 2017 HRS expert consensus statement on cardiovascular implantable electronic device lead management and extraction. Heart Rhythm, 2017; 14: e503-e551.

11. When planning the anesthesia type for the placement of a subcutaneous implantable cardioverter-defibrillator, which of the following is NOT an acceptable technique?
  A. General anesthesia
  B. Regional anesthesia as the primary anesthetic
  C. Monitored anesthesia care with minimal sedation
  D. All of the above are acceptable

Correct Answer: C

Explanation: Compared to placement of transvenous cardiovascular implantable electronic devices, their subcutaneous counterparts require more than local anesthetic infiltration with titrated sedation, as extensive surgical dissection and tunneling are required. Consequently, in this setting, general and/or regional anesthesia should be considered. Deep levels of general anesthesia can have detrimental effects on patients with left ventricular dysfunction and can also raise the defibrillation threshold during device testing. Furthermore, placement is also associated with significant postoperative pain. Because of these reasons, regional anesthesia may offer advantages if included in the anesthetic plan.

References:

1. Rozner MA. Chapter 5, Cardiac Implantable Electrical Devices. In: Kaplan JA, Augoustides JGT, Manecke GR, et al., eds. Kaplan's Cardiac Anesthesia. 7th ed. Elsevier; 2017:118-139.
2. Mittnacht AJC, Shariat A, Weiner MM, et al. Regional techniques for cardiac and cardiac-related procedures. J Cardiothorac Vasc Anesth, 2019; 33: 532-546.

12. When obtaining magnetic resonance imaging (MRI) in patients with cardiovascular implantable electronic devices (CIEDs), all of the following are true, EXCEPT:
  A. MRIs can be obtained safely in most patients with CIEDs
  B. If, under certain conditions, an MRI can be obtained safely, the CIED is referred to as "MRI-conditional"
  C. The prevalence of CIEDs with "MRI-conditional" labeling is increasing
  D. CIEDs with "MRI-safe" labeling are likely in the near future

Correct Answer: D

Explanation: With millions of cardiovascular implantable cardiovascular devices in clinical practice, many patients will need to undergo imaging with magnetic resonance imaging (MRI) at some point during their care. Many of these patients with both permanent pacemakers and cardioverter-defibrillators have undergone MRI without significant incident, and these CIEDs are referred to as "MRI-conditional," where under certain conditions they are safe for this imaging modality. A typical condition includes ensuring that MRI magnet strength does not exceed 1.5 tesla. With ongoing improvements in technology, the list of "MRI-conditional" devices continues to grow. However, current thought leaders believe that "MRI-safe" labeling of CIEDs is unlikely to occur.

References:

1. Rozner MA. Chapter 5, Cardiac Implantable Electrical Devices. In: Kaplan JA, Augoustides JGT, Manecke GR, et al., eds. Kaplan's Cardiac Anesthesia. 7th ed. Elsevier; 2017:118-139.
2. Stawiarski K, Sorajja D, Ramakrishna H. Magnetic resonance and computed tomography imaging in patients with cardiovascular implantable electronic devices: analysis of expert consensus data and implications for the perioperative clinician. J Cardiothorac Vasc Anesth, 2018; 32: 2817-2822.
3. Martin ET, Coman JA, Shellock FG, et al. Magnetic resonance imaging and cardiac pacemaker safety at 1.5-Tesla. J Am Coll Cardiol, 2004; 43: 1315-1324.

13. During the preoperative anesthesia evaluation, which of the following is typically NOT required to determine whether a patient has a cardiovascular implantable electronic device?
  A. Patient interview and review of medical records
  B. Focused physical exam
  C. Obtaining an electrocardiogram
  D. Obtaining a transthoracic echocardiogram

Correct Answer: D

Explanation: According to recent recommendations from American Society of Anesthesiologists, determining whether a patient has a cardiovascular implantable electronic device is typically done by interviewing the patient, performing a focused physical exam to palpate the device and/or identify an implant scar, and reviewing medical records, chest x-rays, and electrocardiograms. Although transthoracic echocardiography can assist in this assessment, it is not routinely required in this setting.

References:

1. Rozner MA. Chapter 5, Cardiac Implantable Electrical Devices. In: Kaplan JA, Augoustides JGT, Manecke GR, et al., eds. Kaplan's Cardiac Anesthesia. 7th ed. Elsevier; 2017:118-139.

2. Practice Advisory for the Perioperative Management of Patients with Cardiac Implantable Electronic Devices: Pacemakers and Implantable Cardioverter–Defibrillators 2020: An Updated Report by the American Society of Anesthesiologists Task Force on Perioperative Management of Patients with Cardiac Implantable Electronic Devices. Anesthesiology, 2020; 132: 225-252.

14. Prior to proceeding with an elective surgical procedure on a patient with a cardiovascular implantable electronic device (CIED), which of the following has NOT been consistently recommended?
   A. Determine CIED type, manufacturer, and primary indication for placement
   B. Determine whether the patient is pacing-dependent
   C. Have a magnet available to enable asynchronous pacing, regardless of CIED device
   D. Determine the CIED's current settings, that it is functioning properly, and that it is optimally programmed for the planned procedure

Correct Answer: C

Explanation: Because there really is no reliable means to confirm magnet response with cardiovascular implantable electronic devices (CIEDs), calling the manufacturer remains the most reliable method for determining magnet response. For implantable cardioverter-defibrillators with pacing capability, magnet application will generally not alter the pacing mode and specifically will not create asynchronous pacing. However, in many cases applying a magnet will suspend the antitachycardia function. In fact, magnet application to some implantable devices may evoke no response, and older devices could be permanently disabled. Thus, if suspending antitachycardia functions is required, this is best accomplished by consulting a specialist for reprogramming.

In general, for permanent pacemakers, magnet application will result in high-rate (85–100 beats per minute) asynchronous pacing in the majority of devices (>90%). However, placement of a magnet in this setting may produce no change in pacing since not all pacemakers switch to a continuous asynchronous mode.

Current recommendations from the American Society of Anesthesiologists include determining the CIED type, manufacturer, and primary indication for placement. Furthermore, it is important to assess whether the patient is pacing-dependent, as well as the current device settings to confirm that it is functioning properly and that it is optimally programmed for the planned procedure.

References:
1. Rozner MA. Chapter 5, Cardiac Implantable Electrical Devices. In: Kaplan JA, Augoustides JGT, Manecke GR, et al., eds. Kaplan's Cardiac Anesthesia. 7th ed. Elsevier; 2017:118-139.
2. Practice Advisory for the Perioperative Management of Patients with Cardiac Implantable Electronic Devices: Pacemakers and Implantable Cardioverter–Defibrillators 2020: An

Updated Report by the American Society of Anesthesiologists Task Force on Perioperative Management of Patients with Cardiac Implantable Electronic Devices. Anesthesiology, 2020; 132: 225-252.

15. All of the following statements regarding electromagnetic interference (EMI) in the operating room are true, EXCEPT:
   A. EMI is much more likely with use of a monopolar electrosurgery unit (ESU) versus a bipolar ESU
   B. EMI is more likely with use of ESU coagulation mode versus cutting mode
   C. EMI can occur during peripheral nerve stimulation for peripheral nerve blocks
   D. The risk of EMI causing interference with cardiovascular implantable electronic devices is highest during surgical procedures performed below the umbilicus

Correct Answer: D

Explanation: Electromagnetic interference (EMI) refers to the potential disruption of a cardiovascular implantable electronic device (CIED) when it is in the vicinity of an electromagnetic field generated by an external source. During surgical procedures, the external source is most commonly an electrosurgery unit (ESU), where monopolar ESU is much more likely to cause EMI than bipolar ESU. Further, the coagulation mode is high-voltage and thus causes more EMI than the cutting mode (low-voltage). A prospective study demonstrated that monopolar ESU caused clinically significant EMI, defined as interference that would have resulted in delivery of inappropriate antitachycardia therapy (i.e., antitachycardia pacing or shock) by an implantable cardioverters-defibrillator if the device was not reprogrammed in 29% of patients during intrathoracic cardiac surgery, 20% during noncardiac surgery above the umbilicus, and 0% during surgery below the umbilicus. EMI may also occur during peripheral nerve stimulation for peripheral nerve blocks, with recommendations during upper extremity blocks including placing the current return electrode from the nerve stimulator as close as possible to the stimulating electrode such as the patient's arm, rather than across the chest, to direct current away from the CIED.

References:
1. Rozner MA. Chapter 5, Cardiac Implantable Electrical Devices. In: Kaplan JA, Augoustides JGT, Manecke GR, et al., eds. Kaplan's Cardiac Anesthesia. 7th ed. Elsevier; 2017:118-139.
2. Schulman PM, Treggiari MM, Yanez ND, et al. Electromagnetic interference with protocolized electrosurgery dispersive electrode positioning in patients with implantable cardioverter defibrillators. Anesthesiology, 2019; 130: 530-540.
3. McKay RE, Rozner MA. Preventing pacemaker problems with nerve stimulators. Anaesthesia, 2008; 63: 554-556.

16. In patients with cardiovascular implantable electronic devices (CIEDs), which of the following is recommended to minimize the intraoperative risk of electromagnetic interference due to an electrosurgery unit (ESU)?

A. Use monopolar ESU instead of bipolar ESU

B. When using an ESU, use short, intermittent, and irregular bursts at the lowest feasible energy levels

C. Position the ESU and dispersive electrode (bovie pad) so the current pathway is through the CIED generator

D. All of the above are recommended

Correct Answer: B

Explanation: During surgical procedures in patients with cardiovascular implantable electronic devices (CIEDs), electromagnetic interference (EMI) is common from the electrosurgery unit (ESU). In patients with CIEDs, it has been generally recommended to select a bipolar ESU if possible. In contrast to monopolar ESUs, bipolar ESUs restrict the energy field to the areas around the cautery probe and thus minimize its spread throughout the body. However, if a monopolar ESU is required, the recommendation is to limit bursts to <4 seconds separated by at least 2 seconds. It is recommended to position the ESU and dispersive electrode (Bovie pad) so the current pathway does not pass through or near the CIED generator or leads.

References:

1. Rozner MA. Chapter 5, Cardiac Implantable Electrical Devices. In: Kaplan JA, Augoustides JGT, Manecke GR, et al., eds. Kaplan's Cardiac Anesthesia. 7th ed. Elsevier; 2017:118-139.
2. Practice Advisory for the Perioperative Management of Patients with Cardiac Implantable Electronic Devices: Pacemakers and Implantable Cardioverter–Defibrillators 2020: An Updated Report by the American Society of Anesthesiologists Task Force on Perioperative Management of Patients with Cardiac Implantable Electronic Devices. Anesthesiology, 2020; 132: 225-252.

17. A patient with a cardiovascular implantable electronic device (CIED) was scheduled for chest wall surgery. After discussion with the surgeon, the team proceeded with the use of a monopolar electrosurgery unit. Which of the following statements is INCORRECT regarding perioperative management in this setting?

A. If the patient is pacing-dependent, it is essential to reprogram the CIED to an asynchronous pacing mode preoperatively

B. If an implantable cardioverter-defibrillator (ICD) is present, apply a magnet as needed intraoperatively

C. If an ICD is present, suspend antitachycardia function preoperatively per the manufacturer's recommendations

D. If suspending antitachycardia function is indicated, ensure the patient is in a monitored environment

Correct Answer: B

Explanation: As-needed (or indiscriminate) application of a magnet to an implantable cardioverter-defibrillator should be avoided because magnet response is variable. Instead, if suspending antitachycardia function is required, it is best accomplished by consulting a specialist for reprogramming. Otherwise, the remaining recommendations are consistent with the latest practice advisory from the American Society of Anesthesiologists Task Force with respect to patients with cardiovascular implantable electronic devices.

References:

1. Rozner MA. Chapter 5, Cardiac Implantable Electrical Devices. In: Kaplan JA, Augoustides JGT, Manecke GR, et al., eds. Kaplan's Cardiac Anesthesia. 7th ed. Elsevier; 2017:118-139.
2. Practice Advisory for the Perioperative Management of Patients with Cardiac Implantable Electronic Devices: Pacemakers and Implantable Cardioverter–Defibrillators 2020: An Updated Report by the American Society of Anesthesiologists Task Force on Perioperative Management of Patients with Cardiac Implantable Electronic Devices. Anesthesiology, 2020; 132: 225-252.

18. Placement of a magnet over a permanent pacemaker generator usually results in which of the following responses?

A. Asynchronous pacing

B. No change in pacing

C. Loss of pacing

D. Generator battery discharge

Correct Answer: A

Explanation: Although placement of a magnet over a permanent pacemaker (PPM) generator might produce no change in pacing, since not all pacemakers switch to a continuous asynchronous mode, more than 90% of PPMs respond with high-rate (85–100 bpm) asynchronous pacing with magnet application. Furthermore, several PPMs can be quickly identified by their consistent and unique magnet responses, known as magnet mode rates, in the range of 85 to 100 beats per minute. However, despite these trends, calling the manufacturer remains the most reliable method for determining magnet response.

References:

1. Rozner MA. Chapter 5, Cardiac Implantable Electrical Devices. In: Kaplan JA, Augoustides JGT, Manecke GR, et al., eds. Kaplan's Cardiac Anesthesia. 7th ed. Elsevier; 2017:118-139.
2. Cronin B, Essandoh MK. Update on cardiovascular implantable electronic devices for anesthesiologists. J Cardiothorac Vasc Anesth, 2018; 32: 1871-1884.

19. Placement of a magnet over an implantable cardioverter-defibrillator with pacing capability usually results in which of the following responses?

A. Asynchronous pacing

B. Suspension of antitachycardia function

C. Suspension of shock therapy only (i.e., cardioversion or defibrillation)

D. Both A and B

Correct Answer: B

Explanation: For implantable cardioverter-defibrillators (ICDs) with pacing capability, magnet application does not alter the pacing mode, but in most cases applying a magnet will suspend the antitachycardia function, which includes both antitachycardia pacing and shock therapies such as cardioversion or defibrillation. However, there really is no reliable means to confirm the magnet response. In fact, magnet application to some ICDs may elicit no response, and older devices could be permanently disabled. Thus, if suspending antitachycardia function is required, it is best accomplished by consulting a specialist for reprogramming.

References:

1. Rozner MA. Chapter 5, Cardiac Implantable Electrical Devices. In: Kaplan JA, Augoustides JGT, Manecke GR, et al., eds. Kaplan's Cardiac Anesthesia. 7th ed. Elsevier; 2017:118-139.
2. Practice Advisory for the Perioperative Management of Patients with Cardiac Implantable Electronic Devices: Pacemakers and Implantable Cardioverter–Defibrillators 2020: An Updated Report by the American Society of Anesthesiologists Task Force on Perioperative Management of Patients with Cardiac Implantable Electronic Devices. Anesthesiology, 2020; 132: 225-252.

20. During an intraoperative emergency in a patient with an implantable cardioverter-defibrillator (ICD), if defibrillation or cardioversion is indicated which of the following should be done first?
   A. Place a magnet on the ICD
   B. If an ICD magnet has been applied, remove it
   C. Begin transcutaneous pacing
   D. Perform external defibrillation or cardioversion immediately

Correct Answer: B

Explanation: An advantage of magnet placement, if indicated, is that it can easily be removed. In the case of ventricular arrhythmias during surgery, before attempting emergency external defibrillation or cardioversion, if a magnet has been applied to an implantable cardioverter-defibrillator (ICD), it should be removed first to permit reactivation of the antitachycardia function of the ICD. However, if magnet removal does not immediately result in reactivation of the device with appropriate defibrillation or cardioversion, an external defibrillator should be employed.

Importantly, it must be kept in mind that, with magnet application, the magnet must be reliably secured over the device and out of the surgical field to ensure that the ICD is disabled. This cannot be taken lightly, because inappropriate antitachycardia pacing and shock therapy can result in significant battery depletion or myocardial injury; thus, proper preoperative preparation is essential prior to determining if magnet application or reprograming should be done.

References:

1. Rozner MA. Chapter 5, Cardiac Implantable Electrical Devices. In: Kaplan JA, Augoustides JGT, Manecke GR, et al., eds. Kaplan's Cardiac Anesthesia. 7th ed. Elsevier; 2017:118-139.

2. Cronin B, Essandoh MK. Update on cardiovascular implantable electronic devices for anesthesiologists. J Cardiothorac Vasc Anesth, 2018; 32: 1871-1884.

21. When reprogramming a permanent pacemaker to asynchronous pacing, all of the following statements are true, EXCEPT:
   A. It is typically required for pacing-dependent patients
   B. It is typically required for procedures above the umbilicus
   C. It could result in R-on-T pacing with the development of a malignant ventricular arrhythmias
   D. It will protect the device from internal damage or reset caused by electromagnetic interference

Correct Answer: D

Explanation: Pacemaker reprogramming to asynchronous pacing is typically required in patients who are pacing-dependent and/or are undergoing major procedures in the chest or abdomen. Perioperative asynchronous pacing at a rate greater than the patient's underlying rate usually ensures that electromagnetic interference will not affect pacing. Although rare, asynchronous pacing can produce detrimental effects such as R-on-T pacing resulting in induced malignant ventricular arrhythmias such as ventricular fibrillation. However, many perioperative patients also have electrolyte abnormalities, myocardial ischemia, or other underlying heart disease that may portend additional risk, and because of this, asynchronous pacing should be used with caution. Asynchronous pacing will not protect the device from internal damage or reset caused by electromagnetic interference.

References:

1. Rozner MA. Chapter 5, Cardiac Implantable Electrical Devices. In: Kaplan JA, Augoustides JGT, Manecke GR, et al., eds. Kaplan's Cardiac Anesthesia. 7th ed. Elsevier; 2017:118-139.
2. Atlee JL, Bernstein AD. Harm associated with reprogramming pacemakers for surgery. Anesthesiology, 2002; 97: 1034-1035.
3. Streckenbach SC, Dalia AA. Perioperative management of cardiac implantable electronic devices: a single-center report of 469 interrogations. J Cardiothorac Vasc Anesth, 2021; 35: 3183-3192.

22. A patient with a permanent pacemaker who is pacing-dependent is undergoing thoracic surgery, and you have been informed that your anesthesia monitors are routinely configured to accentuate the display of pacing spikes on the electrocardiogram (ECG). If ECG artifacts occur during the surgery, which of the following is the BEST additional monitor to ensure the presence of adequate mechanical systoles?
   A. Automated external defibrillator
   B. Noninvasive blood pressure
   C. Pulse oximeter waveform
   D. End-tidal CO_2 waveform

Correct Answer: C

Explanation: Perioperative monitoring in patients with a permanent pacemaker must include the ability to detect mechanical systoles, since electromagnetic interference can interfere with the display of the QRS complex and pacemaker spikes on the electrocardiogram (ECG). Although most modern digital ECG monitors filter high-frequency signals (between 1000 and 2000 Hz), which includes pacemaker spikes (pacemaker signal is about 2000 Hz), accentuation of pacing spikes can be enabled and is routinely done during an anesthetic. However, this accentuation occasionally goes awry and marks artifact as pacing spikes. Ultimately, heart rate counting may be inaccurate, and subsequent misinterpretation of these erroneous heart rates could result in the inappropriate use of anesthetic or chronotropic/vasoactive medications. Thus, it is vital to confirm an adequate peripheral pulse by monitoring with pulse oximetry or an arterial waveform to avoid confusion with ECG artifacts.

References:

1. Rozner MA. Chapter 5, Cardiac Implantable Electrical Devices. In: Kaplan JA, Augoustides JGT, Manecke GR, et al., eds. Kaplan's Cardiac Anesthesia. 7th ed. Elsevier; 2017:118-139.
2. Crossley GH, Poole JE, Rozner MA, et al. The Heart Rhythm Society (HRS)/American Society of Anesthesiologists (ASA) Expert Consensus Statement on the perioperative management of patients with implantable defibrillators, pacemakers and arrhythmia monitors: facilities and patient management this document was developed as a joint project with the American Society of Anesthesiologists (ASA), and in collaboration with the American Heart Association (AHA), and the Society of Thoracic Surgeons (STS). Heart Rhythm, 2011; 8: 1114-1154.

23. Following a surgical procedure, which of the following is NOT an indication for cardiovascular implantable electronic device (CIED) interrogation prior to patient discharge from the postanesthesia care unit?
    A. The patient underwent cardiac or significant vascular surgery
    B. Monopolar electrosurgery unit was used at a site distant from the CIED
    C. CIED was reprogrammed prior to the procedure
    D. Intraoperative cardiac arrest with external electrical cardioversion occurred

Correct Answer: B

Explanation: The rationale for postoperative interrogation of devices is based on whether preoperative reprogramming was performed, if the patient underwent cardiac or significant vascular surgery (i.e., hemodynamically challenging cases), whether electromagnetic interference (EMI) exposure was in close proximity to the generator (e.g., EMI exposure was above the umbilicus), and/or if significant intraoperative events occurred such as cardiac arrest, cardiopulmonary resuscitation, external electrical cardioversion, and/or temporary pacing. During most surgical procedures EMI is frequently encountered from an electrosurgery unit that applies a focused radiofrequency electrical current to produce tissue desiccation for surgical cutting and/or coagulation to control bleeding.

With the described scenarios, postoperative interrogation ensures that the device has not entered a backup safety mode and that functionality is not impaired, and is intended to restore preprocedural programming settings. Although some manufacturers recommended postoperative interrogation if any monopolar electrosurgery unit was used, the expert consensus from the Heart Rhythm Society and American Society of Anesthesiologists has stated that this is only necessary when significant EMI occurs above the umbilicus. For procedures where the above is not applicable, postoperative cardiovascular implantable electronic device evaluation is not necessary and can occur at a later time, such as within 30 days or at routine follow-up.

References:

1. Rozner MA. Chapter 5, Cardiac Implantable Electrical Devices. In: Kaplan JA, Augoustides JGT, Manecke GR, et al., eds. Kaplan's Cardiac Anesthesia. 7th ed. Elsevier; 2017:118-139.
2. Crossley GH, Poole JE, Rozner MA, et al. The Heart Rhythm Society (HRS)/American Society of Anesthesiologists (ASA) Expert Consensus Statement on the perioperative management of patients with implantable defibrillators, pacemakers and arrhythmia monitors: facilities and patient management. Heart Rhythm, 2011; 8: 1114-1154.

24. While preparing for separation from cardiopulmonary bypass with temporary epicardial pacing, pacemaker failure to capture is recognized. Which of the following is LEAST likely to be contributing to this phenomenon?
    A. Dobutamine infusion
    B. Myocardial ischemia
    C. Hyperkalemia
    D. Acidemia

Correct Answer: A

Explanation: Pacemaker failure has three causes: lead failure, generator failure, or failure of capture. Failure of capture occurs when a pacing stimulus is generated but fails to trigger myocardial depolarization. On the electrocardiogram, failure of capture is identified by the presence of pacing spikes without associated myocardial depolarization. Its causes include elevated myocardial pacing thresholds associated with hyperkalemia, alkalosis, acidosis, myocardial ischemia, and/or abnormal levels of antiarrhythmic drugs. Sympathomimetic drugs generally lower the myocardial pacing threshold.

References:

1. Rozner MA. Chapter 5, Cardiac Implantable Electrical Devices. In: Kaplan JA, Augoustides JGT, Manecke GR, et al., eds. Kaplan's Cardiac Anesthesia. 7th ed. Elsevier; 2017:118-139.
2. Chua J, Schwarzenberger J, Mahajan A. Optimization of pacing after cardiopulmonary bypass. J Cardiothorac Vasc Anesth, 2012; 26: 291-301.

25. During cardiac surgery temporary epicardial pacing leads are placed and are connected to a temporary pacemaker. R-on-T pacing leading to malignant ventricular arrhythmias is LEAST likely to occur with which of the following?
   A. Asynchronous ventricular pacing
   B. Demand atrial pacing
   C. DDD pacing without an atrial lead
   D. Pacemaker loss of sensing (i.e., undersensing)

Correct Answer: B

Explanation: R-on-T pacing occurs when a pacing stimulus occurs in the vulnerable period (on the T wave), which can potentially induce malignant ventricular arrhythmias such as polymorphic ventricular tachycardia and ventricular fibrillation. Although actual reports are rare, R-on-T pacing can occur in several perioperative scenarios and with temporary epicardial pacing. Most cases occur with asynchronous ventricular pacing, since the pacemaker is not programed to sense intrinsic cardiac activity and thus delivers electrical stimuli at a selected rate regardless of the underlying native conduction.

It can also occur with demand ventricular pacing if undersensing occurs. Because of the undersensing, electrical stimuli may be delivered regardless of the underlying native conduction, similarly to asynchronous ventricular pacing. Undersensing is identified by the characteristic presence of inappropriate pacing spikes on monitors. Importantly, after cardiac surgery, epicardial pacing wires usually fail to sense and capture after a few days. Furthermore, in the acute postoperative period there is a potential proarrhythmic biochemical and metabolic milieu that can predispose patients to arrhythmias. Because of these factors, some experts suggest avoiding backup pacing modes and turning off the temporary pacemaker when pacing support is no longer required after cardiac surgery.

In addition, when DDD pacing mode is enabled without an atrial lead, some generators cannot detect the lack of an atrial lead. Because of this, it will issue an atrial pacing stimulus when deemed appropriate, and during this atrial pacing the generator cannot simultaneously sense on the ventricular lead (known as postatrial ventricular blanking), which leads to undersensing and its risks.

References:
1. Rozner MA. Chapter 5, Cardiac Implantable Electrical Devices. In: Kaplan JA, Augoustides JGT, Manecke GR, et al., eds. Kaplan's Cardiac Anesthesia. 7th ed. Elsevier; 2017:118-139.
2. Schulman PM, Merkel MJ, Rozner MA. Accidental, unintentional reprogramming of a temporary external pacemaker leading to R-on-T and cardiac arrest. J Cardiothorac Vasc Anesth, 2013; 27: 944-948.
3. Chemello D, Subramanian A, Kumaraswamy N. Cardiac arrest caused by undersensing of a temporary epicardial pacemaker. Can J Cardiol, 2010; 26: e13-e14.

26. Prior to separation from cardiopulmonary bypass, only ventricular temporary epicardial pacing wires are placed. Which temporary pacing mode could result in postatrial ventricular blanking?
   A. VVI
   B. DDD
   C. AAI
   D. AOO

Correct Answer: B

Explanation: When DDD pacing mode is enabled without an atrial lead, some generators cannot detect the lack of an atrial lead. Because of this, the generator will issue an atrial pacing stimulus when deemed appropriate, and during this atrial pacing the generator cannot simultaneously sense on the ventricular lead (known as postatrial ventricular blanking), which leads to undersensing. As a result, any spontaneous ventricular event taking place in proximity (within 20–60 msec) of the atrial pacing will not be sensed; thus, ventricular pacing will be delivered approximately 200 msec later, creating an R-on-T pace that can induce malignant ventricular arrhythmias.

References:
1. Rozner MA. Chapter 5, Cardiac Implantable Electrical Devices. In: Kaplan JA, Augoustides JGT, Manecke GR, et al., eds. Kaplan's Cardiac Anesthesia. 7th ed. Elsevier; 2017:118-139.
2. Schulman PM, Merkel MJ, Rozner MA. Accidental, unintentional reprogramming of a temporary external pacemaker leading to R-on-T and cardiac arrest. J Cardiothorac Vasc Anesth, 2013; 27: 944-948.

27. Which of the following scenarios is LEAST likely to develop an indication for perioperative temporary cardiac pacing?
   A. Bifascicular block on preoperative electrocardiogram prior to planned noncardiac surgery
   B. Noncardiac surgery with the development of symptomatic bradycardia refractory to medical treatment
   C. Separation from cardiopulmonary bypass following orthotopic heart transplantation
   D. Cardiac surgery for aortic valve endocarditis

Correct Answer: A

Explanation: Symptomatic bradycardia refractory to medical treatment is an indication of temporary cardiac pacing. Heart transplantation may be associated with sinus node injury and dysfunction that usually recovers over time. Aortic valve bacterial endocarditis, especially with abscess, may damage the His-Purkinje system, causing atrioventricular block, which may or may not improve following antimicrobial and surgical treatment. The natural progression of asymptomatic bifascicular block to complete heart block (CHB) in patients occurs with a frequency of approximately 1% per year, and the risk of developing CHB in this population under general anesthesia has not been shown to be increased; thus, preoperative permanent pacemaker placement is not recommended. Preoperative electrocardiogram demonstrating bifascicular block in an asymptomatic patient is not reason enough for temporary pacing prior to surgery, given the low risk of progression to complete heart block in patients undergoing general anesthesia. In this setting, consideration can be made for decreasing vagal tone perioperatively with the administration of an anticholinergic such as glycopyrrolate.

References:

1. Rozner MA. Chapter 5, Cardiac Implantable Electrical Devices. In: Kaplan JA, Augoustides JGT, Manecke GR, et al., eds. Kaplan's Cardiac Anesthesia. 7th ed. Elsevier; 2017:118-139.
2. Morozowich ST, Saslow SB. Progression of asymptomatic bifascicular block to complete heart block during upper gastrointestinal endoscopy with propofol sedation. Can J Anaesth, 2009; 56: 83-84.

28. When a transvenous implantable cardioverter-defibrillator (ICD) device detects a sufficient number of short cardiac R-R intervals indicating either ventricular tachycardia (VT) or ventricular fibrillation (VF), which of the following typically occurs next?
  A. Asynchronous pacing
  B. Antibradycardia pacing
  C. The ICD internal computer will reconfirm VT or VF prior to delivering antitachycardia pacing or shock therapy
  D. No therapy is indicated

Correct Answer: C

Explanation: When a transvenous implantable cardioverter-defibrillator (ICD) detects a sufficient number of short cardiac R-R intervals suggesting a ventricular tachyarrhythmia, it will begin an antitachycardia event. Although some ICDs will deliver immediate antitachycardia pacing while charging in preparation for a shock, most are programmed to reconfirm ventricular tachycardia or ventricular fibrillation after charging, to prevent inappropriate shock therapy.

Therapy with overdrive pacing refers to the delivery of short bursts (e.g., eight beats) of rapid ventricular pacing to terminate ventricular tachycardia by pacing the ventricle faster than the tachycardia, which is intended to enter the reentrant circuit, thus leaving it refractory and terminating the arrhythmia. This approach uses less energy than shock therapy and is better tolerated by the patient.

An ICD with antibradycardia pacing capability will begin pacing when the R-R interval is too long. Asynchronous pacing is not typically indicated in this setting, as it is ineffective and can trigger further ventricular arrhythmias.

References:

1. Rozner MA. Chapter 5, Cardiac Implantable Electrical Devices. In: Kaplan JA, Augoustides JGT, Manecke GR, et al., eds. Kaplan's Cardiac Anesthesia. 7th ed. Elsevier; 2017:118-139.
2. Wathen MS, Sweeney MO, DeGroot PJ, et al. Shock reduction using antitachycardia pacing for spontaneous rapid ventricular tachycardia in patients with coronary artery disease. Circulation, 2001; 104: 796-801.

29. Which of the following represents inappropriate shock therapy with an implantable cardioverter-defibrillator?
  A. Defibrillation for ventricular tachycardia (VT)
  B. Defibrillation for supraventricular tachycardia
  C. Defibrillation for ventricular fibrillation
  D. Cardioversion for VT

Correct Answer: B

Explanation: Avoiding inappropriate shock therapy (IST) is important, as elevated troponin levels in the absence of an ischemic event can occur as a result, and even death has been reported. It is recognized that IST may occur in the setting of supraventricular arrhythmias such as atrial flutter and/or atrial fibrillation with rapid ventricular response. Cardioversion is a shock that is synchronized and delivered to organized rhythm at the peak of the R wave. Defibrillation is an unsynchronized shock delivered randomly during the cardiac cycle. Since ventricular tachycardia is typically an organized electrical rhythm, cardioversion prevents shock delivery during the vulnerable period, which may result in further degeneration to ventricular fibrillation. Since ventricular fibrillation is not an organized rhythm, defibrillation is performed. However, defibrillation may also be performed if ventricular tachycardia is rapid and difficult to synchronize (typically resulting in hemodynamic instability as well).

References:

1. Rozner MA. Chapter 5, Cardiac Implantable Electrical Devices. In: Kaplan JA, Augoustides JGT, Manecke GR, et al., eds. Kaplan's Cardiac Anesthesia. 7th ed. Elsevier; 2017:118-139.
2. Wathen MS, Sweeney MO, DeGroot PJ, et al. Shock reduction using antitachycardia pacing for spontaneous rapid ventricular tachycardia in patients with coronary artery disease. Circulation, 2001; 104: 796-801.

30. Which of the of the following conditions is NOT an accepted indication for implantable cardioverter-defibrillator placement for primary prevention of sudden cardiac death due to life-threatening ventricular tachycardia or ventricular fibrillation?
  A. Nonischemic cardiomyopathy with heart failure and left ventricular ejection fraction >35%
  B. Hypertrophic cardiomyopathy
  C. Congenital long QT syndrome
  D. Arrhythmogenic right ventricular cardiomyopathy

Correct Answer: A

Explanation: Implantable cardioverter-defibrillators (ICDs) are indicated for primary prevention in select patients who are deemed to be at high risk for life-threatening ventricular tachyarrhythmias. These conditions include congenital long QT syndrome with recurrent symptoms, hypertrophic cardiomyopathy, and arrhythmogenic right ventricular cardiomyopathy. In addition, several trials have included patients with nonischemic cardiomyopathy and heart failure, demonstrating that ICD placement will lower mortality in those with a left ventricular ejection fraction below 35%.

References:

1. Rozner MA. Chapter 5, Cardiac Implantable Electrical Devices. In: Kaplan JA, Augoustides JGT, Manecke GR, et al., eds. Kaplan's Cardiac Anesthesia. 7th ed. Elsevier; 2017:118-139.

2. Al-Khatib SM, Stevenson WG, Ackerman MJ, et al. 2017 AHA/ACC/HRS Guideline for management of patients with ventricular arrhythmias and the prevention of sudden cardiac death: a report of the American College of Cardiology/American Heart Association Task Force on Clinical Practice Guidelines and the Heart Rhythm Society. J Am Coll Cardiol, 2018; 72: e91-e220.

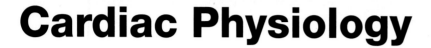

SECTION TWO Cardiovascular Physiology and Pharmacology

CHAPTER 6

Cardiac Physiology

Patrick Hussey and Matthew M. Townsley

KEY POINTS

1. The cartilaginous skeleton, myocardial fiber orientation, valves, blood supply, and conduction system of the heart determine its mechanical capabilities and limitations.

2. The cardiac myocyte is engineered for contraction and relaxation, not protein synthesis.

3. Laplace's law describes the transformation of alterations in muscle tension and length observed during contraction and relaxation in vitro into phasic changes in pressure and volume that occur in the intact heart.

4. The cardiac cycle is a highly coordinated, temporally related series of electrical, mechanical, and valvular events.

5. A time-dependent, two-dimensional projection of continuous pressure and volume during the cardiac cycle creates a phase space diagram that is useful for the analysis of systolic and diastolic function of each cardiac chamber in vivo.

6. Each cardiac chamber is constrained to operate within its end-systolic and end-diastolic pressure-volume relationships when contractile state and compliance are constant.

7. Heart rate, preload, afterload, and myocardial contractility are the main determinants of pump performance.

8. Preload is the quantity of blood that a cardiac chamber contains immediately before contraction begins, and afterload is the external resistance to emptying with which the chamber is confronted after the onset of contraction.

9. Myocardial contractility is quantified using indices derived from pressure-volume relationships, isovolumic contraction, the ejection phase, or power analysis, but these indices have significant limitations because the contractile state and loading conditions are interrelated.

10. Pressure-volume diagrams are useful for describing the mechanical efficiency of energy transfer between elastic chambers, such as the left ventricle and the proximal arterial vasculature.

11. Diastolic function is the ability of a cardiac chamber to effectively collect blood at a normal filling pressure.

12. Left ventricular diastole is a complicated sequence of temporally related, heterogeneous events; no single index of diastolic function completely describes this period of the cardiac cycle.

13. Left ventricular diastolic dysfunction is a primary cause of heart failure in as many as 50% of patients.

14. The left ventricular pressure-volume framework allows the invasive analysis of diastolic function during isovolumic relaxation, early filling, and atrial systole.

15. Transmitral and pulmonary venous blood flow velocities, tissue Doppler imaging, and color M-mode propagation velocity are used to noninvasively quantify the severity of diastolic function.

16. The pericardium exerts important restraining forces on chamber filling and is a major determinant of ventricular interdependence.

17. The atria serve three major mechanical roles, as conduits, reservoirs, and contractile chambers.

1. What provides the skeletal foundation of the heart?
   A. An interstitial collagen fiber network composed of thick type I collagen cross-linked with thin type III collagen
   B. The valve annuli, the aortic and pulmonary roots, the central fibrous body, and the right and left trigone
   C. Atrial and ventricular myocardium
   D. Orthogonally oriented layers of myocardium

Correct Answer: B

Explanation: The valve annuli, the aortic and pulmonary roots, the central fibrous body, and the right and left trigone provide the structural foundation of the heart. These are strong, flexible cartilaginous structures at the base of the heart that allow for support of the cardiac valves, resist the forces of pressure and blood flow, and allow for insertion of superficial subepicardial muscle. Thick type I and thin type III collagen allow for structural support of the atrial and ventricular myocardium, which consists of three layers: interdigitating deep sinospiral muscle, superficial sinospiral muscle, and superficial bulbospiral muscle. The right and left atrium are made of orthogonally oriented layers of myocardium.

References:

1. Pagel P, Freed J. Chapter 6: Cardiac Physiology. In: Kaplan JA, Augoustides JGT, Manecke GR, et al., eds. Kaplan's Cardiac Anesthesia. 7th ed. Elsevier; 2017: 143-178.
2. Khamooshian A, Amador Y, Hai T, et al. Dynamic three-dimensional geometry of the aortic valve apparatus – a feasibility study. J Cardiothorac Vasc Anesth, 2017; 31: 1290-1300.

2. Left ventricular fiber architecture resembles:
   A. Sphere
   B. Perpendicular interwoven streets
   C. Lattice system
   D. Infinity symbol

Correct Answer: D

Explanation: The left ventricular fiber architecture consists of subendocardial and subepicardial interdigitating perpendicular, oblique, and helical muscle running from base to apex in a flattened figure eight pattern. This reverses direction approximately at the left ventricular midpoint. Midmyocardial fibers are circumferentially oriented. A spherical configuration change contributes to reduced systolic function during heart failure. The elastic recoil of the systolic motion pattern is critical for diastolic suction.

References:

1. Pagel P, Freed J. Chapter 6: Cardiac Physiology. In: Kaplan JA, Augoustides JGT, Manecke GR, et al., eds. Kaplan's Cardiac Anesthesia. 7th ed. Elsevier; 2017: 143-178.
2. Buckberg GD, Coghlan HC, Torrent-Guasp F. The structure and function of the helical heart and its buttress wrapping. VI. Geometric concepts of heart failure and use for structural correction. Semin Thorac Cardiovasc Surg, 2001; 13: 386-401.

3. Where is the thickest portion of the left ventricular (LV) wall?
   A. Base
   B. Mid-LV wall
   C. Apex
   D. Consistent thickness throughout

Correct Answer: A

Explanation: There is a decrease in left ventricular mid-myocardial fibers from the base to the apex, causing a progressive decline in thickness from the base to apex of the left ventricle. The apical free wall only consists of subendocardial and subepicardial fibers, and the apical interventricular septum only consists of subendocardial fibers. Right ventricular subendocardial fibers contribute to the interventricular septum. Given this muscle distribution, the basal interventricular septum is commonly ablated or excised in hypertrophic obstructive cardiomyopathy.

References:

1. Pagel P, Freed J. Chapter 6: Cardiac Physiology. In: Kaplan JA, Augoustides JGT, Manecke GR, et al., eds. Kaplan's Cardiac Anesthesia. 7th ed. Elsevier; 2017: 143-178.
2. Addis DA, Townsley MM. Perioperative implications of the 2020 American Heart Association/American College of Cardiology Guidelines for the diagnosis and treatment of patients with hypertrophic cardiomyopathy: a focused review. J Cardiothorac Vasc Anesth, 2022; 36: 2143-2153.

4. What is true about the sinuses of Valsalva?
   A. They promote formation of eddy currents
   B. They provide structural support to the aortic valve
   C. They are also present in the pulmonary artery
   D. They are not named according to the related aortic valve leaflet

Correct Answer: A

Explanation: Sinuses of Valsalva facilitate the formation of eddy currents, preventing the aortic valve leaflets from occluding their respective coronary ostia. These eddy currents also facilitate aortic valve closure during diastole. As there are no ostia adjacent to the pulmonary valve, sinuses of Valsalva are not present in the pulmonary artery. The aortic valve leaflets are named according to coronary ostium and are supported by the aortic annulus. The sinuses of Valsalva are named according to the corresponding aortic valve leaflet, and so typically there are a right, left, and noncoronary sinus of Valsalva.

References:

1. Pagel P, Freed J. Chapter 6: Cardiac Physiology. In: Kaplan JA, Augoustides JGT, Manecke GR, et al., eds. Kaplan's Cardiac Anesthesia. 7th ed. Elsevier; 2017: 143-178.
2. Shimizu H, Yozu R. Valve-sparing aortic root replacement. Ann Thorac Cardiovasc Surg, 2011; 17: 330-336.

5. Tertiary chordae tendineae:
   A. Insert into the mitral valve edge
   B. Insert into the mitral valve smooth zone
   C. Insert into the mitral valve rough zone
   D. Only arise from the posteromedial papillary muscle

Correct Answer: D

Explanation: Tertiary chordae tendineae only arise from the posteromedial papillary muscle and attach to the posterior mitral valve leaflet near the annulus or adjacent myocardium. Primary chordae tendineae attach to the mitral valve edge. Secondary chordae tendineae attach to both the mitral valve smooth and rough zone.

References:

1. Pagel P, Freed J. Chapter 6: Cardiac Physiology. In: Kaplan JA, Augoustides JGT, Manecke GR, et al., eds. Kaplan's Cardiac Anesthesia. 7th ed. Elsevier; 2017: 143-178.
2. Kampaktsis PN, Lebehn M, Wu IY. Mitral regurgitation in 2020: the 2020 focused update of the 2017 American College of Cardiology expert consensus decision pathway on the management of mitral regurgitation. J Cardiothorac Vasc Anesth, 2021; 35: 1678-1690.

6. Differences between the right ventricle (RV) and left ventricle (LV) include:
   A. RV has fine trabecular muscle
   B. The tricuspid valve has a well-defined collagenous annulus
   C. Presence of an anterior papillary muscle can differentiate the RV from the LV
   D. The atrioventricular groove between right atrium and RV contains the proximal right coronary artery

Correct Answer: D

Explanation: The proximal portion of the right coronary artery runs through the atrioventricular groove between right atrium and right ventricle (RV). The RV has coarse trabecular muscle, unlike the fine trabecular muscle of the left ventricle, which contributes to septal papillary muscle found only in the RV. The mitral valve has a well-defined collagenous annulus.

References:

1. Pagel P, Freed J. Chapter 6: Cardiac Physiology. In: Kaplan JA, Augoustides JGT, Manecke GR, et al., eds. Kaplan's Cardiac Anesthesia. 7th ed. Elsevier; 2017: 143-178.
2. Ho SY, Nihoyannopoulos P. Anatomy, echocardiography, and normal right ventricular dimensions. Heart, 2006; 92 Suppl 1: i2-i13.

7. The right coronary artery:
   A. Supplies the posterior left ventricular wall and posterior third of the interventricular septum
   B. Is solely responsible for perfusion of the right ventricle
   C. Is solely responsible for perfusion of the sinoatrial and atrioventricular node
   D. Supplies the posterior descending artery in 20% of patients

Correct Answer: A

Explanation: The right coronary artery supplies the posterior left ventricular wall and posterior third of the interventricular septum. It supplies the posterior descending artery in 80% of patients, labeling the majority as "right-dominant." The left anterior descending coronary artery contributes to right ventricle free wall perfusion. The left circumflex coronary artery supplies the sinoatrial node in 45% of patients and the atrioventricular node less commonly.

References:

1. Pagel P, Freed J. Chapter 6: Cardiac Physiology. In: Kaplan JA, Augoustides JGT, Manecke GR, et al., eds. Kaplan's Cardiac Anesthesia. 7th ed. Elsevier; 2017: 143-178.
2. Vanneman MW. Anesthetic considerations for percutaneous coronary intervention for chronic total occlusions – a narrative review. J Cardiothorac Vasc Anesth, 2022; 36: 2132-2142.

8. What is the order of the fastest to slowest elements of the conduction system of the heart?
   A. Sinoatrial node, atrial myocardium, atrioventricular node, bundle of His, Purkinje fibers, ventricular myocardium
   B. Purkinje fibers, bundle of His, atrial myocardium, ventricular myocardium, atrioventricular node, sinoatrial node
   C. Bundle of His, Purkinje fibers, atrial myocardium, ventricular myocardium, atrioventricular node, sinoatrial node
   D. Bundle of His, Purkinje fibers, atrioventricular node, sinoatrial node, atrial myocardium, ventricular myocardium

Correct Answer: B

Explanation: Conduction through Purkinje fibers and the bundle of His can reach up to 4 m/s. Conduction at the sinoatrial node is the slowest at less than 0.01 m/s. The correct pathway of conduction begins at the sinoatrial node, then atrial myocardium, atrioventricular node, bundle of His, and Purkinje fibers, and terminates through the ventricular myocardium. Table 6.1 provides specific details pertaining to the cardiac electrical activation sequence.

References:

1. Pagel P, Freed J. Chapter 6: Cardiac Physiology. In: Kaplan JA, Augoustides JGT, Manecke GR, et al., eds. Kaplan's Cardiac Anesthesia. 7th ed. Elsevier; 2017: 143-178.
2. Neuburger PJ, Pospishil L, Ibrahim H. Anesthetic management of conduction disturbances following transcatheter aortic valve replacement: a review of the 2020 ACC expert consensus decision pathway. J Cardiothorac Vasc Anesth, 2021; 35: 982-986.

TABLE 6.1

Cardiac Electrical Activation Sequence

Structure	Conduction Velocity (ms)
SA node	<0.01
Atrial myocardium	1.0–1.2
AV node	0.02–0.05
Bundle branches	2.0–4.0
Purkinje network	2.0–4.0
Ventricular myocardium	0.3–1.0

AV, Atrioventricular; *SA*, sinoatrial.
From Katz AM, ed. Physiology of the Heart. 3rd ed. Lippincott Williams & Wilkins; 2001.

9. What is the function of the sarcoplasmic reticulum of each cardiac myocyte?
   A. To store Ca^{2+}
   B. To transport Ca^{2+}
   C. To house ryanodine receptors
   D. To generate protein synthesis

Correct Answer: A

Explanation: The sarcoplasmic reticulum of a cardiac myocyte stores Ca^{2+} until ryanodine receptors in adjacent cisternae allow for gated passage through the cisternae for transportation of Ca^{2+}. The contractile unit and mitochondria of a cardiac myocyte make up 80% of its total volume. Contraction, not protein synthesis, is the primary purpose of the cardiac myocyte.

References:

1. Pagel P, Freed J. Chapter 6: Cardiac Physiology. In: Kaplan JA, Augoustides JGT, Manecke GR, et al., eds. Kaplan's Cardiac Anesthesia. 7th ed. Elsevier; 2017: 143-178.
2. Ren X, Hensley N, Brady MB, et al. The genetic and molecular basis for hypertrophic cardiomyopathy: the role for calcium sensitization. J Cardiothorac Vasc Anesth, 2018; 32: 478-487.

10. How does Ca^{2+} facilitate cardiomyocyte contraction?
   A. Ca^{2+} binds to tropomyosin, changing its structure to allow for actin and myosin binding and subsequent contraction
   B. L-type and T-type Ca^{2+} channels allow for influx of Ca^{2+} in the extracellular space, where actin undergoes receptor-mediated absorption to bind and contract with myosin
   C. Ca^{2+} binds to troponin C, changing the structure of tropomyosin to allow for actin and myosin binding and subsequent contraction
   D. A Ca^{2+}-ATPase and a Na^+/Ca^{2+} exchanger increases Ca^{2+} concentration in the extracellular space, allowing for actin and myosin binding and subsequent contraction

Correct Answer: C

Explanation: Ca^{2+} binds to troponin C, changing the structure of tropomyosin to allow for actin and myosin binding and subsequent contraction. L-type and T-type Ca^{2+} channels do facilitate increased Ca^{2+} concentration, but through troponin C–mediated tropomyosin structural change. Ca^{2+}-ATPase and a Na^+/Ca^{2+} exchanger decrease Ca^{2+} concentration in the extracellular space after cardiomyocyte contraction.

References:

1. Pagel P, Freed J. Chapter 6: Cardiac Physiology. In: Kaplan JA, Augoustides JGT, Manecke GR, et al., eds. Kaplan's Cardiac Anesthesia. 7th ed. Elsevier; 2017: 143-178.
2. Ren X, Hensley N, Brady MB, et al. The genetic and molecular basis for hypertrophic cardiomyopathy: the role for calcium sensitization. J Cardiothorac Vasc Anesth, 2018; 32: 478-487.

11. Regarding wall stress of the left ventricle (LV):
   A. An increase in LV pressure will cause a decrease in wall stress
   B. An increase in LV thickness will cause an increase in wall stress
   C. An increase in LV radius will cause a decrease in wall stress
   D. The constant in the wall stress equation is $\frac{1}{2}$

Correct Answer: D

Explanation: Wall stress, or the law of Laplace, is defined: $\sigma = Pr/2h$, where σ = wall stress, P = pressure, r = radius, and h = wall thickness. There are three considerations regarding the law of Laplace: (1) the chamber is spherical with a uniform wall thickness (h) and internal radius (r); (2) the wall stress (σ) throughout the thickness of the chamber wall is constant; and (3) the chamber must be in static equilibrium (not contracting). Regardless of these limitations, the law of Laplace can be used to predict which patients will have greater myocardial oxygen consumption and could be more susceptible to acute myocardial ischemia.

References:

1. Pagel P, Freed J. Chapter 6: Cardiac Physiology. In: Kaplan JA, Augoustides JGT, Manecke GR, et al., eds. Kaplan's Cardiac Anesthesia. 7th ed. Elsevier; 2017: 143-178.
2. Gilbert JC, Glantz SA. Determinants of left ventricular filling and of the diastolic pressure-volume relation. Circ Res, 1989; 64: 827-852.

12. Which phase of the cardiac cycle is most likely to be eliminated during sinus tachycardia?
   A. Early left ventricular filling
   B. Diastasis
   C. Atrial systole
   D. No phases will be eliminated

Correct Answer: B

Explanation: Diastasis contributes 5% of left ventricular end-diastolic volume and is the period where pulmonary venous blood traverses the left atrium into the left ventricle after early filling has completed. Early ventricular filling often contributes 70% to 75% of left ventricular end-diastolic volume, and atrial systole contributes 15% to 25%.

References:

1. Pagel P, Freed J. Chapter 6: Cardiac Physiology. In: Kaplan JA, Augoustides JGT, Manecke GR, et al., eds. Kaplan's Cardiac Anesthesia. 7th ed. Elsevier; 2017: 143-178.
2. Bombardini T, Sicari R, Blanchini E, et al. Abnormal shortened diastolic time length at increasing heart rates in patients with abnormal exercise-induced increase in pulmonary artery pressure. Cardiovasc Ultrasound, 2011; 9: 36.

13. Regarding the left ventricular pressure-volume loop, in what scenario would the left ventricle have increased end-systolic volume?
   A. Increased preload
   B. Increased afterload
   C. Increased contractility
   D. Decreased compliance

Correct Answer: B

Explanation: Although increased preload would increase end-diastolic volume, left ventricular end-systolic volume would remain the same. Decreased, not increased, contractility would increase left ventricular end-systolic volume. Decreased compliance would increase end-diastolic pressure and, subsequently, could affect left ventricular end-diastolic volume. However, it should not affect left ventricular end-systolic volume.

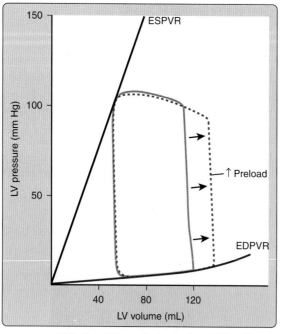

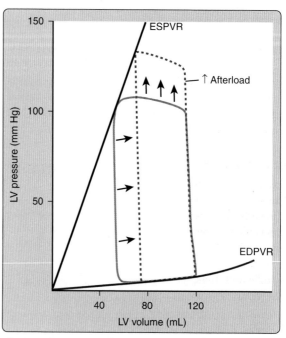

FIG. 6.1 Schematic illustrations of the alterations in the steady-state LV pressure-volume diagram produced by a pure theoretical increase in LV preload *(left)* or afterload *(right)*. Additional preload directly increases stroke volume (SV) and LV end-diastolic pressure, whereas an acute increase in afterload produces greater LV pressure but reduces SV. *EDPVR,* End-diastolic pressure-volume relationship; *ESPVR,* end-systolic pressure-volume relationship; *LV,* left ventricular.

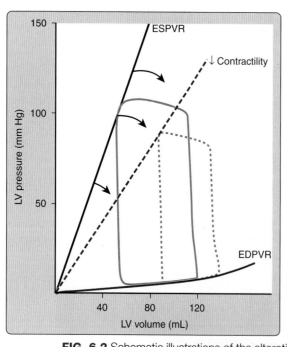

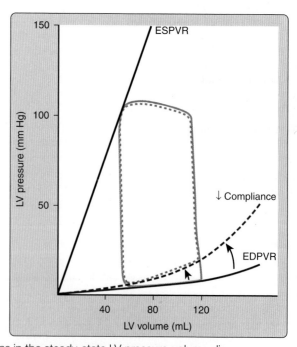

FIG. 6.2 Schematic illustrations of the alterations in the steady-state LV pressure-volume diagram produced by a reduction in myocardial contractility, as indicated by a decrease in the slope of the ESPVR *(left)* and a decrease in LV compliance as indicated by an increase in the position of the EDPVR *(right).* The diagrams emphasize that heart failure may result from LV systolic or diastolic dysfunction independently. *EDPVR,* End-diastolic pressure-volume relationship; *ESPVR,* end-systolic pressure-volume relationship; *LV,* left ventricular.

References:

1. Pagel P, Freed J. Chapter 6: Cardiac Physiology. In: Kaplan JA, Augoustides JGT, Manecke GR, et al., eds. Kaplan's Cardiac Anesthesia. 7th ed. Elsevier; 2017: 143-178.
2. Silbiger JJ. Pathophysiology and echocardiographic diagnosis of left ventricular diastolic dysfunction. J Am Soc Echocardiogr, 2019; 32: 216-232.

14. Heart failure with preserved ejection fraction is characterized by:
    A. Eccentric hypertrophy
    B. Parallel replication of sarcomeres
    C. Left ventricular wall dilation
    D. Increase in end-diastolic volume

Correct Answer: **B**

Explanation: Heart failure with preserved ejection fraction begins due to an increase in ventricular pressure, leading to an increase in end-systolic wall stress, parallel replication of sarcomeres, thickening of the ventricular wall, and concentric hypertrophy. Heart failure with reduced ejection fraction begins due to an increase in ventricular volume leading to an increase in end-systolic wall stress, series replication of sarcomeres, dilation of the ventricular wall, and eccentric hypertrophy.

References:

1. Pagel P, Freed J. Chapter 6: Cardiac Physiology. In: Kaplan JA, Augoustides JGT, Manecke GR, et al., eds. Kaplan's Cardiac Anesthesia. 7th ed. Elsevier; 2017: 143-178.
2. Mohananey D, Heidari-Bateni G, Villablanca PA, et al. Heart failure with preserved ejection fraction-a systematic review and analysis of perioperative outcomes. J Cardiothorac Vasc Anesth, 2018; 32: 2423-2434.

15. Which of the following is not an important component of diastolic function?
    a. Mitral valve integrity
    b. Ventricular compliance
    c. Left atrial function
    d. Ventricular contractility

Correct Answer: **A**

Explanation: Mitral valve integrity, along with pulmonary vein blood flow, left atrial function and relaxation, and ventricular compliance, are all components of left ventricular diastolic function. These components make up the "preload" component of systolic function. Systolic function also consists of afterload (related to arterial mechanics) and contractility to generate cardiac output.

References:

1. Pagel P, Freed J. Chapter 6: Cardiac Physiology. In: Kaplan JA, Augoustides JGT, Manecke GR, et al., eds. Kaplan's Cardiac Anesthesia. 7th ed. Elsevier; 2017: 143-178.
2. Silbiger JJ. Pathophysiology and echocardiographic diagnosis of left ventricular diastolic dysfunction. J Am Soc Echocardiogr, 2019; 32: 216-232.

16. Which of the following is the most commonly derived index of the global left ventricular contractile state during isovolumic contraction?
    A. End-systolic pressure-volume relation (E_{es})
    B. Maximum rate of increase of left ventricular pressure (dP/dt_{max})
    C. Stroke volume
    D. Maximal left ventricular power (PWR_{max})

Correct Answer: **B**

Explanation: Indices of myocardial contractility may be classified into four broad categories: pressure-volume relationships, isovolemic contraction, ejection phase, and power analysis. The maximum rate of increase of left ventricular pressure (dP/dt_{max}) is the most commonly derived index of the global contractile state during isovolumic contraction. The end-systolic pressure-volume relation (E_{es}) represents the slope of the end-systolic pressure-volume relationship and is therefore an index derived from pressure-volume analysis. Stroke volume and maximal left ventricular power (PWR_{max}) are categorized as indices of the ejection phase and ventricular power, respectively.

References:

1. Pagel P, Freed J. Chapter 6: Cardiac Physiology. In: Kaplan JA, Augoustides JGT, Manecke GR, et al., eds. Kaplan's Cardiac Anesthesia. 7th ed. Elsevier; 2017: 143-178.
2. Mor-Avi V, Lang RM, Badano LP, et al. Current and evolving echocardiographic techniques for the quantitative evaluation of cardiac mechanics: ASE/EAE consensus statement on methodology and indications endorsed by the Japanese Society of Echocardiography. J Am Soc Echocardiograph, 2011; 24: 277-313.

17. Which of the following indices of left ventricular contractility is derived from analysis of pressure-volume relationships?
    A. Stroke work-end-diastolic volume relation (M_{SW})
    B. Ejection fraction
    C. Velocity of shortening
    D. Maximum rate of increase of left ventricular pressure (dP/dt_{max})

Correct Answer: **A**

Explanation: Common indices of left ventricular (LV) contractility are grouped into four broad categories, as follows:

1. **Pressure-Volume Analysis**
   End-systolic pressure-volume relation (E_{es})
   Stroke work-end-diastolic volume relation (M_{SW})
2. **Isovolumic Contraction**
   Maximum rate of increase of LV pressure (dP/dt_{max})
   dP/dt_{max} measured at 50 mm Hg ($dP/dt_{max}/50$)
   Ratio of dP/dt_{max} to peak developed LV pressure ($dP/dt_{max}/P$)
   dP/dt_{max}-end-diastolic volume relation (dE/dt_{max})
3. **Ejection Phase**
   Stroke volume
   Cardiac output
   Ejection fraction

Fractional area change

Fractional shortening

Wall thickening

Velocity of shortening

4. Ventricular Power

Maximal LV power (PWR_{max})

Ratio of LV PWR_{max} to the square of end-diastolic volume (PWR_{max}/EDV^2)

References:

1. Pagel P, Freed J. Chapter 6: Cardiac Physiology. In: Kaplan JA, Augoustides JGT, Manecke GR, et al., eds. Kaplan's Cardiac Anesthesia. 7th ed. Elsevier; 2017: 143-178.
2. Mor-Avi V, Lang RM, Badano LP, et al. Current and evolving echocardiographic techniques for the quantitative evaluation of cardiac mechanics: ASE/EAE consensus statement on methodology and indications endorsed by the Japanese Society of Echocardiography. J Am Soc Echocardiograph, 2011; 24: 277-313.

18. In left ventricular systolic heart failure, which of the following patterns of cardiac remodeling would be expected?

A. Decreased end-diastolic volume, decreased end-systolic volume

B. Decreased end-diastolic volume, increased end-systolic volume

C. Increased end-diastolic volume, increased end-systolic volume

D. Increased end-diastolic volume, decreased end-systolic volume

Correct Answer: C

Explanation: Cardiac remodeling in left ventricular (LV) systolic and diastolic heart failure occurs as follows:

	LEFT VENTRICULAR SYSTOLIC HEART FAILURE	LEFT VENTRICULAR DIASTOLIC HEART FAILURE
End-diastolic volume	Increased	Normal
End-systolic volume	Increased	Normal
Left ventricular mass	Increased	Increased
Geometry	Eccentric	Concentric
Cardiac myocyte	Increased length	Increased diameter
Extracellular matrix	Decreased collagen	Increased collagen

References:

1. Pagel P, Freed J. Chapter 6: Cardiac Physiology. In: Kaplan JA, Augoustides JGT, Manecke GR, et al., eds. Kaplan's Cardiac Anesthesia. 7th ed. Elsevier; 2017: 143-178.
2. Mor-Avi V, Lang RM, Badano LP, et al. Current and evolving echocardiographic techniques for the quantitative evaluation of cardiac mechanics: ASE/EAE consensus statement on methodology and indications endorsed by the Japanese Society of Echocardiography. J Am Soc Echocardiograph, 2011; 24: 277-313.

19. Which of the following is most likely to be observed in a patient with left ventricular (LV) diastolic heart failure?

A. Increased stroke work

B. Decreased slope of the LV end-systolic pressure-volume relationship (E_{es})

C. Decreased maximum rate of increase of LV pressure (dP/dt_{max})

D. Limited preload reserve

Correct Answer: D

Explanation: Expected pathophysiologic changes in left ventricular (LV) systolic function in patients with left ventricular systolic and diastolic heart failure are as follows:

	LEFT VENTRICULAR SYSTOLIC HEART FAILURE	LEFT VENTRICULAR DIASTOLIC HEART FAILURE
Stroke volume	Decreased (or normal)	Normal (or decreased)
Stroke work	Decreased	Normal
M_{sw}	Decreased	Normal
E_{es}	Decreased	Normal (or increased)
Ejection fraction	Decreased	Normal
dP/dt_{max}	Decreased	Normal
Preload reserve	Exhausted	Limited

Abbreviations: M_{sw}, Slope of the LV stroke work-end-diastolic volume relationship; E_{es}, slope of the LV end-systolic pressure-volume relationship; dP/dt_{max}, maximum rate of increase of LV pressure.

References:

1. Pagel P, Freed J. Chapter 6: Cardiac Physiology. In: Kaplan JA, Augoustides JGT, Manecke GR, et al., eds. Kaplan's Cardiac Anesthesia. 7th ed. Elsevier; 2017: 143-178.
2. Silbiger JJ. Pathophysiology and echocardiographic diagnosis of left ventricular diastolic dysfunction. J Am Soc Echocardiogr, 2019; 32: 216-232.

20. Early diastolic subendocardial coronary blood flow is compromised in patients with left ventricular (LV) relaxation delays due to:

A. Increased LV end-diastolic volume

B. Decreased LV end-diastolic pressure

C. Compression of intramyocardial coronary arterioles

D. Coronary artery spasm

Correct Answer: C

Explanation: With delays in left ventricular relaxation, early diastolic subendocardial coronary blood flow is reduced, because failure to complete actin-myosin dissociation and facilitate elastic recoil prolongs the compression of intramyocardial coronary arterioles. Increases in left ventricular end-diastolic volume or decreases in end-diastolic pressure do not compromise early diastolic subendocardial coronary blood flow. Coronary artery spasm would compromise coronary blood flow throughout the cardiac cycle and is not related to left ventricular relaxation delays.

References:

1. Pagel P, Freed J. Chapter 6: Cardiac Physiology. In: Kaplan JA, Augoustides JGT, Manecke GR, et al., eds. Kaplan's Cardiac Anesthesia. 7th ed. Elsevier; 2017: 143-178.
2. Silbiger JJ. Pathophysiology and echocardiographic diagnosis of left ventricular diastolic dysfunction. J Am Soc Echocardiogr, 2019; 32: 216-232.

21. An increase in the ventricular relaxation time constant (τ) would be expected in the following scenario:
   A. Administration of sevoflurane
   B. Sinus tachycardia
   C. Continuous infusion of isoproterenol
   D. Calcium chloride administration

Correct Answer: A

Explanation: The time constant (τ) is used to quantify left ventricular (LV) relaxation. It is calculated from the following equation: $P(t) = P_0 e^{-t/\tau}$, where $P(t)$ represents time-dependent LV pressure, P_0 is LV pressure at end-systole, e is the natural exponent, and t is time (ms) after LV end-systole. Increases in τ, corresponding to delays in LV relaxation, may be seen in myocardial ischemia, pressure-overload hypertrophy, or hypertrophic cardiomyopathy, or due to administration of negative inotropic drugs such as volatile anesthetics. A reduction in τ suggests more rapid LV relaxation, which may occur with tachycardia, sympathetic nervous system stimulation, or administration of positive inotropic drugs.

References:

1. Pagel P, Freed J. Chapter 6: Cardiac Physiology. In: Kaplan JA, Augoustides JGT, Manecke GR, et al., eds. Kaplan's Cardiac Anesthesia. 7th ed. Elsevier; 2017: 143-178.
2. McIlroy DR, Lin E, Durkin C. Intraoperative transesophageal echocardiography: a critical appraisal of its current role in the assessment of diastolic dysfunction. J Cardiothorac Vasc Anesth, 2015; 29: 1033-1043.

22. With regards to noninvasive evaluation of diastolic function, the most commonly used surrogate for invasively derived indices of left ventricular (LV) relaxation is the:
   A. Peak rate of LV pressure decrease (dP/dt$_{min}$)
   B. Time constant (τ)
   C. LV ejection time (ET)
   D. Isovolumic relaxation time (IVRT)

Correct Answer: D

Explanation: The isovolumic relaxation time (IVRT), measured using either M-mode or continuous-wave Doppler echocardiography, is the period between aortic valve closure and mitral valve opening. In the absence of mitral or aortic valve pathology, the major determinants of IVRT are the rate of left ventricular (LV) relaxation and the difference between LV end-systolic pressure and left atrial pressure at the time of mitral valve opening. IVRT is dependent on the loading conditions of the heart. Both dP/dt$_{min}$ and τ are

invasive measures of diastolic function, while ejection time assesses LV systolic, not diastolic, function.

References:

1. Pagel P, Freed J. Chapter 6: Cardiac Physiology. In: Kaplan JA, Augoustides JGT, Manecke GR, et al., eds. Kaplan's Cardiac Anesthesia. 7th ed. Elsevier; 2017: 143-178.
2. McIlroy DR, Lin E, Durkin C. Intraoperative transesophageal echocardiography: a critical appraisal of its current role in the assessment of diastolic dysfunction. J Cardiothorac Vasc Anesth, 2015; 29: 1033-1043.

23. Which of the following diagnostic modalities is most useful for distinguishing between constrictive pericarditis and restrictive cardiomyopathy?
   A. Color M-mode echocardiography
   B. Tissue Doppler imaging
   C. Invasive measurement of the time constant (τ)
   D. Continuous-wave Doppler echocardiography

Correct Answer: B

Explanation: Tissue Doppler imaging of septal or lateral mitral annular motion allows for evaluation regarding the relative severity of left ventricular diastolic dysfunction. This form of imaging utilizes low-velocity (10–15 cm/s) pulsed-wave Doppler. In addition, tissue Doppler imaging may also aid in distinguishing between constrictive pericarditis and restrictive cardiomyopathy. Specifically, tissue Doppler e' velocity is normal in constrictive pericarditis but reduced in restrictive cardiomyopathy.

References:

1. Pagel P, Freed J. Chapter 6: Cardiac Physiology. In: Kaplan JA, Augoustides JGT, Manecke GR, et al., eds. Kaplan's Cardiac Anesthesia. 7th ed. Elsevier; 2017: 143-178.
2. Tuck BC, Townsley MM. Clinical update in pericardial diseases. J Cardiothorac Vasc Anesth, 2019; 33: 184-199.

24. The physiologic effects of cardiac tamponade are determined primarily by:
   A. Amount of fluid contained in the pericardial space
   B. Type of fluid contained in the pericardial space
   C. Rate of accumulation of fluid in the pericardial space
   D. Localized compression of the ventricular chambers

Correct Answer: C

Explanation: The pericardium is significantly less compliant than the myocardium. Therefore, the pericardium possesses very limited volume reserve, so that it may only accommodate a small increase in volume before a large increase in pericardial pressure occurs. The volume of pericardial fluid does not necessarily correlate to the hemodynamic significance of the effusion, as chronic fluid accumulation gradually stretches the pericardium, increasing its compliance and attenuating the degree of pressure transmitted to the cardiac chambers. Small effusions may cause tamponade if fluid accumulation occurs quickly. The type of fluid does not have a large role in determining the physiologic effects of the pericardial effusion. Although the rate of fluid accumulation in the pericardial space is the primary driver of the physiologic effects, a small, rapid accumulation can result in localized compression of cardiac chambers such as the right and left atrium.

References:

1. Pagel P, Freed J. Chapter 6: Cardiac Physiology. In: Kaplan JA, Augoustides JGT, Manecke GR, et al., eds. Kaplan's Cardiac Anesthesia. 7th ed. Elsevier; 2017: 143-178.
2. Tuck BC, Townsley MM. Clinical update in pericardial diseases. J Cardiothorac Vasc Anesth, 2019; 33: 184-189.

25. Normal pericardial pressure is normally:
A. −5 to 0 mmHg
B. 0 to 10 mmHg
C. 10 to 15 mmHg
D. 15 to 20 mmHg

Correct Answer: A

Explanation: Normal pericardial pressure is subatmospheric (−5 to 0 mmHg), producing minimal to no mechanical effects on a normal heart under euvolemic loading conditions. Pericardial pressure does vary with changes in intrathoracic pressure.

References:

1. Pagel P, Freed J. Chapter 6: Cardiac Physiology. In: Kaplan JA, Augoustides JGT, Manecke GR, et al., eds. Kaplan's Cardiac Anesthesia. 7th ed. Elsevier; 2017: 143-178.
2. Tuck BC, Townsley MM. Clinical update in pericardial diseases. J Cardiothorac Vasc Anesth, 2019; 33: 184-189.

26. In a patient with cardiac tamponade, which of the following best explains the presence of dramatic changes in systolic blood pressure during the respiratory cycle?
A. Acute reduction in left ventricular systolic function
B. Acute reduction in right ventricular systolic function
C. Impaired atrial contraction
D. Ventricular interdependence

Correct Answer: D

Explanation: The pericardium plays a critical role in ventricular interdependence, which is defined as the influence of the pressure and volume of one ventricle on the mechanical behavior of the other. Exaggerated ventricular interdependence occurs during cardiac tamponade, as the influence of one ventricle exerts on the other during filling becomes pronounced because of the shared septal wall and restraining forces of the pericardium. The compressive effects of a pericardial effusion on the right-sided cardiac chambers subsequently reduces left ventricular compliance and limits left ventricular filling.

References:

1. Pagel P, Freed J. Chapter 6: Cardiac Physiology. In: Kaplan JA, Augoustides JGT, Manecke GR, et al., eds. Kaplan's Cardiac Anesthesia. 7th ed. Elsevier; 2017: 143-178.

2. Tuck BC, Townsley MM. Clinical update in pericardial diseases. J Cardiothorac Vasc Anesth, 2019; 33: 184-189.

27. Compared to the left ventricle, the left atrium:
A. Is more susceptible to afterload mismatch
B. Experiences a greater degree of myocardial depression by volatile anesthetics
C. Experiences a lesser degree of myocardial depression by volatile anesthetics
D. Is more susceptible to changes in parasympathetic function

Correct Answer: A

Explanation: Similar changes occur in both the left atrium and left ventricle due to alterations in the autonomic nervous system and when exposed to negative inotropic agents, such as volatile anesthetics. However, the left atrium is significantly more susceptible to increases in afterload than the left ventricle. Impaired left ventricular filling can lead to increases in left atrial afterload that may result in left atrial hypertrophy, dilation, and eventual contractile failure.

References:

1. Pagel P, Freed J. Chapter 6: Cardiac Physiology. In: Kaplan JA, Augoustides JGT, Manecke GR, et al., eds. Kaplan's Cardiac Anesthesia. 7th ed. Elsevier; 2017: 143-178.
2. Rong LQ, Menon A, Lopes AJ, et al. Left atrial strain quantification by intraoperative transesophageal echocardiography: validation with transthoracic echocardiography. J Cardiothorac Vasc Anesth, 2022; 36: 2412-2417.

28. A unifying feature found in all forms of heart failure with preserved ejection fraction is:
A. Diastolic dysfunction
B. Renal insufficiency
C. Left ventricular volume overload
D. Restrictive cardiomyopathy

Correct Answer: A

Explanation: As many as 50% of patients with heart failure do not have a significant reduction in left ventricular ejection fraction. Heart failure with preserved ejection fraction (HFpEF) is commonly associated with advanced age (>60 years), female gender, poorly controlled essential hypertension, obesity, renal insufficiency, anemia, general deconditioning, and atrial fibrillation. The unifying feature of all forms of HFpEF, regardless of the underlying cause, is diastolic dysfunction.

References:

1. Pagel P, Freed J. Chapter 6: Cardiac Physiology. In: Kaplan JA, Augoustides JGT, Manecke GR, et al., eds. Kaplan's Cardiac Anesthesia. 7th ed. Elsevier; 2017: 143-178.
2. Pagel PS, Tawil JN, Boettcher BT, et al. Heart failure with preserved ejection fraction: a comprehensive review and update of diagnosis, pathophysiology, treatment, and perioperative implications. J Cardiothorac Vasc Anesth, 2021; 35: 1839-1859.

29. The major limitation of all modalities attempting to quantify systolic function is that they are:

A. Not reproducible

B. Dependent on chamber geometry

C. Load-dependent

D. Unreliable in the setting of diastolic dysfunction

Correct Answer: C

Explanation: Myocardial contractility may be assessed by indices based on pressure-volume relationships, isovolumic contraction, ejection phase, and power analysis. However, all contractile indices are limited by the fact that the contractile state and loading conditions are interrelated.

References:

1. Pagel P, Freed J. Chapter 6: Cardiac Physiology. In: Kaplan JA, Augoustides JGT, Manecke GR, et al., eds. Kaplan's Cardiac Anesthesia. 7th ed. Elsevier; 2017: 143-178.
2. Mor-Avi V, Lang RM, Badano LP, et al. Current and evolving echocardiographic techniques for the quantitative evaluation of cardiac mechanics: ASE/EAE consensus statement on methodology and indications endorsed by the Japanese Society of Echocardiography. J Am Soc Echocardiograph, 2011; 24: 277-313.

30. In the evaluation of transmitral blood flow velocities to assess diastolic dysfunction, a pseudonormal pattern of diastolic dysfunction appears indistinguishable from a normal pattern of transmitral blood flow because of:

A. Increased left atrial pressure

B. Exaggerated interventricular independence

C. Decreased left atrial-left ventricular pressure gradient

D. Increased atrial contraction

Correct Answer: A

Explanation: Pulsed-wave Doppler echocardiographic evaluation of the pattern of transmitral blood flow velocity allows for the noninvasive analysis and grading of diastolic dysfunction. The three major patterns of abnormal left ventricular filling, from least to most severe, are delayed relaxation, pseudonormal, and restrictive. Reduced left ventricular filling and an increased contribution of left atrial systole to overall left ventricular filling characterize the delayed relaxation phase. When diastolic dysfunction worsens to reach the pseudonormal stage, further pathologic increases in left atrial pressure restore the normal left atrial-left ventricular pressure gradient on mitral valve opening. This causes the early filling phase, which appears reduced on transmitral blood flow Doppler analysis in the delayed relaxation phase, to appear normal again (despite the continued presence of impaired left ventricular relaxation). Further deterioration in diastolic function leads to the restrictive pattern with severe left atrial hypertension, a pronounced early filling phase, and a minor contribution from atrial contraction.

References:

1. Pagel P, Freed J. Chapter 6: Cardiac Physiology. In: Kaplan JA, Augoustides JGT, Manecke GR, et al., eds. Kaplan's Cardiac Anesthesia. 7th ed. Elsevier; 2017: 143-178.
2. McIlroy DR, Lin E, Durkin C. Intraoperative transesophageal echocardiography: a critical appraisal of its current role in the assessment of diastolic dysfunction. J Cardiothorac Vasc Anesth, 2015; 29: 1033-1043.

CHAPTER 7

Coronary Physiology and Atherosclerosis

Patrick Hussey and Matthew M. Townsley

KEY POINTS

1. To care for patients with coronary artery disease in the perioperative period safely, the clinician must understand how the coronary circulation functions in health and disease.
2. Coronary endothelium modulates myocardial blood flow by producing factors that relax or contract the underlying vascular smooth muscle.
3. Vascular endothelial cells help maintain the fluidity of blood by elaborating anticoagulant, fibrinolytic, and antiplatelet substances.
4. One of the earliest changes in coronary artery disease, preceding the appearance of stenoses, is the loss of the vasoregulatory and antithrombotic functions of the endothelium.
5. The mean systemic arterial pressure, and not the diastolic pressure, may be the most useful and reliable measure of coronary perfusion pressure in the clinical setting.
6. Although sympathetic activation increases myocardial oxygen demand, activation of α-adrenergic receptors causes coronary vasoconstriction.
7. It is unlikely that one substance alone (e.g., adenosine) provides the link between myocardial metabolism and myocardial blood flow under a variety of conditions.
8. As coronary perfusion pressure decreases, the inner layers of myocardium nearest the left ventricular cavity are the first to become ischemic and display impaired relaxation and contraction.
9. The progression of an atherosclerotic lesion is similar to the process of wound healing.
10. Lipid-lowering therapy can help restore endothelial function and prevent coronary events.

---

1. When caring for patients with coronary artery disease, the anesthesiologist must prevent or minimize myocardial ischemia by maintaining optimal conditions for perfusion of the heart.

   What provides the most resistance in the coronary artery circulation?
   A. Larger-conductance vessels visible on coronary angiography
   B. Vessels larger than 100 μm in diameter
   C. Vessels 250 nm to 10 μm in diameter (arterioles)
   D. Veins

Correct answer: B

Explanation: Traditionally, it was thought that arterioles (<50 μm in size) accounted for most coronary resistance; however, close to 50% of total coronary vascular resistance is due to vessels larger than 100 μm in diameter due to the length of these vessels. Inability to regulate tone in these

vessels is one of the early changes in coronary artery atherosclerosis.

References:

1. Hibbert B, Nathan H, Simard T, et al. Chapter 7: Coronary Physiology and Atherosclerosis. In: Kaplan JA, Augoustides JGT, Manecke GR, et al., eds. Kaplan's Cardiac Anesthesia. 7th ed. Elsevier; 2017: 179-205.
2. Daubenspeck D, Chaney M. Clinical importance of quantitative assessment of myocardial blood flow. J Cardiothorac Vasc Anesth, 2022; 36: 1511-1515.

2. Where do the vasa vasorum reside in a coronary artery?
   A. Tunica intima
   B. Tunica media
   C. Tunica adventitia
   D. There are no vasa vasorum in coronary arteries

Correct answer: C

Explanation: The outermost layer of the artery (tunica adventitia) contains the vasa vasorum, which are the small blood vessels necessary for perfusion of the coronary artery. In addition, the adventitia also contains adipocytes, fibroblasts, and nerves. The tunica media consists of smooth muscle cells with variable orientation. The tunica intima can vary from an endothelial monolayer to endothelium overlaying an extracellular matrix with smooth muscle cells. The tunica media is separated from the tunica intima by the internal elastic lamina, and the tunica adventitia by the external elastic lamina.

References:
1. Hibbert B, Nathan H, Simard T, et al. Chapter 7: Coronary Physiology and Atherosclerosis. In: Kaplan JA, Augoustides JGT, Manecke GR, et al., eds. Kaplan's Cardiac Anesthesia. 7th ed. Elsevier; 2017: 179-205
2. Maiellaro K, Taylor WR. The role of the adventitia in vascular inflammation. Cardiovasc Res, 2007; 75: 640-648.

3. What is a characteristic of prostacyclin I_2?
   A. It facilitates production of cyclic guanosine monophosphate
   B. It contracts endothelial smooth muscle
   C. It promotes platelet aggregation
   D. It is activated by shear stress, pulsatility of blood flow, hypoxia, and a variety of vasoactive mediators

Correct answer: D

Explanation: Prostaglandin I_2 is a product of the cyclooxygenase pathway and is activated by shear stress, pulsatility of blood flow, hypoxia, and a variety of vasoactive mediators. Via cyclic adenosine monophosphate, it relaxes endothelial smooth muscle cells and inhibits platelet aggregation.

References:
1. Hibbert B, Nathan H, Simard T, et al. Chapter 7: Coronary Physiology and Atherosclerosis. In: Kaplan JA, Augoustides JGT, Manecke GR, et al., eds. Kaplan's Cardiac Anesthesia. 7th ed. Elsevier; 2017: 179-205.
2. Laflamme M, Perrault LP, Carrier M, et al. Preliminary experience with combined inhaled milrinone and prostacyclin in cardiac surgical patients with pulmonary hypertension. J Cardiothorac Vasc Anesth, 2015; 29: 38-45.

4. Which of the following is an endothelium-derived vascular muscle contracting factor?
   A. Prostaglandin H_2
   B. Prostacyclin
   C. Nitric oxide
   D. Hyperpolarizing factor

Correct answer: A

Explanation: Prostacyclin, nitric oxide, and hyperpolarizing factor are all endothelium-derived vascular muscle relaxing factors. Prostaglandin H_2, thromboxane A_2, and endothelin are all endothelium-derived vascular muscle contracting factors. Although the factors in each group achieve the same effect, the mechanism by which they achieve this effect may vary. For example, prostacyclin is mediated by cyclic adenosine monophosphate, while nitric oxide is mediated by cyclic guanosine monophosphate.

References:
1. Hibbert B, Nathan H, Simard T, et al. Chapter 7: Coronary Physiology and Atherosclerosis. In: Kaplan JA, Augoustides JGT, Manecke GR, et al., eds. Kaplan's Cardiac Anesthesia. 7th ed. Elsevier; 2017: 179-205.
2. Dai B, Cavaye J, Judd M, et al. Perioperative presentations of Kounis syndrome: a systematic literature review. J Cardiothorac Vasc Anesth, 2022; 36: 2070-2076.

5. Which of the following is a primary determinant of coronary blood flow?
   A. Coronary reserve
   B. Autoregulation
   C. Myocardial extravascular compression
   D. Transmural blood flow

Correct answer: C

Explanation: The four major components responsible for coronary blood flow include: (1) perfusion pressure, (2) myocardial extravascular compression, (3) myocardial metabolism, and (4) neurohumoral control. Autoregulation allows for coronary blood flow to remain constant despite changes in perfusion pressure, but it is not a primary determinant of flow. Perfusion pressure is the difference between the aortic root and the ventricular end-diastolic pressures. External compression from the myocardium can contribute 10% to 25% of the coronary vascular resistance. Normally, flow and myocardial metabolism are matched over a wide range of oxygen consumption so that coronary sinus oxygen saturation changes very little. Neurohumoral control includes sympathetic and parasympathetic changes in heart rate, blood pressure, and contractility. Coronary reserve and transmural blood flow are not primary determinants of coronary blood flow.

References:
1. Hibbert B, Nathan H, Simard T, et al. Chapter 7: Coronary Physiology and Atherosclerosis. In: Kaplan JA, Augoustides JGT, Manecke GR, et al., eds. Kaplan's Cardiac Anesthesia. 7th ed. Elsevier; 2017: 179-205.
2. Daubenspeck D, Chaney M. Clinical importance of quantitative assessment of myocardial blood flow. J Cardiothorac Vasc Anesth, 2022; 36: 1511-1515.

6. What provides parasympathetic stimulation of the heart?
   A. Thoracic ganglia 1-4
   B. Superior, middle, and inferior cervical ganglia
   C. Stellate ganglia
   D. Vagus nerve

Correct answer: D

Explanation: The vagus nerve provides efferent cholinergic cardiac stimulation, resulting in a reduction in heart rate, decreased contractility, and a reduction in blood pressure as the effects for parasympathetic stimulation of the heart. Sympathetic stimulation can come from the superior, middle, and inferior cervical sympathetic cervical ganglia, the first four thoracic ganglia, and the stellate ganglia (merging of the inferior cervical and first thoracic ganglia).

References:

1. Hibbert B, Nathan H, Simard T, et al. Chapter 7: Coronary Physiology and Atherosclerosis. In: Kaplan JA, Augoustides JGT, Manecke GR, et al., eds. Kaplan's Cardiac Anesthesia. 7th ed. Elsevier; 2017: 179-205.
2. Deschamps A, Denault A, Rochon A, et al. Evaluation of autonomic reserves in cardiac surgery patients. J Cardiothorac Vasc Anesth, 2013; 27; 485-493.

7. What are alpha-adrenergic effects on the cardiac system?
   A. Feedback inhibition of norepinephrine release
   B. Coronary artery dilation
   C. Increased contractility
   D. Increased heart rate

Correct answer: A

Explanation: Alpha-adrenergic effects of the heart cause vasoconstriction of the coronary arteries. This is likely an attempt to limit the beta-adrenergic effects of increased heart rate, contractility, and coronary vasodilation. Presynaptic nerve terminals mediate feedback inhibition and can decrease norepinephrine release.

References:

1. Hibbert B, Nathan H, Simard T, et al. Chapter 7: Coronary Physiology and Atherosclerosis. In: Kaplan JA, Augoustides JGT, Manecke GR, et al., eds. Kaplan's Cardiac Anesthesia. 7th ed. Elsevier; 2017: 179-205.
2. Seyrek M, Halici Z, Yildiz O, et al. Interaction between dexmedetomidine and α-adrenergic receptors: emphasis on vascular actions. J Cardiothorac Vasc Anesth, 2011; 25: 856-862.

8. In a heart with coronary artery disease, what are the effects of exercise on the coronary artery segments distal to the lesion?
   A. Vasodilation of the artery distal to the stenosis
   B. Vasoconstriction of the artery distal to the stenosis
   C. Vasodilation of the artery proximal to the stenosis
   D. Vasoconstriction of the artery proximal to the stenosis

Correct answer: B

Explanation: In a patient with myocardial ischemia, the sympathetic nervous system relies on predominately alpha-adrenergic signaling from the sympathetic nervous system vasoconstricts post-stenotic coronary artery segments, producing an anti-steal effect as blood flow is restricted at the level of the fixed lesion. Beta-adrenergic stimulation in areas without myocardial ischemia will increase coronary perfusion to areas where tissue is currently functional.

References:

1. Hibbert B, Nathan H, Simard T, et al. Chapter 7: Coronary Physiology and Atherosclerosis. In: Kaplan JA, Augoustides JGT, Manecke GR, et al., eds. Kaplan's Cardiac Anesthesia. 7th ed. Elsevier; 2017: 179-205.
2. Daubenspeck D, Chaney M. Clinical importance of quantitative assessment of myocardial blood flow. J Cardiothorac Vasc Anesth, 2022; 36: 1511-1515.

9. What is a characteristic of histamine's interaction with the coronary vessels?
   A. H_1 receptors are located on large and small coronary artery vascular smooth muscle cells and mediate vasoconstriction
   B. H_2 receptors are located on arteriole smooth muscle cells and mediate vasoconstriction
   C. Histamine does not cause coronary artery vasospasm
   D. H_1 receptors mediate vasoconstriction by stimulation of nitric oxide release

Correct answer: A

Explanation: H_1 receptors located on large and small coronary artery vascular smooth muscle cells mediate vasoconstriction. H_1 receptors located on vascular endothelium mediate vasodilation by stimulation of nitric oxide release. H_2 receptors are located on arteriole smooth muscle cells and mediate vasodilation.

References:

1. Hibbert B, Nathan H, Simard T, et al. Chapter 7: Coronary Physiology and Atherosclerosis. In: Kaplan JA, Augoustides JGT, Manecke GR, et al., eds. Kaplan's Cardiac Anesthesia. 7th ed. Elsevier; 2017: 179-205.
2. Cirkel J, Schutz A, Baumert JH, et al. Arrythmias during CABG-surgery – are they partly histamine-induced? J Cardiothorac Vasc Anesth, 1994; 8: 175.

10. What is true regarding autoregulation of the coronary arteries?
    A. Autoregulation is more effective in the right ventricle than in the left ventricle
    B. Autoregulation can be accurately studied via direct cannulation of the coronary ostium and measurement of coronary sinus saturation
    C. Coronary artery autoregulation occurs between mean arterial pressures of 60- and 140-mm Hg
    D. Autoregulation is not present in transplanted hearts

Correct answer: C

Explanation: Coronary artery blood flow is constant between a mean arterial pressure of 60 mmHg and 140 mmHg. Autoregulation is similar between the right and left ventricles. Despite direct cannulation of the coronary ostium, as perfusion pressure changes myocardial extraction of oxygen changes as well, making accurate measurements challenging. Autoregulation is a local mechanism of control and can be seen in isolated, denervated hearts.

References:

1. Hibbert B, Nathan H, Simard T, et al. Chapter 7: Coronary Physiology and Atherosclerosis. In: Kaplan JA, Augoustides JGT, Manecke GR, et al., eds. Kaplan's Cardiac Anesthesia. 7th ed. Elsevier; 2017: 179-205.
2. Daubenspeck D, Chaney M. Clinical importance of quantitative assessment of myocardial blood flow. J Cardiothorac Vasc Anesth, 2022; 36: 1511-1515.

11. Coronary vasodilation due to myocardial ischemia is called:
   A. Oxygen autoregulation
   B. Myocardial regulation
   C. Myocardial fractional flow reserve
   D. Reactive hyperemia

Correct answer: D

Explanation: Reactive hyperemia occurs when abrupt myocardial ischemia occurs, creating a "debt area" of malperfusion. After reperfusion occurs, there is a restoration of coronary blood flow by five to six times the resting flow rate, which now becomes the "repayment area." Autoregulation in the coronary artery is due to mean arterial pressure, not oxygenation. The myocardial fractional flow reserve is the relationship of coronary pressure distal to a lesion during maximum pharmacologic dilation. Myocardial regulation does not play a major role in coronary vasodilation due to myocardial ischemia.

References:

1. Hibbert B, Nathan H, Simard T, et al. Chapter 7: Coronary Physiology and Atherosclerosis. In: Kaplan JA, Augoustides JGT, Manecke GR, et al., eds. Kaplan's Cardiac Anesthesia. 7th ed. Elsevier; 2017: 179-205.
2. Daubenspeck D, Chaney M. Clinical importance of quantitative assessment of myocardial blood flow. J Cardiothorac Vasc Anesth, 2022; 36: 1511-1515.

12. What is the first portion of the left ventricular wall to become ischemic?
   A. Inner third
   B. Middle third
   C. Outer third
   D. All wall segments become ischemic at the same time

Correct answer: A

Explanation: When coronary perfusion pressure becomes inadequate, the inner third of the left ventricular wall is the first region to experience ischemia. Intramyocardial pressure is highest in the inner layers of the ventricle, which restricts perfusion to that area. This is exaggerated in eccentric hypertrophy.

References:

1. Hibbert B, Nathan H, Simard T, et al. Chapter 7: Coronary Physiology and Atherosclerosis. In: Kaplan JA, Augoustides JGT, Manecke GR, et al., eds. Kaplan's Cardiac Anesthesia. 7th ed. Elsevier; 2017: 179-205.

2. Daubenspeck D, Chaney M. Clinical importance of quantitative assessment of myocardial blood flow. J Cardiothorac Vasc Anesth, 2022; 36: 1511-1515.

13. How do vascular endothelial cells maintain the fluidity of blood?
   A. Process substances such as norepinephrine, serotonin, and prostaglandins
   B. Produce anticoagulant, fibrinolytic, and antiplatelet substances
   C. Neurohumoral control regulates flow and fluidity of blood
   D. Transport coagulant factors originating from the liver

Correct answer: B

Explanation: Vascular endothelial cells produce anticoagulant, fibrinolytic, and antiplatelet substances to maintain the fluidity of blood. These include anticoagulant factors (protein C and thrombomodulin), fibrinolytic factors (tissue-type plasminogen activator), and antiplatelet substances (prostacyclin and nitric oxide). Vascular endothelial cells process norepinephrine, serotonin, and prostaglandins for coronary artery dilation and constriction. Neurohumoral control is a determinant of coronary blood flow constriction and dilation. Coagulant factors do traverse through coronary arteries; however, there is limited interaction with vascular endothelial cells and blood fluidity.

References:

1. Hibbert B, Nathan H, Simard T, et al. Chapter 7: Coronary Physiology and Atherosclerosis. In: Kaplan JA, Augoustides JGT, Manecke GR, et al., eds. Kaplan's Cardiac Anesthesia. 7th ed. Elsevier; 2017: 179-205.
2. Daubenspeck D, Chaney M. Clinical importance of quantitative assessment of myocardial blood flow. J Cardiothorac Vasc Anesth, 2022; 36: 1511-1515.

14. Angiotensin-converting enzyme is responsible for:
   A. Converting angiotensin II to angiotensin III
   B. Degrading substance P
   C. Converting angiotensinogen to angiotensin I
   D. Degrading bradykinin

Correct answer: D

Explanation: Angiotensin-converting enzyme is present on vascular endothelium and converts angiotensin I to angiotensin II, which causes coronary vasoconstriction. This endothelial enzyme also inactivates bradykinin, which attenuates vasoconstriction by nitric oxide stimulation. Angiotensin II facilitates norepinephrine release from presynaptic adrenergic nerve terminals. Despite theoretical possibilities, inhibition of this endothelial enzyme has not been shown to be of benefit in human myocardial ischemia other than through control of afterload.

References:

1. Hibbert B, Nathan H, Simard T, et al. Chapter 7: Coronary Physiology and Atherosclerosis. In: Kaplan JA, Augoustides

JGT, Manecke GR, et al., eds. Kaplan's Cardiac Anesthesia. 7th ed. Elsevier; 2017: 179-205.
2. Yoon U, Setren A, Chen A, et al. Continuation of angiotensin-converting enzyme inhibitors on the day of surgery is not associated with increased risk of hypotension upon induction of general anesthesia in elective noncardiac surgeries. J Cardiothorac Vasc Anesth, 2021; 35: 508-513.

15. Which molecule is suggested as the link between myocardial metabolism and myocardial blood flow?
   A. Oxygen
   B. Carbon dioxide
   C. Adenosine
   D. There is no one molecule responsible

Correct answer: D

Explanation: Although oxygen, reactive oxygen species, carbon dioxide, and adenosine are all suggested to contribute to both myocardial metabolism and blood flow, there is no one responsible molecule. A decrease in oxygen content, an increase in carbon dioxide, or an increase in adenosine contributes to coronary vasodilation and an increase in myocardial blood flow. An increase in reactive oxygen species such as peroxide can increase both myocardial metabolism and myocardial blood flow.

References:

1. Hibbert B, Nathan H, Simard T, et al. Chapter 7: Coronary Physiology and Atherosclerosis. In: Kaplan JA, Augoustides JGT, Manecke GR, et al., eds. Kaplan's Cardiac Anesthesia. 7th ed. Elsevier; 2017: 179-205.
2. Daubenspeck D, Chaney M. Clinical importance of quantitative assessment of myocardial blood flow. J Cardiothorac Vasc Anesth, 2022; 36: 1511-1515.

16. Myocardial extravascular compression normally contributes what percentage of total coronary vascular resistance?
   A. Less than 5%
   B. 10% to 25%
   C. 25% to 40%
   D. More than 40%

Correct answer: B

Explanation: Determining the pressure gradient across the coronary circulation is complicated by the fact that the heart compresses the intramural coronary vessels during systolic contraction. The effects of this systolic myocardial compression are most pronounced in the subendocardial layers, where this force mirrors intraventricular pressure. However, in normal conditions, this extravascular compression contributes only a small component (10%–25%) of the overall coronary vascular resistance.

References:

1. Hibbert B, Nathan H, Simard T, et al. Chapter 7: Coronary Physiology and Atherosclerosis. In: Kaplan JA, Augoustides JGT, Manecke GR, et al., eds. Kaplan's Cardiac Anesthesia. 7th ed. Elsevier; 2017: 179-205.

2. Daubenspeck D, Chaney M. Clinical importance of quantitative assessment of myocardial blood flow. J Cardiothorac Vasc Anesth, 2022; 36: 1511-1515.

17. The most reliable measure of coronary perfusion pressure in the clinical setting is:
   A. Systolic blood pressure
   B. Diastolic blood pressure
   C. Mean systemic arterial pressure
   D. Central venous pressure

Correct answer: C

Explanation: Coronary blood flow is proportional to the pressure gradient across the coronary circulation, which represents the difference in the aortic root pressure and the ventricular end-diastolic pressure. Since coronary perfusion occurs mostly during the period of aortic valve closure, the most accurate reflection of coronary driving pressure is the average pressure of the aortic root during diastole. Although either the aortic diastolic or mean pressure approximate this driving pressure for flow, peripheral diastolic blood pressure measurements in the clinical environment often differ from the central aortic pressure. Therefore, the mean arterial pressure is the most consistently reliable measure of coronary driving pressure in the clinical environment.

References:

1. Hibbert B, Nathan H, Simard T, et al. Chapter 7: Coronary Physiology and Atherosclerosis. In: Kaplan JA, Augoustides JGT, Manecke GR, et al., eds. Kaplan's Cardiac Anesthesia. 7th ed. Elsevier; 2017: 179-205.
2. Daubenspeck D, Chaney M. Clinical importance of quantitative assessment of myocardial blood flow. J Cardiothorac Vasc Anesth, 2022; 36: 1511-1515.

18. Binding of norepinephrine to α_2-receptors on the vascular endothelium promotes the release of:
   A. Prostaglandin H_2
   B. Endothelin
   C. Thromboxane A_2
   D. Nitric oxide

Correct answer: D

Explanation: When norepinephrine binds to α_2-receptors on the surface of the vascular endothelium, this stimulates the release of nitric oxide. The release of nitric oxide then acts to cause vascular smooth muscle relaxation. The endothelium is also capable of metabolizing norepinephrine to limit its effect, thus providing the endothelium with a mechanism to control the effects of alpha-adrenergic stimulation.

References:

1. Hibbert B, Nathan H, Simard T, et al. Chapter 7: Coronary Physiology and Atherosclerosis. In: Kaplan JA, Augoustides JGT, Manecke GR, et al., eds. Kaplan's Cardiac Anesthesia. 7th ed. Elsevier; 2017: 179-205.

2. Seyrek M, Halici Z, Yildiz O, et al. Interaction between dexmedetomidine and α-adrenergic receptors: emphasis on vascular actions. J Cardiothorac Vasc Anesth, 2011; 25: 856-862.

19. The most important early, adverse consequence of atherosclerosis is:
    A. Formation of lipid-filled macrophages
    B. Arterial remodeling
    C. Impairment of endothelial function
    D. Coronary steal

Correct answer: C

Explanation: In addition to serving as a physical barrier between the blood stream and coronary artery wall, the normal endothelium plays a critical role in modulating vascular tone, thrombogenicity, fibrinolysis, platelet function, and inflammation. Impairment of endothelial function is an important early consequence of atherosclerosis and appears to occur before the development of angiographically-visible arterial stenoses. Although the accumulation of intracellular lipid in the subendothelial region to form lipid-filled macrophages ("foam cells") is an early detectable change in the disease process, collections of these cells are encased by intact endothelium and are not associated with significant smooth muscle accumulation. Arterial remodeling refers to the ability of the coronary arteries to undergo compensatory enlargement. This luminal expansion of the arterial wall may occur to a significant extent before narrowing of the arterial lumen occurs. Coronary steal is not an early adverse event of atherosclerosis.

References:

1. Hibbert B, Nathan H, Simard T, et al. Chapter 7: Coronary Physiology and Atherosclerosis. In: Kaplan JA, Augoustides JGT, Manecke GR, et al., eds. Kaplan's Cardiac Anesthesia. 7th ed. Elsevier; 2017: 179-205.
2. Smit M, Coetzee AR, Lochner A. The pathophysiology of myocardial ischemia and perioperative myocardial infarction. J Cardiothorac Vasc Anesth, 2020; 34: 2501-2512.

20. At rest, the diameter of a coronary artery must be reduced by what percentage to result in a decrease in coronary blood flow?
    A. 25%
    B. 50%
    C. 65%
    D. 80%

Correct answer: D

Explanation: At rest, coronary artery flow is unchanged until the coronary diameter is reduced by at least 80%. Resting flow remains constant as the lumen diameter decreases until this point due to progressive dilation of the coronary arterioles. This compensates for the resistance of the stenosis by diminishing the resistance of the distal coronary bed. Blood flow through a stenotic coronary artery produces a loss of energy by entrance effects, frictional losses, and separation losses. Entrance effects are typically negligible, while frictional losses are only pronounced in very long segments of stenosis. Separation losses occur when turbulent flow exits pass the stenotic area. Accordingly, the following equation represents the hemodynamic severity of stenosis:

$$\Delta P = fQ + sQ^2$$

In this equation, ΔP is the pressure drop across the stenosis, Q is the volume flow of blood, f is a factor accounting for frictional effects, and s accounts for separation effects. Note that separation losses increase with the square of blood flow velocity, meaning that the amount of energy loss (drop in pressure) across the obstruction increases exponentially as flow rate increases.

References:

1. Hibbert B, Nathan H, Simard T, et al. Chapter 7: Coronary Physiology and Atherosclerosis. In: Kaplan JA, Augoustides JGT, Manecke GR, et al., eds. Kaplan's Cardiac Anesthesia. 7th ed. Elsevier; 2017: 179-205.
2. Daubenspeck D, Chaney M. Clinical importance of quantitative assessment of myocardial blood flow. J Cardiothorac Vasc Anesth, 2022; 36: 1511-1515.

21. During maximal exercise effort, the diameter of a coronary artery must be reduced by what percentage to result in a decrease in coronary blood flow?
    A. 25%
    B. 50%
    C. 65%
    D. 80%

Correct answer: B

Explanation: Please refer to the explanation for question 20. Because the separation loss (pressure drop) across a stenosis increases exponentially with blood velocity, maximal coronary flow begins to fall when the arterial diameter is reduced by 50%. Therefore, in the presence of severe stenosis, stressors such as exercise, anemia, and arteriolar vasodilators such as dipyridamole are poorly tolerated.

References:

1. Hibbert B, Nathan H, Simard T, et al. Chapter 7: Coronary Physiology and Atherosclerosis. In: Kaplan JA, Augoustides JGT, Manecke GR, et al., eds. Kaplan's Cardiac Anesthesia. 7th ed. Elsevier; 2017: 179-205.
2. Daubenspeck D, Chaney M. Clinical importance of quantitative assessment of myocardial blood flow. J Cardiothorac Vasc Anesth, 2022; 36: 1511-1515.

22. The most important determinant of myocardial oxygen consumption is:
    A. Heart rate
    B. Myocardial contractility
    C. Wall stress
    D. Basal metabolic requirements

Correct answer: B

Explanation: The major determinants of myocardial oxygen consumption are myocardial contractility, heart rate, and wall tension (chamber pressure × radius/wall thickness), while shortening, activation, and basal metabolic requirements are all minor determinants. In isolation, increasing contractility has the most pronounced effect in terms of increasing myocardial oxygen consumption, followed by increasing heart rate, and then increasing wall tension (effects on oxygen consumption: contractility > heart rate > wall tension).

References:

1. Hibbert B, Nathan H, Simard T, et al. Chapter 7: Coronary Physiology and Atherosclerosis. In: Kaplan JA, Augoustides JGT, Manecke GR, et al., eds. Kaplan's Cardiac Anesthesia. 7th ed. Elsevier; 2017: 179-205.
2. Daubenspeck D, Chaney M. Clinical importance of quantitative assessment of myocardial blood flow. J Cardiothorac Vasc Anesth, 2022; 36: 1511-1515.

23. In a patient with a coronary artery fistula (right coronary artery to right atrium) and no significant coronary artery disease detected on angiography, coronary ischemia is most likely to occur as a result of:
    A. Rupture of coronary artery aneurysm
    B. Coronary steal
    C. Coronary vasospasm
    D. Intramural coronary compression

Correct answer: B

Explanation: Coronary artery fistulas are abnormal communications between the coronary arteries and the cardiac chambers, coronary sinus, or other vessels around the heart. Their presence may ultimately lead to coronary dilation or aneurysmal malformation. Coronary artery fistulas may lead to ischemia due to coronary steal. In this presented scenario, coronary steal may occur if the difference in the high-pressure coronary artery and the low-pressure right atrium eventually results in a left-to-right shunt in which flow is diverted (stolen) from the coronary artery to the right atrium.

References:

1. Hibbert B, Nathan H, Simard T, et al. Chapter 7: Coronary Physiology and Atherosclerosis. In: Kaplan JA, Augoustides JGT, Manecke GR, et al., eds. Kaplan's Cardiac Anesthesia. 7th ed. Elsevier; 2017: 179-205.
2. Liu H, Li X, Song H, et al. Anesthesia management for a patient with coronary artery fistula and huge coronary aneurysm undergoing off-pump surgery. J Cardiothorac Vasc Anesth, 2020; 34: 1885-1889.

24. In infants with an anomalous origin of the left coronary artery from the pulmonary artery, what is the reported mortality rate of those who do not undergo surgical repair within the first year of life?
    A. 25%
    B. 50%
    C. 70%
    D. 90%

Correct answer: D

Explanation: Anomalous origin of the left coronary artery from the pulmonary artery (ALCAPA) is the most common variant of an anomalous coronary artery origin from the pulmonary circulation. Surgical repair entails direct reimplantation of the anomalous coronary artery into the aorta. If left untreated, mortality is exceedingly high (90%) in infants who do not have surgical repair within the first year of life. This makes ALCAPA one of the most significant etiologies of myocardial ischemia and heart failure in children. The majority of patients present within the first few weeks of life, as the high pulmonary vascular resistance associated with the fetal circulation begins to naturally decline. Without subsequent development of adequate coronary collateral flow, myocardial ischemia quickly occurs. In rare cases, patients with well-developed coronary collateral circulation may demonstrate a delayed presentation as teenagers or young adults.

References:

1. Hibbert B, Nathan H, Simard T, et al. Chapter 7: Coronary Physiology and Atherosclerosis. In: Kaplan JA, Augoustides JGT, Manecke GR, et al., eds. Kaplan's Cardiac Anesthesia. 7th ed. Elsevier; 2017: 179-205.
2. Addis DR, Townsley MM. Implications of congenital coronary anomalies for the cardiothoracic anesthesiologist: an overview of the 2020 American Society of Echocardiography recommendations for multimodality assessment of congenital coronary anomalies. J Cardiothorac Vasc Anesth, 2020; 34: 2291-2296.

25. Which of the following conditions is characterized by a loss of arterial elasticity and luminal narrowing that may affect the coronary arteries?
    A. Down syndrome
    B. Williams syndrome
    C. Turner syndrome
    D. Edwards syndrome

Correct answer: B

Explanation: Elastin is important for the structural integrity and normal function of arterial walls. Williams syndrome results from a microdeletion at the chromosomal location of the elastin gene (7q11.23), resulting in a profound elastin deficiency that may cause both central (proximal ascending aorta, central pulmonary artery) and peripheral (coronary, carotid, renal, mesenteric arteries) arteriopathies. The hallmark of Williams syndrome is supravalvular aortic stenosis. The pathophysiology of Williams syndrome creates an environment in which profound myocardial oxygen supply and demand mismatch may occur, and these patients carry a high risk for sudden cardiac death (especially when receiving sedation or general anesthesia).

References:

1. Hibbert B, Nathan H, Simard T, et al. Chapter 7: Coronary Physiology and Atherosclerosis. In: Kaplan JA, Augoustides JGT,

Manecke GR, et al., eds. Kaplan's Cardiac Anesthesia. 7th ed. Elsevier; 2017: 179-205.

2. Addis DR, Townsley MM. Implications of congenital coronary anomalies for the cardiothoracic anesthesiologist: an overview of the 2020 American Society of Echocardiography recommendations for multimodality assessment of congenital coronary anomalies. J Cardiothorac Vasc Anesth, 2020; 34: 2291-2296.

26. What is the normal coronary sinus oxygen saturation at rest?
  A. 25% to 30%
  B. 40% to 45%
  C. 50% to 55%
  D. 60% to 65%

Correct answer: A

Explanation: Normal coronary sinus oxygen saturation at rest is 25% to 30%. Because the heart is an obligate aerobic organ, it is completely dependent on coronary perfusion for an uninterrupted blood supply. Under normal conditions, myocardial oxygen demand is met by myocardial oxygen delivery so that normal myocardium does not become ischemic when oxygen consumption is increased. There is a linear relationship of the ability of myocardial oxygen supply to meet increased demand, explained mostly by the capability of the coronary circulation to dilate and increase flow to meet demand. The necessary increase in coronary blood flow during periods of high myocardial oxygen consumption is required because of the high myocardial oxygen extraction under normal conditions. Therefore, the coronary circulation is described as a low flow–high extraction regional circulation, meaning that increases in myocardial oxygen consumption cannot be met by increasing oxygen extraction.

References:

1. Hibbert B, Nathan H, Simard T, et al. Chapter 7: Coronary Physiology and Atherosclerosis. In: Kaplan JA, Augoustides JGT, Manecke GR, et al., eds. Kaplan's Cardiac Anesthesia. 7th ed. Elsevier; 2017: 179-205.
2. Smit M, Coetzee AR, Lochner A. The pathophysiology of myocardial ischemia and perioperative myocardial infarction. J Cardiothorac Vasc Anesth, 2020; 34: 2501-2512.

27. The most common underlying pathophysiology responsible for perioperative myocardial infarction is:
  A. Vulnerable plaque rupture
  B. Coronary artery vasospasm
  C. Myocardial oxygen delivery demand mismatch
  D. Mechanical coronary compression

Correct answer: C

Explanation: Type 1 myocardial infarction (MI) refers to an acute coronary syndrome, which may include unstable angina, non–ST segment elevation myocardial infarction, and ST segment elevation myocardial infarction. This occurs due to rupture of a vulnerable arterial plaque, followed by thrombus formation, arterial spasm, and, ultimately, coronary occlusion.

Type 2 MI occurs due to myocardial oxygen delivery and demand mismatch in the setting of fixed coronary stenosis (stable coronary artery disease). Type 3 MI occurs when there is high suspicion for an acute myocardial ischemic event in the absence of cardiac biomarker evidence of MI (mortality occurred prior to obtaining biomarkers). Type 4 and Type 5 MIs refer to infarction occurring during percutaneous coronary intervention or coronary artery bypass grafting, respectively.

The majority of perioperative MIs are thought to occur as a result of myocardial oxygen delivery and demand mismatch (type 2 MI). This highlights the importance of maximizing myocardial oxygen delivery and minimizing myocardial oxygen consumption during the perioperative period to optimize the myocardial oxygen supply-demand balance. In particular, there is a strong association between tachycardia and ischemia.

References:

1. Hibbert B, Nathan H, Simard T, et al. Chapter 7: Coronary Physiology and Atherosclerosis. In: Kaplan JA, Augoustides JGT, Manecke GR, et al., eds. Kaplan's Cardiac Anesthesia. 7th ed. Elsevier; 2017: 179-205.
2. Smit M, Coetzee AR, Lochner A. The pathophysiology of myocardial ischemia and perioperative myocardial infarction. J Cardiothorac Vasc Anesth, 2020; 34: 2501-2512.

28. The most likely presentation in a patient experiencing a postoperative myocardial infarction is:
  A. Asymptomatic
  B. Shortness of breath
  C. Chest pain
  D. Diaphoresis

Correct answer: A

Explanation: The majority of perioperative myocardial infarctions are asymptomatic. Chest pain is rarely reported, as opposed to when myocardial infarction occurs outside of the perioperative setting, in which chest pain is the most common presenting complaint. Possible explanations include concomitant postoperative analgesia, sedation (leading to underreporting of symptoms), or other distracting sources of pain.

References:

1. Hibbert B, Nathan H, Simard T, et al. Chapter 7: Coronary Physiology and Atherosclerosis. In: Kaplan JA, Augoustides JGT, Manecke GR, et al., eds. Kaplan's Cardiac Anesthesia. 7th ed. Elsevier; 2017: 179-205.
2. Smit M, Coetzee AR, Lochner A. The pathophysiology of myocardial ischemia and perioperative myocardial infarction. J Cardiothorac Vasc Anesth, 2020; 34: 2501-2512.

29. The most prominent risk factor in the development of atherosclerosis is:
  A. High low-density lipoprotein levels
  B. Low high-density lipoprotein levels
  C. Inflammation
  D. Physical inactivity

Correct answer: C

Explanation: High levels of low-density lipoproteins (LDLs) have historically been thought to be the major instigating factor in the development of atherosclerosis; however, recent evidence now suggests that half of all atherosclerotic deaths occur in patients without significant hyperlipidemia. Instead, inflammation is now recognized as a more important risk factor in the development of atherosclerosis than lipid abnormalities. Elevated levels of highly specific C-reactive protein (hs-CRP) are predictive of an increased risk for coronary artery disease. Additionally, beneficial effects of statins appear related to their inherent antiinflammatory effects. Statins have been shown to reduce the incidence of major cardiovascular events by reducing hs-CRP levels in patients with normal levels of LDL.

References:

1. Hibbert B, Nathan H, Simard T, et al. Chapter 7: Coronary Physiology and Atherosclerosis. In: Kaplan JA, Augoustides JGT, Manecke GR, et al., eds. Kaplan's Cardiac Anesthesia. 7th ed. Elsevier; 2017: 179-205.
2. Smit M, Coetzee AR, Lochner A. The pathophysiology of myocardial ischemia and perioperative myocardial infarction. J Cardiothorac Vasc Anesth, 2020; 34: 2501-2512.

30. Blood supply to the basal inferoseptal wall of the left ventricle is predominately provided by which artery?

A. Right coronary

B. Circumflex

C. Left anterior descending

D. Obtuse marginal

Correct answer: A

Explanation: The guidelines from the American Society of Echocardiography outline predominant coronary perfusion patterns to the left ventricular walls (based upon a 17-segment model) as follows:

Right coronary artery: basal inferoseptal, basal inferior, mid inferoseptal, mid inferior, and apical inferior segments

Left anterior descending artery: basal anteroseptal, basal anterior, mid anteroseptal, mid anterior, apical septal, and apical anterior segments. At times, overlap may occur between segments perfused by the left anterior descending and right coronary arteries, especially in the apical region

Circumflex coronary artery: basal inferolateral, basal anterolateral, mid inferolateral, mid anterolateral, apical lateral, and apex segments

References:

1. Hibbert B, Nathan H, Simard T, et al. Chapter 7: Coronary Physiology and Atherosclerosis. In: Kaplan JA, Augoustides JGT, Manecke GR, et al., eds. Kaplan's Cardiac Anesthesia. 7th ed. Elsevier; 2017: 179-205.
2. Hahn RT, Abraham T, Adams MS, et al. Guidelines for performing a comprehensive transesophageal echocardiographic examination: recommendations from the American Society of Echocardiography and the Society of Cardiovascular Anesthesiologists. J Am Soc Echocardiogr, 2013; 26: 921-964.

CHAPTER 8

Molecular and Genetic Cardiovascular Medicine

Patrick Hussey and Matthew M. Townsley

KEY POINTS

1. The rapid development of molecular biologic and genetic techniques has greatly expanded the understanding of cardiac functioning, and these techniques are beginning to be applied clinically.
2. Cardiac ion channels form the machinery behind the cardiac rhythm; cardiac membrane receptors regulate cardiac function.
3. Sodium, potassium, and calcium channels are the main ion channel types involved in the cardiac action potential. Many subtypes exist, and their molecular structure is known in some detail, thus allowing a molecular explanation for phenomena such as voltage sensing, ion selectivity, and inactivation.
4. Muscarinic and adrenergic receptors, both of the G-protein–coupled receptor class, are the main regulators of cardiac function.
5. Adenosine plays important roles in myocardial preconditioning through an action on adenosine triphosphate–regulated potassium channels and is an effective antiarrhythmic drug by its action on G-protein–coupled adenosine receptors.
6. Volatile anesthetic agents significantly affect calcium channels and muscarinic receptors.
7. Powerful genetic analysis techniques are being used to better understand adverse cardiovascular events through molecular approaches. Research using these techniques has begun to explore links between genomics and perioperative adverse cardiovascular events.
8. Treatment through gene therapy is evolving in cardiovascular medicine, although it currently does not have a prominent role in the perioperative setting.

---

1. Which ion is primarily responsible for cardiac membrane depolarization?
    A. Na^+
    B. K^+
    C. Cl^-
    D. Ca^{2+}

Correct answer: A

Explanation: Membrane depolarization occurs primarily from the inflow of Na^+ through ion channels down its electrochemical gradient ($+50$ mV) towards the equilibrium potential (0 mV). The opening and closing of ion channels selective for a single ion results in an individual ionic current. Ion channels are highly selective for a single ion: K^+ is responsible for repolarization, Cl^- has a minor contribution to membrane potential, and Ca^{2+} contributes throughout all phases of the depolarization and repolarization cycle.

References:

1. Fox AA, Sharma S, Mounsey JP, et al. Chapter 8: Molecular and Genetic Cardiovascular Medicine. In: Kaplan JA, Augoustides JGT, Manecke GR, et al., eds. Kaplan's Cardiac Anesthesia. 7th ed. Elsevier; 2017: 206-230.
2. Niimi N, Yuki K, Zaleski K. Long QT syndrome and perioperative torsades de pointes: what the anesthesiologist should know. J Cardiothorac Vasc Anesth 2022; 36: 286-302

2. Which ion is primarily responsible for cardiac membrane repolarization?
    A. Na^+
    B. K^+
    C. Cl^-
    D. Ca^{2+}

Correct answer: B

Explanation: Membrane depolarization occurs primarily from the inflow of Na^+ through ion channels down its electrochemical gradient ($+50$ mV) towards the equilibrium potential (0 mV). The opening and closing of ion channels selective for a single ion results in an individual ionic current. Ion channels are highly selective for a single ion: K^+ is responsible for repolarization, Cl^- has a minor contribution to membrane potential, and Ca^{2+} contributes throughout all phases of the depolarization and repolarization cycle. Membrane repolarization occurs primarily from the outflow of K^+ through ion channels down its electrochemical gradient (-90 mV) toward the equilibrium potential (0 mV).

References:

1. Fox AA, Sharma S, Mounsey JP, et al. Chapter 8: Molecular and Genetic Cardiovascular Medicine. In: Kaplan JA, Augoustides JGT, Manecke GR, et al., eds. Kaplan's Cardiac Anesthesia. 7th ed. Elsevier; 2017: 206-230.
2. Niimi N, Yuki K, Zaleski K. Long QT syndrome and perioperative torsades de pointes: what the anesthesiologist should know. J Cardiothorac Vasc Anesth, 2022; 36: 286-302.

3. Which of the following best describes rectification of an ion channel?
   A. Activation of a channel
   B. Inactivation of a channel
   C. A conformational change in the channel
   D. Current passing more easily in one direction than another across a channel

Correct answer: D

Explanation: Ion channels are selective for a single ion and may pass current in one direction across the membrane more easily than the other in a process known as rectification. Electrical and chemical stimulation can cause opening (activation) and closing (inactivation) of the channel. This process, known as gating, causes a conformational change in the channel molecule.

References:

1. Fox AA, Sharma S, Mounsey JP, et al. Chapter 8: Molecular and Genetic Cardiovascular Medicine. In: Kaplan JA, Augoustides JGT, Manecke GR, et al., eds. Kaplan's Cardiac Anesthesia. 7th ed. Elsevier; 2017: 206-230.
2. Niimi N, Yuki K, Zaleski K. Long QT syndrome and perioperative torsades de pointes: what the anesthesiologist should know. J Cardiothorac Vasc Anesth, 2022; 36: 286-302.

4. What is the difference between voltage clamping and patch clamping?
   A. Patch clamping records ion flow through individual ion channels, voltage clamping records ion flow through individual cardiac cells
   B. Patch clamping inhibits individual ion channels, voltage clamping inhibits individual cardiac cells
   C. Patch clamping inhibits inflow of ion channels, voltage clamping inhibits outflow of ion channels
   D. Patch clamping inhibits outflow of ion channels, voltage clamping inhibits inflow of ion channels

Correct answer: A

Explanation: Patch clamping is a technique for recording ion currents through individual ion channels. This allows for the resolution of events at the single–ion channel level. In this technique, small patches of cell membrane (<1 μm^2) are isolated electrically and physically in the tip of a glass micropipette. Voltage clamping, or whole-cell current, is the sum of the currents through all of the individual channels in the cell membrane.

References:

1. Fox AA, Sharma S, Mounsey JP, et al. Chapter 8: Molecular and Genetic Cardiovascular Medicine. In: Kaplan JA, Augoustides JGT, Manecke GR, et al., eds. Kaplan's Cardiac Anesthesia. 7th ed. Elsevier; 2017: 206-230.
2. Montnach J, Lorenzini M, Lesage A, et al. Computer modeling of whole-cell voltage-clamp analyses to delineate guidelines for good practice of manual and automated patch-clamp. Sci Rep, 2021; 11: 3282.

5. Which phase of the cardiac action potential represents the plateau phase?
   A. Phase 0
   B. Phase 1
   C. Phase 2
   D. Phase 3

Correct answer: C

Explanation: There are five phases of a cardiac action potential. Phase 0 (rapid upstroke) is primarily due to Na^+ channel opening. Phase 1 (early rapid repolarization) occurs from the inactivation of Na^+ current and opening of K^+ channels. Phase 2 (plateau phase) is a balance between K^+ and Ca^{2+} currents. Phase 3 (final rapid repolarization) initiates with the activation of Ca^{2+} channels. Finally, phase 4 (diastolic depolarization) is an equilibrium and balance between Na^+ and K^+ currents.

References:

1. Fox AA, Sharma S, Mounsey JP, et al. Chapter 8: Molecular and Genetic Cardiovascular Medicine. In: Kaplan JA, Augoustides JGT, Manecke GR, et al., eds. Kaplan's Cardiac Anesthesia. 7th ed. Elsevier; 2017: 206-230.
2. Niimi N, Yuki K, Zaleski K. Long QT syndrome and perioperative torsades de pointes: what the anesthesiologist should know. J Cardiothorac Vasc Anesth, 2022; 36: 286-302.

6. Which phase of the cardiac action potential is affected in myocardial hypertrophy and congestive cardiomyopathy?
   A. Phase 0
   B. Phase 1
   C. Phase 2
   D. Phase 3

Correct answer: B

Explanation: Phase 1 is the early, rapid repolarization phase of the action potential, facilitated by a transient outward current (I_{T0}), carried mainly by K^+ ions. I_{T0} has two separate currents: I_{T01}, activated by depolarization and blocked by 4-aminopyridine; and I_{T02}, activated by intracellular Ca^{2+}.

In patients with myocardial hypertrophy and congestive heart failure, I_{T0} has been found to be depressed.

References:

1. Fox AA, Sharma S, Mounsey JP, et al. Chapter 8: Molecular and Genetic Cardiovascular Medicine. In: Kaplan JA, Augoustides JGT, Manecke GR, et al., eds. Kaplan's Cardiac Anesthesia. 7th ed. Elsevier; 2017: 206-230.
2. Dalia AA, Essandoh M, Cronin B, et al. A narrative review for anesthesiologists of the 2017 American Heart Association/ American College of Cardiology/Heart Rhythm Society guideline for management of patients with ventricular arrhythmias and the prevention of sudden cardiac death. J Cardiothorac Vasc Anesth, 2019; 33: 1722-1730.

7. Which cardiac action potential phase is missing in ventricular tissues, but present in atrial and pacemaker tissues?
   A. Phase 0
   B. Phase 1
   C. Phase 2
   D. Phase 3

Correct answer: D

Explanation: Phase 3 is enhanced by a large, outward, repolarizing K^+ current. Given the lack of this phase in ventricular tissue, ventricular action potential can vary greatly. In addition, specialized midmyocardial cells (M cells) have been identified in the normal ventricle that exhibit prolongation of the action potential duration at slow stimulation rates. Therefore, intrinsic pacing capabilities of the ventricle are often nonexistent, as compared to the sinoatrial node, the atrioventricular node, or the atrium.

References:

1. Fox AA, Sharma S, Mounsey JP, et al. Chapter 8: Molecular and Genetic Cardiovascular Medicine. In: Kaplan JA, Augoustides JGT, Manecke GR, et al., eds. Kaplan's Cardiac Anesthesia. 7th ed. Elsevier; 2017: 206-230.
2. Niimi N, Yuki K, Zaleski K. Long QT syndrome and perioperative torsades de pointes: what the anesthesiologist should know. J Cardiothorac Vasc Anesth, 2022; 36: 286-302.

8. Phase 4 of the cardiac action potential is also known as which of the following?
   A. Early rapid repolarization
   B. Plateau phase
   C. Pacemaker current
   D. Final rapid repolarization

Correct answer: C

Explanation: Diastolic depolarization, or pacemaker current, is characteristic of phase 4 of the cardiac action potential. Pacemaker activity results from a slow net gain of positive charge, which depolarizes the cell from its maximal diastolic potential to threshold. Pacemaker cells in the sinus node are relatively depolarized, and a slow inward Na^+ current (I_f) competes with slowly inactivating delayed rectifier K^+ currents to cause diastolic depolarization.

References:

1. Fox AA, Sharma S, Mounsey JP, et al. Chapter 8: Molecular and Genetic Cardiovascular Medicine. In: Kaplan JA, Augoustides JGT, Manecke GR, et al., eds. Kaplan's Cardiac Anesthesia. 7th ed. Elsevier; 2017: 206-230.
2. Niimi N, Yuki K, Zaleski K. Long QT syndrome and perioperative torsades de pointes: what the anesthesiologist should know. J Cardiothorac Vasc Anesth, 2022; 36: 286-302.

9. What is the most important subunit of voltage-gated Na^+, Ca^{2+}, and K^+ channels?
   A. α
   B. β
   C. γ
   D. δ

Correct answer: A

Explanation: The α subunit of voltage-gated Na^+, Ca^{2+}, and K^+ channels is the largest subunit and is usually sufficient alone to induce channel activity in the above biologic membranes. However, the β, γ, and δ subunits can modulate the activity of the α subunit. Na^+ and Ca^{2+} channel α subunits are similar in structure, whereas K^+ channel α subunits are much smaller.

References:

1. Fox AA, Sharma S, Mounsey JP, et al. Chapter 8: Molecular and Genetic Cardiovascular Medicine. In: Kaplan JA, Augoustides JGT, Manecke GR, et al., eds. Kaplan's Cardiac Anesthesia. 7th ed. Elsevier; 2017: 206-230.
2. Dalia AA, Essandoh M, Cronin B, et al. A narrative review for anesthesiologists of the 2017 American Heart Association/ American College of Cardiology/Heart Rhythm Society guideline for management of patients with ventricular arrhythmias and the prevention of sudden cardiac death. J Cardiothorac Vasc Anesth, 2019; 33: 1722-1730.

10. The Cardiac Arrhythmia Suppression Trial demonstrated which of the following findings?
   A. The mortality rate of asymptomatic patients after myocardial infarction decreased after initiation of Na^+ channel–blocking agents
   B. The mortality rate of asymptomatic patients after myocardial infarction increased after initiation of Na^+ channel–blocking agents
   C. The mortality rate of asymptomatic patients after myocardial infarction decreased after initiation of K^+ channel–blocking agents
   D. The mortality rate of asymptomatic patients after myocardial infarction increased after initiation of K^+ channel–blocking agents

Correct answer: B

Explanation: With initiation of encainide and flecainide, both Na^+ channel–blocking agents, asymptomatic patients after myocardial infarction had a twofold increase in mortality rate. These findings were attributed to likely slowing of conduction velocity, with an increase in fatal reentrant arrhythmias.

References:

1. Fox AA, Sharma S, Mounsey JP, et al. Chapter 8: Molecular and Genetic Cardiovascular Medicine. In: Kaplan JA, Augoustides JGT, Manecke GR, et al., eds. Kaplan's Cardiac Anesthesia. 7th ed. Elsevier; 2017: 206-230.
2. Echt DS, Liebson PR, Mitchell LB, et al. Mortality and morbidity in patients receiving encainide, flecainide, or placebo: the Cardiac Arrythmia Suppression Trial. N Engl J Med, 1991; 324: 781-788.

11. Which antiarrhythmic drug class reduces fatal arrhythmias after myocardial infarction?
　A. Na$^+$ channel blockers
　B. Beta blockers
　C. K$^+$ channel blockers
　D. Ca^{2+} channel blockers

Correct answer: B

Explanation: In 1982, the First International Study of Infarct Survival discovered that beta blockers were the only class of antiarrhythmics that prolong survival and reduce fatal arrhythmias. As of 2022, no current research has discovered another class that prolongs survival. Interestingly, beta blockers have no direct effect on cardiac ion channels.

References:

1. Fox AA, Sharma S, Mounsey JP, et al. Chapter 8: Molecular and Genetic Cardiovascular Medicine. In: Kaplan JA, Augoustides JGT, Manecke GR, et al., eds. Kaplan's Cardiac Anesthesia. 7th ed. Elsevier; 2017: 206-230.
2. Hjalmarson A. Effects of beta blockade on sudden cardiac death during acute myocardial infarction and the postinfarction period. Am J Cardiol, 1997; 80: 35J-39J.
3. Dalia AA, Essandoh M, Cronin B, et al. A narrative review for anesthesiologists of the 2017 American Heart Association/American College of Cardiology/Heart Rhythm Society guideline for management of patients with ventricular arrhythmias and the prevention of sudden cardiac death. J Cardiothorac Vasc Anesth, 2019; 33: 1722-1730.

12. With regard to short QT syndrome, the primary electrical mechanism leading to the pathophysiology of this condition is:
　A. Abnormal repolarization
　B. Slow ventricular conduction
　C. Abnormal intracellular calcium homeostasis
　D. Abnormal depolarization

Correct answer: A

Explanation: Genetic cardiac ion channelopathies have a well-documented association with sudden cardiac death in both children and adults, usually caused by sustained ventricular tachycardia. These are a heterogeneous group of multisystem disorders that include Brugada syndrome, catecholaminergic polymorphic ventricular tachycardia, and arrhythmogenic right ventricular cardiomyopathy. The following features are shared by these disorders: (1) a structurally normal heart, (2) genetic basis, and (3) predisposition to fatal arrhythmias. Channelopathies may be associated with abnormalities in Na$^+$, K$^+$, Ca^{2+}, and Cl$^-$ channels. In cardiac ion channelopathies, specific pathophysiologic mechanisms have been demonstrated as follows: (1) abnormal repolarization in long QT, short QT, and Brugada syndromes, (2) slow ventricular conduction in Brugada syndrome, and (3) abnormal intracellular calcium homeostasis in catecholaminergic polymorphic ventricular tachycardia.

References:

1. Fox AA, Sharma S, Mounsey JP, et al. Chapter 8: Molecular and Genetic Cardiovascular Medicine. In: Kaplan JA, Augoustides JGT, Manecke GR, et al., eds. Kaplan's Cardiac Anesthesia. 7th ed. Elsevier; 2017: 206-230.
2. Ramakrishna H, O' Hare M, Mookadam F, et al. Sudden cardiac death and disorders of the QT interval: anesthetic implications and focus on perioperative management. J Cardiothorac Vasc Anesth, 2015; 29: 1723-1733.

13. What is the first line treatment for long QT syndrome?
　A. Na$^+$ channel blockers
　B. Beta blockers
　C. K$^+$ channel blocker
　D. Can vary based on patient characteristics

Correct answer: D

Explanation: The long QT syndrome (LQTS), caused by inherited abnormalities that prolong the cardiac action potential, occurs in roughly 1 in 2000 people. It can result in early afterdepolarizations (oscillations during the plateau phase), which may trigger extrasystoles and death from polymorphic ventricular tachycardia (torsades de pointes). Currently, at least 15 different subtypes of LQTS exist, with three genes accounting for 75% of diagnoses. Beta blockers are the first-line treatment for LQT1 and LQT2, as the mutation involves a loss of function of the slowly activating and rapidly activating delayed rectifier K channels. Na$^+$ channel blockers are the first line treatment for LQT3, as the mutation is a gain-of-function mutation of the cardiac Na$^+$ channel that results in slow or incomplete channel inactivation.

References:

1. Fox AA, Sharma S, Mounsey JP, et al. Chapter 8: Molecular and Genetic Cardiovascular Medicine. In: Kaplan JA, Augoustides JGT, Manecke GR, et al., eds. Kaplan's Cardiac Anesthesia. 7th ed. Elsevier; 2017: 206-230.
2. Niimi N, Yuki K, Zaleski K. Long QT syndrome and perioperative torsades de pointes: what the anesthesiologist should know. J Cardiothorac Vasc Anesth, 2022; 36: 286-302.

14. What is an expected finding on the electrocardiogram of a patient with Brugada syndrome?
　A. Short PR interval and broad QRS complexes
　B. Right axis deviation, dominant R wave in V1, and epsilon wave after each QRS
　C. Broad QRS complexes, dominant R' wave in aVR, and borderline first-degree atrioventricular block
　D. Incomplete right bundle branch block, persistent ST elevation in anterior precordial leads

Correct answer: D

Explanation: Brugada syndrome is diagnosed by incomplete right bundle branch block and persistent ST elevation in the anterior precordial leads. Like long QT syndrome, many different subtypes of Brugada syndrome affect cardiac repolarization and can result in cardiac sudden death from polymorphic ventricular tachycardia and ventricular fibrillation. A short PR interval and broad QRS complexes (delta waves) are seen in Wolff-Parkinson-White syndrome. Arrhythmogenic right ventricular dysplasia is identified by right axis deviation, dominant R wave in V1, and epsilon wave after each QRS complex. Overdose of Na^+-blocking agents or tricyclic antidepressants can result with excessive Na^+ blockade, characterized by broad QRS complexes, dominant R' wave in aVR, and borderline first-degree atrioventricular block.

References:

1. Fox AA, Sharma S, Mounsey JP, et al. Chapter 8: Molecular and Genetic Cardiovascular Medicine. In: Kaplan JA, Augoustides JGT, Manecke GR, et al., eds. Kaplan's Cardiac Anesthesia. 7th ed. Elsevier; 2017: 206-230.
2. Vanneman MW, Madhok J, Weimer JM, et al. Perioperative implications of the 2020 American Heart Association scientific statement on drug-induced arrhythmias: a focused review. J Cardiothorac Vasc Anesth, 2022; 36: 952-961.

15. Phosphorylation is an important step in which receptors?
  A. Protein tyrosine kinase receptors
  B. G-protein–coupled receptors
  C. Beta adrenergic receptors
  D. Muscarinic receptors

Correct answer: A

Explanation: Protein tyrosine kinase receptors and G-protein-coupled receptors (GPCRs) are two broad classes of receptors. Protein tyrosine kinase receptors incorporate phosphorylating enzyme activity via ligand binding. GPCRs are much smaller than protein tyrosine kinase receptors, and ligand binding results in activation of an associated protein (G protein). Beta-adrenergic receptors, alpha-adrenergic receptors, muscarinic acetylcholine receptors, adenosine A1 receptors, adenosine triphosphate receptors, histamine H_2 receptors, vasoactive intestinal peptide receptors, and angiotensin II receptors are all examples of GPCRs.

References:

1. Fox AA, Sharma S, Mounsey JP, et al. Chapter 8: Molecular and Genetic Cardiovascular Medicine. In: Kaplan JA, Augoustides JGT, Manecke GR, et al., eds. Kaplan's Cardiac Anesthesia. 7th ed. Elsevier; 2017: 206-230.
2. Hubbard SR, Till JH. Protein tyrosine kinase structure and function. Annu Rev Biochem, 2000; 69: 373-398.

16. What G protein subunit allows for activation of a G-protein–coupled receptor?
  A. α
  B. β
  C. γ
  D. $\beta\gamma$

Correct answer: A

Explanation: G proteins are heterotrimeric, consisting of α, β, and γ subunits. The β and γ subunits are closely associated and commonly referred to as a singular $\beta\gamma$ subunit. The α subunit contains the guanosine diphosphate (GDP)-guanosine triphosphate (GTP) binding domain. It also possesses hydrolytic activity, which allows for conversion of GDP to GTP, as well as subsequent activation and facilitation of functions within the cell until inactivation by hydrolysis of GTP back to GDP. The $\beta\gamma$ subunit can also have activation features, but not to the extent of the α subunit. There are several classes of heterotrimeric G proteins, indicated by their respective subscripts.

> **BOX 8.1 G protein classes**
>
> - G_s: activates adenylate cyclase
> - G_i: inhibits adenylate cyclase
> - G_q: activates phospholipase C
> - G_o: subtype of G_i, found mostly in brain; activates phospholipase C
> - G_k: subtype of G_i, linked to K^+ channels

References:

1. Fox AA, Sharma S, Mounsey JP, et al. Chapter 8: Molecular and Genetic Cardiovascular Medicine. In: Kaplan JA, Augoustides JGT, Manecke GR, et al., eds. Kaplan's Cardiac Anesthesia. 7th ed. Elsevier; 2017: 206-230.
2. Duc NM, Kim HR, Chung KY. Structural mechanism of G protein activation by G protein-coupled receptor. Eur J Pharmacol, 2015; 763: 214-222.

17. Beta-adrenergic stimulation leads to increases in cardiac contractility via:
  A. Increases in cyclic adenosine monophosphate levels
  B. Increases in cyclic guanosine monophosphate levels
  C. Increases in inositol-1,4,5-triphosphate levels
  D. Increases in diacylglycerol levels

Correct answer: A

Explanation: Both β_1- and β_2-receptors in the heart lead to increased cardiac contractility by initially coupling to G proteins. This activates adenylate cyclase, leading to increased levels of cyclic adenosine monophosphate (cAMP). The inotropic and electrophysiologic effects of beta-adrenergic stimulation are indirect results of the elevated levels of cAMP, which activates a specific protein kinase capable of phosphorylating several important cardiac ion channels. By altering channel functioning, phosphorylation causes changes in cell membrane electrophysiology that modifies myocardial activity. Beta-adrenergic stimulation has not primarily been associated with increases in cyclic guanosine monophosphate, inositol triphosphate, or diacylglycerol with respect to increases in cardiac contractility.

References:

1. Fox AA, Sharma S, Mounsey JP, et al. Chapter 8: Molecular and Genetic Cardiovascular Medicine. In: Kaplan JA, Augoustides JGT, Manecke GR, et al., eds. Kaplan's Cardiac Anesthesia. 7th ed. Elsevier; 2017: 206-230.

2. Harding SE, Brown LA, Wynne DG, et al. Mechanisms of beta adrenoceptor desensitization in the failing human heart. Cardiovasc Res, 1994; 28: 1451-1460.

18. What is the relative ratio of β_1- to β_2-receptors in the heart under normal conditions?
  A. 70:30
  B. 60:40
  C. 40:60
  D. 30:70

Correct answer: A

Explanation: Under normal conditions, the relative ratio of β_1- to β_2-receptors in the heart is roughly 70:30. However, this ratio may change significantly with underlying cardiac disease. Dramatic increases in cardiac output are capable with β-receptor stimulation as a component of the "fight-or-flight" response, but these effects are only beneficial in the short term. Prolonged adrenergic stimulation results in adverse effects on the heart and, ultimately, leads to myocardial cell death and cardiac failure. A primary mechanism for decreasing β-receptor functioning is the downregulation of receptors. In heart failure, receptor levels may be reduced by as much as 50%, with β_1-receptors downregulating more than β_2-receptors. Therefore, the ratio of β_1- to β_2-receptors typically changes to approximately 3:2 in patients with heart failure.

References:

1. Fox AA, Sharma S, Mounsey JP, et al. Chapter 8: Molecular and Genetic Cardiovascular Medicine. In: Kaplan JA, Augoustides JGT, Manecke GR, et al., eds. Kaplan's Cardiac Anesthesia. 7th ed. Elsevier; 2017: 206-230.
2. Harding SE, Brown LA, Wynne DG, et al. Mechanisms of beta adrenoceptor desensitization in the failing human heart. Cardiovasc Res 1994; 28: 1451-1460

19. The stimulation of α_2-receptors results in which of the following consequences?
  A. Decreased diacylglycerol levels
  B. Decreased inositol-1,4,5-triphosphate levels
  C. Decreased cyclic adenosine monophosphate levels
  D. Decreased cyclic guanosine monophosphate levels

Correct answer: C

Explanation: The alpha-adrenergic receptors consist of both α_1- and α_2-receptors. The α_1-receptors couple to G proteins to activate phospholipase C, which leads to an increase in intracellular calcium concentrations. The α_2-receptors couple to G proteins to inhibit adenylate cyclase, which leads to reduced concentrations of intracellular cyclic adenosine monophosphate.

References:

1. Fox AA, Sharma S, Mounsey JP, et al. Chapter 8: Molecular and Genetic Cardiovascular Medicine. In: Kaplan JA, Augoustides JGT, Manecke GR, et al., eds. Kaplan's Cardiac Anesthesia. 7th ed. Elsevier; 2017: 206-230.

2. Seyrek M, Halici Z, Yildiz O, et al. Interaction between dexmedetomidine and α-adrenergic receptors: emphasis on vascular actions. J Cardiothorac Vasc Anesth, 2011; 25: 856-862.

20. Which of the following is true regarding the distribution of muscarinic receptors in the heart?
  A. Most of the muscarinic receptors are present in the atria
  B. Most of the muscarinic receptors are present in the ventricles
  C. Muscarinic receptors are distributed evenly in the both the atria and ventricles
  D. No muscarinic receptors are present in the ventricles

Correct answer: A

Explanation: There are five types of muscarinic receptors; however, only one type (M_2) is present in cardiac tissue. Most muscarinic receptors are found in the atria. Although the ventricles are innervated by the vagus nerve, muscarinic receptors are found in lower concentrations in the ventricles than the atria. The atria contain typically have about twice the concentration of muscarinic receptors as the ventricles. Therefore, as a result of this differential concentration, the primary function of cardiac muscarinic signaling involves heart rate control via actions at the atrial level.

References:

1. Fox AA, Sharma S, Mounsey JP, et al. Chapter 8: Molecular and Genetic Cardiovascular Medicine. In: Kaplan JA, Augoustides JGT, Manecke GR, et al., eds. Kaplan's Cardiac Anesthesia. 7th ed. Elsevier; 2017: 206-230.
2. Deighton NM, Motomura S, Borquez D, et al. Muscarinic cholinoceptors in the human heart: demonstration, subclassification, and distribution. Naunyn Schmiedebergs Arch Pharmacol, 1990; 341: 14-21.
3. Bertolizio G, Yuki K, Odegard K, et al. Cardiac arrest and neuromuscular blockade reversal agents in the transplanted heart. J Cardiothorac Vasc Anesth, 2013; 27: 1374-1378.

21. In a patient with Wolf-Parkinson-White syndrome, what is the most appropriate first-line medication to treat orthodromic atrioventricular re-entrant tachycardia?
  A. Lidocaine
  B. Adenosine
  C. Flecainide
  D. Sotalol

Correct answer: B

Explanation: Orthodromic atrioventricular re-entrant tachycardia is the most common type of arrhythmia encountered in patients with Wolf-Parkinson-White syndrome. It is a regular, narrow, re-entrant tachycardia in which a closed loop of conduction is formed and continues until block occurs in the tachycardia circuit. In this syndrome, the weakest link in the conducting pathway is the atrioventricular node, so increasing refractoriness at this location will terminate the tachycardia. Adenosine is the best first-line pharmacologic agent of the given choices to treat this tachycardia in a titrated fashion to terminate the arrhythmia. By inhibiting adenylate cyclase, adenosine lowers cyclic adenosine monophosphate levels to increase cellular potassium efflux, and subsequently causes cell hyperpolarization. This leads to an increased refractory period at the atrioventricular node.

References:

1. Fox AA, Sharma S, Mounsey JP, et al. Chapter 8: Molecular and Genetic Cardiovascular Medicine. In: Kaplan JA, Augoustides JGT, Manecke GR, et al., eds. Kaplan's Cardiac Anesthesia. 7th ed. Elsevier; 2017: 206-230.
2. Bengali R, Wellens HJJ, Jian Y. Perioperative management of the Wolff-Parkinson-White syndrome. J Cardiothorac Vasc Anesth, 2014; 28: 1375-1386.

22. Which of the following conditions represents a cardiovascular disorder caused directly by a single gene defect?
    A. Coronary artery disease
    B. Hypertension
    C. Atherosclerosis
    D. Hypertrophic cardiomyopathy

Correct answer: D

Explanation: Cardiovascular disorders with a genetic bases are divided into two groups: monogenic and multigenic disorders. In monogenic disorders such as hypertrophic cardiomyopathy, changes in a single gene are implicated in the disease, which usually shows a characteristic inheritance pattern. Multigenic disorders, such as hypertension, coronary artery disease, and atherosclerosis, are characterized by an etiology in which multiple genes influence the disease process. They are more common than monogenic disorders. In these multigenic disorders, a collection of genetic variants interact to enhance disease susceptibility and/or augment the impact of environmental risk factors on the disease process.

BOX 8.2 Examples of important cardiovascular disorders with a genetic basis

- Monogenic disorders
  - Familial hypercholesterolemia
  - Hypertrophic cardiomyopathy
  - Dilated cardiomyopathy
  - Long QT syndrome
- Multigenic disorders
  - Coronary artery disease
  - Hypertension
  - Atherosclerosis

References:

1. Fox AA, Sharma S, Mounsey JP, et al. Chapter 8: Molecular and Genetic Cardiovascular Medicine. In: Kaplan JA, Augoustides JGT, Manecke GR, et al., eds. Kaplan's Cardiac Anesthesia. 7th ed. Elsevier; 2017: 206-230.
2. Fokstuen S, Makrythanasis P, Nikolaev S, et al. Multiplex targeted high-throughput sequencing for mendelian cardiac disorders. Clin Genet, 2014; 85: 365-370.

23. On an electrocardiogram, the sum of ventricular depolarization and repolarization is represented by which of the following intervals?
    A. QRS complex
    B. QT interval
    C. RR interval
    D. Peak of the T wave to the end of T wave interval (TPE)

Correct answer: B

Explanation: The QT interval represents the sum of ventricular depolarization and repolarization and is measured from the beginning of the QRS complex to the end of the T-wave. It is inversely proportional to heart rate and is often corrected (QTc) to a standardized heart rate of 60 beats/minute to improve diagnostic utility. The Bazett formula is the most common method of QTc calculation and is represented as follows:

$$QTc = QT/ (RR\ interval)^{1/2}$$

The normal values for the QT interval depend on both age and gender, with QTc prolongation defined as 450 ms or more in men and 460 ms or more in women.

References:

1. Fox AA, Sharma S, Mounsey JP, et al. Chapter 8: Molecular and Genetic Cardiovascular Medicine. In: Kaplan JA, Augoustides JGT, Manecke GR, et al., eds. Kaplan's Cardiac Anesthesia. 7th ed. Elsevier; 2017: 206-230.
2. Niimi N, Yuki K, Zaleski K. Long QT syndrome and perioperative torsades de pointes: what the anesthesiologist should know. J Cardiothorac Vasc Anesth, 2022; 36: 286-302.

24. Which of the following drugs is considered safest in patients with the long QT syndrome?
    A. Methadone
    B. Ketamine
    C. Propofol
    D. Droperidol

Correct answer: C

Explanation: Numerous classes of medications prolong the QT interval. Some of the most well-known drugs causing this effect are the Vaughan Williams class IA and III antiarrhythmic agents, including disopyramide, quinidine, procainamide, sotalol, ibutilide, dofetilide, and amiodarone. Further examples of QT-prolonging medications commonly encountered in the perioperative setting include ondansetron, droperidol, depolarizing neuromuscular relaxants, methadone, ketamine, and anticholinesterase/anticholinergic drugs such as glycopyrrolate, atropine, and neostigmine.

Common perioperative medications that may be safely administered to patients with long QT syndrome include fentanyl, remifentanil, morphine, midazolam, propofol, etomidate, nondepolarizing neuromuscular relaxants, sugammadex, and dexamethasone.

References:

1. Fox AA, Sharma S, Mounsey JP, et al. Chapter 8: Molecular and Genetic Cardiovascular Medicine. In: Kaplan JA, Augoustides JGT, Manecke GR, et al., eds. Kaplan's Cardiac Anesthesia. 7th ed. Elsevier; 2017: 206-230.
2. Niimi N, Yuki K, Zaleski K. Long QT syndrome and perioperative torsades de pointes: what the anesthesiologist should know. J Cardiothorac Vasc Anesth, 2022; 36: 286-302.

25. Regarding drugs that prolong the QT interval, what is the most well-established mechanism for causing QT prolongation?
   A. Blockade of rapid component of delayed rectifier K^+ current
   B. Blockade of inward Na^+ current
   C. Activation of slow inward Ca^{2+} current
   D. Disruption of balance between K^+ and Ca^{2+} currents

Correct answer: A

Explanation: At the level of the ion channel, myocardial repolarization is primarily mediated by the efflux of potassium. There are two subtypes of a delayed rectifier K^+ current (I_{Kr} [rapid] and I_{Ks} [slow]) that are responsible for repolarization. Almost all drugs that prolong the QT interval block the rapid component of the delayed rectifier K^+ current. Importantly, acquired long QT syndrome and torsades de pointes are triggered at low heart rates.

References:

1. Fox AA, Sharma S, Mounsey JP, et al. Chapter 8: Molecular and Genetic Cardiovascular Medicine. In: Kaplan JA, Augoustides JGT, Manecke GR, et al., eds. Kaplan's Cardiac Anesthesia. 7th ed. Elsevier; 2017: 206-230.
2. Ramakrishna H, O'Hare M, Mookadam F, et al. Sudden cardiac death and disorders of the QT interval: anesthetic implications and focus on perioperative management. J Cardiothorac Vasc Anesth, 2015; 29: 1723-1733.

26. Which of the following agents has been demonstrated to have little to no effect on the QT interval?
   A. Isoflurane
   B. Sevoflurane
   C. Fentanyl
   D. Ketamine

Correct answer: C

Explanation: All volatile anesthetics cause QT prolongation via inhibition of the delayed rectifier K^+ currents. These effects on the QT interval are independent of their other physiologic effects on the autonomic nervous system. However, it is generally agreed that volatile anesthetics are usually safe in patients with long QT syndrome, with an important caveat that these patients receive beta-blockers throughout the perioperative period. Isoflurane is the recommended agent of choice in this scenario. Fentanyl has minimal effects on the QT interval. Ketamine may prolong the QT interval.

References:

1. Fox AA, Sharma S, Mounsey JP, et al. Chapter 8: Molecular and Genetic Cardiovascular Medicine. In: Kaplan JA, Augoustides JGT, Manecke GR, et al., eds. Kaplan's Cardiac Anesthesia. 7th ed. Elsevier; 2017: 206-230.
2. Ramakrishna H, O'Hare M, Mookadam F, et al. Sudden cardiac death and disorders of the QT interval: anesthetic implications and focus on perioperative management. J Cardiothorac Vasc Anesth, 2015; 29: 1723-1733.

27. Of the following agents, which plays the most significant role in myocardial preconditioning?
   A. Procainamide
   B. Adenosine
   C. Amiodarone
   D. Sotalol

Correct answer: B

Explanation: Myocardial preconditioning describes the phenomenon in which temporary exposure of the myocardium to ischemia allows it to better withstand subsequent exposure to longer durations of ischemia. Adenosine, an effective antiarrhythmic drug, has also been shown to play an important role in various adaptive and protective responses to ischemia. It may serve as both a trigger and mediator of cardioprotection. Additionally, it is a coronary vasodilator, and its platelet blocker effects help to maintain the patency of the myocardial microvasculature during reperfusion. Its negative inotropic and chronotropic effects also reduce myocardial oxygen demand, allowing for the replenishment of adenosine triphosphate. Procainamide, amiodarone, and sotalol do not typically have a major role in myocardial preconditioning.

References:

1. Fox AA, Sharma S, Mounsey JP, et al. Chapter 8: Molecular and Genetic Cardiovascular Medicine. In: Kaplan JA, Augoustides JGT, Manecke GR, et al., eds. Kaplan's Cardiac Anesthesia. 7th ed. Elsevier; 2017: 206-230.
2. Ammar A, Mahmoud K, Elkersh A, et al. A randomized controlled trial of intra-aortic adenosine infusion before release of the aortic cross-clamp during coronary artery bypass surgery. J Cardiothorac Vasc Anesth, 2018; 32: 2520-2527.

28. Which of the following conditions is characterized by an increased calcium sensitivity at the cellular level?
   A. Dilated cardiomyopathy
   B. Long QT syndrome
   C. Hypertrophic cardiomyopathy
   D. Brugada syndrome

Correct answer: C

Explanation: Genetic causes of hypertrophic cardiomyopathy include single-point mutations, insertion or deletion mutations, or truncation of myocardial filament proteins. Although the definitive molecular mechanisms leading to disease progression are incompletely understood, increased calcium sensitivity is a universal feature of the disease. At the molecular level in hypertrophic cardiomyopathy, increased cross-bridging enhances force generation, with consequent hypercontractility. This calcium sensitization and resulting hypercontractility are a major stimulus for disease development and the phenotypic expression in hypertrophic cardiomyopathy.

References:

1. Fox AA, Sharma S, Mounsey JP, et al. Chapter 8: Molecular and Genetic Cardiovascular Medicine. In: Kaplan JA, Augoustides JGT, Manecke GR, et al., eds. Kaplan's Cardiac Anesthesia. 7th ed. Elsevier; 2017: 206-230.
2. Ren X, Hensley N, Brady MB, et al. The genetic and molecular bases for hypertrophic cardiomyopathy: the role for calcium sensitization. J Cardiothorac Vasc Anesth, 2018; 32: 478-487.

29. Drug-induced bradycardia requiring treatment with atropine or glycopyrrolate is most likely to occur with which of the following medications?
    A. Ketamine
    B. Morphine
    C. Isoflurane
    D. Dexmedetomidine

Correct answer: D

Explanation: Dexmedetomidine, a central α_2-receptor agonist, may cause bradycardia due to hyperpolarization of noradrenergic neurons, reduced firing, and suppression of norepinephrine release. A multicenter trial in adult noncardiac surgery demonstrated that dexmedetomidine infusion raises the risk of symptomatic bradycardia requiring prompt intervention. Severe bradycardia is not typically associated with ketamine, morphine, or isoflurane.

References:

1. Fox AA, Sharma S, Mounsey JP, et al. Chapter 8: Molecular and Genetic Cardiovascular Medicine. In: Kaplan JA, Augoustides JGT, Manecke GR, et al., eds. Kaplan's Cardiac Anesthesia. 7th ed. Elsevier; 2017: 206-230.
2. Vanneman MW, Madhok J, Weimer JM, et al. Perioperative implications of the 2020 American Heart Association scientific statement on drug-induced arrhythmias: a focused review. J Cardiothorac Vasc Anesth, 2022; 36: 952-961.
3. Beloeil H, Garot M, Lebuffe G, et al. Balanced opioid-free anesthesia with dexmedetomidine versus balanced anesthesia with remifentanil for major or intermediate noncardiac surgery. Anesthesiology, 2021; 134: 541-551.

30. Which of the following ion channel types is most significantly affected by volatile anesthetic agents?
    A. Sodium
    B. Potassium
    C. Calcium
    D. Magnesium

Correct answer: C

Explanation: The cardiac ion channels most significantly affected by volatile anesthetic agents are the voltage-gated calcium channels. Almost all volatile agents inhibit L-type calcium channels. This inhibition is modest, typically in the 25% to 30% range at a 1 minimum alveolar concentration. Although modest, this effect is substantial enough to account for volatile anesthetic–induced physiologic changes.

References:

1. Fox AA, Sharma S, Mounsey JP, et al. Chapter 8: Molecular and Genetic Cardiovascular Medicine. In: Kaplan JA, Augoustides JGT, Manecke GR, et al., eds. Kaplan's Cardiac Anesthesia. 7th ed. Elsevier; 2017: 206-230.
2. Pagel PS, Crystal GJ. The discovery of myocardial preconditioning using volatile anesthetics: a history and contemporary clinical perspective. J Cardiothorac Vasc Anesth, 2018; 32: 1112-1134.

CHAPTER 9

Systemic Inflammation

J. Bradley Meers and Matthew M. Townsley

KEY POINTS

1. Mortality and morbidity are relatively common after major surgical procedures.
2. Postoperative morbidity often involves multiple organ systems, and this implies a systemic process.
3. Excessive systemic inflammation is proposed to be a cause of postoperative organ dysfunction.
4. No interventions that attenuate systemic inflammation have been proved in large, randomized clinical trials to protect patients from morbidity and mortality.

---

1. A 76-year-old man undergoes coronary artery bypass grafting with aortic valve replacement. Which of the following estimates is closest to the rate of complications in patients over the age of 75 years undergoing these cardiac surgical procedures?
   A. 5%
   B. 10%
   C. 25%
   D. 50%

Correct Answer: D

Explanation: Review of "all-comers" undergoing coronary artery bypass grafting or aortic valve surgery who were in the Medicare Claims Database demonstrated a 30-day all-cause mortality rate of 4% to 4.5% after coronary artery bypass grafting and 6.5% to 9.1% after aortic valve replacement. A report by Rady and colleagues about a large series of patients 75 years of age or older who underwent cardiac surgical procedures demonstrated a mortality rate of 8% and a serious complication rate that exceeded 50%. The postoperative complications include delirium, stroke, atrial fibrillation, ventricular dysfunction requiring inotropic agents, acute lung injury, infection, gastrointestinal injuries, and renal dysfunction.

References:

1. Whitlock R, Benett-Guerrero E, Augoustides JGT, Kaplan JA. Chapter 9: Systemic Inflammation. In: Kaplan JA, Augoustides JGT, Manecke GR, et al., eds. Kaplan's Cardiac Anesthesia. 7th ed. Elsevier; 2017:231-246.
2. Rady MY, Ryan T, Starr NJ. Perioperative determinants of morbidity and mortality in elderly patients undergoing cardiac surgery. Crit Care Med, 1998; 26: 225-235.
3. Birkmeyer JD, Stukel TA, Siewers AE, et al. Surgeon volume and operative mortality in the United States. N Engl J Med, 2003; 349: 2117-2127.

2. The diagnostic criteria for systemic inflammatory response syndrome include which of the following?
   A. Heart rate greater than 80 beats per minute
   B. Respiratory rate greater than 20 breaths per minute or $PaCO_2$ less than 32 mmHg
   C. Temperature over 37.5°C
   D. Positive blood cultures

Correct Answer: B

Explanation: The systemic inflammatory response syndrome (SIRS) is a systemic response to a variety of severe clinical insults that is manifested by two or more of the following criteria: (1) temperature over 38°C or under 36°C; (2) heart rate over 90 beats/minute; (3) respiratory rate over 20 breaths/minute or $PaCO_2$ under 32 mmHg; and (4) white blood cell count greater than 12,000/mm³, or less than 4,000/mm³, or more than 10% immune (band) forms. Because infection is not a prerequisite for the development of this inflammation, the criteria for SIRS do not require the presence of infection. Systemic inflammation is a spectrum ranging from mild severity without organ dysfunction to a more severe syndrome characterized by multisystem organ failure and death. Although most patients fulfill the criteria for SIRS after a major surgical procedure, most of these patients do not develop clinically significant organ dysfunction from systemic inflammation.

References:

1. Whitlock R, Benett-Guerrero E, Augoustides JGT, Kaplan JA. Chapter 9: Systemic Inflammation. In: Kaplan JA, Augoustides JGT, Manecke GR, et al., eds. Kaplan's Cardiac Anesthesia. 7th ed. Elsevier; 2017:231-246.
2. Squiccimarro E, Labriola C, Malvindi PG, et al. Prevalence and clinical impact of systemic inflammatory reaction after cardiac surgery. J Cardiothorac Vasc Anesth, 2019; 6: 1682-1690.

3. Sepsis is distinguished from systemic inflammatory response syndrome by which of the following?
   A. Elevated white blood cell count
   B. Hypotension
   C. Infection
   D. Temperature higher than 38°C

Correct Answer: C

Explanation: Sepsis is a systemic response to infection manifested by two or more of the following conditions in response to infection: (1) temperature over 38°C or under 36°C; (2) heart rate over 90 beats/minute; (3) respiratory rate over 20 breaths/minute or $PaCO_2$ under 32 mmHg; and (4) white blood cell count greater than 12,000/mm^3, less than 4,000/mm^3, or more than 10% immune (band) forms. The presence of infection distinguishes sepsis from the systemic inflammatory response syndrome. The interrelations between infection, sepsis, and the systemic inflammatory syndrome are outlined in the box.

BOX 9.1 Definitions related to inflammation

- Infection: microbial phenomenon characterized by an inflammatory response to the presence of microorganisms or the invasion of normally sterile host tissue by those organisms
- Bacteremia: presence of viable bacteria in the blood
- Systemic inflammatory response syndrome (SIRS): systemic inflammatory response to a variety of severe clinical insults that is manifested by two or more of the following conditions: (1) temperature >38°C or <36°C; (2) heart rate >90 beats/minute; (3) respiratory rate >20 breaths/minute or $PaCO_2$ <32 mmHg; and (4) white blood cell count >12,000/mm^3, <4,000/mm^3, or >10% immature (band) forms
- Sepsis: systemic response to infection, manifested by two or more of the following conditions as a result of infection: (1) temperature >38°C or <36°C; (2) heart rate >90 beats/minute; (3) respiratory rate >20 breaths/minute or $PaCO_2$ <32 mmHg; and white blood cell count >12,000/mm^3, <4,000/mm^3, or >10% immune (band) forms

From Bone RC, Balk RA, Cerra FB, et al. Definitions for sepsis and organ failure and guidelines for the use of innovative therapies in sepsis: ACCP/SCCM consensus conference. Chest. 1992;101:1644–1655.

References:

1. Whitlock R, Benett-Guerrero E, Augoustides JGT, Kaplan JA. Chapter 9: Systemic Inflammation. In: Kaplan JA, Augoustides JGT, Manecke GR, et al., eds. Kaplan's Cardiac Anesthesia. 7th ed. Elsevier; 2017:231-246.
2. Squiccimarro E, Labriola C, Malvindi PG, et al. Prevalence and clinical impact of systemic inflammatory reaction after cardiac surgery. J Cardiothorac Vasc Anesth 2019; 6: 1682-1690

4. Sepsis-induced hypotension is defined by what reduction of systolic blood pressure from baseline in the absence of other cases of hypotension?
   A. 40 mmHg or higher
   B. 30 mmHg or higher
   C. 20 mmHg or higher
   D. 10 mmHg or higher

Correct answer: A

Explanation: Sepsis-induced hypotension is defined as systolic blood pressure under 90 mmHg or reduction of 40 mmHg or more from baseline in the absence of other causes of hypotension. Severe sepsis is defined as sepsis associated with organ dysfunction, hypoperfusion, or hypotension. Hypoperfusion and perfusion abnormalities may include, but are not limited to, lactic acidosis, oliguria, or an acute alteration in mental status. Patients who are receiving inotropic or vasopressor agents may not be hypotensive at the time that perfusion abnormalities are measured.

References:

1. Whitlock R, Benett-Guerrero E, Augoustides JGT, Kaplan JA. Chapter 9: Systemic Inflammation. In: Kaplan JA, Augoustides JGT, Manecke GR, et al., eds. Kaplan's Cardiac Anesthesia. 7th ed. Elsevier; 2017:231-246.
2. Paternoster G, Guarracino F. Sepsis after cardiac surgery: from pathophysiology to management. J Cardiothorac Vasc Anesth, 2016; 30: 773-780.

5. Which of the following diagnoses can be made without confirming the presence of a viable organism in the blood?
   A. Bacteremia
   B. Endotoxemia
   C. Septicemia
   D. Fungemia

Correct answer: D

Explanation: Whereas bacteremia refers to the presence of viable bacteria in the blood, endotoxemia refers to the presence of endotoxin in the blood. Endotoxin is also known as lipopolysaccharide, a component of the cell membranes of gram-negative bacteria, and its presence does not require the existence of viable organisms. Septicemia occurs from a bacterial blood stream infection and can lead to both sepsis and septic shock. Sepsis is a systemic response to infection, manifested by two or more of the following conditions as a result of infection: (1) temperature over 38°C or under 36°C; (2) heart rate over 90 beats/minute; (3) respiratory rate over 20 breaths/minute or $PaCO_2$ less than 32 mmHg; and (4) white blood cell count greater than 12,000/mm^3, less than 4,000/mm^3, or more than 10% immune (band) forms.

References:

1. Whitlock R, Benett-Guerrero E, Augoustides JGT, Kaplan JA. Chapter 9: Systemic Inflammation. In: Kaplan JA, Augoustides JGT, Manecke GR, et al., eds. Kaplan's Cardiac Anesthesia. 7th ed. Elsevier; 2017:231-246.
2. Hill GE, Whitten CW, Landers DF. The influence of cardiopulmonary bypass on cytokines and cell-cell communication. J Cardiothorac Vasc Anesth, 1997; 11: 367-375.
3. Warren OJ, Smith AJ, Alexiou C, et al. The inflammatory response to cardiopulmonary bypass: part 1 – mechanisms of pathogenesis. J Cardiothorac Vasc Anesth, 2009; 23: 222-231.

6. Inflammation-induced cellular injury begins with activation of which of the following leukocytes?
   A. Basophil
   B. Eosinophils
   C. Monocytes
   D. Neutrophils

Correct answer: D

Explanation: Neutrophil activation leads to the release of oxygen radicals, intracellular proteases, and fatty acid metabolites that include arachidonic acid. These products of neutrophil activation can cause or exacerbate tissue injury. Activated neutrophils release granules that contain myeloperoxidase, as well as other toxic digestive enzymes such as neutrophil elastase, lactoferrin, B-glucuronidase, and N-acetyl-b-glycosaminidase. The release of these intracellular enzymes causes tissue damage. Activation of neutrophils also leads to adhesion of leukocytes to the endothelium and formation of clumps of inflammatory cells known as microaggregates. Activated leukocytes have less deformability, and this affects their ability to pass through capillaries. The microaggregates can cause organ dysfunction through microvascular occlusion and reductions in blood flow and oxygen at the local level.

References:

1. Whitlock R, Benett-Guerrero E, Augoustides JGT, Kaplan JA. Chapter 9: Systemic Inflammation. In: Kaplan JA, Augoustides JGT, Manecke GR, et al., eds. Kaplan's Cardiac Anesthesia. 7th ed. Elsevier; 2017:231-246.
2. Squiccimarro E, Labriola C, Malvindi PG, et al. Prevalence and clinical impact of systemic inflammatory reaction after cardiac surgery. J Cardiothorac Vasc Anesth, 2019; 6: 1682-1690.

7. Oxygen free radicals cause cellular damage by which of the following mechanisms?
   A. Damage to the lipid membrane
   B. Producing a localized hypoxic environment
   C. Damage to the mitochondria
   D. Reduction in blood flow

Correct answer: A

Explanation: Oxygen free radicals are thought to cause cellular injury through damage to the lipid membrane. Increased levels of lipid peroxidation products such as malondialdehyde are thought to reflect the severity of free radical cellular damage. Reductions in blood flow and oxygen delivery to localized areas can be seen with micro-occlusion of capillaries by leukocytes following neutrophil activation. The mitochondria produce free radicals as by-products during normal metabolism. The mitochondria reduce oxygen to generate free radical superoxide at various sites in the respiratory chain. It is thought that high levels of free radicals can lead to changes in mitochondrial genetic code over time; this is referred to as the mitochondrial free radical theory of aging.

References:

1. Whitlock R, Benett-Guerrero E, Augoustides JGT, Kaplan JA.. Chapter 9: Systemic Inflammation. In: Kaplan JA, Augoustides

JGT, Manecke GR, et al., eds. Kaplan's Cardiac Anesthesia. 7th ed. Elsevier; 2017:231-246.
2. Lotz C, Kehl F. Volatile anesthetic-induced cardiac protection: molecular mechanisms, clinical aspects, and interactions with non-volatile agents. J Cardiothorac Vasc Anesth, 2015; 29: 749-760.
3. Gutierrez J, Ballinger SW, Darley-Usmar VM, et al. Free radicals, mitochondria, and oxidized lipids: the emerging role in signal transduction in vascular cells. Circ Res 2006, 99: 924-932.

8. Which of the following is an effect of leukotrienes?
   A. Arteriolar vasodilation
   B. Increased vascular permeability
   C. Reduced localized edema
   D. Bronchodilation

Correct answer: B

Explanation: Activated leukocytes release leukotrienes, such as leukotriene B4. Leukotrienes are arachidonic acid metabolites generated by the lipoxygenase pathway. They markedly increase vascular permeability and are potent arteriolar vasoconstrictors. These effects account for some of the clinical signs of systemic inflammation, such as generalized edema as well as third space losses. Leukotrienes lead to smooth muscle contraction and can cause bronchoconstriction. Prostaglandins are also generated from arachidonic acid through the cyclooxygenase pathway and act as mediators of the inflammatory process.

References:

1. Whitlock R, Benett-Guerrero E, Augoustides JGT, Kaplan JA. Chapter 9: Systemic Inflammation. In: Kaplan JA, Augoustides JGT, Manecke GR, et al., eds. Kaplan's Cardiac Anesthesia. 7th ed. Elsevier; 2017:231-246.
2. Greeley WJ, Leslie JB, Reves JG. Prostaglandins and the cardiovascular system: a review and update. J Cardiothorac Vasc Anesth, 1987; 1: 331-349.
3. Warren OJ, Smith AJ, Alexiou C, et al. The inflammatory response to cardiopulmonary bypass: part 1 – mechanisms of pathogenesis. J Cardiothorac Vasc Anesth, 2009; 23: 222-231.

9. Which cytokine subtype aids in the communication between white blood cells?
   A. Chemokines
   B. Interferons
   C. Interleukins
   D. Tumor necrosis factor

Correct answer: C

Explanation: Cytokines are proteins released from activated macrophages, monocytes, fibroblasts, and endothelial cells that bind to specific cell-surface receptors. The effects of cytokines are far-reaching. Interleukins are a type of cytokine that aids in communication between leukocytes. Chemokines are a subgroup of cytokines that mediate the attraction of immune system cells to local areas of injury or infection. Interferons are signaling proteins made in response to the presence of viruses. Tumor necrosis factor is an inflammatory cytokine produced by macrophages and monocytes during acute inflammation and is responsible for a diverse range of signaling events within the cell leading to necrosis and apoptosis.

References:

1. Whitlock R, Benett-Guerrero E, Augoustides JGT, Kaplan JA. Chapter 9: Systemic Inflammation. In: Kaplan JA, Augoustides JGT, Manecke GR, et al., eds. Kaplan's Cardiac Anesthesia. 7th ed. Elsevier; 2017:231-246.
2. Hill GE, Whitten CW, Landers DF. The influence of cardiopulmonary bypass on cytokines and cell-cell communication. J Cardiothorac Vasc Anesth, 1997; 11: 367-375.
3. Warren OJ, Smith AJ, Alexiou C, et al. The inflammatory response to cardiopulmonary bypass: part 1 – mechanisms of pathogenesis. J Cardiothorac Vasc Anesth, 2009; 23: 222-231.

10. In the cardiac surgical patient, levels of which of the following cytokines are elevated following a proinflammatory stimulus and then quickly disappear?
   A. Tumor necrosis factor
   B. Interleukin-2
   C. Interleukin-6
   D. Interleukin-8

Correct answer: A

Explanation: Tumor necrosis factor (TNF) is one of the earliest cytokines detected in the blood after activation of macrophages and other proinflammatory cells. It has been demonstrated that the peak concentration of TNF correlates with increased temperature and heart rate, as well as circulating levels of adrenocorticotropic hormone and epinephrine. TNF levels are not increased when they are measured in patients with systemic inflammation. The reason for this is likely because test samples are obtained long after exposure to the primary inflammatory stimulus. This issue of sampling time may partially account for the range of TNF levels detected in various cardiac surgical studies. The cytokines that received the most attention related to cardiac surgical procedures include TNF and the interleukins (ILs), including IL-1, IL-6, IL-8, and IL-10.

References:

1. Whitlock R, Benett-Guerrero E, Augoustides JGT, Kaplan JA. Chapter 9: Systemic Inflammation. In: Kaplan JA, Augoustides JGT, Manecke GR, et al., eds. Kaplan's Cardiac Anesthesia. 7th ed. Elsevier; 2017:231-246.
2. Hill GE, Whitten CW, Landers DF. The influence of cardiopulmonary bypass on cytokines and cell-cell communication. J Cardiothorac Vasc Anesth, 1997; 11: 367-375.
3. Warren OJ, Smith AJ, Alexiou C, et al. The inflammatory response to cardiopulmonary bypass: part 1 – mechanisms of pathogenesis. J Cardiothorac Vasc Anesth, 2009; 23: 222-231.

11. Which of the following cytokines increase following the appearance of tumor necrosis factor and may lead to decreased systemic vascular resistance after cardiopulmonary bypass?
   A. Interleukin-10
   B. Interleukin-9
   C. Interleukin-2
   D. Interleukin-1

Correct answer: D

Explanation: Levels of interleukin-1 increase in cardiac surgical patients following the appearance of tumor necrosis factor. Studies have shown that peak levels of this interleukin occur from several hours to 24 hours after cardiopulmonary bypass. This may explain the inability to detect interleukin-1 during the intraoperative period. This interleukin may decrease systemic vascular resistance after cardiopulmonary bypass by induction of nitric oxide synthesis in vascular endothelial cells. Although it appears that interleukin-1 is important in the initiation and propagation of the inflammatory cascade, it is not clear whether its levels serve as a biomarker for organ dysfunction after cardiac operations. Interleukin-10 is a potent inhibitor of the synthesis of tumor necrosis factor. Interleukin- 2 and interleukin-9 have not been extensively studied in the cardiac surgical population.

References:

1. Whitlock R, Benett-Guerrero E, Augoustides JGT, Kaplan JA.. Chapter 9: Systemic Inflammation. In: Kaplan JA, Augoustides JGT, Manecke GR, et al., eds. Kaplan's Cardiac Anesthesia. 7th ed. Elsevier; 2017:231-246.
2. Hill GE, Whitten CW, Landers DF. The influence of cardiopulmonary bypass on cytokines and cell-cell communication. J Cardiothorac Vasc Anesth, 1997; 11: 367-375.
3. Warren OJ, Smith AJ, Alexiou C, et al. The inflammatory response to cardiopulmonary bypass: part 1 – mechanisms of pathogenesis. J Cardiothorac Vasc Anesth, 2009; 23: 222-231.

12. In the cardiac surgical patient, levels of this anti-inflammatory cytokine have been observed to increase at the same time as proinflammatory cytokines decrease:
   A. Interleukin-6
   B. Interleukin-8
   C. Interleukin-10
   D. Tumor necrosis factor

Correct answer: C

Explanation: The regulation of inflammation is complex and involves a balance between proinflammatory and anti-inflammatory cytokines. Interleukin-10 is a potent inhibitor of multiple cytokines, including tumor necrosis factor, interleukin-1, interleukin-6, and interleukin-8. The levels of interleukin-10 increase in the perioperative period. During cardiopulmonary bypass, increases have been observed in the proinflammatory cytokines such as tumor necrosis factor, interleukin-1, and interleukin-8. As proinflammatory cytokines levels decrease, concomitant increases in anti-inflammatory cytokines such as interleukin-10 have been observed. The balancing effects of cytokines may determine whether a patient suffers from the effects of excessive systemic inflammation such as postoperative organ dysfunction or the effects of inadequate immune system function such as post-operative infection and poor wound healing.

References:

1. Whitlock R, Benett-Guerrero E, Augoustides JGT, Kaplan JA. Chapter 9: Systemic Inflammation. In: Kaplan JA, Augoustides JGT, Manecke GR, et al., eds. Kaplan's Cardiac Anesthesia. 7th ed. Elsevier; 2017:231-246.
2. Hill GE, Whitten CW, Landers DF. The influence of cardiopulmonary bypass on cytokines and cell-cell communication. J Cardiothorac Vasc Anesth, 1997; 11: 367-375.
3. Warren OJ, Smith AJ, Alexiou C, et al. The inflammatory response to cardiopulmonary bypass: part 1 – mechanisms of pathogenesis. J Cardiothorac Vasc Anesth, 2009; 23: 222-231.

13. The alternative pathway of the complement system can be activated by which of the following?
   A. Recognition of circulating factor A
   B. Recognition of bacteria or other activating surfaces
   C. Recognition of antigen-antibody complexes
   D. Recognition of tumor necrosis factor

Correct answer: B

Explanation: The complement system includes at least 20 plasma proteins and is involved in the chemoattraction, activation, opsonization, and lysis of cells. The complement cascade can be triggered by either the classic pathway or the alternative pathway. In the alternative pathway, C3 is activated by contact of complement factors B and D with complex polysaccharides or endotoxin, or exposure of blood to foreign substances such as the cardiopulmonary bypass circuit. Contact activation describes contact of blood with a foreign surface, with resulting adherence of platelets and activation of factor XII (Hageman factor). The classic pathway involves activation of C1 by antibody-antigen complexes. Administration of protamine after separation from CPB has been reported to result in heparin-protamine complexes, which can activate the classic pathway.

References:

1. Whitlock R, Benett-Guerrero E, Augoustides JGT, Kaplan JA. Chapter 9: Systemic Inflammation. In: Kaplan JA, Augoustides JGT, Manecke GR, et al., eds. Kaplan's Cardiac Anesthesia. 7th ed. Elsevier; 2017:231-246.
2. Knudsen F, Andersen PT, Nielsen LK, Jersild C. Complement and leukocyte changes during major vascular surgery. J Cardiothorac Vasc Anesth, 1988; 2: 646-649.
3. Warren OJ, Smith AJ, Alexiou C, et al. The inflammatory response to cardiopulmonary bypass: part 1 – mechanisms of pathogenesis. J Cardiothorac Vasc Anesth, 2009; 23: 222-231.

14. Which of the following are also known as anaphylatoxins?
   A. C3a and C5a
   B. C7a and C9a
   C. C1a and C2a
   D. C4a and C6a

Correct answer: A

Explanation: Activated complement exhibits effects upon mast cells and basophils. Fragments of C3a and C5a (also called anaphylatoxins) lead to release of numerous mediators, including histamine, leukotriene B4, platelet-activating factor, prostaglandins, thromboxanes, and tumor necrosis factor. Complement factors, such as C3b and C5a, complex with microbes and stimulate macrophages to secrete inflammatory mediators. C3b activates neutrophils and macrophages and enhances their ability to phagocytose bacteria. Activated complement factors make invading cells "sticky" such that they bind to one another in a process known as agglutination. The complement-mediated process of capillary dilation, leakage of plasma proteins and fluid, and accumulation and activation of neutrophils make up part of the acute inflammatory response.

References:

1. Whitlock R, Benett-Guerrero E, Augoustides JGT, Kaplan JA. Chapter 9: Systemic Inflammation. In: Kaplan JA, Augoustides JGT, Manecke GR, et al., eds. Kaplan's Cardiac Anesthesia. 7th ed. Elsevier; 2017:231-246.
2. Bengtson A, Millocco I, Heideman M, et al. Altered concentrations of terminal complement complexes, anaphylatoxins, and leukotrienes in the coronary sinus during cardiopulmonary bypass. J Cardiothorac Vasc Anesth, 1989; 3: 305-310.
3. Warren OJ, Smith AJ, Alexiou C, et al. The inflammatory response to cardiopulmonary bypass: part 1 – mechanisms of pathogenesis. J Cardiothorac Vasc Anesth, 2009; 23: 222-231.

15. Evidence suggests that which of the following procedures results in a minimal increase in measurable activated complement?
   A. Acute aortic dissection repair with circulatory arrest
   B. Aortic valve replacement
   C. On-pump coronary artery bypass grafting
   D. Off-pump coronary artery bypass grafting

Correct answer: D

Explanation: Significant evidence demonstrates an increase in complement activation during cardiopulmonary bypass (CPB). Regarding operations in which CPB was not used, C3a levels in 116 patients undergoing cardiac operations with CPB and 12 patients undergoing operations without CPB were examined. Patients undergoing procedures without CPB did not demonstrate increases in complement, suggesting that factors unique to CPB cause activation of complement. In several large randomized clinical trials, complement activation was selectively blocked but did not appear to have an impact on complications such as pulmonary and renal dysfunction and severe vasodilation. These results suggest that complement activation may not play as large a role in the development of systemic inflammation-mediated morbidity as previously thought.

References:

1. Whitlock R, Benett-Guerrero E, Augoustides JGT, Kaplan JA. Chapter 9: Systemic Inflammation. In: Kaplan JA, Augoustides JGT, Manecke GR, et al., eds. Kaplan's Cardiac Anesthesia. 7th ed. Elsevier; 2017:231-246.
2. Segal H, Sheikh S, Kallis P, et al. Complement activation during major surgery: the effect of extracorporeal circuits and high-dose aprotinin. J Cardiothorac Vasc Anesth, 1998; 12: 542-547.

3. Shaefi S, Mittel A, Loberman D, et al. Off-pump versus on-pump coronary artery bypass grafting: a systematic review and analysis of clinical outcomes. J Cardiothorac Vasc Anesth, 2019; 33: 232-244.
4. Warren OJ, Smith AJ, Alexiou C, et al. The inflammatory response to cardiopulmonary bypass: part 1 – mechanisms of pathogenesis. J Cardiothorac Vasc Anesth, 2009; 23: 222-231.

16. Endotoxin is a component of which of the following?
A. Gram-negative bacteria
B. Gram-positive bacteria
C. RNA viruses
D. Fungi

Correct answer: A

Explanation: Endotoxin, also called lipopolysaccharide, is a component of the cell membrane of gram-negative bacteria. Endotoxin is a potent activator of complement and cytokines and appears to be one of the initial triggers of systemic inflammation. Lipid A is embedded in the outer leaflet of the outer membrane, has the same basic structure in practically all gram-negative bacteria and is the toxic component of endotoxin. The O-polysaccharide outer region (O-specific antigen or O-specific side chain) is highly variable and is composed of one or more oligosaccharide repeating units characteristic of the serotype.

References:

1. Whitlock R, Benett-Guerrero E, Augoustides JGT, Kaplan JA. Chapter 9: Systemic Inflammation. In: Kaplan JA, Augoustides JGT, Manecke GR, et al., eds. Kaplan's Cardiac Anesthesia. 7th ed. Elsevier; 2017:231-246.
2. Hill GE, Whitten CW, Landers DF. The influence of cardiopulmonary bypass on cytokines and cell-cell communication. J Cardiothorac Vasc Anesth, 1997; 11: 367-375.
3. Warren OJ, Smith AJ, Alexiou C, et al. The inflammatory response to cardiopulmonary bypass: part 1 – mechanisms of pathogenesis. J Cardiothorac Vasc Anesth, 2009; 23: 222-231.

17. Which of the following is the most likely source for the rise in blood endotoxin levels seen in cardiac surgical patients?
A. Cardiopulmonary bypass circuit tubing
B. Membrane oxygenator
C. Microaspiration
D. Impaired gut barrier

Correct answer: D

Explanation: Although endotoxin can be found in sterile fluids administered to the patient, it is believed that that the majority of endotoxin arises through a patient's impaired gut barrier. Intestinal flora contains a large amount of endotoxin from gram-negative microorganisms. The average human colon contains approximately 25 billion nanograms of endotoxin. Many of the bacteria in the intestine are dead, and endotoxin can enter the blood stream contained within cell membrane fragments of dead bacteria. Endotoxin may initiate a systemic inflammatory response through potent activation of macrophages and other proinflammatory cells.

Endotoxin has been linked to dysfunction in every organ system of the body and may be the key initiating factor in the development of systemic inflammation.

References:

1. Whitlock R, Benett-Guerrero E, Augoustides JGT, Kaplan JA. Chapter 9: Systemic Inflammation. In: Kaplan JA, Augoustides JGT, Manecke GR, et al., eds. Kaplan's Cardiac Anesthesia. 7th ed. Elsevier; 2017:231-246.
2. Oudemans-van Straaten HM, Jansen PG, et al. Intestinal permeability, circulating endotoxin, and postoperative systemic responses in cardiac surgery patients. J Cardiothorac Vasc Anesth, 1996; 10: 187-194.
3. Warren OJ, Smith AJ, Alexiou C, et al. The inflammatory response to cardiopulmonary bypass: part 1 – mechanisms of pathogenesis. J Cardiothorac Vasc Anesth, 2009; 23: 222-231.

18. Serotype-specific antibodies responsible for late tolerance host defense demonstrate a high affinity for which portion of endotoxin?
A. O-specific region
B. Lipid A region
C. Core region
D. P-specific region

Correct answer: A

Explanation: Two distinct types of tolerance to endotoxin exist and are classified as early tolerance and late tolerance. Early tolerance to endotoxin begins within hours of exposure and decreases almost to baseline within 2 days. Early tolerance cannot be transferred with plasma. Early tolerance may protect the host from lethal systemic inflammation after an overwhelming exposure to endotoxin. Late tolerance is caused by the synthesis of immunoglobulins (i.e., antibodies) directed against the offending endotoxin. Late tolerance begins approximately 72 hours following exposure and persists for at least 2 weeks. Serotype specific antibodies exhibit high affinity to and protection from specific serotypes of endotoxin. These serotype (O-specific region) antiendotoxin antibodies do not recognize the many variations of endotoxin O-polysaccharide side chains and are ineffective at conferring protection against the numerous subtypes of endotoxin encountered in the clinical setting. The inner core region is well conserved across endotoxin, and cross-reactivity to this region should theoretically be observed.

References:

1. Whitlock R, Benett-Guerrero E, Augoustides JGT, Kaplan JA. Chapter 9: Systemic Inflammation. In: Kaplan JA, Augoustides JGT, Manecke GR, et al., eds. Kaplan's Cardiac Anesthesia. 7th ed. Elsevier; 2017:231-246.
2. Oudemans-van Straaten HM, Jansen PG, et al. Intestinal permeability, circulating endotoxin, and postoperative systemic responses in cardiac surgery patients. J Cardiothorac Vasc Anesth, 1996; 10: 187-194.
3. Warren OJ, Smith AJ, Alexiou C, et al. The inflammatory response to cardiopulmonary bypass: part 1 – mechanisms of pathogenesis. J Cardiothorac Vasc Anesth, 2009; 23: 222-231.

19. Hypoperfusion to which of the following organ beds is an important cause of systemic inflammation?
   A. Coronary circulation
   B. Pulmonary circulation
   C. Splanchnic circulation
   D. Cerebral circulation

Correct answer: C

Explanation: Splanchnic hypoperfusion appears to be an important cause of systemic inflammation. The gut is very susceptible to hypoperfusion during conditions of trauma or stress. Evidence suggests that, during periods of hypovolemia, the gut vasoconstricts, thus shunting blood toward "more vital organs" such as the heart and brain. In the setting of cardiopulmonary bypass, endogenously released vasoconstrictors such as angiotensin II, thromboxane A_2, and vasopressin may also decrease splanchnic perfusion. Gut perfusion is likely also reduced by vasoconstrictors that may be administered in the setting of hypotension. Additional evidence indicates that systemic endotoxemia may worsen intestinal permeability, thus exacerbating splanchnic hypoperfusion.

References:

1. Whitlock R, Benett-Guerrero E, Augoustides JGT, Kaplan JA. Chapter 9: Systemic Inflammation. In: Kaplan JA, Augoustides JGT, Manecke GR, et al., eds. Kaplan's Cardiac Anesthesia. 7th ed. Elsevier; 2017:231-246.
2. McNicol L, Andersen LW, Liu G, et al. Markers of splanchnic perfusion and intestinal translocation of endotoxins during cardiopulmonary bypass: effects of dopamine and milrinone. J Cardiothorac Vasc Anesth, 1999; 13: 292-298.
3. Warren OJ, Smith AJ, Alexiou C, et al. The inflammatory response to cardiopulmonary bypass: part 1 – mechanisms of pathogenesis. J Cardiothorac Vasc Anesth, 2009; 23: 222-231.

20. Which of the following demonstrates complex interaction with the coagulation cascade, complement system, immunologic system, and inflammatory system?
   A. T lymphocytes
   B. B lymphocytes
   C. Macrophages
   D. Endotoxin

Correct answer: D

Explanation: Many of the complications linked to splanchnic hypoperfusion do not involve the gastrointestinal system. The effects of splanchnic hypoperfusion are far-reaching due to the initiation of systemic inflammation. Endotoxin has been reported to have adverse effects on the pulmonary, renal, cardiac, and vascular systems. Endotoxin effects on the coagulation system can be both antihemostatic and prothrombotic. Activation of the inflammatory cascade has been shown to worsen neurological injury in animal models. Infections are common after cardiac surgical procedures and may arise from translocation of bacteria across the gastrointestinal tract. Infections are likely not caused directly by systemic inflammation, but rather by secondary effects on host immunity. Following cardiac surgical procedures, antibody production by B lymphocytes (plasma cells) is depressed, as is T lymphocyte function. The resulting reduced humoral and cell-mediated immunity may lead to increased infection rates after cardiac procedures.

References:

1. Whitlock R, Benett-Guerrero E, Augoustides JGT, Kaplan JA. Chapter 9: Systemic Inflammation. In: Kaplan JA, Augoustides JGT, Manecke GR, et al., eds. Kaplan's Cardiac Anesthesia. 7th ed. Elsevier; 2017:231-246.
2. Hill GE, Whitten CW, Landers DF. The influence of cardiopulmonary bypass on cytokines and cell-cell communication. J Cardiothorac Vasc Anesth, 1997; 11: 367-375.
3. Warren OJ, Smith AJ, Alexiou C, et al. The inflammatory response to cardiopulmonary bypass: part 1 – mechanisms of pathogenesis. J Cardiothorac Vasc Anesth 2009; 23: 222-231.

21. Steroid administration has been shown to decrease which of the following perioperative cardiac surgical complications?
   A. Death
   B. Renal failure
   C. Stroke
   D. None of the above

Correct answer: D

Explanation: Steroids have been demonstrated to attenuate the release of proinflammatory cytokines, mitigate complement activation, and increase anti-inflammatory mediators during cardiac surgical procedures. The Dexamethasone for Cardiac Surgery Study demonstrated that dexamethasone had no effect on the primary outcomes of death, myocardial infarction, stroke, new renal failure, respiratory failure, new-onset atrial fibrillation, or postoperative cognitive decline. The Steroids in Cardiac Surgery trial failed to demonstrate benefit of methylprednisolone on the risk of death, myocardial injury, stroke, renal failure, or respiratory failure in patients with elevated perioperative risk. No therapies are currently in widespread clinical use to prevent or treat organ dysfunction resulting from systemic inflammation.

References:

1. Whitlock R, Benett-Guerrero E, Augoustides JGT, Kaplan JA. Chapter 9: Systemic Inflammation. In: Kaplan JA, Augoustides JGT, Manecke GR, et al., eds. Kaplan's Cardiac Anesthesia. 7th ed. Elsevier; 2017:231-246.
2. Crawford JH, Townsley MM. Analyzing the data for steroids in cardiac surgery. J Cardiothorac Vasc Anesth, 2020; 34: 106-107.

22. Which of the following beneficial outcomes has been demonstrated with the use of heparin-coated cardiopulmonary bypass circuit tubing?
   A. Decreased rates of blood transfusion
   B. Decreased postoperative infection rates
   C. Decreased incidence of atrial fibrillation
   D. Decreased rates of stroke

Correct answer: A

Explanation: Although heparin-coated circuits have many theoretical advantages, evidence that their use during cardiac operations results in fewer clinically significant adverse complications is scant. No difference in cytokine levels or markers of complement have been observed in patients randomized to heparin-coated circuits compared to traditional circuits. A meta-analysis of 3434 patients from 41 randomized trials demonstrated reductions in blood transfusion and duration of mechanical ventilation, intensive care unit stay, and hospital length of stay with the use of heparin-coated circuits. Although there may be multifactorial etiology to these outcomes, these findings provide some support for use of heparin-coated circuits as an intervention to improve outcomes.

References:

1. Whitlock R, Benett-Guerrero E, Augoustides JGT, Kaplan JA. Chapter 9: Systemic Inflammation. In: Kaplan JA, Augoustides JGT, Manecke GR, et al., eds. Kaplan's Cardiac Anesthesia. 7th ed. Elsevier; 2017:231-246.
2. Kreisler KR, Vance RA, Cruzzavala J, et al. Heparin-bonded cardiopulmonary bypass circuits reduce the rate of red blood cell transfusion during elective coronary artery bypass surgery. J Cardiothorac Vasc Anesth, 2005; 19: 608-611.
3. Warren OJ, Smith AJ, Alexiou C, et al. The inflammatory response to cardiopulmonary bypass: part 1 – mechanisms of pathogenesis. J Cardiothorac Vasc Anesth, 2009; 23: 222-231.
4. Warren OJ, Watret AL, de Wit KL, et al. The inflammatory response to cardiopulmonary bypass: part 2 – anti-inflammatory therapeutic strategies. J Cardiothorac Vasc Anesth, 2009; 23: 384-393.

23. Centrifugal vortex blood pumping has been shown to reduce which of the following parameters?
    A. Neutrophil activation
    B. Systemic inflammation
    C. Perioperative mortality
    D. Cytokine levels

Correct answer: A

Explanation: Centrifugal vortex blood pumping has been shown to result in reduced complement and neutrophil activation, as well as reduced hemolysis, during cardiac surgical procedures compared with standard roller blood pumping. Centrifugal vortex pumping did not significantly prevent increases in cytokines in pediatric patients randomized to this technique. The literature has not demonstrated a significant advantage of centrifugal over roller head pumps in terms of the inflammatory response, neurocognitive deficits, or perioperative mortality.

References:

1. Whitlock R, Benett-Guerrero E, Augoustides JGT, Kaplan JA. Chapter 9: Systemic Inflammation. In: Kaplan JA, Augoustides JGT, Manecke GR, et al., eds. Kaplan's Cardiac Anesthesia. 7th ed. Elsevier; 2017:231-246.
2. Ashraf SS, Tian Y, Cowan D, et al. Proinflammatory cytokine release during pediatric cardiopulmonary bypass: influence of centrifugal and roller pumps. J Cardiothorac Vasc Anesth, 1997; 11: 718-722.

3. Medikinda R, Ong CSO, Vadia R, et al. Trends and updates on cardiopulmonary bypass setup in pediatric cardiac surgery. J Cardiothorac Vasc Anesth, 2019; 33: 2804-2813.

24. Which of the following components of the cardiopulmonary bypass circuit has been associated with better pulmonary function postoperatively?
    A. Bubble oxygenator
    B. Membrane oxygenator
    C. Heparin-coated tubing
    D. Reduced-volume venous reservoir

Correct answer: B

Explanation: The role of membrane oxygenators as a means of reducing systemic inflammation-related complications is controversial. Less complement activation has been observed with the use of membrane oxygenators in some, but not all, studies. The choice of a membrane oxygenator has been associated with better pulmonary function as compared with the use of a bubble oxygenator. Whether this observed difference in pulmonary function reflects reduced systemic inflammation remains unclear.

References:

1. Whitlock R, Benett-Guerrero E, Augoustides JGT, Kaplan JA. Chapter 9: Systemic Inflammation. In: Kaplan JA, Augoustides JGT, Manecke GR, et al., eds. Kaplan's Cardiac Anesthesia. 7th ed. Elsevier; 2017:231-246.
2. Byrick RJ, Noble WH. Postperfusion lung syndrome. Comparison of Travenol bubble and membrane oxygenators. J Thorac Cardiovasc Surg, 1978; 76: 685-693.
3. Medikinda R, Ong CSO, Vadia R, et al. Trends and updates on cardiopulmonary bypass setup in pediatric cardiac surgery. J Cardiothorac Vasc Anesth, 2019; 33: 2804-2813.

25. Which of the following outcomes has been observed in cardiac surgical patients who have undergone ultrafiltration?
    A. Decreased risk of multiorgan dysfunction
    B. Decreased length of hospital stay
    C. Decreased incidence of infection
    D. Decreased incidence of postoperative fever

Correct answer: D

Explanation: Removal of excess fluid with ultrafiltration has been proposed as a method for eliminating proinflammatory mediators during cardiac surgical procedures, particularly in the pediatric surgical population. It is unclear in studies thus far whether the beneficial effects of ultrafiltration are caused by a combination of the following factors: dampening the initiation of inflammation, removal of inflammatory mediators, or removal of excessive fluid alone. Ultrafiltration may reduce perioperative fever, blood loss, time to tracheal extubation, and the alveolar-arterial oxygen gradient, findings that suggest an association between proinflammatory cytokines and clinically meaningful end points. The small sample size of studies related to this topic precludes conclusions regarding further outcomes such as the risk of the multiorgan dysfunction syndrome, incidence of perioperative infection, and/or hospital length of stay.

References:

1. Whitlock R, Benett-Guerrero E, Augoustides JGT, Kaplan JA. Chapter 9: Systemic Inflammation. In: Kaplan JA, Augoustides JGT, Manecke GR, et al., eds. Kaplan's Cardiac Anesthesia. 7th ed. Elsevier; 2017:231-246.
2. Kosour C, Dragosavac D, Antunes N, et al. Effect of ultrafiltration on pulmonary function and interleukins in patients undergoing cardiopulmonary bypass. J Cardiothorac Vasc Anesth, 2016; 30: 884-890.
3. Medikinda R, Ong CSO, Vadia R, et al. Trends and updates on cardiopulmonary bypass setup in pediatric cardiac surgery. J Cardiothorac Vasc Anesth, 2019; 33: 2804-2813.

26. A 71-year-old male with severe peripheral vascular disease is found to have critical left main stenosis and presents for coronary artery bypass grafting. Has received pentoxifylline for intermittent claudication. Continuation of pentoxifylline during the perioperative period is most likely to contribute to which of the following postoperative outcomes?
  A. Decreased mechanical ventilation time
  B. Decreased risk of perioperative myocardial infarction
  C. Decreased risk of graft thrombosis
  D. Improved myocardial ejection fraction

Correct answer: A

Explanation: Pentoxifylline is a nonspecific phosphodiesterase inhibitor that is similar in chemical structure to theophylline. Pentoxifylline has multiple rheologic and anti-inflammatory properties, though the exact mechanism of these effects is incompletely understood. This agent significantly attenuates endothelial damage and generation of oxygen radicals after ischemia-reperfusion. It also may prevent fever after the administration of endotoxin and attenuates bacterial translocation from the gut during shock. A small clinical trial in cardiac surgery demonstrated that exposure to pentoxifylline reduced the duration of mechanical ventilation, the need for hemofiltration, and the length of stay in the intensive care unit. In the lung transplant setting, this agent may also reduce the risk of allograft dysfunction and postoperative mortality. These outcome benefits require confirmation in large, multicenter trials. Perioperative administration of pentoxifylline has not been associated with improvements in left ventricular ejection fraction or the risks for myocardial infarction and graft thrombosis.

References:

1. Whitlock R, Benett-Guerrero E, Augoustides JGT, Kaplan JA. Chapter 9: Systemic Inflammation. In: Kaplan JA, Augoustides JGT, Manecke GR, et al., eds. Kaplan's Cardiac Anesthesia. 7th ed. Elsevier; 2017:231-246.
2. Hall R. Identification of inflammatory mediators and their modulation by strategies for the management of the systemic inflammatory response during cardiac surgery. J Cardiothorac Vasc Anesth, 2013; 27: 983-1033.

27. A 75-year-old woman with a history of hypertension and hypercholesterolemia presents with chest pain and shortness of breath. She is found to have multivessel coronary artery disease and is scheduled for coronary artery bypass grafting. Which of the following may result from the continued administration of her statin therapy in the perioperative period?
  A. Decreased levels of activated complement
  B. Increased serum creatinine
  C. Decreased levels of tumor necrosis factor
  D. Increased bilirubin

Correct answer: C

Explanation: The pleiotropic effects of statins have received significant attention. These widespread effects include improvements in endothelial dysfunction, as well as their antioxidant and anti-inflammatory properties. The clinical benefits of reducing the stress response and inflammation in the perioperative period could potentially decrease postoperative atrial fibrillation, as well as neurologic and pulmonary complications. However, clinical trials have yet to demonstrate these outcome advantages, including effects on length of stay, as well as pulmonary, renal, or neurologic outcomes. Meta-analysis has demonstrated that statin exposure is associated with lower levels of inflammatory markers such as interleukin-6, interleukin-8, C-reactive protein, and tumor necrosis factor.

References:

1. Whitlock R, Benett-Guerrero E, Augoustides JGT, Kaplan JA. Chapter 9: Systemic Inflammation. In: Kaplan JA, Augoustides JGT, Manecke GR, et al., eds. Kaplan's Cardiac Anesthesia. 7th ed. Elsevier; 2017:231-246.
2. Hall R. Identification of inflammatory mediators and their modulation by strategies for the management of the systemic inflammatory response during cardiac surgery. J Cardiothorac Vasc Anesth, 2013; 27: 983-1033.

28. Which of the following agents is most protective for splanchnic circulation?
  A. Epinephrine
  B. Vasopressin
  C. Dopamine
  D. Milrinone

Correct answer: D

Explanation: Inodilators such as milrinone and dobutamine may be more protective for the splanchnic circulation than inoconstrictors such as epinephrine, norepinephrine, and dopamine. Although dopamine is often touted as preserving splanchnic blood flow, clinical responses to this agent vary, with vascular resistance increasing in some patients even at low doses. The vasodilatory properties in concert with increased cardiac output generated with inodilating agents such as milrinone may increase cardiac output to a dilated splanchnic circulation, thereby enhancing oxygen delivery. Vasopressin can cause splanchnic vasoconstriction and worsen perfusion to the splanchnic circulation despite an increase in system blood pressure.

References:
1. Whitlock R, Benett-Guerrero E, Augoustides JGT, Kaplan JA. Chapter 9: Systemic Inflammation. In: Kaplan JA, Augoustides JGT, Manecke GR, et al., eds. Kaplan's Cardiac Anesthesia. 7th ed. Elsevier; 2017:231-246.
2. Hall R. Identification of inflammatory mediators and their modulation by strategies for the management of the systemic inflammatory response during cardiac surgery. J Cardiothorac Vasc Anesth, 2013; 27: 983-1033.

29. Which of the following anesthetic agents has been demonstrated to attenuate interleukin-6 levels after cardiac surgery with cardiopulmonary bypass?
A. Ketamine
B. Isoflurane
C. Propofol
D. Dexmedetomidine

Correct answer: A

Explanation: In an initial study in cardiac surgical patients, administration of a low dose (0.25 mg/kg) of ketamine before cardiopulmonary bypass prevented an increase in interleukin-6 for 7 days postoperatively. In animal models, ketamine administration has inhibited production of tumor necrosis factor and oxygen radicals, as well as decreased the degree of leukocyte adherence. However, despite its anti-inflammatory effects, large trials are still required to test whether these effects improve clinical outcomes. The effects on interleukin-6 of isoflurane, propofol, and dexmedetomidine in cardiac surgery with cardiopulmonary bypass require further investigation.

References:
1. Whitlock R, Benett-Guerrero E, Augoustides JGT, Kaplan JA. Chapter 9: Systemic Inflammation. In: Kaplan JA, Augoustides

JGT, Manecke GR, et al., eds. Kaplan's Cardiac Anesthesia. 7th ed. Elsevier; 2017:231-246.
2. Hall R. Identification of inflammatory mediators and their modulation by strategies for the management of the systemic inflammatory response during cardiac surgery. J Cardiothorac Vasc Anesth, 2013; 27: 983-1033.

30. Selective digestive decontamination with administration of oral nonabsorbable antibiotics has been associated with which of the following postoperative events?
A. Decreased incidence of wound infection
B. Reduced levels of endotoxin and interleukin-6
C. Decreased risk of clinical ileus
D. Reduced levels of tumor necrosis factor

Correct answer: B

Explanation: Selective digestive decontamination represents a possible approach to limit the incidence and severity of systemic inflammation. The technique aims to reduce the reservoir of endotoxin within the gut in an attempt to reduce the total amount of endotoxin exposure. Although this perioperative intervention lowers gut bacterial counts as well as blood levels of endotoxin and interleukin-6, clinical trials have yet to demonstrate that this approach significantly improves clinically meaningful outcomes after cardiac surgery.

References:
1. Whitlock R, Benett-Guerrero E, Augoustides JGT, Kaplan JA. Chapter 9: Systemic Inflammation. In: Kaplan JA, Augoustides JGT, Manecke GR, et al., eds. Kaplan's Cardiac Anesthesia. 7th ed. Elsevier; 2017:231-246.
2. Chan MXF, Buitinck S, Stooker M, et al. Clinical effects of perioperative selective decontamination of the digestive tract (SDD) in cardiac surgery: a propensity score matched analysis. J Cardiothorac Vasc Anesth, 2019; 33: 3001-3009.

CHAPTER 10

Pharmacology of Anesthetic Drugs

J. Bradley Meers and Matthew M. Townsley

KEY POINTS

1. In patients, the observed acute effect of a specific anesthetic agent on the cardiovascular system represents the net effect on the myocardium, coronary blood flow, and vasculature; electrophysiologic behavior; and neurohormonal reflex function. Anesthetic agents within the same class may differ from one another quantitatively and qualitatively. The acute response to an anesthetic agent may be modulated by the patient's underlying pathology or pharmacologic treatment, or both.

2. Volatile agents cause dose-dependent decreases in systemic blood pressure. For halothane and enflurane, this mainly results from depression of contractile function, and for isoflurane, desflurane, and sevoflurane, pressure changes result from decreases in systemic vascular responses. Volatile anesthetics cause dose-dependent depression of contractile function that is mediated at a cellular level by attenuating calcium currents and decreasing calcium sensitivity. Decreases in systemic vascular responses reflect various effects on endothelium-dependent and endothelium-independent mechanisms.

3. Volatile agents determine coronary blood flow by their effect on systemic hemodynamics, myocardial metabolism, and coronary vasculature. When these variables were controlled in studies, the anesthetics exerted only mild direct vasodilatory effects on the coronary vasculature.

4. In addition to causing acute coronary syndromes, myocardial ischemia can manifest as myocardial stunning, preconditioning, or hibernating myocardium. Volatile anesthetics can attenuate myocardial ischemia development through mechanisms that are independent of myocardial oxygen supply and demand and can facilitate functional recovery of stunned myocardium. Volatile agents also can simulate ischemic preconditioning, a phenomenon described as anesthetic preconditioning; the mechanisms of which are similar but not identical.

5. Intravenous induction agents (i.e., hypnotics) belong to various drug classes, including barbiturates, benzodiazepines, N-methyl-D-aspartate receptor antagonists, and α_2-adrenergic receptor agonists. Although they all induce hypnosis, their sites of action and molecular targets are different, and their cardiovascular effects partially depend on the class to which they belong.

6. Studies of isolated cardiac myocytes, cardiac muscle tissue, and vascular tissue have demonstrated that induction agents inhibit cardiac contractility and relax vascular tone by inhibiting the mechanisms that increase intracellular calcium ion (Ca^{2+}) concentration. This may be offset by mechanisms that increase myofilament Ca^{2+} sensitivity in the cardiac myocyte and vascular smooth muscle, which can modulate cardiovascular changes. However, the cumulative effects of induction agents on contractility, vascular resistance, and vascular capacitance are mediated predominantly by their sympatholytic effects. Induction agents should be used judiciously and with extreme caution in patients with shock, heart failure, or other pathophysiologic circumstances in which the sympathetic nervous system is paramount in maintaining myocardial contractility and arterial and venous tone.

7. Opioids have diverse chemical structures, but all retain an essential T-shaped component that is stereochemically necessary for the activation of the µ-, κ-, and δ-opioid receptors. These receptors are not confined to the nervous system and have been identified in the myocardium and blood vessels where endogenous opioid proteins can be synthesized.

8. Acute exogenous opioid administration modulates many determinants of central and peripheral cardiovascular regulation. However, the predominant clinical effect is mediated by attenuation of central sympathetic outflow.

9. Activation of the δ-opioid receptor can elicit preconditioning, which is mediated by signaling pathways that involve G-protein–coupled protein kinases, caspases, nitric oxide, and other chemicals. In contrast with ischemia in homeotherms, hibernation is well tolerated in certain species. This phenomenon may partially depend on mechanisms that are activated by opioids or opioid-like molecules.

1. A 62-year-old man with nonischemic cardiomyopathy presents for left ventricular assist device placement. The baseline left ventricular ejection fraction is 20%. He then undergoes inhalational induction with sevoflurane. Which of the following parameters is expected to decrease?
   A. Heart rate
   B. Myocardial contractility
   C. Cerebral blood flow
   D. Coronary blood flow

Correct Answer: B

Explanation: The influence of volatile anesthetics on contractile function has been investigated extensively in humans and in animal models. Although it is widely agreed that volatile agents can cause dose-dependent depression of contractile function, different volatile anesthetics vary in this regard. Sevoflurane, isoflurane, and desflurane produce reflex sympathetic activation that minimizes myocardial depression, as compared to halothane and enflurane, which lack such a response. In the setting of preexisting myocardial depression, volatile agents have a greater effect on contractility than in normal myocardium. The vasodilatory properties of the current volatile anesthetics (sevoflurane, isoflurane, and desflurane) lead to increased blood flow to numerous vascular beds, including the coronary and cerebral circulation. Systemic vasodilation can produce reflex tachycardia, leading to an increased, not decreased, heart rate.

References:

1. Lester L, Mitter N, Berkowitz DE, Augoustides JGT, Kaplan JA. Chapter 10: Pharmacology of Anesthetic Drugs. In: Kaplan JA, Augoustides JGT, Manecke GR, et al., eds. Kaplan's Cardiac Anesthesia. 7th ed. Elsevier; 2017:247-291.
2. Pagel PS, Nijhawan N, Warltier DC, et al. Quantitation of volatile anesthetic-induced depression of myocardial contractility using a single beat index derived from maximal ventricular power. J Cardiothorac Vasc Anesth, 1993; 7: 688-695.
3. DeTraglia MC, Komai H, Rusy BF. Differential effects of inhalation anesthetics on myocardial potentiated-state contractions in vitro. Anesthesiology, 1988; 68: 534-540.
4. Pagel PS. Myocardial protection by volatile anesthetics in patients undergoing cardiac surgery: a critical review of the laboratory and clinical evidence. J Cardiothorac Vasc Anesth, 2013; 27: 972-982.

2. As related to myocardial performance, volatile anesthetics mainly exert their inotropic effects on what receptor?
   A. Sodium
   B. Potassium
   C. Hydrogen
   D. Calcium

Correct Answer: D

Explanation: At the cellular level, volatile anesthetics exert negative inotropic effects primarily by modulating sarcolemmal L-type Ca^{2+} channels, the sarcoplasmic reticulum, and contractile proteins. The L-type Ca^{2+} currents are decreased and the release of calcium from the sarcoplasmic reticulum is depressed by volatile agents. In the presence of volatile anesthetics, the contractile response to reduced Ca^{2+} levels is further attenuated. The contractile response is decreased by volatile agents at any given calcium level because volatile agents decrease Ca^{2+} sensitivity. The mechanism by which anesthetic agents modify ion channels is not completely understood, as channels are usually studied under *ex vivo* circumstances. Volatile agents demonstrate numerous sites of action with ion channels in the *ex vivo* myocyte, but it is the Ca^{2+} channel upon which volatile agents exhibit their negative inotropic effects.

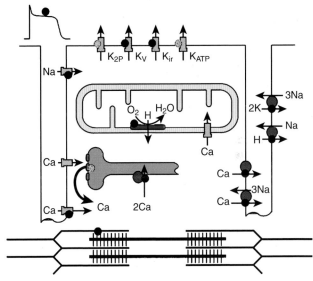

FIGURE 10.1 Sites of action of volatile anesthetics in a ventricular myocyte. *Black circles* indicate inhibitory actions; *small green circles* indicate stimulatory actions. (From Hanley PJ, ter Keurs HEDJ, Cannell MB, Excitation-contraction in the heart and the negative inotropic action of volatile anesthetics. Anesthesiology. 2004;101:999.)

References:

1. Lester L, Mitter N, Berkowitz DE, Augoustides JGT, Kaplan JA. Chapter 10: Pharmacology of Anesthetic Drugs. In: Kaplan JA, Augoustides JGT, Manecke GR, et al., eds. Kaplan's Cardiac Anesthesia. 7th ed. Elsevier; 2017:247-291.
2. Pagel PS, Crystal GJ. The discovery of myocardial preconditioning using volatile anesthetics: a history and contemporary clinical perspective. J Cardiothorac Vasc Anesth, 2018; 32: 1112-1134.

3. Volatile anesthetic agents have been demonstrated to prolong which portion of the cardiac cycle?
   A. Isovolumetric relaxation
   B. Isovolumetric contraction
   C. Ejection
   D. Diastasis

Correct Answer: A

Explanation: Diastolic dysfunction is an important cause of congestive heart failure. The mechanisms underlying diastolic dysfunction are categorized as those involving alterations in myocardial relaxation (i.e., calcium handling by the sarcoplasmic reticulum), those related to intrinsic properties of myocardial tissue (i.e., myocyte cytoskeletal elements), and those that are extramyocardial (i.e., loading conditions). Because indices of diastolic function were not readily available in the past, there remains a relative paucity of literature detailing the modulating effects of volatile agents on diastolic function. However, there is reasonable agreement in the literature that volatile agents prolong isovolumetric relaxation in a dose-dependent manner. At the molecular level, alterations in relaxation likely reflect modulation of calcium currents, including sarcoplasmic reticulum calcium reuptake mechanisms.

References:

1. Lester L, Mitter N, Berkowitz DE, Augoustides JGT, Kaplan JA. Chapter 10: Pharmacology of Anesthetic Drugs. In: Kaplan JA, Augoustides JGT, Manecke GR, et al., eds. Kaplan's Cardiac Anesthesia. 7th ed. Elsevier; 2017:247-291.
2. Yamada T, Takeda J, Koyama K, et al. Effects of sevoflurane, isoflurane, enflurane, and halothane on left ventricular diastolic performance in dogs. J Cardiothorac Vasc Anesth, 1994; 8: 618-624.

4. A 55-year-old woman with severe mitral regurgitation secondary to a flail posterior leaflet presents for robotic mitral valve repair. The maintenance of anesthesia is achieved with isoflurane. Which of the following is the expected effect of isoflurane on the coronary vasculature of this patient?
   A. Coronary vasoconstriction
   B. Coronary vasodilation
   C. Coronary steal
   D. No change in coronary vasoregulation

Correct Answer: B

Explanation: Volatile anesthetics modulate several determinants of myocardial oxygen supply and demand. They also directly modulate the myocyte response to ischemia. Under normal hemodynamic conditions, coronary blood flow is controlled by coronary vascular smooth muscle tone, which is modulated via the endothelium either directly (endothelial independent) or indirectly (endothelial dependent). Volatile agents can modulate mechanisms underlying vascular tone by receptor-dependent and receptor-independent mechanisms. Several volatile agents cause coronary vasodilation though mechanisms dependent on ATP-sensitive K^+ (K^+_{ATP}) channels. Sevoflurane-induced K^+ and Ca^{+2} channel–mediated effects increase coronary blood flow. The effects in vivo are typically modest because local control mechanisms of coronary blood flow likely predominate. Studies of isoflurane, sevoflurane, and desflurane demonstrated mild direct coronary vasodilatory effects of these agents. When potential confounding variables were controlled, there was no evidence these agents lead to coronary steal syndrome.

References:

1. Lester L, Mitter N, Berkowitz DE, Augoustides JGT, Kaplan JA. Chapter 10: Pharmacology of Anesthetic Drugs. In: Kaplan JA,

Augoustides JGT, Manecke GR, et al., eds. Kaplan's Cardiac Anesthesia. 7th ed. Elsevier; 2017:247-291.
2. Hartman JC, Kampine JP, Schmeling WT, et al. Actions of isoflurane on myocardial perfusion in chronically instrumented dogs with poor, moderate, or well-developed coronary collaterals. J Cardiothorac Vasc Anesth, 1990; 4: 715-725.
3. Iannou CV, Stergiopoulos N, Georgakarakos E, et al. Effects of isoflurane anesthesia on aortic compliance and systemic hemodynamics in compliant and noncompliant aortas. J Cardiothorac Vasc Anesth, 2013; 27: 1282-1288.

5. Currently available volatile anesthetics (isoflurane, sevoflurane, and desflurane) primarily decrease systemic arterial pressure by which of the following mechanisms?
   A. Decreased cardiac stroke volume
   B. Decreased cardiac output
   C. Decreased heart rate
   D. Decreased systemic vascular resistance

Correct Answer: D

Explanation: Volatile agents modulate vascular tone. The specific effect is influenced by the agent utilized, the vascular bed, vessel size and tone within the vascular bed, the level of preexisting tone, patient age, and indirect effects of the agents, such as anesthesia-induced hypotension and reflex autonomic nervous system activity. All volatile anesthetics decrease systemic blood pressure in a dose-dependent manner. Halothane and enflurane decrease systemic blood pressure primarily through decreases in stroke volume and cardiac output. Isoflurane, sevoflurane, and desflurane decrease systemic blood pressure by decreasing overall systemic vascular resistance while maintaining cardiac output.

References:

1. Lester L, Mitter N, Berkowitz DE, Augoustides JGT, Kaplan JA. Chapter 10: Pharmacology of Anesthetic Drugs. In: Kaplan JA, Augoustides JGT, Manecke GR, et al., eds. Kaplan's Cardiac Anesthesia. 7th ed. Elsevier; 2017:247-291.
2. Rödig G, Wild K, Behr R, et al. Effects of desflurane and isoflurane on systemic vascular resistance during hypothermic cardiopulmonary bypass. J Cardiothorac Vasc Anesth, 1997; 11: 54-57.

6. Which of the following time intervals for ischemic duration is consistent with reversible myocardial ischemia?
   A. 20 minutes
   B. 1 hour
   C. 3 hours
   D. 6 hours

Correct Answer: A

Explanation: Prolonged ischemia results in irreversible myocardial damage and necrosis. Depending on the duration and sequence of ischemic insults, shorter durations of myocardial ischemia can lead to preconditioning or myocardial stunning. Stunning occurs after a brief period of ischemia and is characterized by myocardial dysfunction in the setting

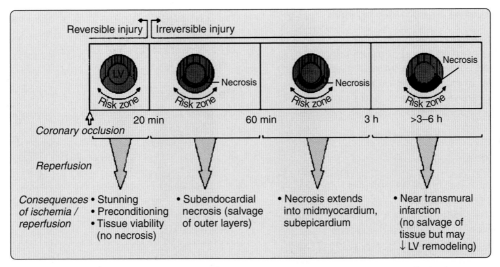

FIGURE 10.2 Effects of ischemia and reperfusion on the heart based on studies using an anesthetized canine model of proximal coronary artery occlusion. Periods of ischemia of less than 20 minutes followed by reperfusion are not associated with development of necrosis (ie, reversible injury). Brief ischemia and reperfusion results in stunning and preconditioning. If the duration of coronary occlusion is extended beyond 20 minutes, necrosis develops from the subendocardium to subepicardium over time. Reperfusion before 3 hours of ischemia salvages ischemic but viable tissue. Salvaged tissue may demonstrate stunning. Reperfusion beyond 3 to 6 hours in this model does not reduce myocardial infarct size. Late reperfusion may still have a beneficial effect on reducing or preventing myocardial infarct expansion and left ventricular (*LV*) remodeling. (From Kloner RA, Jennings RB. Consequences of brief ischemia: stunning, preconditioning, and their clinical implications, part I. Circulation. 2001; 104: 2981.).

of normal restored blood flow and an absence of myocardial necrosis. Ischemic preconditioning is characterized by an attenuation of infarct size after sustained ischemia if the period of sustained ischemia is preceded by a period of brief ischemia. Periods of ischemia of less than 20 minutes, followed by reperfusion, are not associated with the development of necrosis. If the duration of coronary occlusion extends beyond 20 minutes, necrosis develops from the subendocardium to the subepicardium over time. Reperfusion before 3 hours of ischemia salvages ischemic but viable tissue. Reperfusion beyond 3 to 6 hours does not reduce myocardial infarct size. Late reperfusion may still have a beneficial effect on reducing or preventing myocardial infarct expansion.

References:

1. Lester L, Mitter N, Berkowitz DE, Augoustides JGT, Kaplan JA. Chapter 10: Pharmacology of Anesthetic Drugs. In: Kaplan JA, Augoustides JGT, Manecke GR, et al., eds. Kaplan's Cardiac Anesthesia. 7th ed. Elsevier; 2017:247-291.
2. Kloner RA, Jennings RB. Consequences of brief ischemia: stunning, preconditioning, and their clinical implications: part 2. Circulation, 2001; 104: 3158-3167.
3. Lin S, Neelankavil J, Wang Y. Cardioprotective effect of anesthetics: translating science to practice. J Cardiothorac Vasc Anesth, 2021; 35: 730-740.

7. Ischemic preconditioning requires which of the following?
   A. Collateral blood flow
   B. Reperfusion

   C. Inhalational anesthetic use
   D. Systemic arterial hypotension

Correct Answer: B

Explanation: Ischemic preconditioning, first described in 1986, is characterized by an attenuation of infarct size after sustained ischemia if the period of sustained ischemia is preceded by a period of brief ischemia. This effect is independent of collateral flow. In the absence of reperfusion, there is subendocardial ischemia followed by mid- and subepicardial ischemia and, ultimately, necrosis if perfusion is not restored. Volatile anesthetic agents have been found to limit myocardial infarct size and lactate production after prolonged ischemia. This effect appears to be independent of the main determinants of myocardial oxygen supply and demand, suggesting that volatile agents may exert a beneficial effect at the level of the myocyte. Isoflurane has been shown to facilitate recovery of contractile function in stunned myocardium. Nearly 10 years after ischemic preconditioning was first described, the term anesthetic preconditioning was introduced to describe the effects of volatile agents on preconditioning.

References:

1. Lester L, Mitter N, Berkowitz DE, Augoustides JGT, Kaplan JA. Chapter 10: Pharmacology of Anesthetic Drugs. In: Kaplan JA, Augoustides JGT, Manecke GR, et al., eds. Kaplan's Cardiac Anesthesia. 7th ed. Elsevier; 2017:247-291.
2. Pagel PS, Crystal GJ. The discovery of myocardial preconditioning using volatile anesthetics: a history and contemporary clinical perspective. J Cardiothorac Vasc Anesth, 2018; 32: 1112-1134.

BOX 10.1   Volatile anesthetic agents

- All volatile anesthetic agents cause dose-dependent decreases in systemic blood pressure, which for halothane and enflurane predominantly result from attenuation of myocardial contractile function and which for isoflurane, desflurane, and sevoflurane predominantly result from decreases in systemic vascular resistance.
- Volatile agents obtund all components of the baroreceptor reflex arc.
- The effects of volatile agents on myocardial diastolic function are not well characterized and await the application of emerging technologies that have the sensitivity to quantitate indices of diastolic function.
- Volatile anesthetics lower the arrhythmogenic threshold to catecholamines. However, the underlying molecular mechanisms are not well understood.
- When confounding variables are controlled (e.g., systemic blood pressure), isoflurane does not cause coronary steal by a direct effect on coronary vasculature.
- The effects of volatile agents on systemic regional vascular beds and on the pulmonary vasculature are complex and depend on many variables, including the specific anesthetic, precise vascular bed, and vessel size and whether endothelial-dependent or endothelial-independent mechanisms are being investigated.

---

8. The phenomenon of ischemic preconditioning exhibits which of the following characteristics?

   A. It is unique to humans
   B. It provides biphasic cardiac protection
   C. Its effects are limited to cardiac tissue
   D. It is triggered only by ischemia

Correct Answer: B

Explanation: The phenomenon of ischemic preconditioning (IPC) and its underlying mechanisms are a focus of extensive investigation. IPC results in two periods of protection. The first (i.e., early or classic) occurs at 1 to 3 hours, and the second (i.e., late or delayed) occurs 24 to 96 hours after the preconditioning stimulus. IPC is ubiquitous across species, though it is more pronounced in larger species with lower metabolism and slower heart rates. IPC is mediated by multiple endogenous signaling pathways and also occurs in noncardiac tissue (i.e., brain, kidney). Preconditioning can be triggered by events other than ischemia, such as cellular stressors, pharmacologic agonists, and anesthetic agents. The benefits of IPC depend on the specific trigger, the species under study, and the type (i.e., classic or delayed) of IPC. For example, rapid pacing affords protection against arrythmias but not against infarct evolution. In contrast, cytokine-induced IPC limits infarct size but has no effect on arrhythmias. These various triggers of IPC, capable of modulating different end points, suggest that there are also mechanistic differences among triggers. Anesthetic preconditioning may not be identical to IPC mechanistically.

Induced ischemia in a region of the body away from the heart (i.e., remote ischemic preconditioning) has myocardial-protective effects in animals and has shown promising results in humans.

References:

1. Lester L, Mitter N, Berkowitz DE, Augoustides JGT, Kaplan JA. Chapter 10: Pharmacology of Anesthetic Drugs. In: Kaplan JA, Augoustides JGT, Manecke GR, et al., eds. Kaplan's Cardiac Anesthesia. 7th ed. Elsevier; 2017:247-291.
2. Healy DA, Kahn WA, Wong CS, et al. Remote preconditioning and major clinical complications following adult cardiovascular surgery: systematic review and meta-analysis. Int J Cardiol, 2014; 176: 20-31.
3. Vroom MB, van Wezel HB. Myocardial stunning, hibernation, and ischemic preconditioning. J Cardiothorac Vasc Anesth, 1996; 10: 789-799.

BOX 10.2   Volatile agents and myocardial ischemia

- Volatile anesthetic agents can attenuate the effects of myocardial ischemia (i.e., acute coronary syndromes).
- Nonacute manifestations of myocardial ischemia include hibernating myocardium, stunning, and preconditioning.
- Halothane and isoflurane facilitate the recovery of stunned myocardium.
- Preconditioning, an important adaptive and protective mechanism in biologic tissues, can be provoked by protean nonlethal stresses, including ischemia.
- Volatile anesthetic agents can mimic preconditioning (i.e., anesthetic preconditioning), which can have important clinical implications and provide insight into the cellular mechanisms of action of these volatile agents.

---

9. Which of the following ion channels plays a critical role in ischemic preconditioning and anesthetic preconditioning?

   A. H^+
   B. Na^+
   C. Ca^{2+}
   D. K^+

Correct Answer: D

Explanation: Mitochondrial potassium channels play a critical role in ischemic preconditioning. Volatile agents that exhibit anesthetic preconditioning activate mitochondrial potassium channels. Specific antagonists of these mitochondrial potassium channels can block anesthetic preconditioning. Furthermore, protein kinase C and mitogen-activated protein kinase are important signaling pathways in preconditioning. Volatile anesthetics have been shown to modulate the translocation of protein kinase C from the cytosol to the cell membrane.

Oxidant stress is also a central feature of reperfusion. Current evidence indicates that volatile agents can increase oxidant stress to levels that trigger preconditioning. Mitochondrial activation can also attenuate ischemia-induced oxidant stress, decrease the release of cytochrome c into the cytoplasm, and attenuate cellular calcium overload. Mitochondrial cytochrome c release is an important mechanism in the apoptotic process. Although the mechanisms of mitochondrial activation have been aggressively studied, they remain incompletely understood.

References:

1. Lester L, Mitter N, Berkowitz DE, Augoustides JGT, Kaplan JA. Chapter 10: Pharmacology of Anesthetic Drugs. In: Kaplan JA, Augoustides JGT, Manecke GR, et al., eds. Kaplan's Cardiac Anesthesia. 7th ed. Elsevier; 2017:247-291.
2. Healy DA, Kahn WA, Wong CS, et al. Remote preconditioning and major clinical complications following adult cardiovascular surgery: systematic review and meta-analysis. Int J Cardiol, 2014; 176: 20-31.
3. Pagel PS, Crystal GJ. The discovery of myocardial preconditioning using volatile anesthetics: a history and contemporary clinical perspective. J Cardiothorac Vasc Anesth, 2018; 32: 1112-1134.

10. In cardiac surgical patients, which of the following anesthetic techniques has been associated with significant reductions in length of stay in the intensive care unit and hospital?
    A. Total intravenous anesthesia
    B. Volatile anesthetic use
    C. Opioid-free anesthesia
    D. High-dose opioid anesthesia

Correct Answer: B

Explanation: The use of volatile anesthetics has been shown to affect outcomes after cardiac surgery. Meta-analysis has demonstrated that exposure to volatile anesthetics is associated with a significant reduction in length of stay both in the intensive care unit and in the hospital. These beneficial effects were enhanced by a longer duration of volatile anesthetic exposure throughout the cardiac surgical procedure. Compared to total intravenous anesthesia, recent meta-analysis has suggested a volatile anesthetic technique in cardiac surgery does not reduce cardiac troponin release, time to tracheal extubation, or survival in the first year.

References:

1. Lester L, Mitter N, Berkowitz DE, Augoustides JGT, Kaplan JA. Chapter 10: Pharmacology of Anesthetic Drugs. In: Kaplan JA, Augoustides JGT, Manecke GR, et al., eds. Kaplan's Cardiac Anesthesia. 7th ed. Elsevier; 2017:247-291.
2. Beverstock J, Park T, Alston RP, et al. A comparison of volatile anesthesia and total intravenous anesthesia (TIVA) effects on outcome from cardiac surgery: a systematic review and meta-analysis. J Cardiothorac Vasc Anesth, 2021; 35: 1096-1105.
3. Bignami E, Biondi-Zoccai G, Landoni G, et al. Volatile anesthetics reduce mortality in cardiac surgery. J Cardiothorac Vasc Anesth, 2009; 23: 594-599.

11. Which of the following sites bind propofol with a consequent effect on cardiac contractility?
    A. Myosin heads
    B. Mitochondria
    C. Troponin
    D. Beta receptors

Correct Answer: A

Explanation: The studies of propofol remain controversial about whether there is a direct effect on myocardial contractile function at clinically relevant concentrations. The weight of evidence suggests that propofol has a modest negative inotropic effect, which may be mediated by inhibition of L-type Ca^{2+} channels or modulation of Ca^{2+} release. The effect of propofol may be mediated at multiple sites in the cardiac myocyte, including the actin and myosin filaments. Propofol binds to the myosin heads of the myosin filaments, including both the essential light chain and the regulatory light chain. Furthermore, direct actions on myofilaments results in myocardial depression independent of Ca^{2+} concentration. Clinically relevant concentrations of propofol attenuate beta-adrenergic signal transduction in cardiac myocytes by inhibition of cyclic adenosine monophosphate production. The site of action for these inhibitory effects of propofol is upstream of the adenylyl cyclase and involves activation of protein kinase C alpha. Propofol does not appear to affect cardiac contractility through binding to mitochondria, troponin, or beta receptors.

References:

1. Lester L, Mitter N, Berkowitz DE, Augoustides JGT, Kaplan JA. Chapter 10: Pharmacology of Anesthetic Drugs. In: Kaplan JA, Augoustides JGT, Manecke GR, et al., eds. Kaplan's Cardiac Anesthesia. 7th ed. Elsevier; 2017:247-291.

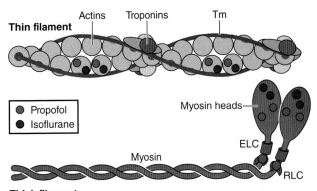

FIGURE 10.3 Multiple binding sites are shown for isoflurane and propofol on actin and myosin. The direct actions on myofilaments result in myocardial depression that is independent of calcium concentration. Identification of specific binding sites for volatile and intravenous anesthetics may lead to development of agents that produce less myocardial depression. *ELC,* Essential light chain; *RLC,* regulatory light chain; *Tm,* tropomyosin. (From Gao WD, Meng T, Bu W, et al. Molecular mechanism of anesthetic-induced depression of myocardial contraction. FASEB J. 2016;30(8):2915–2925.)

2. Gao WD, Meng T, Bu W, et al. Molecular mechanism of anesthetic-induced depression of myocardial contraction. FASEB J, 2016; 30: 2915-2925.
3. Ririe DG, Lundell JC, Neville MJ. Direct effects of propofol on myocardial and vascular tissue from mature and immature rats. J Cardiothorac Vasc Anesth, 2001; 15: 745-749.

12. Which of the following anesthetic agents demonstrates a negative inotropic effect at clinically relevant concentrations?
   A. Midazolam
   B. Etomidate
   C. Fentanyl
   D. Ketamine

Correct Answer: D

Explanation: The inotropic effects of induction agents may be species-dependent, which further confounds the literature in this regard. In a human study of isolated atrial muscle tissue, no inhibition of myocardial contractility was found in the clinical concentration ranges of midazolam or etomidate. Thiopental showed strong negative inotropic properties, whereas ketamine showed slight negative inotropic properties. These negative inotropic effects may partially explain the cardiovascular depression on induction of anesthesia with thiopental. The noted improvement in hemodynamics after induction of anesthesia with ketamine is likely due to the concomitant sympathoexcitation rather than its intrinsic myocardial effects.

References:

1. Lester L, Mitter N, Berkowitz DE, Augoustides JGT, Kaplan JA. Chapter 10: Pharmacology of Anesthetic Drugs. In: Kaplan JA, Augoustides JGT, Manecke GR, et al., eds. Kaplan's Cardiac Anesthesia. 7th ed. Elsevier; 2017:247-291.
2. Gelissen HP, Epema AH, Henning RH, et al. Inotropic effects of propofol, thiopental, midazolam, etomidate, and ketamine on isolated human atrial muscle. Anesthesiology, 1996; 84: 397-403.
3. Gursoy S, Berkan O, Bagcivan I, et al. Effects of intravenous anesthetics on the human radial artery used as a coronary artery bypass graft. J Cardiothorac Vasc Anesth, 2007; 21: 41-44.

13. Which of the following sedative agents has been shown to act as a free radical scavenger?
   A. Propofol
   B. Dexmedetomidine
   C. Ketamine
   D. Fentanyl

Correct Answer: A

Explanation: Oxidative stress remains an important pathophysiologic mechanism for cellular injury in critically ill patients and represents an imbalance between the production of free radicals and the enzymatic defense system that removes them. Propofol and midazolam act as free radical scavengers at near-therapeutic doses and suggest a role for propofol in modulating injury. Propofol has a chemical structure similar to that of phenol-based free radical scavengers such as vitamin E. Propofol also impairs the activity of neutrophils by inhibiting the oxidative burst and may modulate injury at the critical phase of reperfusion by reducing free radicals, calcium influx, and neutrophil activation. The current evidence suggests that dexmedetomidine, ketamine, and fentanyl are not associated with free radical scavenging.

References:

1. Lester L, Mitter N, Berkowitz DE, Augoustides JGT, Kaplan JA. Chapter 10: Pharmacology of Anesthetic Drugs. In: Kaplan JA, Augoustides JGT, Manecke GR, et al., eds. Kaplan's Cardiac Anesthesia. 7th ed. Elsevier; 2017:247-291.
2. Krzych LJ, Szurlej D, Bochenek A. Rationale for propofol use in cardiac surgery. J Cardiothorac Vasc Anesth, 2009; 23: 878-885.
3. Murphy PG, Myers DS, Davies MJ, et al. The antioxidant potential of propofol (2,6-diisopropylphenol). Br J Anaesth, 1992; 68: 613-618.

14. A 55-year-old female with severely reduced left ventricular systolic function presents for aortic valve replacement for severe acute aortic insufficiency due to endocarditis. The patient undergoes induction of a general anesthesia with propofol and becomes profoundly hypotensive. The mechanism of hypotension in this patient is most likely due to?
   A. Sepsis-induced vasodilation
   B. Activation of the parasympathetic nervous systems by propofol
   C. Suppression of the sympathetic nervous system by propofol
   D. Immune-mediated vasodilation

Correct Answer: C

Explanation: The physiologic actions of an anesthetic in the cardiovascular system represent a summation of its effects on the autonomic nervous system, as well as direct effects on the heart and vascular smooth muscle. Propofol decreases systemic vascular resistance in humans. This effect is predominately mediated by reduced sympathetic tone, but in isolated arteries propofol has been shown to decrease vascular tone and agonist-induced contraction. Propofol mediates these effects by inhibiting calcium influx into the cell and inhibition of calcium release from the intracellular stores. Propofol administration has been associated with a profound decrease in sympathetic activity with a reciprocal increase in blood flow due to consequent vasodilation. Sympathetic baroreflex sensitivities were also depressed by propofol, highlighting the profound effect on central sympathetic modulation of integrated cardiovascular function. Propofol inhibits the vasomotor mechanisms in the medulla to affect its hypotensive actions. This sympathoinhibition is amplified in patients with baseline high sympathetic activity, including conditions such as circulatory shock and heart failure.

References:

1. Lester L, Mitter N, Berkowitz DE, Augoustides JGT, Kaplan JA. Chapter 10: Pharmacology of Anesthetic Drugs. In: Kaplan JA, Augoustides JGT, Manecke GR, et al., eds. Kaplan's Cardiac Anesthesia. 7th ed. Elsevier; 2017:247-291.
2. Sellgren J, Ejnell H, Elam M, et al. Sympathetic muscle nerve activity, peripheral blood flows and baroreceptor reflexes in humans during propofol anesthesia and surgery. Anesthesiology, 1994; 80: 534-544.
3. Tritapepe L, Voci P, Marino P, et al. Calcium chloride minimizes the hemodynamic effects of propofol in patients undergoing coronary artery bypass grafting. J Cardiothorac Vasc Anesth, 1999; 13: 150-153.

15. In which of the following vascular beds does propofol act as a vasoconstrictor?
  A. Neurologic
  B. Mesenteric
  C. Pulmonary
  D. Renal

Correct Answer: C

Explanation: Propofol decreases systemic vascular resistance in humans. In the mesenteric vascular bed, propofol attenuates norepinephrine-induced vasoconstriction through reductions in intracellular calcium. In pulmonary circulation, propofol attenuates vasodilation through mechanisms involving nitric oxide and increases the sensitivity of the contractile myofilaments to calcium. Furthermore, propofol does not inhibit hypoxic pulmonary vasoconstriction. Propofol does not appear to cause vasoconstriction in the cerebral and renal vasculature.

References:

1. Lester L, Mitter N, Berkowitz DE, Augoustides JGT, Kaplan JA. Chapter 10: Pharmacology of Anesthetic Drugs. In: Kaplan JA, Augoustides JGT, Manecke GR, et al., eds. Kaplan's Cardiac Anesthesia. 7th ed. Elsevier; 2017:247-291.
2. Horibe M, Ogawa K, Sohn JT, et al. Propofol attenuates acetylcholine-induced pulmonary vasorelaxation: role of nitric oxide and endothelium-derived hyperpolarizing factors. Anesthesiology, 2000; 93: 447-455.
3. Kondo U, Kim SO, Nakayama M, et al. Pulmonary vascular effects of propofol at baseline, during elevated vasomotor tone, and in response to sympathetic alpha- and beta-adrenoreceptor activation. Anesthesiology, 2001; 94: 815-823.
4. Tarry D, Powell M. Hypoxic pulmonary vasoconstriction. BJA Education, 2017; 17: 209-213.

16. Which of the following statements is true regarding midazolam administration in patients undergoing cardiac surgery with cardiopulmonary bypass (CPB)?
  A. It is recommended for routine premedication
  B. It decreases systemic vascular resistance more than diazepam during CPB
  C. It enhances the analgesic effects of fentanyl
  D. It affects capacitance vessels more than diazepam during CPB

Correct Answer: D

Explanation: Midazolam is benzodiazepine with a rapid onset, short duration of action, and relatively rapid plasma clearance. It is cleared more rapidly than other benzodiazepines due to rapid redistribution and a high rate of liver clearance. This rapid clearance results in brief hypnotic and hemodynamic effects. Overall, only small hemodynamic changes occur after intravenous administration of midazolam. However, it has been shown to increase the risk for postoperative delirium, so it is not recommended for routine preoperative premedication in all patients and should be avoided in those at high risk for delirium. Midazolam appears to affect the venous capacitance vessels more than diazepam during cardiopulmonary bypass, with consequent decreases in venous reservoir pump volume. Diazepam decreases systemic vascular resistance to a greater extent than midazolam during cardiopulmonary bypass. Although its hypnotic effects are well-proven, midazolam does not possess any analgesic properties.

References:

1. Lester L, Mitter N, Berkowitz DE, Augoustides JGT, Kaplan JA. Chapter 10: Pharmacology of Anesthetic Drugs. In: Kaplan JA, Augoustides JGT, Manecke GR, et al., eds. Kaplan's Cardiac Anesthesia. 7th ed. Elsevier; 2017:247-291.
2. Aldecoa C, Bettelli G, Bilotta F, et al. European Society of Anaesthesiology evidence-based and consensus-based guideline on postoperative delirium. Eur J Anaesthesiol, 2017; 34: 192-214.

17. Which of the following statements is true regarding etomidate?
  A. It stimulates 11-β-hydroxylase
  B. It may cause histamine release at high doses
  C. It may be associated with myoclonus
  D. It does not induce adrenal suppression

Correct Answer: C

Explanation: Etomidate is a carboxylated imidazole derivative targeting the γ-aminobutyric acid type A receptor in the central nervous system. It possesses many favorable characteristics such as rapid onset, short duration, stable hemodynamic profile, and lack of histamine release. This favorable profile has led to its selection as an especially suitable induction agent for critically ill cardiac surgery patients. At a recommended induction dose range, it has pronounced hypnotic effects, but is commonly associated with myoclonic movements that are not associated with epileptic activity on the electroencephalogram.

Both infusions and single-dose administrations of etomidate have been shown to directly suppress adrenocortical function. Inhibition of 11-β-hydroxylase by the imidazole radical of etomidate leads to diminished biosynthesis of cortisol and aldosterone. Despite historical concerns for increased morbidity and mortality due to etomidate-induced adrenal insufficiency, current evidence, including a recent meta-analysis, does not suggest worse outcomes in cardiac surgery patients receiving etomidate.

References:

1. Lester L, Mitter N, Berkowitz DE, Augoustides JGT, Kaplan JA. Chapter 10: Pharmacology of Anesthetic Drugs. In: Kaplan JA, Augoustides JGT, Manecke GR, et al., eds. Kaplan's Cardiac Anesthesia. 7th ed. Elsevier; 2017:247-291.
2. Yao Y, He L, Fang N, et al. Anesthetic induction with etomidate in cardiac surgical patients: a PRISMA-compliant systematic review and meta-analysis. J Cardiothorac Vasc Anesth, 2021; 35: 1073-1085.

18. Preliminary data suggest a potentially protective effect against postoperative cognitive dysfunction in patients undergoing cardiac surgery with which of the following agents?
   A. Midazolam
   B. Ketamine
   C. Sevoflurane
   D. Isoflurane

Correct Answer: B

Explanation: A growing body of evidence suggests the possibility of a protective effect against postoperative cognitive dysfunction linked to perioperative ketamine administration. There are also data to suggest that ketamine may attenuate postoperative delirium in cardiac surgical patients. Although the exact mechanism remains unclear, concomitant reductions in serum C-reactive protein linked to ketamine administration suggest that this potential neuroprotective effect may be linked to anti-inflammatory actions of the drug. Current evidence does not suggest that midazolam, sevoflurane, or isoflurane has a protective effect in cognitive dysfunction after cardiac surgery.

References:

1. Lester L, Mitter N, Berkowitz DE, Augoustides JGT, Kaplan JA. Chapter 10: Pharmacology of Anesthetic Drugs. In: Kaplan JA, Augoustides JGT, Manecke GR, et al., eds. Kaplan's Cardiac Anesthesia. 7th ed. Elsevier; 2017:247-291.
2. Hudetz JA, Patterson KM, Iqbal Z, et al. Ketamine attenuated delirium after cardiac surgery with cardiopulmonary bypass. J Cardiothorac Vasc Anesth, 2009; 23: 651-657.
3. Trabold B, Metterlein T. Postoperative delirium: risk factors, prevention, and treatment. J Cardiothorac Vasc Anesth, 2014; 28: 1352-1360.

19. Following a 1 μg/kg bolus dose of dexmedetomidine in a healthy 22-year-old male patient, which of the following effects is most likely?
   A. Increase in heart rate
   B. Increase in blood pressure
   C. Decrease in blood pressure
   D. Respiratory depression

Correct Answer: B

Explanation: Administration of a 1 μg/kg bolus of dexmedetomidine induces an initial transient increase in blood pressure, with a reflex decrease in heart rate, due to peripheral stimulation of the alpha-2B-adrenergic receptors of the vascular smooth muscle. This effect may be particularly prominent in young, healthy individuals. This effect may be attenuated with a slow infusion of the loading dose over 10–15 minutes. Dexmedetomidine provides sedation and analgesia without causing respiratory depression.

References:

1. Lester L, Mitter N, Berkowitz DE, Augoustides JGT, Kaplan JA. Chapter 10: Pharmacology of Anesthetic Drugs. In: Kaplan JA, Augoustides JGT, Manecke GR, et al., eds. Kaplan's Cardiac Anesthesia. 7th ed. Elsevier; 2017:247-291.
2. Gallego-Ligorit L, Vives M, Valles-Torres J, et al. Use of dexmedetomidine in cardiothoracic and vascular anesthesia. J Cardiothorac Vasc Anesth, 2018; 32: 1426-1438.

20. Which of the following mechanisms is most responsible for hypotension following administration of a single dose of intravenous morphine?
   A. Depletion of intracellular free calcium
   B. Antagonism of μ-opioid receptors
   C. Stimulation of κ-opioid receptors
   D. Histamine release

Correct Answer: D

Explanation: Hypotension may occur after even small doses of morphine, an agonist of the μ-opioid receptor. This is mostly due to a decrease in systemic vascular resistance caused by histamine release. Pretreatment with histamine blockade can attenuate the hypotensive response in this setting. Morphine administration does not appear to stimulate the κ-opioid receptors or directly deplete intracellular free calcium.

References:

1. Lester L, Mitter N, Berkowitz DE, Augoustides JGT, Kaplan JA. Chapter 10: Pharmacology of Anesthetic Drugs. In: Kaplan JA, Augoustides JGT, Manecke GR, et al., eds. Kaplan's Cardiac Anesthesia. 7th ed. Elsevier; 2017:247-291.
2. Wehrfritz A, Senger AS, Just P, et al. Patient-controlled analgesia after cardiac surgery with median sternotomy: no advantages of hydromorphone when compared to morphine. J Cardiothorac Vasc Anesth, 2022; 36: 3587-3595.

21. Which statement below is true regarding the consequences of acute hemodilution by the cardiopulmonary bypass pump prime on drug disposition?
   A. Volume of distribution is significantly increased
   B. Free drug concentrations in plasma do not return back to equilibrium
   C. Effects of heparin may lead to displacement of drugs bound to plasma proteins
   D. Blood and plasma clearance of drugs all bear the same relationship after hemodilution

Correct Answer: C

TABLE 10.1

Effects of cardiopulmonary bypass on drug disposition

Pharmacokinetic Process	Pathophysiology	Pharmacokinetic Sequelae
Absorption	Hypotension and alterations in regional blood flow or perfusion	Reduced oral or intramuscular absorption
Distribution	Lung sequestration	Decreased volume of distribution
	Decreased pulmonary blood flow	Decreased pulmonary drug distribution and increased systemic drug levels
	Hypotension, altered regional blood flow	Decreased volume of distribution
	Decreased protein binding	Increased volume of distribution
	Hemodilution	
	Dilution of binding proteins	
	Postoperative increased α_1-acid glycoprotein	Decreased volume of distribution
	Postoperative increased protein binding	Interpretation of postoperative drug levels difficult
Elimination	Decreased hepatic blood flow	Decreased drug clearance
	Hypothermia	Decreased intrinsic clearance (decreased hepatic metabolism)
	Decreased renal blood flow and hypothermia	Decreased renal function

Explanation: There are major consequences of acute hemodilution by the pump prime on drug distribution during cardiopulmonary bypass. Plasma drug concentration is reduced with no change in the amount of drug in the body, which leads to an acute increase in the apparent volume of distribution. This increase is typically by a relatively small amount. Following acute hemodilution, drug redistribution from the tissues allows free drug concentrations in plasma and tissues to return back into equilibrium. The relative amounts of drug in the tissues and plasma, as well as the degree of protein binding, affect the magnitude of this flux. A focus on total drug concentration of the free fraction and free concentration change may give misleading information on the anticipated change in the drug effect. Regarding drugs whose plasma and red cell partitioning is not equal, blood and plasma clearance do not bear the same relationship to each other after hemodilution and must be distinguished. Heparin has an effect on the measurement of drug-protein binding by causing release of lipoprotein lipase and hepatic lipase. This hydrolyzes plasma triglycerides into nonesterified fatty acids, which can bind competitively to plasma proteins and lead to displacement of the bound drug and an increase in the concentration of the unbound fraction.

References:

1. Lester L, Mitter N, Berkowitz DE, Augoustides JGT, Kaplan JA. Chapter 10: Pharmacology of Anesthetic Drugs. In: Kaplan JA, Augoustides JGT, Manecke GR, et al., eds. Kaplan's Cardiac Anesthesia. 7th ed. Elsevier; 2017:247-291.
2. Skacel M, Knott C, Reynolds F, et al. Extracorporeal circuit sequestration of fentanyl and alfentanil. Br J Anaesth, 1986; 58: 947-949.

22. In patients undergoing cardiac surgery with cardiopulmonary bypass (CPB), which of the following events is most likely to result in an increase of plasma fentanyl concentrations?
    A. Initiation of mechanical ventilation in preparation for separation from CPB
    B. Addition of albumin to the pump prime during CPB
    C. Increase in the pump flow rate during CPB
    D. Initiation of moderate systemic hypothermia early during CPB

Correct Answer: A

Explanation: During cardiopulmonary bypass, the lungs are isolated from the circulation with interruption of pulmonary artery blood flow. Basic drugs such as fentanyl, lidocaine, propranolol are taken up by the lung and sequestered during cardiopulmonary bypass. The lungs may therefore serve as a reservoir for drug release upon re-establishment of systemic reperfusion. Following institution of cardiopulmonary bypass, plasma fentanyl concentrations decrease acutely, then plateau. Once mechanical ventilation of the lungs resumes prior to separation from cardiopulmonary bypass, plasma fentanyl concentrations increase, suggesting that fentanyl is being washed out from the lungs. When normothermia is reestablished during cardiopulmonary bypass, tissue reperfusion may lead to washout of drugs sequestered during the hypothermic period, resulting in an increase in plasma drug levels during the rewarming period. The addition of albumin to the pump prime and increasing the pump flow rate do not directly affect fentanyl concentrations significantly during cardiopulmonary bypass.

References:

1. Lester L, Mitter N, Berkowitz DE, Augoustides JGT, Kaplan JA. Chapter 10: Pharmacology of Anesthetic Drugs. In: Kaplan JA, Augoustides JGT, Manecke GR, et al., eds. Kaplan's Cardiac Anesthesia. 7th ed. Elsevier; 2017:247-291.
2. Bentley JB, Conahan TJ 3rd, Cork RC, et al. Fentanyl sequestration in lungs during cardiopulmonary bypass. Clin Pharmacol Ther, 1983; 34: 703-706.

23. Which opioid demonstrates the most stable free concentrations during cardiopulmonary bypass?
- **A.** Fentanyl
- **B.** Alfentanil
- **C.** Sufentanil
- **D.** Morphine

Correct Answer: B

Explanation: Free alfentanil concentrations remain relatively stable throughout cardiopulmonary bypass, and the pharmacologically active concentrations remain unchanged. Based upon its pharmacokinetic profile, alfentanil may be the most suitable opioid for cardiopulmonary bypass since its free concentrations are stable and its half-life is significantly less prolonged than other opioids such as fentanyl or morphine.

References:

1. Lester L, Mitter N, Berkowitz DE, Augoustides JGT, Kaplan JA. Chapter 10: Pharmacology of Anesthetic Drugs. In: Kaplan JA, Augoustides JGT, Manecke GR, et al., eds. Kaplan's Cardiac Anesthesia. 7th ed. Elsevier; 2017:247-291.
2. Hug CC Jr, Burm AG, de Lange S. Alfentanil pharmacokinetics in cardiac surgical patients. Anesth Analg, 1994; 78: 231-239.

24. Which of the following statements is true regarding the effect of cardiopulmonary bypass with induced hypothermia on the uptake of volatile anesthetics administered via the oxygenator?
- **A.** Cooling decreases the blood/gas solubility of volatile agents
- **B.** Hemodilution increases the blood/gas solubility of volatile agents
- **C.** Hypothermia increases solubility in tissue of volatile agents
- **D.** Uptake of volatile agents by the oxygenator has minimal effect

Correct Answer: C

Explanation: There are several factors that determine the effect of cardiopulmonary bypass with induced hypothermia on the uptake of volatile anesthetics administered via the oxygenator. The first consideration is the blood/gas solubility of the agent. Systemic cooling during cardiopulmonary bypass will increase blood/gas solubility of volatile anesthetics, whereas hemodilution will decrease the solubility of volatile agents due to changes in lipid concentration, osmolarity, and hematocrit. The onset of systemic hypothermia during cardiopulmonary bypass will increase the tissue solubility of volatile anesthetics. Lastly, the uptake of volatile anesthetics by the oxygenator can be significant.

References:

1. Lester L, Mitter N, Berkowitz DE, Augoustides JGT, Kaplan JA. Chapter 10: Pharmacology of Anesthetic Drugs. In: Kaplan JA, Augoustides JGT, Manecke GR, et al., eds. Kaplan's Cardiac Anesthesia. 7th ed. Elsevier; 2017:247-291.
2. Nussmeier N, Cohen NH, Moskowitz G, et al. Washin and washout of three volatile anesthetics concurrently administered during cardiopulmonary bypass. Anesthesiology, 1988; 69: 657-662.
3. Yeoh CJ, Hwang NC. Volatile anesthesia versus total intravenous anesthesia during cardiopulmonary bypass: a narrative review on the technical challenges and considerations. J Cardiothorac Vasc Anesth, 2020; 34: 2181-2188.

25. Which intravenous anesthetic induction agent produces the least change in the balance of myocardial oxygen demand and supply?
- **A.** Ketamine
- **B.** Etomidate
- **C.** Propofol
- **D.** Thiopental

Correct Answer: B

Explanation: Etomidate is the intravenous anesthetic agent that minimally changes the hemodynamic variables that affect myocardial oxygen balance such as heart rate, contractility, and systemic blood pressure. Compared with ketamine, propofol, and thiopental, etomidate produces the smallest change in these factors and therefore affects the balance of myocardial oxygen demand and supply the least.

References:

1. Lester L, Mitter N, Berkowitz DE, Augoustides JGT, Kaplan JA. Chapter 10: Pharmacology of Anesthetic Drugs. In: Kaplan JA, Augoustides JGT, Manecke GR, et al., eds. Kaplan's Cardiac Anesthesia. 7th ed. Elsevier; 2017:247-291.
2. Yao Y, He L, Fang N, et al. Anesthetic induction with etomidate in cardiac surgical patients: a PRISMA-compliant systematic review and meta-analysis. J Cardiothorac Vasc Anesth, 2021; 35: 1073-1085.

26. Which intravenous anesthetic agent has the most potential to facilitate the induction of ventricular arrhythmias during electrophysiologic procedures?
- **A.** Propofol
- **B.** Etomidate
- **C.** Ketamine
- **D.** Dexmedetomidine

Correct Answer: C

Explanation: In contrast to other intravenous anesthetic drugs, ketamine possesses stimulatory effects on the cardiovascular system. Although these effects are related to several mechanisms, one of the most important is central sympathetic nervous system stimulation and the subsequent release of norepinephrine. Although ketamine is also reported to

BOX 10.3 Intravenous anesthetics

Thiopental

- Thiopental decreases cardiac output by:
  - A direct negative inotropic action
  - Decreased ventricular filling resulting from increased venous capacitance
  - Transiently decreasing sympathetic outflow from the central nervous system
- Because of these effects, caution should be used when thiopental is given to patients who have left or right ventricular failure, cardiac tamponade, or hypovolemia.

Midazolam

- Small hemodynamic changes occur after the intravenous administration of midazolam.

Etomidate

- Etomidate is the drug that changes hemodynamic variables the least. Studies in noncardiac patients and patients who have heart disease document remarkable hemodynamic stability after administration of etomidate.
- Patients who have hypovolemia, cardiac tamponade, or low cardiac output probably represent the population for whom etomidate is better than other induction drugs, with the possible exception of ketamine.

Ketamine

- A unique feature of ketamine is stimulation of the cardiovascular system with the most prominent hemodynamic changes, including significant increases in heart rate, cardiac index, systemic vascular resistance, pulmonary artery pressure, and systemic artery pressure. These circulatory changes increase myocardial oxygen consumption with an appropriate increase in coronary blood flow.
- Studies have demonstrated the safety and efficacy of induction with ketamine in hemodynamically unstable patients, and it is the induction drug of choice for patients with cardiac tamponade physiology.

Dexmedetomidine

- Dexmedetomidine is a highly selective, specific, and potent adrenoreceptor agonist.
- α_2-Adrenergic agonists can safely reduce anesthetic requirements and improve hemodynamic stability. They can enhance sedation and analgesia without producing respiratory depression or prolonging the recovery period.

cause inhibition of serotonin and norepinephrine reuptake, there remains debate about the mechanism of norepinephrine reuptake. Ketamine administration has been associated with maintenance of sympathetic tone that facilitates the induction of ventricular arrhythmias in electrophysiologic procedures under general anesthesia. It was speculated that, in this scenario, ketamine's sympathomimetic properties may synergistically enhance the induction of ventricular tachyarrhythmias in concert with isoproterenol.

References:

1. Lester L, Mitter N, Berkowitz DE, Augoustides JGT, Kaplan JA. Chapter 10: Pharmacology of Anesthetic Drugs. In: Kaplan JA, Augoustides JGT, Manecke GR, et al., eds. Kaplan's Cardiac Anesthesia. 7th ed. Elsevier; 2017:247-291.
2. Atiyeh RH, Arthur ME, Berman AE, et al. The utility of ketamine in facilitating the induction of isoproterenol-refractory idiopathic ventricular tachyarrhythmias. J Cardiothorac Vasc Anesth, 2009; 23: 373-378.

27. Which anesthetic drug has shown promise for improving renal outcomes in cardiac surgery patients?
   A. Dexmedetomidine
   B. Isoflurane
   C. Propofol
   D. Ketamine

Correct Answer: A

Explanation: Several studies have demonstrated findings that perioperative dexmedetomidine may improve renal outcomes in surgical patients, potentially due to its anti-inflammatory properties. Clinical trials have shown positive effects on renal transplant outcomes with the administration of perioperative dexmedetomidine, as well as suggesting that renal outcomes may be improved with dexmedetomidine in the setting of cardiac surgery. Although the exact mechanism by which dexmedetomidine may improve renal outcomes is not fully understood, this topic is currently under active investigation. Isoflurane, propofol, and ketamine have not received much attention for renal protection in cardiac surgery.

References:

1. Lester L, Mitter N, Berkowitz DE, Augoustides JGT, Kaplan JA. Chapter 10: Pharmacology of Anesthetic Drugs. In: Kaplan JA, Augoustides JGT, Manecke GR, et al., eds. Kaplan's Cardiac Anesthesia. 7th ed. Elsevier; 2017:247-291.
2. Hong E, Alfadhel A, Ortoleva J. Perioperative dexmedetomidine and renal protection: promising and more investigation is warranted. J Cardiothorac Vasc Anesth, 2022; 36: 3725-3726.
3. Li B, Li Y, Tian S, et al. Anti-inflammatory effects of perioperative dexmedetomidine administered as an adjunct to general anesthesia: a meta-analysis. Sci Rep, 2015; 5: 12342.
4. Shan X, Hu L, Wang Y, et al. Effect of perioperative dexmedetomidine on delayed graft function following a donation-after-cardiac-death kidney transplant: a randomized clinical trial. JAMA Netw Open, 2022; 5: e2215217.
5. Peng K, Li D, Applegate RL, et al. Effect of dexmedetomidine on cardiac surgery-associated acute kidney injury: a meta-analysis with trial sequential analysis of randomized controlled trials. J Cardiothorac Vasc Anesth, 2020; 34: 603-613.

28. The inhibitory actions of opioids are primarily due to their interactions with which ion?
A. Sodium
B. Potassium
C. Calcium
D. Magnesium

Correct Answer: C

Explanation: The actions of opioids are mainly inhibitory. Opioids close N-type, voltage-operated calcium channels and open calcium-dependent inwardly rectifying potassium channels. This leads to hyperpolarization and a reduction in neuronal excitability. Calcium ions have essential roles in the processes of nociception.

References:

1. Lester L, Mitter N, Berkowitz DE, Augoustides JGT, Kaplan JA. Chapter 10: Pharmacology of Anesthetic Drugs. In: Kaplan JA, Augoustides JGT, Manecke GR, et al., eds. Kaplan's Cardiac Anesthesia. 7th ed. Elsevier; 2017:247-291.
2. McFadzean I. The ionic mechanisms underlying opioid actions. Neuropeptides, 1988; 11: 173-180.

29. The estimated number of deaths from opioid overdoses in the United States and Canada since 1999 is:
A. 100,000
B. 200,000
C. 500,000
D. >600,000

Correct Answer: D

Explanation: The opioid epidemic is a crisis in contemporary clinical practice and society at large. It is estimated that more than 600,000 people have died from opioid overdoses in the United States and Canada since 1999. The disruption of medical services and support care during the COVID-19 pandemic in 2020 further exacerbated this crisis. Cardiac anesthesiologists are some of the largest users of opioids in medicine, and opioid use remains indispensable in the perioperative cardiac surgical environment. The potential of opioids to cause harm should not lead to overtly restrictive usages (as that would also cause substantial patient harm); however, evidence clearly links the possibility of perioperative opioid use as a contributory factor to the opioid crisis. Approximately 10% of patients undergoing coronary artery bypass grafting and 8% of patients undergoing valve surgery who received an opioid prescription after discharge developed persistent opioid usage. This underscores the importance of cardiac anesthesiologists embracing innovative approaches to pain management, including multimodal nonopioid approaches with respect to both systemic medications and fascial plane blocks. Clearly, further large-scale studies are needed to help better determine strategies for addressing the opioid crisis without compromising quality of pain relief and comfort provided to cardiac surgery patients.

References:

1. Lester L, Mitter N, Berkowitz DE, Augoustides JGT, Kaplan JA. Chapter 10: Pharmacology of Anesthetic Drugs. In: Kaplan JA, Augoustides JGT, Manecke GR, et al., eds. Kaplan's Cardiac Anesthesia. 7th ed. Elsevier; 2017:247-291.
2. Tempe DK. Opioid stewardship in cardiac anesthesia practice. J Cardiothorac Vasc Anesth, 2022; 36: 2262-2264.
3. Brown CR, Chen Z, Khurshan F, et al. Development of persistent opioid use after cardiac surgery. JAMA Cardiology, 2020; 5: 889-896.

30. In a patient receiving isoflurane delivered during cardiac surgery with cardiopulmonary bypass, which of the following interventions would be expected to increase plasma concentrations of isoflurane?
A. Addition of red blood cells
B. Addition of crystalloid
C. Rewarming during cardiopulmonary bypass
D. Administration of cardioplegia solution

Correct Answer: A

Explanation: Crystalloid and colloid prime solutions cause hemodilution during cardiopulmonary bypass, which reduces the blood solubility of volatile anesthetics. Conversely, the addition of red blood cells to the prime increases the plasma concentration of volatile agents. The uptake and plasma solubility of volatile agents increase during hypothermia; however, during the rewarming phase prior to separation from cardiopulmonary bypass the temperature increase is typically more rapid than the increase in hematocrit. This decreases the blood/gas solubility to low levels, which promotes washout of volatile anesthetic and an abrupt decrease in the depth of anesthesia.

References:

1. Lester L, Mitter N, Berkowitz DE, Augoustides JGT, Kaplan JA. Chapter 10: Pharmacology of Anesthetic Drugs. In: Kaplan JA, Augoustides JGT, Manecke GR, et al., eds. Kaplan's Cardiac Anesthesia. 7th ed. Elsevier; 2017:247-291.
2. Yeoh CJ, Hwang NC. Volatile anesthesia versus total intravenous anesthesia during cardiopulmonary bypass: a narrative review on the technical challenges and considerations. J Cardiothorac Vasc Anesth, 2020; 34: 2181-2188.

Cardiovascular Pharmacology

J. Bradley Meers and Matthew M. Townsley

KEY POINTS

1. Ischemia during the perioperative period demands immediate attention by the anesthesiologist. The impact of ischemia may be acute (i.e., impending infarction or hemodynamic compromise) and chronic (i.e., marker of previously unknown cardiac disease or prognostic indicator of poor outcome).

2. Nitroglycerin is indicated in most cases of perioperative myocardial ischemia. Mechanisms of action include coronary vasodilation and favorable alterations in preload and afterload. Nitroglycerin is contraindicated in cases of hypotension.

3. Perioperative β-blockade may reduce the incidence of perioperative myocardial ischemia by several mechanisms when initiated at an appropriate time in the preoperative period. Favorable hemodynamic changes associated with β-blockade include blunting of the stress response and reduced heart rate, blood pressure, and contractility. All of these conditions improve myocardial oxygen supply-to-demand ratios.

4. Calcium channel blockers reduce myocardial oxygen demand by depression of contractility, reduction of heart rate, and decrease in arterial blood pressure. Calcium channel blockers are often administered in the perioperative period for long-term antianginal symptomatic control.

5. Current guidelines suggest seeking a target blood pressure of less than 150/90 mmHg in patients 60 years of age or older to minimize the long-term risk of adverse cardiovascular morbidity and mortality.

6. For patients younger than 60 years of age or those with diabetes or chronic kidney disease, blood pressures lower than 140/90 mmHg are recommended.

7. Mild or moderate hypertension does not represent an independent risk factor for perioperative complications, but a diagnosis of hypertension necessitates preoperative assessment for target organ damage.

8. Patients with poorly controlled preoperative hypertension experience more labile blood pressures in the perioperative setting with a greater potential for hypertensive and hypotensive episodes.

9. The signs, symptoms, and treatment of chronic heart failure are related to the neurohormonal response and underlying ventricular dysfunction.

10. Treatments for chronic heart failure are aimed at prolonging survival, along with relief of symptoms.

11. The pathophysiology, treatment, and prognosis of low cardiac output syndrome seen after cardiac surgery are different from those of chronic heart failure, with which it is sometimes compared.

12. Physicians must be cautious in administering antiarrhythmic drugs, because their proarrhythmic effects can increase mortality for certain subgroups of patients.

13. Amiodarone has become a popular intravenous antiarrhythmic drug for use in the operating room and critical care areas because it has a broad range of effects for ventricular and supraventricular arrhythmias.

14. β-Receptor antagonists are effective but underused antiarrhythmics in the perioperative period because many arrhythmias are adrenergically mediated due to the stress of surgery and critical illness.

15. Managing electrolyte abnormalities and treating underlying disease processes such as hypervolemia and myocardial ischemia are critical treatment steps before the administration of any antiarrhythmic agent.

1. A 47-year-old man presents for coronary artery bypass grafting. On arrival at the preoperative holding area, he complains of crushing chest pain with shortness of breath and diaphoresis. His systemic blood pressure is 130/70 mmHg, heart rate 85 beats per minute, and oxygen saturation 98% on 2 liters of nasal cannula oxygen. Administration of which of the following medications is the most appropriate choice to treat his symptoms?

A. Phenylephrine
B. Metoprolol
C. Ranitidine
D. Nitroglycerin

Correct Answer: D

Explanation: This patient's symptoms are concerning for myocardial ischemia. Myocardial ischemia results from alterations in the oxygen supply-to-demand balance (see Table 11.1). The clinical management in this setting should include additional history from the patient and physical exam. Angina and its variants including Prinzmetal angina due to coronary vasospasm, as well as silent ischemia, respond to nitroglycerin administration. Nitroglycerin therapy decreases the incidence of anginal attacks and improves exercise tolerance before angina symptoms occur. During therapy with intravenous nitroglycerin, if hypotension occurs and ischemia is not relieved, the addition of phenylephrine allows coronary perfusion pressure to be maintained while allowing higher doses of nitroglycerin to be used for ischemia relief.

TABLE 11.1

Myocardial ischemia: factors governing oxygen supply and demand

Oxygen Supply	Oxygen Demand
Heart rate[a]	Heart rate[a]
O_2 content	Contractility
Hgb, SAT%, PaO_2	Wall tension
Coronary blood flow	Afterload
CPP = DP − LVEDP[a]	Preload (LVEDP)[a]
CVR	

[a]Affects supply and demand.
CPP, Coronary perfusion pressure; CVR, coronary vascular resistance; DP, diastolic blood pressure; Hgb, hemoglobin; LVEDP, left ventricular end-diastolic pressure; PaO_2, partial pressure of oxygen; SAT, percent oxygen saturation.
Modified from Royster RL. Intraoperative administration of inotropes in cardiac surgery patients. J Cardiothorac Anesth, 1990; 6: 17.

References:

1. Royster RL, Groban L, Slaughter TF, Augoustides JGT, Kaplan JA. Chapter 11: Cardiovascular Pharmacology. In: Kaplan JA, Augoustides JGT, Manecke GR, et al., eds. Kaplan's Cardiac Anesthesia. 7th ed. Elsevier; 2017:292-354.
2. Horowitz JD. Role of nitrates in unstable angina pectoris. Am J Cardiol, 1992; 70: 64B
3. Mikhail MS, Thangathurai D, Thaker KB, et al. Echocardiographic assessment of coronary blood flow velocity during controlled hypotensive anesthesia with nitroglycerin. J Cardiothorac Vasc Anesth, 2000; 14: 565-570.

2. A 65-year-old woman with previous percutaneous coronary interventions to the left anterior descending and right coronary arteries is receiving nitroglycerin for angina treatment and prevention. Nitroglycerin exhibits vasodilatory effects through acting on which of the following cell signaling pathways?

A. Ion channel-linked receptors
B. G-protein–coupled receptors
C. Enzyme-linked receptors
D. Steroid hormone receptors

Correct Answer: B

Explanation: Nitrates, organic nitrites, and other nitric oxide donors such as sodium nitroprusside enter the smooth muscle vascular cells and are converted to nitric oxide or S-nitrosothiols, which stimulate guanylate cyclase metabolism via the G-protein–coupled receptor pathway. A cyclic guanosine monophosphate–dependent protein kinase is stimulated, with resultant protein phosphorylation in the smooth muscle. This leads to a dephosphorylation of the myosin light chain and smooth muscle relaxation. Cell surface receptors play an essential role in the transmission of information from the exterior of a cell to the interior. These transmembrane receptors change conformation when specific ligands, including drugs, ions, or proteins, bind to the receptor. Genetic variations may affect the pharmacological response to a given drug class such as nitrates through pharmacokinetic and pharmacodynamic effects. The relative selectivity of nitroglycerin compounds as preferential venodilators at low doses remains to be elucidated but may be related to enhanced uptake of these compounds by veins as compared to arteries.

References:

1. Royster RL, Groban L, Slaughter TF, Augoustides JGT, Kaplan JA. Chapter 11: Cardiovascular Pharmacology. In: Kaplan JA, Augoustides JGT, Manecke GR, et al., eds. Kaplan's Cardiac Anesthesia. 7th ed. Elsevier; 2017:292-354.
2. Kertai MD, Fontes M, Podgoreanu MV. Pharmacogenomics of β-blockers and statins: possible implications for perioperative cardiac complications. J Cardiothorac Vasc Anesth, 2012; 26: 1101-1114.
3. Ferdinand KC, Elkayan U, Mancini D, et al. Use of isosorbide dinitrate and hydralazine in African-Americans with heart failure 9 years after the Arican-American Heart Failure Trial. Am J Cardiol, 2014; 114: 151-159.

3. A 70-year-old male patient has received nitroglycerin to treat increasingly frequent anginal symptoms, but he has developed tolerance to its effects. Which of the following mechanisms explains this loss of effectiveness with prolonged exposure to nitroglycerin?

A. Upregulation of the calcium-hydrogen exchange channel
B. Increased metabolism of nitroglycerin
C. Increased metabolism of sulfhydryl groups
D. Increased metabolism of nitric oxide

Correct Answer: C

Explanation: Nitroglycerin is converted to reactive nitric oxide or to S-nitrosothiols, which both stimulate guanylate

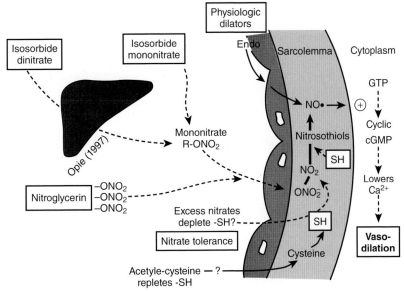

FIGURE 11.1 Mechanisms of nitrates *(ONO$_2$)* in the generation of the free radical nitric oxide *(NO•)* and stimulation of guanylate cyclase cyclic guanosine monophosphate *(cGMP)*, which mediates vasodilation. Sulfhydryl *(SH)* groups are required for the formation of NO• and the stimulation of guanylate cyclase. Isosorbide dinitrate is metabolized by the liver, whereas this route of metabolism is bypassed by the mononitrates. *Endo*, Endothelium; *GTP*, guanosine triphosphate. (Modified from Opie LH. 1995.)

cyclase metabolism to produced cyclic guanosine monophosphate (cGMP). Thereafter, a cGMP-dependent protein kinase is stimulated, with resultant protein phosphorylation in the smooth muscle. This leads to dephosphorylation of the myosin light chain and smooth muscle relaxation. Vasodilation is associated with a reduction of intracellular calcium. Sulfhydryl groups are required for formation of nitric oxide and the stimulation of cGMP. When excessive amounts of sulfhydryl groups are metabolized by prolonged exposure to nitroglycerin, vascular tolerance occurs. The addition of N-acetylcysteine, a donor of sulfhydryl groups, reverses nitroglycerin tolerance.

References:

1. Royster RL, Groban L, Slaughter TF, Augoustides JGT, Kaplan JA. Chapter 11: Cardiovascular Pharmacology. In: Kaplan JA, Augoustides JGT, Manecke GR, et al., eds. Kaplan's Cardiac Anesthesia. 7th ed. Elsevier; 2017:292-354.
2. Parker JD, Farrell B, Fenton T, et al. Counter-regulatory responses to continuous and intermittent therapy with nitroglycerin. Circulation, 1991; 84: 2336.

---

4. A 55-year-old female patient is receiving a low-dose nitroglycerin infusion for treatment of chest pain in the cardiac intensive care unit while awaiting a coronary artery bypass grafting operation. Which of the following parameters is expected to decrease in this patient?
A. Ventricular pressure
B. Aortic pressure
C. Cerebral pressure
D. Intraocular pressure

Correct Answer: A

Explanation: Two important physiologic effects of nitroglycerin are systemic and regional venous dilation. Venodilation can markedly reduce venous pressure, venous return to the heart, and cardiac filling pressures. Prominent venodilation occurs at lower doses and does not further increase as the nitroglycerin dose increases. Venodilation results primarily in pooling of blood in the splanchnic capacitance system. Mesenteric blood volume increases as ventricular size, ventricular pressures, and intrapericardial pressure decrease. Nitroglycerin increases the distensibility and conductance of large arteries without changing systemic vascular resistance at low doses. Improved compliance of the large arteries does not necessarily imply afterload reduction. At higher doses, nitroglycerin dilates small arterioles and resistance vessels, reducing afterload and blood pressure. Reductions in cardiac dimensions and pressure reduce myocardial oxygen consumption and improve myocardial ischemia. Nitroglycerin may preferentially reduce cardiac preload while maintaining systemic perfusion pressure. In hypovolemic states, higher doses of nitroglycerin may reduce systemic blood pressure to dangerous levels. Nitroglycerin can cause vasodilation of the cerebral vasculature, leading to headaches and increased intracranial pressure.

References:

1. Royster RL, Groban L, Slaughter TF, Augoustides JGT, Kaplan JA. Chapter 11: Cardiovascular Pharmacology. In: Kaplan JA, Augoustides JGT, Manecke GR, et al., eds. Kaplan's Cardiac Anesthesia. 7th ed. Elsevier; 2017:292-354.
2. Smith ER, Smiseth OA, Kingma I, et al. Mechanism of action of nitrates. Role of changes in venous capacitance and in the left ventricular diastolic pressure-volume relation. Am J Med, 1984; 76: 14-2.

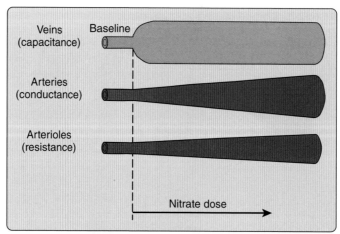

FIGURE 11.2 Actions of organic nitrates on the major vascular beds and relation of vasodilation to the size of the administered dose. The venous capacitance system dilates maximally with very low doses of organic nitrates. Increasing the amount of drug does not cause appreciable additional venodilation. Arterial dilation and enhanced arterial conductance begin at low doses of nitrates, with further vasodilation as the dosage is increased. With high plasma concentrations of nitrates, the arteriolar resistance vessels dilate, decreasing systemic and regional vascular resistance. (Modified from Abrams J. Hemodynamic effects of nitroglycerin and long-acting nitrates. Am Heart J. 1985;110(pt 2):216.)

3. Kieler-Jensen N, Houltz E, Milocco I, et al. Central hemodynamics and right ventricular function after coronary artery bypass surgery. A comparison of prostacyclin, sodium nitroprusside, and nitroglycerin for treatment of postcardiac surgical hypertension. J Cardiothorac Vasc Anesth, 1993; 7: 555-559.

5. Which region of the myocardium is most prone to ischemia and benefits most from nitroglycerin administration?
   A. Epicardium
   B. Subepicardium
   C. Endocardium
   D. Subendocardium

Correct Answer: D

Explanation: Nitroglycerin is a potent epicardial coronary artery vasodilator in normal and diseased vessels. Stenotic lesions dilate with nitroglycerin, reducing the resistance to coronary blood flow and improving myocardial ischemia. Smaller coronary arteries dilate relatively more than larger coronary vessels, but the degree of dilation may depend on the baseline tone of the vessel. Nitroglycerin effectively reverses or prevents coronary vasospasm. Although total coronary blood flow may initially increase, it eventually decreases over time with nitroglycerin despite coronary vasodilation. Autoregulatory mechanisms likely decrease total flow as a result of reductions in wall tension and myocardial oxygen consumption. However, regional blood flow may be improved by vasodilation of intercoronary collateral vessels or reduction of subendocardial compressive forces. Improvement in blood flow to the subendocardium, the area most vulnerable to development of ischemia, results from improvement in collateral flow and reductions in left ventricular end-diastolic pressure, which

reduce subendocardial resistance to blood flow. The ratio of endocardial to epicardial blood in transmural segments is enhanced with nitroglycerin.

References:
1. Royster RL, Groban L, Slaughter TF, Augoustides JGT, Kaplan JA. Chapter 11: Cardiovascular Pharmacology. In: Kaplan JA, Augoustides JGT, Manecke GR, et al., eds. Kaplan's Cardiac Anesthesia. 7th ed. Elsevier; 2017:292-354.
2. Smit M, Coetzee AR, Lochner A. The pathophysiology of myocardial ischemia and perioperative myocardial infarction. J Cardiothorac Vasc Anesth, 2020; 34: 2501-2512.

6. A 65-year-old patient presents to the cardiac catheterization lab with an ST segment elevation myocardial infarction. He received sublingual nitroglycerin at the time of transport with relief of chest pain. Upon moving to the procedural table, the patient notes worsening chest pain. The duration of action of sublingual nitroglycerin is expected to be which of the following?
   A. 5 to 10 minutes
   B. 10 to 15 minutes
   C. 15 to 30 minutes
   D. 30 to 45 minutes

Correct Answer: D

Explanation: Sublingual nitroglycerin (0.15–0.6 mg tablets) achieves blood levels adequate to cause hemodynamic changes within several minutes, with the physiologic effects lasting 30 to 45 minutes. Sublingual bioavailability is approximately 80% and bypasses the high (90%) first-pass biodegradation in the liver by nitrate reductase to glycerol dinitrate and nitrite, which are renally excreted. The plasma half-life of sublingual nitroglycerin is 4 to 7 minutes. Nitroglycerin spray has pharmacokinetics and pharmacodynamics equivalent to those of a 0.4 mg sublingual tablet but has a longer shelf half-life compared with the tablets, which decompose in air and at warm temperatures. A tablet that adheres to the buccal area between the upper lip and teeth has a rapid onset and has the advantage of a longer half-life than sublingual tablets. Although nitroglycerin is readily absorbed through the gastric mucosa, the high rate of liver metabolism makes oral administration highly unpredictable. Nitroglycerin is readily absorbed through the skin and available as an ointment. Topical nitroglycerin provides longer lasting effects, with a duration of action of 4 to 6 hours. The surface area of the ointment application, not the amount administered, determines the blood level achieved.

References:

1. Royster RL, Groban L, Slaughter TF, Augoustides JGT, Kaplan JA. Chapter 11: Cardiovascular Pharmacology. In: Kaplan JA, Augoustides JGT, Manecke GR, et al., eds. Kaplan's Cardiac Anesthesia. 7th ed. Elsevier; 2017:292-354.
2. Armstrong PW, Armstrong JA, Marks GS. Blood levels after sublingual nitroglycerin. Circulation, 1979; 59: 585.

7. Administration of which of the following antihypertensive agents can contribute to the generation of increased methemoglobin levels?
   A. Nitroprusside
   B. Nitroglycerin
   C. Nicardipine
   D. Clevidipine

Correct Answer: B

Explanation: The metabolism of nitroglycerin by liver nitrate reductases produces a nitrite that oxidizes the ferrous iron of hemoglobin to the ferric form of methemoglobin. The ferric iron does not bind or release oxygen. Methemoglobin is formed normally and is reduced by enzyme systems within the red blood cell. Normally, methemoglobin levels do not exceed 1%, but may increase when direct oxidants such as nitrates are present in the serum. Methemoglobinemia with levels up to 20% is not a clinical problem. Documented increases in methemoglobin blood levels occur with intravenous nitroglycerin administration, averaging 1.5% in one study of 50 patients receiving nitroglycerin for longer than 48 hours. Nitroglycerin doses of 5 mg/kg per day and higher should be avoided to prevent significant methemoglobinemia. Prolonged infusions of nitroprusside can lead to generation of cyanide. Nitrates are effective in producing methemoglobin, which binds cyanide to form cyanomethemoglobin. Nicardipine and clevidipine therapy have not been associated with the development of methemoglobinemia.

References:

1. Royster RL, Groban L, Slaughter TF, Augoustides JGT, Kaplan JA. Chapter 11: Cardiovascular Pharmacology. In: Kaplan JA, Augoustides JGT, Manecke GR, et al., eds. Kaplan's Cardiac Anesthesia. 7th ed. Elsevier; 2017:292-354.
2. Kaplan KJ, Taber M, Teagarden JR, et al. Association of methemoglobinemia and intravenous nitroglycerin administration. Am J Cardiol, 1985; 55: 181.
3. Williams RS, Mickell JJ, Young ES, et al. Methemoglobin levels during prolonged combined nitroglycerin and sodium nitroprusside infusions in infants after cardiac surgery. J Cardiothorac Vasc Anesth, 1994; 8: 658-662.

8. Which of the following coagulation effects has been observed in patients receiving a nitroglycerin infusion?
   A. No effect on coagulation
   B. Increased responsiveness to the anticoagulant effects of heparin
   C. Decreased platelet aggregation
   D. Increase in partial thromboplastin time

Correct Answer: C

Explanation: Nitroglycerin interferes with platelet aggregation. The ability of platelets to adhere to damaged intima is reduced, and the primary and secondary wave aggregation of platelets is also attenuated. Previously formed platelet plugs are disaggregated. In a small study of 10 patients with coronary artery disease, a mean nitroglycerin dose of 1.19 mcg/kg/minute inhibited platelet aggregation by 50%, with a return to baseline platelet aggregation 15 minutes after the infusion was discontinued. Nitroglycerin exposure enhances nitric oxide production with increases in cyclic guanosine monophosphate, leading to modulation of intracellular platelet calcium and reductions in platelet secretion of proaggregatory factors. The clinical significance of these actions, however, remains unclear.

Nitroglycerin may induce resistance to the anticoagulant effects of heparin. During simultaneous infusions of nitroglycerin and heparin, an increase in the nitroglycerin infusion results in a decrease in partial thromboplastin time. Nitroglycerin-induced heparin resistance at infusion rates greater than 350 mcg/min have been reported. The mechanism has been suggested to be a qualitative problem with antithrombin III, because in this setting the levels of this protein did not decrease. Nitroglycerin may interfere with the interaction of antithrombin III with heparin by N-desulfation of the heparin molecule at its binding site for antithrombin III.

References:

1. Royster RL, Groban L, Slaughter TF, Augoustides JGT, Kaplan JA. Chapter 11: Cardiovascular Pharmacology. In: Kaplan JA, Augoustides JGT, Manecke GR, et al., eds. Kaplan's Cardiac Anesthesia. 7th ed. Elsevier; 2017:292-354.
2. Diodati J, Theroux P, Latour JG, et al. Effects of nitroglycerin at therapeutic doses on platelet aggregation in unstable angina pectoris and acute myocardial infarction. Am J Cardiol, 1990; 66: 683.
3. Reich DL, Hammerschlag BC, Rand JH, et al. Modest doses of nitroglycerin do not interfere with beef lung heparin anticoagulation in patients taking nitrates. J Cardiothorac Vasc Anesth, 1992; 6: 677-679.
4. Becker RC, Corrao JM, Bovill EG, et al. Intravenous nitroglycerin-induced heparin resistance: a qualitative antithrombin III abnormality. Am Heart J, 1990; 119: 1254.

9. A 75-year-old patient presents with unstable angina. Vital signs demonstrate a heart rate of 95 beats per minute, systemic blood pressure of 100/50 mmHg, and oxygen saturation of 100% on 2 liters of nasal cannula oxygen. Bedside transthoracic echocardiography demonstrates preserved biventricular systolic function with mild anterior wall hypokinesis. Administration of which of the following agents is most appropriate?

A. Nitroglycerin
B. Metoprolol
C. Dobutamine
D. Epinephrine

Correct Answer: B

Explanation: Beta-adrenergic blockers have multiple favorable effects treating the ischemic heart. Beta blockers reduced oxygen consumption by decreasing heart rate, blood pressure, and myocardial contractility. Heart rate reduction increases diastolic coronary blood flow. Increased collateral blood flow and redistribution of blood to ischemic areas may occur with beta blockers. Microcirculatory oxygen delivery improves, and oxygen dissociates more easily from hemoglobin after beta-adrenergic blockade. Platelet aggregation is inhibited. Beta blockers should be started early in ischemic patients in the absence of contraindications. If the hemodynamics prevent concomitant nitroglycerin and beta blocker use, beta blockers should receive precedence. In this patient with an elevated heart rate and borderline systemic blood pressure, metoprolol represents the most appropriate agent. Epinephrine and dobutamine are beta agonists, and, while they may increase the systemic blood pressure, the heart rate would likely increase, further worsening ischemia. Nitroglycerin administration could lead to worsening hypotension with reflex tachycardia, leading to more ischemia in the setting of worsening hypotension and tachycardia. Beta blockers without intrinsic sympathomimetic activity are preferable when treating acute myocardial ischemia. Beta blockers administered during myocardial infarction reduce myocardial infarct size. Morbidity has been reduced by acute intravenous metoprolol administration during myocardial infarction with reductions in mortality extending up to 3 years thereafter.

BOX 11.2   ACC/AHA guidelines for early therapeutic use of β-adrenoceptor blocking agents after STEMI

Class I[a]

1. Oral beta blocker therapy should be initiated in the first 24 hours for patients who do not have any of the following: (1) signs of heart failure, (2) evidence of low output state, (3) increased risk[a] of cardiogenic shock, or (4) other relative contraindications to beta blockade (PR interval >0.24 s, second- or third-degree heart block, active asthma, or reactive airway disease) (level of evidence [LOE] B).
2. Patients with contraindications within the first 24 hours of STEMI should be reevaluated for candidacy for beta blocker therapy as secondary prevention (LOE C).
3. Patients with moderate or severe left ventricular failure should receive beta blocker therapy as secondary prevention with a gradual titration scheme (LOE B).

Class IIa

1. It is reasonable to administer an intravenous beta blocker at the time of presentation to STEMI patients who are hypertensive and who do not have any of the following: (1) signs of heart failure, (2) evidence of a low-output state, (3) increased risk[a] for cardiogenic shock, or (4) other relative contraindications to beta blockade (PR interval > 0.24 s, second- or third-degree heart block, active asthma, or reactive airway disease) (LOE B).

Class III

1. Intravenous beta blockers should not be administered to STEMI patients who have any of the following: (1) signs of heart failure, (2) evidence of a low-output state, (3) increased risk[a] of cardiogenic shock, or (4) other relative contraindications to beta blockade (PR interval > 0.24 s, second- or third-degree heart block, active asthma, or reactive airway disease) (LOE A).

[a]Risk factors for cardiogenic shock (the greater the number of risk factors, the higher the risk of developing cardiogenic shock) are age older than 70 years, systolic blood pressure less than 120 mmHg, sinus tachycardia greater than 110 beats/minute or heart rate less than 60 beats/minute, and increased time since the onset of symptoms of STEMI.
ACC, American College of Cardiology; *AHA*, American Heart Association; *STEMI*, ST-segment elevation myocardial infarction.
Reprinted with permission Circulation. 2008;117:296-329. © 2008 American Heart Association, Inc.

BOX 11.1   **Effects of beta adrenergic blockers on myocardial ischemia**

- Reductions in myocardial oxygen consumption
- Improvements in coronary blood flow
- Prolonged diastolic perfusion period
- Improved collateral flow
- Increased flow to ischemic areas
- Overall improvement in the supply-to-demand ratio
- Stabilization of cellular membranes
- Improved oxygen dissociation from hemoglobin
- Inhibition of platelet aggregation
- Reduced mortality rate after myocardial infarction

References:

1. Royster RL, Groban L, Slaughter TF, Augoustides JGT, Kaplan JA. Chapter 11: Cardiovascular Pharmacology. In: Kaplan JA, Augoustides JGT, Manecke GR, et al., eds. Kaplan's Cardiac Anesthesia. 7th ed. Elsevier; 2017:292-354.
2. Smit M, Coetzee AR, Lochner A. The pathophysiology of myocardial ischemia and perioperative myocardial infarction. J Cardiothorac Vasc Anesth, 2020; 34: 2501-2512.
3. Antman EM, Hand M, Armstrong PW, et al. 2007 Focused Update of the ACC/AHA 2004 Guidelines for the Management of Patients With ST-Elevation Myocardial Infarction: a report of the American College of Cardiology/American Heart Association Task Force on Practice Guidelines: developed in collaboration with the Canadian Cardiovascular Society endorsed by the American Academy of Family Physicians: 2007 Writing Group to Review New Evidence and Update the ACC/AHA 2004 Guidelines for the Management of Patients With ST-Elevation Myocardial Infarction, writing on behalf of the 2004 Writing Committee [published correction appears in Circulation. 2008 Feb 12;117(6):e162]. Circulation, 2008; 117: 296-329.

10. Initiation of beta blocker therapy immediately prior to surgery in patients who are intermediate to high risk for coronary artery disease complications has demonstrated which of the following effects?
    A. Lower rates of death
    B. Higher rates of acute kidney injury
    C. Lower rates of hypotension
    D. Higher rates of stroke

Correct Answer: D

Explanation: Studies investigating the role of perioperative beta blockade have generated conflicting results. The PeriOperative Ischemic Evaluation (POISE) trial examined the outcome effects of metoprolol started in patients with or at risk for atherosclerotic disease on the day of noncardiac surgery. The results of this trial demonstrated an increased perioperative risk of stroke and mortality. A meta-analysis concluded that perioperative beta blockade started less than a day before noncardiac surgery prevented nonfatal myocardial infarction but increased the perioperative risks of bradycardia, hypotension, stroke, and death.

References:

1. Royster RL, Groban L, Slaughter TF, Augoustides JGT, Kaplan JA. Chapter 11: Cardiovascular Pharmacology. In: Kaplan JA, Augoustides JGT, Manecke GR, et al., eds. Kaplan's Cardiac Anesthesia. 7th ed. Elsevier; 2017:292-354.
2. Leibowitz AB, Porter SB. Perioperative beta-blockade in patients undergoing noncardiac surgery: a review of the major randomized clinical trials. J Cardiothorac Vasc Anesth, 2009; 23: 684-693.
3. Wijeysundera DN, Duncan D, Nkonde-Price C, et al. Perioperative beta blockade in noncardiac surgery: a systematic review for the 2014 ACC/AHA guideline on perioperative cardiovascular evaluation and management of patients undergoing noncardiac surgery: a report of the American College of Cardiology/American Heart Association Task Force on practice guidelines. J Am Coll Cardiol, 2014; 64: 2406-2425.

11. Which receptor subtype is found at a higher density at the sinus node, atrioventricular node, and left and right bundle branches and in the Purkinje system?
    A. β_1
    B. α_1
    C. β_2
    D. α_2

Correct Answer: C

Explanation: The beta receptors have a multitude of responses. The β_1 and β_2 forms of stimulation primarily involve cardiac function. Endogenous norepinephrine produces inotropic responses in the myocardium by β_1 receptor stimulation. Epinephrine produces its maximal inotropic effects on the atria by β_2 receptor stimulation and up to 50% of its maximal inotropic response in the ventricles by β_2 receptor stimulation. The sinus node, atrioventricular node, left and right bundle branches, and Purkinje system contain higher densities of β_2 receptors. Both receptor subtypes have cardiac inotropic, chronotropic, and dromotropic properties. The β_2 receptors comprise 93% of the total population of beta receptors in arterioles and 100% of receptors in the epicardium, vena cava, aorta, and pulmonary artery. β_2 receptors are found on the internal mammary artery, but not the saphenous vein. β_2 receptor stimulation results in vascular smooth muscle relaxation and vasodilation.

References:

1. Royster RL, Groban L, Slaughter TF, Augoustides JGT, Kaplan JA. Chapter 11: Cardiovascular Pharmacology. In: Kaplan JA, Augoustides JGT, Manecke GR, et al., eds. Kaplan's Cardiac Anesthesia. 7th ed. Elsevier; 2017:292-354.
2. Molenaar P, Russell FD, Shimada T, et al. Function, characterization and autoradiographic localization and quantitation of beta-adrenoceptors in cardiac tissues. Clin Exp Physiol Pharmacol, 1989; 16: 529.

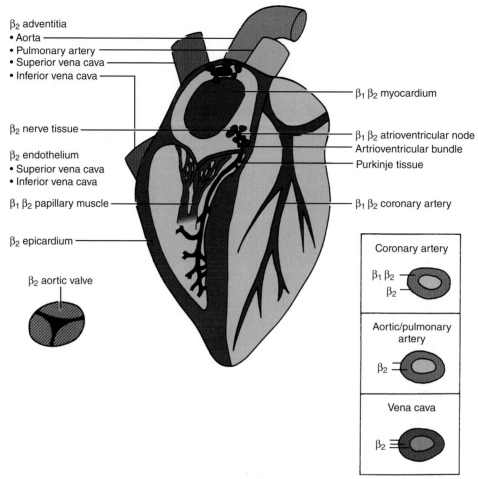

β₂ adventitia
- Aorta
- Pulmonary artery
- Superior vena cava
- Inferior vena cava

β₂ nerve tissue

β₂ endothelium
- Superior vena cava
- Inferior vena cava

β₁ β₂ papillary muscle

β₂ epicardium

β₂ aortic valve

β₁ β₂ myocardium

β₁ β₂ atrioventricular node
Artrioventricular bundle
Purkinje tissue

β₁ β₂ coronary artery

Coronary artery
β₁ β₂
β₂

Aortic/pulmonary artery
β₂

Vena cava
β₂

FIGURE 11.3 Locations of β_1- and β_2-adrenoceptors in rat, guinea pig, dog, and human hearts, as determined by autoradiography. The β_1- and β_2-adrenoceptors are located on myocardium and specialized conducting tissue. A greater density of β_2-adrenoceptors is found on the atrioventricular node, bundle of His, and left and right bundle branches compared with surrounding myocardium in guinea pig. The β_2-adrenoceptors are located on blood vessels, nerve tissue, epicardium, and the aortic valve. In large canine coronary arteries (0.5–2 mm in diameter), β_1-adrenoceptors account for 85% of the total population of β-adrenoceptors; in small arterioles (16–55 μm), β_2-adrenoceptors comprise 93% of the total population. (Modified from Summers RJ, Molenaar P, Stephenson JA. Autoradiographic localization of receptors in the cardiovascular system. Trends Pharmacol Sci, 1987; 8: 272; Jones CR. New views of human cardiac β-adrenoceptors. J Mol Cell Cardiol, 1989; 21: 519.)

12. Which of the following signaling pathways is utilized by both beta agonists and beta antagonists?
- **A.** Cyclic adenosine monophosphate signal pathway
- **B.** Phosphatidylinositol signal pathway
- **C.** Direct activation of membrane voltage-gated ion channels
- **D.** Cyclic guanosine monophosphate signal pathway

Correct Answer: C

Explanation: The beta receptor is a polypeptide chain of approximately 50,000 to 60,000 kilodaltons that is embedded in the cellular membrane. There are seven transmembrane crossings with two extramembranous terminal ends. Three extracellular and intracellular loops connect the intramembranous portion of the receptor. Agonist-antagonist binding occurs at the intramembranous portion, and the intracellular loops modulate interaction with the G-protein complex. The terminal intracellular end contains amino acid residues that undergo phosphorylation, which is related to desensitization and downregulation of the receptor. Receptor stimulation activates a G-protein, which stimulates adenylyl cyclase. Adenylyl cyclase converts adenosine triphosphate to cyclic adenosine monophosphate, which phosphorylates a protein kinase and produces the appropriate cellular response.

Cyclic guanosine monophosphate is a key intracellular signaling molecule in signal transduction pathways activated by nitric oxide. Phosphatidylinositol signal pathways may be activated after an extracellular signal molecule binds with the

G-protein receptor but is not the pathway utilized for signaling following beta receptor binding.

References:

1. Royster RL, Groban L, Slaughter TF, Augoustides JGT, Kaplan JA. Chapter 11: Cardiovascular Pharmacology. In: Kaplan JA, Augoustides JGT, Manecke GR, et al., eds. Kaplan's Cardiac Anesthesia. 7th ed. Elsevier; 2017:292-354.
2. Oprea AD, Lombard FW, Kertai MD. Perioperative β-adrenergic blockade in noncardiac and cardiac surgery: a clinical update. J Cardiothorac Vasc Anesth, 2019; 33: 817-832.
3. Gilman AG. G proteins: transducers of receptor-generated signals. Annu Rev Biochem, 1987; 56: 615.

13. Following implantation of a left ventricular assist device, a 55-year-old patient is receiving infusions of epinephrine and dobutamine for pharmacologic right ventricular function augmentation. An arterial blood gas immediately following separation from cardiopulmonary bypass demonstrates a serum K^+ level of 3.7 mEq/L. Which of the following changes in K^+ level is eventually expected to occur?
A. Decreased measured serum K^+ on arterial blood gas 2 hours later
B. Decreased total body K^+ levels
C. Increased measured serum K^+ on arterial blood gas 2 hours later
D. Increased total body K^+ levels

Correct Answer: A

Explanation: Dobutamine and epinephrine are beta receptor agonists with stimulatory effects on both β_1 and β_2 receptors. β_1 receptor stimulation increases plasma renin production and aqueous humor production. β_2 receptor stimulation increases insulin secretion, glycogenolysis, and lipolysis. β_2 receptor stimulation also shifts extracellular potassium to intracellular locations. This β_2 receptor stimulation would be expected to decrease the measured serum K^+ in this patient receiving beta agonist stimulation, while the total body potassium would acutely remain unchanged. β_2 receptor stimulation increases renal potassium loss. In this patient with a left ventricular assist device (LVAD), right ventricular systolic function is of paramount importance to generate output to fill the left heart for the LVAD to function. Arrhythmias from electrolyte disorders must be avoided and require careful monitoring of and treatment with electrolytes. With cessation of beta agonist therapy, K^+ may shift out of the intracellular space.

References:

1. Royster RL, Groban L, Slaughter TF, Augoustides JGT, Kaplan JA. Chapter 11: Cardiovascular Pharmacology. In: Kaplan JA, Augoustides JGT, Manecke GR, et al., eds. Kaplan's Cardiac Anesthesia. 7th ed. Elsevier; 2017:292-354.
2. Campbell NG, Allen E, Montgomery H, et al. Maintenance of serum potassium levels ≥3.6 mEq/L versus ≥4.5 mEq/L after isolated elective coronary artery bypass grafting and the incidence of new-onset atrial fibrillation: pilot and feasibility study results. J Cardiothorac Vasc Anesth, 2022; 36: 847-854.

TABLE 11.2
Physiologic effects of β_1- and β_2-receptor stimulation

Physiologic Effect	β_1 Response	β_2 Response
Cardiovascular Effects		
Increased heart rate	++	++
Increased contractility		
Atrium	+	++
Ventricle	++	++
Increased Automaticity and Conduction Velocity		
Nodal tissue	++	++
His-Purkinje	++	++
Arterial relaxation	—	
Coronary	—	++
Skeletal muscle	—	++
Pulmonary	—	+
Abdominal	—	+
Renal	+	+
Venous relaxation	—	++
Smooth Muscle Relaxation		
Trachea and bronchi	—	+
Gastrointestinal system	—	+
Bladder	—	+
Uterus	—	+
Splenic capsule	—	+
Ciliary muscle	—	+
Metabolic Effects		
Renin release	++	—
Lipolysis	++	+
Insulin secretion	—	+
Glycogenolysis, gluconeogenesis	—	++
Cellular K^+ uptake	—	+
ADH secretion (pituitary)	+	—

ADH, Antidiuretic hormone; +, response; ++, greater response; —, no response.
Modified from Lefkowitz RJ, Hoffman BB, Taylor P. Neurohumoral transmission: the autonomic and somatic motor nervous systems. In: Gilman AG, Rall TW, Niew AS, et al., eds. Goodman and Gilman's the Pharmacological Basis of Therapeutics. Pergamon Press; 1990:84-121.

14. Which of the following beta blockers demonstrates the most lipid solubility?
A. Labetalol
B. Esmolol
C. Metoprolol
D. Propranolol

Correct Answer: D

Explanation: Lipid-soluble beta blockers such as propranolol, metoprolol, and labetalol are well absorbed after oral administration and attain high concentrations in the brain. Lipid-soluble agents produce a high incidence of central nervous system effects, such as depression, sleep disturbances, and impotence. The rate of first-pass hepatic metabolism after oral ingestion can be very high but varies from patient to patient and affects daily dosing schedules. Cirrhosis, congestive heart failure, and cigarette smoking may reduce hepatic metabolism. Lipophilic agents are highly protein bound. The hepatic metabolism of lipophilic agents is independent of protein binding, which is different from most drugs for which hepatic metabolism occurs only with the unbound drug.

Propranolol is the most lipid-soluble beta blocker and has the most side effects in the central nervous system. Because the rate of first-pass liver metabolism is very high (90%), it requires much higher oral doses than intravenous doses for pharmacodynamic effect. Metoprolol is lipid-soluble, with 50% of the drug metabolized during first-pass hepatic metabolism and only 3% excreted renally. Labetalol is moderately lipid soluble and is completely absorbed after oral administration. Renal excretion of unchanged labetalol is minimal.

References:

1. Royster RL, Groban L, Slaughter TF, Augoustides JGT, Kaplan JA. Chapter 11: Cardiovascular Pharmacology. In: Kaplan JA, Augoustides JGT, Manecke GR, et al., eds. Kaplan's Cardiac Anesthesia. 7th ed. Elsevier; 2017:292-354.
2. Nies AS, Shand DG. Clinical pharmacology of propranolol. Circulation, 1975; 52: 6.
3. Fumargalli C, Maurizi N, Marchionni N, et al. β-blockers: their new life from hypertension to cancer and migraine. Pharmacol Res, 2020; 151: 104587.

15. Which of the following β-blockers demonstrates organ independent metabolism?
   A. Esmolol
   B. Sotalol
   C. Atenolol
   D. Metoprolol

Correct Answer: A

Explanation: Lipid-soluble beta blockers (propranolol, labetalol, metoprolol) undergo varying degrees of first-pass metabolism and undergo hepatic degradation. Lipid-insoluble or water-soluble agents (atenolol, nadolol, acebutolol, sotalol) are less absorbed orally and are not hepatically metabolized. These water-soluble agents are almost entirely eliminated by renal excretion and must be used cautiously in renal insufficiency. The chemical structure of esmolol is similar to metoprolol and propranolol except that it has a methyl ester group in the *para*-position of the phenyl ring, making it susceptible to rapid hydrolysis by red blood cell esterases. Esmolol is not metabolized by plasma cholinesterase.

References:

1. Royster RL, Groban L, Slaughter TF, Augoustides JGT, Kaplan JA. Chapter 11: Cardiovascular Pharmacology. In: Kaplan JA, Augoustides JGT, Manecke GR, et al., eds. Kaplan's Cardiac Anesthesia. 7th ed. Elsevier; 2017:292-354.
2. Jaramillo RP, Monaco F, Zangrillo A, et al. Ultra-short-acting β-blockers (esmolol and landiolol) in the perioperative period and in critically ill patients. J Cardiothorac Vasc Anesth, 2018; 32: 1415-1425.

16. Which of the following agents may exacerbate variant or vasospastic angina?
   A. Calcium channel blockers
   B. Beta blockers
   C. Angiotensin converting enzyme inhibitors
   D. Angiotensin receptor blockers

Correct Answer: B

Explanation: Calcium channel blockers are used primarily for symptom control in patients with stable angina pectoris. In the setting of acute ischemia, calcium channel blockers such as verapamil or diltiazem may be used for rate control when beta blockers are contraindicated. An important effect of calcium channel blockers is the treatment of variant angina. These drugs can attenuate ergonovine-induced coronary vasoconstriction in patients with variant angina, suggesting protection by coronary dilation. All calcium channel blockers are effective at reversing coronary spasm, reducing ischemic episodes, and reducing nitroglycerin consumption in patients with variant or Prinzmetal angina. Beta blockers may aggravate anginal episodes in some patients with vasospastic angina and should be used with caution. Preservation of coronary blood flow with calcium channel blockers is a significant difference from the predominant anti-ischemic effects of beta blockers.

References:

1. Royster RL, Groban L, Slaughter TF, Augoustides JGT, Kaplan JA. Chapter 11: Cardiovascular Pharmacology. In: Kaplan JA, Augoustides JGT, Manecke GR, et al., eds. Kaplan's Cardiac Anesthesia. 7th ed. Elsevier; 2017:292-354.
2. Robertson RH, Wood AJJ, Vaughan WK, et al. Exacerbation of vasotonic angina pectoris by propranolol. Circulation, 1982; 65: 281.
3. Turlapaty P, Vary R, Kaplan JA. Nicardipine, a new intravenous calcium antagonist: a review of its pharmacology, pharmacokinetics, and perioperative applications. J Cardiothorac Anesth, 1989; 3: 344-355.
4. Lord MS, Augoustides JG. Perioperative management of pheochromcytoma: focus on magnesium, cleviidpine, and vasopressin. J Cardiothorac Vasc Anesth, 2012; 26: 526-531.

17. Which of the following voltage-gated calcium channels is blocked by calcium antagonists?
   A. T channel
   B. C channel
   C. L channel
   D. N channel

Correct Answer: C

Explanation: There are three types of voltage-dependent calcium channels: the transient (T), long-lasting (L), and neuronal (N) channels. The T and L channels are located in cardiac and smooth muscle tissue, whereas the N channels are located only in neuronal tissue. The T channel is activated at low voltages (–50 mV) in cardiac tissue, plays a major role in cardiac depolarization (phase 0), and is not blocked by calcium antagonists. The L channels are the classic slow channels, are activated at higher voltages (–30 mV), and are responsible for phase 2 of the cardiac action potential. The L-type calcium channel has specific receptors that bind to each of the different chemical classes of calcium channel blockers. There are no described C voltage-gated calcium channels.

References:

1. Royster RL, Groban L, Slaughter TF, Augoustides JGT, Kaplan JA. Chapter 11: Cardiovascular Pharmacology. In: Kaplan JA, Augoustides JGT, Manecke GR, et al., eds. Kaplan's Cardiac Anesthesia. 7th ed. Elsevier; 2017:292-354.
2. Nowycky MC, Fox AP, Tsien RW. Three types of neuronal calcium channel with different calcium agonist sensitivity. Nature, 1985; 316: 440.
3. Colson P, Médioni P, Saussine M, et al. Hemodynamic effect of calcium channel blockade during anesthesia for coronary artery surgery. J Cardiothorac Vasc Anesth, 1992; 6: 424-428.

18. Which of the following agents does not suppress sinoatrial and atrioventricular node conduction?
 A. Diltiazem
 B. Verapamil
 C. Sotalol
 D. Nifedipine

Correct Answer: D

Explanation: Calcium channel blockers exert their primary electrophysiologic effects on tissue of the conducting system that depends on calcium for generation of the action potential, primarily at the sinoatrial and atrioventricular nodes. Nifedipine does not depress nodal conduction, whereas verapamil and diltiazem slow conduction velocity and prolong refractoriness of nodal tissue. Cautious use of intravenous verapamil with beta blockers is necessary because of an increased risk for atrioventricular block and/or severe myocardial depression. Sotalol is a beta blocker that slows nodal conduction.

References:

1. Royster RL, Groban L, Slaughter TF, Augoustides JGT, Kaplan JA. Chapter 11: Cardiovascular Pharmacology. In: Kaplan JA, Augoustides JGT, Manecke GR, et al., eds. Kaplan's Cardiac Anesthesia. 7th ed. Elsevier; 2017:292-354.
2. Rowland E, Evans T, Krikler D. Effect of nifedipine on atrioventricular conduction as compared with verapamil. Intracardiac electrophysiological study. Br Heart J, 1979; 42: 124.
3. van Wezel HB, Bovill JG, Visser CA, et al. Myocardial metabolism, catecholamine balance, and left ventricular function during coronary artery surgery: effects of nitroprusside and nifedipine. J Cardiothorac Anesth, 1987; 1: 408-417.

19. Which of following calcium channel blockers demonstrates non–organ-dependent degradation?
 A. Clevidipine
 B. Verapamil
 C. Diltiazem
 D. Nicardipine

Correct Answer: A

Explanation: Clevidipine is a dihydropyridine agent with a unique chemical structure that renders it inactive by cleavage of an ester linkage by nonspecific esterases in the blood and tissue. This unique property makes it an extremely short-acting drug, similar to other agents such as esmolol that are metabolized via this pathway. In patients receiving a clevidipine infusion, the clinical effects are fully reversed in 5 to 15 minutes following discontinuation of the infusion. Nicardipine has a plasma half-life of 8 to 9 hours and undergoes extensive hepatic metabolism, with less than 1% of the drug excreted renally, though plasma levels may increase in patients with renal failure. Verapamil and diltiazem undergo hepatic metabolism. The metabolism of verapamil may decrease in the presence of histamine receptor blockers.

References:

1. Royster RL, Groban L, Slaughter TF, Augoustides JGT, Kaplan JA. Chapter 11: Cardiovascular Pharmacology. In: Kaplan JA, Augoustides JGT, Manecke GR, et al., eds. Kaplan's Cardiac Anesthesia. 7th ed. Elsevier; 2017:292-354.
2. Lord MS, Augoustides JG. Perioperative management of pheochromocytoma: focus on magnesium, clevidipine, and vasopressin. J Cardiothorac Vasc Anesth, 2012; 26: 526-531.

20. Based on data from the Framingham Heart study, the lifetime risk for the subsequent development of hypertension in a patient who is normotensive at age 55 years is:
 A. 10%
 B. 25%
 C. 70%
 D. 90%

Correct Answer: D

Explanation: Systemic hypertension, long recognized as a leading cause of cardiovascular morbidity and mortality, accounts for enormous healthcare-related expenditures. Almost one-fourth of the US population has hypertensive vascular disease, but 30% of these individuals are unaware of their condition, and another 30% to 50% are inadequately treated. Based on data from the Framingham Heart Study, normotensive patients at age 55 years can expect a 90% lifetime risk for subsequent development of hypertension. Hypertension is the single most treatable risk factor for myocardial infarction, stroke, peripheral vascular disease, congestive heart failure, renal failure, and aortic dissection. Successful treatment of hypertension has been associated with a 35% to 40% reduction in the incidence of stroke, a 50% reduction in congestive heart failure, and a 25% reduction in myocardial infarction.

References:

1. Royster RL, Groban L, Slaughter TF, Augoustides JGT, Kaplan JA. Chapter 11: Cardiovascular Pharmacology. In: Kaplan JA, Augoustides JGT, Manecke GR, et al., eds. Kaplan's Cardiac Anesthesia. 7th ed. Elsevier; 2017:292-354.
2. Hunt SA, Baker DW, Chin MH, et al. ACC/AHA guidelines for the evaluation and management of chronic heart failure in the adult: executive summary. A report of the American College of Cardiology/American Heart Association task force on practice guidelines (committee to revise the 1995 guidelines for the evaluation and management of heart failure). J Am Coll Cardiol, 2001; 38: 2101.

21. Which of the following medications is capable of attenuating insulin resistance?
    A. Metoprolol
    B. Enalapril
    C. Valsartan
    D. Hydrochlorothiazide

Correct Answer: B

Explanation: Angiotensin-converting enzyme (ACE) inhibitors, such as enalapril, have several beneficial effects in patients with chronic heart failure. Through inhibition of ACE (which decreases levels of angiotensin II and norepinephrine while increasing levels of bradykinin, nitric oxide, and prostacyclin) they are potent vasodilators. ACE inhibitors reduce renal salt and water reabsorption, as well as release of norepinephrine from sympathetic nerves. They also play an important role in cardiac remodeling and reducing mortality in patients with chronic heart failure. Independent of angiotensin II activity, ACE inhibitors have also been shown to attenuate insulin resistance. Angiotensin receptor antagonists such as valsartan have not demonstrated a similar effect in attenuating insulin resistance. Metoprolol and hydrochlorothiazide have not been associated with attenuation of insulin resistance.

References:

1. Royster RL, Groban L, Slaughter TF, Augoustides JGT, Kaplan JA. Chapter 11: Cardiovascular Pharmacology. In: Kaplan JA, Augoustides JGT, Manecke GR, et al., eds. Kaplan's Cardiac Anesthesia. 7th ed. Elsevier; 2017:292-354.
2. Yoon U, Setren A, Chen A, et al. Continuation of angiotensin-converting enzyme inhibitors on the day of surgery is not associated with increased risk of hypotension upon induction of general anesthesia in elective noncardiac surgeries. J Cardiothorac Vasc Anesth, 2021; 35: 508-513.

22. Levosimendan increases cardiac contractility via which of the following mechanisms?
    A. Directly increasing cyclic adenosine monophosphate (cAMP) levels
    B. Indirectly increasing cAMP levels
    C. Causing calcium sensitization
    D. Directly increasing cyclic guanosine monophosphate levels

Correct Answer: C

Explanation: Cardiac anesthesiologists routinely manage acute heart failure, particularly when encountering low cardiac output syndrome during weaning from cardiopulmonary bypass. Positive inotropic drugs are a mainstay in treating this condition. In general, positive inotropes can be divided into two broad classifications: agents that increase cyclic adenosine monophosphate (cAMP) and agents that do not. Medications that increase cAMP levels indirectly include phosphodiesterase inhibitors such as milrinone, whereas beta adrenergic agents such as epinephrine and dobutamine do so directly. There are a number of medications that do not depend on cAMP to improve cardiac contractility, including: cardiac glycosides, calcium salts, thyroid hormone, and calcium sensitizers. Levosimendan is a calcium-sensitizing inodilator that activates adenosine triphosphate-sensitive potassium channels. Importantly, levosimendan improves myocardial contractility without increasing myocardial oxygen consumption.

References:

1. Royster RL, Groban L, Slaughter TF, Augoustides JGT, Kaplan JA. Chapter 11: Cardiovascular Pharmacology. In: Kaplan JA, Augoustides JGT, Manecke GR, et al., eds. Kaplan's Cardiac Anesthesia. 7th ed. Elsevier; 2017:292-354.
2. Faisal SA, Apatov DA, Ramakrishna H, et al. Levosimendan in cardiac surgery: evaluating the evidence. J Cardiothorac Vasc Anesth, 2019; 33: 1146-1158.

23. Milrinone increases cardiac contractility via which of the following mechanisms?
    A. Directly increasing cyclic adenosine monophosphate (cAMP) levels
    B. Indirectly increasing cAMP levels
    C. Causing calcium sensitization
    D. Directly increasing cyclic guanosine monophosphate levels

Correct Answer: A

Explanation: Milrinone inhibits phosphodiesterase III, which decreases the degradation of cyclic adenosine monophosphate (cAMP), leading indirectly to increases in intracellular cAMP. In addition to its effects as a positive inotrope, milrinone also improves diastolic relaxation. It is a potent vasodilator, producing reductions in preload, afterload, and pulmonary vascular resistance. Although a valuable treatment option for cardiac surgical patients with low cardiac output syndrome, it is important to appreciate the systemic vasodilatory effects of milrinone, which may require concomitant administration of a systemic vasopressor such as norepinephrine or vasopressin to ensure adequate systemic perfusion pressure.

References:

1. Royster RL, Groban L, Slaughter TF, Augoustides JGT, Kaplan JA. Chapter 11: Cardiovascular Pharmacology. In: Kaplan JA, Augoustides JGT, Manecke GR, et al., eds. Kaplan's Cardiac Anesthesia. 7th ed. Elsevier; 2017:292-354.
2. Ushio M, Egi M, Wakabayashi J, et al. Impact of milrinone administration in adult cardiac surgery patients: updated meta-analysis. J Cardiothorac Vasc Anesth, 2016; 30: 1454-1460.

24. Regarding beta-adrenergic receptor agonists, which of the following statements is true regarding their use in the perioperative cardiac surgical setting?
   A. Dopamine has a predominant effect on stroke volume rather than heart rate
   B. Dobutamine causes more tachycardia and hypotension than isoproterenol
   C. Dobutamine increases heart rate more than epinephrine
   D. Dobutamine has a predominant effect on stroke volume rather than heart rate

Correct Answer: C

Explanation: Similar to phosphodiesterase inhibitors, beta-adrenergic receptor agonists also augment cardiac contractility via cyclic adenosine monophosphate–dependent pathways. In the setting of cardiac surgery, the most commonly used beta-adrenergic receptor agonists include epinephrine, dobutamine, isoproterenol, and dopamine. Dopamine is a relatively weak inotrope with a more prominent effect on heart rate than stroke volume. Data suggest that dobutamine causes less tachycardia and hypotension than isoproterenol. Dobutamine does appear to have a more predominant effect on heart rate compared to stroke volume. Epinephrine is a powerful adrenergic agonist. Despite historical assumptions that epinephrine increases heart rate more than dobutamine in the setting of cardiac surgery, dobutamine has been demonstrated to increase heart rate more than epinephrine.

References:
1. Royster RL, Groban L, Slaughter TF, Augoustides JGT, Kaplan JA. Chapter 11: Cardiovascular Pharmacology. In: Kaplan JA, Augoustides JGT, Manecke GR, et al., eds. Kaplan's Cardiac Anesthesia. 7th ed. Elsevier; 2017:292-354.
2. Butterworth JF IV, Prielipp RC, Royster RL, et al. Dobutamine increases heart rate more than epinephrine in patients recovering from aortocoronary bypass surgery. J Cardiothorac Vasc Anesth, 1992; 6: 535.

25. In the Vaughan-Williams classification of antiarrhythmic drugs, Class IA agents exert their effects by which of the following mechanisms?
   A. Decreased slow-channel Ca^{2+} conductance
   B. Interference with Na^+ and Ca^{2+} exchange
   C. Beta-adrenergic receptor blockade
   D. Fast channel (Na^+) blockade

Correct Answer: D

TABLE 11.3
Classification of antiarrhythmic drugs

Effects	Type of Antiarrhythmic Drug			
	I (Membrane Stabilizers)	II (β-Adrenergic Receptor Antagonists)	III (Drugs Prolonging Repolarization)	IV (Calcium Antagonists)
Pharmacologic	Fast channel (Na^+) blockade	Beta-adrenergic receptor blockade	Uncertain: possible interference with Na^+ and Ca^{2+} exchange	Decreased slow-channel calcium conductance
Electrophysiologic	Decreased rate of V_{max}	Decreased V_{max}, increased APD, increased ERP, and increased ERP:APD ratio	Increased APD, increased ERP, increased ERP:ADP ratio	Decreased slow-channel depolarization; decreased ADP

APD, Action potential duration; *ERP*, effective refractory period; V_{max}, maximal rate of depolarization.

TABLE 11.4
Subgroup of Class I antiarrhythmic drugs

Electrophysiologic Activity	Subgroup		
	IA	IB	IC
Phase 0	Decreased	Slight effect	Marked decrease
Depolarization	Prolonged	Slight effect	Slight effect
Conduction	Decreased	Slight effect	Markedly slowed
ERP	Increased	Slight effect	Slight prolongation
APD	Increased	Decreased	Slight effect
ERP:APD ratio	Increased	Decreased	Slight effect
QRS duration	Increased	No effect during sinus rhythm	Marked increase
Prototype drugs	Quinidine, procainamide, disopyramide, diphenylhydantoin	Lidocaine, mexiletine, tocaine	Lorcainide, encainide, flecainide, aprinidine

APD, Action potential duration; *ERP*, effective refractory period.

Explanation: The Vaughan-Williams classification scheme is commonly utilized to describe the effects of different anti-arrhythmic drugs. However, it is important to understand that there is substantial overlap in the pharmacologic and electrophysiologic effects of specific agents among the different classes. In general, the mechanisms of action of the four Vaughan-Williams classes of drugs are as follows: Class I drugs inhibit the fast inward depolarizing current carried by Na^+ ions; Class II drugs block beta-adrenergic receptors; Class III drugs prolong cardiac repolarization; and Class IV drugs antagonize Ca^{2+} channels.

References:

1. Royster RL, Groban L, Slaughter TF, Augoustides JGT, Kaplan JA. Chapter 11: Cardiovascular Pharmacology. In: Kaplan JA, Augoustides JGT, Manecke GR, et al., eds. Kaplan's Cardiac Anesthesia. 7th ed. Elsevier; 2017:292-354.
2. Sharma A, Arora L, Subramani S, et al. Analysis of the 2018 American Heart Association focused update on advanced cardiovascular life support use of antiarrhythmic drugs during and immediately after cardiac arrest. J Cardiothorac Vasc Anesth, 2020; 34: 537-544.

26. In addition to amiodarone, the updated 2018 American Heart Association guidelines also recommend what other drug for treatment of ventricular fibrillation or pulseless ventricular tachycardia that does not respond to initial defibrillation?
    A. Procainamide
    B. Lidocaine
    C. Magnesium
    D. Mexiletine

Correct Answer: B

Explanation: Lidocaine is a Class IB antiarrhythmic agent that inactivates sodium channels in both the conduction system and myocardium, which raises the depolarization threshold and decreases arrhythmogenesis. In their updated guidelines for advanced cardiac life support, the American Heart Association recommended either lidocaine or amiodarone for treatment of ventricular fibrillation or pulseless ventricular tachycardia that does not respond to initial defibrillation. Amiodarone is a Class III antiarrhythmic agent that acts by blocking potassium rectifier currents responsible for repolarization of the heart during phase 3 of the cardiac action potential. By this mechanism, amiodarone decreases myocyte excitability, which prevents re-entry mechanisms and ectopic foci from perpetuating tachyarrhythmias.

References:

1. Royster RL, Groban L, Slaughter TF, Augoustides JGT, Kaplan JA. Chapter 11: Cardiovascular Pharmacology. In: Kaplan JA, Augoustides JGT, Manecke GR, et al., eds. Kaplan's Cardiac Anesthesia. 7th ed. Elsevier; 2017:292-354.
2. Sharma A, Arora L, Subramani S, et al. Analysis of the 2018 American Heart Association focused update on advanced cardiovascular life support use of cantiarrhythmic drugs during and immediately after cardiac arrest. J Cardiothorac Vasc Anesth, 2020; 34: 537-544.

27. Which of the following statements is true regarding amiodarone?
    A. It may cause significant negative inotropic effects
    B. It has a short elimination half-life
    C. Mortality from amiodarone-induced pulmonary toxicity is 5% to 10%
    D. Heart rate is not increased during amiodarone-associated hyperthyroidism

Correct Answer: D

Explanation: Amiodarone is a Class III antiarrhythmic drug effective at treating both supraventricular and ventricular arrhythmias. The pharmacokinetic profile of amiodarone demonstrates a low bioavailability, very long elimination half-life, relatively low clearance, and a large volume of distribution. It possesses very little negative inotropic activity, which makes it particularly attractive for use in patients with compromised ventricular function. Amiodarone unfortunately has a significant adverse reaction profile. Amiodarone-induced pulmonary toxicity is one of the most serious complications and leading causes of mortality associated with its use. Reported mortality rates from pulmonary toxicity range as high as 20% to 25%. Thyroid abnormalities are also common with amiodarone, with the frequencies of hyper- and hypothyroidism ranging from 1% to 5% and 1% to 2%, respectively. Heart rate is not increased during amiodarone-associated hyperthyroidism, most likely due to its antiadrenergic effects.

References:

1. Royster RL, Groban L, Slaughter TF, Augoustides JGT, Kaplan JA. Chapter 11: Cardiovascular Pharmacology. In: Kaplan JA, Augoustides JGT, Manecke GR, et al., eds. Kaplan's Cardiac Anesthesia. 7th ed. Elsevier; 2017:292-354.
2. Feduska ET, Thoma BN, Torjman MC, et al. Acute amiodarone pulmonary toxicity. J Cardiothorac Vasc Anesth, 2021; 35: 1485-1494.

28. Which of the following is considered a first-line drug treatment option for achieving rate control in a hemodynamically stable patient with atrial fibrillation?
    A. Digoxin
    B. Sotalol
    C. Diltiazem
    D. Amlodipine

Correct Answer: C

Explanation: Both beta blockers and nondihydropyridine calcium channel blockers such as diltiazem are useful first-line agents for attempting rate control therapy in hemodynamically stable patients with atrial fibrillation. In general, these agents are preferred over digoxin due to their more rapid onset and effectiveness in patients with a high sympathetic tone. Of note, combination therapy may often be required. Although digoxin is not effective in patients with a high sympathetic drive, it does not possess the negative inotropic effects of beta blockers and nondihydropyridine calcium channel blockers. Amiodarone may be considered as a

BOX 11.3 **Intravenous supraventricular antiarrhythmic therapy**

Class I Drugs

- Procainamide (IA): converts acute atrial fibrillation, suppresses PACs and precipitation of atrial fibrillation or flutter, converts accessory pathway SVT; 100 mg IV loading dose every 5 minutes until arrhythmia subsides or total dose of 15 mg/kg (rarely needed) with continuous infusion of 2–6 mg/min.

Class II Drugs

- Esmolol: converts or maintains slow ventricular response in acute atrial fibrillation; 0.5–1 mg/kg loading dose with each 50 µg/kg per minute increase in infusion, with infusions of 50–300 µg/kg per minute. Hypotension and bradycardia are limiting factors.

Class III Drugs

- Amiodarone: converts acute atrial fibrillation to sinus rhythm; 5 mg/kg IV over 15 minutes.
- Ibutilide (Convert): converts acute atrial fibrillation and flutter.
  - Adults (>60 kg): 1 mg IV given over 10 minutes; may repeat once.
  - Adults (<60 kg) and children: 0.01 mg/kg IV given over 10 minutes; may repeat once.
- Vernakalant: 3 mg/kg over 10 minutes in acute-onset atrial fibrillation; if no conversion, wait 15 minutes and then repeat with 2 mg/kg over 10 minutes. Hypotension may occur in a few patients.

Class IV Drugs

- Verapamil: slow ventricular response to acute atrial fibrillation; converts AV node reentry SVT; 75–150 µg/kg IV bolus.
- Diltiazem: slow ventricular response in acute atrial fibrillation; converts AV node reentry SVT; 0.25 µg/kg bolus, then 100–300 µg/kg/h infusion.

Other Therapy

- Adenosine: converts AV node reentry SVT and accessory pathway SVT; aids in diagnosis of atrial fibrillation and flutter. Increased dosage required with methylxanthines; decreased use required with dipyridamole.
  - Adults: 3–6 mg IV bolus, repeat with 6–12 mg bolus.
  - Children: 100 µg/kg bolus, repeat with 200 µg/kg bolus.
- Digoxin: maintenance IV therapy for atrial fibrillation and flutter; slows ventricular response.
  - Adults: 0.25 mg IV bolus followed by 0.125 mg every 1–2 hours until rate is controlled; not to exceed 10 µg/kg in 24 hours.
  - Children (<10 years): 10–30 µg/kg load given in divided doses over 24 hours.
  - Maintenance: 25% of loading dose.

AV, Atrioventricular; *IV*, intravenous; *PACs*, premature atrial contractions. *SVT*, supraventricular tachycardia.

treatment option for rate control in critically ill patients and those with severely reduced left ventricular systolic function. It may also be considered as an option when combination therapy is ineffective. In hemodynamically unstable patients, electric cardioversion is the initial management option of choice. Amlodipine is a dihydropyridine calcium channel blocker and is not a recommended treatment option for rate control in atrial fibrillation. Sotalol is an oral beta blocker that can be utilized in the long-term management of atrial fibrillation in select patients, but it is not typically considered a first-line agent for acute rate control in atrial fibrillation.

References:

1. Royster RL, Groban L, Slaughter TF, Augoustides JGT, Kaplan JA. Chapter 11: Cardiovascular Pharmacology. In: Kaplan JA, Augoustides JGT, Manecke GR, et al., eds. Kaplan's Cardiac Anesthesia. 7th ed. Elsevier; 2017:292-354.
2. Nelson JA, Gue YX, Christensen JM, et al. Analysis of the ESC/ EACTS 2020 atrial fibrillation guidelines with perioperative implications. J Cardiothorac Vasc Anesth, 2022; 36: 2177-2295.

29. A 57-year-old male undergoes combined aortic valve and mitral valve replacement. Approximately 4 hours following surgery he develops atrial fibrillation. His hemodynamics are stable, and rhythm control therapy is being considered by the intensive care unit team. Which of the following agents would be least indicated in this setting?

- **A.** Procainamide
- **B.** Amiodarone
- **C.** Flecainide
- **D.** Sotalol

Correct Answer: C

Explanation: When attempting to achieve rhythm control in patients with atrial fibrillation following cardiac surgery, it is important to appreciate that early recurrence is common. Therefore, ongoing antiarrhythmic drug therapy to prevent relapse is typically preferred over isolated cardioversion in hemodynamically stable patients. Class IA (quinidine, procainamide, disopyramide), Class IC (flecainide, propafenone), and Class III (amiodarone, sotalol, ibutilide, dofetilide) agents have all been demonstrated to be more effective than placebo. However, since Class IC agents are contraindicated in patients with structural heart disease, they would be contraindicated in this scenario due to their high proarrhythmic risk.

References:

1. Royster RL, Groban L, Slaughter TF, Augoustides JGT, Kaplan JA. Chapter 11: Cardiovascular Pharmacology. In: Kaplan JA, Augoustides JGT, Manecke GR, et al., eds. Kaplan's Cardiac Anesthesia. 7th ed. Elsevier; 2017:292-354.

2. Boons J, Van Biesen S, Fivez T, et al. Mechanisms, prevention, and treatment of atrial fibrillation after cardiac surgery: a narrative review. J Cardiothorac Vasc Anesth, 2021; 35: 3394-3403.
3. Andrikopoulos GK, Patromas S, Tzeis S. Flecainide: current status and perspectives in arrhythmia management. Word J Cardiol, 2015; 7: 76-85.

30. Following separation from cardiopulmonary bypass for combined coronary artery bypass grafting and mitral valve repair, a 54-year-old male is experiencing severe vasoplegia refractory to treatment with multiple vasopressor infusions. Prior to the administration of intravenous methylene blue, a review of the patient's history suggested a possible adverse reaction with one of his medications. Methylene blue may precipitate a significant adverse reaction when co-administered with which of the following drugs?
   A. Gabapentin
   B. Fluoxetine
   C. Digoxin
   D. Valsartan

Correct Answer: B

Explanation: Vasoplegia after cardiopulmonary bypass is a common, and potentially fatal, complication of cardiac surgery. Proposed mechanisms for its occurrence include an increased production of nitric oxide and endothelial dysfunction due to systemic inflammation. Methylene blue inhibits nitric oxide synthase and guanylate cyclase to decrease effects of nitric oxide on vascular smooth muscle relaxation. It may be considered as a treatment option for profound vasoplegia refractory to other therapies. Methylene blue is structurally similar to both tricyclic antidepressants and interferes with the uptake of serotonin. Patients taking serotonergic agents such as fluoxetine may be at increased risk for the development of serotonin syndrome when administered methylene blue. Methylene blue does not appear to have adverse reactions in the setting of therapy with gabapentin, digoxin, or valsartan.

References:

1. Royster RL, Groban L, Slaughter TF, Augoustides JGT, Kaplan JA. Chapter 11: Cardiovascular Pharmacology. In: Kaplan JA, Augoustides JGT, Manecke GR, et al., eds. Kaplan's Cardiac Anesthesia. 7th ed. Elsevier; 2017:292-354.
2. Hohlfelder B, Douglas A, Wang L, et al. Association of methylene blue dosing with hemodynamic response for the treatment of vasoplegia. J Cardiothorac Vasc Anesth, 2022; 36: 3543-3550.

CHAPTER 12

Electrocardiographic Monitoring

Gerard Manecke and Joel A. Kaplan

KEY POINTS

1. The electrocardiogram reflects differences in transmembrane voltages in myocardial cells that occur during depolarization and repolarization within each cycle.
2. Processing of the electrocardiogram occurs in a series of steps.
3. Where and how electrocardiographic (ECG) electrodes are placed on the body are critical determinants of the morphology of the ECG signal.
4. ECG signals must be amplified and filtered before display.
5. How accurately the clinician places ECG leads on the patient's torso is probably the single most important factor influencing clinical utility of the electrocardiogram.
6. The ST segment is the most important portion of the QRS complex for evaluating ischemia.
7. Use of inferior leads (II, III, aVF) allows superior discrimination of P-wave morphology and facilitates visual diagnosis of arrhythmias and conduction disorders.
8. Electrolyte abnormalities typically cause changes in repolarization (ST-T-U waves).

---

1. The P wave on the electrocardiogram monitor is produced by:
   A. Sinoatrial node depolarization
   B. Atrioventricular node depolarization
   C. Atrial depolarization
   D. Atrial repolarization

Correct Answer: C

Explanation: Although the sinoatrial node normally generates the spontaneous action potential that is then propagated to the atrial tissue, its action potential is too small to be detected by clinical electrocardiogram monitors. The atrial depolarization generates a larger current, producing the "P wave" on the monitor. The clinical significance of this is that, although P waves on the monitor indicate atrial depolarization, they may not be resulting from sinus rhythm. When P waves are present, other atrial foci could be generating an action potential that is then propagated to atrial tissue.

References:

1. Freudzon L, Akhtar S, London MJ, et al. Chapter 12: Electrocardiographic Monitoring. In: Kaplan JA, Augoustides JGT, Manecke GR, et al., eds. Kaplan's Cardiac Anesthesia. 7th ed. Elsevier; 2017:357-389.
2. Douedi S, Douedi H. P Wave. In: StatPearls [Internet]. Treasure Island (FL): StatPearls Publishing; 2022.

2. Channels for which ions account for the electrical activity of the heart:
   A. Sodium
   B. Potassium
   C. Chloride
   D. All of the above

Correct Answer: D

Explanation: Sodium, potassium, chloride, and calcium channels are present in the heart, accounting for depolarization, repolarization, and propagation of action potentials.

References:

1. Freudzon L, Akhtar S, London MJ, et al. Chapter 12: Electrocardiographic Monitoring. In: Kaplan JA, Augoustides JGT, Manecke GR, et al., eds. Kaplan's Cardiac Anesthesia. 7th ed. Elsevier; 2017:357-389.
2. Oberman R, Bhardwaj A. Cardiac Physiology. In: StatPearls [Internet]. Treasure Island (FL): StatPearls Publishing; 2022.

3. The power spectrum of the electrocardiogram monitor waveform is used for:
A. Amplification
B. Filtering
C. Analog to digital conversion
D. Analog signal detection

Correct Answer: B

Explanation: The power spectrum of the electrocardiogram is a component of digital signal processing. After the electrical signal has been digitized (analog to digital conversion), it undergoes mathematical process called the Fourier transform. The Fourier transform is a type of frequency analysis, allowing a variety of digital signal processing techniques—the most notable being filtering.

References:

1. Freudzon L, Akhtar S, London MJ, et al. Chapter 12: Electrocardiographic Monitoring. In: Kaplan JA, Augoustides JGT, Manecke GR, et al., eds. Kaplan's Cardiac Anesthesia. 7th ed. Elsevier; 2017:357-389.
2. Chavan MS, Agarwala RA, Uplane MD. Suppression of baseline wander and power line interference in ECG using digital IIR filter. International J Circuit, 2008; 2: 356-365.

4. The ECG waveform component with the highest intrinsic frequency (Hz) is:
A. QRS complex
B. T wave
C. Pacemaker spike
D. S-T segment

Correct Answer: C

Explanation: Pacemaker spikes are very high–intrinsic frequency, short-duration events (1.5–5 kHz). These characteristics make them problematic for automatic assessment of

TABLE 12.1

Range of signal frequencies included in different phases of processing in an electrocardiographic monitor

Processing	Frequency Range
Display	0.5 (or 0.05)–40 Hz
QRS detection	5–30 Hz
Arrhythmia detection	0.05–60 Hz
ST-segment monitoring	0.05–60 Hz
Pacemaker detection	1.5–5 kHz

heart rate. Thus, automatic heart rate determination usually relies on QRS complexes, and not pacemaker spikes.

References:

1. Freudzon L, Akhtar S, London MJ, et al. Chapter 12: Electrocardiographic Monitoring. In: Kaplan JA, Augoustides JGT, Manecke GR, et al., eds. Kaplan's Cardiac Anesthesia. 7th ed. Elsevier; 2017:357-389.
2. Tsibulko VV, Iliev IT, Jekova II. Methods for detecting pacemaker pulses in ECG signal: a review. Ann J Electron, 2014.

5. The electrocardiogram sampling rate recommended by the American Heart Association for detection of myocardial ischemia is:
A. 0.5 to 10 Hz
B. 0.05 to 100 Hz
C. 0.5 to 1 kHz
D. 5 to 10 MHz

Correct Answer: B

Explanation: The American Heart Association recommends an electrocardiogram (ECG) sampling rate of 0.05 to 100 Hz for detection of myocardial ischemia. Although the frequencies of the components of the ECG are usually below 100 Hz, some portions of the waveform reach or exceed 100 Hz.

References:

1. Freudzon L, Akhtar S, London MJ, et al. Chapter 12: Electrocardiographic Monitoring. In: Kaplan JA, Augoustides JGT, Manecke GR, et al., eds. Kaplan's Cardiac Anesthesia. 7th ed. Elsevier; 2017:357-389.
2. Fleisher LA, Beckman JA, Brown KA, et al. ACC/AHA 2007 guidelines on perioperative cardiovascular evaluation and care for noncardiac surgery: a report of the American College of Cardiology/American Heart Association Task Force on Practice Guidelines (Writing Committee to Revise the 2002 Guidelines on Perioperative Cardiovascular Evaluation for Noncardiac Surgery): developed in collaboration with the American Society of Echocardiography, American Society of Nuclear Cardiology, Heart Rhythm Society, Society of Cardiovascular Anesthesiologists, Society for Cardiovascular Angiography and Interventions, Society for Vascular Medicine and Biology, and Society for Vascular Surgery. Circulation, 2007; 116: e418-e499.

6. Noise reduction for the electrocardiogram waveform on monitor systems is accomplished by:
A. Digital filtering
B. Beat alignment
C. Signal averaging
D. All of the above

Correct Answer: D

Explanation: Digital low-pass filtering allows the removal of high frequency noise. Also, during processing, electrocardiogram data bits are inspected by a microprocessor using a form of mathematical construct to determine where reference points ("fiducial points") are located. A common method locates the point of most rapid change in amplitude (located on the down slope of the R wave). This process characterizes the baseline QRS complex (QRS recognition) and provides a "template" on which subsequent beats are overlaid (beat alignment) and averaged (signal averaging). This not only allows visual display of the QRS complex and quantification of its components, but also eliminates random electrical noise and wide complex beats that fail to meet criteria established by the fiducial points. QRS waveform amplitudes and durations are subject to beat-to-beat variability and to respiratory variability between beats. Digital electrocardiograms can adjust for respiratory variability and decrease beat-to-beat noise to improve the measurement precision in individual leads by forming a representative complex for each lead. Signal averaging is a critical component of this process.

References:

1. Freudzon L, Akhtar S, London MJ, et al. Chapter 12: Electrocardiographic Monitoring. In: Kaplan JA, Augoustides JGT, Manecke GR, et al., eds. Kaplan's Cardiac Anesthesia. 7th ed. Elsevier; 2017:357-389.
2. Froelicher VF. Special methods: computerized exercise ECG analysis. In: Exercise and the Heart. Year Book; 1987:36.

7. On electrocardiogram monitors, S-T segment elevation is tracked using:

   A. J point assessment

   B. Fiducial points to identify ST segments

   C. Fourier transform

   D. QRS slopes

Correct Answer: B

Explanation: "Fiducial points" are determined by the electrocardiogram (ECG) microprocessors and used to identify various components of the ECG waveform. A feature incorporated into most monitors is a visual trend line from which deviations in the position of the ST segment can be rapidly detected, a feature that can aid online detection of ischemia. In addition, nearly all monitors display on-screen numeric values for the position of the ST segment used for ischemia detection (generally 60–80 ms after the J point), although the specific fiducial point used (based on heart rate) can be adjusted by the clinician.

References:

1. Freudzon L, Akhtar S, London MJ, et al. Chapter 12: Electrocardiographic Monitoring. In: Kaplan JA, Augoustides JGT, Manecke GR, et al., eds. Kaplan's Cardiac Anesthesia. 7th ed. Elsevier; 2017:357-389.
2. Lee S, Jeong Y, Park D, et al. Efficient fiducial point detection of ECG QRS complex based on polygonal approximation. Sensors (Basel). 2018;18(12):4502. doi: 10.3390/s18124502. PMID: 30572644; PMCID: PMC6308480.

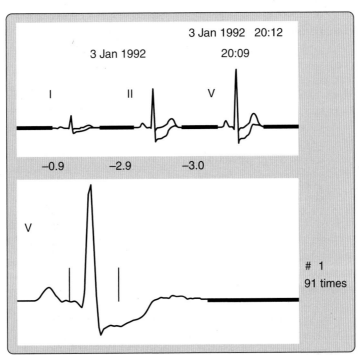

FIGURE 12.1 The graphic output of the ST-segment adjustment window from a Marquette Electronics Series 7010 monitor (Milwaukee, WI) ST-segment analyzer. This software allows trending and display of three leads (i.e., I, II, and any single V lead). In this window, the initial complex ("learned" when the program was activated) is displayed along with the current complex. Two complexes are superimposed with different intensities to facilitate comparison. ST-segment analysis is performed automatically at 80 ms after the J point, although the user can manually adjust this. The number of QRS complexes that are input to the monitor is displayed. (From Reich DL, Mittnacht A, London M, Kaplan J. Monitoring of the Heart and Vascular System. In: Kaplan JA, Konstadt SN, Reich DL, eds. Kaplan's Cardiac Anesthesia. 5th ed. Philadelphia: Saunders; 2006.)

8. Which of the following is NOT associated with electrocardiogram (ECG) artifact caused by the cardiopulmonary bypass pump?
  A. The electrical energy required to drive the roller pumps
  B. Low ambient temperature
  C. Low relative humidity
  D. ECG baseline variability at 1 to 4 Hz

Correct Answer: A

Explanation: Surprisingly, the electrical energy driving the roller pump is not the cause of the electrocardiogram (ECG) interference. Rather, static electricity resulting from the pump rotation is thought to be the cause of ECG artifact during cardiopulmonary bypass (CPB). This artifact has been noted when the roller pump is hand-cranked. Low ambient temperature and low relative humidity have been associated with CPB-induced ECG artifact.

References:

1. Freudzon L, Akhtar S, London MJ, et al. Chapter 12: Electrocardiographic Monitoring. In: Kaplan JA, Augoustides JGT, Manecke GR, et al., eds. Kaplan's Cardiac Anesthesia. 7th ed. Elsevier; 2017:357-389.
2. Khambatta HJ, Stone JG, Wald A, et al. Electrocardiographic artifacts during cardiopulmonary bypass. Anesth Analg, 1990; 71: 88-91

9. In which situation is deterioration to complete heart block when placing a pulmonary artery catheter a particular concern?
  A. Sinus bradycardia
  B. Frequent premature ventricular contractions
  C. Right bundle branch block
  D. Left bundle branch block

Correct Answer: D

Explanation: Sinus bradycardia and frequent premature ventricular contractions may be concerns during placement of a pulmonary artery catheter. Left bundle branch block, however, poses the unique risk of complete heart block if conduction via the right His-Purkinje bundle is disrupted by mechanical disturbance by the catheter as it is passed through the right ventricle. Thus, the distinct risk of complete heart block should be considered when placing a pulmonary artery catheter in a patient with left bundle branch block.

References:

1. Freudzon L, Akhtar S, London MJ, et al. Chapter 12: Electrocardiographic Monitoring. In: Kaplan JA, Augoustides JGT, Manecke GR, et al., eds. Kaplan's Cardiac Anesthesia. 7th ed. Elsevier; 2017:357-389.
2. Abernathy WS. Complete heart block caused by the Swan-Ganz catheter. Chest, 1974; 65: 349.

10. During cardiovascular surgery, which electrocardiogram monitoring lead combination has been shown to be the most sensitive in detecting intraoperative myocardial ischemia?
  A. II only
  B. V5 only
  C. II and V4
  D. aVL only

Correct Answer: C

Explanation: Of those listed, the combination of leads II and V4 has been shown to be the most sensitive in detecting myocardial ischemia using electrocardiogram monitoring.

TABLE 12.2

Sensitivity for different electrocardiographic lead combinations

Number of Leads	Combination	Sensitivity (%)
1 lead	II	33
	V_4	61
	V_5	75
2 leads	II/V_5	80
	II/V_4	82
	V_4/V_5	90
3 leads	V_3/V_4/V_5	94
	II/V_4/V_5	96
4 leads	II/V_2–V_5	100

Data from London MJ, Hollenberg M, Wong MG, et al. Intraoperative myocardial ischemia: localization by continuous 12-lead electrocardiography. Anesthesiology, 1988; 69: 232.

References:

1. Freudzon L, Akhtar S, London MJ, et al. Chapter 12: Electrocardiographic Monitoring. In: Kaplan JA, Augoustides JGT, Manecke GR, et al., eds. Kaplan's Cardiac Anesthesia. 7th ed. Elsevier; 2017:357-389.
2. London MJ, Hollenberg M, Wong MG, et al. Intraoperative myocardial ischemia: localization by continuous 12-lead electrocardiography. Anesthesiology, 1988; 69: 232-241.

11. The single electrocardiogram monitoring lead that is most sensitive in detecting the onset of prolonged myocardial ischemia is:
  A. V3
  B. V6
  C. II
  D. V2

Correct Answer: A

Explanation: Lead V3 has been shown to be the most sensitive electrocardiogram monitoring lead for detecting the onset of prolonged myocardial ischemia.

References:

1. Freudzon L, Akhtar S, London MJ, et al. Chapter 12: Electrocardiographic Monitoring. In: Kaplan JA, Augoustides JGT,

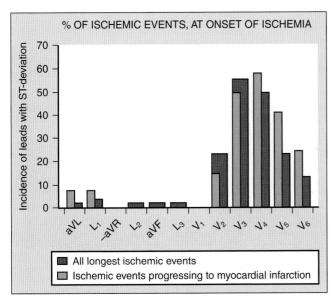

FIGURE 12.2 Histogram showing the incidence in which prolonged ischemia was first noted by each lead at the onset of ischemia in all 38 longest ischemic events and in the 12 ischemic events that progressed to myocardial infarction. (Reproduced with permission from Landesberg G, Mosseri M, Wolf Y, et al. Perioperative myocardial ischemia and infarction: identification by continuous 12-lead electrocardiogram with online ST-segment monitoring. Anesthesiology, 2002; 96: 264–270.)

Manecke GR, et al., eds. Kaplan's Cardiac Anesthesia. 7th ed. Elsevier; 2017:357-389.

2. Landesberg G, Mosseri M, Wolf Y, et al. Perioperative myocardial ischemia and infarction: identification by continuous 12-lead electrocardiogram with online ST-segment monitoring. Anesthesiology, 2002; 96: 264-270.

12. Perioperative T wave changes in noncardiac surgery are associated with:
    A. Myocardial ischemia
    B. Potassium abnormalities
    C. Acute cholecystitis
    D. All of the above

Correct Answer: D

Explanation: T-wave changes are associated with a variety of stimuli, including changes in serum glucose, elevated catecholamines, acute hyperventilation, and upper gastrointestinal disease. Potassium abnormalities are also associated with T wave changes, an example being the tall or "peaked" T waves seen in hyperkalemia.

References:

1. Freudzon L, Akhtar S, London MJ, et al. Chapter 12: Electrocardiographic Monitoring. In: Kaplan JA, Augoustides JGT, Manecke GR, et al., eds. Kaplan's Cardiac Anesthesia. 7th ed. Elsevier; 2017:357-389.
2. Breslow MJ, Miller CF, Parker SD, et al. Changes in T-wave morphology following anesthesia and surgery: a common recovery-room phenomenon. Anesthesiology, 1986; 64: 398-402.

13. A 41-year-old woman with mitral valve prolapse has undergone a mitral valve repair utilizing cardiopulmonary bypass (CPB), aortic cross clamping, and high potassium cardioplegia. Her serum [K+] immediately prior to separation from CPB is 6.5 meq/L. You observe the electrocardiogram monitor to determine if there are cardiac electrical abnormalities associated with her hyperkalemia. Which are NOT associated with hyperkalemia?
    A. U waves
    B. "Peaked" T waves
    C. Prolonged QRS complex
    D. Prolonged P-R interval

Correct Answer: A

Explanation: Hyperkalemia is common immediately following cardiopulmonary bypass during which high potassium cardioplegia was administered. Electrocardiogram changes associated with hyperkalemia typically start with narrowing and peaking of the T waves. Further elevation of extracellular potassium leads to prolongation of the QRS complex. The reason is delayed atrioventricular (AV) conduction, and an AV block may appear. These changes are typically followed by prolongation of the PR interval, flattening of the P waves, and loss of the P wave because the high potassium levels delay the spread of the cardiac activating impulse through the myocardium. Further increase in plasma potassium levels cause sine waves, which can progress to asystole or ventricular fibrillation. Hyperkalemia may also reduce the myocardial response to artificial pacemaker stimulation. U waves are not associated with hyperkalemia; they are associated with hypokalemia.

References:

1. Freudzon L, Akhtar S, London MJ, et al. Chapter 12: Electrocardiographic Monitoring. In: Kaplan JA, Augoustides JGT, Manecke GR, et al., eds. Kaplan's Cardiac Anesthesia. 7th ed. Elsevier; 2017:357-389.
2. Levis JT. ECG diagnosis: hyperkalemia. Perm J, 2013; 17: 69.

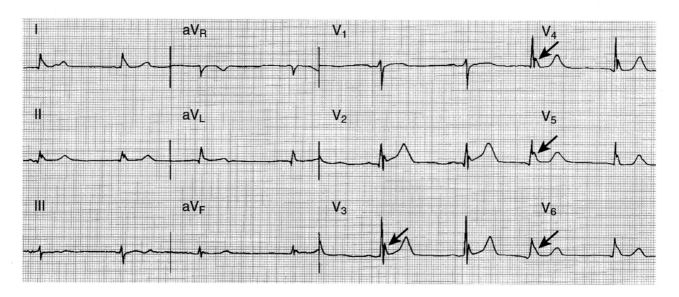

14. Immediately following cardiac surgery utilizing hypothermic cardiopulmonary bypass, the upward deflections in the figure (arrows) are noted on the initial postoperative 12-lead electrocardiogram. Which of the following is (are) true?
  A. They are often associated with hypothermia
  B. When present, they are most apparent in the limb and precordial leads
  C. They may be associated with severe hypercalcemia
  D. All of the above

Correct Answer: D

Explanation: The depicted waves are known as "Osborn waves" or "J waves." They are positive deflections at the J point, most apparent in the limb leads I, II, and III and in the precordial leads. Most commonly associated with hypothermia, they may also be seen in severe hypercalcemia.

References:

1. Freudzon L, Akhtar S, London MJ, et al. Chapter 12: Electrocardiographic Monitoring. In: Kaplan JA, Augoustides JGT, Manecke GR, et al., eds. Kaplan's Cardiac Anesthesia. 7th ed. Elsevier; 2017:357-389.
2. Jain AG, Zafar H, Jain S, et al. Osborn waves: differential diagnosis. Tex Heart Inst J, 2019; 46: 231-232.

15. Which of the following cause shortening of the Q-T interval?
  A. Droperidol
  B. Digoxin
  C. Amiodarone
  D. Procainamide

Correct Answer: B

Explanation: Cardiac glycosides cause shortening of the Q-T interval and "scooping" of the ST segment. Droperidol may cause prolongation of the Q-T interval. Amiodarone and procainamide have both been reported to cause Q-T interval prolongation as well.

References:

1. Freudzon L, Akhtar S, London MJ, et al. Chapter 12: Electrocardiographic Monitoring. In: Kaplan JA, Augoustides JGT, Manecke GR, et al., eds. Kaplan's Cardiac Anesthesia. 7th ed. Elsevier; 2017:357-389.
2. Farzam K, Tivakaran VS. Q-T prolonging drugs. In: StatPearls [Internet]. Treasure Island (FL): StatPearls Publishing; 2022.

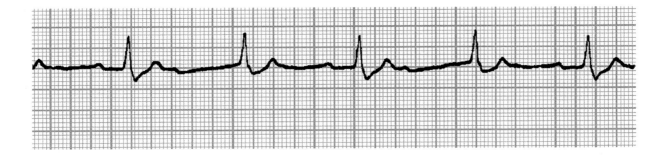

16. The above tracing was obtained in a 78-year-old man undergoing aortic valve replacement immediately prior to separation from cardiopulmonary bypass. The rhythm is most consistent with:
  A. Third degree heart block
  B. Sinus arrhythmia
  C. First degree heart block
  D. AV nodal rhythm

Correct Answer: A

Explanation: Third-degree heart block is characterized by lack of association between P waves and QRS complexes, bradycardia, and the P wave rate faster than the QRS rate. The QRS complex may be prolonged, depending on where the QRS is initiated. Electrical pacing should be instituted if the patient is hemodynamically unstable.

17. Please refer to the figure in question 16: The above rhythm is best treated with:
  A. Atropine
  B. Dual-chamber cardiac pacing
  C. Intravenous dopamine
  D. Intravenous epinephrine infusion

Correct Answer: B

Explanation: The tracing above demonstrates third degree heart block. The most reliable treatment is cardiac pacing. Atrial pacing will be ineffective, since atrial depolarizations are not transmitted to the ventricles. Likewise, atropine may increase the atrial rate while having little or no effect on the ventricular rate. Epinephrine may increase the heart rate, but the most reliable method of increasing the heart rate while providing AV synchrony is dual-chamber pacing.

References:

1. Freudzon L, Akhtar S, London MJ, et al. Chapter 12: Electrocardiographic Monitoring. In: Kaplan JA, Augoustides JGT, Manecke GR, et al., eds. Kaplan's Cardiac Anesthesia. 7th ed. Elsevier; 2017:357-389.
2. Wallenhaupt SL, Rogers AT. Intraoperative use of dual-chamber demand pacemakers for open heart operations. Ann Thorac Surg, 1989; 48: 579-581.

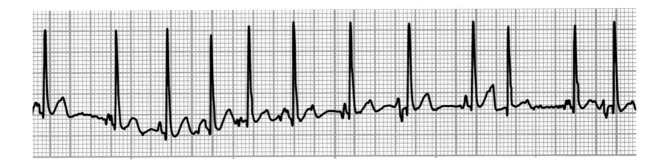

18. In the figure, the electrocardiogram abnormality is most commonly associated with:
  A. Right coronary artery disease
  B. Left anterior descending coronary artery disease
  C. Severe lung disease
  D. Hypertrophic cardiomyopathy

Correct Answer: C

Explanation: This is an example of multifocal atrial tachycardia (MFAT), which is most commonly associated with severe lung disease. MFAT is characterized by heart rate 100 to 200 beats per minute, irregular rhythm, and consecutive P waves of varying shape.

References:

1. Freudzon L, Akhtar S, London MJ, et al. Chapter 12: Electrocardiographic Monitoring. In: Kaplan JA, Augoustides JGT, Manecke GR, et al., eds. Kaplan's Cardiac Anesthesia. 7th ed. Elsevier; 2017:357-389.
2. Custer AM, Yelamanchili VS, Lappin SL. Multifocal atrial tachycardia. In: StatPearls [Internet]. Treasure Island (FL): StatPearls Publishing; 2022.

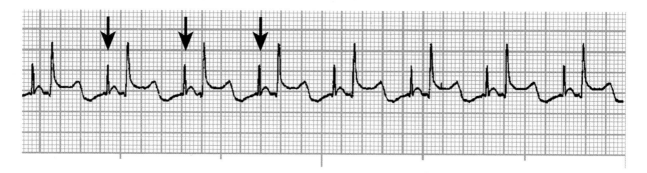

19. The type of cardiac pacing seen in the figure is most commonly used for:
   A. Atrial stimulation when atrioventricular (AV) conduction is intact
   B. Emergency pacing in which AV conduction is failing
   C. Asynchronous support in atrial fibrillation
   D. Dual-chamber stimulation

Correct Answer: A

Explanation: The tracing in the figure depicts atrial pacing. Atrial pacing is often used when atrioventricular conduction is intact. It is particularly useful when the patient benefits from the atrial contraction to enhance stroke volume. The arrows indicate atrial pacing spikes; a P wave with associated QRS complex follows each spike.

References:

1. Freudzon L, Akhtar S, London MJ, et al. Chapter 12: Electrocardiographic Monitoring. In: Kaplan JA, Augoustides JGT, Manecke GR, et al., eds. Kaplan's Cardiac Anesthesia. 7th ed. Elsevier; 2017:357-389.
2. Reade MC. Temporary epicardial pacing after cardiac surgery: a practical review. Anaesthesia, 2007; 62: 364-373.

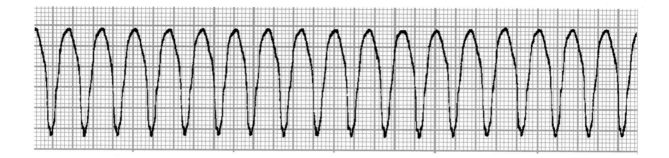

20. A 66-year-old woman underwent coronary artery bypass surgery. Postoperatively, upon arrival to the intensive care unit, her monitor suddenly shows the tracing seen in the figure. Her blood pressure is 71/33 mmHg, and the pulse oximeter, placed on the right index finger, senses a pulse. The most appropriate first step in treating the patient is:
   A. Defibrillation
   B. Synchronous DC cardioversion
   C. Adenosine, 6 mg IV
   D. Lidocaine 100 mg IV

Correct Answer: B

Explanation: The above rhythm is ventricular tachycardia. The wide QRS complex and absence of P waves are the most notable characteristics. In the presence of hemodynamic compromise with a pulse, as in this case, immediate direct current synchronized cardioversion is required. If the patient is pulseless, defibrillation is indicated. If the patient is stable, pharmacologic management is preferred. Ventricular tachycardia should be differentiated from supraventricular tachycardia with aberrancy (SVT-A). The presence of P waves and response to vagal maneuvers such as carotid massage would suggest SVT-A.

References:

1. Freudzon L, Akhtar S, London MJ, et al. Chapter 12: Electrocardiographic Monitoring. In: Kaplan JA, Augoustides JGT, Manecke GR, et al., eds. Kaplan's Cardiac Anesthesia. 7th ed. Elsevier; 2017:357-389.
2. Goyal A, Sciammarella JC, Chhabra L, et al. Synchronized electrical cardioversion. In: StatPearls [Internet]. Treasure Island (FL): StatPearls Publishing; 2022.

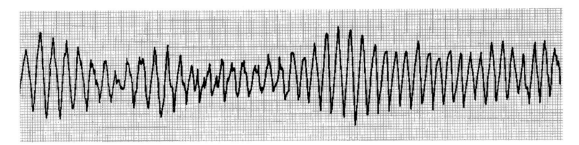

21. The rhythm seen in the figure:
   A. Should prompt the administration of intravenous (IV) magnesium sulfate
   B. May be prevented by avoiding medications that cause decreases in the QTc interval
   C. May respond to IV epinephrine
   D. All of the above

Correct Answer: A

Explanation: The rhythm depicted in the figure is torsades de pointes. A risk factor for this type of ventricular tachycardia is prolonged QT interval. Administering standard antiarrhythmic agents (e.g., lidocaine, procainamide) may worsen torsades de pointes. Prevention includes treating the electrolyte disturbances and avoiding medications that prolong the QTc interval. Treatment includes administration of intravenous magnesium sulfate (2 g over 1–2 minutes), and DC cardioversion may be necessary in unstable patients.

References:

1. Freudzon L, Akhtar S, London MJ, et al. Chapter 12: Electrocardiographic Monitoring. In: Kaplan JA, Augoustides JGT, Manecke GR, et al., eds. Kaplan's Cardiac Anesthesia. 7th ed. Elsevier; 2017:357-389.
2. Cohagan B, Brandis D. Torsades de pointes. In: StatPeals [Internet]. Treasure Island (FL): StatPearls Publishing; 2022.

22. A 58-year-old man is undergoing aortic valve replacement using cardiopulmonary bypass (CPB). The aorta is crossclamped, and cardioplegia has been administered. You become concerned that there may still be cardiac electrical activity because you note rhythmic activity on the electrocardiogram monitor at 3 Hz. Methods to determine if this phenomenon is artifactual include:
   a. Temporarily change or discontinue CPB flow
   b. Observe the heart using transesophageal echocardiography
   c. Directly observe the heart in the surgical field
   d. All of the above

Correct Answer: D

Explanation: Bypass pump artifact during cardiopulmonary bypass (CPB) is common, characterized by wandering electrocardiogram baseline at 0 to 4 Hz. Because it results from electrical signals from the roller pump, changing the speed of the roller pump (pump flow) or temporarily stopping CPB flow will change the frequency of or eliminate the artifact. Thus, changing or discontinuing pump flow may change the frequency of the artifact. The heart can also be observed directly in the surgical field or by using transesophageal echocardiography to detect evidence of cardiac contractions.

References:

1. Freudzon L, Akhtar S, London MJ, et al. Chapter 12: Electrocardiographic Monitoring. In: Kaplan JA, Augoustides JGT, Manecke GR, et al., eds. Kaplan's Cardiac Anesthesia. 7th ed. Elsevier; 2017:357-389.
2. Khambatta HJ, Stone JG, Wald A, et al. Electrocardiographic artifacts during cardiopulmonary bypass. Anesth Analg, 1990; 71: 88-91.

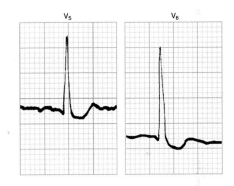

23. A 73-year-old man with history of congestive heart failure and coronary artery disease presents for coronary artery bypass surgery. Upon application of the electrocardiogram (ECG) monitor prior to anesthetic induction, the ECG tracing (seen in the figure) is noted. The abnormality is most likely associated with:
   A. Evolving transmural myocardial infarction
   B. Left bundle branch block
   C. Digoxin therapy
   D. Beta blockade withdrawal

Correct Answer: C

Explanation: The "scooping" of the ST segments is characteristic of "digitalis effect." An easy way to remember this is to envision a digoxin pill "sitting" in the scooped portion of the ST segment.

References:

1. Freudzon L, Akhtar S, London MJ, et al. Chapter 12: Electrocardiographic Monitoring. In: Kaplan JA, Augoustides JGT, Manecke GR, et al., eds. Kaplan's Cardiac Anesthesia. 7th ed. Elsevier; 2017:357-389.
2. Djohan AH, Sia CH, Singh D, et al. A myriad of electrocardiographic findings associated with digoxin use. Singapore Med J, 2020; 61: 9-14.

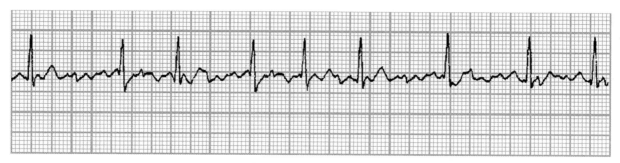

24. A 55-year-old, 68-kg man presents for coronary artery bypass surgery. His preoperative 12-lead electrocardiogram (ECG), performed 2 months prior to admission, demonstrated normal sinus rhythm and left ventricular hypertrophy. He has no history of cardiac rhythm abnormalities, and baseline monitoring of his ECG in the operating room reveals normal sinus rhythm. Immediately after anesthetic induction, the ECG tracing (seen in the figure) is obtained. His blood pressure is 132/88 mmHg, arterial oxygen saturation is 98%, and his end-tidal CO_2 is 35 mmHg. The most appropriate next step is to:

A. Perform synchronized DC cardioversion

B. Administer amiodarone 150 mg intravenously over 10 minutes

C. Administer diltiazem 10 mg intravenously

D. Perform transesophageal echocardiography

Correct Answer: D

Explanation: The irregularly irregular rhythm, normal QRS duration, and absence of P waves all lead to the diagnosis of atrial fibrillation. This may represent new atrial fibrillation, although it is possible that he had asymptomatic bouts of atrial fibrillation previously that were not detected on 12-lead electrocardiogram. Since atrial fibrillation may have been present prior to this event, and the patient is hemodynamically stable, the first item of business is to obtain an echocardiogram to rule out thrombus in the left atrium (most commonly left atrial appendage). Because transesophageal echocardiography (TEE) is more sensitive than transthoracic echocardiography for the diagnosis of left atrial pathology, TEE is the preferred method to rule out left atrial thrombus. Cardioversion in a stable patient with atrial fibrillation should not be performed until left atrial thrombus has been ruled out because of the risk of thrombotic stroke upon cardioversion.

References:

1. Freudzon L, Akhtar S, London MJ, et al. Chapter 12: Electrocardiographic Monitoring. In: Kaplan JA, Augoustides JGT, Manecke GR, et al., eds. Kaplan's Cardiac Anesthesia. 7th ed. Elsevier; 2017:357-389.
2. January CT, Wann, LS, Calkins H, et al. 2019 AHA/ACC/HRS focused update of the 2014 AHA/ACC/HRS Guideline for the Management of Patients With Atrial Fibrillation: A Report of the American College of Cardiology/American Heart Association Task Force on Clinical Practice Guidelines and the Heart Rhythm Society in collaboration with the Society of Thoracic Surgeons. Circulation, 2019; 140: e125-e151.

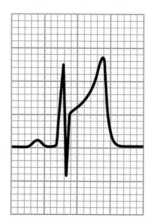

25. A 76-year-old man is undergoing coronary artery bypass. During attempted separation from cardiopulmonary bypass the tracing in the figure is observed in lead V4. Of the following, the most likely diagnosis is:

A. Air in the right coronary artery

B. Inferior wall myocardial infarction

C. Air in the left coronary artery

D. Normal J point elevation

Correct Answer: C

Explanation: The elevated ST segment in V4, a precordial lead, suggests severe perfusion deficit to the anterior wall of the left ventricle. Retained air in the left coronary artery is a possible etiologic factor. This usually resolves with supportive care, nitroglycerin, and blood pressure support. If the situation does not resolve with supportive care, surgical removal of the air may be required (air can often be visualized in saphenous vein grafts). Further, there may be a coronary occlusion or some other cause, such as thrombosis, kinked graft, or ineffective coronary anastomosis. These problems often necessitate further revascularization.

References:

1. Freudzon L, Akhtar S, London MJ, et al. Chapter 12: Electrocardiographic Monitoring. In: Kaplan JA, Augoustides JGT, Manecke GR, et al., eds. Kaplan's Cardiac Anesthesia. 7th ed. Elsevier; 2017:357-389.
2. Bashir H, Adroja S, Jabri A, et al. Improved acute ST-segment elevation due to air embolism after coronary artery bypass graft procedure. Chest, 2020; 158: A273.

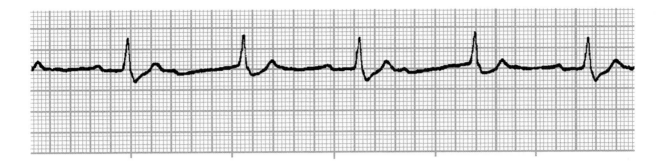

26. In the figure the electrocardiogram abnormality results from a surgical complication most commonly associated with:
   A. Transcutaneous aortic valve replacement
   B. Transvascular abdominal aortic aneurysm repair
   C. Left coronary artery bypass surgery
   D. Right coronary artery bypass surgery

Correct Answer: A

Explanation: The tracing demonstrates complete heart block, which is characterized by P waves and QRS complexes independent of one another, with atrial rate faster than the ventricular rate. Because of close proximity of the atrioventricular (AV) conduction system to the aortic valve, AV block is a common complication of aortic valve surgery (open and transvascular).

References:

1. Freudzon L, Akhtar S, London MJ, et al. Chapter 12: Electrocardiographic Monitoring. In: Kaplan JA, Augoustides JGT, Manecke GR, et al., eds. Kaplan's Cardiac Anesthesia. 7th ed. Elsevier; 2017:357-389.
2. Rodés-Cabau J, Ellenbogen KA, Krahn AD, et al. Management of conduction disturbances associated with transcatheter aortic valve replacement: JACC Scientific Expert Panel. J Am Coll Cardiol, 2019: 74: 1086-1106.

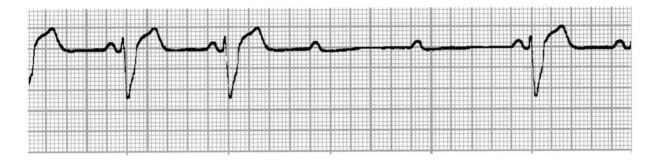

27. A 67-year-old man is undergoing an aortic root repair utilizing hypothermic cardiopulmonary bypass (CPB). Immediately prior to separation from CPB the rhythm (seen in the figure) is noted on the electrocardiogram monitor. The most appropriate first step in management of this is:
   a. Ventricular pacing at 80 beats per minute
   b. Atrial pacing at 80 beats per minute
   c. Atrioventricular pacing at 80 beats per minute
   d. Continue current management without cardiac pacing, but ensure that emergency epicardial pacing leads have been placed and a function portable pacemaker unit is attached

Correct Answer: D

Explanation: The tracing is representative of Mobitz II second degree heart block. It is characterized by occasional "dropped" QRS complexes. Cardiac pacing is usually not necessary, since most atrial depolarizations are conducted normally to the ventricles. This type of heart block is indicative of myocardial injury and may degenerate to complete heart block. For that reason, emergency pacing should be made available.

References:

1. Freudzon L, Akhtar S, London MJ, et al. Chapter 12: Electrocardiographic Monitoring. In: Kaplan JA, Augoustides JGT, Manecke GR, et al., eds. Kaplan's Cardiac Anesthesia. 7th ed. Elsevier; 2017:357-389.
2. Shigematsu-Locatelli M, Kawano T. Nishigaki A. General anesthesia in a patient with asymptomatic second-degree two-to-one atrioventricular block. JA Clin Rep, 2017; 3: 27.

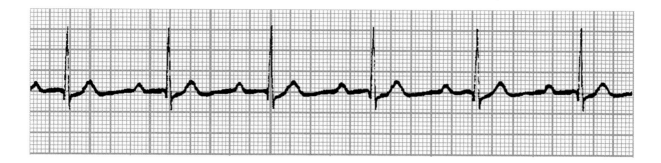

28. A 56-year-old woman with a history of hypertension and coronary artery disease presents for coronary artery bypass surgery. Upon placement of monitors, prior to anesthetic induction, the electrocardiogram tracing (seen in the figure) is obtained. True statements about the abnormality include:

   A. It usually does not require treatment

   B. It may be caused by beta blocker therapy

   C. It may be caused by dexmedetomidine

   D. All of the above

Correct Answer: D

Explanation: The tracing illustrates first degree heart block. First degree heart block is characterized by a prolonged P-R interval (>0.20 ms), regular heart rate, and intact atrioventricular conduction. It is usually clinically innocuous, although it may be a sign of myocardial damage. Various medications can cause first-degree heart block, including beta blockers and dexmedetomidine.

References:

1. Freudzon L, Akhtar S, London MJ, et al. Chapter 12: Electrocardiographic Monitoring. In: Kaplan JA, Augoustides JGT, Manecke GR, et al., eds. Kaplan's Cardiac Anesthesia. 7th ed. Elsevier; 2017:357-389.

2. Takata K, Adachi YU, Suzuki K, et al. Dexmedetomidine-induced atrioventricular block followed by cardiac arrest during atrial pacing: a case report and review of the literature. J Anesth, 2014; 28: 116-120.

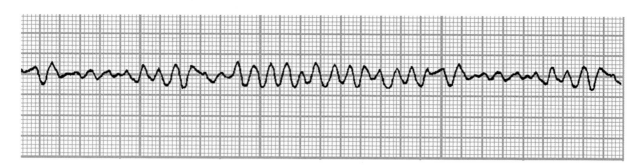

29. The tracing seen in the figure was obtained in an 81-year-old man who had undergone an aortic valve replacement, immediately after he was moved from the operating room table to the intensive care unit bed. The first step in managing this situation is:

   A. Electrical defibrillation

   B. Lidocaine 100 mg intravenous (IV)

   C. Check for pulse and/or arterial blood pressure tracing

   D. Epinephrine 1 mg IV

Correct Answer: C

Explanation: The tracing is strongly suggestive of ventricular fibrillation. Although the first step in treatment of ventricular fibrillation is electrical defibrillation, the anesthesiologist should quickly check for a pulse or arterial blood pressure tracing, since a displaced electrocardiogram lead could result in artifact with similar characteristics to ventricular fibrillation. Electrical defibrillation should be performed only if the patient is pulseless.

References:

1. Freudzon L, Akhtar S, London MJ, et al. Chapter 12: Electrocardiographic Monitoring. In: Kaplan JA, Augoustides JGT, Manecke GR, et al., eds. Kaplan's Cardiac Anesthesia. 7th ed. Elsevier; 2017:357-389.

2. Lieb M, Orr T, Gallagher C, et al. A case of intra-operative ventricular fibrillation: Electro-cauterization, undiagnosed Takotsubo cardiomyopathy or long QT syndrome? Int J Surg Case Rep, 2012; 3: 155-157.

30. A 37-year-old woman with mitral valve prolapse presented for mitral valve repair. After anesthetic induction and intubation, while positive pressure ventilation is applied, pronounced variation in amplitude of the QRS wave in lead II of the electrocardiogram is noted. This variation may be a sign of:

   A. Mitral regurgitation

   B. Volume responsiveness

C. Congestive heart failure

D. Esophageal intubation

Correct Answer: B

Explanation: A promising application of the electrocardiogram is to correlate respiratory variation in wave amplitude with patients' volume responsiveness. The R wave, especially in lead II (RII), shows consistent respiratory amplitude variation during positive-pressure mechanical ventilation. This variation is likely caused by the "Brody effect," a theoretical analysis of left ventricular volume and electrical conductance. RII wave amplitude variation may be used as a dynamic index of volume responsiveness in a mechanically ventilated patient, similar to the use of arterial pulse contour analysis and esophageal Doppler monitoring to derive pulse pressure and stroke volume variation as dynamic measures of fluid responsiveness.

References:

1. Lorne E, Mahjoub Y, Guinot PG, et al. Respiratory variations of R-wave amplitude in lead II are correlated with stroke volume variations evaluated by transesophageal Doppler echocardiography. J Cardiothorac Vasc Anesth, 2012; 26: 381-386.

2. Giraud R, Siegenthaler N, Morel DR, et al. Respiratory change in ECG-wave amplitude is a reliable parameter to estimate intravascular volume status. J Clin Monit Comput, 2013; 27: 107-111.

CHAPTER 13

Cardiovascular Monitoring

Gerard Manecke and Joel A. Kaplan

KEY POINTS

1. Normally, arterial pressure readings differ according to the site of monitoring. As one moves distally in the arterial tree, the systolic pressure increases, the diastolic pressure decreases, and the mean arterial pressure remains approximately constant.

2. After cardiopulmonary bypass, the arterial pressure wave may be damped in the periphery (e.g., radial artery). This is particularly common following extended periods of bypass with hypothermia. In some cases, the peripheral mean arterial pressure will be less than the central mean arterial pressure. If the gradients are large and persist, it may be necessary to insert a more central arterial catheter (e.g., femoral arterial catheter).

3. Underdamping and overdamping of pressure waveforms generated by fluid-filled systems are common. Recognizing and understanding reasons for underdamped and overdamped waveforms is important to assure accurate pressure data for patient care.

4. Understanding the surgical plan and approach to cardiopulmonary bypass for surgeries on the aortic arch and distal aorta is critical for determining sites of arterial pressure monitoring.

5. The use of surface ultrasound for insertion of arterial and central venous catheters has become a very common, invaluable technique. The skilled use of surface ultrasound decreases the number of attempts, time to insertion, and complications.

6. Inspection of the waveform is important in the interpretation of the central venous pressure. Variations in the components of the wave can assist in the diagnosis of such abnormalities as tricuspid regurgitation, junctional rhythm, and constrictive pericarditis.

7. Increased intrathoracic pressure from any cause, including the use of positive end expiratory pressure, may cause increases in central venous pressure, pulmonary artery pressure, and pulmonary capillary wedge pressure. This should be considered when using these parameters to guide therapy. Echocardiography can be useful to determine cardiac chamber volume status when the intrathoracic pressure is elevated.

8. All vascular access procedures have associated contraindications and complications. The anesthesiologist should be well versed in them to make informed risk/benefit assessments when deciding on monitoring modalities and vascular access.

9. Minimally invasive and noninvasive cardiac output and volume responsiveness assessment tools continue to be developed. Although they are not yet sufficiently accurate for management of the critically ill, they may be useful in hemodynamic management of a subgroup of cardiac and vascular surgery patients who are relatively healthy.

1. Normally, the systolic pressure is highest in the:
- **A.** Aorta
- **B.** Femoral artery
- **C.** Brachial artery
- **D.** Radial artery

Correct Answer: **D**

Explanation: The systolic pressure is progressively higher, as it is measured more distally in the arterial tree. This likely results from wave reflections. The proximal aortic wave tends to be sinusoidal, with little impact of wave reflections. In contrast, the radial artery and the dorsalis pedis artery tracings have high peaks, indicative of wave reflections in the vascular tree.

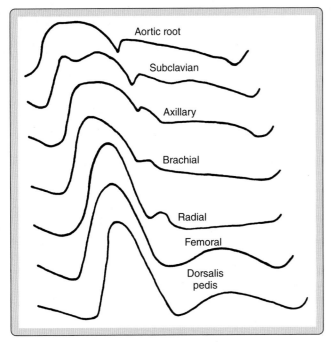

FIGURE 13.1 The waveform of the arterial pressure changes significantly according to the site of the intraarterial catheter. These changes are shown as a progression from central monitoring *(top)* through peripheral monitoring *(bottom)*. These changes are thought to be caused by forward wave propagation and wave reflection. In the periphery, systolic pressure is higher, diastolic pressure is lower, and mean pressure is minimally lower. (Modified from Bedford RF. Invasive blood pressure monitoring. In: Blitt CD, ed. Monitoring in Anesthesia and Critical Care. Churchill Livingstone; 1985:505.)

References:

1. Mittnacht AJC, Reich DL, Sander M, et al. Chapter 13: Monitoring of the Heart and Vascular System. In: Kaplan JA, Augoustides JGT, Manecke GR, et al., eds. Kaplan's Cardiac Anesthesia. 7th ed. Elsevier; 2017:390-426.
2. Remington JW. Contour changes of the aortic pulse during propagation. Am J Physiol, 1960; 199: 331-334.

2. At the conclusion of hypothermic cardiopulmonary bypass, the mean arterial pressure (MAP) in the radial artery is often:
   A. Higher than aortic root MAP
   B. Equal to aortic cannula MAP
   C. Lower than aortic root MAP
   D. Equal to aortic cardioplegia cannula MAP

Correct Answer: C

Explanation: Normally, the mean arterial pressure is similar between proximal and distal arteries. After separation from cardiopulmonary bypass, however, the mean arterial pressure measured in a peripheral artery such as the radial artery may be lower than central aortic pressure. This pressure gradient may be particularly pronounced following extended periods of hypothermic cardiopulmonary bypass.

References:

1. Carmona MJ, Barboza Junior LC, Buscatti RY, et al. Evaluation of the aorta-to-radial artery pressure gradient in patients undergoing surgery with cardiopulmonary bypass. Rev Bras Anesthesiol, 2007; 57: 618-629.
2. Bouchard-Dechene V, Couture P, Su A, et al. Risk factors for radial-to-femoral artery pressure gradient in patients undergoing cardiac surgery with cardiopulmonary bypass. J Cardiothorac Vasc Anesth, 2018; 32: 692-698.

3. Adding 20 cm of stiff tubing to an invasive arterial pressure transducing system will:
   A. Result in underdamping of the waveform
   B. Result in overdamping of the waveform
   C. Cause no change in the waveform because the tubing is stiff
   D. Decrease the mean arterial pressure reading

Correct Answer: A

Explanation: Fluid-filled transducing systems are designed such that their natural frequency is much higher than the natural frequency of the patients' arterial system. As tubing length is added to a transducer system, the natural frequency of the system decreases. As the natural frequency of the system becomes similar to the natural frequency of the patients' arterial system, resonance occurs. The resonance results in amplification of various aspects of the waveform (underdamping). Underdamping results in falsely high systolic blood pressure readings and falsely low diastolic blood pressure readings, with the mean arterial pressure largely unaffected.

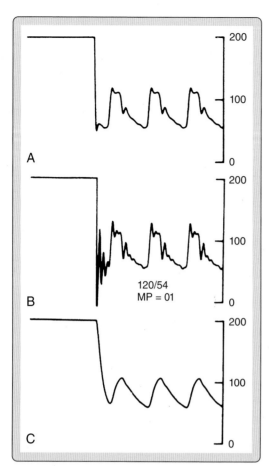

FIGURE 13.2 The fast-flush test demonstrates the harmonic characteristics of a pressure monitoring system (i.e., transducer, fluid-filled tubing, and intra-arterial catheter). In an optimally damped system (A), the pressure waveform returns to baseline after only one oscillation. In an underdamped system (B), the pressure waveform oscillates above and below the baseline several times. In an overdamped system (C), the pressure waveform returns to the baseline slowly with no oscillations. (A–C, Adapted from Gibbs NC, Gardner RM. Dynamics of invasive pressure monitoring systems: clinical and laboratory evaluation. Heart Lung, 1988; 17: 43–51.)

References:

1. Mittnacht AJC, Reich DL, Sander M, et al. Chapter 13: Monitoring of the Heart and Vascular System. In: Kaplan JA, Augoustides JGT, Manecke GR, et al., eds. Kaplan's Cardiac Anesthesia. 7th ed. Elsevier; 2017:390-426.
2. Todorovic M, Jensen EW, Thogersen C. Evaluation of dynamic performance in liquid-filled catheter systems for measuring invasive blood pressure. Int J Clin Monit Comput, 1996; 13: 173.

4. Fluid-filled electronic transducers use:
  A. Piezoelectric crystals to convert pressure signals to voltage signals
  B. Wheatstone bridges to convert pressure signals to changes in resistance
  C. Silicon matrices
  D. Wavelength spectroscopy for high resolution pressure sensors

Correct Answer: B

Explanation: Wheatstone bridges in the transducers are used to detect changes in resistance to current applied to the transducer system. The change in resistance in the Wheatstone bridge is caused by pressure on the transducer diaphragm. The change in resistance is then mathematically converted to a pressure wave that is digitized, processed, and displayed on the monitor.

References:

1. Mittnacht AJC, Reich DL, Sander M, et al. Chapter 13: Monitoring of the Heart and Vascular System. In: Kaplan JA, Augoustides JGT, Manecke GR, et al., eds. Kaplan's Cardiac Anesthesia. 7th ed. Elsevier; 2017:390-426.
2. Moxham IM. Physics of invasive blood pressure monitoring. S Africa J Anaesth Analges, 2003; 9: 33-38.

5. The "fast flush" test of fluid filled transducer systems is useful for determining:
  A. Pressure sensitivity
  B. Damping characteristics
  C. Fluid resistance
  D. Response time

Correct Answer: B

Explanation: The "fast flush" is used to determine the harmonic characteristics of a transducer system. These characteristics include the damping coefficient and the natural frequency. The test consists of holding the flush valve of a transducer open and suddenly releasing it, allowing the valve to close. Upon closure, oscillations are produced on the monitor by the resonance of the transducer, tubing, and catheter. The frequency of the oscillations is the natural frequency of the system, and the amplitudes and number of oscillations are used to determine the damping coefficient (see Figure 13.2).

References:
1. Mittnacht AJC, Reich DL, Sander M, et al. Chapter 13: Monitoring of the Heart and Vascular System. In: Kaplan JA, Augoustides JGT, Manecke GR, et al., eds. Kaplan's Cardiac Anesthesia. 7th ed. Elsevier; 2017:390-426.
2. Kleinman B, Powell S, Kumar P, et al. The fast-flush test measures the dynamic response of the entire blood pressure monitoring system. Anesthesiology, 1992; 77: 1215.

6. Which of the following results in underdamping of a fluid filled transducer system?
   A. Adding 18 inches of rigid tubing
   B. Removing 6 inches of rigid tubing
   C. Increasing the natural frequency of the system
   D. Replacing rigid tubing with soft tubing

Correct Answer: A

Explanation: Fluid transducer systems are designed to have natural frequencies at least eight times higher than the natural frequency of the human cardiovascular system. If the natural frequency of the transducer system is too low, it overlaps with the natural frequency of the cardiovascular system, resulting in resonance (ringing). This resonance results in amplification of components of the pressure wave (underdamping). Longer rigid transducer tubing results in lower natural frequency, and thus underdamping. Shortening the tubing length has the opposite effect. Replacing the rigid transducer tubing with soft tubing has a damping effect.

References:
1. Mittnacht AJC, Reich DL, Sander M, et al. Chapter 13: Monitoring of the Heart and Vascular System. In: Kaplan JA, Augoustides JGT, Manecke GR, et al., eds. Kaplan's Cardiac Anesthesia. 7th ed. Elsevier; 2017:390-426.
2. Gibbs NC, Gardner RM. Dynamics of invasive pressure monitoring systems: Clinical and laboratory evaluation. Heart Lung, 1988; 17: 43.

7. Direct axillary artery cannulation for cardiopulmonary bypass results in:
   A. Decreased arterial pressure readings in the ipsilateral radial artery
   B. Hyperperfusion of the ipsilateral arm
   C. Greater pump flow capability compared to aortic cannula
   D. All of the above

Correct Answer: A
Explanation: Direct cannulation of the axillary artery often results in decreased blood flow to the ipsilateral arm because of distal flow obstruction by the cannula (flow from the cannula is directed proximal). For this reason, end-to side cannulation using a vascular graft is often used. This, however, can result in hyperperfusion of the ipsilateral arm.

References:
1. Mittnacht AJC, Reich DL, Sander M, et al. Chapter 13: Monitoring of the Heart and Vascular System. In: Kaplan JA, Augoustides JGT, Manecke GR, et al., eds. Kaplan's Cardiac Anesthesia. 7th ed. Elsevier; 2017:390-426.
2. Sinclair MC, Singer RL, Manley NJ, et al. Cannulation of the axillary artery for cardiopulmonary bypass: safeguards and pitfalls. Ann Thorac Surg, 2003; 75: 931.

8. Axillary artery cannulation for cardiopulmonary bypass:
   A. Is necessary for retrograde cerebral perfusion
   B. May be useful in surgeries involving antegrade cerebral perfusion
   C. Is used for aortic root replacement surgeries
   D. Is used for descending aortic dissection repairs

Correct Answer: B

Explanation: Axillary artery cannulation is often used for surgeries involving the aortic arch. Such surgeries often require periods of hypothermic circulatory arrest. Axillary artery cannulation may facilitate antegrade cerebral perfusion, a useful technique for brain protection during circulatory arrest. Retrograde cerebral perfusion is performed via central venous cannulation.

References:
1. Mittnacht AJC, Reich DL, Sander M, et al. Chapter 13: Monitoring of the Heart and Vascular System. In: Kaplan JA, Augoustides JGT, Manecke GR, et al., eds. Kaplan's Cardiac Anesthesia. 7th ed. Elsevier; 2017:390-426.
2. Qu JZ, Kao LW, Smith JE, et al. Brain protection in aortic arch surgery: an evolving field. J Cardiothorac Vasc Anesth, 2021; 35: 1176-1188.

9. Hyperextension of the wrist in placement and management of a radial arterial catheter should be avoided because of potential injury to the:
   A. Radial artery
   B. Radial nerve
   C. Median nerve
   D. Ulnar nerve

Correct Answer: C

Explanation: Hyperextension of the wrist may cause median nerve damage by stretching the nerve over the wrist.

References:
1. Chowet AL, Lopez JR, Brock-Utne JG, et al. Wrist hyperextension leads to median nerve conduction block: implications for intra-arterial catheter placement. Anesthesiology, 2004; 100: 287-291.
2. Mittnacht AJC, Reich DL, Sander M, et al. Chapter 13: Monitoring of the Heart and Vascular System. In: Kaplan JA, Augoustides JGT, Manecke GR, et al., eds. Kaplan's Cardiac Anesthesia. 7th ed. Elsevier; 2017:390-426.

10. True statements about using ultrasound for cannulation of the radial artery include:
   A. In-plane technique is associated with a higher success rate than out-of-plane approach
   B. Low frequency, curvilinear probe should be used
   C. When providers experienced in using ultrasound are studied, the number of attempts when using ultrasound is less than the number of attempts without ultrasound
   D. Ultrasound should not be used in pediatrics because the radial artery is too small for adequate visualization

Correct Answer: C

Explanation: Levin and associates randomized patients in a prospective study to ultrasound-guided (UG) radial artery cannulation versus the classic palpation technique. The use of UG resulted in a higher success rate on the first attempt, and fewer subsequent attempts were required to place the arterial catheter. The overall time for catheter placement was not significantly different between the two groups (trend for shorter overall time in UG group). In a similar study, Shiver and colleagues randomized patients in the emergency department to UG versus the traditional palpation technique of placing the arterial catheter. Patients in the UG group required a significantly shorter time (107 vs. 314 seconds; $P = .0004$), fewer placement attempts (1.2 vs. 2.2; $P = .001$), and fewer sites required for successful arterial catheter placement. High-frequency linear probes are recommended because the radial artery is shallow, and the higher frequency provides higher resolution. Ultrasound is often used successfully for radial artery cannulation in infants and children.

BOX 13.1   Ultrasound-guided arterial cannulation

Benefits
- Higher success rate on first attempt
- Fewer overall attempts
- Increased patient comfort (fewer attempts)
- Fewer complications (e.g., anticoagulated patients)
- Demonstration of vessel patency, anatomic variants
- Low pulsatile or nonpulsatile flow (e.g., nonpulsatile assist devices, extracorporeal membrane oxygenation, shock)
- Nonpalpable or weakly palpable pulses (e.g., peripheral edema, hematoma)
- Emergency access (e.g., catheter placement during resuscitation)

Concerns
- Risk of catheter-related infections if poor aseptic technique is applied
- Additional training required
- Costs involved with equipment required

References:

1. Levin PH, Sheinin O, Gozal Y. Use of ultrasound guidance in the insertion of radial artery catheters. Crit Care Med, 2003; 31: 481-484.
2. Shiver S, Blaivas M, Lyon M. A prospective comparison of ultrasound-guided and blindly placed radial arterial catheters. Acad Emerg Med, 2006; 13: 1275-1279.
3. Ganesh A, Kaye R, Cahill AM, et al. Evaluation of ultrasound-guided radial artery cannulation in children. Pediatr Crit Care Med, 2009; 10: 45-48.
4. Mittnacht AJC, Reich DL, Sander M, et al. Chapter 13: Monitoring of the Heart and Vascular System. In: Kaplan JA, Augoustides JGT, Manecke GR, et al., eds. Kaplan's Cardiac Anesthesia. 7th ed. Elsevier; 2017:390-426.

11. Complications of arterial catheterization include:
   A. Infection
   B. Incorrect management because of arterial stenosis
   C. Incorrect management because of "zero drift"
   D. All of the above

Correct Answer: D

Explanation: Infection, thrombosis, embolus, hematoma, and incorrect management because of zeroing issues, proximal arterial stenosis, and leveling are all potential complications of arterial catheter placement. Such potential complications should be considered when invasive arterial pressure monitoring is contemplated.

References:

1. Mittnacht AJC, Reich DL, Sander M, et al. Chapter 13: Monitoring of the Heart and Vascular System. In: Kaplan JA, Augoustides JGT, Manecke GR, et al., eds. Kaplan's Cardiac Anesthesia. 7th ed. Elsevier; 2017:390-426.
2. Garg K, Howell BW, Saltzberg SS, et al. Open surgical management of complications from indwelling radial artery catheters. J Vasc Surg, 2013; 58: 1325-1330.

12. In a 73-year-old man undergoing coronary artery bypass, following anesthetic induction and placement of a central venous catheter, tall, "cannon" A waves are noted on the central venous pressure tracing. These are most likely indicative of:
   A. Premature atrial contractions
   B. Atrial fibrillation
   C. Junctional rhythm
   D. Tricuspid regurgitation

Correct Answer: C

Explanation: Junctional rhythm results in the contraction of the atria and ventricles at the same time, with the right atrium contracting against a closed tricuspid valve. This results in a tall, "cannon" A wave. This characteristic wave can be useful in the diagnosis of junctional rhythm, although it may also be observed when premature ventricular contractions or complete heart block occur.

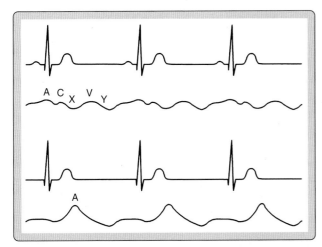

FIGURE 13.3 Relationship of the central venous pressure tracing to the electrocardiogram during junctional (atrioventricular nodal) rhythm. The contraction of the atrium against the closed tricuspid valve results in the cannon A waves. Note that the P wave is hidden within the QRS complex of the electrocardiogram.

References:

1. Mittnacht AJC, Reich DL, Sander M, et al. Chapter 13: Monitoring of the Heart and Vascular System. In: Kaplan JA, Augoustides JGT, Manecke GR, et al., eds. Kaplan's Cardiac Anesthesia. 7th ed. Elsevier; 2017:390-426.
2. Mark JB. Central venous pressure monitoring: clinical insights beyond the numbers. J Cardiothorac Vasc Anesth, 1991; 5: 163-173.

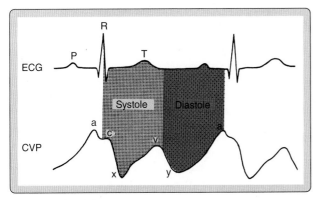

FIGURE 13.4 Relationship of the central venous pressure (*CVP*) tracing to the electrocardiogram (*ECG*) in normal sinus rhythm. The normal CVP waveform consists of three upward deflections (A, C, and V waves) and two downward deflections (X and Y descents). The A wave is produced by right atrial contraction and occurs just after the P wave on the ECG. The C wave occurs because of the isovolumic ventricular contraction forcing the tricuspid valve to bulge upward into the right atrium (RA). The pressure within the RA then decreases as the tricuspid valve is pulled away from the atrium during right ventricular ejection, forming the X descent. The RA continues to fill during late ventricular systole, forming the V wave. The Y descent occurs when the tricuspid valve opens and blood from the RA empties rapidly into the right ventricle during early diastole. (Adapted from Mark JB. Central venous pressure monitoring: clinical insights beyond the numbers. J Cardiothorac Vasc Anesth. 1991;5:163–173.)

13. The "V" wave in the central venous pressure tracing seen in the Figure 13.3 is associated with:
   A. Tricuspid regurgitation
   B. Ventricular contraction
   C. Relaxation of the right ventricle
   D. Filling of the right atrium

Correct Answer: D

Explanation: The normal central venous pressure waveform consists of three upward deflections (A, C, and V waves) and two downward deflections (X and Y descents). The A wave is produced by right atrial contraction and occurs just after the P wave on the electrocardiogram. The C wave occurs because of the isovolumic ventricular contraction forcing the tricuspid valve to bulge upward into the right atrium (RA). The pressure within the RA then decreases as the tricuspid valve is pulled away from the atrium during right ventricular ejection, forming the X descent. The RA continues to fill during late ventricular systole, forming the V wave. The Y descent occurs when the tricuspid valve opens and blood from the RA empties rapidly into the right ventricle during early diastole. Tricuspid regurgitation is associated with systolic filling of the RA, causing pronounced CV waves.

References:

1. Mittnacht AJC, Reich DL, Sander M, et al. Chapter 13: Monitoring of the Heart and Vascular System. In: Kaplan JA, Augoustides JGT, Manecke GR, et al., eds. Kaplan's Cardiac Anesthesia. 7th ed. Elsevier; 2017:390-426.
2. Mark JB. Central venous pressure monitoring: clinical insights beyond the numbers. J Cardiothorac Vasc Anesth, 1991; 5: 163-173.

14. The central venous pressure tracing seen in the Figure 13.5 is most consistent with:
   A. Constrictive pericarditis
   B. Tricuspid regurgitation
   C. Cardiac tamponade
   D. Mitral stenosis

Correct Answer: A

Explanation: In constrictive pericarditis, the venous return is decreased because of the inability of the heart chambers to dilate as a result of the constriction. This causes prominent A and V waves and steep X and Y descents (creating an M configuration) resembling those observed with diseases that cause decreased right ventricular compliance. Egress of blood from the right atrium to the right ventricle is initially rapid during early diastolic filling of the right ventricle (creating a steep Y descent) but is short-lived and abruptly halted by the restrictive, noncompliant right ventricle. The right atrial pressure then increases rapidly and reaches a plateau until the end of the A wave, at the end of diastole. With pericardial tamponade, the X descent is steep, but the Y descent is not present because early diastolic run-off is impaired by the pericardial fluid collection. In the central venous pressure tracing, a characteristic M configuration with prominent

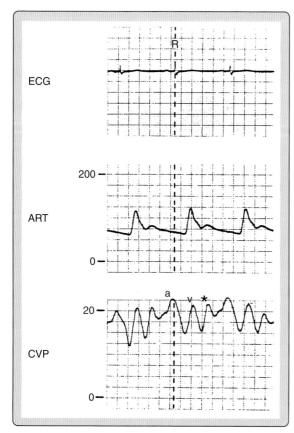

FIGURE 13.5 Central venous pressure *(CVP)* waveform during pericardial constriction. The characteristic M configuration with prominent *a* and *v* waves, accompanied by steep x and y descents, is evident. An additional wave *(asterisk)* is present because of an impairment of ventricular filling by the rigid pericardial shell. *ART,* Arterial pressure; *ECG,* electrocardiogram. (Adapted from Mark JB. Central venous pressure monitoring: clinical insights beyond the numbers. J Cardiothorac Vasc Anesth. 1991;5:163–173.)

A and V waves, accompanied by steep X and Y descents, is evident. An additional wave is present because of an impairment of ventricular filling by the rigid pericardial shell.

References:

1. Mittnacht AJC, Reich DL, Sander M, et al. Chapter 13: Monitoring of the Heart and Vascular System. In: Kaplan JA, Augoustides JGT, Manecke GR, et al., eds. Kaplan's Cardiac Anesthesia. 7th ed. Elsevier; 2017:390-426.
2. Mark JB. Central venous pressure monitoring: clinical insights beyond the numbers. J Cardiothorac Vasc Anesth, 1991; 5: 163-173.

15. In a 47-year-old man with biventricular congestive heart failure, the central venous pressure:
   A. Is often useful because it reflects left ventricular filling
   B. Is often useful because it reflects right ventricular volume
   C. May be useful when responses to fluid boluses are observed
   D. Is not useful for intravascular volume management in patients with congestive heart failure

Correct Answer: C

Explanation: The central venous pressure (CVP) is a useful monitor if the factors affecting it are recognized and its limitations are understood. Thromboses of the vena cavae and alterations of intrathoracic pressure, such as those induced by positive end-expiratory pressure, affect measurement of the CVP. The correlation with left-sided heart filling pressures and assessment of left ventricular preload is poor. Clinically, following serial measurements as a trend rather than isolated observations is often more relevant. The response of the CVP to a volume infusion, however, is a useful test. For example, if administration of a fluid bolus results in an increase in cardiac output but the CVP does not increase, the patient likely responded appropriately to the fluid bolus and may benefit from another one. In contrast, an increase in CVP without an increase in stroke volume after a fluid bolus is an ominous sign. This often indicates that the right side of the heart is unable to accommodate increases in volume.

BOX 13.2   Indications for central venous catheter placement

- Major operative procedures involving large fluid shifts or blood loss in patients with good heart function
- Intravascular volume assessment when urine output is not reliable or unavailable (e.g., renal failure)
- Major trauma
- Surgical procedures with a high risk of air embolism, such as sitting-position craniotomies during which the central venous pressure catheter may be used to aspirate intracardiac air
- Frequent venous blood sampling
- Venous access for vasoactive or irritating drugs
- Chronic drug administration
- Inadequate peripheral intravenous access
- Rapid infusion of intravenous fluids (only when using large-bore cannulae)
- Total parenteral nutrition

References:

1. Mittnacht AJC, Reich DL, Sander M, et al. Chapter 13: Monitoring of the Heart and Vascular System. In: Kaplan JA, Augoustides JGT, Manecke GR, et al., eds. Kaplan's Cardiac Anesthesia. 7th ed. Elsevier; 2017:390-426.
2. Godje O, Peyerl M, Seebauer T, et al. Central venous pressure, pulmonary capillary wedge pressure and intrathoracic blood volumes as preload indicators in cardiac surgery patients. Eur J Cardiothorac Surg, 1998; 13: 533.

16. A 71-year-old man presents for aortic valve replacement. While performing surface ultrasound prior to cannulation of the right internal jugular vein, you notice what appears to be thrombus in the vessel. You then decide to cannulate the left internal jugular vein instead. Which of the following complications are more likely when cannulating the left internal jugular vein as compared to the right internal jugular vein?

A. Difficulty placing the tip of the catheter at the superior vena cava–right atrium junction
B. Trauma to the carotid artery
C. Trauma to the thoracic duct
D. A and C

Correct Answer: D

Explanation: Placing a central venous catheter via the left internal jugular (LIJ) vein may be challenging because, during placement, the tip of the catheter must enter the left subclavian vein and traverse the midline to the superior vena cava (SVC). In contrast, the right internal jugular vein (RIJ) enters the SVC directly, in a straight path. The thoracic duct lies in close proximity to the LIJ and may be traumatized when cannulation of the LIJ is attempted. Trauma to the carotid artery is a risk when attempting to cannulate the RIJ vein or the LIJ vein.

References:

1. Mittnacht AJC, Reich DL, Sander M, et al. Chapter 13: Monitoring of the Heart and Vascular System. In: Kaplan JA, Augoustides JGT, Manecke GR, et al., eds. Kaplan's Cardiac Anesthesia. 7th ed. Elsevier; 2017:390-426.
2. Muralidhar K. Left internal versus right internal jugular vein access to central venous circulation using the Seldinger technique. J Cardiothorac Anesth, 1995; 9: 115.

> ### BOX 13.3 **Complications of central venous catheterization**
>
> **Complications of Central Venous Access and Cannulation**
> * Arterial puncture with hematoma
> * Arteriovenous fistula
> * Hemothorax
> * Chylothorax
> * Pneumothorax
> * Nerve injury
> * Brachial plexus injury
> * Stellate ganglion injury (Horner syndrome)
> * Air embolus
> * Catheter or wire shearing
> * Guide wire loss and embolization
> * Right atrial or right ventricular perforation
>
> **Complications of Catheter Presence**
> * Thrombosis, thromboembolism
> * Infection, sepsis, endocarditis
> * Arrhythmias
> * Hydrothorax

17. Reliable methods of confirming correct venous access prior to placing a large bore catheter in the internal jugular vein include all the following EXCEPT:

A. Transducing a small-bore catheter placed in the vessel and observing the pressure and waveform on the monitor
B. Drawing blood from a small catheter and comparing its color to that of arterial blood
C. Observing the guidewire in the superior vena cava using transesophageal echocardiography
D. Attaching a small-bore catheter to clear tubing, allowing blood return, then holding the tubing up to observe venous pressure

Correct Answer: B

Explanation: Various techniques have been suggested for confirming venous access prior to placing a large bore venous catheter or sheath. A small-bore catheter can be attached to a transducer by sterile tubing to observe the pressure waveform. Another option is to attach the cannula to sterile tubing and allow blood to flow retrograde into the tubing. The tubing is then held upright as a venous manometer, and the height of the blood column is observed. If the catheter is in a vein, it will stop rising at a level consistent with the central venous pressure and demonstrate respiratory variation. Despite its reported use in the past, color comparison and observation of nonpulsatile flow are notoriously inaccurate methods of determining that the catheter is not in the carotid artery. With the more widespread use of echocardiography, the correct intravenous position can also be confirmed by following the Seldinger wire along its course in the internal jugular vein more distally by handheld transcutaneous probes or demonstrated within the right atrium if the transesophageal probe was inserted before central venous cannulation. The use of more than one technique to confirm the venous location of the guidewire may provide additional reassurance of correct placement before cannulation of the vein with a larger catheter or introducer.

References:

1. Mittnacht AJC, Reich DL, Sander M, et al. Chapter 13: Monitoring of the Heart and Vascular System. In: Kaplan JA, Augoustides JGT, Manecke GR, et al., eds. Kaplan's Cardiac Anesthesia. 7th ed. Elsevier; 2017:390-426.
2. Fabian JA, Jesudian MC. A simple method for improving the safety of percutaneous cannulation of the internal jugular vein. Anesth Analg, 1985; 64: 1032.

18. Disadvantages of using ultrasound guidance in performing internal jugular venipuncture in adults include:

A. Greater number of attempts necessary
B. Steep learning curve with additional training required
C. Increased complication rate
D. Increased time necessary to perform the procedure

Correct Answer: B

Explanation: Ultrasound guidance in placing internal jugular catheters has consistently been associated with decreased number of attempts, decreased complication rate, and decreased time to cannulation. Disadvantages include the cost of the ultrasound equipment and the time and training necessary to learn ultrasound guidance technique.

References:

1. Mittnacht AJC, Reich DL, Sander M, et al. Chapter 13: Monitoring of the Heart and Vascular System. In: Kaplan JA, Augoustides JGT, Manecke GR, et al., eds. Kaplan's Cardiac Anesthesia. 7th ed. Elsevier; 2017:390-426.
2. Serafimidis K, Sakorafas GH, Konstantoudakis G, et al. Ultrasound-guided catheterization of the internal jugular vein in oncologic patients; comparison with the classical landmark technique: a prospective study. Int J Surg, 2009; 7: 526-528.

19. A 68-year-old woman presented for elective aortic valve replacement using cardiopulmonary bypass. Unfortunately, attempted right internal jugular vein cannulation resulted in a large-bore sheath placed in the right carotid artery. Which of the following management approaches is most appropriate?
    A. Remove the catheter and hold pressure on the wound for 20 minutes
    B. Leave the catheter in place, with a plan to remove it following the surgery, after reversal of heparinization
    C. Leave the catheter in place, delay surgery, and consult a vascular surgeon
    D. Remove the catheter and immediately apply a pressure dressing

Correct Answer: C

Explanation: Inadvertent arterial puncture during central venous cannulation is not uncommon. The primary reasons this phenomenon occurs are that most veins commonly used for cannulation lie in close proximity to arteries and the venous anatomy is quite variable. Localized hematoma formation is the usual consequence, which may be minimized if a small-gauge needle is initially used to localize the vein or if ultrasound guidance is employed. If the arterial puncture is large or if the patient has a coagulopathy, then a massive hematoma may form. In the neck, this may lead to airway obstruction requiring urgent tracheal intubation. If the artery is cannulated with a large-bore catheter, then leaving the catheter or introducer sheath in place and requesting surgical consultation for further management and possible surgical repair are recommended.

References:

1. Eckhardt W, Iaconetti D, Kwon J, et al. Inadvertent carotid artery cannulation during pulmonary artery catheter insertion. J Cardiothorac Vasc Anesth, 1996; 10: 283.
2. Guilbert MC, Elkouri S, Bracco D, et al. Arterial trauma during central venous catheter insertion: case series, review and proposed algorithm. J Vasc Surg, 2008; 48: 918-925.
3. Mittnacht AJC, Reich DL, Sander M, et al. Chapter 13: Monitoring of the Heart and Vascular System. In: Kaplan JA, Augoustides JGT, Manecke GR, et al., eds. Kaplan's Cardiac Anesthesia. 7th ed. Elsevier; 2017:390-426.

20. Access sites used for central venous pressure monitoring include:
    A. Basilic vein
    B. External jugular vein
    C. Internal jugular vein
    D. All of the above

Correct Answer: D

Explanation: The external jugular vein can be used as means of reaching the central circulation. The success rate with this approach is lower than the internal jugular approach because of the tortuous path followed by the vein. A valve is usually present at the point where the external jugular vein perforates the fascia to join with the subclavian vein, making this approach challenging. The primary advantage of this technique is that advancing a needle into the deeper structures of the neck is not needed. Another route for central venous monitoring is via the antecubital basilic or cephalic veins. The advantages of this approach are the low likelihood of complications and the ease of access if the arm is exposed. The major disadvantage is that placement of the catheter in a central vein is often difficult to ensure. Chest radiographs are usually necessary to confirm that the tip of the catheter has been appropriately placed.

References:

1. Martin AK, Renew JR, Ramakrishna H. Practice guideline for central venous access: latest report from the American Society of Anesthesiologists. J Cardiothorac Vasc Anesth, 2020; 34: 2012-2014.
2. Roth S, Aronson S. Placement of a right atrial air aspiration catheter guided by transesophageal echocardiography. Anesthesiology, 1995; 83: 1359.
3. Mittnacht AJC, Reich DL, Sander M, et al. Chapter 13: Monitoring of the Heart and Vascular System. In: Kaplan JA, Augoustides JGT, Manecke GR, et al., eds. Kaplan's Cardiac Anesthesia. 7th ed. Elsevier; 2017:390-426.

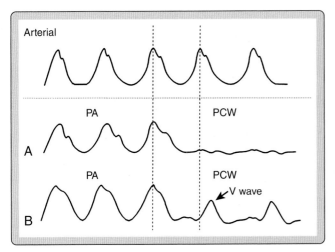

FIGURE 13.6 The relationship of the systemic arterial waveform, the pulmonary arterial *(PA)* waveform, and the pulmonary capillary wedge *(PCW)* waveform in the normal situation (A) and in the presence of V waves (B). Note the widening of the PA waveform and the loss of the dicrotic notch in the presence of V waves. The peak of the V wave *(arrow)* occurs after the peak of the systemic arterial waveform.

21. A 59-year-old man is undergoing coronary artery bypass without the use of cardiopulmonary bypass ("off-pump"). Following anesthetic induction and placement of a pulmonary artery catheter, the pulmonary artery tracing and the pulmonary capillary wedge tracing were normal, as depicted in tracing "A" of Figure 13.6. While the heart is being positioned for an obtuse marginal coronary artery distal anastomosis, the tracing labeled "B" is observed. The changes noted are most likely the result of:

A. Volume overload

B. Acute drug reaction resulting in pulmonary hypertension

C. Tricuspid regurgitation

D. Mitral regurgitation

Correct Answer: **D**

Explanation: The tracing labeled "B" shows new V waves, indicated by the arrow. Note that they occur late in systole (see the arterial tracing), and probably result from mitral regurgitation. Myocardial ischemia is common during manipulation of the heart, especially during extreme positioning such as that for the obtuse marginal anastomosis. The ischemia may involve the papillary muscles, resulting in acute mitral regurgitation. The diagnosis should be confirmed using transesophageal echocardiography, and the surgeon should be notified. Treatment options include repositioning the heart, releasing the cardiac vessel stabilizer, administering intravenous nitroglycerin, and administering intravenous phenylephrine to enhance coronary perfusion pressure.

References:

1. Moore RA, Neary MJ, Gallagher HD, et al. Determination of the pulmonary capillary wedge position in patients with giant left atrial V waves. J Cardiothorac Anesth, 1987; 1: 108.

2. Schmitt EA, Brantigan CO. Common artifacts of pulmonary artery pressures: recognition and interpretation. J Clin Monit, 1986; 2: 44.

3. Mittnacht AJC, Reich DL, Sander M, et al. Chapter 13: Monitoring of the Heart and Vascular System. In: Kaplan JA, Augoustides JGT, Manecke GR, et al., eds. Kaplan's Cardiac Anesthesia. 7th ed. Elsevier; 2017:390-426.

22. A 48-year-old obese man (body mass index = 44) is undergoing coronary artery bypass surgery. After anesthetic induction and placement of pulmonary artery catheter, 20 cmH$_2$O of positive end-expiratory pressure is applied. His pulmonary artery pressure is 50/28 mmHg, his central venous pressure is 22 mmHg, and his pulmonary capillary wedge pressure is 23 mmHg. His cardiac index is 1.6 L/min/m^2, and his heart rate is 64 beats per minute. Transesophageal echocardiography reveals a small left atrium and an underfilled left ventricle. There are no wall motion abnormalities, and the left ventricular ejection fraction is 60%. This hemodynamic profile is most likely caused by:

A. Diastolic left ventricular failure

B. Diastolic right ventricular failure

C. Hypervolemia

D. Positive end-expiratory pressure, resulting in decreased left ventricular filling

Correct Answer: **D**

Explanation: High levels of positive end-expiratory pressure (PEEP) decrease venous return, potentially resulting in underfilling of the heart. The high levels of PEEP may be transmitted within the thorax to the pulmonary vasculature and great veins, resulting in increased measured central filling pressure. Conditions resulting in discrepancies between pulmonary capillary wedge pressure and left ventricular end diastolic pressure are summarized in the box 13.4.

BOX 13.4 Conditions resulting in discrepancies between pulmonary capillary wedge pressure and left ventricular end diastolic pressure

PCWP > LVEDP

- Positive pressure ventilation
- High levels of PEEP
- Increased intrathoracic pressure
- Non-west lung zone III PAC placement
- Chronic obstructive pulmonary disease
- Increased pulmonary vascular resistance
- Left atrial myxoma
- Mitral valve disease (e.g., stenosis, regurgitation)

PCWP < LVEDP

- Noncompliant left ventricle (e.g., ischemia, hypertrophy)
- Aortic regurgitation (premature closure of the mitral valve)

LVEDP, Left ventricular end diastolic pressure; *PAC,* pulmonary artery catheter; *PCWP,* pulmonary capillary wedge pressure; *PEEP,* positive end-expiratory pressure.
Adapted from Tuman KJ, Carroll GC, Ivankovich AD. Pitfalls in interpretation of pulmonary artery catheter data. J Cardiothorac Vasc Anesth. 1989;3:625-641.

References:

1. Tuman KJ, Carroll GC, Ivankovich AD. Pitfalls in interpretation of pulmonary artery catheter data. J Cardiothorac Vasc Anesth, Update. 1991; 2: 1-24.
2. Mittnacht AJC, Reich DL, Sander M, et al. Chapter 13: Monitoring of the Heart and Vascular System. In: Kaplan JA, Augoustides JGT, Manecke GR, et al., eds. Kaplan's Cardiac Anesthesia. 7th ed. Elsevier; 2017:390-426.

23. A 27-year-old man for surgical excision of a mobile right atrial mass utilizing cardiopulmonary bypass. The surgeon requests that you place a pulmonary artery catheter (PAC) so that she can closely monitor cardiac function and pulmonary artery pressures postoperatively. Of the following, the most appropriate response is to:

A. Place PAC after induction via the right internal jugular vein, advancing the catheter slowly

B. Strongly recommend against PAC placement because of the risk of tumor embolization

C. Place an introducer sheath in the right internal jugular vein and place a PAC only as far as the superior vena cava. After the mass is excised, and the heart is beating and ejecting, advance the PAC into the pulmonary artery with surgical and echocardiographic guidance

D. Ask the surgeon to have the cardiology team place the PAC preoperatively with fluoroscopic guidance

Correct Answer: C

Explanation: The presence of a mobile right atrial mass presents a contraindication to pulmonary artery catheter (PAC) placement because of possible dislodgement of the mass and pulmonary embolization. If the surgeon believes that cardiac output and pulmonary artery pressure monitoring are necessary for postoperative care, a solution is to place the PAC after induction, advancing only to the superior vena cava. Prior to the separation from bypass after tumor excision, with the heart ejecting blood, the PAC can be advanced into the pulmonary artery. Prior to excision, the PAC can be placed carefully, using echocardiographic guidance to

attempt to steer the catheter away from the tumor. This approach, in most cases, is probably not worth the risk of dislodging the tumor.

References:

1. Mittnacht AJC, Reich DL, Sander M, et al. Chapter 13: Monitoring of the Heart and Vascular System. In: Kaplan JA, Augoustides JGT, Manecke GR, et al., eds. Kaplan's Cardiac Anesthesia. 7th ed. Elsevier; 2017:390-426.
2. Esandoh M. Is pulmonary artery catheter placement in the setting of right atrial tumor thrombus worth the risk? J Cardiothorac Vasc Anesth, 2018; 32: e1-e34.

24. Contraindications to the placement of a pulmonary artery catheter include all of the following EXCEPT:

A. Severe pulmonary hypertension

B. Recently placed right atrial and right ventricle pacemaker wires

C. Severe dysrhythmias

D. Friable tricuspid valve vegetations

Correct Answer: A

Explanation: Recently placed endocardial pacemaker wires and severe dysrhythmias are relative contraindications to placement of a pulmonary arterial catheter (PAC). Friable tumor, vegetation, or thrombus in the right atrium or right ventricle are absolute contraindications. Although placement of a PAC in the setting of severe pulmonary hypertension may be challenging and has been associated with increased risk of pulmonary artery bleeding, it is not a contraindication to PAC placement.

References:

1. Mittnacht AJC, Reich DL, Sander M, et al. Chapter 13: Monitoring of the Heart and Vascular System. In: Kaplan JA, Augoustides JGT, Manecke GR, et al., eds. Kaplan's Cardiac Anesthesia. 7th ed. Elsevier; 2017:390-426.
2. Kelly CR, Rabbani LE. Pulmonary artery catheterization. N Engl J Med, 2013; 369: e35.

BOX 13.6   Contraindications for pulmonary artery catheterization

Absolute Contraindications
- Severe tricuspid or pulmonary stenosis
- Right atrial or right ventricular mass
- Tetralogy of Fallot

Relative Contraindications
- Severe arrhythmias
- Left bundle branch block (consider pacing PAC)
- Newly inserted pacemaker wires, AICD, or CRT
- Severe coagulopathy

AICD, Automatic implantable cardioverter defibrillator; *CRT,* cardiac resynchronization therapy; *PAC,* pulmonary artery catheter.

BOX 13.5   Possible clinical indications for pulmonary artery catheter monitoring

Major Procedures Involving Large Fluid Shifts or Blood Loss in Patients With:
- Right-sided heart failure, pulmonary hypertension
- Severe left-sided heart failure not responsive to therapy
- Cardiogenic or septic shock or with multiple-organ failure
- Orthotopic heart transplantation
- Left ventricular–assist device implantation

BOX 13.7   **American society of anesthesiologists' practice guidelines for pulmonary artery catheter use**

Opinions

- PA catheterization provides new information that may change therapy, with poor clinical evidence of its effect on clinical outcome or mortality.
- There is no evidence from large, controlled studies that preoperative PA catheterization improves outcome regarding hemodynamic optimization.
- Perioperative PAC monitoring of hemodynamic parameters leading to goal-directed therapy has produced inconsistent data in multiple studies and clinical scenarios.
- Having immediate access to PAC data allows important preemptive measures for selected subgroups of patients who encounter hemodynamic disturbances that require immediate and precise decisions about fluid management and drug treatment.
- Experience and understanding are the major determinants of PAC effectiveness.
- PA catheterization is inappropriate as routine practice in surgical patients and should be limited to cases in which the anticipated benefits of catheterization outweigh the potential risks.
- PA catheterization can be harmful.

Recommendations

- The appropriateness of PA catheterization depends on a combination of patient-, surgery-, and practice setting–related factors.

- Perioperative PA catheterization should be considered in patients with significant organ dysfunction or major comorbidity that poses an increased risk for hemodynamic disturbances or instability (e.g., ASA IV or V patients).
- Perioperative PA catheterization in surgical settings should be considered based on the hemodynamic risk of the individual case rather than generalized surgical setting–related recommendations. High-risk surgical procedures are those during which large fluid changes or hemodynamic disturbances can be anticipated and procedures that are associated with a high risk of morbidity and mortality.
- Because of the risk of complications from PA catheterization, the procedure should not be performed by clinicians or nursing staff or in practice settings in which competency in safe insertion, accurate interpretation of results, and appropriate catheter maintenance cannot be guaranteed.
- Routine PA catheterization is not recommended when the patient, procedure, or practice setting poses a low or moderate risk for hemodynamic changes.

ASA, American Society of Anesthesiologists; *PA,* pulmonary artery; *PAC,* pulmonary artery catheter.
Adapted from American Society of Anesthesiologists. Practice guidelines for pulmonary artery catheterization. Available at: http://www.asahq.org/~/media/sites/asahq/files/public/resources/standards-guidelines/practice-guidelines-for-pulmonary-artery-catheterization.pdf

25. Which of the following is NOT required for calculating cardiac output using the Fick equation?
   A. Blood temperature
   B. Oxygen consumption
   C. Arterial oxygen content
   D. Venous oxygen content

Correct Answer: A

Explanation: The Fick equation is based on the principle that total body oxygen consumption (VO_2) is equal to the cardiac output (CO) times difference in oxygen content between arterial (CaO_2) and venous blood (CvO_2):

$$VO_2 = CO(CaO_2 - CvO_2)$$

This equation is easily rearranged for calculation of the cardiac output:

$$CO = VO_2/(CaO_2 - CvO_2)$$

In the direct Fick method, oxygen consumption is measured by calorimetry using algorithms based on inspired and expired oxygen concentrations and volumes. Oxygen consumption can be calculated when the rate of fresh gas flow, respiratory rate, and change of oxygen concentration are known. Arterial oxygen content is measured from an arterial blood sample, and mixed venous oxygen content can be obtained from the pulmonary artery catheter. Oxygen content differences must be measured at steady state because the Fick principle is valid only when tissue oxygen uptake equals lung oxygen uptake.

References:

1. Mittnacht AJC, Reich DL, Sander M, et al. Chapter 13: Monitoring of the Heart and Vascular System. In: Kaplan JA, Augoustides JGT, Manecke GR, et al., eds. Kaplan's Cardiac Anesthesia. 7th ed. Elsevier; 2017:390-426.
2. Taylor K, La Rotta G, McCrindle BW, et al. A comparison of cardiac output by thoracic impedance and direct Fick in children with congenital heart disease undergoing diagnostic cardiac catheterization. J Cardiothorac Vasc Anesth, 2011; 25: 776-779.

26. Inaccuracies in the calculation of cardiac output using thermodilution with a pulmonary arterial catheter include:
   A. Overestimation of the cardiac output if room temperature fluid is being rapidly infused in the central catheter
   B. Overestimation of the cardiac output if too little fluid is injected

C. Overestimation of the cardiac output if the fluid is injected too slowly

D. None of the above

Correct Answer: B

Explanation: When a thermal indicator is used, the modified Stewart-Hamilton equation is used to calculate cardiac output (CO):

$$CO = \frac{V(T_B - T_I) \times K_1 \times K_2}{\int_0^\infty \Delta T_B(t)dt}$$

in which CO is the cardiac output (L/min), V is the volume of injectate (mL), T_B is the initial blood temperature (degrees Celsius), T_I is the initial injectate temperature (degrees Celsius), K_1 is the density factor, K_2 is the computation constant, and the denominator is the integral of blood temperature change over time. A computer that integrates the area under the temperature versus time curve performs the calculation. Cardiac output is inversely proportional to the area under the curve. Injection of too little injectate results in a temperature change cure with less area, leading to overestimation of the cardiac output. Conversely, room air fluid running into the same central line as the injectate will result in a larger temperature change curve, and thus an underestimation of cardiac output. Slow injection of thermal indicator may result in a larger (longer) temperature change curve with consequent underestimation of the cardiac output, although computer-embedded algorithms will usually reject these attempts as artifactual.

References:

1. Mittnacht AJC, Reich DL, Sander M, et al. Chapter 13: Monitoring of the Heart and Vascular System. In: Kaplan JA, Augoustides JGT, Manecke GR, et al., eds. Kaplan's Cardiac Anesthesia. 7th ed. Elsevier; 2017:390-426.
2. Weisel RD, Berger RL, Hechtman HB, et al. Measurement of cardiac output by thermodilution. N Engl J Med, 1975; 292: 682.

BOX 13.8   Common errors in pulmonary artery catheter thermodilution cardiac output measurements

Underestimation of True Cardiac Output
- Injectate volume greater than programmed volume (typically 10 mL)
- Large amounts of fluid administered simultaneous to cardiac output measurement (rapid infusions should be stopped)
- Injectate colder than measured temperature injectate (injectate temperature probe next to heat-emitting hardware instead of injectate fluid)

Overestimation of True Cardiac Output
- Injectate volume less than programmed volume
- Injectate warmer than measured temperature injectate

Other Considerations
- Surgical manipulation of the heart
- Fluid administration from aortic CPB cannula
- Arrhythmias

CPB, Cardiopulmonary bypass.

27. A 33-year-old woman with chronic thromboembolic pulmonary hypertension presents for pulmonary thromboendarterectomy. Her preoperative transthoracic echocardiogram reveals severe tricuspid regurgitation. True statements about her severe tricuspid regurgitation include:

A. It causes a falsely low cardiac output as assessed by the Fick principle

B. It causes a falsely low cardiac output as assessed by arterial pressure pulse contour analysis

C. It causes a falsely low cardiac output as assessed by thermodilution

D. All of the above

Correct Answer: C

Explanation: Severe tricuspid regurgitation has been reported to cause a falsely low measurement of cardiac output with the thermodilution technique. It has no effect on measurements using the Fick principle, or measurements on the left side of the circulation such as arterial pulse contour analysis.

References:

1. Mittnacht AJC, Reich DL, Sander M, et al. Chapter 13: Monitoring of the Heart and Vascular System. In: Kaplan JA, Augoustides JGT, Manecke GR, et al., eds. Kaplan's Cardiac Anesthesia. 7th ed. Elsevier; 2017:390-426.
2. Balik M, Pachl J, Hendl J, et al. Effect of the degree of tricuspid regurgitation on cardiac output measurements by thermodilution. Intensive Care Med, 2002; 28: 1117.

28. Arterial pulse contour analysis can potentially reveal all of the following EXCEPT:

A. Stroke volume variation

B. Pulse pressure variation

C. Left-sided stroke volume index

D. Pulmonary vascular resistance

Correct Answer: D

Explanation: Stroke volume variation, pulse pressure variation, and left-sided stroke volume index are all parameters that can be assessed by arterial pulse contour analysis systems. Because they assess events only on the left side of the circulation, they are unable to assess right-sided parameters such as pulmonary vascular resistance or right-sided cardiac output.

References:

1. Mittnacht AJC, Reich DL, Sander M, et al. Chapter 13: Monitoring of the Heart and Vascular System. In: Kaplan JA, Augoustides JGT, Manecke GR, et al., eds. Kaplan's Cardiac Anesthesia. 7th ed. Elsevier; 2017:390-426.
2. Slagt C, Malagon I, Groeneveld AB. Systematic review of uncalibrated arterial pressure waveform analysis to determine cardiac output and stroke volume variation. Br J Anaesth, 2014; 112: 626-637.

BOX 13.9 **Parameters derived from pulse contour analysis**

Continuous Parameters (Not for All Monitoring Devices)

- Pulse contour/pulse wave cardiac index and stroke volume index
- Stroke volume variation (SVV)
- Pulse pressure variation (PPV)
- Systemic vascular resistance (SVR)
- Cardiac power index (CPI)
- Left ventricular contractility (dPmax)

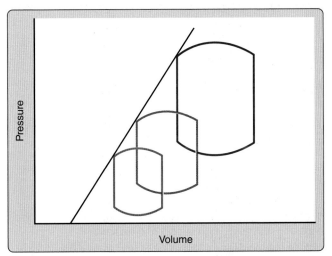

FIGURE 13.7 The end-systolic pressure-volume relationship, also known as end-systolic elastance, is the line connecting the end-systolic points of multiple pressure-volume loops that are obtained at various preloads. An increased slope (i.e., steeper line) represents increased contractility, and a decreased slope represents decreased contractility. This measurement is relatively insensitive to variations in afterload.

29. In the plot of cardiac work loops (seen in the Figure 13.7), the straight line indicated by the arrow:
    A. Is an indicator of diastolic function
    B. Has a steeper slope when contractility increases
    C. Can be used to calculate total cardiac work
    D. Has a decreased slope when the left ventricle is underfilled

Correct Answer: B

Explanation: The end-systolic pressure-volume relationship, also known as end-systolic elastance, is the line connecting the end-systolic points of multiple pressure-volume loops that are obtained at various preloads. An increased slope (steeper line) represents increased contractility, and a decreased slope represents decreased contractility. This measurement is relatively insensitive to variations in preload and afterload. Since the

end-systolic elastance consists of end-systolic pressure/volume points, it contains no information about diastolic function. Cardiac work for any given cycle is calculated by determining the area within the cardiac work loop.

References:

1. Mittnacht AJC, Reich DL, Sander M, et al. Chapter 13: Monitoring of the Heart and Vascular System. In: Kaplan JA, Augoustides JGT, Manecke GR, et al., eds. Kaplan's Cardiac Anesthesia. 7th ed. Elsevier; 2017:390-426.
2. Schreuder JJ, Biervliet JD, van der Velde ET, et al. Systolic and diastolic pressure-volume relationships during cardiac surgery. J Cardiothorac Vasc Anesth, 1991; 5: 539.
3. Bombardini T, Constantino MF, Sicari R, et al. End-systolic elastance and ventricular-arterial coupling reserve predict cardiac events in patients with negative stress echocardiography. Biomed Res Int, 2013; 2013: 235194.

30. Noninvasive technologies for determining cardiac output use which of the following techniques?
    A. Volume clamp method
    B. Transpulmonary thermodilution
    C. Infrared plethysmography
    D. Lithium dilution

Correct Answer: A

Explanation: Certain current noninvasive arterial pulse contour systems employ the volume clamp method to calculate cardiac output. The principle of this technology is based on the idea that blood volume in the arterial vascular bed varies during the cardiac cycle. The blood volume in the respective finger can be held constant using a rapid response finger pressure cuff (volume clamping). The cuff pressure and volume required correlates with blood pressure and stroke volume changes and allows reconstructing a continuous beat-to-beat curve for blood pressure and cardiac output measurement. Alternative noninvasive systems employ thoracic impedance and bioreactance to determine cardiac output. Transpulmonary thermodilution and lithium dilution are invasive techniques for assessment of cardiac output that require arterial and/or venous access. Infrared plethysmography is utilized for pulse oximetry but is not currently used for cardiac output assessment.

References:

1. Mittnacht AJC, Reich DL, Sander M, et al. Chapter 13: Monitoring of the Heart and Vascular System. In: Kaplan JA, Augoustides JGT, Manecke GR, et al., eds. Kaplan's Cardiac Anesthesia. 7th ed. Elsevier; 2017:390-426.
2. Bogert LWJ, Wesseling KH, Schraa O, et al. Pulse contour cardiac output derived from non-invasive arterial pressure in cardiovascular disease. Anaesthesia, 2010; 65: 1119-1125.
3. Maas SWMC, Roekkaerts PMHJ, Lance MD. Cardiac output measurement by bioimpedance and non-invasive pulse contour analysis compared with the continuous pulmonary artery thermodilution technique. J Cardiothorac Vasc Anesth, 2014; 28; 534-539.

CHAPTER 14

Central Nervous System Monitoring

Gerard Manecke and Joel A. Kaplan

KEY POINTS

1. Cardiac surgery–associated brain injury is common, multifactorial, and often preventable.
2. Electroencephalography can detect cerebral ischemia or hypoxia and seizures and can measure hypnotic effect.
3. Middle-latency auditory-evoked potentials objectively document inadequate hypnosis.
4. Brainstem auditory-evoked potentials measure the effects of cooling and rewarming on deep brain structures.
5. Somatosensory-evoked potentials may detect developing injury in cortical and subcortical brain structures and peripheral nerves.
6. Transcranial electric motor-evoked potentials monitor function of the descending motor pathways.
7. Transcranial Doppler ultrasound examination assesses the direction and character of blood flow through large intracranial arteries and identifies microemboli.
8. Cerebral oximetry, using spatially resolved transcranial near-infrared spectroscopy, provides a continuous measure of change in the balance of cerebral oxygen supply and demand.
9. Used in concert, these technologies can reduce the incidence of brain injury and ensure the adequacy of hypnosis.

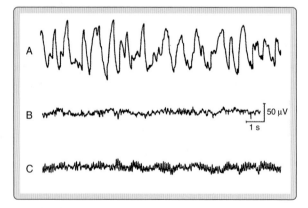

Correct Answer: D

Explanation: Delta waves on the electroencephalogram have a high amplitude and low frequency, as shown in tracing A. These delta waves may indicate various cerebral states, including deep non–rapid eye movement sleep, the anesthetized state, cerebral ischemia, or cerebral hypoxia. Immediately prior to circulatory arrest, the electroencephalogram should be isoelectric (quiescent). Delta waves are not typically seen in the awake state or after conscious sedation.

1. The electroencephalographic tracing A in the figure that shows high voltage and low frequency (1 Hz, Delta waves) is characteristic of:
   A. Coronary artery bypass patient in the preoperative area prior to sedation
   B. Coronary artery bypass patient after administration of sedation prior to anesthetic induction
   C. Aortic arch surgery patient under general anesthesia immediately prior to circulatory arrest
   D. Coronary artery bypass patient under general anesthesia

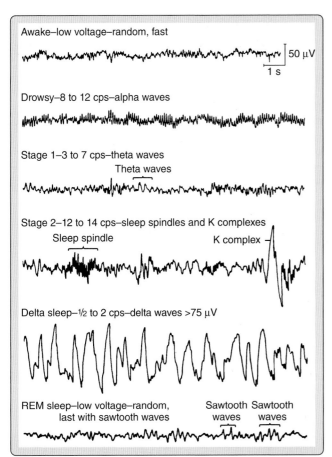

Awake–low voltage–random, fast

50 µV

1 s

Drowsy–8 to 12 cps–alpha waves

Stage 1–3 to 7 cps–theta waves

Theta waves

Stage 2–12 to 14 cps–sleep spindles and K complexes

Sleep spindle

K complex

Delta sleep–½ to 2 cps–delta waves >75 µV

REM sleep–low voltage–random,
last with sawtooth waves

Sawtooth   Sawtooth
waves   waves

FIGURE 14.1 Specific electroencephalographic characteristics of human sleep-wakefulness cycle stages. Note the appearance of the four most common frequency bands, from the lowest frequency delta through theta and alpha to high-frequency beta. An even higher gamma frequency band (25–55 cps) is also described. *REM,* Rapid-eye-movement. (Modified from Yli-Hankala A, ed. Handbook of Four-Channel EEG in Anesthesia and Critical Care. Helsinki, Finland: GE HealthCare; 2004:5, with permission of the publisher.)

References:

1. Edmonds HL, Gordon EK, Levy WJ. Chapter 14: Central Nervous System Monitoring. In: Kaplan JA, Augoustides JGT, Manecke GR, et al., eds. Kaplan's Cardiac Anesthesia. 7th ed. Elsevier; 2017:677-697.
2. Yli-Hankala A, ed. Handbook of Four-Channel EEG in Anesthesia and Critical Care. GE Medical Datex-Ohmeda Division; 2004:5.
3. Montlupil JM, Defresne A, Bonhomme V, et al. The raw and processed electroencephalogram as a monitoring and diagnostic tool. J Cardiothorac Vasc Anesth, 2019; 33: S3-S10.

2. Electroencephalographic tracing B (see figure), which shows low voltage, high frequency (>15 Hz), and random contour, is characteristic of:
   A. Coronary artery bypass patient in the preoperative area prior to sedation
   B. Coronary artery bypass patient after administration of sedation prior to anesthetic induction
   C. Aortic arch surgery patient under general anesthesia immediately prior to circulatory arrest
   D. Coronary artery bypass patient under general anesthesia

Correct Answer: A

Explanation: An electroencephalographic tracing with high frequency, low amplitude, and random-appearing contour is characteristic of the awake state (see figure in question 1). Delta waves, as illustrated by tracing A, are characteristic of the anesthetized state, as explained in question 1. The electroencephalogram is typically isoelectric immediately prior to hypothermic circulatory arrest for aortic arch surgery. The sedated state is not associated with a high-frequency, low-amplitude, and random-contour electroencephalographic pattern (See figure, page 150).

References:

1. Edmonds HL, Gordon EK, Levy WJ. Chapter 14: Central Nervous System Monitoring. In: Kaplan JA, Augoustides JGT, Manecke GR, et al., eds. Kaplan's Cardiac Anesthesia. 7th ed. Elsevier; 2017:677-697.
2. Yli-Hankala A, ed. Handbook of Four-Channel EEG in Anesthesia and Critical Care. GE Medical Datex-Ohmeda Division; 2004:5.
3. Montlupil JM, Defresne A, Bonhomme V, et al. The raw and processed electroencephalogram as a monitoring and diagnostic tool. J Cardiothorac Vasc Anesth, 2019; 33: S3-S10.

3. The electroencephalographic tracing C in the figure that shows frequency of 8–12 Hz with alpha waves is characteristic of:
   A. Coronary artery bypass patient in the preoperative area prior to sedation
   B. Coronary artery bypass patient after administration of sedation prior to anesthetic induction
   C. Aortic arch surgery patient under general anesthesia immediately prior to circulatory arrest
   D. Coronary artery bypass patient under general anesthesia

Correct Answer: B

Explanation: An electroencephalographic tracing with a frequency of 8 to 12 Hz and alpha waves is characteristic of drowsiness. Such drowsiness may occur naturally, or result from administration of sedatives (see figure in question 1). The awake state and the anesthetized state are not typically associated with alpha waves. The electroencephalogram is typically isoelectric immediately prior to circulatory arrest for aortic arch surgery (See figure, page 150).

References:

1. Edmonds HL, Gordon EK, Levy WJ. Chapter 14: Central Nervous System Monitoring. In: Kaplan JA, Augoustides JGT, Manecke GR, et al., eds. Kaplan's Cardiac Anesthesia. 7th ed. Elsevier; 2017:677-697.
2. Yli-Hankala A, ed. Handbook of Four-Channel EEG in Anesthesia and Critical Care. GE Medical Datex-Ohmeda Division; 2004:5.
3. Montlupil JM, Defresne A, Bonhomme V, et al. The raw and processed electroencephalogram as a monitoring and diagnostic tool. J Cardiothorac Vasc Anesth, 2019; 33: S3-S10.

4. Factors shown to cause cerebral injury during cardiac surgery include all the following EXCEPT:

   A. Microemboli from the cardiopulmonary bypass pump
   B. Macroemboli from aortic plaques
   C. Cerebral hypoperfusion
   D. Deep anesthesia

Correct Answer: D

Explanation: Microemboli, macroemboli, and cerebral perfusion have all been shown to cause cerebral injury during cardiac surgery. Although deep anesthesia has been implicated as a possible contributor to poor postoperative neurocognitive outcomes, this has not been conclusively shown.

BOX 14.1   factors contributing to brain injury during cardiac surgical procedures

- Atheromatous emboli from aorta manipulation
- Lipid microemboli from recirculation of unwashed cardiotomy suction
- Gaseous microemboli from air leakage and cavitation.
- Cerebral hypoperfusion or hyperperfusion.
- Cerebral hyperthermia.
- Cerebral dysoxygenation.

(Adapted from the Kaplan's Cardiac Anesthesia 7th edition, Joel A. Kaplan, John G.T. Augoustides, and Gerard R. Manecke et al., from chap 18, page 678.)

References:

1. Edmonds HL, Gordon EK, Levy WJ. Chapter 14: Central Nervous System Monitoring. In: Kaplan JA, Augoustides JGT, Manecke GR, et al., eds. Kaplan's Cardiac Anesthesia. 7th ed. Elsevier; 2017:677-697.
2. Hogue CW, Gottesman RF, Stearns J. Mechanisms of cerebral injury from cardiac surgery. Crit Care Clin, 2008; 24: 83-98.
3. Milne B, Gilbey T, Gautel L, et al. Neuromonitoring and neurocognitive outcomes in cardiac surgery: a narrative review. J Cardiothorac Vasc Anesth, 2022; 36: 2098-2113.

5. The International 10–20 system of electrode placement for an electroencephalogram:

   A. Requires bipolar leads to consistently detect abnormalities in discrete areas of the cortex
   B. Detects voltages similar to those of electrocardiographic electrodes
   C. Uses bispectral analysis for level of consciousness monitoring
   D. Is less sensitive to artifact than electrocardiographic electrodes

Correct Answer: A

Explanation: The International 10–20 system for electroencephalogram electrode placement is the current standard for formal electroencephalography. It permits uniform spacing of electrodes, independent of head circumference, in scalp regions known to correlate with specific areas of cerebral cortex. Four anatomic landmarks are used—the nasion, inion, and preauricular points. Electrodes are located at 10% or 20% segments of the distance between two of these landmarks. The alphanumeric label for each site uses an initial upper-case letter to signify the skull region (i.e., frontal, central, temporal, parietal, occipital, auricular, and mastoid). Second and sometimes third letters, in lowercase, further delineate position (e.g., "p" represents frontal pole, whereas "z" indicates zero or midline). Subscripted numbers represent left (odd) or right (even) and specific hemispheric location, with the lowest numbers closest to the midline. The prime notation (′) is used to signify specialized locations designed for certain evoked potential applications (e.g., C3′ and C4′ represent 2 cm posterior to C3 and C4, directly over the upper limb sensory cortex).

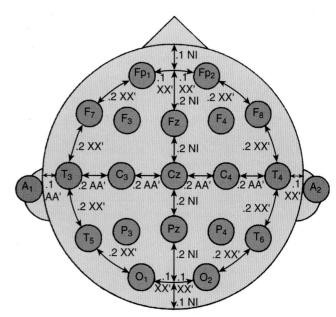

FIGURE 14.2 Electroencephalographic electrode positions in the International 10–20 system. The sagittal hemicircumference (labeled AA′) is measured from the root of one zygoma (just anterior to the ear) to the other, across the vertex. The third measurement is the ipsilateral hemicircumference (XX′) measured from a point 10% of the coronal hemicircumference above the zygoma. Through these intersecting lines all the scalp electrodes may be located, except the frontal (F3, F4) and parietal (P3, P4) electrodes. The frontal and parietal electrodes are placed along the frontal or parietal coronal line midway between the middle electrode and the electrode marked in the circumferential ring.

References:

1. Edmonds HL, Gordon EK, Levy WJ. Chapter 14: Central Nervous System Monitoring. In: Kaplan JA, Augoustides JGT, Manecke GR, et al., eds. Kaplan's Cardiac Anesthesia. 7th ed. Elsevier; 2017:677-697.
2. Goldensohn ES, Legatt AD, Koszer S, et al., eds. Goldensohn's EEG Interpretation. 2nd ed. Futura; 1999:16.
3. Montlupil JM, Defresne A, Bonhomme V, et al. The raw and processed electroencephalogram as a monitoring and diagnostic tool. J Cardiothorac Vasc Anesth, 2019; 33: S3-S10.

BIPOLAR RECORDING

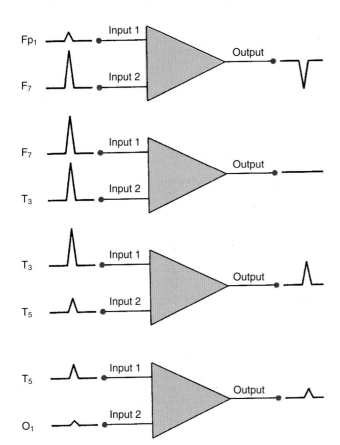

FIGURE 14.3 Detection of focal electroencephalographic (EEG) abnormalities. Their accurate characterization requires that one of the amplifier's inputs be outside the field distribution of the transient EEG abnormality. If both inputs lie within the transient field, the signal may become invisible because of in-phase cancellation. (Modified from Goldensohn ES, Legatt AD, Koszer S, et al., eds. Goldensohn's EEG Interpretation. 2nd ed. Futura; 1999, with permission of the publisher.)

6. Simultaneous amplitude and frequency increases during electroencephalographic monitoring may be a sign of:
   A. Light anesthesia
   B. Cerebral ischemia
   C. Seizure activity
   D. High-dose fentanyl administration

Correct Answer: C

Explanation: Light anesthesia (wakefulness) is indicated by high frequency with low amplitude. Cerebral ischemia and high-dose fentanyl administration are both associated with low-frequency, high-amplitude tracings known as delta waves. Seizure activity often shows high frequency and high amplitude on the electroencephalogram.

References:

1. Edmonds HL, Gordon EK, Levy WJ. Chapter 14: Central Nervous System Monitoring. In: Kaplan JA, Augoustides JGT, Manecke GR, et al., eds. Kaplan's Cardiac Anesthesia. 7th ed. Elsevier; 2017:677-697.

2. Emmady PD, Anilkumar AC. EEG Abnormal Waveforms. In: StatPearls [Internet]. Treasure Island (FL): StatPearls Publishing; 2022.
3. Montlupil JM, Defresne A, Bonhomme V, et al. The raw and processed electroencephalogram as a monitoring and diagnostic tool. J Cardiothorac Vasc Anesth, 2019; 33: S3-S10.

7. In digitizing an electroencephalographic signal, if the highest frequency of interest is 50 Hz, the sampling rate necessary to avoid aliasing must be at LEAST:
   A. 25 Hz
   B. 50 Hz
   C. 75 Hz
   D. 100 Hz

Correct Answer: D

Explanation: Modern electroencephalographic monitors use digital microprocessors to analyze the amplified analog biopotentials. Digitization converts a continuously varying biopotential into a series or sample of discrete quantal values. This process of digitization is at risk for conversion inaccuracies and aliasing that can create false, low frequencies. At least two samples per period are required to minimize these errors. The sampling (Nyquist) frequency must be greater than twice the highest frequency of interest. For example, with an electroencephalographic bandwidth of 50 Hz, the minimum acceptable sampling frequency is 100 Hz.

References:

1. Edmonds HL, Gordon EK, Levy WJ. Chapter 14: Central Nervous System Monitoring. In: Kaplan JA, Augoustides JGT, Manecke GR, et al., eds. Kaplan's Cardiac Anesthesia. 7th ed. Elsevier; 2017:677-697.
2. Nilsson J, Panizza M, Hallett M. Principles of digital sampling of a physiologic signal. Electroencephalogr Clin Neurophysiol, 1993; 89: 349-358.
3. Montlupil JM, Defresne A, Bonhomme V, et al. The raw and processed electroencephalogram as a monitoring and diagnostic tool. J Cardiothorac Vasc Anesth, 2019; 33: S3-S10.

8. Which of the following are "time domain" displays?
   A. Compressed spectral array (waterfall) plot during carotid endarterectomy
   B. Arterial pressure wave during coronary artery surgery
   C. Power spectrum plot of electroencephalographic data during aortic surgery
   D. Color density spectral array during aortic valve surgery

Correct Answer: B

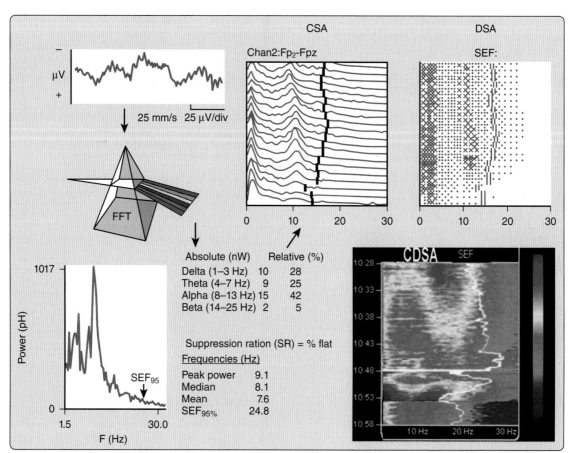

FIGURE 14.4 Comparison of time- and frequency-domain electroencephalographic (EEG) displays. The traditional analog EEG signal shown in the upper left is a time-domain graph of scalp-recorded amplitude (μV) as a function of time. Digitized EEG segments (epochs) are computer processed using the fast Fourier transform (FFT), which, like a prism, decomposes a complex electromagnetic signal into a series of sinusoids, each with a discrete frequency. The instantaneous relationship is then graphically depicted by the power spectrum (lower left), a frequency-domain plot of power (μV2 or pW) as a function of frequency. The spectral edge frequency (SEF) defines the signal amplitude upper boundary. The three-dimensional compressed spectral array (CSA) plots successive power spectra with time on the z-axis (upper middle). The density-modulated spectral array (DSA; upper right) improves data compression by using dot density to represent signal amplitude (i.e., power). Amplitude resolution is improved through color coding in the color density spectral array (CDSA) shown at the lower right. The SEF is shown as the white vertical line. Note the EEG suppression at the bottom of each spectral trend. (Courtesy Dr. Mark Moehring, Broadview Labs, Seattle, Wash.)

Explanation: "Time domain" displays refer to plots in which calculated or measured values are displayed and analyzed as a function of time. For example, arterial pressure waves consist of amplitude (pressure) plotted on the y axis, and time is on the x axis. "Frequency domain" displays refer to plots in which calculated values are displayed as a function of frequency. Compressed spectral array ("waterfall") plots, power spectral displays, and color density spectral array are all examples of "frequency domain" displays.

References:

1. Edmonds HL, Gordon EK, Levy WJ. Chapter 14: Central Nervous System Monitoring. In: Kaplan JA, Augoustides JGT, Manecke GR, et al., eds. Kaplan's Cardiac Anesthesia. 7th ed. Elsevier; 2017:677-697.
2. Dressler O, Schneider G. Stockmanns G, et al. Awareness and the EEG power spectrum: analysis of frequencies. Br J Anesth, 2004; 93: 806-809.
3. Montlupil JM, Defresne A, Bonhomme V, et al. The raw and processed electroencephalogram as a monitoring and diagnostic tool. J Cardiothorac Vasc Anesth, 2019; 33: S3-S10.

9. Which of the following electroencephalographic findings is associated with cerebral ischemia?
 A. Increased median dominant frequency
 B. Decreased spectral edge 95%
 C. Decreased amplitude with increasing frequency
 D. Spindle waves

Correct Answer: B

Explanation: A decreasing spectral edge 95% indicates decreasing overall frequency. This may be a sign of cerebral ischemia. An increased median dominant frequency is not associated with ischemia. A decreased amplitude with increasing frequency is associated with the awake state, and spindle waves are associated with sleep.

References:

1. Edmonds HL, Gordon EK, Levy WJ. Chapter 14: Central Nervous System Monitoring. In: Kaplan JA, Augoustides JGT, Manecke GR, et al., eds. Kaplan's Cardiac Anesthesia. 7th ed. Elsevier; 2017:677-697.
2. Foreman B, Claassen J. Quantitative EEG for the detection of brain ischemia. Crit Care, 2012; 16: 216.
3. Milne B, Gilbey T, Gautel L, et al. Neuromonitoring and neurocognitive outcomes in cardiac surgery: a narrative review. J Cardiothorac Vasc Anesth, 2022; 36: 2098-2113.

10. A 68-year-old man is undergoing an open repair of a descending thoracic aortic aneurysm. Monitoring which of the following is the most useful in detecting decreased perfusion from the anterior spinal artery during the procedure?

A. Somatosensory-evoked potentials
B. Motor-evoked potentials
C. Femoral arterial blood pressure
D. Lower extremity near-infrared spectroscopy

Correct Answer: B

Explanation: Because the anterior spinal artery supplies blood flow to the motor areas of the spinal cord, anterior spinal artery perfusion deficits typically manifest as motor deficits. By relying on the delivery of a rapid stimulus pulse train, it is possible to monitor the integrity of descending motor pathways continuously by using transcranial electric motor-evoked potentials. The most frequent application of this monitoring modality for cardiothoracic surgical procedures currently is during open surgical or endovascular repair of the descending aorta. The need for improved spinal cord protection remains critical because, even with modern spinal cord preservation techniques, the infarction rate during type I and II aneurysm repairs in patients remains disturbingly high.

References:

1. Edmonds HL, Gordon EK, Levy WJ. Chapter 14: Central Nervous System Monitoring. In: Kaplan JA, Augoustides JGT, Manecke GR, et al., eds. Kaplan's Cardiac Anesthesia. 7th ed. Elsevier; 2017:677-697.
2. Jameson LC. Transcranial motor evoked potentials. In: Koht A, Sloan TB, Toleikis JR, eds. Monitoring the Nervous System for Anesthesiologists and Other Health Care Professionals. Springer; 2012:27-46.

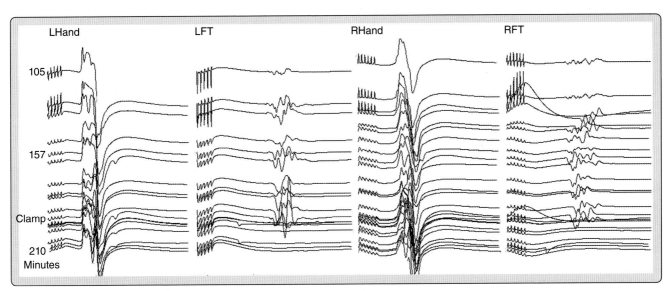

FIGURE 14.5 Motor-evoked potential (MEP) detection of spinal cord hypoperfusion. Changes are shown in hand (LHand and RHand) and foot (LFT and RFT) MEP responses to clamping of the descending aorta during surgical repair of a thoracoabdominal aneurysm. Note the bilateral loss of lower-limb MEP with clamp application. MEP monitoring helped guide management of left-sided heart bypass and reimplantation of the superior mesenteric and renal arteries into the aortic graft.

3. Miller LK, Patel VI, Wagener G. Spinal cord protection for thoracoabdominal aortic surgery. J Cardiothorac Vasc Anesth, 2022; 36: 577-586.

11. Transcranial motor evoked potentials may be used to monitor which of the following?

A. C fiber pain transmission
B. Dorsal horn postsynaptic transmission
C. Neuromuscular function
D. Latency indicating posterior spinal cord ischemia

Correct Answer: C

Explanation: Motor-evoked potentials are used to monitor the function of upper and lower motor neurons and can also be used to monitor neuromuscular function. C fibers are sensory, and somatosensory-evoked potentials are used for monitoring of the sensory function of the spinal cord, including the dorsal horn.

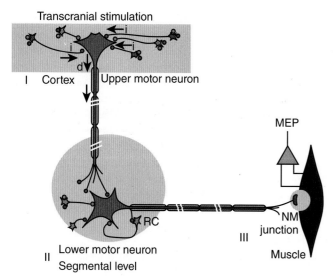

Transcranial stimulation

I   Cortex

Upper motor neuron

MEP

NM junction

III

Muscle

RC

II   Lower motor neuron

Segmental level

FIGURE 14.6 Neural generators of transcranial motor-evoked potentials (MEPs). High-intensity transcranial electric or magnetic stimulation results in direct (d) activation of upper motor neurons. In addition, indirect motor neuron activation (i) results from transcranial activation of horizontally oriented excitatory (light) and inhibitory (dark) neuronal axons. Descending motor potentials are conducted unidirectionally through the corticospinal, rubrospinal, tectospinal, vestibulospinal, and cerebellospinal tracts to lower (alpha) motor neurons in the lateral and anterior spinal cord. In the absence of complete pharmacologic neuromuscular (NM) blockade, alpha motor neuron action potentials then produce muscle fiber contraction that is recorded by electromyography. (Modified from Journee JL. Motor EP physiology, risks and specific anesthetic effects. In: Nuwer MR, ed. Handbook of Clinical Neurophysiology. Vol. 8. Intraoperative Monitoring of Neural Function. Elsevier; 2008:219.)

References:

1. Edmonds HL, Gordon EK, Levy WJ. Chapter 14: Central Nervous System Monitoring. In: Kaplan JA, Augoustides JGT, Manecke GR, et al., eds. Kaplan's Cardiac Anesthesia. 7th ed. Elsevier; 2017:677-697.
2. Jameson LC. Transcranial motor evoked potentials. In: Koht A, Sloan TB, Toleikis JR, eds. Monitoring the Nervous System for Anesthesiologists and Other Health Care Professionals. Springer; 2012:27-46.
3. Miller LK, Patel VI, Wagener G. Spinal cord protection for thoracoabdominal aortic surgery. J Cardiothorac Vasc Anesth, 2022; 36: 577-586.

12. A 66-year-old man is undergoing aortic root repair, and transcranial Doppler monitoring is utilized for detection of cerebral emboli. The vessel most commonly monitored with transcranial Doppler is:
    A. Internal carotid artery
    B. Vertebral artery
    C. External carotid artery
    D. Middle cerebral artery

Correct Answer: D

Explanation: Ultrasonic probes of a clinical transcranial Doppler sonograph contain an electrically activated piezoelectric crystal that transmits low-power 1- to 2-MHz acoustic vibrations (insonation signal) through the thinnest portion of temporal bone to yield an acoustic window into brain tissue. The frequency differences between the insonation signal and each echo in the series are proportional to the associated velocity, and this velocity is determined from the Doppler equation. Although several large intracranial arteries may be insonated through the temporal window, the middle cerebral artery is generally monitored during cardiac operations because it carries approximately 40% of the hemispheric blood flow. Transcranial Doppler monitoring of the middle cerebral artery may be useful for quantification of cerebral embolic load.

References:

1. Edmonds HL, Gordon EK, Levy WJ. Chapter 14: Central Nervous System Monitoring. In: Kaplan JA, Augoustides JGT, Manecke GR, et al., eds. Kaplan's Cardiac Anesthesia. 7th ed. Elsevier; 2017:677-697.
2. Georgiadis D, Siebler M. Detection of microembolic signals with transcranial Doppler ultrasound. Front Neurol Neurosci, 2006; 21: 194-205.
3. Finucane E, Jooste E, Machovec KA. Neuromonitoring modalities in pediatric cardiac anesthesia: a review of the literature. J Cardiothorac Vasc Anesth, 2020; 34: 3420-3428.

13. A 70-year-old woman is undergoing aortic arch repair, and transcranial Doppler monitoring is utilized for detection of cerebral emboli, as depicted in the figure. In the Doppler M mode and spectral displays in the figure, labels a, b, c, and d indicate:
    A. Movement artifact
    B. Premature ventricular contractions
    C. Erythrocyte rouleaux reflection
    D. Microemboli

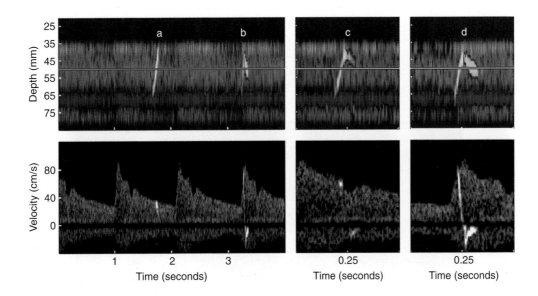

Correct Answer: D

Explanation: Labels a, b, c, and d indicate embolic signals detected by the transcranial Doppler M-mode and spectral displays. The appearance of emboliform high-intensity transient signals is compared using the M-mode and frequency spectral displays. The white horizontal line at a depth of 50 mm depicts the site of the spectral measurement along the axis of the vessel. A high-intensity transient signal represents linear migration of an embolus in the M2 segment of the ipsilateral middle cerebral artery. This embolus (white dot) is noted on the spectral display as it passes through the 50-mm measurement site. In contrast, emboli in the remaining panels suddenly change direction as they pass into a smaller branch vessel. The emboli b and d have direction changes that are noted on the spectral displays as the characteristic "lambda" sign. However, the embolus c is misidentified as two emboli because the direction change occurs outside the spectral sample volume.

References:

1. Edmonds HL, Gordon EK, Levy WJ. Chapter 14: Central Nervous System Monitoring. In: Kaplan JA, Augoustides JGT, Manecke GR, et al., eds. Kaplan's Cardiac Anesthesia. 7th ed. Elsevier; 2017:677-697.
2. Georgiadis D, Siebler M. Detection of microembolic signals with transcranial Doppler ultrasound. Front Neurol Neurosci, 2006; 21: 194-205.
3. Milne B, Gilbey T, Gautel L, et al. Neuromonitoring and neurocognitive outcomes in cardiac surgery: a narrative review. J Cardiothorac Vasc Anesth, 2022; 36: 2098-2113.

14. Jugular venous bulb oximetry may be useful for:
  A. Detecting regional deficiencies in cerebral oxygenation
  B. Assessing the cerebral oxygenation effects of hyperthermia
  C. Identifying a transfusion trigger
  D. B and C

Correct Answer: D

Explanation: Jugular venous bulb oxygenation monitoring provides a global assessment of brain oxygen balance. One of its weaknesses is that, because cerebral perfusion is heterogeneous, it does not detect small, regional deficiencies in cerebral perfusion. Global cerebral oxygen balance, as determined by jugular venous bulb oximetry, has been used successfully as a transfusion trigger and to document the deleterious effect of even modest cerebral hyperthermia. Furthermore, the trending of this monitor can guide the conduct of deep hypothermia for aortic arch repair, as well as to compare the frequency of cerebral oxygen desaturation during myocardial revascularization with and without cardiopulmonary bypass.

References:

1. Edmonds HL, Gordon EK, Levy WJ. Chapter 14: Central Nervous System Monitoring. In: Kaplan JA, Augoustides JGT, Manecke GR, et al., eds. Kaplan's Cardiac Anesthesia. 7th ed. Elsevier; 2017:677-697.
2. Diephuis JC, Moons KG, Nierich AN, et al. Jugular bulb desaturation during coronary artery surgery: a comparison of off-pump and on-pump procedures. Br J Anesth, 2005; 94: 715.
3. Milne B, Gilbey T, Gautel L, et al. Neuromonitoring and neurocognitive outcomes in cardiac surgery: a narrative review. J Cardiothorac Vasc Anesth, 2022; 36: 2098-2113.

15. Near-infrared spectroscopy of the brain measures:
  A. Tissue oxygenation
  B. 30% venous blood oxygenation, 70% arterial oxygenation
  C. 50% venous blood oxygenation, 50% arterial oxygenation
  D. 70% venous blood oxygenation, 30% arterial oxygenation

Correct Answer: D

Explanation: Because the human skull is translucent to infrared light, intracranial intravascular regional saturation (rSO2) may be measured noninvasively with transcranial near-infrared spectroscopy (NIRS). An infrared light source contained in a self-adhesive patch affixed to glabrous skin of the scalp transmits photons through underlying tissues to the outer layers of the cerebral cortex. Adjacent sensors separate photons reflected from the skin, muscle, skull, and dura from those of the brain tissue. NIRS measures all hemoglobin, pulsatile and nonpulsatile, in a mixed microvascular bed composed of gas-exchanging vessels with a diameter of less than 1 mm. The measurement is thought to reflect approximately 70% venous blood.

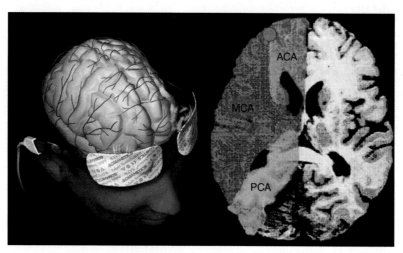

FIGURE 14.7 Cerebral oximetry monitors the anterior arterial watershed region. The frontal cortex anterior cerebral artery (ACA) and middle cerebral artery (MCA) watershed region may be sampled bilaterally by cerebral oximeter sensors located on the forehead above each eye. The diagram at the right illustrates the anterior (green) and middle cerebral artery (pink) flow distributions and the approximate size and location of the oximetric sampling region (red dot). *PCA,* Posterior cerebral artery. (© 2023 Medtronic. All rights reserved. Used with the permission of Medtronic.)

References:

1. Edmonds HL, Gordon EK, Levy WJ. Chapter 14: Central Nervous System Monitoring. In: Kaplan JA, Augoustides JGT, Manecke GR, et al., eds. Kaplan's Cardiac Anesthesia. 7th ed. Elsevier; 2017:677-697.
2. Ferrari M, Quaresima V. Near infrared brain and muscle oximetry: from the discovery to current applications. J Near Infrared Spectrosc, 2012; 20: 1.
3. Milne B, Gilbey T, Gautel L, et al. Neuromonitoring and neurocognitive outcomes in cardiac surgery: a narrative review. J Cardiothorac Vasc Anesth, 2022; 36: 2098-2113.

16. A 44-year-old woman is undergoing pulmonary thromboendarterectomy with hypothermic circulatory arrest. Of the following, the most effective means of determining regional oxygenation during cardiopulmonary bypass and during circulatory arrest is:
   A. Near-infrared spectroscopy
   B. Transcranial Doppler
   C. Jugular venous bulb saturation
   D. Bispectral index monitoring

Correct Answer: A

Explanation: Cerebral oximetry appears both to quantify change reliably from an individualized baseline and to offer an objective measure of regional hypoperfusion. Unlike pulse and jugular bulb oximetry, cerebral oximetry may be used during nonpulsatile cardiopulmonary bypass and circulatory arrest. Transcranial Doppler and bispectral monitoring, while potentially useful, do not directly measure regional oxygenation.

References:

1. Edmonds HL, Gordon EK, Levy WJ. Chapter 14: Central Nervous System Monitoring. In: Kaplan JA, Augoustides JGT, Manecke GR, et al., eds. Kaplan's Cardiac Anesthesia. 7th ed. Elsevier; 2017:677-697.
2. Zheng F, Sheinberg R, Yee M-S, et al. Cerebral near-infrared spectroscopy monitoring and neurologic outcomes in adult cardiac surgery patients: a systematic review. Anesth Analg, 2013; 116: 198.
3. Ali J, Cody J, Maldonado Y, et al. Near-infrared spectroscopy (NIRS) for cerebral and tissue oximetry: analysis of evolving applications. J Cardiothorac Vasc Anesth, 2022; 36: 2758-2766.

17. Which of the following statements is true about normal values in near-infrared spectroscopy?
   A. They are consistent across devices produced by different companies
   B. They are in the same range both for infants presenting for congenital heart surgery and for healthy infants
   C. They are the same in adult cardiac surgery patients as in healthy volunteers
   D. They may change depending upon the placement of the sensors on the skull

Correct Answer: D

Explanation: The normative value of 71% ± 6% for near-infrared spectroscopy reported for healthy adults is significantly higher than that obtained from cardiac surgical patients. An even larger difference is observed between healthy infants and infants with congenital heart disease. Because of the technical differences among competing oximeters, clinicians should appreciate that these normative values are device-dependent and not always interchangeable. Furthermore, the normal values are also dependent on the position of the sensors on the skull.

References:

1. Edmonds HL, Gordon EK, Levy WJ. Chapter 14: Central Nervous System Monitoring. In: Kaplan JA, Augoustides JGT, Manecke GR, et al., eds. Kaplan's Cardiac Anesthesia. 7th ed. Elsevier; 2017:677-697.
2. Heringlake M, Garbers C, Käbler J-H, et al. Preoperative cerebral oxygen saturation and clinical outcomes in cardiac surgery. Anesthesiology, 2011; 114: 58.
3. Ali J, Cody J, Maldonado Y, et al. Near-infrared spectroscopy (NIRS) for cerebral and tissue oximetry: analysis of evolving applications. J Cardiothorac Vasc Anesth, 2022; 36: 2758-2766.

18. The circle of Willis is completely normal in what percentage of the population?
   A. 10%
   B. 25%
   C. 50%
   D. 100%

Correct Answer: B

Explanation: The circle of Willis is completely normal in only 25% of the population. There is considerable variation, with more than 80 variations in five continuous groups. The spectrum of variations include hypoplastic segments, absent segments, and accessory segments. These variations become important during hypothermic circulatory arrest for aortic arch repair, as they can influence the conduct of cerebral perfusion.

References:

1. Edmonds HL, Gordon EK, Levy WJ. Chapter 14: Central Nervous System Monitoring. In: Kaplan JA, Augoustides JGT, Manecke GR, et al., eds. Kaplan's Cardiac Anesthesia. 7th ed. Elsevier; 2017:677-697.
2. Ayre JR, Bazira P, Abumattar M, et al. A new classification system for the anatomical variations of the human circle of Willis: a systematic review. J Anat, 2022; 240: 1187-1204.

19. What percentage of patients have abnormalities of their circle of Willis that predispose them to cerebral ischemia when hypothermic circulatory arrest with unilateral antegrade cerebral perfusion is performed?
   A. 22%
   B. 42%
   C. 62%
   D. 82%

Correct Answer: B

Explanation: As many as 42% of patients will likely have circle of Willis abnormalities predisposing them to cerebral ischemia when unilateral antegrade cerebral perfusion is performed for cerebral protection during aortic arch repair. This high prevalence suggests that regional cerebral oxygenation monitoring, such as near-infrared spectroscopy, should be considered in these settings to guide the conduct of antegrade cerebral perfusion. If there is contralateral cerebral desaturation detected by cerebral oximetry monitoring, then bilateral antegrade cerebral perfusion might be indicated to restore adequate cerebral oxygenation.

References:

1. Edmonds HL, Gordon EK, Levy WJ. Chapter 14: Central Nervous System Monitoring. In: Kaplan JA, Augoustides JGT, Manecke GR, et al., eds. Kaplan's Cardiac Anesthesia. 7th ed. Elsevier; 2017:677-697.
2. Papantchev V, Hristove S, Todorova D, et al. Some variations of the circle of Willis, important for cerebral protection in aortic surgery: a study in Eastern Europeans. Eur J Cardiothorac Surg, 2007; 31: 982.

20. Which of the following monitors is fully reliable in detecting an isoelectric electroencephalogram (EEG)?
   A. Level of consciousness processed EEG monitor
   B. Multichannel EEG monitor with complete array
   C. Somatosensory-evoked potentials
   D. A and B

Correct Answer: B

Explanation: The complete array electroencephalogram (EEG) is the most reliable monitor to confirm cerebral isoelectricity. The processed EEG monitor is not particularly adept for detection of cerebral electrical silence. This discordance with the processed EEG monitor occurs because the intrinsic algorithm considers EEG activity to be suppressed when the amplitude is less than 5 μV, whereas voltages lower than 2 μV are generally considered isoelectric. Cooling prolongs peak and interpeak latencies and suppresses amplitude of the cortical response predominantly during monitoring of somatosensory-evoked potentials (SSEP). Consequently, SSEP responses can also be used to assess the extent of cooling. However, because subcortical SSEP responses involve far fewer synapses than the electroencephalogram, these responses often persist when cortical neuronal activity is totally cold suppressed.

References:

1. Edmonds HL, Gordon EK, Levy WJ. Chapter 14: Central Nervous System Monitoring. In: Kaplan JA, Augoustides JGT, Manecke GR, et al., eds. Kaplan's Cardiac Anesthesia. 7th ed. Elsevier; 2017:677-697.
2. Stecker MM, Cheung AT, Pochettino A, et al. Deep hypothermic circulatory arrest. I. Effects of cooling on electroencephalogram and evoked potentials. Ann Thorac Surg, 2001; 71: 14-21.
3. Milne B, Gilbey T, Gautel L, et al. Neuromonitoring and neurocognitive outcomes in cardiac surgery: a narrative review. J Cardiothorac Vasc Anesth, 2022; 36: 2098-2113.

21. A 53-year-old woman presents for ascending aortic arch surgery. Which of the following monitoring modalities would not require added personnel with specific training?
   A. Multichannel electroencephalographic monitoring
   B. Near-infrared spectroscopy
   C. Somatosensory-evoked potentials
   D. Transcranial Doppler

Correct Answer: B

Explanation: Multichannel electroencephalography, somatosensory-evoked potential monitoring, and transcranial Doppler all require added personnel with specific training in utilizing these devices. This limits their potential utility to specific clinical circumstances in cardiac surgery. Special circumstances might include electroencephalographic guidance during hypothermic circulatory arrest for aortic arch surgery, spinal cord monitoring with somatosensory- and motor-evoked potentials during descending thoracic aortic surgery, and patients at high risk for stroke where embolic load measurement is desired with transcranial Doppler monitoring. Near-infrared spectroscopy is an attractive alternative for assessing regional oxygenation because it is simple to apply and does not require significant added expertise for interpretation.

References:

1. Edmonds HL, Gordon EK, Levy WJ. Chapter 14: Central Nervous System Monitoring. In: Kaplan JA, Augoustides JGT, Manecke GR, et al., eds. Kaplan's Cardiac Anesthesia. 7th ed. Elsevier; 2017:677-697.
2. Deschamps A, Lambert J, Cuture P, et al. Reversal of decreases in cerebral saturation in high-risk cardiac surgery. J Cardiothorac Vasc Anesth, 2013; 27: 1260.
3. Milne B, Gilbey T, Gautel L, et al. Neuromonitoring and neurocognitive outcomes in cardiac surgery: a narrative review. J Cardiothorac Vasc Anesth, 2022; 36: 2098-2113.
4. Rasulo FA, Bertuetti R. Transcranial Doppler and optic nerve sonography. J Cardiothoracic Vasc Anesth, 2019; 33: S38-S52.

22. Near-infrared spectroscopy of the brain is possible:
   A. Because the skull is translucent to red light
   B. Because brain tissue absorbs red and infrared light differentially
   C. Because the skull is translucent to infrared light
   D. Because the skull is opaque to infrared light

Correct Answer: C

Explanation: Because the human skull is translucent to infrared light, intracranial intravascular regional oxygen saturation may be measured noninvasively with transcranial near-infrared spectroscopy. An infrared light source contained in a self-adhesive patch affixed to glabrous skin of the scalp transmits photons through underlying tissues to the outer layers of the cerebral cortex. Adjacent sensors separate photons reflected from the skin, muscle, skull, and dura from those of the brain tissue. This technique measures all hemoglobin, with pulsatile and nonpulsatile flow, in a mixed microvascular bed composed of gas-exchanging vessels with a diameter of less than 1 mm. The measurement is thought to reflect approximately 70% venous blood.

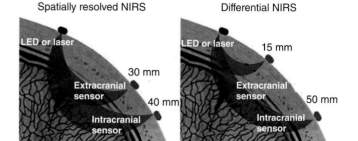

FIGURE 14.8 Comparison of transcranial spatially resolved near-infrared spectroscopy (NIRS) and differential NIRS. Unabsorbed photons travel a parabolic (i.e., banana-shaped) path through the adult cranium from scalp-mounted infrared sources to nearby sensors. The average penetration depth of these reflected photons is given by the square root of the source-detector separation. Spatially resolved NIRS uses a pair of sensors located at sufficient distances from the light source to ensure that both signals detect photons reflected from extracranial and intracranial tissue (left panel). Two-point extracranial and intracranial measurement permits partial suppression of both the extracranial signal and the interpatient variance in intracranial photon scatter. The resultant cerebral oxygen saturation measurement appears to be approximately 65% intracranial. In contrast, differential NIRS uses a sensor placed very near the light source to record exclusively extracranial signal and another more distant sensor for extracranial and intracranial measurement (right panel). Single-point subtraction suppresses much of the extracranial signal, but not the intersubject variation in intracranial photon scatter. Mitigation of this confounding influence is attempted through the use of additional infrared wavelengths. The proportion of the differential regional hemoglobin oxygen saturation signal that represents intracranial tissue has not been established. *LED*, Light-emitting diode. (© 2023 Medtronic. All rights reserved. Used with the permission of Medtronic.)

References:

1. Edmonds HL, Gordon EK, Levy WJ. Chapter 14: Central Nervous System Monitoring. In: Kaplan JA, Augoustides JGT, Manecke GR, et al., eds. Kaplan's Cardiac Anesthesia. 7th ed. Elsevier; 2017:677-697.
2. Ferrari M, Quaresima V. Near infrared brain and muscle oximetry: from the discovery to current applications. J Near Infrared Spectrosc, 2012; 20: 1.
3. Denault A, Ali MS, Couture EJ, et al. A practical approach to cerebro-somatic near-infrared spectroscopy and whole-body ultrasound. J Cardiothorac Vasc Anesth, 2019; 33: S11-S37.

23. Barriers to adoption of multimodal central nervous system (CNS) monitoring include:
   A. CNS outcomes are currently good, even without incurring the cost of new technologies
   B. The incidence of awareness is very low during cardiac surgery
   C. The myriad of data and types of displays from multiple CNS monitors is unwieldy for the cardiac anesthesiologist
   D. The data generated from CNS monitors are unlikely to change practice or improve outcomes

Correct Answer: C

Explanation: Because each monitoring modality may evaluate only a portion of the central nervous system, multimodal monitoring would appear to be desirable to monitor neurologic wellness more completely. The variety of techniques for neuromonitoring and the plethora of display formats provide visually confusing information for the anesthesiologist trying to understand the data in the context of the anesthetic regimen and the surgical procedure. Considerable improvement is needed in ergonomics or the development of alternative display technologies for effective and facile intraoperative use of multimodal central nervous system monitoring by the cardiac anesthesiologist.

References:

1. Edmonds HL, Gordon EK, Levy WJ. Chapter 14: Central Nervous System Monitoring. In: Kaplan JA, Augoustides JGT, Manecke GR, et al., eds. Kaplan's Cardiac Anesthesia. 7th ed. Elsevier; 2017:677-697.
2. Hemphill J, Andrews P, De Georgia M. Multimodal monitoring and neurocritical care bioinformatics. Nat Rev Neurol, 2011; 7: 451-460.
3. Schraag S. Combined monitoring – brain function monitoring and cerebral oximetry. J Cardiothorac Vasc Anesth, 2019; 33: S53-S57.

24. The incidence of awareness during cardiac surgical procedures compared to general surgery is approximately:
   A. 10 times greater
   B. The same
   C. Two times less
   D. Two times greater

Correct Answer: A

Explanation: Reported rates of intraoperative awareness during cardiac operations range from 0.2% to 2%, a 10-fold increase in risk compared with the general surgical population.

References:

1. Avidan MS, Jacobsohn E, Glick D, et al. Prevention of intraoperative awareness in a high-risk surgical population. N Engl J Med, 2011; 365: 591-600.
2. Dowd NP, Cheng DC, Karski JM, et al. Intraoperative awareness in fast-track cardiac anesthesia. Anesthesiology, 1998; 89: 1068-1073.
3. Groesdonk HV, Pietzner J, Borger MA, et al. The incidence of intraoperative awareness in cardiac surgery fast-track treatment. J Cardiothorac Vasc Anesth, 2010; 24: 785-789.

25. Limitations of brain oxygenation monitoring with near infrared spectroscopy include which of the following?
   A. Hair causes "light piping," interfering with spectroscopy
   B. Devices from different companies differ in clinical performance
   C. Hematomas and placement over a venous sinus can confound the data
   D. All of the above

Correct Answer: D

Explanation: The technical limitations of cerebral oximetry primarily involve factors influencing photon migration. Sensor placement is currently limited to glabrous skin because hair may compromise the measurement as a result of environmental light piping. The clinical performance of cerebral oximetry systems appears to be device-specific. Supporting evidence for one device does not necessarily apply to competing products. Objective comparison of these devices remains difficult because of the lack of a universally accepted direct reference standard measure of regional brain microcirculatory oxygen saturation. Weak signals may result from hematoma or sensor placement over a venous sinus. In either case, the large hemoglobin volume acts as a photon sink.

References:

1. Edmonds HL, Gordon EK, Levy WJ. Chapter 14: Central Nervous System Monitoring. In: Kaplan JA, Augoustides JGT, Manecke GR, et al., eds. Kaplan's Cardiac Anesthesia. 7th ed. Elsevier; 2017:677-697.
2. Mutoh T, Ishikawa T, Suzuki A, Yasui N. Continuous cardiac output and near-infrared spectroscopy monitoring to assist in management of symptomatic cerebral vasospasm after subarachnoid hemorrhage. Neurocrit Care, 2010; 13: 331.
3. Schraag S. Combined monitoring – brain function monitoring and cerebral oximetry. J Cardiothorac Vasc Anesth, 2019; 33: S53-S57.

26. Which of the following agents has the LEAST suppressive effect on monitoring with motor-evoked potentials?
   A. Isoflurane
   B. Sevoflurane
   C. Ketamine
   D. Desflurane

Correct Answer: C

Explanation: In the presence of neuromonitoring with motor-evoked potentials, the anesthetic should be designed to provide minimal interference with this sensitive modality. Of the listed anesthetics, ketamine has the least suppressive effect on motor-evoked potentials.

References:

1. Edmonds HL, Gordon EK, Levy WJ. Chapter 14: Central Nervous System Monitoring. In: Kaplan JA, Augoustides JGT, Manecke GR, et al., eds. Kaplan's Cardiac Anesthesia. 7th ed. Elsevier; 2017:677-697.
2. Sloan TB, Jäntti V. Anesthetic effects on evoked potentials. In: Nuwer MR, ed. Handbook of Clinical Neurophysiology. Vol. 8. Intraoperative Monitoring of Neural Function. Elsevier; 2008:94-126.
3. Milne B, Gilbey T, Gautel L, et al. Neuromonitoring and neurocognitive outcomes in cardiac surgery: a narrative review. J Cardiothorac Vasc Anesth, 2022; 36: 2098-2113.

TABLE 14.1
Anesthetic[a] effects on sensory- and motor-evoked responses

Pharmacologic Class	Agent	SSEP	AEP	MEP
Nonspecific inhibitor	Isoflurane	Suppression	Suppression	Suppression
	Sevoflurane	Suppression	Suppression	Suppression
	Desflurane	Suppression	Suppression	Suppression
	Barbiturates	Suppression	Suppression	Suppression
GABA-specific agonist	Propofol	Suppression[b]	Suppression	Suppression[b]
α_2 agonist	Clonidine	Suppression[b]	?	Suppression[b]
	Dexmedetomidine	Suppression[b]	?	Suppression[b]
NMDA antagonist	Nitrous oxide	Suppression	—	Suppression
	Ketamine	Increase	—	Suppression[b]
	Xenon	Suppression[b]	Suppression[b]	Suppression[b]

[a]1 MAC-equivalent dose.
[b]Slight to minimal effect.

AEP, Auditory-evoked potential; *GABA,* γ-aminobutyric acid; *MAC,* minimum alveolar concentration; *MEP,* motor-evoked potential; *NMDA,* N-methyl-D-aspartate; *SSEP,* somatosensory-evoked potential.

Modified from Sloan TB, Jäntti V. Anesthetic effects on evoked potentials. In: Nuwer MR, ed. Handbook of Clinical Neurophysiology. Vol. 8. Intraoperative Monitoring of Neural Function. Elsevier; 2008:94-126.

TABLE 14.2
Multimodality neuromonitoring for cardiac surgical procedures

Modality	Function
Electroencephalography	Cortical synaptic activity
Brainstem auditory-evoked potentials	Cochlear, auditory nerve, and brainstem auditory pathway function
Middle latency auditory-evoked potentials	Subcortical-cortical afferent auditory pathway function
Somatosensory-evoked potentials	Peripheral nerve, spinal cord, and brain somatosensory afferent pathway function
Transcranial motor-evoked potentials	Cortical, subcortical, spinal cord, and peripheral nerve efferent motor pathway function
Transcranial Doppler ultrasonography	Cerebral blood flow change and emboli detection
Tissue oximetry	Regional tissue oxygen balance

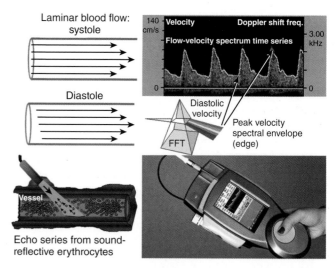

FIGURE 14.9 Physiologic basis of the transcranial Doppler (TCD) ultrasound display. Large-vessel laminar flow results in a cross-sectional series of erythrocyte velocities, with the lowest values nearest the vessel wall. Ultrasonic vessel insonation produces a series of erythrocyte echoes. The frequency differences (i.e., Doppler-shift frequencies) between the insonating signal and its echoes are proportional to erythrocyte velocity and flow direction. Fast Fourier transform (FFT) analysis of this complex echo produces an instantaneous power spectrum analogous to that used in electroencephalographic analysis. The time series of successive Doppler-shift spectra (upper right) resembles an arterial pressure waveform but represents fluctuating erythrocyte velocities during each cardiac cycle. Some modern TCD sonographs are small enough to be handheld or incorporated into multimodal neurophysiologic signal analyzers. (Image of the 500P Pocket Transcranial Doppler courtesy Multigon Industries, Inc, Yonkers, NY.)

27. Which of the following can be calculated from the spectral time series generated by transcranial Doppler?
   A. Systolic arterial pressure
   B. Mean arterial pressure
   C. Mean blood flow velocity
   D. Ischemic threshold for cerebral blood flow

Correct Answer: C

Explanation: Transcranial Doppler is used to measure blood flow velocity in cerebral vessels. It does not measure pressure. Determining the ischemic threshold (cerebral blood flow or velocity below which cerebral ischemia occurs) would require a measure of cerebral oxygenation with jugular venous bulb oxygen saturation or near-infrared spectroscopy (see figure).

References:

1. Edmonds HL, Gordon EK, Levy WJ. Chapter 14: Central Nervous System Monitoring. In: Kaplan JA, Augoustides JGT, Manecke GR, et al., eds. Kaplan's Cardiac Anesthesia. 7th ed. Elsevier; 2017:677-697.

2. Purkayastha S, Sorond F. Transcranial Doppler ultrasound: technique and application. Semin Neurol, 2012; 32: 411-420.

3. Milne B, Gilbey T, Gautel L, et al. Neuromonitoring and neurocognitive outcomes in cardiac surgery: a narrative review. J Cardiothorac Vasc Anesth, 2022; 36: 2098-2113.

28. A 54-year-old man with an aneurysm of the ascending aorta involving the aortic arch presents for surgical repair with hypothermic circulatory arrest and antegrade cerebral perfusion via the right subclavian artery. Which of the following would be most useful in monitoring the effectiveness of the antegrade cerebral perfusion?
    A. Right radial arterial catheter
    B. Femoral arterial catheter
    C. Regional near-infrared spectroscopy
    D. Left radial arterial catheter

Correct Answer: C

Explanation: Management of aortic surgical procedures using antegrade cerebral perfusion through the right subclavian artery typically involves only moderate hypothermia. However, the potential for cerebral ischemia secondary to an incomplete circle of Willis emphasizes the need for the early detection of ischemia with some form of neuromonitoring. The circle of Willis is completely normal in only a small fraction (25%) of patients, although many of the anomalies consist of hypoplasia (not absence) of a single segment and may not predispose patients to ischemia. Although theoretical arguments favor a multichannel electroencephalogram montage because the region of malperfusion cannot be predicted with certainty, in practice transcranial Doppler and near-infrared spectroscopy appear capable of demonstrating asymmetry in the presence of such malperfusion should it occur in the region monitored. The acute occurrence of asymmetry in any monitored modality coincident with initiation of perfusion through the right subclavian artery would suggest a need to adapt surgical technique with a low threshold for institution of bilateral antegrade cerebral perfusion to address the possibility of an incomplete circle of Willis.

References:

1. Edmonds HL, Gordon EK, Levy WJ. Chapter 14: Central Nervous System Monitoring. In: Kaplan JA, Augoustides JGT, Manecke GR, et al., eds. Kaplan's Cardiac Anesthesia. 7th ed. Elsevier; 2017:677-697.

2. Agostini M, Di Gregorio V, Bertora M, et al. Near-infrared spectroscopy-detected cerebral ischemia resolved by cannulation of an axillo-femoral graft during surgical repair of type A aortic dissection. Heart Surg Forum, 2012; 15: E221.

3. Qu JZ, Kao LW, Smith JE, et al. Brain protection in aortic arch surgery: an evolving field. J Cardiothorac Vasc Anesth, 2021; 35: 1176-1188.

29. A 48-year-old man with chronic thromboembolic pulmonary hypertension is undergoing pulmonary thromboendarterectomy with hypothermic circulatory arrest. Which of the following is the most effective means of achieving cerebral protection prior to circulatory arrest?
    A. Cooling the patient such that the electroencephalogram is isoelectric
    B. Cooling the patient such that the nasopharyngeal temperature is 18°C
    C. Administering propofol 200 mg intravenous
    D. Cooling the patient such that burst suppression appears

Correct Answer: A

Explanation: When the planned technique includes circulatory arrest, with or without retrograde cerebral perfusion, the first imperative is to ensure that the brain is adequately cooled to withstand the necessary period of cerebral ischemia. Optimal protection of cerebral cortical tissue by cooling occurs when electrical silence has occurred on the electroencephalogram, because more than 60% of the brain's metabolic effort is expended in the generation of electrical signals. Cooling slows the electroencephalogram in a dose-dependent fashion, with recovery following a similar pattern but not necessarily following the same curve or returning completely to baseline. The actual temperature at which electrical silence occurs can vary from 11 to 18°C.

References:

1. Edmonds HL, Gordon EK, Levy WJ. Chapter 14: Central Nervous System Monitoring. In: Kaplan JA, Augoustides JGT, Manecke GR, et al., eds. Kaplan's Cardiac Anesthesia. 7th ed. Elsevier; 2017:677-697.

2. Banks DA, Pretorius GV, Kerr KM, et al. Pulmonary endarterectomy: Part II. Operation, anesthetic management, and postoperative care. Semin Cardiothorac Vasc Anesth, 2014; 18: 331-340.

30. A 55-year-old man with right ventricular failure is receiving venoarterial extracorporeal membrane oxygenation. The drainage cannula is in the right femoral vein, and the return cannula is in the left femoral artery. The most effective means of detecting maldistribution of oxygenated blood is:
    A. Pulse oximeter probe on the left upper extremity
    B. Pulse oximeter probe on the right lower extremity
    C. Near-infrared spectroscopy probe on the right side of the head
    D. Near-infrared spectroscopy probe on the left side of the head

Correct Answer: C

Explanation: Venoarterial extracorporeal membrane oxygenation (ECMO) is becoming more common for the support of patients with failing cardiac or pulmonary function. The magnitude of the support can encompass complete bypass of the native cardiopulmonary function; however, some cardiac ejection commonly occurs even though ECMO flows are providing essentially all systemic needs. This small cardiac output consists of blood that has gone through the lungs and may be inadequately oxygenated if the patient has respiratory failure. This blood preferentially perfuses the innominate artery, and thus the right side of the brain may be receiving hypoxic blood even though arterial blood gas measurements (obtained from an indwelling catheter in the groin or left radial artery) appear normal. Although application of pulse oximeters to fingers of both hands may detect such right-sided desaturation, the pulse waveform during ECMO is often inadequate for detection of the saturation by pulse oximetry. Cerebral oximetry is well suited for assessing the development of unilateral desaturation in these patients who may need to be monitored continuously for days or weeks.

References:

1. Edmonds HL, Gordon EK, Levy WJ. Chapter 14: Central Nervous System Monitoring. In: Kaplan JA, Augoustides JGT, Manecke GR, et al., eds. Kaplan's Cardiac Anesthesia. 7th ed. Elsevier; 2017:677-697.
2. Winiszewski H, Guinot, PG, Schmidt M. et al. Optimizing PO2 during peripheral veno-arterial ECMO: a narrative review. Crit Care, 2022; 26: 226.
3. Denault A, Ali MS, Couture EJ, et al. A practical approach to cerebro-somatic near-infrared spectroscopy and whole-body ultrasound. J Cardiothorac Vasc Anesth, 2019; 33: S11-S37.

CHAPTER 15

Coagulation Monitoring

Gerard Manecke and Joel A. Kaplan

KEY POINTS

1. Monitoring the effect of heparin is done using the activated coagulation time (ACT), a functional test of heparin anticoagulation. The ACT is susceptible to prolongation because of hypothermia and hemodilution and to reduction because of platelet activation or thrombocytopathy.

2. Heparin resistance can be congenital or acquired. Pretreatment heparin exposure predisposes a patient to altered heparin responsiveness because of antithrombin III depletion, platelet activation, or activation of extrinsic coagulation.

3. Heparin-induced thrombocytopenia is a prothrombotic disorder caused by an abnormal immunologic response to the heparin–platelet factor 4 complex and is sometimes associated with overt thrombosis.

4. Protamine neutralization of heparin can be associated with "protamine reactions," which include vasodilatory hypotension, anaphylactoid reactions, and pulmonary hypertensive crises (types 1, 2, and 3, respectively).

5. Before considering a transfusion of plasma, it is important to document that the effect of heparin has been neutralized. This can be done using a heparinase-neutralized test or a protamine-neutralized test.

6. Point-of-care tests are available for use in transfusion algorithms that can measure coagulation factor activity (normalized ratio, activated partial thromboplastin time) and platelet function.

7. Fibrinolysis is common after cardiopulmonary bypass when antifibrinolytic therapy is not used.

8. Newer thrombin inhibitor drugs are available for anticoagulation in patients who cannot receive heparin. These can be monitored using the ecarin clotting time or a modified ACT. Bivalirudin and hirudin are the two direct thrombin inhibitors that have been used most often in cardiac surgical procedures.

9. Platelet dysfunction is the most common reason for bleeding after cardiopulmonary bypass. Point-of-care tests can be used to measure specific aspects of platelet function.

10. The degree of platelet inhibition as measured by standard or point-of-care instruments has been shown to correlate with decreased ischemic outcomes after coronary intervention. However, cardiac surgical patients who are receiving antiplatelet medication are at increased risk for postoperative bleeding.

---

1. During cardiac surgery, the major components of blood clotting are all of the following, EXCEPT:
   A. Platelets
   B. Vascular endothelium
   C. Fibrinolysis
   D. Coagulation glycoproteins

Correct Answer: C

Explanation: Hemostasis is the body's normal response to vascular injury, and it involves a complex interplay of systems within the body that helps to seal the endovascular defect and prevent exsanguination. The three major components of hemostasis are as follows: (1) the vascular endothelium; (2) the platelets, which constitute primary hemostasis; and (3) the coagulation cascade glycoproteins, which constitute secondary hemostasis. Fibrinolysis, the normal physiologic response to clot formation, ensures that coagulation remains localized to the area of vascular injury.

References:

1. Shore-Lesserson L, Enriquez LJ, and Weitzel N. Chapter 19: Coagulation Monitoring. In: Kaplan JA, Augoustides JGT, Manecke GR, et al., eds. Kaplan's Cardiac Anesthesia. 7th ed. Elsevier; 2017:698-727.
2. Fabbro M, Patel P, Henderson R, et al. Coagulation and transfusion update from 2021. J Cardiothorac Vasc Anesth, 2022: 36: 3447-3458.

2. The activated coagulation time is usually used during cardiac surgery and cardiopulmonary bypass. This important test is:
  A. Normally less than 80 seconds
  B. Activated by glass beads and rotation
  C. Warmed to 32°C
  D. A functional test of clotting

Correct Answer: D

Explanation: The activated clotting time (ACT) was first introduced by Hattersley in 1966 and is still the most widely used monitor of heparin effect during cardiac surgical procedures. Whole blood is added to a test tube containing an activator, either diatomaceous earth (celite) or kaolin. The presence of an activator augments the contact activation phase of coagulation, which stimulates the intrinsic coagulation pathway. The ACT can be performed manually, whereby the operator measures the time interval from when blood is injected into the test tube to when clot is seen along the sides of the tube. More commonly, the ACT is automated, and the test tube is placed in a device that warms the sample to 37°C. Normal ACT values range from 80 to 120 seconds, and it is a functional test of overall coagulation.

References:

1. Shore-Lesserson L, Enriquez LJ, and Weitzel N. Chapter 19: Coagulation Monitoring. In: Kaplan JA, Augoustides JGT, Manecke GR, et al., eds. Kaplan's Cardiac Anesthesia. 7th ed. Elsevier; 2017:698-727.
2. Bosch Y, Weerwind P. An evaluation of factors affecting the ACT. J Cardiothor Vasc Anesth, 2012; 26: 563-568.

3. An increasing activated clotting time can be due to any of the following, EXCEPT:
  A. Increasing body temperature
  B. Preoperative aspirin use and prolonged cardiopulmonary bypass
  C. Hypothermia during cardiopulmonary bypass
  D. Autologous hemodilution and added colloid during bypass

Correct Answer: A

Explanation: The monitoring of heparinization with the activated clotting time (ACT) is not without pitfalls, and its use has been criticized because of the extreme variability of the ACT and the absence of a correlation with plasma heparin levels. Many factors have been suggested to alter the ACT, and these factors are prevalent during cardiac surgical procedures. When the extracorporeal circuit prime is added to the patient's blood volume, hemodilution occurs and may theoretically increase the ACT. This hemodilution combined with hypothermia significantly increase the ACT of a heparinized blood sample. Hypothermia increases the ACT in a "dose-related" fashion. Platelet counts less than 30,000 to 50,000/μL can also prolong the ACT. During cardiopulmonary bypass, heparin decay also varies substantially, and its measurement is problematic because hemodilution and hypothermia alter the metabolism of heparin.

References:

1. Shore-Lesserson L, Enriquez LJ, and Weitzel N. Chapter 19: Coagulation Monitoring. In: Kaplan JA, Augoustides JGT, Manecke GR, et al., eds. Kaplan's Cardiac Anesthesia. 7th ed. Elsevier; 2017:698-727.
2. Patel P, Henderson R, Bollinger D, et al. The year in coagulation. J Cardiothorac Vasc Anesth, 2021; 35: 2266-2272.

4. During cardiopulmonary bypass, heparin resistance can be seen with:
  A. High activated coagulation test values
  B. Preoperative fresh frozen plasma administration
  C. Coumadin prophylaxis for a mechanical valve
  D. Antithrombin deficiency

Correct Answer: D

Explanation: Heparin resistance is documented by an inability to increase the activated clotting time (ACT) of blood to expected levels despite an adequate dose and plasma concentration of heparin. Many clinical conditions are associated with heparin resistance. Sepsis, liver disease,

TABLE 15.1
Disease states associated with heparin resistance

Disease State or Condition	Comment
Newborn status	Decreased AT III levels until 6 months of age
Venous thromboembolism	May have increased factor VIII level
	Accelerated clearance of heparin
Pulmonary embolism	Accelerated clearance of heparin
Congenital AT III deficiency	40%–60% of normal AT III concentration
Type I	Reduced synthesis of normal/abnormal AT III
Type II	Molecular defect within the AT III molecule
Acquired AT III deficiency	<25% of normal AT III concentration
Preeclampsia	Levels unchanged in normal pregnancy
Cirrhosis	Decreased protein synthesis
Nephrotic syndrome	Increased urinary excretion of AT III
DIC	Increased consumption of AT III
Heparin pretreatment	85% of normal AT III concentration because of accelerated clearance
Estrogen therapy	Decreased postheparin triglyceride hydrolase activity
Cytotoxic drug therapy (L-Asparaginase)	Decreased protein synthesis

AT III, Antithrombin III; *DIC,* disseminated intravascular coagulation.

BOX 15.1 **Heparin resistance**

- It is primarily caused by antithrombin III deficiency in pediatric patients.
- It is multifactorial in adult cardiac surgical patients.
- The critical activated coagulation time value necessary in patients who demonstrate acquired heparin resistance is not yet determined.
  Heparin resistance also can be a sign of heparin-induced thrombocytopenia.

BOX 15.2 **Heparin neutralization**

- The most benign form of bleeding after cardiac surgical procedures results from residual heparinization.
- Treatment is with either protamine or another heparin-neutralizing product.
- Transfusion of allogeneic blood products is rarely indicated.
- Residual heparin can be measured by using the following:
  - A protamine titration assay
  - A heparin neutralized thrombin time assay
  - A heparinase activated coagulation time (ACT) compared with ACT
  - Any other heparinase test that compares itself with the test without heparinase added

and pharmacologic agents represent just a few of the conditions associated with heparin resistance. In general, decreased levels of antithrombin III are the usual cause of heparin resistance. The inadequate prolongation of the ACT can be managed with additional heparin doses or administration of fresh frozen plasma or antithrombin III concentrates.

References:

1. Shore-Lesserson L, Enriquez LJ, and Weitzel N. Chapter 19: Coagulation Monitoring. In: Kaplan JA, Augoustides JGT, Manecke GR, et al., eds. Kaplan's Cardiac Anesthesia. 7th ed. Elsevier; 2017:698-727.
2. Chen Y, Phoon P, Hwang N. Heparin resistance during cardiopulmonary bypass in adults. J Cardiothorac Vasc Anesth, 2022; 36: 4150-4160.

5. The "4 Ts" test for heparin-induced thrombocytopenia includes all of the following, EXCEPT:

   A. Thrombocytosis
   B. Thrombosis
   C. Timing of platelet fall
   D. Thrombocytopenia

Correct Answer: A

Explanation: Heparin-induced thrombocytopenia (HIT) is a potentially life-threatening disorder that occurs in patients receiving unfractionated heparin. The incidence is between 0.2% and 5% in patients exposed to heparin, with reports of incidence as high as 15% to 20% in patients undergoing cardiac surgical procedures. HIT most often occurs 5 to 14 days after heparin administration and is mediated by antibodies binding to the complex formed between heparin and PF4. This complex binds to platelets, thereby causing platelet activation and subsequently thrombocytopenia.

Aiding in the diagnosis of HIT is a scoring system called the "4 Ts." This systematic method estimates the probability of HIT based on clinical presentation and has the following criteria: thrombocytopenia, timing of platelet count decline, thrombosis, and possible other causes of thrombocytopenia. When combined with a laboratory test, this scoring system provides the highest predictivity for HIT.

TABLE 15.2

Pretest scoring system for heparin-induced thrombocytopenia: the "4 Ts"

"4 Ts"	2 Points	1 Point	0 Points
Thrombocytopenia	Platelet count fall >50% and platelet nadir ≥20%[a]	Platelet count fall 30%–50% or platelet nadir 10%–19%	Platelet count fall <30% and platelet nadir <10%
Timing of platelet count fall	Clear onset between days 5–10 or platelet fall ≤1 day (previous heparin exposure within 30 days)[b]	Consistent with days 5–10 fall, but not clear (e.g., missing platelet counts); onset after day 10[c]; or fall ≤1 day (previous heparin exposure 30–100 days ago)	Platelet count fall <4 days without recent exposure
Thrombosis or other sequelae	New thrombosis (confirmed); skin necrosis[d]; acute systemic reaction postintravenous unfractionated heparin bolus	Progressive or recurrent thrombosis[e]; non-necrotizing erythematous skin lesions[d]; suspected thrombosis (not proven)[f]	None
Thrombocytopenia of other causes	None apparent	Possible[c]	Definite[c]

[a]Greifswald, Germany (GW): platelet count fall >50% or nadir 20%–100%; Hamilton, Canada (but not GW): platelet count fall >50% directly resulting from surgical procedure counts as 1 point, rather than 2 points.
[b]GW: onset from days 5–14 (rather than days 5–10); platelet fall within 1 day (heparin exposure within 100 days).
[c]GW: onset after day 14.
[d]Skin lesions at heparin injection sites.
[e]Progression refers to objectively documented increase in thrombus size (usually, extension of deep vein thrombosis by ultrasonography); recurrence refers to newly formed thromboembolus in previously affected region (usually, new perfusion defects in a patient with previous pulmonary embolism).
[f]In GW, suspected thrombosis (not proven) was not included as a criterion. Determination of whether the presence of another apparent cause of thrombocytopenia was possible or definite was at the discretion of the investigator.

References:

1. Shore-Lesserson L, Enriquez LJ, and Weitzel N. Chapter 19: Coagulation Monitoring. In: Kaplan JA, Augoustides JGT, Manecke GR, et al., eds. Kaplan's Cardiac Anesthesia. 7th ed. Elsevier; 2017:698-727.
2. Kram S, Hamid A, Kram B, et al. The predictive value of the 4 Ts and HEP score. J Cardiothorac Vasc Anesth, 2022: 36; 1873-1879.

6. The test that correlates best with heparin levels on cardiopulmonary bypass is the:
   A. Activated coagulation time
   B. Activated clotting time with added heparinase
   C. Factor X levels
   D. High-dose thrombin time

Correct Answer: D

Explanation: A functional test of heparin-induced anticoagulation that correlates well with heparin levels is the high-dose thrombin time (HiTT; International Technidyne Corp., Edison, NJ). The thrombin time is a clotting time that measures the conversion of fibrinogen to fibrin by thrombin. The thrombin time is prolonged by the presence of heparin and by hypofibrinogenemias or dysfibrinogenemias. Because the thrombin time is sensitive to very low levels of heparin, a high dose of thrombin is necessary in the thrombin time test to assay accurately the high doses of heparin during cardiopulmonary bypass. In-vitro assays indicate that the HiTT is equivalent to the activated clotting time (ACT) in evaluation of the anticoagulant effects of heparin at heparin concentrations in the range of 0 to 4.8 IU/mL. Unlike the ACT, the HiTT is not altered by hemodilution and hypothermia and has been shown to correlate better with heparin concentration than the ACT during cardiopulmonary bypass. The heparin concentration and the HiTT decrease during cardiopulmonary bypass, whereas the Hemochron and the Hepcon ACTs increase.

References:

1. Shore-Lesserson L, Enriquez LJ, and Weitzel N. Chapter 19: Coagulation Monitoring. In: Kaplan JA, Augoustides JGT, Manecke GR, et al., eds. Kaplan's Cardiac Anesthesia. 7th ed. Elsevier; 2017:698-727.
2. Isaacs J, Welsby J, Schroder J, et al. ACT and heparin-protamine devices to manage heparin on CPB. J Cardiothorac Vasc Anesth, 2021: 35; 3299-3302.

7. Following cardiopulmonary bypass, heparin neutralization can be measured by:
   A. Thromboelastograph platelet function assay
   B. Protamine titration assay
   C. Protamine neutralized thrombin time
   D. Normal prothrombin time and partial thromboplastin time

Correct Answer: B

Explanation: To administer the appropriate dose of protamine at the conclusion of cardiopulmonary bypass, it would

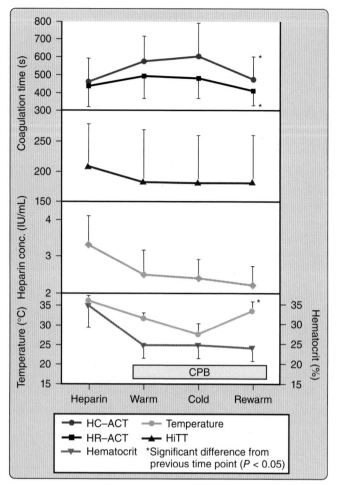

FIGURE 15.1 Changes over time in the Hemochron (International Technidyne Corp., Edison, NJ) activated coagulation time (ACT) *(HC-ACT; gray circles),* Hepcon (Medtronic Perfusion Services, Minneapolis, MN) ACT *(HR-ACT; squares),* and high-dose thrombin time *(HiTT; upward triangles)* in cardiac surgical patients. HiTT is unaffected by the changes in temperature *(pink circles)* and hematocrit *(downward triangles)* during cardiopulmonary bypass *(CPB).* The HC-ACT and HR-ACT increase with the initiation of CPB, and the heparin concentration *(Heparin conc.)* and HiTT decrease. (From Wang JS, Lin CY, Karp RB. Comparison of high-dose thrombin time with activated clotting time for monitoring of anticoagulant effects of heparin in cardiac surgical patients. Anesth Analg, 1994;79: 9–13.)

be ideal to measure the concentration of heparin present and give the dose of protamine necessary to neutralize only the circulating heparin. As a result of heparin metabolism and elimination, which vary considerably among individual patients, the dose of protamine required to reverse a given dose of heparin decreases over time. Administration of a large fixed dose of protamine or a dose based on the total heparin dose given is no longer the standard of care and may result in an increased incidence of protamine-related adverse effects. An optimal dose of protamine is desired because non-neutralized heparin results in clinical bleeding, and an excess of protamine may produce undesired coagulopathy. The use of individualized protamine dose-response curves uniformly results in a reduced protamine dose and has been shown to reduce postoperative bleeding.

The activated clotting time (ACT) has a high predictive value for adequate anticoagulation when the ACT is longer than 225 seconds but is poorly predictive for inadequate anticoagulation when the ACT is shorter than 225 seconds. The low levels of heparin present when heparin is incompletely neutralized are best measured by other, more sensitive tests of heparin-induced anticoagulation, such as heparin concentration, activated partial thromboplastin time, and thrombin time. Thus, after cardiopulmonary bypass, confirmation of return to the unanticoagulated state should be performed with a sensitive test for heparin anticoagulation such as a protamine titration assay.

BOX 15.3 Thrombin inhibitors

- These anticoagulant drugs are superior to heparin.
- They inhibit both clot-bound and soluble thrombin.
- They do not require a cofactor, activate platelets, or cause immunogenicity.
- These drugs include hirudin, argatroban, and bivalirudin.
- Heparin remains an attractive drug because of its long history of safe use and the presence of a specific drug antidote, protamine.

References:

1. Shore-Lesserson L, Enriquez LJ, and Weitzel N. Chapter 19: Coagulation Monitoring. In: Kaplan JA, Augoustides JGT, Manecke GR, et al., eds. Kaplan's Cardiac Anesthesia. 7th ed. Elsevier; 2017:698-727.
2. Abvelkasem E, Mazzeffi M, Henderson R, et al. Clinical impact of protamine titration-based heparin neutralization in CABG. J Cardiothorac Vasc Anesth, 2019: 33; 2153-2160.

8. Fibrinolysis during a heart transplantation procedure in the post–cardiopulmonary bypass phase in the operating room is best assessed by:
   A. Activated coagulation time
   B. Point of care fibrin split products
   C. Clotting time test
   D. Viscoelastic test

Correct Answer: D

Explanation: During cardiopulmonary bypass, fibrinolysis is most likely secondary to the microvascular coagulation that is occurring despite attempts at suppression using high doses of heparin. Fibrinolysis can be identified through either direct measurement of the clot lysis time (manual or viscoelastic tests) or measurement of the end products of fibrin degradation. The manual clot lysis time simply involves the placement of whole blood into a test tube. This blood clots in a matter of minutes. Visual inspection determines the end

point for observation of clot lysis, and this time period is the clot lysis time. This technique is time-consuming and requires constant observation by the person performing the test. Viscoelastic tests measure the unique properties of the clot as it is forming, organizing, strengthening, and lysing. As a result, fibrinolysis determination by this method requires that time elapse during which clot formation is occurring. Clot lysis parameters can be measured subsequent to clot formation and platelet-fibrin linkages. For this reason, viscoelastic tests often require longer than 1 hour to detect the initiation of fibrinolysis; however, if fibrinolysis is enhanced, results often can be obtained in 30 minutes. Other methods for quantifying fibrinolysis include measurement of the end products of fibrin degradation. Fibrin degradation products are the result of the cleavage of fibrin monomers and polymers and can be measured using a latex agglutination assay. When plasmin cleaves cross-linked fibrin, dimeric units are formed that comprise one D-domain from each of two adjacent fibrin units. These "D-dimers" are frequently measured by researchers in clinical and laboratory investigations. They are measured by either enzyme-linked immunosorbent assays or latex agglutination techniques and thus are not available for on-site use.

References:

1. Shore-Lesserson L, Enriquez LJ, and Weitzel N. Chapter 19: Coagulation Monitoring. In: Kaplan JA, Augoustides JGT, Manecke GR, et al., eds. Kaplan's Cardiac Anesthesia. 7th ed. Elsevier; 2017:698-727.
2. Lanigan M, Siers D, Wilkey A, et al. The use of viscoelastic–based transfusion algorithms reduces transfusions after LVAD or heart transplants. J Cardiothorac Vasc Anesth, 2022: 36; 3038-3046.

9. For adult cardiac surgery, bivalirudin is:
   A. An anticoagulant with a 2-hour plasma half-life
   B. A thrombin inhibitor of clot-bound soluble thrombin
   C. A drug that requires a cofactor to work in humans
   D. Superior to heparin in deep hypothermic circulatory arrest

Correct Answer: B

Explanation: Bivalirudin is a small, 20–amino acid molecule with a plasma half-life of 24 minutes. It is a synthetic derivative of hirudin and acts as a direct thrombin inhibitor. Bivalirudin binds to both the catalytic binding site and the anion-binding exosite on fluid-phase and clot-bound thrombin. The drug does not require a cofactor such as antithrombin III. The part of the molecule that binds to thrombin is actually cleaved by thrombin itself, so the elimination of bivalirudin activity is independent of specific organ metabolism. Bivalirudin has been used successfully as an anticoagulant agent in interventional cardiology procedures and cardiac surgery as a replacement for heparin therapy. Multicenter clinical trials comparing bivalirudin with heparin in off-pump coronary artery bypass operations and in procedures with cardiopulmonary bypass demonstrated "noninferiority" of bivalirudin. Efficacy of

BOX 15.4   Platelet function

- Patients frequently have extreme degrees of thrombocytopenia but do not bleed because they have adequate platelet function.
- The measure of platelet function correlates temporally with the bleeding course seen after cardiac surgical procedures.
- The thromboelastogram maximal amplitude, mean platelet volume, and other functional platelet tests are useful in transfusion algorithms.

anticoagulation and markers of blood loss were similar in the two groups, a finding suggesting that bivalirudin can be a safe and effective anticoagulant agent in cardiopulmonary bypass. Bivalirudin has not been found to be superior to heparin, but may be satisfactory when heparin is not available for use in the patient.

References:

1. Shore-Lesserson L, Enriquez LJ, and Weitzel N. Chapter 19: Coagulation Monitoring. In: Kaplan JA, Augoustides JGT, Manecke GR, et al., eds. Kaplan's Cardiac Anesthesia. 7th ed. Elsevier; 2017:698-727.
2. Erdoes G, Ortman E, Reid C, et al. Role of bivalirudin for anticoagulation in perioperative cardiothoracic practice. J Cardiothorac Vasc Anesth, 2020: 34; 2207-2214.

10. In the post–cardiopulmonary bypass phase of surgery and in the intensive care unit, platelet function can be best measured by:
   A. Complete blood count with platelet smear
   B. Bleeding time
   C. Aggregometry or thromboelastometry
   D. Platelet count

Correct Answer: C

Explanation: Qualitative platelet defects occur more commonly than thrombocytopenia during cardiopulmonary bypass (CPB). The range of possible causes of platelet dysfunction includes traumatic extracorporeal techniques, pharmacologic therapy, hypothermia, and fibrinolysis; the hemostatic insult increases with the duration of CPB. The use of bubble oxygenators (although infrequent), noncoated extracorporeal circulation, and cardiotomy suctioning causes various degrees of platelet activation, initiates the release reaction, and partly depletes platelets of the contents of their α granules.

The bleeding time becomes abnormal during CPB and does not return to baseline even by 72 hours postoperatively, whereas markers of platelet activation return to baseline by 24 hours postoperatively. Although data on the bleeding time exists, it is considered by most investigators to be an antiquated test and is rarely used clinically. Aggregometry is a useful research tool for measuring platelet responsiveness to a variety of different agonists. The end result, platelet aggregation, is an objective measure of platelet activation. The inability of this test to be performed easily in the clinical setting has usually restricted platelet aggregometry to use as a research tool, with occasional clinical applications. Thromboelastography is a useful tool for diagnosing and treating perioperative coagulopathy in patients undergoing cardiac surgical procedures because of a variety of potential coagulation defects that may exist. Within 15 to 30 minutes, on-site information is available regarding the integrity of the coagulation system, the platelet function, fibrinogen function, and fibrinolysis. A new application of thromboelastography (TEG) in the clinical setting is its use in monitoring platelet receptor blockade in patients treated with specific antiplatelet agents. TEG with platelet mapping has been shown to be useful in prediction of bleeding after multiple small-scale studies of cardiopulmonary bypassing, mostly in patients receiving antiplatelet medications.

References:

1. Shore-Lesserson L, Enriquez LJ, and Weitzel N. Chapter 19: Coagulation Monitoring. In: Kaplan JA, Augoustides JGT, Manecke GR, et al., eds. Kaplan's Cardiac Anesthesia. 7th ed. Elsevier; 2017:698-727.
2. Aggarwal S, Johnson R, Kirmani B. Pre and post-CPB platelet function tests with aggregometry and TEG platelet mapping. J Cardiothorac Vasc Anesth, 2015: 29; 1272-1276.

11. Viscoelastic tests of coagulation include all of the following, EXCEPT:
   A. Sonoclot analyzer
   B. HMS heparin management system
   C. Thromboelastography (TEG)
   D. Thromboelastometry (ROTEM)

Correct Answer: B

Explanation: In the late 19th century, investigators first began to explore the possibility that viscoelastic tests of blood could yield information on coagulation status. The changes that occur in the viscosity of blood as it clots could be studied and measured, and this information would reflect certain aspects of coagulation function. Bedside coagulation tests based on these principles demonstrate utility in real-time diagnostic decision making such as treating coagulopathy after cardiopulmonary bypass, and they also show promise in risk stratification and bleeding risk prediction.

The Thrombelastograph (TEG) can be used on site either in the operating room or in a laboratory and provides rapid whole-blood analysis that yields information about clot formation and clot dissolution. TEG is a useful tool for diagnosing and treating perioperative coagulopathy in patients undergoing cardiac surgical procedures because of a variety of potential coagulation defects that may exist. Rotational thrombelastometry (ROTEM) gives a viscoelastic measurement of clot strength in whole blood. Another test of viscoelastic properties of blood is

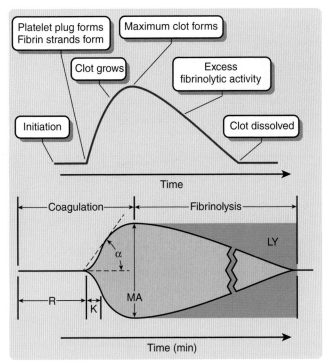

FIGURE 15.2 Normal Thrombelastograph (TEG, Haemonetics, Braintree, MA) tracing with standard parameters. *R* is the reaction time or the latency time from placing blood in the cup until the clot begins to form and the tracing opens to 2 mm (typically relates to function or amount of coagulation factors). *K* is a parameter arbitrarily assigned as the time between the TEG trace reaching 2 mm and going up to 20 mm (thought to reflect fibrinogen levels). *α* is the angle between the line in the middle of the TEG tracing and the line tangential to the developing TEG tracing (predictive of maximal amplitude). *MA* is maximal amplitude (largest measured width on the TEG tracing) and is considered to represent maximal thrombin-induced platelet activity and clot formation (total clot strength representing platelet function and clot interactions); *LY* is lysis index, which is the percent of lysis, typically measured as LY30 or 30 minutes after achieving MA.

the Sonoclot, which is a coagulation analyzer that measures the changing impedance on an ultrasonic probe immersed in a coagulating blood sample. Sonoclot has been studied in the clinical setting. As with other point-of-care devices, frequent applications include the perioperative setting, the catheterization laboratory, intensive care unit, and specialty clinics.

References:

1. Shore-Lesserson L, Enriquez LJ, and Weitzel N. Chapter 19: Coagulation Monitoring. In: Kaplan JA, Augoustides JGT, Manecke GR, et al., eds. Kaplan's Cardiac Anesthesia. 7th ed. Elsevier; 2017:698-727.
2. Meco M, Montisci A, Greco M, et al. Viscoelastic test use in adult cardiac surgery. J Cardiothorac Vasc Anesth, 2020: 34; 119-127.

12. In an adult patient with congenital heart disease, which part of the thromboelastograph shown will be maximally altered by a heparin dose of 300 IU/kg?
  A. Alpha angle
  B. K factor
  C. Maximum amplitude
  D. R time

Correct Answer: D

Explanation: Characteristic Thrombelastograph tracings can be recognized to indicate particular coagulation defects. A prolonged R value indicates a deficiency in coagulation factor activity or level and is seen typically in patients with liver disease and in patients receiving anticoagulant agents such as warfarin or heparin. The maximum amplitude (MA) is reduced in states associated with platelet dysfunction or thrombocytopenia, and the alpha-angle is reduced in the presence of a fibrinogen defect. LY30, or the lysis index at 30 minutes after MA, is increased in conjunction with fibrinolysis.

References:

1. Shore-Lesserson L, Enriquez LJ, and Weitzel N. Chapter 19: Coagulation Monitoring. In: Kaplan JA, Augoustides JGT, Manecke GR, et al., eds. Kaplan's Cardiac Anesthesia. 7th ed. Elsevier; 2017:698-727.
2. Fang Z, Berrnier R, Emani S, et al. TEG profile of patients with congenital heart disease. J Cardiothorac Vasc Anesth, 2018: 32; 1657-1663.

13. Which statement is TRUE regarding the use of the Thromboelastograph in a patient with Covid-19 undergoing cardiac surgery?
  A. The width of the maximum amplitude represents thrombin-induced clot
  B. The alpha angle does not reflect the speed of clot formation
  C. Fibrinolysis is measured over 10 minutes
  D. The sample in the cup remains at room temperature

Correct Answer: A

Explanation: The maximal amplitude (MA; normal is 50–60 mm) is an index of clot strength as determined by platelet function, the cross-linkage of fibrin, and the interactions of platelets with polymerizing fibrin. The percentage reduction in MA after 30 minutes reflects the fibrinolytic activity present and normally is not more than 7.5%. The α angle, an index of speed of clot formation, is the angle formed between the horizontal axis of the tracing and the tangent to the tracing at 20-mm amplitude. The α values normally range from 45 to 55 degrees. The sample in the thromboelastograph cup is measured at 37°C.

References:

1. Shore-Lesserson L, Enriquez LJ, and Weitzel N. Chapter 19: Coagulation Monitoring. In: Kaplan JA, Augoustides JGT, Manecke GR, et al., eds. Kaplan's Cardiac Anesthesia. 7th ed. Elsevier; 2017:698-727.
2. Wang J, Hajizadeth N, Shore-Lesserson L. The value of TEG in COVID 19 critical illness. J Cardiothroac Vasc Anesth, 2022: 36; 2536-2543.

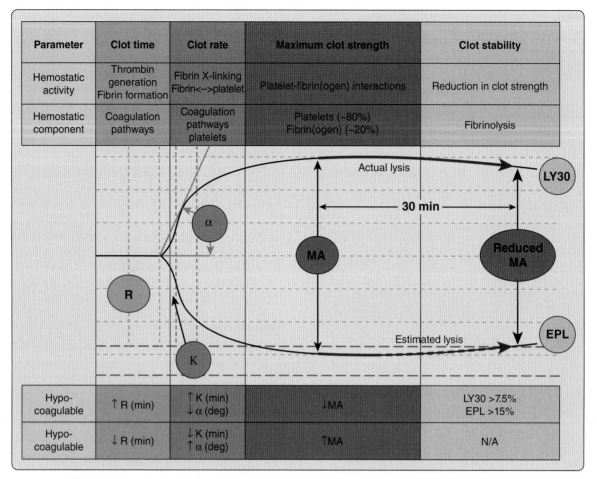

Parameter	Clot time	Clot rate	Maximum clot strength	Clot stability
Hemostatic activity	Thrombin generation Fibrin formation	Fibrin X-linking Fibrin<-->platelet	Platelet-fibrin(ogen) interactions	Reduction in clot strength
Hemostatic component	Coagulation pathways	Coagulation pathways platelets	Platelets (~80%) Fibrin(ogen) (~20%)	Fibrinolysis
Hypo-coagulable	↑ R (min)	↑ K (min) ↓ α (deg)	↓MA	LY30 >7.5% EPL >15%
Hypo-coagulable	↓ R (min)	↓ K (min) ↑ α (deg)	↑MA	N/A

FIGURE 15.3 Normal Thrombelastograph (TEG, Haemonetics, Braintree, Mass) tracing with standard parameters. α, An angle between the line in the middle of the TEG tracing and the line tangential to the developing TEG tracing (predictive of maximal amplitude); K, a parameter arbitrarily assigned as the time between the TEG trace reaching 2 mm and going up to 20 mm (may represent fibrinogen levels); LY, lysis index; MA, maximal amplitude, considered to represent maximal thrombin-induced platelet activity and clot formation (total clot strength representing platelet function and clot interactions); R, reaction time or the latency time from placing blood in the cup until the clot begins to form, reaching a TEG tracing amplitude of 2 mm (typically relates to function or amount of coagulation factors).

14. In regards to use of the thromboelastograph during cardiac surgery, which of the following statements is true?
   A. It was developed by cardiac anesthesiologists for use in cardiac surgery
   B. It can differentiate novel oral anticoagulant versus heparin effects
   C. It is more precise than the activated coagulation time for measuring heparin and protamine effects
   D. It can help diagnose the cause of coagulopathies within 15–30 minutes

Correct Answer: D

Explanation: The coaguloviscometers developed in the 1920s formed the basis of viscoelastic coagulation testing that is now known as thromboelastography. Thromboelastography in its current form was developed by Hartert in 1948 and has been used in many different clinical situations to diagnose coagulation abnormalities. The Thrombelastograph can be used on site either in the operating room or in a laboratory and provides rapid whole-blood analysis that yields information about clot formation and clot dissolution. Within minutes, information on the integrity of the coagulation cascade, platelet function, platelet-fibrin interactions, and fibrinolysis is obtained.

References:

1. Shore-Lesserson L, Enriquez LJ, and Weitzel N. Chapter 19: Coagulation Monitoring. In: Kaplan JA, Augoustides JGT, Manecke GR, et al., eds. Kaplan's Cardiac Anesthesia. 7th ed. Elsevier; 2017:698-727.
2. Raphael J, Mazer C, Subramani S, et al. SCA clinical practice improvement advisory for management of bleeding and hemostasis in cardiac surgery. J Cardiothorac Vasc Anesth, 2019: 33; 2887-2899.

TABLE 15.3

Mechanisms of point-of-care platelet function monitors

Instrument	Mechanism	Platelet Agonist	Clinical Utility
Thrombelastograph (Haemonetics, Braintree, MA)	Viscoelastic	Thrombin (native), ADP, arachidonic acid	Post-CPB, liver transplant, pediatrics, obstetrics, drug efficacy
Sonoclot (Sienco, Arvada, CO)	Viscoelastic	Thrombin (native)	Post-CPB, liver transplant
ROTEM (TEM Systems, Durham, NC)	Viscoelastic	Thrombin (native)	Post-CPB, transfusion algorithm
HemoSTATUS (Medtronic Perfusion Services, Minneapolis, MN)	ACT reduction	PAF	Post-CPB, DDAVP, transfusion algorithm
Plateletworks (Helena Laboratories, Beaumont, TX)	Platelet count ratio	ADP, collagen	Post-CPB, drug therapy
PFA-100 (Siemens Medical Solutions USA, Malvern, PA)	In vitro bleeding time	ADP, epinephrine	vWD, congenital disorder, aspirin therapy, post CPB
VerifyNow (Accriva Diagnostics, Accumetrics, San Diego, CA)	Agglutination	TRAP, ADP	GpIIb/IIIa receptor blockade therapy, drug therapy, post-CPB
Clot Signature Analyzer (Xylum, Scarsdale, NY)	Shear-induced in vitro bleeding time	Collagen (one channel only)	Post-CPB, drug effects
Whole-blood aggregometry	Electrical impedance	Multiple	Post-CPB
Impact Cone and Plate(let) Analyzer (Matis Medical, Beersel, Belgium)	Shear-induced platelet function	None	Post-CPB, congenital disorder, drug effects
Multiplate Analyzer (Roche Diagnostics, Indianapolis, IN)	Electrical impedance	ADP, arachidonic acid, collagen, ristocetin, TRAP-6	Drug therapy, congenital disorder, post CPB

ACT, Activated clotting time; *ADP*, adenosine diphosphate; *CPB*, cardiopulmonary bypass; *DDAVP*, desmopressin; *Gp*, glycoprotein; *PAF*, platelet-activating factor; *ROTEM*, rotational thrombelastometry; *TRAP*, thrombin receptor agonist peptide; *vWD*, von Willebrand disease.

---

15. During complex cardiac surgical procedures with cardiopulmonary bypass at 28°C, the thromboelastograph:

A. Can be used during cardiopulmonary bypass with heparinase added to the cup

B. Cannot be used during cardiopulmonary bypass, only afterwards following protamine administration

C. Cannot be used to measure platelet function

D. Can measure factor Xa to assess the adequacy of anticoagulation

Correct Answer: A

Explanation: Thromboelastography (TEG) is a useful tool for diagnosing and treating perioperative coagulopathy in patients undergoing cardiac surgical procedures because of a variety of potential coagulation defects that may exist. Within 15 to 30 minutes, on-site information is available regarding the integrity of the coagulation system, including an assessment of the platelet function, fibrinogen function, and fibrinolysis. With the addition of heparinase in the cup, TEG can be performed during cardiopulmonary bypass and can provide valuable and timely information regarding coagulation status. Because TEG is a viscoelastic test and evaluates whole-blood hemostasis interactions, proponents suggest that TEG is a more accurate predictor of postoperative hemorrhage than are routine coagulation tests. The TEG does not measure individual coagulation factors.

References:

1. Shore-Lesserson L, Enriquez LJ, and Weitzel N. Chapter 19: Coagulation Monitoring. In: Kaplan JA, Augoustides JGT, Manecke GR, et al., eds. Kaplan's Cardiac Anesthesia. 7th ed. Elsevier; 2017:698-727.
2. Tuman K, McCarthy R, Rizzo V, et al. Evaluation of coagulation during CPB with a heparinase modified TEG. J Cardiothorac Vasc Anesth, 1994: 8; 144-149.
3. Raphael J, Mazer C, Subramani S, et al. SCA clinical practice improvement advisory for management of bleeding and hemostasis in cardiac surgery. J Cardiothorac Vasc Anesth, 2019: 33; 2887-2899.

16. A 69-year-old man is scheduled for coronary revascularization. He was taking prasugrel for his left anterior descending coronary stent until 2 days ago. Which of the following thromboelastographic values can be used to show the effect of the drug?

A. R value

B. Maximal amplitude

C. K value

D. Clot lysis index

Correct Answer: B

Explanation: Characteristic thromboelastographic (TEG) tracings can be recognized to indicate particular coagulation defects. A prolonged R value indicates a deficiency in

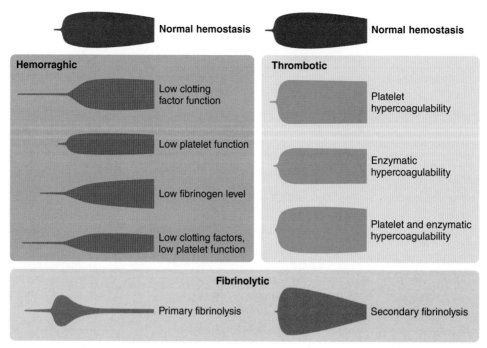

FIGURE 15.4 Thrombelastograph (TEG, Haemonetics, Braintree, MA) tracings in various coagulation states.

coagulation factor activity or level and is seen typically in patients with liver disease and in patients receiving anticoagulant agents such as heparin. Maximal amplitude (MA) and the α angle are reduced in states associated with platelet dysfunction or thrombocytopenia and are reduced even further in the presence of a fibrinogen defect. LY30, or the lysis index at 30 minutes after MA, is increased in conjunction with fibrinolysis. These particular signature tracings are depicted. More precise measures of platelet function can be obtained with modifications of the TEG including the TEG Platelet Mapping System.

References:

1. Shore-Lesserson L, Enriquez LJ, and Weitzel N. Chapter 19: Coagulation Monitoring. In: Kaplan JA, Augoustides JGT, Manecke GR, et al., eds. Kaplan's Cardiac Anesthesia. 7th ed. Elsevier; 2017:698-727.
2. Bollinger D, Lance M, Siegemond M. Point of care platelet function testing implications with platelet inhibitors in cardiac surgery. J Cardiothorac Vasc Anesth, 2021; 35; 1049-1059.

17. Platelet mapping with thromboelastography (TEG) can be done during off-pump coronary artery surgery:
   A. With full or partial heparinization
   B. Only if heparinase is added to the TEG cup
   C. Only if novel oral anticoagulants have been discontinued for more than 5 days
   D. With discontinuation of Coumadin for 3 days in patients with mechanical valves

Correct Answer: A

Explanation: PlateletMapping is a modification of thromboelastography that assesses platelet function by comparing the maximal amplitude (MA) tracing induced by activation

with arachidonic acid (AA) or ADP receptors (MA_{pi}) to the MA achieved with no platelet activity (MA_f), and with maximal platelet activation (MA_{kh}). For PlateletMapping, the reaction is carried out in the setting of heparinized blood, thus inhibiting thrombin platelet activation. The following formula calculates the percentage reduction in platelet activity using this assay:

$$\% \text{ inhibition} = 100 - \left[\left(MA_{pi} - MA_f\right)/\left(MAkh - MA_f\right) \times 100\right]$$

PlateletMapping has demonstrated consistent correlation with optical platelet aggregation assays. The percentage of inhibition, as well as the MA_{ADP} was shown to predict postoperative chest tube output following cardiac surgery.

References:

1. Shore-Lesserson L, Enriquez LJ, and Weitzel N. Chapter 19: Coagulation Monitoring. In: Kaplan JA, Augoustides JGT, Manecke GR, et al., eds. Kaplan's Cardiac Anesthesia. 7th ed. Elsevier; 2017:698-727.
2. Chowdhury M, Shore-Lesserson L, Mais A, Leyvi R. TEG and platelet mapping predicts postoperative chest tube drainage after CABG. J Cardiothorac Vasc Anesth, 2014: 28; 217-223.

18. Normal thromboelastograph values include all of the following, EXCEPT:
   A. K value is 3 to 6 minutes
   B. R value is 7 to 14 minutes
   C. Maximal amplitude (MA) is 50 to 60 mm
   D. MA is greater than 80 mm

Correct Answer: D

Explanation: The R value represents the time for initial fibrin formation and measures the intrinsic coagulation pathway, the extrinsic coagulation pathway, and the final common pathway. Normal values vary by activator, but they range from 7 to 14 minutes using celite activator. The K value is a measure of the speed of clot formation and is measured from the end of the R time to the time the amplitude reaches 20 mm. Normal values (3–6 minutes) also vary with the type of activators used. The maximal amplitude (MA) normal value is 50 to 60 mm and is an index of clot strength as determined by platelet function, the cross-linkage of fibrin, and the interactions of platelets with polymerizing fibrin. A larger MA represents hypercoagulability.

References:

1. Shore-Lesserson L, Enriquez LJ, and Weitzel N. Chapter 19: Coagulation Monitoring. In: Kaplan JA, Augoustides JGT, Manecke GR, et al., eds. Kaplan's Cardiac Anesthesia. 7th ed. Elsevier; 2017:698-727.
2. Fabbro M, Jain R. Hemodilution on CPB and impact of the TEG. J Cardiothorac Vasc Anesth, 2017: 31; 1564-1566.
3. Fabbro M, Patel P, Henderson R, et al. Coagulation and transfusion updates from 2021. J Cardiothorac Vasc Anesth, 2022: 36; 3447-3458.

19. During cardiac surgery, the Sonoclot:
   A. Is more accurate than the thromboelastograph (TEG) in the operating room
   B. Cannot measure platelet function
   C. Can be used to help diagnose and treat coagulopathies
   D. Takes much longer than the TEG

Correct Answer: C

Explanation: Another test of viscoelastic properties of blood is the Sonoclot. The Sonoclot signature reflects coagulation in real time, from the start of fibrin formation, to fibrin cross-linkage, platelet-mediated clot strengthening, and, eventually, to clot retraction and fibrinolysis. Early studies along with thromboelastography (TEG) demonstrated an accuracy of 74% using Sonoclot and an accuracy of 88% using TEG to predict bleeding after cardiac surgical

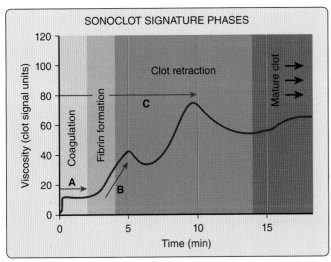

FIGURE 15.5 Sonoclot (Sienco, Arvada, CO) Signature phases. *(A)* Onset time or activated clotting time; *(B)* clot rate; and *(C)* time to peak, also known as platelet function time.

procedures. Significant correlations have been documented between specific Sonoclot parameters and platelet count and coagulation factor assays. Published studies indicate Sonoclot's utility in the setting of coagulopathy from cardiopulmonary bypass, monitoring the use of recombinant factor VIIa, and coagulation changes associated with the use of colloid starches.

References:

1. Shore-Lesserson L, Enriquez LJ, and Weitzel N. Chapter 19: Coagulation Monitoring. In: Kaplan JA, Augoustides JGT, Manecke GR, et al., eds. Kaplan's Cardiac Anesthesia. 7th ed. Elsevier; 2017:698-727.
2. Bischof D, Gantar M, Shore-Lesserson L, et al. Viscoelastic blood measurement with Sonoclot predicts postoperative bleeding. J Cardiothorac Vasc Anesth, 2015: 29; 715-722.

20. Rotational thrombelastometry (ROTEM) for assessment of coagulation during cardiac surgery:
   A. Includes the clotting time that equals the activated clotting time
   B. Includes the maximum clot firmness that measures fibrinogen level
   C. Is approved by the US Food and Drug Administration in the United States
   D. Does not measure platelet function

Correct Answer: C

Explanation: Rotational thrombelastometry (ROTEM) gives a viscoelastic measurement of clot strength in whole blood. ROTEM has been used extensively in Europe and increasingly in the United States after receiving approval from the US Food and Drug Administration in 2011. The main descriptive parameters associated with the standard ROTEM tracing are the following:

Clotting time: corresponding to the time in seconds from the beginning of the reaction to an increase in amplitude of the tracing of 2 mm. It represents the initiation of clotting, thrombin formation, and start of clot polymerization.

Maximum clot firmness: the maximum amplitude in millimeters reached in the tracing that correlates with platelet count, platelet function, and concentration of fibrinogen.

References:

1. Shore-Lesserson L, Enriquez LJ, and Weitzel N. Chapter 19: Coagulation Monitoring. In: Kaplan JA, Augoustides JGT, Manecke GR, et al., eds. Kaplan's Cardiac Anesthesia. 7th ed. Elsevier; 2017:698-727.
2. Tanaka K, Bollinger D, Vadlamura R, et al. ROTEM blood coagulation monitoring in cardiac surgery. J Cardiothorac Vasc Anesth, 2012: 26; 1083-1093.

21. During adult cardiac surgery, point-of-care testing with thromboelastography or rotational thromboelastometry has been shown to:
   A. Correlate with fibrinogen levels
   B. Decrease the cost of cardiac surgery
   C. Shorten the duration of cardiac surgery
   D. Reduce the time on cardiopulmonary bypass

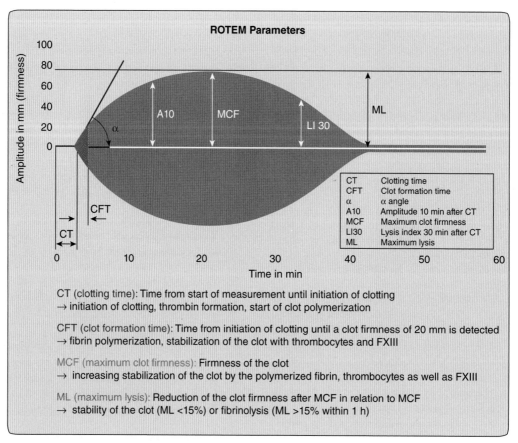

ROTEM Parameters

CT (clotting time): Time from start of measurement until initiation of clotting
→ initiation of clotting, thrombin formation, start of clot polymerization

CFT (clot formation time): Time from initiation of clotting until a clot firmness of 20 mm is detected
→ fibrin polymerization, stabilization of the clot with thrombocytes and FXIII

MCF (maximum clot firmness): Firmness of the clot
→ increasing stabilization of the clot by the polymerized fibrin, thrombocytes as well as FXIII

ML (maximum lysis): Reduction of the clot firmness after MCF in relation to MCF
→ stability of the clot (ML <15%) or fibrinolysis (ML >15% within 1 h)

FIGURE 15.6 Rotational thrombelastometry (ROTEM, TEM Systems, Durham, NC) parameters.

Correct Answer: A

Explanation: In a comparison of thromboelastography (TEG) and rotational thromboelastometry (ROTEM) in patients undergoing elective coronary artery bypass grafting with sample collection before bypass, 1 hour postoperatively, and at 24 hours, all of the TEG and ROTEM parameters showed differences after bypass and could be used to track changes in hemostasis during surgical procedures. Plasma fibrinogen level correlated well with TEG and ROTEM at all of the time points. Correlations with standard laboratory tests were difficult to interpret and underscore the difference in using point-of-care whole-blood testing versus plasma-based tests.

References:

1. Shore-Lesserson L, Enriquez LJ, and Weitzel N. Chapter 19: Coagulation Monitoring. In: Kaplan JA, Augoustides JGT, Manecke GR, et al., eds. Kaplan's Cardiac Anesthesia. 7th ed. Elsevier; 2017:698-727.

2. Momeni M, Carlier C, Baele P, et al. Fibrinogen concentration significantly decreases after CABG via ROTEM analysis. J Cardiothorac Vasc Anesth, 2013: 27; 5-11.

22. During complex cardiac surgery, institution of transfusion algorithms based on thromboelastography (TEG) monitoring resulted in:

A. Increased incidence of mediastinal exploration
B. Increased use of rFVIIa
C. Reduced use of protamine
D. Reduced transfusions of blood products

Correct Answer: D

Explanation: The largest impact of this type of point-of-care testing has been in the development of goal-directed transfusion algorithms based on the results. Initial research in the 1990s in more than 1000 patients found that the institution of a transfusion algorithm using thromboelastography resulted in a significant reduction in the incidence of mediastinal exploration and in the rate of transfusion of allogeneic blood products. A review in 2013 quantified 16 studies including both retrospective and prospective trials totaling 8507 patients. The authors reported benefits including consistent reductions in re-exploration for bleeding, massive transfusion, and overall hospital costs as well as transfusion products using viscoelastic-guided algorithms, with the greatest effect in patients with more complex coagulopathy.

References:

1. Shore-Lesserson L, Enriquez LJ, and Weitzel N. Chapter 19: Coagulation Monitoring. In: Kaplan JA, Augoustides JGT, Manecke GR, et al., eds. Kaplan's Cardiac Anesthesia. 7th ed. Elsevier; 2017:698-727.

2. Lanigan M, Siers D, Wilkey A, et al. Use of a viscoelastic – based transfusion algorithm reduces transfusions in patients undergoing LVAD insertion or heart transplantation. J Cardiothorac Vasc Anesth, 2022: 36; 3038-3046.

23. Following repair of a Type A aortic dissection on cardiopulmonary bypass with deep hypothermic circulatory arrest, the rotational thromboelastometry values are clotting time greater than 75 sec, α angle more than 60 degrees, and maximum clot firmness under 50 mm. Based on these results the proper treatment would be:

A. Platelet concentrate
B. Fresh frozen plasma
C. Packed red blood cells
D. Tranexamic acid

Correct Answer: B

Explanation: Point-of-care testing is likely to have the greatest clinical impact in patients with complex coagulopathies and in guiding transfusion practices in cardiac surgery. Important considerations beyond the use of algorithms include the content of the algorithm itself. In addition to allogeneic blood products, various pharmacologic hemostatic agents and recombinant agents, such as fibrinogen concentrate, prothrombin complex concentrate, and factor VIIa, are being introduced into algorithms guided by point-of-care testing.

References:

1. Shore-Lesserson L, Enriquez LJ, and Weitzel N. Chapter 19: Coagulation Monitoring. In: Kaplan JA, Augoustides JGT, Manecke GR, et al., eds. Kaplan's Cardiac Anesthesia. 7th ed. Elsevier; 2017:698-727.
2. Karrar S, Reniers T, Filns A, et al. ROTEM-guided transfusion algorithm in aortic surgery with DHCA. J Cardiothorac Vasc Anesth, 2022: 36; 1029-1039.

24. The VerifyNow test can be used in preoperative cardiac surgery patients to measure:

A. Platelet activity of GpIIb/IIIa inhibitors
B. Precise platelet counts
C. Clotting times in patients with abnormal international normalized ratio and prothrombin time tests
D. All of the above

Correct Answer: A

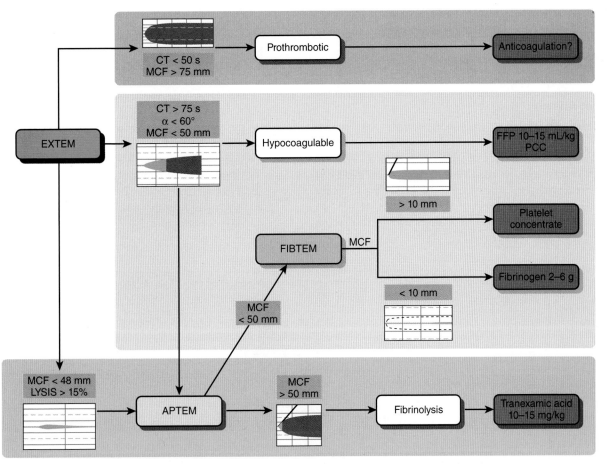

FIGURE 15.7 Coagulation management algorithm guided by rotational thrombelastometry (ROTEM, TEM Systems, Durham, NC). *α*, α Angle; *APTEM*, tissue factor activation + tranexamic acid/aprotinin; *CT*, clotting time; *EXTEM*, extrinsic system; *FFP*, fresh frozen plasma; *FIBTEM*, measure of fibrinogen activity; *MCF*, maximum clot firmness; *PCC*, prothrombin complex concentrate.

Explanation: VerifyNow is a point-of-care monitor designed to measure platelet response and is approved as a platelet function assay. Since antiplatelet drug effects cause diminished agglutination measured by light transmittance, this test can quantify the degree of platelet inhibition. VerifyNow has agonists to examine the antiplatelet activity of GpIIb/IIIa inhibitors, aspirin, and clopidogrel to assess platelet inhibition in a fashion that correlates well as standard laboratory agglutination tests. However, this testing system may be less sensitive than TEG PlateletMapping for assessment of aspirin resistance. It is not a test of the overall coagulation system.

References:

1. Shore-Lesserson L, Enriquez LJ, and Weitzel N. Chapter 19: Coagulation Monitoring. In: Kaplan JA, Augoustides JGT, Manecke GR, et al., eds. Kaplan's Cardiac Anesthesia. 7th ed. Elsevier; 2017:698-727.
2. Bollinger D, Lance M, Siegomund A. Point of care platelet function testing: Implications for platelet inhibitors in cardiac surgery. J Cardiothorac Vasc Anesth, 2021: 35; 1049-1059.

25. Using the rotational thromboelastometry coagulation system during cardiac surgery, the HEPTEM test:
   A. Measures the extrinsic clotting system
   B. Measures the intrinsic clotting system in the presence of heparin
   C. Uses aprotinin as a reagent
   D. Measures heparin and fibrinogen levels

Correct Answer: B

Explanation: Rotational thromboelastometry tests coagulation by using various reagents. The most common tests include INTEM (intrinsic system), EXTEM (extrinsic system), HEPTEM (intrinsic system in presence of heparin), FIBTEM (measures fibrinogen activity), and APTEM (tissue factor activation + tranexamic acid or aprotinin). The HEPTEM test consists of the INTEM test of the intrinsic coagulation

TABLE 15.4

Standard rotational thrombelastometry reagents and assessment pattern

EXTEM	Tissue factor activation; factors VII, X, V, II, I, platelets, and fibrinolysis
INTEM	Contact phase activation; factors XII, XI, IX, VIII, II, I, platelets, and fibrinolysis
FIBTEM	EXTEM + cytochalasin D (platelet blocking); assessment of fibrinogen
APTEM	EXTEM plus aprotinin; useful to rule out fibrinolysis when compared to EXTEM
HEPTEM	INTEM plus heparinase; useful to detect residual heparin

APTEM, Tissue factor activation + tranexamic acid/aprotinin; *EXTEM,* extrinsic system; *FIBTEM,* measure of fibrinogen activity; *HEPTEM,* intrinsic system in presence of heparin; *INTEM,* intrinsic system.

system with added heparinase and is used to detect residual heparin.

References:

1. Shore-Lesserson L, Enriquez LJ, and Weitzel N. Chapter 19: Coagulation Monitoring. In: Kaplan JA, Augoustides JGT, Manecke GR, et al., eds. Kaplan's Cardiac Anesthesia. 7th ed. Elsevier; 2017:698-727.
2. Son K, Yamada T, Tarac K, et al. Effects of cardiac surgery and salvaged blood on coagulation factors assessed by ROTEM. J Cardiothorac Vasc Anesth, 2020: 34; 2375-2382.

26. In the Sonoclot tracing shown in the figure, what is the diagnosis in the right-sided tracing following 2 hours on cardiopulmonary bypass for a double-valve redo procedure?
   A. Inadequate protamine administered
   B. Normal tracing after bypass compared to control
   C. Persistent hypothermia
   D. Poor platelet function

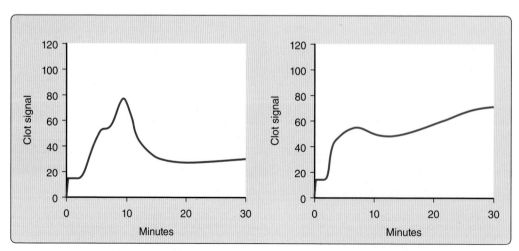

FIGURE 15.8 Comparison of a normal Sonoclot (Sienco, Arvada, CO) tracing with a tracing in the setting of poor platelet function. Notice the lack of clot retraction and the slow uptrending curve on the right tracing.

Correct Answer: D

Explanation: The Sonoclot signature is defined by three distinct parameters: the onset or ACT, the clot rate (CR), and the time to peak (TP), which is also referred to as platelet function (see figure in question 19) The CR phase encompasses two peaks on the signature trace, and the CR represents the maximal slope based on the rate of fibrin formation. The rate of rise of the first peak represented by point B is expressed as the percentage of the peak amplitude per unit time (normal values, 18%–45%). Typically, a shoulder or a dip occurs before the second rise in amplitude and subsequent peak that results from the action of platelets and fibrin in producing clot retraction. As the clot retracts from the walls of the cuvette, the impedance to vibration briefly decreases. As fibrinogen converts to fibrin and fibrin polymerizes, the speed of clot formation and the platelet-fibrin interactions are represented by the TP, which is represented by point C. In the presence of greater concentrations of fibrinogen, a larger clot mass is represented by a greater amplitude. The amplitude of this peak is related to the concentration of normal functional fibrinogen. The subsequent downward slope that occurs results from platelet-mediated clot retraction that causes plasma expulsion and clot size diminution and thus reduced impedance. The magnitude of the clot retraction reflects platelet number and function.

References:

1. Shore-Lesserson L, Enriquez LJ, and Weitzel N. Chapter 19: Coagulation Monitoring. In: Kaplan JA, Augoustides JGT, Manecke GR, et al., eds. Kaplan's Cardiac Anesthesia. 7th ed. Elsevier; 2017:698-727.
2. Bishof D, Ganter M, Shore-Lesserson L, et al. Viscoelastic blood coagulation with Sonoclot. J Cardiothorac Vasc Anesth, 2015: 29; 715-722.

27. Platelet function after cardiopulmonary bypass is very important in postoperative bleeding. Which of the following statements is TRUE?
    A. The platelet count correlates well with postoperative bleeding
    B. Patients may have low platelet counts and not bleed after cardiac surgery
    C. Bleeding time often correlates with postoperative bleeding in the first 6 hours
    D. Thromboelastographic measurements of fibrinolysis frequently correlate with postoperative bleeding

Correct Answer: B

Explanation: It is essential to understand the complex array of hemostatic insults that result from extracorporeal circulation before selecting an appropriate coagulation or hemostasis monitor as well as treatment during and after cardiac surgical procedures. Preoperative, intraoperative, and postoperative testing may be mandated for patients in whom a coagulation defect may predispose to serious degrees of postoperative coagulopathy. Even in hemostatically normal patients, exposure to cardiopulmonary bypass induces a heparin effect, as well as platelet dysfunction, fibrinolysis, and coagulation factor defects for which many clinical laboratory tests are available for accurate diagnoses. With the increase in prescriptions for antithrombotic and platelet inhibitors, the hemostatic defect after cardiopulmonary bypass is even more pronounced. Platelet dysfunction has been the hardest deficiency to measure, but many new tests are now available to analyze for this problem along with the platelet count.

References:

1. Shore-Lesserson L, Enriquez LJ, and Weitzel N. Chapter 19: Coagulation Monitoring. In: Kaplan JA, Augoustides JGT, Manecke GR, et al., eds. Kaplan's Cardiac Anesthesia. 7th ed. Elsevier; 2017:698-727.
2. Tian L, Gao X, Yang J. Assessing ADP-induced platelet amplitude and postoperative bleeding in CABG. J Cardiothorac Vasc Anesth, 2021: 35; 421-428.

28. The Bull heparin dose-response curve:
    A. Requires one measurement before and after cardiopulmonary bypass with heparin administration of 400 IU/kg
    B. Is done automatically by an activated clotting time machine
    C. Is cumbersome to perform manually and usually is not done prior to cardiopulmonary bypass
    D. Is the standard of care for all cardiac surgical cases with cardiopulmonary bypass

Correct Answer: C

Explanation: Bull documented a threefold range of ACT response to a 200 IU/kg heparin dose and similar discrepancy in heparin decay rates and recommended the use of individual patient dose-response curves to determine the optimal heparin dose. A heparin dose-response curve can be generated manually by using the baseline activated clotting time (ACT) and the ACT response to a dose of heparin. Extrapolation to the desired ACT provides the additional heparin dose required for that ACT. Once the actual ACT response to the heparin dose is plotted, further dose-response calculations are made based on the average of the target ACT and the actual ACT.

References:

1. Shore-Lesserson L, Enriquez LJ, and Weitzel N. Chapter 19: Coagulation Monitoring. In: Kaplan JA, Augoustides JGT, Manecke GR, et al., eds. Kaplan's Cardiac Anesthesia. 7th ed. Elsevier; 2017:698-727.
2. Slight R, Buell R, Nzewi O, et al. A comparison of ACT-based techniques for anticoagulation during cardiac surgery with CPB. J Cardiothorac Vasc Anesth, 2008: 22; 47-52.

29. An automated activated clotting time (ACT) test is preferred to a manual test because:
    A. It is more accurate
    B. It routinely does a protamine titration
    C. It is more convenient in the operating room
    D. Heparinase is used to increase the ACT accuracy

Correct Answer: C

Explanation: Even in the absence of heparin resistance, patients' responses to an intravenous bolus of heparin are

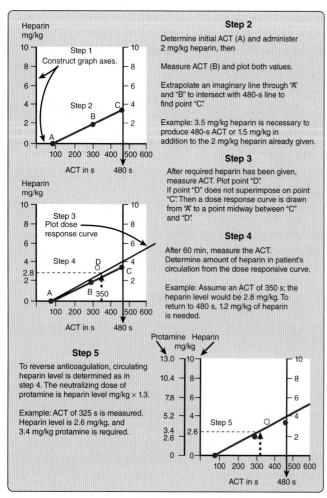

Step 1
Construct graph axes.

Step 2

Determine initial ACT (A) and administer 2 mg/kg heparin, then

Measure ACT (B) and plot both values.

Extrapolate an imaginary line through "A" and "B" to intersect with 480-s line to find point "C".

Example: 3.5 mg/kg heparin is necessary to produce 480-s ACT or 1.5 mg/kg in addition to the 2 mg/kg heparin already given.

Step 3

After required heparin has been given, measure ACT. Plot point "D".
If point "D" does not superimpose on point "C". Then a dose response curve is drawn from "A" to a point midway between "C" and "D".

Step 4

After 60 min, measure the ACT. Determine amount of heparin in patient's circulation from the dose responsive curve.

Example: Assume an ACT of 350 s; the heparin level would be 2.8 mg/kg. To return to 480 s, 1.2 mg/kg of heparin is needed.

Step 5

To reverse anticoagulation, circulating heparin level is determined as in step 4. The neutralizing dose of protamine is heparin level mg/kg × 1.3.

Example: ACT of 325 s is measured. Heparin level is 2.6 mg/kg, and 3.4 mg/kg protamine is required.

FIGURE 15.9 Construction of a dose-response curve for heparin. *ACT*, Activated coagulation time. (From Bull BS, Huse WM, Brauer FS, et al. Heparin therapy during extracorporeal circulation. II. The use of a dose-response curve to individualize heparin and protamine dosage. J Thorac Cardiovasc Surg, 1975; 69: 685–689.)

extremely variable. The variability stems from different concentrations of various endogenous heparin-binding proteins such as vitronectin and platelet factor 4. This variability exists whether measuring heparin concentration or the activated clotting time (ACT); however, variability seems to be greater when measuring the ACT. Because of the large interpatient variation in heparin responsiveness and the potential for heparin resistance, it is critical that a functional monitor of heparin anticoagulation (with or without a measure of

heparin concentration) be used in the cardiac surgical patient. The routine ACT is a standard of care for monitoring heparinization in the operating room. Automated versions of this test are more convenient, and some systems can do additional tests for further analysis. Helpful systems are used by some practitioners that incorporate a protamine titration to determine the protamine dose after bypass, or heparinase to detect residual heparin in the postoperative period.

References:

1. Shore-Lesserson L, Enriquez LJ, and Weitzel N. Chapter 19: Coagulation Monitoring. In: Kaplan JA, Augoustides JGT, Manecke GR, et al., eds. Kaplan's Cardiac Anesthesia. 7th ed. Elsevier; 2017:698-727.
2. Maslow A, Chambers A, Cheeves T, et al. Assessment of heparin anticoagulation by iStat and Hemachron ACTs. J Cardiothorac Vasc Anesth, 2018: 32; 1603-1608.

30. During cardiac surgery in a 57-year-old woman with coronary disease and mitral regurgitation, heparin resistance is most often due to:
   A. Liver disease secondary to heart failure
   B. Infective endocarditis
   C. Heparin-induced thrombocytopenia
   D. Antithrombin III deficiency

Correct Answer: **D**

Explanation: Many clinical conditions are associated with heparin resistance. Sepsis, liver disease, and pharmacologic agents represent just a few (see table in question 4). Many investigators have documented decreased levels of antithrombin III (AT III) secondary to heparin pretreatment, whereas others have not found decreased AT III levels. Patients receiving preoperative heparin therapy traditionally require larger heparin doses to achieve a given level of anticoagulation when that anticoagulation is measured by the activated clotting time (ACT). Presumably, this "heparin resistance" is the result of deficiencies in the level or activity of AT III.

References:

1. Shore-Lesserson L, Enriquez LJ, and Weitzel N. Chapter 19: Coagulation Monitoring. In: Kaplan JA, Augoustides JGT, Manecke GR, et al., eds. Kaplan's Cardiac Anesthesia. 7th ed. Elsevier; 2017:698-727.
2. Levy JH. Heparin resistance and antithrombin: Should it still be called heparin resistance? J Cardiothorac Vasc Anesth, 2004: 18; 129-130.

CHAPTER 16

Anesthesia for Myocardial Revascularization

Iwan Sofjan and Alexander Mittnacht

KEY POINTS

1. Guideline updates emphasize the efficacy of surgical approaches to myocardial revascularization in patients with multivessel coronary artery disease.

2. Perioperative risk reduction includes careful consideration of all of the patient's relevant antihypertensive, antiplatelet, and antianginal medications.

3. Significant valvular abnormalities in patients scheduled for coronary revascularization should be evaluated and considered in surgical planning.

4. Off-pump coronary artery bypass surgery is an established alternative to on-pump myocardial revascularization (i.e., coronary artery bypass grafting [CABG]). The choice and outcomes of either approach are highly surgeon dependent. Despite apparent advantages of avoiding cardiopulmonary bypass (CPB), evidence from large prospective trials enrolling mostly low-risk patients has not shown clear reductions in mortality with an off-pump approach.

5. Mitral valve repair for ischemic mitral regurgitation (MR) at the time of coronary revascularization is still controversial; however, it should probably be considered in patients who have a dilated annulus and at least moderate ischemic MR.

6. Possible indications for pulmonary artery catheter use in CABG surgery include patients with pulmonary hypertension, right-sided heart failure, or severely impaired ventricular function, particularly those who require postoperative cardiac output monitoring.

7. Fast-tracking, including early extubation and mobilization, has been almost universally adopted for patients undergoing myocardial revascularization.

8. Anesthetic drugs, especially inhaled anesthetic agents, may help to ameliorate myocardial injury associated with CPB and aortic cross-clamping by their preconditioning and postconditioning effects. However, the magnitude of these effects on outcome remains controversial.

---

1. Atrioventricular node dysfunction secondary to coronary artery disease is most likely due to a significant occlusion of the:
   A. Right coronary artery
   B. Left anterior descending artery
   C. Left circumflex artery
   D. Obtuse marginal artery

Correct Answer: A

Explanation: The anatomy of the coronary artery system is important. The right coronary artery originates from the right sinus of Valsalva and includes branches such as the acute marginal artery, sinus node artery (in 60% of patients), atrioventricular node artery (in 85% of patients), and posterior descending artery (in 80%–85% of patients). The left main coronary artery splits into the left anterior descending artery and the circumflex artery. Major branches of the left anterior descending artery include the diagonal arteries and the septal perforators. The left circumflex artery gives rise to obtuse marginal arteries, and, in a minority of patients, the posterior descending artery. When the posterior descending artery originates from the circumflex artery, the coronary circulation is called left dominant. In this case, the left coronary circulation supplies the entire interventricular septum and the atrioventricular node.

References:

1. Mittnacht AJC, London MJ, Puskas JD, et al. Chapter 16: Anesthesia for Myocardial Revascularization. In: Kaplan JA, Augoustides JGT, Manecke GR, et al., eds. Kaplan's Cardiac Anesthesia. 7th ed. Elsevier; 2017:731-769.
2. Smit M, Coetzee AR, Lochner A. The pathophysiology of myocardial ischemia and perioperative myocardial infarction. J Cardiothorac Vasc Anesth, 2020; 34: 2501-2512.

2. During discontinuation of cardiopulmonary bypass, the coronary artery most prone to air emboli is the:
   A. Right coronary artery
   B. Left anterior descending artery
   C. Circumflex artery
   D. Left main coronary artery

Correct Answer: A

Explanation: In the supine position, the right coronary artery is the most superior coronary artery and thus most likely to entrap air bubbles during aortic cannulation, cardiopulmonary bypass, or open valve surgery. The left main coronary artery may also be affected but less likely compared to the right coronary artery because its origin is typically more inferior during open-heart surgery. The clinical findings associated with coronary air embolism may include concomitant ST segment changes and wall motion abnormalities. These ischemic changes are typically self-limiting, as the air is often cleared with subsequent myocardial recovery.

References:

1. Mittnacht AJC, London MJ, Puskas JD, et al. Chapter 16: Anesthesia for Myocardial Revascularization. In: Kaplan JA, Augoustides JGT, Manecke GR, et al., eds. Kaplan's Cardiac Anesthesia. 7th ed. Elsevier; 2017: 731-769.
2. Gerstein NS, Pannikath PV, Mirrakhimov AE, et al. Cardiopulmonary bypass emergencies and intraoperative issues. J Cardiothorac Vasc Anesth, 2022; 36: v4505-4522.

3. In a left-dominant coronary circulation, the posterior interventricular septum is mostly supplied by the:
   A. Right coronary artery
   B. Posterior descending artery
   C. Left anterior descending
   D. Diagonal branches

Correct Answer: B

Explanation: The posterior interventricular septum is supplied by the posterior descending artery, regardless of coronary dominance. More than 80% of patients have a right-dominant circulation, in which the posterior descending artery originates from the right coronary artery. The rest of patients have a left-dominant circulation, where the posterior descending artery is derived from the circumflex artery. In a minority of patients, the coronary circulation can be codominant, in which the

posterior descending artery is derived both from the right coronary and circumflex arteries.

References:

1. Mittnacht AJC, London MJ, Puskas JD, et al. Chapter 16: Anesthesia for Myocardial Revascularization. In: Kaplan JA, Augoustides JGT, Manecke GR, et al., eds. Kaplan's Cardiac Anesthesia. 7th ed. Elsevier; 2017:731-769.
2. Huard P, Couture P, Chauvette V, et al. Intraoperative new regional wall motion abnormalities following aortic or mitral valve surgery: a case series and management algorithm. J Cardiothorac Vasc Anesth, 2022; 36: 3167-3174.

4. Myocardial ischemia may be alleviated by an increase in:
   A. Preload
   B. Afterload
   C. Heart rate
   D. Aortic root pressure

Correct Answer: D

Explanation: In patients with coronary artery disease, myocardial ischemia results from increases in myocardial oxygen demand that exceeds the capacity of stenosed coronary arteries to increase oxygen supply. Oxygen demand increases with higher contractility, preload, afterload, and heart rate. Oxygen supply increases with higher coronary blood flow and arterial oxygen content. Coronary artery blood flow will depend on the coronary artery diameter and the coronary artery perfusion pressure. The coronary perfusion pressure is the difference between the aortic diastolic pressure and the left ventricular end-diastolic pressure. Therefore, increases in the aortic root pressure will boost coronary artery perfusion pressure and consequently coronary perfusion to alleviate myocardial ischemia.

References:

1. Mittnacht AJC, London MJ, Puskas JD, et al. Chapter 16: Anesthesia for Myocardial Revascularization. In: Kaplan JA, Augoustides JGT, Manecke GR, et al., eds. Kaplan's Cardiac Anesthesia. 7th ed. Elsevier; 2017:731-769.
2. Goodwill AG, Dick GM, Kiel AM, et al. Regulation of coronary blood flow. Compr Physiol, 2017; 16:321-382.

5. Which of the following occurs in coronary artery atherosclerosis?
   A. Higher lipid plaque vulnerability with thicker fibrous caps and smooth muscle cells
   B. Distal vasoconstriction from the stenotic region to improve coronary blood flow
   C. Coronary steal through the collaterals during exercise
   D. Vasodilation from substances secreted by platelets and leukocytes

Correct Answer: C

Explanation: In atherosclerotic heart disease, characteristics of the vulnerable plaque include a high lipid content, a thin fibrous cap, a reduced number of smooth muscle cells, and increased macrophage activity. Acute plaque rupture causes the release of vasoactive substances from platelets and leukocytes, resulting in endothelial dysfunction and vasoconstriction, further reducing coronary blood flow. Two important compensatory mechanisms to improve coronary blood flow in the presence of a coronary artery stenosis include formation of collaterals and distal vasodilation. Collaterals may also develop between the nonischemic and ischemic myocardial regions. Despite these compensatory responses, blood may be shunted away from the ischemic myocardium during periods of increased demand to areas with intact coronary autoregulation, resulting in coronary steal.

References:

1. Mittnacht AJC, London MJ, Puskas JD, et al. Chapter 16: Anesthesia for Myocardial Revascularization. In: Kaplan JA, Augoustides JGT, Manecke GR, et al., eds. Kaplan's Cardiac Anesthesia. 7th ed. Elsevier; 2017:731-769.
2. Smit M, Coetzee AR, Lochner A. The pathophysiology of myocardial ischemia and perioperative myocardial infarction. J Cardiothorac Vasc Anesth, 2020; 34: 2501-2512.

6. The Society of Thoracic Surgeons risk calculator for clinical outcomes after coronary artery bypass grafting includes the prediction of postoperative:
   A. Liver failure
   B. Bypass graft failure
   C. Permanent stroke
   D. Inotropic support

Correct Answer: C

Explanation: The Society of Thoracic Surgeons (STS) is a massive clinical database system that tracks and benchmarks outcomes of common open-heart surgeries such as coronary artery bypass grafting and valve procedures. The STS risk calculator is free and available online through the STS website. The current version considers various patient demographics, cardiovascular-relevant comorbidities, and laboratory data to estimate perioperative outcome risk. The predicted outcomes include mortality, and morbidities such as renal failure, permanent stroke, prolonged ventilation, deep sternal wound infection, reoperation, and prolonged length of stay.

References:

1. Mittnacht AJC, London MJ, Puskas JD, et al. Chapter 16: Anesthesia for Myocardial Revascularization. In: Kaplan JA, Augoustides JGT, Manecke GR, et al., eds. Kaplan's Cardiac Anesthesia. 7th ed. Elsevier; 2017:731-769.
2. Del Rio JM, Abernathy J, Taylor MA, et al. The adult cardiac anesthesiology section of the STS adult cardiac surgery database: 2020 update on quality and outcomes. J Cardiothorac Vasc Anesth, 2021; 35: 22-34.

7. Predictors of acute outcome complications after coronary artery bypass grafting of include:
   A. A 45% occlusion of the right carotid artery
   B. Left ventricular ejection fraction of 45%
   C. Pre-existing neurologic deficit
   D. A 95% occlusion of the right coronary artery

Correct Answer: C

Explanation: The risk of adverse complications after coronary artery bypass grafting can be estimated through consideration of preoperative risk factors. The following features have been identified as significant risk factors for these complications: acute unstable angina, acute myocardial infarction, left ventricular dysfunction with an ejection fraction below 35%, cardiogenic shock, left main high-grade coronary stenosis, concomitant significant valvular disease, age above 70 years, porcelain aorta, and high-grade occlusive carotid artery disease, as well as pre-existing neurologic deficits.

References:

1. Mittnacht AJC, London MJ, Puskas JD, et al. Chapter 16: Anesthesia for Myocardial Revascularization. In: Kaplan JA, Augoustides JGT, Manecke GR, et al., eds. Kaplan's Cardiac Anesthesia. 7th ed. Elsevier; 2017:731-769.
2. Mehta A, Choxi R, Gleason T, et al. Carotid artery disease as a predictor of in-hospital postoperative stroke after coronary artery bypass grafting from 1999 to 2011. J Cardiothorac Vasc Anesth, 2018; 32: 1587-1596.

8. A 67-year-old male with triple-vessel coronary artery disease, a left ventricular ejection fraction of 30%, chronic kidney disease stage 3, and hypertension is scheduled for a coronary artery bypass grafting tomorrow. Which of the following chronic medications can be withheld?
   A. Beta blocker
   B. Aspirin
   C. Lisinopril
   D. Statin

Correct Answer: C

Explanation: The current evidence base suggests that beta blockers reduce the risk of morbidity and mortality in patients at risk for myocardial ischemia. Beta blockers should be continued perioperatively and given within 24 hours before coronary artery bypass grafting to all patients without contraindications such as hypotension, third-degree heart block, and bronchospasm. If there is such a contraindication, beta blockers should be restarted as soon as possible in the postoperative period. Further medications that should be continued perioperatively include statins, calcium channel blockers, and aspirin. Angiotensin-converting enzyme inhibitors such as lisinopril can be held in the immediate preoperative period as they may increase the risk of significant perioperative vasoplegia with risk of vital organ injury.

References:

1. Mittnacht AJC, London MJ, Puskas JD, et al. Chapter 16: Anesthesia for Myocardial Revascularization. In: Kaplan JA, Augoustides JGT, Manecke GR, et al., eds. Kaplan's Cardiac Anesthesia. 7th ed. Elsevier; 2017:731-769.

2. Schonberger RB, Lukens CL, Turkoglu OD, et al. Beta-blocker withdrawal among patients presenting for surgery from home. J Cardiothorac Vasc Anesth, 2012; 26: 1029-1033.
3. Lomivorotov VV, Effremov SM, Abubakirov MN, et al. Perioperative management of cardiovascular medications. J Cardiothorac Vasc Anesth, 2018; 32: 2289-2302.

9. Immediately after prolonged hypothermic cardiopulmonary bypass, which of the following arterial cannulation sites is most inaccurate?

A. Radial
B. Brachial
C. Axillary
D. Femoral

Correct Answer: A

Explanation: Radial arterial pressures may be significantly inaccurate immediately after hypothermic cardiopulmonary bypass due to clinically relevant vasospasm. Substantially low radial arterial pressure compared to the central aortic pressure may last up to 60 minutes or longer after separation from cardiopulmonary bypass. When there is doubt about the radial arterial pressure data, temporary transduction of a central aortic cannula can guide hemodynamic management during separation from cardiopulmonary bypass. In general, more central arterial sites such as the femoral or axillary arteries tend to closer approximate the central aortic pressure.

References:

1. Mittnacht AJC, London MJ, Puskas JD, et al. Chapter 16: Anesthesia for Myocardial Revascularization. In: Kaplan JA, Augoustides JGT, Manecke GR, et al., eds. Kaplan's Cardiac Anesthesia. 7th ed. Elsevier; 2017:731-769.
2. Bouchard-Dechene V, Couture P, Su A, et al. Risk factors for radial-to-femoral artery pressure gradient in patients undergoing cardiac surgery with cardiopulmonary bypass. J Cardiothorac Vasc Anesth, 2018; 32: 692-698.

10. In a patient undergoing coronary artery bypass grafting, the presence of which of the following would make a pulmonary artery catheter most useful?

A. Severe aortic stenosis
B. Small pericardial effusion
C. Severely reduced right ventricular function
D. Diastolic dysfunction

Correct Answer: C

Explanation: The use of pulmonary artery catheters has declined steadily in contemporary practice. The possible downsides of this invasive monitoring include excessive fluid resuscitation, longer time to extubation, longer length of stay, and higher total cost. Possible indications for a pulmonary artery catheter in coronary artery bypass grafting include coronary artery bypass grafting, pulmonary hypertension, right-sided heart failure, severely reduced ventricular function, cardiogenic shock, and hemodynamic instability.

References:

1. Mittnacht AJC, London MJ, Puskas JD, et al. Chapter 16: Anesthesia for Myocardial Revascularization. In: Kaplan JA, Augoustides JGT, Manecke GR, et al., eds. Kaplan's Cardiac Anesthesia. 7th ed. Elsevier; 2017:731-769.
2. Stawiarski K, Ramakrishna H. The pulmonary arterial catheter in cardiogenic and post-cardiotomy shock – analysis of recent data. J Cardiothorac Vasc Anesth, 2022; 36: 2780-2782.

11. Which of the following is TRUE regarding neuromonitoring during coronary artery bypass grafting?

A. High-opioid–based maintenance reduces awareness
B. Cerebral oximetry is reliable during cardiopulmonary bypass
C. The processed electroencephalogram (bispectral index) reduces recall
D. Stroke risk is negligible in off-pump coronary artery bypass grafting

Correct Answer: B

Explanation: Stroke and neurocognitive dysfunction still occur at concerning clinical rates after coronary artery bypass grafting, whether conducted with cardiopulmonary bypass or not. Cerebral oximetry can monitor regional tissue oxygenation, even during periods of nonpulsatile flow during cardiopulmonary bypass. Though there are possible benefits, further high-quality data are required to demonstrate that this technology can reduce the risk of perioperative brain injury. Processed electroencephalography (bispectral index) is commonly used in cardiac surgery in an attempt to decrease intraoperative awareness, but current data remain inconclusive. Fortunately, recent trials have shown a decreased incidence of awareness overall, likely attributed to less use of high-dose, opioid-based anesthetics, and the frequent use of inhalation agents and short-acting benzodiazepines.

References:

1. Mittnacht AJC, London MJ, Puskas JD, et al. Chapter 16: Anesthesia for Myocardial Revascularization. In: Kaplan JA, Augoustides JGT, Manecke GR, et al., eds. Kaplan's Cardiac Anesthesia. 7th ed. Elsevier; 2017:731-769.
2. Ali J, Cody J, Maldonaldo Y, et al. Near-infrared spectroscopy (NIRS) for cerebral and tissue oximetry: analysis of evolving applications. J Cardiothorac Vasc Anesth, 2022; 36: 2758-2766.

12. A significant coronary artery occlusion in which of the following vessels has the highest risk of hemodynamic instability during induction of anesthesia?

A. Proximal right coronary
B. Proximal left anterior descending
C. Proximal left circumflex
D. Obtuse marginal

Correct Answer: B

Explanation: Induction of anesthesia in patients presenting for coronary artery bypass grafting is associated with a significant risk of hemodynamic instability. Tight control of hemodynamic parameters to preserve the coronary perfusion pressure and to minimize myocardial oxygen demand is crucial, especially in patients with significant left main or proximal disease of the left anterior descending artery. Patients with this pattern of coronary artery disease are at high risk for acute left ventricular ischemia during anesthetic induction as the left anterior descending artery perfuses the left ventricular anterior wall that is essential to maintain cardiac output. This acute ischemia of the left ventricle can manifest as cardiogenic shock with or without ventricular arrhythmias.

References:

1. Mittnacht AJC, London MJ, Puskas JD, et al. Chapter 16: Anesthesia for Myocardial Revascularization. In: Kaplan JA, Augoustides JGT, Manecke GR, et al., eds. Kaplan's Cardiac Anesthesia. 7th ed. Elsevier; 2017:731-769.
2. Smit M, Coetzee AR, Lochner A. The pathophysiology of myocardial ischemia and perioperative myocardial infarction. J Cardiothorac Vasc Anesth, 2020; 34: 2501-2512.

13. Which of the following opioids as part of a balanced anesthetic technique for coronary artery bypass grafting is most likely to cause vasodilation secondary to histamine release, increased fluid and vasopressor requirements, and prolonged respiratory depression?
  A. Morphine
  B. Fentanyl
  C. Hydromorphone
  D. Remifentanil

Correct Answer: A

Explanation: Morphine was previously widely used in cardiac surgeries to provide adequate anesthesia without significant direct myocardial depression. However, high-dose morphine has largely become obsolete in modern cardiac anesthesia because it tends to cause vasodilation from histamine release, increased fluid and vasoconstrictor requirements, and prolonged respiratory depression. Compared to morphine, fentanyl causes minimal histamine release and has largely become the most commonly used opioid in cardiac anesthesia for its efficacy and low cost. Furthermore, common opioids such as remifentanil and hydromorphone can also be used to achieve adequate perioperative analgesia.

References:

1. Mittnacht AJC, London MJ, Puskas JD, et al. Chapter 16: Anesthesia for Myocardial Revascularization. In: Kaplan JA, Augoustides JGT, Manecke GR, et al., eds. Kaplan's Cardiac Anesthesia. 7th ed. Elsevier; 2017:731-769.
2. Kwanten LE, O'Brien B, Anwar S, et al. Opioid-based anesthesia and analgesia for adult cardiac surgery: history and narrative review of the literature. J Cardiothorac Vasc Anesth, 2019; 33: 808-816.

14. Intravenous heparin is given prior to aortic cannulation for coronary artery bypass grafting with cardiopulmonary bypass. Which of the following activated clotting time target ranges is appropriate for the initiation of cardiopulmonary bypass?
  A. 250 to 299 seconds
  B. 300 to 349 seconds
  C. 350 to 399 seconds
  D. 400 seconds or more

Correct Answer: D

Explanation: Heparinization prior to aortic cannulation and cardiopulmonary bypass initiation is absolutely critical in avoiding potentially lethal bypass circuit clotting. In most institutions, heparin is given at 300 to 400 international units per kilogram (or as calculated by heparin titration) with a target activated clotting time of at least 400 seconds or greater or heparin level over 2.5 units per milliliter. There is still significant variation across leading institutions in the defined anticoagulation threshold for the initiation and conduct of cardiopulmonary bypass. In patients with contraindications to heparin, adequate anticoagulation for cardiopulmonary bypass can be achieved with a direct thrombin inhibitor such as bivalirudin.

References:

1. Mittnacht AJC, London MJ, Puskas JD, et al. Chapter 16: Anesthesia for Myocardial Revascularization. In: Kaplan JA, Augoustides JGT, Manecke GR, et al., eds. Kaplan's Cardiac Anesthesia. 7th ed. Elsevier; 2017:731-769.
2. Hessel EA. What's new in cardiopulmonary bypass? J Cardiothorac Vasc Anesth, 2019; 33: 2296-2326.

15. The use of dexmedetomidine as a component of a balanced anesthetic technique during coronary artery bypass grafting may increase which of the following?
  A. Pulmonary artery pressure
  B. Tachycardia and hypertension during induction
  C. Plasma norepinephrine
  D. Hypotension during cardiopulmonary bypass

Correct Answer: D

Explanation: Alpha-2 agonists such as dexmedetomidine can prevent hypertension and tachycardia during intubation, surgical stimulation, and emergence from anesthesia and can decrease plasma catecholamine levels. Furthermore, exposure to dexmedetomidine can lower plasma norepinephrine levels and stabilize hemodynamics with attenuation of tachycardia. Despite titration, dexmedetomidine does carry a risk of systemic hypotension in adult cardiac surgery both intraoperatively and postoperatively.

References:

1. Mittnacht AJC, London MJ, Puskas JD, et al. Chapter 16: Anesthesia for Myocardial Revascularization. In: Kaplan JA,

Augoustides JGT, Manecke GR, et al., eds. Kaplan's Cardiac Anesthesia. 7th ed. Elsevier; 2017:731-769.
2. Abowali HA, Paganini M, Enten G, et al. Critical review and meta-analysis of postoperative sedation after adult cardiac surgery: dexmedetomidine versus propofol. J Cardiothorac Vasc Anesth, 2021; 35: 1134-1142.

16. Which of the following is TRUE regarding ischemic preconditioning?
  A. Brief ischemic episodes prior to long coronary artery occlusion increase myocardial injury
  B. It cannot be induced by propofol
  C. This protective effect can be induced remotely
  D. Isoflurane reduces the preconditioning effect

Correct Answer: C

Explanation: Short periods of ischemia before a prolonged period of coronary artery occlusion significantly reduces infarction size after myocardial reperfusion. This concept is referred to as ischemic preconditioning. The brief ischemic periods are thought to initiate signaling pathways that render the myocardium more resistant to subsequent periods of ischemia. Exposure to inhalational and intravenous anesthetics may produce changes similar to ischemic preconditioning. Ischemic myocardial preconditioning can also be induced remotely with short cycles of ischemia in the upper or lower extremity with a device such as a sphygmomanometer. Over the last several decades, various protocol-based clinical trials and subsequent meta-analyses have attempted to study the actual clinical benefits of ischemic preconditioning. Unfortunately, many of the positive trials have not been consistently replicable. Thus, despite the possible benefits, the role of ischemic preconditioning in at-risk patients undergoing cardiac surgery remains yet to be determined.

References:

1. Mittnacht AJC, London MJ, Puskas JD, et al. Chapter 16: Anesthesia for Myocardial Revascularization. In: Kaplan JA, Augoustides JGT, Manecke GR, et al., eds. Kaplan's Cardiac Anesthesia. 7th ed. Elsevier; 2017:731-769.
2. Maldonaldo Y, Weiner MM, Ramakrishna H. Remote ischemic preconditioning in cardiac surgery: is there a proven clinical benefit? J Cardiothorac Vasc Anesth, 2017; 31: 1910-1915.
3. Pagel PS, Crystal GJ. The discovery of myocardial preconditioning using volatile anesthetics: a history and contemporary clinical perspective. J Cardiothorac Vasc Anesth, 2018; 32: 1112-1134.

17. Which of the following is TRUE regarding thoracic epidural anesthesia in cardiac surgery?
  A. It cannot be utilized as the primary anesthetic
  B. It is associated with high rate of neuraxial complications
  C. Thoracic sympathectomy has unfavorable effects on coronary circulation
  D. It is not associated with improved mortality or major morbidity

Correct Answer: D

Explanation: Thoracic epidural anesthesia is rarely utilized during cardiac anesthesia in the United States due to concerns including the risks of epidural hematoma. Nevertheless, thoracic sympathectomy has favorable vasodilating effects on coronary circulation. There are trials from Europe and Asia reporting the feasibility of this technique as the primary anesthetic. For example, high thoracic epidural anesthesia has been successfully applied for conscious off-pump coronary surgery with low risk for conversion to general anesthesia. Furthermore, this technique enhances the quality of analgesia and facilitates fast-track tracheal extubation. Despite these benefits, this anesthetic technique is not associated with significant reductions in mortality, major morbidity, or length of stay.

References:

1. Mittnacht AJC, London MJ, Puskas JD, et al. Chapter 16: Anesthesia for Myocardial Revascularization. In: Kaplan JA, Augoustides JGT, Manecke GR, et al., eds. Kaplan's Cardiac Anesthesia. 7th ed. Elsevier; 2017:731-769.
2. Sarica F, Erturk E, Kutanis D, et al. Comparison of thoracic epidural analgesia and traditional intravenous analgesia with respect to postoperative respiratory effects in cardiac surgery. J Cardiothoracic Vasc Anesth, 2021; 35: 1800-1805.

18. After induction of anesthesia for myocardial revascularization, new ST segment depression and acute hypertension develop. Titration of a nitroglycerin infusion at a low dose in this setting may decrease which of the following?
  A. Coronary arterial resistance
  B. Cardiac contractility
  C. Systemic venous resistance
  D. Cardiac chronotropy

Correct Answer: C

Explanation: Nitroglycerin therapy decreases systemic venous tone at lower doses and decreases arterial and epicardial coronary arterial resistance at higher doses. It is effective in treating acute myocardial ischemia accompanied by acute rises in left ventricular preload and afterload. High wall tension may worsen perfusion deficits in the ischemic subendocardium that will respond favorably to therapy with nitroglycerin. Preoperatively, nitroglycerin is also indicated in the multimodal management of patients with unstable angina.

References:

1. Mittnacht AJC, London MJ, Puskas JD, et al. Chapter 16: Anesthesia for Myocardial Revascularization. In: Kaplan JA, Augoustides JGT, Manecke GR, et al., eds. Kaplan's Cardiac Anesthesia. 7th ed. Elsevier; 2017:731-769.
2. Freiling TP, Dhawan R, Balkhy HH, et al. Myocardial bridge: diagnosis, treatment, and challenges. J Cardiothorac Vasc Anesthesia, 2022; 36: 3955-3963.

19. Which of the following is TRUE regarding applications of perioperative nitroglycerin in coronary artery bypass grafting?
  A. Causes more intracoronary steal compared to sodium nitroprusside
  B. Efficacy can be affected by cardiopulmonary bypass
  C. May increase myocardial oxygen consumption
  D. Prophylactic use significantly reduces myocardial ischemic events

Correct Answer: B

Explanation: In the period before cardiopulmonary bypass, nitroglycerin may be indicated for the treatment of myocardial ischemia, uncontrolled hypertension, and coronary artery spasm. During cardiopulmonary bypass, nitroglycerin may control systemic hypertension but also may be ineffective in up to 40% of patients due to alterations in pharmacokinetics and pharmacodynamics. These alterations include binding to the cardiopulmonary bypass circuit, variations in regional blood flow, hemodilution, hypothermia, as well as sequestration in the oxygenators and filters. After myocardial revascularization, nitroglycerin may treat residual ischemia or coronary artery spasm, as well as reduce preload and afterload. Prophylactic nitroglycerin for prevention of perioperative myocardial ischemia has had little impact, with most studies showing minimal effect in this setting. Although nitroglycerin and nitroprusside control hypertension and decrease myocardial oxygen consumption, the risk of intracoronary steal was significantly increased with exposure to nitroprusside therapy.

References:
  1. Mittnacht AJC, London MJ, Puskas JD, et al. Chapter 16: Anesthesia for Myocardial Revascularization. In: Kaplan JA, Augoustides JGT, Manecke GR, et al., eds. Kaplan's Cardiac Anesthesia. 7th ed. Elsevier; 2017:731-769.
  2. Agrawal V, Hosey C, Smith GT, et al. Detrimental effects of nitroglycerin use during regadenoson vasodilator stress testing: a cautionary tale. J Nucl Cardiol, 2018; 25: 1718-1723.

20. Which of the following is TRUE regarding dihydropyridine calcium channel blockers?
  A. They have a significant effect on both vascular smooth muscle and the conduction system
  B. They relax vascular venous smooth muscle more than arterial smooth muscle
  C. Clevidipine has longer half-life than nicardipine
  D. Nicardipine augments coronary blood flow better than nifedipine

Correct Answer: D

Explanation: Calcium channel blockers inhibit calcium flow through the slow channels of the cell membrane. The main clinical effects are systemic arterial vasodilation and slowing of electrical conduction at the level of the atrioventricular node, depending on the class of calcium channel blockers. Verapamil and diltiazem primarily slow down the conduction system at the level of the atrioventricular node with less effect on the vasculature. In contrast, nicardipine, nifedipine, and clevidipine act primarily on vascular smooth muscle and have little effect on the atrioventricular node. Nicardipine is short-acting and similar to nifedipine. Compared to nifedipine, nicardipine is unique in its consistent augmentation of coronary blood flow and its ability to induce potent vasodilator responses in the coronary bed. Clevidipine is an ultra–short-acting calcium channel blocker, with the fastest onset and offset, and a unique milky white appearance similar to propofol.

References:
  1. Mittnacht AJC, London MJ, Puskas JD, et al. Chapter 16: Anesthesia for Myocardial Revascularization. In: Kaplan JA, Augoustides JGT, Manecke GR, et al., eds. Kaplan's Cardiac Anesthesia. 7th ed. Elsevier; 2017:731-769.
  2. Lord MS, Augoustides JG. Perioperative management of pheochromocytoma: focus on magnesium, clevidipine, and vasopressin. J Cardiothorac Vasc Anesth, 2012; 26: 526-531.

21. Which of the following beta blocker is BEST used intraoperatively during coronary artery bypass grafting?
  A. Carvedilol
  B. Esmolol
  C. Labetalol
  D. Metoprolol

Correct Answer: B

Explanation: Beta blockers can effectively treat hypertension, tachycardia, arrhythmias, and myocardial ischemia in the perioperative period. Despite these benefits, intraoperative beta blockade in coronary artery bypass grafting was limited by relatively long half-lives with a prolonged duration of action. This changed with the advent of the ultra–short-acting beta blockers such as esmolol that is effective in alleviating chest pain while increasing cardiac output in patients with unstable angina. Titration of esmolol can effectively decrease heart rate and systemic blood pressure to treat acute myocardial ischemia and to facilitate off-pump myocardial revascularization.

References:
  1. Mittnacht AJC, London MJ, Puskas JD, et al. Chapter 16: Anesthesia for Myocardial Revascularization. In: Kaplan JA, Augoustides JGT, Manecke GR, et al., eds. Kaplan's Cardiac Anesthesia. 7th ed. Elsevier; 2017:731-769.
  2. Poveda-Jaramilo R, Monaco F, Zangrillo A, et al. Ultra-short-acting beta-blockers (esmolol and landiolol) in the perioperative period and in critically ill patients. J Cardiothorac Vasc Anesth, 2018; 32: 1415-1425.

22. When given at a high loading dose (at least 10 mcg/kg), dexmedetomidine increases which of the following?
  A. Opioid requirement
  B. Coronary vascular resistance
  C. Shivering
  D. Heart rate

Correct Answer: B

Explanation: Dexmedetomidine is a selective alpha2-adrenoceptor agonist that exhibits central sympatholytic and peripheral vasoconstrictive effects. A continuous infusion (0.2–0.8 mcg/kg/hour) has dose-dependent hemodynamic effects such as decreases in heart rate, plasma catecholamine levels, and systemic mean arterial pressure. In addition to raising mean arterial pressure and systemic vascular resistance, higher doses of dexmedetomidine (≥ 10 mcg/kg) may also increase pulmonary arterial and coronary vascular resistance. At the recommended loading (0.5–2 mcg/kg) and maintenance (0.2–0.7 mcg/kg per hour) doses, dexmedetomidine most likely has a favorable effect on myocardial perfusion. Dexmedetomidine is also a useful postoperative sedative because of its minimal respiratory depression and appears to mimic natural sleep patterns. Patients are usually sedated but still arousable and cooperative in response to verbal stimulation. Its analgesic properties significantly reduced additional opioid analgesia requirements in mechanically ventilated patients. Dexmedetomidine has also been used successfully to treat postoperative delirium, alcohol or illicit drug withdrawal, and shivering.

References:

1. Mittnacht AJC, London MJ, Puskas JD, et al. Chapter 16: Anesthesia for Myocardial Revascularization. In: Kaplan JA, Augoustides JGT, Manecke GR, et al., eds. Kaplan's Cardiac Anesthesia. 7th ed. Elsevier; 2017:731-769.
2. Likhvantsev VV, Lndoni G, Grbenchikov OA, et al. Perioperative dexmedetomidine supplement decreases delirium incidence after adult cardiac surgery: a randomized, double-blind, controlled study. J Cardiothorac Vasc Anesth, 2021; 35: 449-457.

23. In the postoperative period, in what way is dexmedetomidine superior to propofol?
    A. Less bradycardia
    B. Shorter time to extubation
    C. Less hypotension
    D. Lower opioid use

Correct Answer: D

Explanation: Compared to propofol in the surgical cardiac intensive care setting, dexmedetomidine typically reduces the use of opioids due to its analgesic properties. The time to tracheal extubation, rate of adverse events, and quality of sedation are all comparable. Dexmedetomidine is also more expensive and has a higher incidence of bradycardia. Hypotension also occurs more often when dexmedetomidine is given with a large loading dose (1-mcg/kg range). These adverse hemodynamic effects can be minimized by starting a low-dose continuous infusion early in the intraoperative phase. In summary, although dexmedetomidine is effective for postoperative sedation after coronary artery bypass grafting, propofol is also a reasonable choice in this setting.

References:

1. Mittnacht AJC, London MJ, Puskas JD, et al. Chapter 16: Anesthesia for Myocardial Revascularization. In: Kaplan JA,

Augoustides JGT, Manecke GR, et al., eds. Kaplan's Cardiac Anesthesia. 7th ed. Elsevier; 2017:731-769.
2. Abowali HA, Paganini M, Enten G, et al. Critical review and meta-analysis of postoperative sedation after adult cardiac surgery: dexmedetomidine versus propofol. J Cardiothorac Vasc Anesth, 2021; 35: 1134-1142.

24. A few hours after surgical myocardial revascularization, a patient develops systemic hypotension in the intensive care unit with ST segment elevation and new left ventricular dysfunction. Assuming this is coronary artery spasm, which of the following interventions will most likely be effective?
    A. Norepinephrine
    B. Thromboxane
    C. Nitroglycerin
    D. Hypothermia

Correct Answer: C

Explanation: Coronary artery spasm is typically associated with profound ST segment elevation, systemic hypotension, acute ventricular dysfunction, and myocardial irritability. The underlying mechanism may be similar to the coronary spasm seen with Prinzmetal variant angina. Effective treatment includes a wide range of vasodilators such as nitroglycerin, calcium channel blockers such as nicardipine, and/or milrinone. Radial artery grafts are prone to spasm after revascularization, making recognition and prevention crucial to prevent serious complications. Potent constrictors of arterial coronary grafts include thromboxane, norepinephrine, and phenylephrine. Nitroglycerin, papaverine, milrinone, and nicardipine are all effective agents for relief of arterial conduit spasm. Hypothermia typically is associated with vasoconstriction and so will exacerbate coronary graft vasospasm.

References:

1. Mittnacht AJC, London MJ, Puskas JD, et al. Chapter 16: Anesthesia for Myocardial Revascularization. In: Kaplan JA, Augoustides JGT, Manecke GR, et al., eds. Kaplan's Cardiac Anesthesia. 7th ed. Elsevier; 2017:731-769.
2. del Valle M, Holland K. Diffuse coronary artery spasm after coronary artery bypass graft surgery. J Cardiothorac Vasc Anesth, 2022; 36: 2575-2577.

25. Which of the following parameters are decreased in fast-track management after coronary artery bypass grafting?
    A. Risk of tracheal reintubation
    B. Length of stay in the intensive care unit
    C. Postoperative myocardial ischemia
    D. Mortality

Correct Answer: B

Explanation: Fast-tracking was introduced to reduce costs. Core themes are protocol-driven care with a multidisciplinary approach, same-day admission when possible, early tracheal extubation, multimodal analgesia, rapid mobilization, intraoperative fluid restriction, and reduction of length of stay both in the intensive care unit and hospital. Meta-analysis has demonstrated that fast-tracking had shorter times to tracheal extubation, and reduced stay in the intensive care unit, with no significant differences in mortality and major morbidity, including risks of tracheal reintubation and postoperative myocardial ischemia.

References:

1. Mittnacht AJC, London MJ, Puskas JD, et al. Chapter 16: Anesthesia for Myocardial Revascularization. In: Kaplan JA, Augoustides JGT, Manecke GR, et al., eds. Kaplan's Cardiac Anesthesia. 7th ed. Elsevier; 2017:731-769.
2. Hendrikx J, Timmers MA, Timimi L, et al. Fast-track failure after cardiac surgery: risk factors and outcome with long-term follow-up. J Cardiothorac Vasc Anesth, 2022; 36: 2463-2472.

26. During an off-pump coronary artery bypass grafting, distal anastomosis of which of the following vessels will most likely cause hemodynamic instability?
    A. Left anterior descending
    B. Diagonal
    C. Acute marginal
    D. Posterior descending

Correct Answer: D

Explanation: Hemodynamic changes encountered during off-pump myocardial revascularization mainly involve the distortion of the cardiac chambers during the grafting process. Stabilizing devices are used to suspend the heart in various positions needed to reach the target coronary vessels. The posterior descending and the circumflex coronary arteries are typically the hardest to reach because of their posterior locations and are thus associated with a significant risk of hemodynamic instability. Lifting of the heart to work on the posterior vessels is commonly referred to as verticalization, in contrast to displacement for the left anterior descending and diagonal anastomoses.

References:

1. Mittnacht AJC, London MJ, Puskas JD, et al. Chapter 16: Anesthesia for Myocardial Revascularization. In: Kaplan JA, Augoustides JGT, Manecke GR, et al., eds. Kaplan's Cardiac Anesthesia. 7th ed. Elsevier; 2017:731-769.
2. Bianco V, Kilic A, Gelzinis T, et al. Off-pump coronary artery bypass grafting: closing the communication gap across the ether screen. J Cardiothorac Vasc Anesth, 2020; 34: 258-266.

27. During verticalization of the heart during off-pump myocardial revascularization, which of the following parameters will most likely increase?
    A. Stroke volume
    B. Mean arterial pressure
    C. Heart rate
    D. Central venous pressure

Correct Answer: D

Explanation: The effects of positional maneuvers, including verticalization of the heart, have been investigated in humans and animal models. During verticalization, there are significant reductions in stroke volume, cardiac output, mean arterial pressure, heart rate, and coronary blood flow, accompanied by increases in the central venous and pulmonary arterial pressures. All of these deleterious hemodynamic changes were alleviated with a 20% head-down tilt of the procedural table to increase cardiac preload. Patients with left ventricular dysfunction may have decreased reserve to tolerate these acute compromises in hemodynamics. During verticalization, there may be heart chamber compression and regional wall motion abnormalities. In addition to a head-down tilt, further management strategies include fluid administration, inotropes, intra-aortic balloon counter pulsation, and conversion to cardiopulmonary bypass.

References:

1. Mittnacht AJC, London MJ, Puskas JD, et al. Chapter 16: Anesthesia for Myocardial Revascularization. In: Kaplan JA, Augoustides JGT, Manecke GR, et al., eds. Kaplan's Cardiac Anesthesia. 7th ed. Elsevier; 2017:731-769.
2. Bianco V, Kilic A, Gelzinis T, et al. Off-pump coronary artery bypass grafting: closing the communication gap across the ether screen. J Cardiothorac Vasc Anesth, 2020; 34: 258-266.

28. Compared to on-pump techniques, off-pump coronary artery bypass grafting is associated with:
    A. Lower mortality
    B. Higher stroke incidence
    C. Improved graft patency
    D. Similar renal failure rate

Correct Answer: D

Explanation: Owing to the technical difficulties, outcomes tend to be highly surgeon-dependent after off-pump myocardial revascularization. Meta-analysis of randomized trials revealed no significant differences in mortality, stroke, myocardial infarction, acute kidney injury, wound infection, or reoperation for bleeding. Of note, the trials excluded high-risk patients with low ejection fraction, repeat procedures, and complex lesions. On the positive side, off-pump techniques were associated with significant reductions in atrial fibrillation, transfusion, respiratory infections, inotropic exposure, mechanical ventilation time, and length of stay. The important issue of graft patency has not been adequately determined in randomized trials. The risk for conversion from off-pump to on-pump revascularization is in the 5% to 10% range. This conversion risk is probably even more substantial in high-risk patients. In summary, off-pump coronary artery bypass grafting can be performed safely and may benefit certain patient subpopulations. Remaining concerns include incomplete revascularization, especially in patients with poor targets, the significant learning curve, and the critical importance of appropriate patient selection.

References:

1. Mittnacht AJC, London MJ, Puskas JD, et al. Chapter 16: Anesthesia for Myocardial Revascularization. In: Kaplan JA, Augoustides JGT, Manecke GR, et al., eds. Kaplan's Cardiac Anesthesia. 7th ed. Elsevier; 2017:731-769.

2. Bianco V, Kilic A, Gelzinis T, et al. Off-pump coronary artery bypass grafting: closing the communication gap across the ether screen. J Cardiothorac Vasc Anesth, 2020; 34: 258-266.

29. Which of the following combinations of coronary lesions are amenable to a hybrid revascularization with a coronary stent and minimally invasive direct coronary artery bypass?
  A. Posterior descending artery and left main
  B. Proximal left circumflex and obtuse marginal
  C. Proximal left anterior descending and right coronary artery
  D. Diagonal and right acute marginal

Correct Answer: C

Explanation: Minimally invasive direct coronary artery bypass was first performed with a limited left thoracotomy that permitted harvesting of the left internal mammary artery and subsequent anastomosis of this arterial graft to the left anterior descending artery on a beating heart. Since then, various techniques have been developed, all with the common goal of fewer complications, smaller incisions, faster recovery, and earlier discharge. The options include access via a thoracoscopic or robotic approach, as well as off-pump and on-pump techniques with femoral cannulation. Because of the limited access to the coronary artery system, this surgical approach is often combined with percutaneous revascularization including placement of coronary stents. A common approach for this hybrid coronary revascularization is typically a proximal stenosis of the left anterior descending artery and one other coronary lesion that can be easily stented.

References:

1. Mittnacht AJC, London MJ, Puskas JD, et al. Chapter 16: Anesthesia for Myocardial Revascularization. In: Kaplan JA, Augoustides JGT, Manecke GR, et al., eds. Kaplan's Cardiac Anesthesia. 7th ed. Elsevier; 2017:731-769.
2. Leyvi G, Dabas A, Leff JD. Hybrid coronary revascularization – current state of the art. J Cardiothorac Vasc Anesth, 2019; 33: 3437-3445.

30. In minimally invasive direct coronary artery bypass, thoracic insufflation with carbon dioxide will likely increase:
  A. Heart rate
  B. Mean arterial pressure
  C. Pulmonary artery pressure
  D. End-tidal oxygen

Correct Answer: C

Explanation: Compared with a standard approach, minimally invasive direct coronary artery bypass presents several unique anesthetic challenges. Selective lung ventilation is typically required, and can be done with a double-lumen tube or a bronchial blocker. Typical preoperative workup and considerations to estimate tolerance for one-lung ventilation apply. Thoracic insufflation with carbon dioxide (CO_2) is also needed to maximize surgical access and typically is associated with relative pulmonary hypertension with possible decreases in systemic blood pressure and cardiac output. Regional wall motion abnormalities may also be seen with transesophageal echocardiography at higher insufflation pressures. Typical treatments include fluid challenges, as well as titrated vasoconstrictor and inotropic support. In cases of resistant hemodynamic instability, femoral-femoral cardiopulmonary bypass should be rapidly instituted. Of note, increased end-tidal CO_2 may be from CO_2 absorption from the thoracic insufflation. Sudden decreases in end-tidal CO_2 have also been reported associated with positive-pressure CO_2 insufflation, and maybe due to a massive CO_2 embolization.

References:

1. Mittnacht AJC, London MJ, Puskas JD, et al. Chapter 16: Anesthesia for Myocardial Revascularization. In: Kaplan JA, Augoustides JGT, Manecke GR, et al., eds. Kaplan's Cardiac Anesthesia. 7th ed. Elsevier; 2017:731-769.
2. Leyvi G, Dabas A, Leff JD. Hybrid coronary revascularization – current state of the art. J Cardiothorac Vasc Anesth, 2019; 33: 3437-3445.

CHAPTER 17

Valvular Heart Disease

Alexander Mittnacht

KEY POINTS

1. Although various valvular lesions generate different physiologic changes, all valvular heart disease is characterized by abnormalities of ventricular loading.

2. The left ventricle normally compensates for increases in afterload by increases in preload. This increase in end-diastolic fiber stretch or radius further increases wall tension in accordance with Laplace's law, resulting in a reciprocal decline in myocardial fiber shortening. The stroke volume is maintained because the contractile force is augmented at the higher preload level.

3. Factors that influence heart function include afterload stress, preload reserve, ventricular compliance, contractility, and the existence of pathology such as valve lesions and hypertrophy.

4. Treatment modalities for hypertrophic obstructive cardiomyopathy, a relatively common genetic malformation of the heart, include β-adrenoceptor antagonists, calcium channel blockers, and myectomy of the septum. Newer approaches include dual-chamber pacing and septal reduction (i.e., ablation) therapy with ethanol.

5. The severity and duration of symptoms of aortic regurgitation may correlate poorly with the degree of hemodynamic and contractile impairment.

6. Mitral regurgitation causes left ventricular volume overload. Treatment depends on the underlying etiology and mechanism among other factors, and includes medical, interventional, and surgical options.

7. Rheumatic disease and congenital abnormalities of the mitral valve are the main causes of mitral stenosis, a slowly progressive disease.

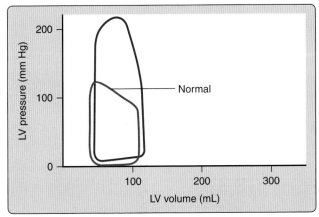

(From Jackson JM, Thomas SJ, Lowenstein E. Anesthetic management of patients with valvular heart disease. Semin Anesth. 1982;1:239.)

1. The pressure-volume loop depicted in the figure is associated with which of the following valvular lesions?
   A. Aortic stenosis
   B. Mitral stenosis
   C. Aortic regurgitation (chronic)
   D. Mitral regurgitation (chronic)

Correct Answer: A

Explanation: Aortic stenosis results in progressive systolic obstruction to blood flow from the left ventricle that significantly affects the normal pressure-volume loop. The peak pressure generated during systole is much greater than normal because of the high transvalvular pressure gradient. Furthermore, the slope of the diastolic limb is steeper, reflecting the reduced left ventricular diastolic compliance that is correlated with the associated left ventricular hypertrophy due to the pressure overload. The systolic limb of the pressure-volume loop shows preservation of pump function, as evidenced by maintenance of the stroke volume and ejection fraction. Although the initial ventricular response to this valvular lesion is hypertrophy, the progressive pressure overload can precipitate left ventricular failure with chamber dilation and adverse clinical outcome.

References:

1. Ramakrishna H, Craner RC, Devaleria PA, et al. Chapter 17: Valvular Heart Disease: Replacement and Repair. In: Kaplan JA, Augoustides JGT, Manecke GR, et al., eds. Kaplan's Cardiac Anesthesia. 7th ed. Elsevier; 2017:770-817.
2. Cormican DS, Czerny M, Ramakrishna H. The dilemma of moderate aortic stenosis in patients with heart failure and reduced ejection fraction: are we waiting too long to intervene or should we wait for more evidence? J Cardiothorac Vasc Anesth, 2022; 36: 15-17.

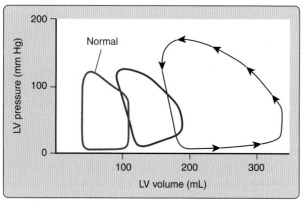

(Modified from Jackson JM, Thomas SJ, Lowenstein E. Anesthetic management of patients with valvular heart disease. Semin Anesth. 1982;1:239.)

2. The pressure-volume loop depicted in the figure (black line with arrows) is associated with which of the following valvular lesions?
   A. Aortic stenosis
   B. Mitral stenosis
   C. Aortic regurgitation (chronic)
   D. Aortic regurgitation (acute)

Correct Answer: C

Explanation: Chronic aortic regurgitation results in left ventricular volume and pressure overload. Progressive volume overload increases cavitary radius (eccentric hypertrophy) and end-diastolic wall tension (ventricular afterload), stimulating some concentric hypertrophy to normalize the ratio of ventricular wall thickness to cavitary radius. The eccentric hypertrophy results in significant cardiomegaly with shifting of the diastolic pressure-volume curve far to the right, thus allowing increases in end-diastolic volume with minimal changes in filling pressure. This accounts for the apparent paradox of high ventricular volumes at relatively low filling pressures. Because the increase in preload is compensated for by ventricular hypertrophy, cardiac output is maintained by

the Frank-Starling mechanism to permit clinical tolerance of significant chronic aortic regurgitation. There is virtually no isovolumic diastolic phase because the ventricle is filling throughout diastole. The isovolumic phase of systole is also brief because of the low aortic diastolic pressure. Minimal impedance to the forward ejection of a large stroke volume permits maximal myocardial work at a minimum of oxygen consumption. Eventually, progressive volume overload overwhelms this ventricular compensation, and a decline in systolic function occurs. In compensated chronic regurgitation, the eccentrically dilated ventricle maintains cardiac output due to the preload reserve with only slight increases in wall stress. In contrast, acute aortic regurgitation as shown in the middle pressure-volume loop, results in sudden diastolic volume overload of a nonadapted left ventricle with a precipitous increase in end-diastolic pressure. In this setting, the end-diastolic pressure can equilibrate with aortic diastolic pressure and exceed the left atrial pressure in late diastole, resulting in diastolic mitral regurgitation.

References:

1. Ramakrishna H, Craner RC, Devaleria PA, et al. Chapter 17: Valvular Heart Disease: Replacement and Repair. In: Kaplan JA, Augoustides JGT, Manecke GR, et al., eds. Kaplan's Cardiac Anesthesia. 7th ed. Elsevier; 2017:770-817.
2. Martin AK, Mohananey D, Ramka S, et al. The 2017 European Society of Cardiology (ESC)/European Association of Cardiothoracic Surgeons (EACTS) guidelines for the management of valvular heart disease - highlights and perioperative implications. J Cardiothorac Vasc Anesth, 2018; 38, 2810-2816.

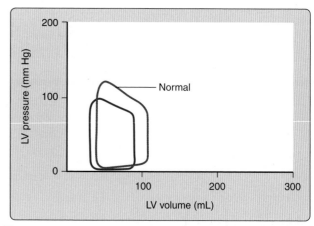

(From Jackson JM, Thomas SJ, Lowenstein E. Anesthetic management of patients with valvular heart disease. Semin Anesth. 1982;1:239.)

3. The pressure-volume loop depicted in the figure is associated with which of the following valvular lesions?
   A. Aortic stenosis
   B. Mitral stenosis
   C. Aortic regurgitation (acute)
   D. Mitral regurgitation (acute)

Correct Answer: B

Explanation: Mitral stenosis results in an underfilled left ventricle due to obstruction of blood flow across the mitral valve during diastole. As shown in the pressure-volume loop, the left ventricular end-diastolic volume and pressure are reduced, with an accompanying decline in stroke volume. Although left ventricular contractility may be preserved, it may also be decreased in about a third of patients. Aortic stenosis results in pressure overload with significant increases rather than decreases in systolic pressures generated by the left ventricle. Aortic and mitral regurgitation are associated with diastolic volume overload, and so shift the pressure-volume loop to the right rather than the leftward shift seen in mitral stenosis.

References:

1. Ramakrishna H, Craner RC, Devaleria PA, et al. Chapter 17: Valvular Heart Disease: Replacement and Repair. In: Kaplan JA, Augoustides JGT, Manecke GR, et al., eds. Kaplan's Cardiac Anesthesia. 7th ed. Elsevier; 2017:770-817.
2. Martin AK, Mohananey D, Ramka S, et al. The 2017 European Society of Cardiology (ESC)/European Association of Cardiothoracic Surgeons (EACTS) guidelines for the management of valvular heart disease - highlights and perioperative implications. J Cardiothorac Vasc Anesth, 2018; 38, 2810-2816.

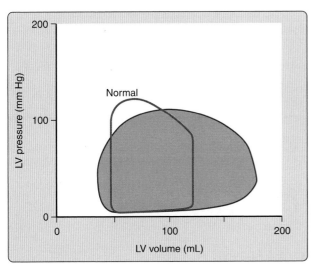

(From Jackson JM, Thomas SJ, Lowenstein E. Anesthetic management of patients with valvular heart disease. Semin Anesth. 1982;1:239.)

4. The pressure-volume loop depicted in the figure is associated with which of the following valvular lesions?
A. Aortic stenosis
B. Mitral stenosis
C. Aortic regurgitation (chronic)
D. Mitral regurgitation (chronic)

Correct Answer: D

Explanation: Mitral regurgitation causes left ventricular volume overload. The regurgitant volume combines with the normal left atrial volume and returns to the left ventricle during diastole. Chronic volume overload triggers left ventricular cavity enlargement by promoting eccentric hypertrophy. Increased preload continues to augment left ventricular systolic performance. At the same time, the left atrium dilates due to the ongoing regurgitation. Although left atrial dilation

maintains a low-pressure circuit that facilitates left ventricular systolic ejection, the increased radius of the left ventricular cavity leads to increased wall tension according to Laplace's law. The isovolumic contraction phase is shortened as the blood is ejected into the low-pressure left atrium early in ventricular systole. With the eventual decline in left ventricular systolic function, patients enter a decompensated phase. Progressive left ventricular dilation increases wall stress and afterload, causing further deterioration in left ventricular performance. The increased left ventricular filling pressures result in increased left atrial pressures with eventual pulmonary vascular congestion, pulmonary hypertension, and right ventricular dysfunction. Aortic stenosis typically causes left ventricular pressure overload, rather than volume overload. Mitral stenosis restricts left ventricular end-diastolic volume, shifting the pressure-volume curve to the right. Although chronic aortic regurgitation also causes volume overload like mitral regurgitation, it also causes relatively higher diastolic pressures and greater degrees of left ventricular dilation due to the progressive diastolic regurgitation.

References:

1. Ramakrishna H, Craner RC, Devaleria PA, et al. Chapter 17: Valvular Heart Disease: Replacement and Repair. In: Kaplan JA, Augoustides JGT, Manecke GR, et al., eds. Kaplan's Cardiac Anesthesia. 7th ed. Elsevier; 2017:770-817.
2. Mohananey D, Aljadah M, Smith AAH, et al. The 2020 ACC/AHA guidelines for management of patients with valvular heart disease: highlights and perioperative implications. J Cardiothorac Vasc Anesth, 2022; 36: 1467-1476.

5. Which of the following is a class I indication for aortic valve replacement in patients with aortic stenosis (AS)?
A. AS with a mean gradient of 32 mmHg
B. AS with a valve area of 1.7 square centimeters
C. Asymptomatic AS with a valve area of 1.2 square centimeters
D. Symptomatic AS with a maximal transvalvular velocity of 4.2 meters per second

Correct Answer: D

Explanation: Symptomatic severe aortic stenosis is a class I indication for aortic valve replacement. Severe aortic stenosis is characterized by features that include the following: a maximal transvalvular velocity of 4 meters per second or higher; a mean pressure gradient of 40 mmHg or higher; and an aortic valve area of 1.0 square centimeter or less. The transvalvular pressure gradient is dependent on flow and ejection fraction. Patients with severe aortic stenosis may have a low-pressure gradient across the aortic valve in the setting of left ventricular dysfunction. Furthermore, patients with severe aortic stenosis and advanced left ventricular hypertrophy may have a low end-diastolic volume that leads to low flow and a consequent low gradient across the aortic valve, despite a normal left ventricular ejection fraction. Further indications for valve replacement in advanced aortic stenosis can be found in the recent guidelines for the management of valvular heart disease.

References:

1. Ramakrishna H, Craner RC, Devaleria PA, et al. Chapter 17: Valvular Heart Disease: Replacement and Repair. In: Kaplan JA, Augoustides JGT, Manecke GR, et al., eds. Kaplan's Cardiac Anesthesia. 7th ed. Elsevier; 2017:770-817.
2. Otto CM, Nishimura RA, Bonow RO, et al. 2020 ACC/AHA guideline for the management of patients with valvular heart disease: A report of the American College of Cardiology/American Heart Association Joint Committee on Clinical Practice Guidelines. J Thorac Cardiovasc Surg, 2021; 162: e183-e353.

6. Which of the following is a class I indication for aortic valve replacement in patients with aortic regurgitation (AR)?
- **A.** Symptomatic AR with an effective regurgitant orifice area of 0.35 square centimeters
- **B.** AR with a regurgitant volume of 45 mL and an ejection fraction of 65%
- **C.** Asymptomatic AR with a regurgitant volume of 70 mL
- **D.** Asymptomatic AR with holodiastolic aortic flow reversal with an ejection fraction of 70%

Correct Answer: A

Explanation: Severe symptomatic aortic regurgitation is a class I indication for aortic valve replacement. Quantitative measures of regurgitation severity such as regurgitant volume, regurgitant fraction, and effective regurgitant orifice area are better predictors of clinical outcome compared to qualitative measures. Severe aortic regurgitation is typically associated with features that include the following: vena contracta over 6 millimeters; holodiastolic aortic flow reversal; a regurgitant volume of 60 mL or more; a regurgitant fraction of 50% or higher; and an effective regurgitant orifice area of 0.3 square centimeters or more. Asymptomatic severe aortic regurgitation is a class II indication, even if the left ventricular ejection fraction is preserved.

References:

1. Ramakrishna H, Craner RC, Devaleria PA, et al. Chapter 17: Valvular Heart Disease: Replacement and Repair. In: Kaplan JA, Augoustides JGT, Manecke GR, et al., eds. Kaplan's Cardiac Anesthesia. 7th ed. Elsevier; 2017:770-817.
2. Otto CM, Nishimura RA, Bonow RO, et al. 2020 ACC/AHA guideline for the management of patients with valvular heart disease: A report of the American College of Cardiology/American Heart Association Joint Committee on Clinical Practice Guidelines. J Thorac Cardiovasc Surg, 2021; 162: e183-e353.

7. Which of the following is consistent with severe mitral stenosis (MS) according to the 2020 guidelines for valvular heart disease from the American Heart Association?
- **A.** MS with a valve area of 1.4 square centimeters
- **B.** MS with a mean gradient of 6 mmHg
- **C.** MS with left atrial enlargement and a pulmonary artery systolic pressure of 41 mmHg
- **D.** MS with a diastolic pressure half time of 140 milliseconds

Correct Answer: A

Explanation: Symptomatic severe mitral stenosis is a class I indication for mitral valve replacement. According to the 2020 guidelines from the American Heart Association, a mitral valve area of 1.5 square centimeters or less is considered severe. Further criteria for severe mitral stenosis include a severe left atrial enlargement with a pulmonary artery systolic pressure of more than 50 mmHg as well as a diastolic pressure half-time of more than 150 milliseconds. Although the mean gradient may vary significantly, typically greater than 10 mmHg is considered severe. Since the mean gradient can vary significantly depending on loading conditions, the 2020 valvular heart disease guidelines have not included transmitral mean pressure gradient in the definition of severe mitral stenosis.

References:

1. Ramakrishna H, Craner RC, Devaleria PA, et al. Chapter 17: Valvular Heart Disease: Replacement and Repair. In: Kaplan JA, Augoustides JGT, Manecke GR, et al., eds. Kaplan's Cardiac Anesthesia. 7th ed. Elsevier; 2017:770-817.
2. Otto CM, Nishimura RA, Bonow RO, et al. 2020 ACC/AHA guideline for the management of patients with valvular heart disease: A report of the American College of Cardiology/American Heart Association Joint Committee on Clinical Practice Guidelines. J Thorac Cardiovasc Surg, 2021; 162: e183-e353.

8. Which of the following is a class I indication for mitral valve repair/replacement in patients with mitral regurgitation (MR)?
- **A.** MR with posterior leaflet prolapse, a regurgitant volume of 70 mL, and an ejection fraction of 45%
- **B.** MR with ischemic cardiomyopathy, restricted leaflet motion, and an effective regurgitant orifice area of 0.5 square centimeters
- **C.** Rheumatic MR with a regurgitant volume of 30 mL
- **D.** Patient undergoing coronary artery bypass grafting with secondary MR that has a vena contracta of 4 millimeters

Correct Answer: A

Explanation: Mitral regurgitation can be classified as primary where there is structural damage to the mitral valve apparatus or as secondary where there are functional abnormalities such as a dilated annulus and/or restricted leaflet motion. Quantitative markers of severe mitral regurgitation include a regurgitant volume of 60 mL or more, a regurgitant fraction of 50% or more, an effective regurgitant orifice area of 0.4 square centimeters or more, and a vena contracta of 7 millimeters or more. Severe primary mitral regurgitation with posterior leaflet prolapse is a class I indication for mitral valve intervention. Severe secondary mitral regurgitation due to an underlying condition such as ischemic cardiomyopathy is a class II indication for mitral valve intervention. Patients with a history of rheumatic heart disease and moderate mitral regurgitation as the leading valve abnormality do not meet class I criteria for valve repair/replacement. Moderate secondary mitral regurgitation in patients undergoing coronary artery bypass surgery is also not a class I indication for mitral valve repair/replacement.

References:
1. Ramakrishna H, Craner RC, Devaleria PA, et al. Chapter 17: Valvular Heart Disease: Replacement and Repair. In: Kaplan JA, Augoustides JGT, Manecke GR, et al., eds. Kaplan's Cardiac Anesthesia. 7th ed. Elsevier; 2017:770-817.
2. Mohananey D, Aljadah M, Smith AAH, et al. The 2020 ACC/AHA guidelines for management of patients with valvular heart disease: highlights and perioperative implications. J Cardiothorac Vasc Anesth, 2022; 36: 1467-1476.

9. Which of the following is a class I indication for tricuspid valve repair/replacement in patients with tricuspid regurgitation (TR)?
A. Severe TR at the time of left-sided valve surgery
B. Severe primary TR
C. Severe TR with progressive right ventricular dilation
D. TR with annular dilation >40 mm at time of left-sided valve surgery

Correct Answer: A

Explanation: Tricuspid regurgitation can be classified as primary where there is structural damage to the tricuspid valve apparatus or as secondary where there are functional abnormalities such as a dilated annulus and/or restricted leaflet motion. Quantitative markers of severe tricuspid regurgitation include a regurgitant volume of 45 mL or more, a regurgitant fraction of 50% or more, an effective regurgitant orifice area of 0.4 square centimeters or more, and a vena contracta of 7 millimeters or more. Severe tricuspid valve regurgitation at time of left-sided valve surgery is a class I indication for repair/replacement. Severe primary tricuspid regurgitation is currently a class IIa indication, while severe tricuspid regurgitation with progressive right ventricular dilation is a class IIb indication. Progressive tricuspid regurgitation with annular dilation at time of left-sided surgery is a class IIa indication for valve intervention.

References:
1. Ramakrishna H, Craner RC, Devaleria PA, et al. Chapter 17: Valvular Heart Disease: Replacement and Repair. In: Kaplan JA, Augoustides JGT, Manecke GR, et al., eds. Kaplan's Cardiac Anesthesia. 7th ed. Elsevier; 2017:770-817.
2. Mohananey D, Aljadah M, Smith AAH, et al. The 2020 ACC/AHA guidelines for management of patients with valvular heart disease: highlights and perioperative implications. J Cardiothorac Vasc Anesth, 2022; 36: 1467-1476.

10. A 78-year-old patient (75 kg, 178 cm) is scheduled for coronary artery bypass grafting surgery. After anesthetic induction, transesophageal echocardiography shows a calcified aortic valve with generalized restricted leaflet motion and a mean gradient of 17 mmHg across his aortic valve. Which step of the following is indicated next?
A. Recommend replacing the aortic valve
B. Recommend inspecting the aortic valve on cardiopulmonary bypass
C. Measure a cardiac output
D. Proceed only with coronary artery bypass grafting

Correct Answer: C

Explanation: Patients with severe aortic stenosis may have a low transvalvular gradient that may be due to severe left ventricular dysfunction. Some patients with low-flow, low-gradient aortic stenosis have a decreased aortic valve area as a result of inadequate forward stroke volume rather than anatomic stenosis. Surgical therapy is unlikely to benefit these patients, because the underlying pathology is a weakly contractile myocardium. However, patients with severe anatomic aortic stenosis may benefit from valve replacement despite the increased operative risk associated with the low-flow, low-gradient hemodynamic state. In this setting, dobutamine echocardiography can differentiate patients with fixed anatomic aortic stenosis from those with flow-dependent aortic stenosis associated with left ventricular dysfunction. Low-flow, low-gradient aortic stenosis has been defined as a mean gradient of less than 30 mmHg and a calculated aortic valve area less than 1.0 square centimeter. In the operating room setting, measuring cardiac output can assist with the interpretation of these echocardiographic findings. If the cardiac output is in the normal range, then this calcified aortic valve with restriction of all three cusps and a low transvalvular gradient is consistent with mild aortic stenosis.

References:
1. Ramakrishna H, Craner RC, Devaleria PA, et al. Chapter 17: Valvular Heart Disease: Replacement and Repair. In: Kaplan JA, Augoustides JGT, Manecke GR, et al., eds. Kaplan's Cardiac Anesthesia. 7th ed. Elsevier; 2017:770-817.
2. Mohananey D, Aljadah M, Smith AAH, et al. The 2020 ACC/AHA guidelines for management of patients with valvular heart disease: highlights and perioperative implications. J Cardiothorac Vasc Anesth, 2022; 36: 1467-1476.

11. In pregnant women with mechanical heart valves, which of the following statements is correct about the anticoagulation management?
A. Warfarin continued throughout pregnancy has the lowest maternal but high fetal morbidity
B. Aspirin is adequate for the first and second trimesters
C. All anticoagulation should be stopped during pregnancy
D. Low-molecular-weight heparin crosses the placenta

Correct Answer: A

Explanation: There is no one best anticoagulation strategy for pregnant women with mechanical heart valves. Pregnant women with mechanical heart valves are at increased risk of serious maternal complications, including valve thrombosis, thromboembolism, hemorrhage, and death. Uninterrupted therapeutic anticoagulation is required throughout pregnancy. Warfarin is safest for the mother, but crosses placenta and is associated with fetal morbidity, including teratogenic complications in the first trimester. Unfractionated heparin and low-molecular-weight heparin do not cross the placenta.

Aspirin as monotherapy is not adequate to protect against thrombosis of mechanical heart valves in pregnancy.

References:

1. Ramakrishna H, Craner RC, Devaleria PA, et al. Chapter 17: Valvular Heart Disease: Replacement and Repair. In: Kaplan JA, Augoustides JGT, Manecke GR, et al., eds. Kaplan's Cardiac Anesthesia. 7th ed. Elsevier; 2017:770-817.
2. Mohananey D, Aljadah M, Smith AAH, et al. The 2020 ACC/AHA guidelines for management of patients with valvular heart disease: highlights and perioperative implications. J Cardiothorac Vasc Anesth, 2022; 36: 1467-1476.

12. A 48-year-old patient with hypertrophic obstructive cardiomyopathy and a resting left ventricular outflow tract gradient of 60 mmHg undergoes septal myectomy. Before cardiopulmonary bypass, the gradient increases to 130 mmHg with isoproterenol challenge with concomitant severe mitral regurgitation. After separation from cardiopulmonary bypass, the resting gradient across the left ventricular outflow tract is 40 mmHg and increases to 70 mmHg with isoproterenol challenge with concomitant moderate mitral regurgitation. Which of the following statements is CORRECT?

A. These hemodynamic parameters are consistent with an adequate result
B. Consider additional septal myectomy
C. Transfer to the intensive care unit and assess further after tracheal extubation
D. Commence norepinephrine therapy and evaluate for increases in the gradient and associated mitral regurgitation

Correct Answer: B

Explanation: In this setting, gradients across the left ventricular outflow tract are typically reduced under general anesthesia. Pharmacological provocative testing with isoproterenol can be part of the intraoperative assessment in patients with hypertrophic obstructive cardiomyopathy. After initial myectomy, a residual gradient of more than 30 mmHg as well as systolic anterior motion of the mitral valve apparatus with significant mitral regurgitation should prompt consideration for additional septal resection on cardiopulmonary bypass. Norepinephrine therapy will increase afterload and improve left ventricular outflow obstruction with reduced gradients and less dynamic mitral regurgitation. These beneficial effects can mask surgical results.

References:

1. Ramakrishna H, Craner RC, Devaleria PA, et al. Chapter 17: Valvular Heart Disease: Replacement and Repair. In: Kaplan JA, Augoustides JGT, Manecke GR, et al., eds. Kaplan's Cardiac Anesthesia. 7th ed. Elsevier; 2017:770-817.
2. Elsayes AB, Basura A, Zahedi F, et al. Intraoperative provocative testing in patients with obstructive hypertrophic cardiomyopathy undergoing septal myectomy. J Am Soc Echocardiogr, 2020; 33: 182-190.

13. A 68-year-old patient (body surface area 2.3 square meters) undergoes aortic valve replacement with a size 21 mechanical valve. After cardiopulmonary bypass, the cardiac index is 1.9 L per square meter, the systemic blood pressure is 110/65 mmHg, and the transvalvular gradient with an otherwise normal functioning prosthetic valve is 50 mmHg. Which of the following best describes the findings and/or next steps?

A. Consider patient-prosthesis mismatch
B. These are normal findings
C. Commence dobutamine to increase cardiac output
D. Titrate norepinephrine to increase blood pressure

Correct Answer: A

Explanation: Patient-prosthesis mismatch describes the situation when an implanted prosthetic valve is too small for the patient. Severe patient-prosthesis mismatch has been defined as an indexed effective orifice area of less than 0.65 square centimeters per square meter of body surface area. Patients with a small aortic annulus should be assessed for possible patient-prosthesis mismatch. With an expected indexed effective orifice area of 0.85 (or less) square centimeters per square meter of body surface area, a larger aortic valve prosthesis and/or aortic root enlarging techniques should be considered. In this scenario, the factors that suggest patient-prosthesis mismatch include the valve size that is relatively small compared to the body surface area, and the low cardiac index with a relatively high transvalvular gradient.

References:

1. Ramakrishna H, Craner RC, Devaleria PA, et al. Chapter 17: Valvular Heart Disease: Replacement and Repair. In: Kaplan JA, Augoustides JGT, Manecke GR, et al., eds. Kaplan's Cardiac Anesthesia. 7th ed. Elsevier; 2017:770-817.
2. Bilkhu R, Jahangiri M, Otto CM. Patient-prosthesis mismatch following aortic valve replacement. Heart, 2019; 105: s28-s33.

14. A 52-year-old patient with hypertrophic obstructive cardiomyopathy presents for septal myectomy. After anesthetic induction, the systemic blood pressure is 92/58 mmHg, the heart rate is 93 beats per minute, and the pulmonary artery pressure tracing shows large tented pressure curves with a pulmonary artery pressure of 54/23 mmHg.

14.1 Which of the following best describes the cause of these hemodynamic findings?

A. Systolic anterior motion of a mitral valve leaflet
B. Intracavitary obstruction within the left ventricle
C. The hemodynamics are due to primary mitral regurgitation
D. There is right ventricular strain

Correct Answer: A

14.2 Which of the following interventions is reasonable in this scenario?
- **A.** No intervention
- **B.** Phenylephrine
- **C.** Epinephrine
- **D.** Milrinone

Correct Answer: B

Explanation: Systolic anterior motion of the anterior mitral leaflet in hypertrophic obstructive cardiomyopathy is typically associated with dynamic mitral regurgitation and left ventricular outflow tract obstruction with relative systemic hypotension. This dynamic obstruction can be exacerbated by anesthetic induction due to factors such as lowering of preload, systemic vasodilation, and consequent tachycardia. Systolic anterior motion of the anterior mitral leaflet may be associated with worsening of mitral regurgitation, explaining pulmonary arterial hypertension. Therapeutic interventions to open the left ventricular outflow tract and encourage forward flow include intravascular volume expansion, increasing afterload, decreasing the heart rate, and avoiding an increase in contractility. Phenylephrine is particularly effective since it both increases afterload and decreases heart rate. Epinephrine will exacerbate the left ventricular outflow obstruction due to increased contractility. Milrinone will also worsen the hemodynamics due to increased contractility and decreased afterload from systemic vasodilation. Although the right ventricular afterload is increased due to the associated pulmonary hypertension, this is a result rather than the cause of the described scenario.

References:

1. Ramakrishna H, Craner RC, Devaleria PA, et al. Chapter 17: Valvular Heart Disease: Replacement and Repair. In: Kaplan JA, Augoustides JGT, Manecke GR, et al., eds. Kaplan's Cardiac Anesthesia. 7th ed. Elsevier; 2017:770-817.
2. Jain P, Patel PA, Fabbro M. Hypertrophic cardiomyopathy and left ventricular outflow tract obstruction: expecting the unexpected. J Cardiothorac Vasc Anesth, 2018; 32: 467-477.

15. In a 42-year-old patient with bicuspid aortic valve and aortic valve stenosis presenting for surgery, which of the following interventions has the lowest expected transvalvular gradient?
- **A.** Transcatheter aortic valve replacement
- **B.** Mechanical aortic valve replacement
- **C.** Bioprosthetic valve replacement
- **D.** Ross procedure

Correct Answer: D

Explanation: The Ross procedure entails the placement of a pulmonary valve autograft in the aortic position, and implantation of an aortic homograft in the pulmonary position. Prosthetic valves all have a higher transvalvular gradient based as compared to a normal functioning native heart valve in the aortic position, accounting for valve size and orifice area. Amongst the prosthetic valves, transcatheter aortic valves tend to have the lowest transvalvular gradients.

References:

1. Ramakrishna H, Craner RC, Devaleria PA, et al. Chapter 17: Valvular Heart Disease: Replacement and Repair. In: Kaplan JA, Augoustides JGT, Manecke GR, et al., eds. Kaplan's Cardiac Anesthesia. 7th ed. Elsevier; 2017:770-817.
2. Ibrahim M, Spelde AE, Carter TI, et al. The Ross operation in the adult: what, why, and when. J Cardiothoracic Vasc Anesth, 2018; 32: 1885-1891.

16. A bicuspid aortic valve is most strongly associated with which of the following additional findings?
- **A.** Left ventricular outflow tract obstruction
- **B.** Pulmonary artery aneurysm
- **C.** Coarctation of the aorta
- **D.** Mitral valve prolapse

Correct Answer: C

Explanation: Bicuspid aortic valve is a common congenital cardiac abnormality that also has a high incidence of associated lesions, including coarctation and hypoplasia of the aorta and aortic aneurysm and dissection. It is important for the cardiac anesthesiologist to consider these associated lesions in perioperative management and to look for their presence during intraoperative transesophageal echocardiography in this setting. Although bicuspid aortic valve may coexist with left ventricular outflow tract obstruction and/or mitral valve prolapse, this is not a common occurrence.

References:

1. Ramakrishna H, Craner RC, Devaleria PA, et al. Chapter 17: Valvular Heart Disease: Replacement and Repair. In: Kaplan JA, Augoustides JGT, Manecke GR, et al., eds. Kaplan's Cardiac Anesthesia. 7th ed. Elsevier; 2017:770-817.
2. Mohananey D, Aljadah M, Smith AAH, et al. The 2020 ACC/AHA guidelines for management of patients with valvular heart disease: highlights and perioperative implications. J Cardiothorac Vasc Anesth, 2022; 36: 1467-1476.

17. A 73-year-old patient with severe aortic stenosis and left ventricular hypertrophy undergoes surgical aortic valve replacement. After separation from cardiopulmonary bypass, the patient has a perfusing junctional rhythm. By approximately what percentage would the initiation of atrial epicardial pacing increase cardiac output?
- **A.** Less than 10%
- **B.** 10% to 20%
- **C.** 20% to 30%
- **D.** More than 30%

Correct Answer: D

Explanation: The contribution of left atrial systole in left ventricular filling is highly dependent on left ventricular compliance, which gradually decreases with factors such as hypertrophy and advanced age. Atrial contraction in the normal heart accounts for approximately 10% to 20% of ventricular filling. In patients with a hypertrophied left ventricle this percentage typically increases to above 40%. In patients with hypertrophic cardiomyopathy, this percentage may increase to as much as 75% of total stroke volume. In the described case, atrial or, if necessary, atrioventricular pacing may significantly improve left ventricular end-diastolic volume and cardiac output.

References:

1. Ramakrishna H, Craner RC, Devaleria PA, et al. Chapter 17: Valvular Heart Disease: Replacement and Repair. In: Kaplan JA, Augoustides JGT, Manecke GR, et al., eds. Kaplan's Cardiac Anesthesia. 7th ed. Elsevier; 2017:770-817.
2. Mohananey D, Aljadah M, Smith AAH, et al. The 2020 ACC/AHA guidelines for management of patients with valvular heart disease: highlights and perioperative implications. J Cardiothorac Vasc Anesth, 2022; 36: 1467-1476.

18. A patient with severe aortic stenosis presented for aortic valve replacement. After anesthetic induction and placement of a pulmonary arterial catheter, the cardiac index is calculated at 1.9 L per minute per square meter with a heart rate of 82 beats per minute. Which of the following interventions is reasonable to increase the cardiac index?
   A. Nitroglycerine
   B. Nicardipine
   C. Dobutamine
   D. Volume administration

Correct Answer: D

Explanation: The use of vasodilators is traditionally contraindicated for patients with severe aortic stenosis because cardiac output is relatively fixed across a narrowed orifice. Vasodilation reduces systemic vascular tone with a limited possibility for a compensatory increase in cardiac output. Systemic hypotension and coronary ischemia may result. Administering volume to compensate for anesthesia related venodilation, and an alpha agonist to maintain systemic perfusion are typically first-choice responses in patients with severe aortic stenosis. The hemodynamic goals for this valvular lesion are to preserve preload and diastolic filling, maintain sinus rhythm at a slower rate when possible, maintain or increase afterload, and avoid myocardial depression. Tachycardia will not only interfere with ventricular filling due to a shortened diastolic time, but will also increase myocardial oxygen demand, and may precipitate myocardial ischemia.

References:

1. Ramakrishna H, Craner RC, Devaleria PA, et al. Chapter 17: Valvular Heart Disease: Replacement and Repair. In: Kaplan JA, Augoustides JGT, Manecke GR, et al., eds. Kaplan's Cardiac Anesthesia. 7th ed. Elsevier; 2017:770-817.
2. Mohananey D, Aljadah M, Smith AAH, et al. The 2020 ACC/AHA guidelines for management of patients with valvular heart disease: highlights and perioperative implications. J Cardiothorac Vasc Anesth, 2022; 36: 1467-1476.

19. A patient with severe aortic stenosis has undergone surgical aortic valve replacement. After separation from cardiopulmonary bypass, the cardiac index is 2.1 L per minute per square meter. Which of the following is the most reliable measure to guide volume administration?
   A. End-diastolic volume determination by echocardiography
   B. Direct inspection of the heart
   C. Central venous pressure
   D. pulmonary capillary wedge pressure

Correct Answer: A

Explanation: End-diastolic volume as assessed with transesophageal echocardiography is the most reliable measure of preload. This is particularly relevant in patients with left ventricular hypertrophy where pressure measurements may not directly correlate with intravascular volume status due to the reduced compliance and accompanying diastolic dysfunction. Direct inspection of the heart typically cannot reliably assess left ventricular parameters, as the left ventricle lies posterior and is often hidden from direct view.

References:

1. Ramakrishna H, Craner RC, Devaleria PA, et al. Chapter 17: Valvular Heart Disease: Replacement and Repair. In: Kaplan JA, Augoustides JGT, Manecke GR, et al., eds. Kaplan's Cardiac Anesthesia. 7th ed. Elsevier; 2017:770-817.
2. Mohananey D, Aljadah M, Smith AAH, et al. The 2020 ACC/AHA guidelines for management of patients with valvular heart disease: highlights and perioperative implications. J Cardiothorac Vasc Anesth, 2022; 36: 1467-1476.

20. A patient with advanced hypertrophic obstructive cardiomyopathy presents for septal myectomy. After anesthesia induction, the systemic blood pressure rapidly decreases quickly to 76/48 mmHg. Which of the following interventions is indicated?
   A. Ephedrine
   B. Epinephrine
   C. Dopamine
   D. Phenylephrine

Correct Answer: D

Explanation: Hemodynamic instability in patients with hypertrophic obstructive cardiomyopathy during anesthetic induction is typically related to decreased left ventricular filling due to systemic venodilation. The decreased end-diastolic volume can precipitate left ventricular outflow tract obstruction and lead to acute mitral exacerbation due to systolic anterior motion of the anterior mitral leaflet. The hemodynamic goals in this setting to promote cardiac output include maintaining preload and afterload, and avoiding increases in inotropy, tachycardia, and vasodilation. Ephedrine, epinephrine, and dopamine worsen hemodynamics due to tachycardia and increased contractility. Phenylephrine is an ideal agent in this setting, as it restores systemic vascular tone and decreases the heart rate to allow more diastolic filling time.

References:

1. Ramakrishna H, Craner RC, Devaleria PA, et al: Chapter 17: Valvular Heart Disease: Replacement and Repair. In: Kaplan JA, Augoustides JGT, Manecke GR, et al., eds. Kaplan's Cardiac Anesthesia. 7th ed. Elsevier; 2017:770-817.
2. Jain P, Patel PA, Fabbro M. Hypertrophic cardiomyopathy and left ventricular outflow tract obstruction: expecting the unexpected. J Cardiothorac Vasc Anesth, 2018; 32: 467-477.

21. Premature mitral valve closure before atrial systole can most likely be seen with which of the following valvular lesions?
    A. Aortic regurgitation (acute)
    B. Aortic regurgitation (chronic)
    C. Mitral regurgitation (acute)
    D. Mitral regurgitation (chronic)

Correct Answer: A

Explanation: In acute aortic regurgitation, sudden diastolic volume overloading of a nonadapted left ventricle results in a precipitous increase in the end-diastolic pressure because the ventricle is operating on the steepest portion of the diastolic pressure-volume curve. In severe acute aortic regurgitation, the left ventricular end-diastolic pressure can equilibrate with aortic diastolic pressure and exceed the left atrial pressure in late diastole. This may be sufficient to cause closure of the mitral valve before atrial systole and may even lead to mitral regurgitation. In chronic aortic regurgitation, the left ventricle adapts to the chronic increase in end-diastolic volume with progressive chamber dilation that avoids acute increases in diastolic pressure. In both acute and chronic mitral regurgitation, there is inadequate closure of the mitral valve that leads to the valvular regurgitation.

References:

1. Ramakrishna H, Craner RC, Devaleria PA, et al. Chapter 17: Valvular Heart Disease: Replacement and Repair. In: Kaplan JA, Augoustides JGT, Manecke GR, et al., eds. Kaplan's Cardiac Anesthesia. 7th ed. Elsevier; 2017:770-817.
2. Otto CM, Nishimura RA, Bonow RO, et al. 2020 ACC/AHA guideline for the management of patients with valvular heart disease: A report of the American College of Cardiology/American Heart Association Joint Committee on Clinical Practice Guidelines. J Thorac Cardiovasc Surg, 2021; 162: e183-e353.

22. A patient with severe aortic regurgitation presents for surgical aortic valve replacement. After anesthetic induction, the systemic blood pressure decreases to 91/32 mmHg with an associated heart rate of 72 beats per minute. Which of the following drugs is indicated as an initial intervention?
    A. Epinephrine
    B. Nicardipine
    C. Phenylephrine
    D. Vasopressin

Correct Answer: A

Explanation: Increases in systemic afterload with titrated phenylephrine or vasopressin may be counterproductive as it typically worsens aortic regurgitation. Although a decrease in afterload with nicardipine therapy would improve forward flow, it may further decrease systemic blood pressure and hence coronary perfusion pressure. Epinephrine can help break a vicious cycle of increases in diastolic pressure and ventricular distension from severe aortic regurgitation to promote forward flow and restore blood pressure through increased contractility and a relative tachycardia. The hemodynamic goals in patients with aortic regurgitation are to maintain or increase contractility, avoid bradycardia, decrease afterload (within normal blood pressure goals), and maintain preload.

References:

1. Ramakrishna H, Craner RC, Devaleria PA, et al. Chapter 17: Valvular Heart Disease: Replacement and Repair. In: Kaplan JA, Augoustides JGT, Manecke GR, et al., eds. Kaplan's Cardiac Anesthesia. 7th ed. Elsevier; 2017:770-817.
2. Otto CM, Nishimura RA, Bonow RO, et al. 2020 ACC/AHA guideline for the management of patients with valvular heart disease: A report of the American College of Cardiology/American Heart Association Joint Committee on Clinical Practice Guidelines. J Thorac Cardiovasc Surg, 2021; 162: e183-e353.

23. A patient with severe mitral regurgitation presents for mitral valve repair. After anesthetic induction, the systemic blood pressure decreases to 78/51 mmHg with an associated heart rate of 72 beats per minute. Which of the following drugs is indicated as an initial intervention?
    A. Epinephrine
    B. Nicardipine
    C. Phenylephrine
    D. Vasopressin

Correct Answer: A

Explanation: Increases in left ventricular afterload with phenylephrine and vasopressin may be counterproductive as forward stroke volume may further decrease with an increase in regurgitant flow. This worsening mitral regurgitation may increase left atrial pressure with pulmonary hypertension to cause right ventricular strain and potentially precipitate acute right ventricular failure. Although a decrease in afterload with nicardipine therapy would improve forward flow, it may further decrease systemic blood pressure and hence coronary perfusion pressure. Mixed alpha- and beta-adrenergic drugs such as ephedrine and epinephrine can help restore cardiac output and blood pressure in this scenario due to increases in contractility and heart rate. The hemodynamic goals in patients with mitral regurgitation are to maintain preload, avoid bradycardia and increases in afterload, and maintain contractility.

References:

1. Ramakrishna H, Craner RC, Devaleria PA, et al. Chapter 17: Valvular Heart Disease: Replacement and Repair. In: Kaplan JA, Augoustides JGT, Manecke GR, et al., eds. Kaplan's Cardiac Anesthesia. 7th ed. Elsevier; 2017:770-817.
2. Otto CM, Nishimura RA, Bonow RO, et al. 2020 ACC/AHA guideline for the management of patients with valvular heart

disease: A report of the American College of Cardiology/American Heart Association Joint Committee on Clinical Practice Guidelines. J Thorac Cardiovasc Surg, 2021; 162: e183-e353.

24. Which of the following is a typical etiology for functional mitral regurgitation?
  A. Endocarditis
  B. Fibroelastic deficiency
  C. Ischemic heart disease
  D. Rheumatic heart disease

Correct Answer: C

Explanation: The term functional (or secondary) mitral regurgitation (MR) describes MR that occurs despite structurally normal leaflets and chordae tendineae and is often due to an underlying disease. The underlying etiology, for example coronary artery disease, is the cause of myocardial ischemia or infarction, with subsequent left ventricular remodeling resulting in leaflet tethering and secondary mitral regurgitation. Functional MR often occurs in the setting of ischemic heart disease, and the term ischemic MR is sometimes used interchangeably with functional MR. However, functional mitral regurgitation can occur in patients without coronary artery disease, such as in those with idiopathic dilated cardiomyopathy. In primary MR, the underlying disease process affects the mitral valve (MV) leaflets apparatus, and MV leaflets are abnormal, for example in degenerative mitral valve disease (fibroelastic deficiency), rheumatic heart disease, or endocarditis.

References:

1. Ramakrishna H, Craner RC, Devaleria PA, et al. Chapter 17: Valvular Heart Disease: Replacement and Repair. In: Kaplan JA, Augoustides JGT, Manecke GR, et al., eds. Kaplan's Cardiac Anesthesia. 7th ed. Elsevier; 2017:770-817.
2. Otto CM, Nishimura RA, Bonow RO, et al. 2020 ACC/AHA guideline for the management of patients with valvular heart disease: A report of the American College of Cardiology/American Heart Association Joint Committee on Clinical Practice Guidelines. J Thorac Cardiovasc Surg, 2021; 162: e183-e353.

25. Which of the following is the typical mechanism for tricuspid regurgitation in a patient with carcinoid syndrome?
  A. Myocardial ischemia
  B. Excessive leaflet motion
  C. Dilated cardiomyopathy
  D. Restricted leaflet motion

Correct Answer: D

Explanation: Carcinoid tumors are neuroendocrine tumors that arise from the small bowel. Manifestations of carcinoid syndrome occur primarily in patients with liver metastasis. Carcinoid heart disease may occur in 20% to 50% of patients with carcinoid syndrome. Carcinoid heart disease characteristically produces tricuspid regurgitation and mixed pulmonic stenosis and regurgitation resulting in severe right-sided heart failure. Carcinoid plaques composed of myofibroblasts, collagen, and myxoid matrix are deposited primarily on the tricuspid and pulmonary valves, bringing about immobility and thickening of the valve leaflets, causing the distinctive valvular changes. The mechanism of tricuspid regurgitation in this syndrome is restricted rather than excessive leaflet motion. Although myocardial ischemia and dilated cardiomyopathy can cause tricuspid regurgitation, they are not typically associated with carcinoid syndrome.

References:

1. Ramakrishna H, Craner RC, Devaleria PA, et al. Chapter 17: Valvular Heart Disease: Replacement and Repair. In: Kaplan JA, Augoustides JGT, Manecke GR, et al., eds. Kaplan's Cardiac Anesthesia. 7th ed. Elsevier; 2017:770-817.
2. Castillo J, Silvay G, Weiner M. Anesthetic management of patients with carcinoid syndrome and carcinoid heart disease: the Mount Sinai algorithm. J Cardiothorac Vasc Anesth, 2018; 32: 1023-1031.

26. A patient with a history of rheumatic heart disease and severe mitral stenosis is presenting for mitral valve replacement. After anesthesia induction, the blood pressure decreases to 92/53 mmHg, with a heart rate of 88 beats per minute, and a pulmonary artery pressure of 78/38 mmHg. Which of the following drugs is indicated as an initial intervention?
  A. Dobutamine
  B. Nicardipine
  C. Nitroglycerine
  D. Norepinephrine

Correct Answer: D

Explanation: Mitral stenosis results in diminished left ventricular preload and a relatively fixed cardiac output, the hallmark of stenotic lesions. Contractility should be preserved, but may increasingly be affected as well, through ventricular interdependence, as right ventricular function and pulmonary artery hypertension worsen. Compared to the normal heart, left ventricular filling increasingly depends on atrial contraction, and a loss in normal sinus rhythm can cause sudden hemodynamic deterioration. Any further increases in pulmonary vascular resistance must be avoided, while maintaining adequate systemic vascular resistance to maintain coronary perfusion. The hemodynamic goals in patients with mitral stenosis are to maintain preload, afterload, and sinus rhythm as well as to avoid excessive tachycardia and pulmonary vasoconstriction. In this scenario, dobutamine will further increase heart rate and contractility; however, stroke volume is relatively fixed, and the systemic vasodilatory effect of dobutamine may offset any increases in cardiac output. Although nitroglycerine may help decrease right ventricular afterload, in advanced mitral stenosis pulmonary vascular resistance is often fixed and typically has minimal response to pulmonary vasodilators. Additionally, systemic vasodilation will further decrease vital perfusion pressure. Norepinephrine will increase systemic blood pressure and coronary perfusion pressure to help avoid further hemodynamic deterioration, although it may increase pulmonary vascular resistance. Vasopressin may be superior to norepinephrine in this scenario because it will increase systemic vascular resistance to restore blood pressure but typically does not increase pulmonary vascular resistance.

References:
1. Ramakrishna H, Craner RC, Devaleria PA, et al. Chapter 17: Valvular Heart Disease: Replacement and Repair. In: Kaplan JA, Augoustides JGT, Manecke GR, et al., eds. Kaplan's Cardiac Anesthesia. 7th ed. Elsevier; 2017:770-817.
2. Otto CM, Nishimura RA, Bonow RO, et al. 2020 ACC/AHA guideline for the management of patients with valvular heart disease: A report of the American College of Cardiology/American Heart Association Joint Committee on Clinical Practice Guidelines. J Thorac Cardiovasc Surg, 2021; 162: e183-e353.

27. A 63-year-old patient is scheduled for aortic valve replacement. Following the release of the aortic cross-clamp, sinus bradycardia rhythm with a heart rate of 48 beats per minute ensues. The surgical team detects left ventricular distention in the operative field. Which of the following maneuvers is indicated next?
A. Commence an epinephrine infusion
B. Initiate ventricular pacing at 90 beats per minute
C. Check for a paravalvular leak
D. Insert a left ventricular vent

Correct Answer: C

Explanation: Left ventricular distension after removal of the aortic cross clamp in this scenario should prompt a search for aortic regurgitation, either with a native aortic valve or with a prosthetic valve that may have a paravalvular leak. In the presented case, with a slow but beating heart, a large paravalvular leak should be ruled out even before separation from cardiopulmonary bypass. Once the aortic cross clamp is off and the aortic root pressurizes, aortic regurgitation due to paravalvular leaks may be diagnosed by transesophageal echocardiography in the midesophageal short-and long-axis views of the aortic valve. Although inotropic support and epicardial pacing may ultimately assist separation from cardiopulmonary bypass, an immediate issue such a large paravalvular leak that requires surgical intervention should be ruled out first. A left ventricular vent is not immediately required since the heart is beating and is being perfused. It may ultimately be required if the heart is arrested to address a large paravalvular leak. Ongoing refinements in bioprosthetic aortic valve design, such as in the Inspiris Resilia aortic valve, result in signature temporary intravalvular leaks immediately after valve implantation that may be difficult to distinguish echocardiographically from paravalvular leaks that require intervention.

References:
1. Ramakrishna H, Craner RC, Devaleria PA, et al. Chapter 17: Valvular Heart Disease: Replacement and Repair. In: Kaplan JA, Augoustides JGT, Manecke GR, et al., eds. Kaplan's Cardiac Anesthesia. 7th ed. Elsevier; 2017:770-817.
2. Vanneman MW, Dalia AA. Perioperative and echocardiographic considerations for the Inspiris Resilia aortic valve – current and future. J Cardiothorac Vasc Anesth, 2020; 34: 2807-2812.

28. A 64-year-old patient with chronic mitral regurgitation presents for mitral valve repair. The left ventricular end-systolic diameter and ejection fraction were quantified by preoperative transthoracic echocardiography to be 45 millimeters and 57%, respectively. Which of the following pairs correctly describe left ventricular size and function?
A. Normal size and function
B. Normal size with abnormal function
C. Abnormal size with normal function
D. Abnormal size and function

Correct Answer: D

Explanation: Because of the chronic volume load and late ejection into a lower-impedance left atrium, the reference ranges for normal values are higher in chronic mitral regurgitation. The left ventricular end-systolic diameter should exceed 40 millimeters to be considered abnormal. The normal left ventricular ejection fraction in patients with chronic mitral regurgitation should exceed 60%. Some studies have even suggested that even with these adjusted ranges, left ventricular dysfunction has already occurred, prompting discussion about consideration of even higher normal values for ejection fraction and lower normal values for end-systolic diameter. The ultimate management goal is to intervene at the optimal time to minimize left ventricular damage due to the mitral regurgitation.

References:
1. Ramakrishna H, Craner RC, Devaleria PA, et al. Chapter 17: Valvular Heart Disease: Replacement and Repair. In: Kaplan JA, Augoustides JGT, Manecke GR, et al., eds. Kaplan's Cardiac Anesthesia. 7th ed. Elsevier; 2017:770-817.
2. Otto CM, Nishimura RA, Bonow RO, et al. 2020 ACC/AHA guideline for the management of patients with valvular heart disease: A report of the American College of Cardiology/American Heart Association Joint Committee on Clinical Practice Guidelines. J Thorac Cardiovasc Surg, 2021; 162: e183-e353.

29. A 65-year-old patient with chronic mitral regurgitation presents for mitral valve repair. The preoperative mechanism of the mitral regurgitation was assessed as isolated prolapse of the middle scallop of the posterior leaflet. During comprehensive intraoperative imaging with transesophageal echocardiography, multiple mechanisms were identified, including a dilated valve annulus, mild annular calcification, and bileaflet multisegmental prolapse, as well as thickened leaflets. Which of the following best describes the planned surgical intervention?
A. Mitral valve repair is recommended
B. Isolated mitral annuloplasty will address these mechanisms of mitral regurgitation
C. Mitral valve replacement is a reasonable choice
D. Mitral edge-to-edge leaflet repair is recommended

Correct Answer: C

Explanation: It is important to discuss unexpected findings during intraoperative transesophageal echocardiography with the procedural team. In the described case, the planned procedure was mitral valve repair, which is the procedure of choice in isolated severe primary mitral regurgitation limited to less than one-half of the posterior leaflet. The intraoperative findings, however, are consistent with Barlow's disease. The surgical approach is significantly more complex, and surgical outcomes inconsistent, due to the multiple mitral abnormalities that contribute to the mitral regurgitation. There is increasing evidence that mitral valve repair in these more complex repairs is not necessarily associated with improved long-term outcomes compared to mitral valve replacement. In the described scenario, the echocardiographic findings must be accurately reviewed with the procedural team to facilitate the optimal intervention for a given patient.

References:

1. Ramakrishna H, Craner RC, Devaleria PA, et al. Chapter 17: Valvular Heart Disease: Replacement and Repair. In: Kaplan JA, Augoustides JGT, Manecke GR, et al., eds. Kaplan's Cardiac Anesthesia. 7th ed. Elsevier; 2017:770-817.
2. Otto CM, Nishimura RA, Bonow RO, et al. 2020 ACC/AHA guideline for the management of patients with valvular heart disease: A report of the American College of Cardiology/American Heart Association Joint Committee on Clinical Practice Guidelines. J Thorac Cardiovasc Surg, 2021; 162: e183-e353.

30. A 67-year-old patient with advanced coronary artery disease presents for coronary artery bypass surgery. The systemic blood pressure is 101/62 mmHg, with a heart rate of 86 beats per minute. Intraoperative imaging with transesophageal echocardiography reveals moderate mitral regurgitation with posterior and anterior mitral valve leaflet tethering. Which of the following maneuvers is best indicated in this clinical scenario?

A. Increase the systemic vascular resistance and re-evaluate the mitral regurgitation
B. Proceed only with coronary artery bypass grafting
C. Recommend concomitant mitral valve replacement
D. Recommend concomitant mitral valve repair

Correct Answer: A

Explanation: It is important to review unexpected findings during intraoperative echocardiography with the surgical team to inform clinical decision-making. In the presented scenario, the planned procedure did not include mitral valve intervention. However, the detected mitral regurgitation was moderate in severity in the setting of ventricular unloading due to general anesthesia and decreased afterload, as indicated by the relatively low systemic blood pressure. Mitral valve surgery for significant mitral regurgitation in patients presenting for coronary artery bypass grafting is a reasonable consideration if the detected regurgitation is severe. Given the relative low loading conditions in this setting, it is reasonable to increase left ventricular loading as a provocative maneuver to assess for the possibility of severe mitral regurgitation, which may prompt a discussion about possible mitral valve intervention. In the setting of ischemic mitral regurgitation with leaflet tethering, mitral valve repair has had limited efficacy, prompting greater consideration of mitral replacement.

References:

1. Ramakrishna H, Craner RC, Devaleria PA, et al. Chapter 17: Valvular Heart Disease: Replacement and Repair. In: Kaplan JA, Augoustides JGT, Manecke GR, et al., eds. Kaplan's Cardiac Anesthesia. 7th ed. Elsevier; 2017:770-817.
2. Mohananey D, Aljadah M, Smith AAH, et al. The 2020 ACC/AHA guidelines for management of patients with valvular heart disease: highlights and perioperative implications. J Cardiothorac Vasc Anesth, 2022; 36: 1467-1476.

31. A 63-year-old patient with hypertrophic obstructive cardiomyopathy presents for septal myectomy. Intraoperative echocardiographic imaging reveals a resting gradient of 45 mmHg across the left ventricular outflow tract with moderate mitral regurgitation. Provocative testing with an isoproterenol challenge resulted in a gradient that increased to 100 mmHg with concomitant severe mitral regurgitation. The jet of mitral regurgitation is anteriorly directed and is associated with systolic anterior motion of the mitral valve apparatus. Which of the following actions is best indicated after this provocative test?

A. Assess for primary mitral regurgitation.
B. Commence norepinephrine therapy and reassess the mitral valve
C. Administer an intravascular volume bolus and reassess the mitral valve
D. Proceed with septal myectomy only

Correct Answer: A

Explanation: The typical mitral regurgitation in hypertrophic cardiomyopathy is posteriorly directed due to the systolic anterior migration of the anterior mitral leaflet into the left ventricular outflow tract. An anteriorly directed jet may occur if there is an additional mechanism for primary mitral regurgitation such as posterior leaflet prolapse. Primary mitral regurgitation should be excluded in this setting, as its presence may prompt mitral valve repair/replacement in addition to the planned septal myectomy. In the described case, increases in afterload with norepinephrine or preload with volume loading will likely improve the mitral regurgitation secondary to systolic anterior motion of the mitral valve apparatus. The important issue, however, is not only the severity of the mitral regurgitation but also its underlying mechanisms. Septal myectomy typically addresses the mitral regurgitation that is secondary to left ventricular outflow tract obstruction but does not address an additional mechanism for primary mitral regurgitation.

References:

1. Ramakrishna H, Craner RC, Devaleria PA, et al. Chapter 17: Valvular Heart Disease: Replacement and Repair. In: Kaplan JA, Augoustides JGT, Manecke GR, et al., eds. Kaplan's Cardiac Anesthesia. 7th ed. Elsevier; 2017:770-817.
2. Hong JH, Schaff HV, Nishimura RA, et al. Mitral regurgitation in patients with hypertrophic obstructive cardiomyopathy: implications for concomitant valve procedures. J Am Coll Cardiol, 2016; 68: 1497-504.

CHAPTER 18

Congenital Heart Disease in Adults

Alexander Mittnacht

KEY POINTS

1. Because of successes in treating congenital cardiac lesions, there are currently as many or more adults than children with congenital heart disease (CHD).
2. Noncardiac anesthesiologists will see these patients for a vast array of ailments and injuries requiring cardiac or non-cardiac surgery.
3. If at all possible, noncardiac surgery on adult patients with moderate-to-complex CHD should be performed at an adult congenital heart center with the consultation of an anesthesiologist experienced with adult CHD.

---

1. What is a typical indication for pulmonary valve replacement in an adult patient with a history of tetralogy of Fallot that was repaired with a transannular patch technique at 5 months of age?
   A. Right ventricular end-diastolic volume index of 180 mL/m^2
   B. Holodiastolic flow reversal in the pulmonary artery
   C. Mean pulmonary valve gradient of 18 mmHg
   D. Residual ventricular septal defect with a pulmonary to systemic blood flow (Qp/Qs) ratio of 1.2/1

Correct Answer: A

Explanation: Pulmonary valve replacement after tetralogy of Fallot repair in infancy is a relatively common procedure in adult congenital heart surgery. The resulting pulmonary regurgitation gradually results in right ventricular dilation and eventual failure if not corrected. There are several indications for this procedure, including the patient's symptoms, right ventricular dilation with an end-diastolic volume index greater than 160 mL/m^2, and right ventricular systolic dysfunction with an ejection fraction less than 45%. Further indications for intervention in this setting include right ventricular outflow tract pathology such as aneurysm or obstruction as well as a residual ventricular septal defect with a pulmonary to systemic blood flow ratio (Qp/Qs) greater than 1.5/1. These patients are typically followed clinically

and with serial echocardiographic and magnetic resonance imaging to time surgical intervention before significant right ventricular dysfunction or dilation occurs. In the described scenario, only the right ventricular dilation stands out. Although holodiastolic flow reversal indicates significant pulmonary regurgitation, this is expected with a transannular patch technique and can be clinically tolerated for many years. The given pulmonary valve gradient is not particularly high, and unless there is residual mechanical outflow tract obstruction this amount of transvalvular gradient is most likely flow related, indicating the degree of pulmonary regurgitation. The residual ventricular septal defect with a Qp/Qs of 1.2/1 is too small to warrant surgery.

References:

1. Baum VC, de Souza DG. Chapter 18: Congenital Heart Disease in Adults. In: Kaplan JA, Augoustides JGT, Manecke GR, et al., eds. Kaplan's Cardiac Anesthesia. 7th ed. Elsevier; 2017: 818-842.
2. Mosca R. Pulmonary valve replacement after repair of tetralogy of Fallot: evolving strategies. J Thorac Cardiovasc Surg, 2016; 151: 623-625.
3. Geva T. Indications for pulmonary valve replacement in repaired tetralogy of Fallot. Circulation, 2013; 128: 1855-1857.
4. Townsley MM, Windsor J, Briston D, et al. Tetralogy of Fallot: perioperative management and analysis of outcomes. J Cardiothorac Vasc Anesth, 2019; 33: 556-565.

2. Which anomalous pulmonary vein connection is most commonly associated with a sinus venosus atrial septal defect?
   A. Right upper
   B. Right lower
   C. Left upper
   D. Left lower

Correct Answer: A

Explanation: There are several anatomic types of atrial septal effect (ASD). The most common type is the secundum type located in the midseptum. The secundum ASD is a defect of the septum primum. Primum ASD is often associated with endocardial cushion defects, particularly atrioventricular canal defects. The sinus venosus ASD, commonly the superior type, is located near the orifice of the superior vena cava and is associated with partial anomalous pulmonary venous return, most frequently drainage of the right upper pulmonary vein to the low superior vena cava. The superior type sinus venosus ASD is more common compared to the inferior type sinus venosus ASD that is associated with the inferior vena cava. Lastly, an uncommon atrial septal type defect occurs when blood passes from the left to the right atrium via an unroofed coronary sinus.

References:

1. Baum VC, de Souza DG. Chapter 18: Congenital Heart Disease in Adults. In: Kaplan JA, Augoustides JGT, Manecke GR, et al., eds. Kaplan's Cardiac Anesthesia. 7th ed. Elsevier; 2017:818-842.
2. Williams T, Lluri G, Boyd EK, et al. Perioperative echocardiography in the adult with congenital heart disease. J Cardiothorac Vasc Anesth, 2020; 34: 1292-1308.

3. What is typically associated with a primum atrial septal defect?
   A. Cleft mitral valve
   B. Anomalous pulmonary vein drainage
   C. Situs inversus
   D. Ebstein anomaly

Correct Answer: A

Explanation: There are several anatomic types of atrial septal defect (ASD). The most common type is the secundum type located in the midseptum. The secundum ASD is a defect of the septum primum. The primum ASD is often associated with endocardial cushion defects, particularly atrioventricular canal defects including a partial atrioventricular canal, which includes a cleft in the anterior leaflet of the mitral valve. The sinus venosus ASD is most commonly located near the orifice of the superior vena cava and is associated with partial anomalous pulmonary venous return, most frequently drainage of the right upper pulmonary vein to the low superior vena cava. The superior type sinus venosus ASD is more common compared to the inferior type sinus venosus ASD that is associated with the inferior vena cava. Lastly, an uncommon atrial septal type defect occurs when blood passes from the left to the right atrium via an unroofed coronary sinus. Situs inversus and the Ebstein anomaly are not typically associated with a primum ASD.

References:

1. Baum VC, de Souza DG. Chapter 18: Congenital Heart Disease in Adults. In: Kaplan JA, Augoustides JGT, Manecke GR, et al., eds. Kaplan's Cardiac Anesthesia. 7th ed. Elsevier; 2017:818-842.
2. Williams T, Lluri G, Boyd EK, et al. Perioperative echocardiography in the adult with congenital heart disease. 2020; 34: 1292-1308.

4. Which valve leaflet is most frequently displaced apically in patients with an Ebstein anomaly?
   A. Septal
   B. Anterior
   C. Posterior
   D. Thebesian

Correct Answer: A

Explanation: In Ebstein's anomaly of the tricuspid valve, part of the tricuspid valve tissue is displaced apically typically by more than 8 mm/m^2. Downward displacement is seen most with the septal leaflet, followed by the posterior leaflet and the anterior leaflet. The anterior leaflet tends to be large and redundant. The defect is associated with a patent foramen ovale or a secundum atrial septal defect. There is "atrialization" of part of the right ventricle. The displacement of the tricuspid valve toward the right ventricular apex results in a portion of the right ventricle being above the tricuspid valve and becoming functionally part of the right atrium.

References:

1. Baum VC, de Souza DG. Chapter 18: Congenital Heart Disease in Adults. In: Kaplan JA, Augoustides JGT, Manecke GR, et al., eds. Kaplan's Cardiac Anesthesia. 7th ed. Elsevier; 2017:818-842.
2. Qureshi MY, O'Leary PW, Connolly HM. Cardiac imaging in Ebstein anomaly. Trends Cardiovasc Med, 2018; 28: 403-409.
3. Williams T, Lluri G, Boyd EK, et al. Perioperative echocardiography in the adult with congenital heart disease. J Cardiothorac Vasc Anesth, 2020; 34: 1292-1308.

5. What is found most frequently in patients with Ebstein's anomaly?
   A. Atrial septal defect
   B. Ventricular septal defect
   C. Cleft mitral valve
   D. Anomalous pulmonary vein

Correct Answer: A

Explanation: In Ebstein's anomaly of the tricuspid valve, part of the tricuspid valve tissue is displaced apically by more than 8 mm/m^2. Downward displacement is seen most with the septal leaflet, followed by the posterior leaflet and the anterior leaflet. The anterior leaflet tends to be large and redundant. The defect is associated with a patent foramen ovale or a secundum atrial septal defect. There is "atrialization" of part of the right ventricle. The displacement of the tricuspid valve toward the right ventricular apex results in a portion of the right ventricle being above the tricuspid valve and becoming functionally part of the right atrium. Although a ventricular septal defect can be found in few patients, an atrial septal defect is present in 80% to 94% of Epstein patients. A cleft mitral valve and anomalous pulmonary veins are not typically associated with an Ebstein anomaly.

References:

1. Baum VC, de Souza DG. Chapter 18: Congenital Heart Disease in Adults. In: Kaplan JA, Augoustides JGT, Manecke GR, et al., eds. Kaplan's Cardiac Anesthesia. 7th ed. Elsevier; 2017: 818-842.
2. Qureshi MY, O'Leary PW, Connolly HM. Cardiac imaging in Ebstein anomaly. Trends Cardiovasc Med, 2018; 28: 403-409
3. Williams T, Lluri G, Boyd EK, et al. Perioperative echocardiography in the adult with congenital heart disease. J Cardiothorac Vasc Anesth, 2020; 34: 1292-1308.

6. A 54-year-old patient with a history of levo-transposition of the great arteries presents for tricuspid valve repair. Which anatomic correlation is correct?
   A. The tricuspid valve is associated with the right ventricle
   B. The aortic valve is associated with the left ventricle
   C. The pulmonic valve is associated with the right ventricle
   D. The inferior vena cava is associated with the left atrium

Correct Answer: A

Explanation: Regardless of any specific type of congenital heart disease, the tricuspid valve is always in continuity with the right ventricle, and the mitral valve with the left ventricle. In levo-transposition of the great arteries, as a consequence of the embryonic heart tube rotating to the left (levo) rather than to the right, the flow of blood is through normal vena cava to the right atrium, through a mitral valve to a right-sided morphologic left ventricle, to the pulmonary artery, through the pulmonary circulation, to the left atrium, through a tricuspid valve to a left-sided morphologic right ventricle, and thence to the aorta. Although anatomically altered, the physiologic flow of blood is appropriate, and there are no mandatory associated shunts. L-transposition of the great arteries is very frequently associated with other cardiac lesions, most commonly a ventricular septal defect, subpulmonic stenosis, heart block, or systemic atrioventricular (tricuspid) valve regurgitation. In the absence of any of these associated cardiac defects, it will usually be asymptomatic through infancy and childhood. When levo-transposition is an isolated lesion, most patients maintain normal biventricular function through early adulthood and can attain a normal life span. However, the relatively thin-walled morphologic right ventricle is not well suited to eject blood against systemic pressure. Over a lifetime, the right ventricle can fail, and the patient will develop heart failure. Systemic atrioventricular (tricuspid) valve insufficiency may not develop until later in life, resulting in approximately 60% of patients being diagnosed as adults. By the age of 45 years, heart failure will

be present in 67% of those patients with associated lesions and 25% of those without.

References:

1. Baum VC, de Souza DG. Chapter 18: Congenital Heart Disease in Adults. In: Kaplan JA, Augoustides JGT, Manecke GR, et al., eds. Kaplan's Cardiac Anesthesia. 7th ed. Elsevier; 2017:818-842.
2. Akpek EA, Miller-Hance WC, Stayer SA, et al. Anesthetic management and outcome of complex late arterial-switch operations for patients with transposition of the great arteries and a systemic right ventricle. J Cardiothorac Vasc Anesth, 2005; 19: 322-328.

7. A 34-year-old patient with a history of hypoplastic left heart syndrome and Fontan palliation is presenting for conduit revision for conduit stenosis. Which is the most likely cause for his baseline saturation of 86% on room air?
   A. Atrial septal defect
   B. Ventricular septal defect
   C. Veno-venous collaterals
   D. Aorto-pulmonary collaterals

Correct Answer: C

Explanation: The specific reasons for a failing Fontan circulation may differ, but the common denominator in these patients is a marked limitation of functional status. They will typically manifest with refractory arrhythmias, protein-losing enteropathy, liver dysfunction, hypoxemia, and/or congestive heart failure. The hallmark of the failing Fontan is typically an elevated central venous pressure, although the underlying etiologies may include a failing single right or left ventricle, significant atrioventricular valve regurgitation, and elevated pulmonary vascular resistance, among others. The resulting dysfunction may involve various major organ systems, including the liver. Liver cirrhosis can result in synthetic dysfunction and affect the coagulation system in many ways. Interestingly, patients are often hypercoagulable with thrombosis occurring in up to 30% of Fontan patients. Warfarin is often administered, and the anesthesiologist must consider complex coagulation disorders and drug effects in case a neuraxial technique is planned.

A mild degree of oxygen desaturation is present in most Fontan patients. This is typically due to coronary sinus blood draining into the common atrium. A small fenestration in the extracardiac conduit at the time of Fontan surgery allows for maintaining cardiac output if pulmonary vascular resistance increases will also be responsible for right-to-left shunting. If the central venous pressure is chronically elevated, large collaterals may form between the central venous and pulmonary venous system or pulmonary artery and pulmonary venous system with right-to-left shunting causing cyanosis. Aorto-pulmonary venous shunts are left-to-right shunts and cause volume load and heart failure symptoms. During the preoperative evaluation, desaturation at baseline should alert the practitioner to the presence of shunts, and most importantly elevated central venous pressure and failing Fontan physiology. In the above-described scenario, an atrial or ventricular septal defect is typically present in a single ventricle patient but is not the cause of cyanosis after Fontan palliation with both pulmonary and systemic circulation in series. Aortopulmonary collaterals cause left-to-right shunt and heart failure and not cyanosis.

References:

1. Baum VC, de Souza DG. Chapter 18: Congenital Heart Disease in Adults. In: Kaplan JA, Augoustides JGT, Manecke GR, et al., eds. Kaplan's Cardiac Anesthesia. 7th ed. Elsevier; 2017:818-842.
2. Eagle SS, Daves SM. The adult with Fontan physiology: systematic approach to perioperative management for noncardiac surgery. J Cardiothorac Vasc Anesth, 2011; 25: 320-334.
3. McNamara JR, McMahon A, Griffin M. Perioperative management of the Fontan patient for cardiac and non-cardiac surgery. J Cardiothorac Vasc Anesth, 2022; 36: 275-285.

8. In a patient with a persistent left superior vena cava, a pulmonary artery catheter inserted into the left internal jugular vein will most likely enter the atrium via which structure?
 A. Coronary sinus
 B. Superior vena cava
 C. Foramen ovale
 D. Thebesian vein

Correct Answer: A

Explanation: A persistent left superior vena cava (LSVC) is a venous vascular anomaly and can be found in 0.1% to 0.5% of the general population. The prevalence is higher in patients with congenital heart disease, and it is reported in up to 13% in certain forms of congenital heart disease. The prevalence also varies significantly based on the patient population and imaging techniques. A persistent LSVC most commonly drains into the right atrium via a dilated coronary sinus, although variations have been described. A bridging vein may connect the LSVC and right superior vena cava with variations of central venous drainage. In the vast majority of cases, a persistent LSVC drains into the right atrium via the coronary sinus, and a pulmonary artery catheter inadvertently inserted into the left internal jugular vein will follow the course of the LSVC and enter via the coronary sinus into the right atrium.

References:

1. Baum VC, de Souza DG. Chapter 18: Congenital Heart Disease in Adults. In: Kaplan JA, Augoustides JGT, Manecke GR, et al., eds. Kaplan's Cardiac Anesthesia. 7th ed. Elsevier; 2017:818-842.
2. Hang D, Pagryzinski AR, Zdanaovec A, et al. Dilated coronary sinus: the usual persistent left superior vena cava or a less common etiology. J Cardiothorac Vasc Anesth, 2022; 36; 2240-2243.

9. An 18-year-old patient with Williams syndrome presents for orthopedic surgery. Following anesthetic induction and endotracheal intubation, the heart rate increases to 154 beats per minute, the systemic blood pressure is 164/93 mmHg, and ST segment depressions develop on the electrocardiogram. What intervention is indicated next?
 A. Esmolol bolus
 B. Nitroglycerine bolus
 C. Sevoflurane increase
 D. Phenylephrine bolus

Correct Answer: A

Explanation: Williams syndrome is a genetic disorder caused by a deletion involving chromosome 7. Cardiac involvement includes supravalvular aortic stenosis, pulmonary artery stenosis, and coronary ostial stenosis in up to 45% of cases. The risk of sudden cardiac death is up to 100 times higher compared to control groups. Patients with Williams syndrome have some of the highest risks of perioperative cardiac events, and meticulous planning of the anesthetic and monitoring is imperative to prevent adverse events. Cardiac arrest can occur suddenly and, based on the multiple stenotic lesions that may be present, can be difficult to treat.

In the described scenario, the patient's level of anesthesia was not adequate, the patient is tachycardic, and the blood pressure is normal. Patients with Williams syndrome may have unrecognized coronary ostial stenosis, and acute coronary ischemia and imminent cardiac arrest may ensue. The key is an immediate decrease in oxygen demand. Although deepening the level of anesthesia is eventually required, increasing sevoflurane may further decrease blood pressure (BP) and cardiac function. The mechanical ostial stenosis is not amenable to coronary dilation, and in a patient who is tachycardic with normal BP, nitroglycerin may further decrease coronary perfusion. Esmolol as a short-acting beta blocker will decrease the heart rate and oxygen demand. Phenylephrine will help increase perfusion pressure and may also be indicated, but the main cause of hemodynamic compromise in the described scenario is the increased heart rate in the setting of coronary ostial stenosis.

References:

1. Baum VC, de Souza DG. Chapter 18: Congenital Heart Disease in Adults. In: Kaplan JA, Augoustides JGT, Manecke GR, et al., eds. Kaplan's Cardiac Anesthesia. 7th ed. Elsevier; 2017: 818-842.
2. Collins RT. Cardiovascular disease in Williams Syndrome. Circulation, 2013; 127: 2125-2134.
3. Staudt GE, Eagle SS. Anesthetic considerations for patients with Williams syndrome. J Cardiothorac Vasc Anesth, 2021; 35: 176-186.

10. Which of the aortic valve cusps are most commonly fused in the bicuspid aortic valve phenotype?
 A. Left-right fusion with a single raphe
 B. Non-right fusion with a single raphe
 C. Non-left fusion with a single raphe
 D. Left-right and right-non fusion with a double raphe

Correct Answer: A

Explanation: The bicuspid aortic valve is a common congenital cardiac anomaly, with an estimated incidence of 1% to 2% in the general population. The Sievers classification distinguishes various subtypes based on the presence or absence of a raphe. Type 0 is characterized by the absence of a raphe and typically has two symmetrical leaflets. Type 1 has a single raphe, with leaflet fusion to yield a conjoint leaflet as follows: most frequently left-right fusion, followed by right-non fusion, and then non-left fusion. Type 2 has a double raphe such as seen in left-right and right-non fusion.

References:

1. Baum VC, de Souza DG. Chapter 18: Congenital Heart Disease in Adults. In: Kaplan JA, Augoustides JGT, Manecke GR, et al., eds. Kaplan's Cardiac Anesthesia. 7th ed. Elsevier; 2017:818-842.
2. Ridley CH, Vallabhajosyula P, Bavaria JE, et al. The Sievers classification of the bicuspid aortic valve for the perioperative echocardiographer: the importance of valve phenotype for aortic valve repair in the era of the functional aortic annulus. J Cardiothorac Vasc Anesth, 2016; 30: 1142-1151.
3. Sievers HH, Schmidtke C. A classification system for the bicuspid aortic valve from 304 surgical specimens. J Thorac Cardiovasc Surg, 2007; 133: 1226-1233.

11. Which finding has been associated with a bicuspid aortic valve?
   A. Coarctation of aorta
   B. Atrial septal defect
   C. Pulmonary valve stenosis
   D. Abdominal aortic aneurysm

Correct Answer: A

Explanation: A bicuspid aortic valve presents most commonly in isolation in adults with approximately 15% of cases associated with congenital heart abnormalities versus about 50% in young children. The associated cardiovascular manifestations include coarctation of the aorta, Shone complex, ventricular septal defect, ascending aortic aneurysm, and aortic dissection. A bicuspid aortic valve is not typically associated with an atrial septal defect or an abdominal aortic aneurysm. The Shone complex is a constellation of a congenital mitral valve abnormality such as a parachute mitral valve in association with left-sided obstructive lesions such as aortic stenosis and aortic coarctation.

References:

1. Baum VC, de Souza DG. Chapter 18: Congenital Heart Disease in Adults. In: Kaplan JA, Augoustides JGT, Manecke GR, et al., eds. Kaplan's Cardiac Anesthesia. 7th ed. Elsevier; 2017:818-842.
2. Michelena HI. Speaking a common language: the international consensus on bicuspid aortic valve nomenclature and classification. Ann Cardiothorac Surg, 2022; 11: 402-417.
3. Rehfeldt KH, Mauermann WJ, Suri RM, et al. The diagnosis of Shone's anomaly by intraoperative transesophageal echocardiography. J Cardiothorac Vasc Anesth, 2009; 23: 75-76.
4. Ridley CH, Vallabhajosyula P, Bavaria JE, et al. The Sievers classification of the bicuspid aortic valve for the perioperative echocardiographer: the importance of valve phenotype for aortic valve repair in the era of the functional aortic annulus. J Cardiothorac Vasc Anesth, 2016; 30: 1142-1151.

12. A 19-year-old patient who was recently diagnosed with a ventricular septal defect presents for closure. The superior vena cava saturation is 69%, the radial artery saturation is 100%, the oxygen saturation drawn from the pulmonary artery catheter is 83%. What is the estimated pulmonary to systemic flow ratio (Qp:Qs)?
   A. 1.6/1
   B. 1.8/1
   C. 2/1
   D. 2.2/1

Correct Answer: B

Explanation: A quick, simplified way to estimate the intracardiac shunt fraction in patients is calculating the pulmonary to systemic flow ratio using the following formula: QP/QS = (aortic saturation − systemic venous saturation)/(pulmonary venous saturation − pulmonary arterial saturation). With a normal cardiac index, the arterio-venous oxygen difference is around 25%. Not accounting for a physiological intrapulmonary shunt, the pulmonary venous saturation can be assumed to be 100%. The venous saturation must be drawn from the superior vena cava (central venous saturation), as a mixed venous saturation (i.e., pulmonary artery) will by definition include blood from the intracardiac shunt, and a sample drawn from the right atrium may also show a step-up in saturation in case an atrial septal defect is present.

A normal pulmonary artery saturation in healthy individuals is typically 70% to 75% (assuming 25%–30% oxygen extraction). A normal central venous saturation is 70%. The oxygen saturation in the superior vena cava is typically 2% to 5% higher compared to a sample from the pulmonary artery. A step-up in mean oxygen saturation of 7% between the caval chambers and the right atrium is diagnostic of an atrial septal defect. A step-up of 5% between the right atrium and right ventricle is diagnostic for a ventricular septal defect.

In the question asked, the QP/QS ratio is as follows:

$$(100 − 69) / (100 − 83) = 31/17 = 1.8/1$$

References:

1. Baum VC, de Souza DG. Chapter 18: Congenital Heart Disease in Adults. In: Kaplan JA, Augoustides JGT, Manecke GR, et al., eds. Kaplan's Cardiac Anesthesia. 7th ed. Elsevier; 2017:818-842.
2. Chassot PG, Bettex DA. Anesthesia and adult congenital heart disease. J Cardiothorac Vasc Anesth, 2006; 20: 414-437.

13. A 27-year-old patient presents for primum atrial septal defect repair. What is a typical associated finding?
   A. Mitral regurgitation
   B. Tricuspid regurgitation
   C. Aortic regurgitation
   D. Pulmonic regurgitation

Correct Answer: A

Explanation: A primum atrial septal defect is a defect in the endocardial cushion. The typical representative of these defects is a complete atrioventricular canal defect that includes an atrial septal defect, a ventricular septal defect, and a common atrioventricular valve. A partial or incomplete atrioventricular canal defect has a very small or no ventricular septal defect, a primum atrial septal defect, and associated defects of the atrioventricular valves. A cleft of the anterior mitral valve is often present. Although a complete atrioventricular canal defect typically manifests at birth and is repaired early in infancy, a partial atrioventricular canal defect with a small primum atrial septal defect may only present in adulthood with mitral regurgitation due to a cleft mitral valve. The perioperative echocardiographer may also detect a small primum atrial septal defect with or without a small ventricular septal defect at the time of the cleft mitral valve repair.

References:

1. Baum VC, de Souza DG. Chapter 18: Congenital Heart Disease in Adults. In: Kaplan JA, Augoustides JGT, Manecke GR, et al., eds. Kaplan's Cardiac Anesthesia. 7th ed. Elsevier; 2017:818-842.
2. Williams T, Lluri G, Boyd EK, et al. Perioperative echocardiography in the adult with congenital heart disease. J Cardiothorac Vasc Anesth, 2020; 34: 1292-1308.
3. Chassot PG, Bettex DA. Anesthesia and adult congenital heart disease. J Cardiothorac Vasc Anesth, 2006; 20: 414-437.

14. Which arrhythmia is most frequently seen as a long-term consequence in patients with Fontan palliation?
   A. Ventricular fibrillation
   B. Monomorphic ventricular tachycardia
   C. Atrial fibrillation
   D. Intra-atrial reentrant tachycardia

Correct Answer: D

Explanation: Fontan patients show a steady increase in atrial tachyarrhythmias with an incidence of over 50% at 20 years. Changes in surgical technique evolved in part to decrease the rate of atrial arrhythmias. Although initial results were promising, unfortunately much of this benefit is lost with longer-term follow-up. Fontan patients tolerate tachycardia very poorly, and acute episodes usually require urgent medical intervention to control ventricular rate and/or to achieve cardioversion to sinus rhythm. Late-onset atrial tachyarrhythmias usually occur between 6 to 10 years after Fontan completion. The most common tachyarrhythmia is right intra-atrial reentrant tachycardia. Over time, episodic attacks of tachycardia become more frequent. Frequently, atrial fibrillation occurs, and the loss of atrioventricular synchrony results in decreased effort tolerance. The onset of atrial tachyarrhythmias often prompts an evaluation of the Fontan pathway with attention turned to relieving any significant obstructions. The management options for chronic atrial arrhythmias in this setting include medical control, catheter ablation, and/or surgical intervention. Given the complex anatomy, chronically dilated atrial morphology, and atrial scar with suture lines from prior surgeries, it is not surprising that atrial arrhythmias can become refractory to standard treatment in many patients. Although catheter ablation typically has a high initial success rate, this therapeutic effect may not be durable in the long term.

References:

1. Baum VC, de Souza DG. Chapter 18: Congenital Heart Disease in Adults. In: Kaplan JA, Augoustides JGT, Manecke GR, et al., eds. Kaplan's Cardiac Anesthesia. 7th ed. Elsevier; 2017:818-842.
2. Eagle SS, Daves SM. The adult with Fontan physiology: systematic approach to perioperative management for noncardiac surgery. J Cardiothorac Vasc Anesth, 2011; 25: 320-334.
3. McNamara JR, McMahon A, Griffin M. Perioperative management of the Fontan patient for cardiac and non-cardiac surgery. J Cardiothorac Vasc Anesth, 2022; 36: 275-285.

15. What is a typical consequence in adulthood after an arterial switch operation for dextro-transposition of great arteries as a newborn?
   A. Normal life expectancy
   B. Atrial arrhythmias
   C. Aorto-pulmonary collaterals
   D. Right ventricular dysfunction

Correct Answer: A

Explanation: Dextro-transposition of the great arteries, unlike levo-transposition of the great arteries, is not compatible with prolonged life as a newborn, prompting surgical correction with the arterial switch operation within the first few days of life. The pulmonary artery and ascending aorta are reconnected to their respective ventricles, and the coronary arteries are moved into correct position as well. Consequently, the left ventricle will pump systemic, and the right ventricle pulmonary blood flow. The native aortic valve will remain connected to the right ventricle, and the pulmonic valve will continue to serve as the "neoaortic valve." After the initial perioperative morbidity and mortality, these patients have an almost normal life expectancy based on currently available long-term outcome data. Long-term consequences in this setting include aortic regurgitation and/or coronary implantation issues that may necessitate transcatheter and/or surgical intervention. Before the arterial switch operation, patients typically had an atrial switch type repair (Mustard or Senning procedure). After a Mustard or Senning operation as an infant, the right ventricle continues to serve as the systemic ventricle, thus explaining the higher likelihood of systemic ventricular failure later in life. The complex atrial suture lines also put the patients at risk for atrial arrhythmias. Aorto-pulmonary collaterals are not a typical complication following surgery for dextro-transposition of the great arteries.

References:

1. Baum VC, de Souza DG. Chapter 18: Congenital Heart Disease in Adults. In: Kaplan JA, Augoustides JGT, Manecke GR, et al., eds. Kaplan's Cardiac Anesthesia. 7th ed. Elsevier; 2017:818-842.

2. Fricke TA, Buratto E, Weintraub RG, et al. Long-term outcomes of the arterial switch operation. J Thorac Cardiovasc Surg, 2022; 163: 212-219.
3. Akpek EA, Miller-Hance WC, Stayer SA, et al. Anesthetic management and outcome of complex late arterial-switch operations for patients with transposition of the great arteries and a systemic right ventricle. J Cardiothorac Vasc Anesth, 2005; 19: 322-328.
4. Chassot PG, Bettex DA. Anesthesia and adult congenital heart disease. J Cardiothorac Vasc Anesth, 2006; 20: 414-437.

16. In patients with Fontan palliation for tricuspid atresia, what is a typical consequence later in life?
   A. Right ventricular failure
   B. Hypercoagulability
   C. Aortic regurgitation
   D. Tricuspid regurgitation

Correct Answer: B

Explanation: Fontan palliation may result in marked limitation of functional status. Patients may manifest refractory arrhythmias, protein-losing enteropathy, liver dysfunction, hypoxemia, and/or congestive heart failure. The hallmark of the failing Fontan is typically an elevated central venous pressure, with a failing single right or left ventricle, significant atrioventricular valve regurgitation, and elevated pulmonary vascular resistance. The resulting dysfunction can affect major organ systems, including the liver. Liver cirrhosis can result in synthetic dysfunction and affect the coagulation system in many ways. Interestingly, patients are often hypercoagulable, with thrombosis occurring in up to 30% of Fontan patients. Warfarin is often administered, and the anesthesiologist must consider complex coagulation disorders and drug effects in case a neuraxial technique is planned. In patients with tricuspid atresia, the functional ventricle is the left ventricle; thus, right ventricular failure is not an option. The aortic valve is the native aortic valve and regurgitation is not a typical complication. The tricuspid valve is atretic. Even in functional Fontan patients, thromboembolic events are not uncommon, and patients are frequently anticoagulated for this reason. The mechanisms for hypercoagulabilty include low levels of antithrombotic proteins such as antithrombin, protein C, and protein S.

References:
1. Baum VC, de Souza DG. Chapter 18: Congenital Heart Disease in Adults. In: Kaplan JA, Augoustides JGT, Manecke GR, et al., eds. Kaplan's Cardiac Anesthesia. 7th ed. Elsevier; 2017:818-842.
2. Eagle SS, Daves SM. The adult with Fontan physiology: systematic approach to perioperative management for noncardiac surgery. J Cardiothorac Vasc Anesth, 2011; 25: 320-334.
3. McNamara JR, McMahon A, Griffin M. Perioperative management of the Fontan patient for cardiac and non-cardiac surgery. J Cardiothorac Vasc Anesth, 2022; 36: 275-285.

17. A pulmonary artery catheter is placed in an adult patient with a large atrial septal defect. Which statement with regards to the measured thermodilution cardiac output is correct?
   A. Systemic flow overestimated
   B. Pulmonic flow overestimated
   C. Systemic flow underestimated
   D. Pulmonic flow underestimated

Correct Answer: A

Explanation: A pulmonary arterial catheter is not typically indicated in patients with an atrial septal defect; however, in selected adult cases it may guide treatment options in case of right ventricular failure after repair. Prior to repair, the atrial level of shunting will cause a more rapid dilution of the injectate. The area under the temperature change time curve will be smaller, and the measured cardiac output will not be reflective of systemic cardiac output. The measured cardiac output will overestimate the systemic cardiac output.

References:
1. Baum VC, de Souza DG. Chapter 18: Congenital Heart Disease in Adults. In: Kaplan JA, Augoustides JGT, Manecke GR, et al., eds. Kaplan's Cardiac Anesthesia. 7th ed. Elsevier; 2017:818-842.
2. Bootsma IT, Boerma EC, Scheeren TWL, et al. The contemporary pulmonary artery catheter. Part 2: measurements, limitations, and clinical applications. J Clin Monit Comp, 2022; 36: 17-31.

18. A 45-year-old patient with levo-transposition of the great arteries presents for tricuspid valve repair for severe tricuspid regurgitation. What is a common consequence in these patients?
   A. Ascites
   B. Coagulation disorders
   C. Pulmonary congestion
   D. Dilation of the ascending aorta

Correct Answer: C

Explanation: In levo-transposition of the great arteries, the deoxygenated venous blood enters the right atrium and from there flows through the mitral valve and left ventricle to the pulmonary artery trunk. The pulmonary venous blood enters the left atrium and flows through the tricuspid valve and right ventricle to the aorta. Thus, a parallel circulation and "normal" systemic and pulmonary circuits allow for oxygenated systemic blood flow. However, since the ventricles are reversed, the right ventricle pumps systemic blood, and the left ventricle pulmonary blood. Patients with this condition can reach adulthood relatively asymptomatic until the systemic right ventricle starts failing from the increased afterload and they present with congestive heart failure.

References:
1. Baum VC, de Souza DG. Chapter 18: Congenital Heart Disease in Adults. In: Kaplan JA, Augoustides JGT, Manecke GR, et al., eds. Kaplan's Cardiac Anesthesia. 7th ed. Elsevier; 2017:818-842.
2. Akpek EA, Miller-Hance WC, Stayer SA, et al. Anesthetic management and outcome of complex late arterial-switch

operations for patients with transposition of the great arteries and a systemic right ventricle. J Cardiothorac Vasc Anesth, 2005; 19: 322-328.

19. A 38-year-old patient presents for surgery for a supravalvular mitral ring. What is frequently seen in these patients?
A. Pulmonary hypertension
B. Primum atrial septal defect
C. Ascending aorta aneurysm
D. Mitral valve stenosis

Correct Answer: A

Explanation: The supramitral ring is functionally a type of mitral valve stenosis. A membrane or ridge of connective tissue is located just above the mitral valve annulus and inferior to the left atrial appendage. An opening of variable size allows blood flow from the larger upper chamber to the smaller lower chamber enclosed between the supramitral membrane above and the mitral valve apparatus below. In cases where the opening is small, the typical symptoms and findings of mitral stenosis including pulmonary hypertension can be seen. With the supramitral ring, unlike the intramitral type, the mitral valve itself is typically normal, and not stenotic. Although it can exist as an isolated defect, in the majority of cases a supramitral ring is associated with other congenital heart defects, mostly left-sided obstructive lesions including subvalvular aortic stenosis, aortic coarctation as well as ventricular septal defects, and tetralogy of Fallot.

References:

1. Baum VC, de Souza DG. Chapter 18: Congenital Heart Disease in Adults. In: Kaplan JA, Augoustides JGT, Manecke GR, et al., eds. Kaplan's Cardiac Anesthesia. 7th ed. Elsevier; 2017:818-842.
2. Burbano N. Congenital mitral stenosis. J Cardiothorac Vasc Anesth, 2020; 34: 2272-2273.

20. A 28-year-old patient with a ventricular septal defect and Eisenmenger syndrome presents for noncardiac surgery. Baseline saturation is 91%. Immediately after anesthesia induction, the saturation drops to 79%. What intervention will most likely help improve his saturation?
A. Increasing the inspired oxygen concentration
B. Vasopressin bolus
C. Inhaled nitric oxide
D. Fluid bolus

Correct Answer: B

Explanation: Eisenmenger syndrome typically refers to the end stage of a large left-to-right shunt resulting in increased pulmonary vascular resistance and irreversible pulmonary vascular changes. Ultimately, severe pulmonary hypertension results in right-to-left shunting with cyanosis, progressive hypoxemia, and heart failure. In general, at the end stage, the pulmonary vasculature will not be responsive to pulmonary vasodilators, and any drop in systemic vascular resistance will further increase the right-left shunt and cyanosis. In the described case, an immediate desaturation following

anesthesia induction is most likely related to the decrease in blood pressure from systemic vasodilation. Most patients are induced with 100% oxygen, and even if a lower fraction of inspired oxygen (FiO_2) was chosen, increasing the FiO_2 with a large right-to-left shunt will not have the same effect as restoring systemic vascular resistance and thereby decreasing the shunt. Vasopressin may have the least effect on pulmonary vascular resistance, although with the mostly fixed pulmonary vascular resistance, the choice of vasoconstrictor may not be as important.

References:

1. Baum VC, de Souza DG. Chapter 18: Congenital Heart Disease in Adults. In: Kaplan JA, Augoustides JGT, Manecke GR, et al., eds. Kaplan's Cardiac Anesthesia. 7th ed. Elsevier; 2017:818-842.
2. Lopez BM, Malhame I, Davies LK, et al. Eisenmenger syndrome in pregnancy: a management conundrum. J Cardiothorac Vasc Anesth, 2020; 34: 2813-2822.

21. A 31-year-old patient with a history of complex congenital heart disease and Fontan palliation presents for knee surgery. Which anesthesia technique is most appropriate?
A. Spinal
B. General
C. Regional block with moderate sedation
D. Epidural

Correct Answer: B

Explanation: The anesthetic goals are maintaining preload, afterload, contractility (cardiac output), and normal sinus rhythm. There is no one best anesthetic or drug in patients with Fontan physiology. There is no consensus about what anesthetic drug or technique is associated with the best outcomes in Fontan patients. Although spontaneous ventilation theoretically will help maintain pulmonary blood flow, hypercapnia and atelectasis from shallow breathing may further increase pulmonary vascular and offset any potential benefits associated with spontaneous ventilation. Most experienced practitioners will choose a general anesthetic, avoid sudden decreases in preload and venous blood return, and choose a ventilation strategy with a low-level positive end-expiratory pressure to avoid atelectasis. Neuraxial techniques, and in particular spinal anesthesia, can cause a sudden decrease in blood pressure and venous blood return and are typically best avoided. Although epidural catheters can be titrated slowly and may be ideal for postoperative pain management, neuraxial catheters can be problematic in patients with Fontan physiology who may present with complex coagulation disorders. Equally important to intraoperative management is an appropriate plan for postoperative analgesia. Postoperative pain resulting in humoral stress response with tachycardia and hypercapnia should be avoided.

References:

1. Baum VC, de Souza DG. Chapter 18: Congenital Heart Disease in Adults. In: Kaplan JA, Augoustides JGT, Manecke GR,

et al., eds. Kaplan's Cardiac Anesthesia. 7th ed. Elsevier; 2017:818-842.

2. Eagle SS, Daves SM. The adult with Fontan physiology: systematic approach to perioperative management for noncardiac surgery. J Cardiothorac Vasc Anesth, 2011; 25: 320-334.

3. McNamara JR, McMahon A, Griffin M. Perioperative management of the Fontan patient for cardiac and non-cardiac surgery. J Cardiothorac Vasc Anesth, 2022; 36: 275-285.

22. A 28-year-old patient with a ventricular septal defect and Eisenmenger syndrome presents for noncardiac surgery. Baseline saturation is 91%. After anesthetic induction, the saturation drops to 85%. Which intervention will likely help improve his saturation?

A. Increasing inspired oxygen concentration

B. Norepinephrine

C. Nitric oxide

D. Fluid bolus

Correct Answer: B

Explanation: Eisenmenger syndrome with a ventricular septal defect implies an end stage of a large left-to-right shunt resulting in severe pulmonary vascular resistance that progresses to right-to-left shunting with cyanosis, progressive hypoxemia, and heart failure. In general, at the end stage, the pulmonary vasculature will be minimally responsive to pulmonary vasodilators to reduce the right-to-left shunt such as hyperoxia, hypocarbia, and inhaled pulmonary vasodilators such as nitric oxide. Acute decreases in systemic vascular resistance will further increase the right-to-left shunt and worsen hypoxia with increasing degrees of cyanosis. In the described case, an immediate desaturation following anesthesia induction is most likely related to systemic vasodilation. Vasopressin may have the least effect on pulmonary vascular resistance, although with the mostly fixed pulmonary vascular resistance the choice of systemic vasoconstrictor may not be as important. Norepinephrine will also increase the systemic vascular resistance and restore oxygenation with reduced right-to-left shunting.

References:

1. Baum VC, de Souza DG. Chapter 18: Congenital Heart Disease in Adults. In: Kaplan JA, Augoustides JGT, Manecke GR, et al., eds. Kaplan's Cardiac Anesthesia. 7th ed. Elsevier; 2017:818-842.

2. Lopez BM, Malhame I, Davies LK, et al. Eisenmenger syndrome in pregnancy: a management conundrum. J Cardiothorac Vasc Anesth, 2020; 34: 2813-2822.

23. A 19-year-old patient with limited effort tolerance and no history of cyanotic spells presents for surgical correction of a large membranous ventricular septal defect associated with pulmonary stenosis. Following anesthetic induction, the patient develops severe hypotension and significant hypoxia. Which intervention is most indicated to restore the blood pressure and improve oxygen saturation?

A. Nitric oxide

B. Milrinone

C. Volume bolus

D. Norepinephrine

Correct Answer: D

Explanation: The described scenario describes an adult patient with tetralogy type ventricular septal defect (VSD) and pulmonary stenosis. Tetralogy of Fallot (TOF) is a spectrum of congenital abnormalities, with a TOF-type VSD and left-to-right shunt on one end of the spectrum and a VSD with pulmonary atresia at the other end. Most commonly, TOF includes the following elements: a VSD with overriding aorta (malalignment VSD); various degrees of subvalvular (infundibular), valvular, and supravalvular pulmonary stenosis; and right ventricular hypertrophy. The shunt in these patients is right-to-left and may include dynamic right ventricular outflow obstruction, predisposing the patient to cyanotic spells. These patients present with cyanosis early in life and typically undergo surgical correction during infancy. However, a few patients with a large VSD, unobstructed right ventricular outflow tract, and valvular pulmonary stenosis may survive into adulthood, despite a large VSD. The pulmonary stenosis "protects" the lungs from the otherwise systemic pressure. In the described patient, the "pulmonary vascular resistance" is fixed (due to valvular stenosis) and not amenable to pulmonary vasodilators. The likely cause of desaturation is a decrease in systemic vascular resistance, causing an increase in right-to-left shunting. Restoring the systemic vascular resistance will decrease the shunting and force more blood through the stenotic pulmonary valve and pulmonary circulation.

References:

1. Baum VC, de Souza DG. Chapter 18: Congenital Heart Disease in Adults. In: Kaplan JA, Augoustides JGT, Manecke GR, et al., eds. Kaplan's Cardiac Anesthesia. 7th ed. Elsevier; 2017:818-842.

2. Chassot PG, Bettex DA. Anesthesia and adult congenital heart disease. J Cardiothorac Vasc Anesth, 2006; 20: 414-437.

24. A 46-year-old patient with a history of dextro-transposition of the great arteries and a Mustard correction presents for an ablation procedure in the electrophysiology lab. What is a typical concern in these patients later in life and should be considered in the preprocedural anesthesia assessment?

A. Right ventricular failure

B. Pulmonary arterial hypertension

C. Aorto-pulmonary collaterals

D. Protein-losing enteropathy

Correct Answer: A

Explanation: Patients with dextro-transposition of the great arteries (unlike levo-transposition of the great arteries) typically requires surgical intervention in early infancy. The pulmonary and systemic circulation are separate, and unless there is adequate shunting from an associated patent ductus arteriosus, atrial septal defect, and/or ventricular septal defect, the lesion is not compatible with life. The standard contemporary approach is the arterial switch operation that has excellent long-term outcomes. However, a few adult patients may present who had an atrial switch operation (Mustard or Senning) prior to the surgical introduction of the arterial switch operation in the mid-1980s. In these patients, the morphologic right ventricle will provide systemic blood flow, with right ventricular failure and tricuspid regurgitation as consequences in later adult life. Furthermore, many of these patients present with atrial arrhythmias.

References:

1. Baum VC, de Souza DG. Chapter 18: Congenital Heart Disease in Adults. In: Kaplan JA, Augoustides JGT, Manecke GR, et al., eds. Kaplan's Cardiac Anesthesia. 7th ed. Elsevier; 2017:818-842.
2. Chassot PG, Bettex DA. Anesthesia and adult congenital heart disease. J Cardiothorac Vasc Anesth, 2006; 20: 414-437.
3. Akpek EA, Miller-Hance WC, Stayer SA, et al. Anesthetic management and outcome of complex late arterial-switch operations for patients with transposition of the great arteries and a systemic right ventricle. J Cardiothorac Vasc Anesth, 2005; 19: 322-328.

25. A 27-year-old patient with a history of tetralogy of Fallot repaired in infancy presents for pulmonary valve replacement. During dissection, there are acute inferior ST segment changes that rapidly progress to ventricular fibrillation. What is the most likely cause?
    A. Injury to the right coronary artery
    B. Coronary air embolization
    C. Right ventricle to pulmonary artery conduit compression
    D. Dynamic obstruction of the right ventricular outflow tract

Correct Answer: A

Explanation: Anomalous coronary arteries have a high prevalence in patients with tetralogy of Fallot with an incidence of 2% to 23%. These anomalies may result in a coronary artery crossing the right ventricular outflow tract that may not be immediately visible even during initial repair, due to myocardial bridging and overlying epicardial fat. When patients present for pulmonary valve reoperation later in life, additional challenges arise from pericardial adhesions due to previous surgery. During surgical dissection in this setting, there is a high risk of coronary injury, with subsequent myocardial ischemia and adverse surgical outcomes. The presence of a significant coronary artery or its branch crossing the right ventricular outflow tract necessitates a change in the surgical strategy. The coronary anatomy is therefore typically defined before surgical intervention with appropriate imaging to facilitate adaptation of the surgical approach to the pulmonary valve.

References:

1. Baum VC, de Souza DG. Chapter 18: Congenital Heart Disease in Adults. In: Kaplan JA, Augoustides JGT, Manecke GR, et al., eds. Kaplan's Cardiac Anesthesia. 7th ed. Elsevier; 2017:818-842.
2. Talwar S, Sengupta S, Marathe S, et al. Tetralogy of Fallot with coronary crossing the right ventricular outflow tract: a tale of a bridge and the artery. Ann Pediatr Cardiol, 2021; 14: 53-62.
3. Koppel CJ, Jongbloed MRM, Kies P, et al. Coronary anomalies in tetralogy of Fallot – a meta-analysis. Int J Cardiol, 2020; 306: 78-85.

26. What is a typical consequence of a persistent left superior vena cava in adulthood?
    A. Right ventricular failure
    B. Left ventricular failure
    C. Pulmonary arterial hypertension
    D. No pathophysiological findings

Correct Answer: D

Explanation: A persistent left superior vena cava (LSVC) is prevalent in 0.1% to 0.3% of the general population. This incidence increases significantly to 5% to 11% in patients with congenital heart disease. The LSVC in the majority of cases drains into the coronary sinus, which is typically dilated. There are typically no pathophysiological consequences, as a persistent LSVC is typically asymptomatic and is often an incidental finding. It does not cause ventricular failure or pulmonary arterial hypertension. However, there are implications for central venous access and in particular placement of a pulmonary artery catheter. The left internal jugular vein is typically larger compared to the right internal jugular vein (reverse from normal). The insertion of a pulmonary artery into the left internal jugular vein should be avoided if the presence of a persistent LSVC is known. If unknown, the pulmonary artery catheter will follow the course of the coronary sinus to reach the right heart, and the typical waveforms are typically appreciated at higher insertion depths than expected. The surgeons must also consider the presence of a LSVC, as retrograde cardioplegia is not feasible because an adequate retrograde cardioplegia pressure cannot be achieved and it will drain into the LSVC rather than the coronary venous system. Furthermore, the excessive venous blood return in the surgical field will persist despite bicaval venous cannulation. The presence of a LSVC may be diagnosed with preoperative imaging. It can also be diagnosed by intraoperative transesophageal echocardiography with the appearance of agitated saline contrast entering the right atrium via the coronary sinus after its injection into a left upper extremity vein.

References:

1. Baum VC, de Souza DG. Chapter 18: Congenital Heart Disease in Adults. In: Kaplan JA, Augoustides JGT, Manecke GR, et al., eds. Kaplan's Cardiac Anesthesia. 7th ed. Elsevier; 2017:818-842.
2. Chassot PG, Bettex DA. Anesthesia and adult congenital heart disease. J Cardiothorac Vasc Anesth, 2006; 20: 414-437.
3. Hang D, Pagryzinski AR, Zdanaovec A, et al. Dilated coronary sinus: the usual persistent left superior vena cava or a less common etiology. J Cardiothorac Vasc Anesth, 2022; 36: 2240-2243.

27. A 54-year-old patient presents for mitral valve repair for mitral regurgitation. Following the start of cardiopulmonary bypass and opening of the atrium, the surgeon complains about excessive blood in the surgical field. Aside from problems related to cardiopulmonary bypass, what should be considered as a cause?
   A. Persistent left superior vena cava
   B. Aortic regurgitation
   C. Persistent foramen ovale
   D. Anomalous left coronary artery origin

Correct Answer: A

Explanation: A persistent left superior vena cava (LSVC) is present in 0.1% to 0.3% of the general population, and is typically an incidental finding. This incidence increases significantly to 5% to 11% in patients with congenital heart disease. The LSVC in the majority of cases drains into the coronary sinus, which is typically dilated. The left as compared to the right internal jugular vein is also typically enlarged compared to the right internal jugular vein. The presence of a LSVC may be diagnosed with preoperative imaging. It can also be diagnosed by intraoperative transesophageal echocardiography with the appearance of agitated saline contrast entering the right atrium via the coronary sinus after its injection into a left upper extremity vein. If inserted via the left internal jugular vein, a pulmonary artery catheter will follow the course of the coronary sinus to reach the right heart, and the typical waveforms are typically appreciated at higher insertion depths than expected. The presence of a LSVC can also affect the conduct of the surgical procedure. Despite bicaval cannulation, the excessive blood return from the coronary sinus can interfere with surgical exposure in the heart. This may necessitate cannulation of the dilated coronary sinus for additional venous drainage to create a bloodless field and restore surgical exposure. Furthermore, retrograde cardioplegia is not feasible because an adequate retrograde cardioplegia pressure cannot be achieved and it will drain into the LSVC rather than the coronary venous system. Aortic regurgitation, a patent foramen ovale, and an anomalous origin of a left coronary origin do not typically increase venous return to obscure the surgical field during cardiac surgery.

References:

1. Baum VC, de Souza DG. Chapter 18: Congenital Heart Disease in Adults. In: Kaplan JA, Augoustides JGT, Manecke GR, et al., eds. Kaplan's Cardiac Anesthesia. 7th ed. Elsevier; 2017:818-842.
2. Chassot PG, Bettex DA. Anesthesia and adult congenital heart disease. J Cardiothorac Vasc Anesth, 2006; 20: 414-437.
3. Hang D, Pagryzinski AR, Zdanaovec A, et al. Dilated coronary sinus: the usual persistent left superior vena cava or a less common etiology. J Cardiothorac Vasc Anesth, 2022; 36; 2240-2243.

28. A 54-year-old patient presents for mitral valve repair for mitral regurgitation. Transesophageal echocardiography shows a large billowing mitral valve with a single papillary muscle. What should be assessed for as a potential additional finding?
   A. Subvalvular aortic stenosis
   B. Aorto-pulmonary collaterals
   C. Descending aortic aneurysm
   D. Pulmonary stenosis

Correct Answer: A

Explanation: Shone's anomaly (complex) consists of congenital mitral anomalies associated with left-sided obstructive lesions. The congenital mitral anomalies include a supravalvular ring and a parachute mitral valve. A parachute mitral valve has all the chordal apparatus attached to a single large papillary valve, as described in this clinical vignette. It may be associated with a syndrome or may occur in isolation. It can present as an incidental finding, or with advanced mitral regurgitation or stenosis. In the described case with a parachute mitral valve, the practitioner should assess the patient for these additional left-sided findings such as subvalvular aortic stenosis, bicuspid aortic valve, and aortic coarctation. The Shone complex does not include aorto-pulmonary collaterals, descending aortic aneurysm, or pulmonary stenosis.

References:

1. Baum VC, de Souza DG. Chapter 18: Congenital Heart Disease in Adults. In: Kaplan JA, Augoustides JGT, Manecke GR, et al., eds. Kaplan's Cardiac Anesthesia. 7th ed. Elsevier; 2017:818-842.
2. Rehfleldt KH, Mauermann WJ, Suri RM, et al. The diagnosis of Shone's anomaly by intraoperative transesophageal echocardiography. J Cardiothorac Vasc Anesth, 2009; 23: 75-76.
3. Misra S, Koshy T, Dash PKl. Diagnosis of Shone's anomaly by intraoperative transesophageal echocardiography in an adult patient undergoing repair of coarctation of the aorta. J Cardiothorac Vasc Anesth, 2011; 25: 838-840.
4. Aslam S, Khairy P, Shohoudi A, et al. Shone complex: an underrecognized congenital heart disease with substantial morbidity in adulthood. Can J Cardiol, 2017; 33: 253-259.

29. What coronary abnormality is associated with the highest risk of sudden cardiac death?
   A. Circumflex coronary artery from right sinus of Valsalva
   B. Single coronary artery
   C. Anomalous right coronary artery from left sinus of Valsalva
   D. Anomalous left coronary artery from right sinus of Valsalva

Correct Answer: D

Explanation: The anomalous origin of the circumflex coronary artery from the right sinus or right coronary artery is the most frequent coronary anomaly. However, both the right-from-left and left-from-right anomalies are associated with a much higher incidence of sudden cardiac death. The anomalous left coronary artery from the right sinus is considered more malignant and found more frequently in autopsies of patients with sudden cardiac death because of the large amount of left ventricular myocardium involved.

References:

1. Baum VC, de Souza DG. Chapter 18: Congenital Heart Disease in Adults. In: Kaplan JA, Augoustides JGT, Manecke GR, et al., eds. Kaplan's Cardiac Anesthesia. 7th ed. Elsevier; 2017:818-842.
2. Finocchiaro G, Behr ER, Tanzarella G, et al. Anomalous coronary artery origin and sudden cardiac death: clinical and pathological insights from a national pathology registry. JACC: Clinical Electrophysiology, 2019; 5: 516-522.
3, Bêique F, De Tran QH, Ma F, et al. Anomalous right coronary artery originating from the left sinus of Valsalva. J Cardiothorac Vasc Anesth, 2004; 18: 788-798.
4. Addis DR, Townsley MM. Implications of congenital coronary anomalies for the cardiothoracic anesthesiologist: overview of the 2020 ASE recommendations for the multimodality assessment of congenital coronary anomalies. J Cardiothorac Vasc Anesth, 2020; 34: 2291-2296.

30. What is the most common cyanotic congenital heart disease in adults?
   A. Tetralogy of Fallot
   B. Epstein's anomaly
   C. Atrial septal defect
   D. Pulmonary stenosis

Correct Answer: A

Explanation: A bicuspid aortic valve, certain types of degenerative mitral valve disease, and coronary anomalies may have a higher incidence, but are often not included when assessing the prevalence of congenital heart disease in the general population. In adult congenital heart disease, a secundum atrial septal defect often has the highest incidence. However, the most common cyanotic congenital heart disease across most age groups is the tetralogy of Fallot. This condition has an estimated incidence of 421 cases per million live births. It is defined by anterior deviation of the interventricular septum resulting in a ventricular septal defect, overriding aorta, right ventricular outflow tract obstruction, and consequent right ventricular hypertrophy.

References:

1. Baum VC, de Souza DG. Chapter 18: Congenital Heart Disease in Adults. In: Kaplan JA, Augoustides JGT, Manecke GR, et al., eds. Kaplan's Cardiac Anesthesia. 7th ed. Elsevier; 2017: 818-842.
2. Chassot PG, Bettex DA. Anesthesia and adult congenital heart disease. J Cardiothorac Vasc Anesth, 2006; 20: 414-437.

CHAPTER 19

Thoracic Aorta

Alexander Mittnacht

KEY POINTS	1. Aortic surgery is complex, and therefore it requires an anesthetic tailored to the specific goals for hemodynamics, neuromonitoring, and cerebral/spinal cord perfusion.
	2. Multidisciplinary guidelines for the diagnosis and management of thoracic aortic disease summarize the evidence and expert consensus for this challenging group of important diseases.
	3. Deliberate hypothermia is the most important therapeutic intervention to prevent cerebral ischemia during temporary interruption of cerebral perfusion during aortic arch reconstruction.
	4. Early detection and interventions to increase spinal cord perfusion pressure are effective for the treatment of delayed-onset spinal cord ischemia after thoracic or thoracoabdominal aortic aneurysm repair.
	5. Stanford type A dissection, involving the ascending aorta and aortic arch, is a surgical emergency. Stanford type B dissection, confined to the descending thoracic or abdominal aorta, should be managed medically when possible.
	6. Endovascular approaches to the management of thoracic aortic disease continue to evolve and have a great impact on both elective and emergent aortic surgery.

---

1. Which pressure monitoring site is indicated for blood pressure monitoring when selective antegrade cerebral perfusion via right axillary artery cannulation is planned for aortic arch repair?
   A. Right radial
   B. Right axillary
   C. Left radial
   D. Left axillary

Correct Answer: C

Explanation: When aortic arch surgery with selective antegrade perfusion via axillary cannulation is planned, typically the left radial (or brachial) artery is the most appropriate monitoring site, as it reflects cerebral blood pressure during antegrade selective perfusion. Some practitioners opt to place bilateral radial artery lines, most commonly if a side-graft to axillary artery cardiopulmonary bypass cannulation surgical technique is used, versus direct cannulation of the right axillary artery. With a side-graft technique, overperfusion of the low-resistance right arm may go unnoticed when only a left-sided arterial line is used. However, a right-sided arterial line would not reflect cerebral blood pressure with either technique. The left axillary site is less commonly used, also because the tip of a long catheter may actually be too close to the anastomosis.

In pediatric cardiac surgery for aortic arch repair, the surgeon typically sews a graft to the right innominate artery, and a right-sided arterial line is used to monitor selective cerebral perfusion pressure.

Ultimately, there are many variations in surgical techniques and institutional practices. The most common site to measure blood pressure during adult aortic arch surgery is the left radial artery.

References:
1. Patel PA, Augoustides JGT, Pantin EJ, et al. Chapter 19: Thoracic Aorta. In: Kaplan JA, Augoustides JGT, Manecke GR, eds. Kaplan's Cardiac Anesthesia. 7th ed. Elsevier; 2017: 843-882.
2. Qu JZ, Kao LW, Smith JE, et al. Brain protection in aortic arch surgery: an evolving field. J Cardiothorac Vasc Anesth, 2021; 35: 1176-1188.

2. Which anesthetic agent interferes the most with somato-sensory-evoked potential monitoring?
   A. Dexmedetomidine infusion
   B. Sevoflurane at 1 minimum alveolar concentration
   C. Propofol infusion
   D. Remifentanil infusion

Correct Answer: B

Explanation: With concomitant electroencephalographic and/or somatosensory-evoked potential (SSEP) monitoring, anesthetic signal interference is minimized with the avoidance of barbiturates, bolus propofol, and doses of inhaled anesthetic greater than 0.5 minimum alveolar concentration. Some practitioners opt not to use any inhaled anesthetic agents at all. Propofol infusion, narcotics, and neuromuscular blocking drugs do not interfere with SSEP monitoring. With intraoperative motor-evoked potential monitoring, high-quality signals are obtained when the anesthetic technique comprises total intravenous anesthesia without neuromuscular blockade, including agents such as propofol, dexmedetomidine, and remifentanil.

References:

1. Patel PA, Augoustides JGT, Pantin EJ, et al. Chapter 19: Thoracic Aorta. In: Kaplan JA, Augoustides JGT, Manecke GR, eds. Kaplan's Cardiac Anesthesia. 7th ed. Elsevier; 2017: 843-882.
2. Sloan TB, Edmonds HL, Koht A. Intraoperative electrophysiologic monitoring in aortic surgery. J Cardiothorac Vasc Anesth, 2013; 27: 1364-1373.

3. Which pharmacologic agent is best avoided when motor-evoked potential monitoring is planned?
   A. Dexmedetomidine
   B. Succinylcholine
   C. Propofol
   D. Cisatracurium

Correct Answer: D

Explanation: With intraoperative motor-evoked potential (MEP) monitoring, high-quality signals are obtained when the anesthetic technique comprises total intravenous anesthesia with propofol and a narcotic such as remifentanil without neuromuscular blockade. Succinylcholine is often used to facilitate endotracheal intubation, although with the availability of sugammadex, rocuronium and vecuronium can be used and then readily reversed if their effects have not subsided when MEP monitoring is started.

References:

1. Patel PA, Augoustides JGT, Pantin EJ, et al. Chapter 19: Thoracic Aorta. In: Kaplan JA, Augoustides JGT, Manecke GR, eds. Kaplan's Cardiac Anesthesia. 7th ed. Elsevier; 2017: 843-882.
2. Sloan TB, Edmonds HL, Koht A. Intraoperative electrophysiologic monitoring in aortic surgery. J Cardiothorac Vasc Anesth, 2013; 27: 1364-1373.

4. What has been associated with an ascending aorta aneurysm?
   A. Bicuspid aortic valve
   B. Mitral valve prolapse
   C. Infrarenal aortic aneurysm
   D. Takotsubo cardiomyopathy

Correct Answer: A

Explanation: Besides acquired risk factors such as hypertension, hypercholesterolemia, and smoking, current evidence points to the strong influence of genetic inheritance for the development of thoracic aortic aneurysms. Aneurysms of the aortic root and/or ascending aorta are commonly associated with a bicuspid aortic valve. Inflammatory causes for thoracic aortic aneurysms include syphilis, mycotic aneurysm from endocarditis, giant-cell arteritis, and Takayasu arteritis. Mitral valve prolapse and Takotsubo cardiomyopathy are not typically associated with ascending aortic aneurysms.

References:

1. Patel PA, Augoustides JGT, Pantin EJ, et al. Chapter 19: Thoracic Aorta. In: Kaplan JA, Augoustides JGT, Manecke GR, eds. Kaplan's Cardiac Anesthesia. 7th ed. Elsevier; 2017: 843-882.
2. Borger MA, Fedak PWM, Stephens EH, et al. The American Association for Thoracic Surgery consensus guidelines on bicuspid aortic valve-related aortopathy. J Thorac Cardiovasc Surg, 2018; 156: e41-e74.

5. What has been associated the most with paraplegia following repair of descending thoracic aortic aneurysms?
   A. Aortic atheroma
   B. Patient age
   C. Multisegment aneurysm
   D. Intraoperative temperature

Correct Answer: C

Explanation: Aneurysms of the descending thoracic aorta are classified by considering which third(s) of the descending thoracic aorta is (are) involved. Extent A involves the proximal third, extent B involves the middle third, and extent C involves the distal third. If more than one-third is involved, then the extent is classified according to which thirds are involved. Essentially, multisegment aneurysms such as AB and ABC have a high risk for spinal cord ischemia after surgical repair, whether open or endovascular. This is due to the significant compromise of the spinal cord collateral arterial network through the loss of the intercostal arterial supply at multiple levels. The number of segments sacrificed (extent of aneurysm) is a strong predictor of perioperative spinal cord injury in this setting. Aortic atheroma, patient age, and intraoperative temperature may also influence the risk of spinal cord ischemia, but in contemporary practice, with a multimodal approach to spinal cord protection, the number of segments sacrificed (extent of aneurysm) is the strongest predictor of spinal cord injury (paraplegia).

References:

1. Patel PA, Augoustides JGT, Pantin EJ, et al. Chapter 19: Thoracic Aorta. In: Kaplan JA, Augoustides JGT, Manecke GR, eds. Kaplan's Cardiac Anesthesia. 7th ed. Elsevier; 2017: 843-882.
2. Zoli S, Roder F, Etz CD, et al. Predicting the risk of paraplegia after thoracic and thoracoabdominal aneurysm repair. Ann Thorac Surg, 2010; 90: 1237-1244.

6. What is an indication for medical therapy in patients with an ascending aortic aneurysm?
   A. Ascending aorta diameter 4.4 cm
   B. Ascending aorta 4.8 cm up from 4.1 cm 1 year ago
   C. Ascending aorta 4.5 cm and bicuspid aortic valve
   D. Ascending aorta diameter 5.6 cm

Correct Answer: A

Explanation: Clinical decision-making for asymptomatic ascending aorta aneurysm repair depends on multiple considerations, including diameter, location, expansion rate, family history of rupture/dissection, and aortic valve anatomy and function, as well as the presence of contributing etiologies such as connective tissue disorders. Without contributing factors, an ascending aortic diameter under 5 cm is often treated medically. Ascending aorta diameter of 5 cm or more and ascending aorta 4.0 to 4.9 cm with existing contributing factors are indications for surgery in asymptomatic patients.

References:

1. Patel PA, Augoustides JGT, Pantin EJ, et al. Chapter 19: Thoracic Aorta. In: Kaplan JA, Augoustides JGT, Manecke GR, eds. Kaplan's Cardiac Anesthesia. 7th ed. Elsevier; 2017: 843-882.
2. Saeyeldin A, Zafar MA, Li Y, et al. Decision-making algorithm for ascending aortic aneurysm: effectiveness in clinical application? J Thorac Cardiovasc Surg, 2019; 157: 1733-1745.

7. What is supported by the best evidence to be effective in protecting the brain during circulatory arrest during aortic arch repair?
   A. Prearrest intravenous thiopental
   B. Prearrest intravenous magnesium
   C. Topical ice on head
   D. Deliberate hypothermia

Correct Answer: D

Explanation: Various surgical techniques exist for the conduct of aortic arch repair, ranging from complete hypothermic cerebral circulatory arrest to almost no or only brief interruption of cerebral blood flow with modern selective antegrade cerebral perfusion techniques. Hypothermia is the only and the most effective way to allow for any prolonged interruption of cerebral blood flow to occur. Cooling for systemic hypothermia is accomplished using the cardiopulmonary bypass heat-exchanger. Topical ice, contrary to popular belief, contributes very little to effective cerebral cooling, and its hypothermic effect typically does not reach the deep structures of the brain. Topical ice mostly serves to avoid rewarming during hypothermic circulatory arrest when the brain is not perfused, and thus would slowly warm up from the ambient room temperature. Pharmacologic neuroprotection with thiopental and magnesium has not achieved widespread adoption in this clinical setting due to very weak evidence of benefit. Cerebral hyperthermia prevention during rewarming is also an important measure to help prevent adverse neurological outcomes.

References:

1. Patel PA, Augoustides JGT, Pantin EJ, et al. Chapter 19: Thoracic Aorta. In: Kaplan JA, Augoustides JGT, Manecke GR, eds. Kaplan's Cardiac Anesthesia. 7th ed. Elsevier; 2017: 843-882.
2. Svyatets M, Tolani K, Zhang M, et al. Perioperative management of deep hypothermic circulatory arrest. J Cardiothorac Vasc Anesth, 2010; 24: 644-655.

8. Which temperature gradient between the set temperature on the heat exchanger and the patient temperature should not be exceeded to help avoid ischemia/reperfusion injury to the brain?
   A. Greater than 2°C
   B. Greater than 6°C
   C. Greater than 8°C
   D. Greater than 10°C

Correct Answer: D

Explanation: Rewarming increases cerebral metabolic rate and can aggravate neuronal injury during ischemia/reperfusion. Consequently, it is important to rewarm gradually by maintaining a temperature gradient of no more than 10°C in the heat exchanger and avoiding cerebral hyperthermia, defined as a nasopharyngeal temperature greater than 37.5°C. Avoiding cerebral hyperthermia is one of the strategies for brain protection during aortic arch repair.

References:

1. Patel PA, Augoustides JGT, Pantin EJ, et al. Chapter 19: Thoracic Aorta. In: Kaplan JA, Augoustides JGT, Manecke GR, eds. Kaplan's Cardiac Anesthesia. 7th ed. Elsevier; 2017: 843-882.
2. Svyatets M, Tolani K, Zhang M, et al. Perioperative management of deep hypothermic circulatory arrest. J Cardiothorac Vasc Anesth, 2010; 24: 644-655.

9. Which temperature on cardiopulmonary bypass falls in the moderate hypothermia range?
   A. 14°C
   B. 18°C
   C. 25°C
   D. 29°C

Correct Answer: C

Explanation: Recent expert consensus has defined levels of hypothermia during the conduct of aortic arch repair. Mild hypothermia was categorized as 28.1°C to 34°C. Moderate hypothermia has a temperature range of 20.1°C to 28°C. Deep hypothermia was defined as a temperature range of 14.1°C to 20°C, and profound hypothermia was categorized as a temperature of 14°C or less.

References:

1. Patel PA, Augoustides JGT, Pantin EJ, et al. Chapter 19: Thoracic Aorta. In: Kaplan JA, Augoustides JGT, Manecke GR, eds. Kaplan's Cardiac Anesthesia. 7th ed. Elsevier; 2017: 843-882.
2. Yan TD, Bannon PG, Bavaria JE, et al. Consensus on hypothermia in aortic arch surgery. Ann Cardiothorac Surg, 2013; 2: 163-168.

10. Retrograde selective cerebral perfusion provides cold oxygenated blood to the brain via which vascular structure?
   A. Coronary sinus
   B. Carotid artery
   C. Superior vena cava
   D. Vertebral artery

Correct Answer: C

Explanation: Retrograde cerebral perfusion (RCP) is a cerebral perfusion technique performed by infusing cold oxygenated blood into the superior vena cava cannula at a temperature of 8°C to 14°C during hypothermic circulatory arrest. The internal jugular venous pressure is maintained at less than 25 mmHg to prevent cerebral edema, with typical flow rates of 200 to 600 mL/minute. The potential benefits of RCP include partial supply of cerebral metabolic substrate, cerebral embolic washout, and maintenance of cerebral hypothermia. However, there is evidence from animal studies that much of the blood is shunted at a lower level, and oxygen cannot be supplied to the brain reliably via the venous system in a retrograde fashion. Because of these limitations, antegrade cerebral perfusion has become much more popular in most institutions.

References:

1. Patel PA, Augoustides JGT, Pantin EJ, et al. Chapter 19: Thoracic Aorta. In: Kaplan JA, Augoustides JGT, Manecke GR, eds. Kaplan's Cardiac Anesthesia. 7th ed. Elsevier; 2017: 843-882.
2. Svyatets M, Tolani K, Zhang M, et al. Perioperative management of deep hypothermic circulatory arrest. J Cardiothorac Vasc Anesth, 2010; 24: 644-655.
3. Ziganshin BA, Elefteriades JA. Deep hypothermic circulatory arrest. Ann Cardiothorac Surg, 2013; 2: 303-315.

11. During selective antegrade cerebral perfusion (ACP) via right axillary artery cannulation, bilateral cerebral oximetry monitoring is most useful to help assess which of the following?
    A. ACP flow rate
    B. ACP temperature
    C. Cerebral perfusion pressure
    D. Cerebral cross perfusion

Correct Answer: D

Explanation: Unilateral antegrade cerebral perfusion (ACP) via right axillary arterial cannulation is a popular technique for adult aortic repair. This technique assumes an adequate circle of Willis; however, the anatomic completeness of the circle of Willis does not guarantee adequate cerebral cross perfusion during aortic arch repair. Consequently, it remains essential to monitor the contralateral hemisphere in unilateral ACP with modalities such as cerebral oximetry or transcranial Doppler. Although cerebral oximetry can also contribute information that helps guide ACP management, including flow and pressure, its value in detecting meaningful changes diminishes at lower temperatures. During deliberate hypothermia, cerebral oximetry readings will be increasingly high as metabolic demand decreases, and potentially harmful increases (causing cerebral edema) or decreases (ischemia) in ACP flow and pressure will not be discriminated adequately by cerebral oximetry only.

References:

1. Patel PA, Augoustides JGT, Pantin EJ, et al. Chapter 19: Thoracic Aorta. In: Kaplan JA, Augoustides JGT, Manecke GR, eds. Kaplan's Cardiac Anesthesia. 7th ed. Elsevier; 2017: 843-882.
2. Murkin JM. NIRS: a standard of care for CPB vs. an evolving standard for selective cerebral perfusion? J Extra Corpor Technol, 2009; 41: 11-14.
3. Qu JZ, Kao LW, Smith JE, et al. Brain protection in aortic arch surgery: an evolving field. J Cardiothorac Vasc Anesth, 2021; 35: 1176-1188.

12. The artery of Adamkiewicz most reliably originates from which thoracic or lumbar segment?
    A. T2–T5
    B. T6–T8
    C. T9–T11
    D. T12–L2

Correct Answer: C

Explanation: The thoracolumbar spinal cord typically has multiple arterial sources. An important blood supply is derived from a large radicular artery, the artery of Adamkiewicz, that arises from intercostal arteries T9–T12 in 75%, T8–L3 in 15%, and L1–L2 in 10% of patients. A large meta-analysis has demonstrated that 89% of arteries of Adamkiewicz originate between T8 and L1. The most frequent level of origin was T9 (22.2%), followed by T10 (21.7%) and T11 (18.7%). Unfortunately, reimplantation of this large intercostal artery has yielded limited benefit in preventing spinal cord injury after descending thoracic or thoracoabdominal aortic repair. Advances in vascular imaging of the spinal cord blood supply have suggested a dense network and collateralization of multiple arterial blood sources, rather than just a select few arteries.

References:

1. Patel PA, Augoustides JGT, Pantin EJ, et al. Chapter 19: Thoracic Aorta. In: Kaplan JA, Augoustides JGT, Manecke GR, eds. Kaplan's Cardiac Anesthesia. 7th ed. Elsevier; 2017: 843-882.
2. Taterra D, Skinningsrud B, Pekala PA, et al. Artery of Adamkiewicz: a meta-analysis of anatomical characteristics. Spinal Neuroradiology, 2019; 61: 869-880.

13. During lumbar cerebrospinal fluid (CSF) drainage catheter insertion blood is aspirated mixed with CSF. After a short discussion with the surgeon the decision is made to proceed with surgery. How soon after insertion can heparin be administered?
    A. 30 minutes
    B. 60 minutes
    C. 90 minutes
    D. 120 minutes

Correct Answer: B

Explanation: The recommendation is 60 minutes between neuraxial manipulation and systemic heparinization.

References:

1. Horlocker TT, Vandermeulen E, Kopp SL, et al. Regional anesthesia in the patient receiving antithrombotic or thrombolytic therapy: American Society of Regional Anesthesia and Pain Medicine Evidence-Based Guidelines (Fourth Edition). Reg Anesth Pain Med, 2018; 43: 263-309.

14. Oxygenated blood supply to the brain during thoracoabdominal aortic aneurysm repair with left heart bypass is established via cannulation of which structure?
  A. None
  B. Pulmonary veins
  C. Inferior vena cava
  D. Right axillary artery

Correct Answer: A

Explanation: Various surgical techniques exist for repair of thoracoabdominal aortic aneurysms, including deep hypothermic circulatory arrest, and left heart bypass with or without an oxygenator. Although left heart bypass provides oxygenated blood to the lower body with distal aortic perfusion, the heart is beating and provides blood supply to the area proximal to the aortic clamp, including the brain. Ventilation of the lungs is thus required, although usually permitting left lung collapse to enhance surgical exposure. For perfusion of the lower body, and, if required, renal and mesenteric arteries via direct cannulation, the cannulation technique depends on the use of an oxygenator in the left heart bypass setup. If no oxygenator is used, then blood is drained from the pulmonary veins (see figure for further details). The use of an oxygenator allows cannulation of the inferior vena cava instead. Right axillary artery is used for selective antegrade cerebral perfusion during aortic arch repair, not thoracoabdominal aortic aneurysm repair.

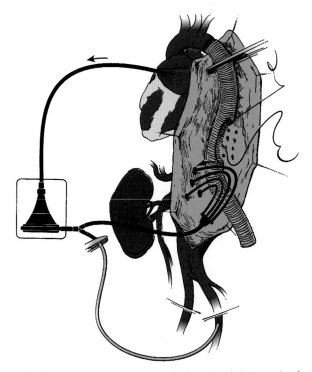

FIGURE 19.1 Extracorporeal perfusion circuit for repair of an extensive thoracoabdominal aortic aneurysm. Cannulation of the left atrium and femoral artery provides distal aortic perfusion by partial left heart bypass. Visceral perfusion can be provided by selective cannulation of the celiac, superior mesenteric, and renal arteries. (Modified from Coselli JS. Descending Thoracoabdominal Aortic Aneurysms. In: Edmunds LH, ed. Cardiac Surgery in the Adult. McGraw-Hill; 1997:1237.)

References:
  1. Patel PA, Augoustides JGT, Pantin EJ, et al. Chapter 19: Thoracic Aorta. In: Kaplan JA, Augoustides JGT, Manecke GR, eds. Kaplan's Cardiac Anesthesia. 7th ed. Elsevier; 2017: 843-882.
  2. Swerdlow NJ, Wu WW, Schermerhorn ML. Open and endovascular management of aortic aneurysms. Circ Res, 2019; 124: 647-661.

15. In the current classification of endoleaks related to endovascular aortic aneurysm repair, what is classified as a type II endoleak?
  A. Inadequate seal at proximal and/or distal landing zone
  B. Structural failure of stent (perforation, fracture)
  C. Stent graft fabric porosity
  D. Retrograde flow from aortic branches into aneurysm

Correct Answer: D

Explanation: Endoleaks are a common complication related to endovascular aortic repair. With an endoleak, blood flow persists in the aneurysm sac. Endoleaks are categorized by the source of this flow. In type I endoleak there is an inadequate seal between the endograft and the landing zones, whether proximal and/or distal. In type II endoleaks, there is residual flow in the aneurysm from aortic side branches. In type III endoleaks, there is a defect or structural failure of the endograft, including perforation and fracture. In type IV endoleaks, blood flow into the aneurysm sac occurs because of the porosity of graft material. Type I and III endoleaks represent direct arterial flow into the sac and warrant prompt treatment. Type II endoleaks may require transcatheter intervention, including selective embolization of culprit aortic side branches. Type IV endoleaks are rarely seen with contemporary endovascular grafts.

References:
  1. Patel PA, Augoustides JGT, Pantin EJ, et al. Chapter 19: Thoracic Aorta. In: Kaplan JA, Augoustides JGT, Manecke GR, eds. Kaplan's Cardiac Anesthesia. 7th ed. Elsevier; 2017: 843-882.
  2. Swerdlow NJ, Wu WW, Schermerhorn ML. Open and endovascular management of aortic aneurysms. Circ Res, 2019; 124: 647-661.

16. Arterial pressure monitoring at which site is usually preferred in surgical intervention for thoracoabdominal aneurysm repair?
  A. Left radial
  B. Right radial
  C. Left axillary
  D. Direct aortic

Correct Answer: B

Explanation: Right radial arterial pressure monitoring typically is preferred, especially if the aortic repair involves clamping the left subclavian artery or gaining surgical endovascular access via the left brachial artery. Femoral arterial pressure monitoring is typically required when distal aortic perfusion is planned, either with left heart bypass or a passive shunt. If there is extensive femoral arterial disease, direct pressure monitoring in the distal abdominal aorta below the distal clamp site can be considered. In these complex cases, it is prudent to discuss the anesthetic plan in detail with the surgical team, including the preferred site(s) for arterial pressure monitoring for a given case.

References:

1. Patel PA, Augoustides JGT, Pantin EJ, et al. Chapter 19: Thoracic Aorta. In: Kaplan JA, Augoustides JGT, Manecke GR, eds. Kaplan's Cardiac Anesthesia. 7th ed. Elsevier; 2017: 843-882.
2. Fort ACP, Rubin LA, Meltzer AJ, et al. Perioperative management of endovascular thoracoabdominal aortic aneurysm repair. J Cardiothorac Vasc Anesth, 2017; 31: 1440-1459.

17. Which of the following measures is most effective in preventing the risk of paraplegia after thoracoabdominal aortic aneurysm repair?
   A. Performing evoked potential monitoring
   B. Reimplanting large intercostal arteries
   C. Increasing spinal cord perfusion pressure
   D. Administering steroids

Correct Answer: C

Explanation: Evoked potential monitoring is often used intraoperatively to help detect spinal cord ischemia, but monitoring will not impact outcome unless it is associated with an intervention that has been shown to improve outcomes. Reimplantation of intercostal arteries, unfortunately, has not been shown to improve the risk of spinal cord ischemia, nor have steroids. The most important intervention associated with outcome is maintaining or increasing spinal cord perfusion pressure.

References:

1. Patel PA, Augoustides JGT, Pantin EJ, et al. Chapter 19: Thoracic Aorta. In: Kaplan JA, Augoustides JGT, Manecke GR, eds. Kaplan's Cardiac Anesthesia. 7th ed. Elsevier; 2017: 843-882.
2. Kemp CM, Feng Z, Aftab M, Reece TB. Preventing spinal cord injury following thoracoabdominal aortic aneurysm repair: the battle to eliminate paraplegia. JTCVS Tech, 2021; 8: 11-15.

18. What cerebrospinal fluid pressure range is typically maintained during repair of a thoracoabdominal aneurysm?
   A. 6–9 mmHg
   B. 10–12 mmHg
   C. 13–15 mmHg
   D. 16–19 mmHg

Correct Answer: B

Explanation: Lumbar cerebrospinal fluid (CSF) drainage is a strongly recommended strategy for protecting the spinal cord during and after repair of thoracoabdominal aortic aneurysms. The physiologic rationale is that reduction of CSF pressure improves spinal cord perfusion pressure, given that spinal cord perfusion pressure is determined by the difference between mean arterial pressure and CSF pressure (or central venous pressure if higher than CSF pressure). Furthermore, CSF drainage may also counter CSF pressure increases caused by aortic cross-clamping, reperfusion, increased central venous pressure, and/or spinal cord edema. Typically, in this setting, CSF should be drained, using a closed-circuit reservoir, when the lumbar CSF pressure exceeds 10 to 12 mmHg, although exact thresholds may vary between institutions. The complications of lumbar CSF drainage are significant and include neuraxial hematoma, catheter fracture, and meningitis, as well as the spectrum of intracranial hypotension, including spinal headache.

References:

1. Patel PA, Augoustides JGT, Pantin EJ, et al. Chapter 19: Thoracic Aorta. In: Kaplan JA, Augoustides JGT, Manecke GR, eds. Kaplan's Cardiac Anesthesia. 7th ed. Elsevier; 2017: 843-882.
2. Kemp C, Ikeno Y, Aftab M, et al. Cerebrospinal fluid drainage in thoracic endovascular aortic repair: mandatory access but tailored placement. Ann Cardiothorac Surg, 2022; 11: 53-55.
3. Oftadeh M, Ural N, LeVan P, et al. The evolution and future of spinal drains for thoracic aortic aneurysm repair: a review. J Cardiothorac Vasc Anesth, 2021; 35: 3362-3373.

19. A 63-year-old patient presents for repair of an extensive thoracoabdominal aortic aneurysm. As part of a multimodal spinal cord protection strategy, a lumbar spinal drain catheter is placed. Postoperatively in the intensive care unit, the patient suddenly develops new-onset lower extremity weakness and loss of reflexes. The cerebrospinal fluid pressure is 10 mmHg, and the systemic pressure is 117/69 mmHg. Which intervention is indicated next?
   A. Start norepinephrine infusion
   B. Drain cerebrospinal fluid
   C. Induce general anesthesia
   D. Administer steroid bolus

Correct Answer: A

Explanation: The new onset of spinal cord ischemia after thoracoabdominal aneurysm repair requires immediate intervention. Since surgical intervention has been completed, multimodal efforts in this setting include intensive clinical neuromonitoring and augmentation of spinal cord perfusion pressure (see teaching box for further detail). In the described scenario, further drainage of cerebrospinal fluid is not the first choice because 10 mmHg already is the lower end of the target range. A systemic blood pressure of 117/69 mmHg in this setting with clinical signs of cord ischemia is relatively low. A systemic vasopressor such as norepinephrine is typically titrated for a goal mean arterial pressure of 90 to 100 mmHg and at times even much higher to restore spinal cord perfusion via the collateral arterial network. The induction of general anesthesia is not indicated in this setting for multiple reasons, including its tendency to induce relative systemic hypotension and compromise spinal cord perfusion. Bolus steroid therapy may be helpful, but the evidence for this intervention is weak at best, and this therapy may have risks such as infection and hyperglycemia.

References:

1. Patel PA, Augoustides JGT, Pantin EJ, et al. Chapter 19: Thoracic Aorta. In: Kaplan JA, Augoustides JGT, Manecke GR, eds. Kaplan's Cardiac Anesthesia. 7th ed. Elsevier; 2017: 843-882.
2. Kemp CM, Feng Z, Aftab M, Reece TB. Preventing spinal cord injury following thoracoabdominal aortic aneurysm repair: The battle to eliminate paraplegia. JTCVS Tech, 2021; 8: 11-15.
3. Oftadeh M, Ural N, LeVan P, et al. The evolution and future of spinal drains for thoracic aortic aneurysm repair: a review. J Cardiothorac Vasc Anesth, 2021; 35: 3362-3373.

20. A patient presents to the emergency room with acute, severe pain radiating to the back. Computed tomographic imaging of the thoracic aorta reveals a dissection entry site just distal to the origin of the left subclavian artery. An intramural hematoma is noticed with retrograde extension through the aortic arch into the ascending aorta, and the patient develops deterioration of mental status. Which management strategy is indicated based on current recommendations?
    A. Emergency surgery
    B. Medical treatment
    C. Monitoring and repeat imaging after 24 hours
    D. Endovascular repair

Correct Answer: A

Explanation: Aortic dissection has traditionally been classified based on the involvement of the ascending and descending aorta with the Stanford and DeBakey systems (see teaching boxes for further detail). A recent revised classification for aortic dissection from the Society for Vascular Surgery and Society of Thoracic Surgeons considers the location of the entry tear, as well as proximal and distal extents, for the suggested classification. Distinguishing between type A and type B dissection is based on entry tear location alone. The retrograde and distal extension is then further described. Although the entry site in the described scenario is past the left subclavian artery, it extends in a retrograde fashion into the aortic arch and ascending aorta. The management of proximal extension is more controversial and an evolving field, and endovascular options may soon be the therapy of choice. Although a watch-and-wait approach may be indicated in patients without neurological symptoms, the latter would most likely prompt emergent surgical intervention in the majority of cases.

References:

1. Patel PA, Augoustides JGT, Pantin EJ, et al. Chapter 19: Thoracic Aorta. In: Kaplan JA, Augoustides JGT, Manecke GR, eds. Kaplan's Cardiac Anesthesia. 7th ed. Elsevier; 2017: 843-882.
2. Lombardi JV, Hughes GC, Appoo JJ, et al. Society for Vascular Surgery (SVS) and Society of Thoracic Surgeons (STS) reporting standards for type B aortic dissections. J Vasc Surg, 2020; 71: 723-747.

21. After aortic cannulation for aortic valve replacement with cardiopulmonary bypass (CPB), the anesthesiologist notices a dissection flap in the ascending aorta extending through the arch and descending aorta. Replacement of the ascending aorta is planned in addition to the primary procedure, and the surgeon proceeds with cannulation of the femoral artery for cardiopulmonary bypass. Immediately after CPB is initiated, the cerebral oximeter readings continue to decrease. Which management strategy is indicated next?
    A. No intervention, as this finding is expected on CPB
    B. Administer phenylephrine to increase blood pressure
    C. Reassess true-lumen cannulation
    D. Cool down to 25°C

Correct Answer: C

Explanation: Acute aortic dissection from aortic cannulation for cardiopulmonary bypass is a well-recognized complication that typically requires replacement of the proximal thoracic aorta. Alternative sites for arterial cannulation include the right axillary and femoral arteries. However, monitoring for adequate bilateral cerebral perfusion in this scenario remains essential because cerebral malperfusion can result from the presence of an intimal flap with true and false lumens. In the described case, the surgeon may have inadvertently cannulated the false lumen. Cerebral oximetry as well as transesophageal echocardiography can assist in detecting cerebral malperfusion during femoral cannulation for cardiopulmonary bypass. In the presented case, a prompt reassessment is indicated to verify true lumen perfusion with cannula revision as needed. Increasing blood pressure and systemic cooling are not indicated at this stage to correct the cerebral ischemia, which is likely due to malperfusion.

References:

1. Patel PA, Augoustides JGT, Pantin EJ, et al. Chapter 19: Thoracic Aorta. In: Kaplan JA, Augoustides JGT, Manecke GR, eds. Kaplan's Cardiac Anesthesia. 7th ed. Elsevier; 2017: 843-882.
2. Ayyash B, Tranquilli M, Elefteriades JA. Femoral artery cannulation for thoracic aortic surgery: safe under transesophageal echocardiographic control. J Thorac Cardiovasc Surg, 2011; 142: 1478-1481.
3. Ram H, Dwarakanath S, Green AE, et al. Iatrogenic aortic dissection associated with cardiac surgery: a narrative review. J Cardiothorac Vasc Anesth, 2021; 35: 3050-3066.

22. A patient presents to the emergency room with severe thoracic pain after a fall from a ladder. Computed tomographic imaging of the thoracic aorta reveals a large intramural hematoma near the aortic isthmus. Furthermore, the aortic wall shows a clear break in the intima and a mural flap with minimal extension past the intimal tear. The history and findings are highly suspicious for which of the following?
    A. Aortic ulcer
    B. Aortic dissection
    C. Aortic transection
    D. Intramural hematoma

Correct Answer: C

Explanation: The features described and the history of a high fall point to traumatic focal aortic injury consistent with aortic transection. The clinical sequence of events and related imaging make a penetrating aortic ulcer unlikely. The lack of a dissection flap extending further into the descending aorta rules out a true dissection. A true intramural hematoma typically does not have a visible intimal tear. The clear intimal disruption makes an extended break of the aortic wall highly likely. In contemporary practice, this focal traumatic lesion can often be managed with endovascular aortic repair.

References:

1. Patel PA, Augoustides JGT, Pantin EJ, et al. Chapter 19: Thoracic Aorta. In: Kaplan JA, Augoustides JGT, Manecke GR, eds. Kaplan's Cardiac Anesthesia. 7th ed. Elsevier; 2017: 843-882.
2. Latif RK, Clifford SP, Ghafghazi S, et al. Echocardiography and management for cardiac trauma. J Cardiothorac Vasc Anesth, 2022; 36: 3265-3277.

23. The use of motor-evoked in addition to somatosensory-evoked potential monitoring during repair of a thoracoabdominal aortic aneurysm mainly offers which potential benefit?
    A. Higher concentrations of inhaled anesthetic agents can be used
    B. Added cerebral ischemia monitoring
    C. Higher amplitude changes during ischemic events
    D. Monitoring of the anterior spinal column

Correct Answer: D

Explanation: Monitoring of somatosensory-evoked potentials (SSEPs) is performed by applying electrical stimuli to peripheral nerves and recording the evoked potential that is generated at the level of the peripheral nerves, spinal cord, brainstem, thalamus, and cerebral cortex. The SSEP monitoring profiles provide information about posterior spinal column integrity. Monitoring of motor-evoked potentials (MEPs) has also been used during repair of thoracoabdominal aneurysms because MEPs monitor the anterior spinal columns, which are typically at risk in this clinical setting. This monitoring is performed by applying paired stimuli to the scalp and recording the evoked potential that is generated in the anterior tibialis muscle. Although SSEPs can reliably exclude spinal cord ischemia with a negative predictive value of 99.2%, their sensitivity for its detection is only 62.5%, with a limited predictive value for delayed-onset paraplegia. Despite the theoretical advantages of MEPs for monitoring the at-risk anterior spinal columns, in practice data suggest that SSEPs alone suffice for clinical purposes. The addition of MEP monitoring does, however, extend the monitoring profile for spinal cord rather than cerebral ischemia. MEP monitoring does not change the amplitude response to neural ischemia and does not allow higher concentrations of inhaled anesthetics, as the MEP signals are very sensitive to these agents.

References:

1. Patel PA, Augoustides JGT, Pantin EJ, et al. Chapter 19: Thoracic Aorta. In: Kaplan JA, Augoustides JGT, Manecke GR, eds. Kaplan's Cardiac Anesthesia. 7th ed. Elsevier; 2017: 843-882.
2. Hattori K, Yoshitani K, Kato S, et al. Association between motor-evoked potentials and spinal cord damage diagnosed with magnetic resonance imaging after thoracoabdominal and descending aortic aneurysm repair. J Cardiothorac Vasc Anesth, 2019; 33: 1835-1842.
3. Sloan TB, Edmonds HL, Koht A. Intraoperative electrophysiologic monitoring in aortic surgery. J Cardiothorac Vasc Anesth, 2013; 27: 1364-1373.

24. A 62-year-old patient is presenting for an extent II thoracoabdominal aneurysm repair. A lumbar spinal catheter is placed with a strategy to drain cerebrospinal fluid (CSF) when the CSF pressure exceeds 10 mmHg. Which CSF drainage rate in mL/hour should typically not be exceeded?
    A. 20-30
    B. 30-50
    C. 50-70
    D. 70-100

Correct Answer: A

Explanation: Typical thresholds for draining cerebrospinal fluid in an effort to improve spinal perfusion pressure during and after thoracoabdominal aneurysm repair are in the range of 10 to 12 mmHg, although exact thresholds may vary between institutions. Typically, a drainage rate of 20 to 30 mL/hour should not be exceeded. Draining larger volumes of cerebrospinal fluid over a prolonged period can cause rare but serious complications including intracranial hematoma and brain stem herniation.

References:

1. Patel PA, Augoustides JGT, Pantin EJ, et al. Chapter 19: Thoracic Aorta. In: Kaplan JA, Augoustides JGT, Manecke GR, eds. Kaplan's Cardiac Anesthesia. 7th ed. Elsevier; 2017: 843-882.
2. Fort ACP, Rubin LA, Meltzer AJ, et al. Perioperative management of endovascular thoracoabdominal aortic aneurysm repair. J Cardiothorac Vasc Anesth, 2017; 31: 1440-1459.
3. Kemp C, Ikeno Y, Aftab M, Reece TB. Cerebrospinal fluid drainage in thoracic endovascular aortic repair: mandatory access but tailored placement. Ann Cardiothorac Surg, 2022; 11: 53-55.
4. Oftadeh M, Ural N, LeVan P, et al. The evolution and future of spinal drains for thoracic aortic aneurysm repair: a review. J Cardiothorac Vasc Anesth, 2021; 35: 3362-3373.

25. What has been shown to decrease the incidence of renal failure following repair of thoracoabdominal aortic aneurysms?
    A. Mannitol
    B. Furosemide
    C. Dopamine
    D. Partial left heart bypass

Correct Answer: D

Explanation: The administration of furosemide, mannitol, or dopamine for the sole purpose of renal preservation is not strongly recommended in distal thoracic aortic repairs. The maintenance of distal aortic pressure and selective renal artery perfusion can help ameliorate the detrimental effects of renal ischemia during aortic cross-clamping for repair of thoracoabdominal aortic aneurysms.

References:

1. Patel PA, Augoustides JGT, Pantin EJ, et al. Chapter 19: Thoracic Aorta. In: Kaplan JA, Augoustides JGT, Manecke GR, eds. Kaplan's Cardiac Anesthesia. 7th ed. Elsevier; 2017: 843-882.
2. Bhamidipati CM, Coselli JS, LeMaire SA. Perfusion techniques for renal protection during thoracoabdominal aortic surgery. J Extra Corpor Technol, 2012; 44: 31-37.

26. Which antihypertensive drug is relatively contraindicated to lower the blood pressure during aortic cross clamping during repair of thoracoabdominal aortic aneurysms?
    A. Esmolol
    B. Labetalol
    C. Nitroprusside
    D. Nitroglycerine

Correct Answer: C

Explanation: The administration of nitroprusside is often considered with caution during repair of thoracoabdominal aortic aneurysms. Nitroprusside is a potent arterial vasodilator and may consequently affect spinal perfusion pressure unfavorably. The risk of administering an antihypertensive drug with mostly arterial vasodilatory properties is that it lowers perfusion pressure in the spinal cord collateral arterial network during cross-clamping even further. Due to this concern, beta blockers are reasonable in treating proximal (upper extremity and head) elevation of blood pressure during aortic clamping in this clinical setting. However, since mild hypothermia is almost universally used, the accompanying bradycardia may limit this application of beta blockers. Nitroglycerine may be preferable over a pure arterial vasodilator if beta blockers are contraindicated, or the heart rate is too low.

References:

1. Patel PA, Augoustides JGT, Pantin EJ, et al. Chapter 19: Thoracic Aorta. In: Kaplan JA, Augoustides JGT, Manecke GR, eds. Kaplan's Cardiac Anesthesia. 7th ed. Elsevier; 2017: 843-882.
2. Marini CP, Levison J, Caliendo F, et al. Control of proximal hypertension during aortic cross-clamping: its effect on cerebrospinal fluid dynamics and spinal cord perfusion pressure. Semin Thorac Cardiovasc Surg, 1998; 10: 51-56.

27. What imaging modality is typically preferable to diagnose an acute type A dissection?
    A. Magnetic resonance imaging
    B. Computed tomography
    C. Transesophageal echocardiography
    D. Cardiac catheterization

Correct Answer: B

Explanation: Practices and circumstances may vary significantly, but in general computed tomographic aortography is the imaging of choice because of its reliability and procedural time in the emergency setting when patients are clinically stable. In the setting of hemodynamic instability, patients at high risk for type A aortic dissection may be admitted to the operating room for clinical stabilization and confirmation of the diagnosis with transesophageal echocardiography. Although magnetic resonance imaging has excellent sensitivity and specificity for acute type A aortic dissection, the logistics for this imaging modality preclude its routine application in the emergency setting. Cardiac catheterization is not the typical first-line imaging modality for acute aortic syndromes due to its invasive nature but can make the diagnosis unexpectedly when a patient with type A dissection presents with myocardial infarction, or when type A dissection is a complication of this procedure.

References:

1. Patel PA, Augoustides JGT, Pantin EJ, et al. Chapter 19: Thoracic Aorta. In: Kaplan JA, Augoustides JGT, Manecke GR, eds. Kaplan's Cardiac Anesthesia. 7th ed. Elsevier; 2017: 843-882.
2. MacKnight BM, Maldonado Y, Augoustides JG, et al. Advances in imaging for the management of acute aortic syndromes: focus on transesophageal echocardiography and type A aortic dissection for the perioperative echocardiographer. J Cardiothorac Vasc Anesth, 2016; 30: 1129-1141.

28. In patients undergoing open repair of thoracoabdominal aortic aneurysms, which perioperative adverse event has the highest incidence?
    A. Renal insufficiency
    B. Paraplegia
    C. Bleeding requiring reoperation
    D. Pulmonary complications

Correct Answer: D

Explanation: Open repairs of extensive thoracoabdominal aneurysms are complicated procedures that carry a substantial risk of perioperative mortality and morbidity, including spinal cord ischemia, bleeding, acute kidney injury, and pulmonary complications. In large observational studies, the rates of adverse outcomes can be in the 10% to 20% range, with a perioperative mortality rate in the 5% to 10% range. The most common complications typically involve the pulmonary system and include prolonged mechanical ventilation, tracheostomy, diaphragmatic dysfunction, and hospital-acquired pneumonia. Permanent paraplegia or paraparesis from spinal cord ischemia may occur in up to 10% of cases, with an immediate onset in 30% to 40% and a delayed onset in 50% to 60% of cases. Acute kidney injury is also common, with an incidence in the 10% to 20% range and a risk of renal replacement therapy in at least a third of patients with renal complications. The perioperative risk of these procedures depends significantly on patient comorbidities, the extent of the thoracoabdominal aneurysm, and the institutional expertise in perioperative management for these procedures.

References:

1. Patel PA, Augoustides JGT, Pantin EJ, et al. Chapter 19: Thoracic Aorta. In: Kaplan JA, Augoustides JGT, Manecke GR, eds. Kaplan's Cardiac Anesthesia. 7th ed. Elsevier; 2017: 843-882.
2. LeMaire SA, Price MD, Green SY, et al. Results of open thoracoabdominal aortic aneurysm repair. Ann Cardiothorac Surg, 2012; 1: 286-292.

29. Which endoleak has the highest incidence after thoracic endovascular repair?
   A. Types I and II
   B. Types I and III
   C. Types II and III
   D. Types II and IV

Correct Answer: A

Explanation: Endoleaks are more commonly seen following endovascular repair of the abdominal aorta and occur in 15% to 30% of patients in the first 30 days after the procedure. They are seen less commonly with thoracic endovascular aortic repair, occurring in 4% to 15% of cases. The most commonly occurring types of endoleaks following both thoracic and abdominal endovascular aortic repair are types I and II. These common endoleaks can often be addressed with repeat endovascular intervention, depending on the severity and clinical presentation.

References:

1. Patel PA, Augoustides JGT, Pantin EJ, et al. Chapter 19: Thoracic Aorta. In: Kaplan JA, Augoustides JGT, Manecke GR, eds. Kaplan's Cardiac Anesthesia. 7th ed. Elsevier; 2017: 843-882.
2. Daye D, Walker TG. Complications of endovascular aneurysm repair of the thoracic and abdominal aorta: evaluation and management. Cardiovasc Diagn Ther, 2018; 8: S138-S156.

3. Mansukhani NA, Haleem MS, Eskandari MK. Thoracic endovascular aortic repair adverse events reported in the Food and Drug Administration manufacturer and user facility device experience database. Med Devices (Auckl), 2019; 12: 461-467.

30. Compared to open repair of thoracoabdominal aortic aneurysms, spinal cord ischemia after endovascular intervention for these extensive aneurysms occurs more often:
   A. Before the procedure
   B. During the procedure
   C. Immediately after the procedure
   D. Somewhat delayed after the procedure

Correct Answer: D

Explanation: Compared to open repair, spinal cord ischemia after endovascular repair for thoracoabdominal aneurysms is more often delayed and may present 24 hours following the procedure. Given this presentation profile, it remains important to monitor these patients closely in a systematic fashion in the postoperative period with a multimodal intervention protocol in place should spinal cord ischemia develop.

References:

1. Patel PA, Augoustides JGT, Pantin EJ, et al. Chapter 19: Thoracic Aorta. In: Kaplan JA, Augoustides JGT, Manecke GR, eds. Kaplan's Cardiac Anesthesia. 7th ed. Elsevier; 2017: 843-882.
2. Awad H, Ramadan ME, et al. Spinal cord injury after thoracic endovascular aortic aneurysm repair. Can J Anaesth, 2017; 64: 1218-1235.
3. Maeda T, Yoshitani K, Sato S, et al. Spinal cord ischemia after endovascular aortic repair versus open surgical repair for descending thoracic and thoracoabdominal aortic aneurism. J Anesth, 2012; 26: 805-811.

CHAPTER 20

Uncommon Cardiac Diseases

Iwan Sofjan and Alexander Mittnacht

KEY POINTS

1. Patients with uncommon cardiac diseases frequently have complicated medical conditions, the treatment for which should take place in the context of an institution capable of providing coordinated multidisciplinary care.

2. Cardiac tumors are rare. In general, a cardiac mass is more likely a vegetation or a thrombus than a tumor. Secondary (metastatic) tumors are far more common than primary cardiac tumors. Among primary cardiac tumors, benign lesions are more common than malignant tumors. Anesthetic management for tumor resection is likely to depend more on a patient's comorbidities and tumor location than on the tumor's pathologic condition.

3. Cardiac myxomas historically have been considered the most common benign cardiac tumor. Although most commonly solitary, sporadic, and located on the left atrial side of the fossa ovalis, they may also occur as multiple, simultaneous tumors inherited in cases of Carney complex. Patients with myxomas typically exhibit signs and symptoms attributable to one of the triad of intracardiac obstruction, embolism, or constitutional symptoms.

4. Papillary fibroelastomas are the most common valvular cardiac tumor and may be the most common benign lesion as well. Typically solitary, fibroelastomas occur most frequently on the mitral and aortic valve leaflets. Once considered an incidental, benign finding, they have a high incidence of coronary and cerebral embolization.

5. Primary malignant cardiac tumors are less common than benign tumors. The overwhelming majority of primary malignant tumors are sarcomas.

6. Metastatic cardiac tumors are far more common than primary tumors. Metastatic tumors may involve the heart by direct extension (breast, lung, esophageal), by venous extension (renal cell carcinoma, hepatocellular carcinoma), or by hematogenous (melanoma) or lymphatic (lymphoma, leukemia) spread. Although metastatic cardiac tumors may affect the pericardium, epicardium, myocardium, or endocardium, pericardial involvement is the most common.

7. Carcinoid tumors are metastasizing neuroendocrine tumors. In patients with carcinoid syndrome, carcinoid heart disease is common and characterized by tricuspid regurgitation, mixed pulmonic regurgitation and stenosis, and right-sided heart failure. The management of patients with carcinoid heart disease, similar to the management of many patients with uncommon cardiac conditions, is complex and requires coordinated care at specialty referral centers. The mainstays of treatment are symptom management with somatostatin analogs, antitumor therapy, and cardiac surgical intervention. Successful perioperative management depends on optimal preoperative symptom control with long-acting somatostatin analogs.

8. Renal cell carcinomas are the most common renal tumors. Clear cell carcinomas are the most common subtype of renal cell carcinoma and tend to produce venous extension into the renal veins and the inferior vena cava. Surgical resection of tumor thrombus extending into the intrahepatic inferior vena cava (New York Heart Association [NYHA] level III tumor) or above the diaphragm (NYHA level IV tumor) may require cardiac surgical and anesthesia involvement, although some institutions are now performing resections of proximal lesions involving the right-sided heart without the assistance of cardiopulmonary bypass.

9. Cardiomyopathies are a heterogeneous group of diseases that may be acquired or genetic and may be confined to the heart (primary) or may be part of a systemic disorder (secondary). The American Heart Association classifies cardiomyopathies as primary or secondary and subclassifies primary processes as genetic, acquired, or mixed. The European Society of Cardiology, however, classifies the cardiomyopathies morphologically and functionally into hypertrophic, dilated, arrhythmogenic, restrictive, and unclassified, each of which, in turn, may be considered genetic or nongenetic.

10. Dilated cardiomyopathy is the most common of the cardiomyopathies and may be acquired, hereditary, or idiopathic. Hearts affected with dilated cardiomyopathy show four-chamber dilatation, myocyte hypertrophy, and disproportionate impairment of systolic heart function. The goals of perioperative management of patients with dilated cardiomyopathy, who most frequently require correction of tricuspid or mitral regurgitation, device implantation, or transplantation, include minimizing further myocardial depression, reducing afterload, and maintaining preload.

11. The first case series of patients with hypertrophic cardiomyopathy was published in 1957 and highlights both the understandings and misunderstandings that continue to affect the current thinking of the disease. Contrary to common belief, hypertrophic cardiomyopathy need not be obstructive, need not be fatal, and need not entail massive left ventricular hypertrophy.

12. Hypertrophic cardiomyopathy is likely the most common inherited cardiac disease and may progress along one or more of three pathways: (1) sudden cardiac death, (2) heart failure, or (3) atrial fibrillation, with or without cardioembolic stroke. Hypertrophic cardiomyopathy is morphologically heterogeneous and includes variants with asymmetric basal septal hypertrophy, midventricular hypertrophy, and apical hypertrophy. Surgical intervention may require transaortic and/or transapical approaches. Anesthetic management requires an intimate knowledge of the patient's anatomy and physiologic characteristics and may differ considerably, depending on whether the patient has a basal lesion with dynamic obstruction or an apical lesion with significant impairment of ventricular filling.

13. The restrictive cardiomyopathies, less common than either the dilated or the hypertrophic cardiomyopathies, are heterogeneous and characterized by impaired myocardial relaxation and decreased ventricular compliance. Although diastolic dysfunction is the hallmark of restrictive cardiomyopathies, systolic function may not be normal, although gross indicators of systolic function such as ejection fraction may be unimpaired. Considering that their treatments are significantly different, restrictive cardiomyopathy and constrictive pericarditis must be distinguished. The patients with restrictive cardiomyopathy who are most likely seen in a cardiac surgical unit are patients with cardiac amyloidosis.

14. Mitral valve prolapse is a relatively common cardiac condition. Most patients remain clinically asymptomatic with normal life expectancies. Progression of mitral valve disease and the development of severe mitral regurgitation are rare; however, severe regurgitation represents a common indication for cardiac surgery. Current approaches to mitral valve prolapse are reviewed, including the range of clinical presentations from mitral valve prolapse syndrome to degenerative valve disease and severe mitral regurgitation.

15. Management of patent foramen ovale has received considerable attention with the widespread use of percutaneous closure devices. Determining the superiority of percutaneous device closure to medical management is heavily debated. The management of an incidental patent foramen ovale found during cardiac surgery via transesophageal echocardiography continues to evolve; however, few data suggest that closure offers morbidity or mortality benefit and may actually increase the risk of postoperative stroke.

16. The definitive approach to a patient with both carotid and coronary artery disease requires a large multicenter, randomized trial; however, the many approaches to the surgical management of combined procedures are described.

17. Heart disease continues to be the leading cause of maternal and fetal death during pregnancy; consequently, the important features of managing the pregnant patient who requires cardiopulmonary bypass and cardiac surgery is updated.

18. With newly developed therapies, the incubation time to develop acquired immune deficiency syndrome after infection and the life expectancy of those with human immunodeficiency virus have been extended; therefore the likelihood of cardiac surgery is greater. Consequently, the rates of exposure, types of procedures, and the precautions of the individuals are addressed.

19. The number of individuals with chronic renal failure, not necessarily dialysis dependent before surgery, are more frequently undergoing cardiac surgery and are likely to develop worsening renal function after cardiopulmonary bypass; therefore the identification of steps that may improve outcome are discussed.

20. Anesthetic concerns for patients with hematologic problems who undergo cardiac surgery are further complicated by the stress cardiopulmonary bypass places on coagulation and oxygen-carrying systems and require special considerations and techniques.

1. A 45-year-old male patient has an incidental finding of a possible cardiac tumor. Assuming the mass is a primary cardiac tumor, it is most likely a:
A. Myxoma
B. Sarcoma
C. Lymphoma
D. Lipoma

Correct Answer: A

Explanation: All the answers listed are primary cardiac tumors, which are much less common than secondary cardiac tumors. Among the primary tumors, benign lesions are more common than malignant ones. In adults, the most common primary benign tumors are myxomas, although several series now suggest that papillary fibroelastomas may be more common. In children, rhabdomyomas are the most common benign tumor. Common symptoms of myxoma include dizziness, palpitations, dyspnea, congestive heart failure, fever, fatigue, and loss of weight. Coronary and cerebral embolisms have also been reported with myxoma, but are rare.

References:
1. Fox JF, Smith MM, Nuttall GA, et al. Chapter 20: Uncommon Cardiac Diseases. In: Kaplan JA, Augoustides JGT, Manecke GR, et al., eds. Kaplan's Cardiac Anesthesia. 7th ed. Elsevier; 2017:883-973.
2. Waikar HD, Jayakrishnan AG, Bandusena BSN, et al. Left atrial myxoma presenting as cerebral embolism. J Cardiothorac Vasc Anesth, 2020; 34: 3452-3461.

2. In a 6-year-old male patient, which cardiac tumor is the most common primary malignant cardiac tumor?
A. Sarcoma
B. Lymphoma
C. Mesothelioma
D. AV nodal tumor

Correct Answer: A

Explanation: Approximately 15% to 25% of primary cardiac tumors are malignant, with sarcomas being the most common in both adults and children. Tumors with high rates of cardiac metastases include pleural mesothelioma, melanoma, lung adenocarcinoma and squamous cell carcinoma, and breast carcinoma. Cardiac sarcomas carry a poor prognosis. Chemotherapy or radiotherapy has been used but is usually not effective. Complete surgical resection is often not feasible, and the recurrence rate is high.

References:
1. Fox JF, Smith MM, Nuttall GA, et al. Chapter 20: Uncommon Cardiac Diseases. In: Kaplan JA, Augoustides JGT, Manecke GR, et al., eds. Kaplan's Cardiac Anesthesia. 7th ed. Elsevier; 2017:883-973.
2. Vallés-Torres J, Izquierdo-Villarroya MB, Vallejo-Gil JM, et al. Cardiac undifferentiated pleomorphic sarcoma mimicking left atrial myxoma. J Cardiothorac Vasc Anesth, 2019; 33: 493-496.

3. Cardiac metastasis from a secondary tumor most likely involves the:
A. Endocardium
B. Myocardium
C. Epicardium
D. Pericardium

Correct Answer: D

Explanation: Cardiac metastases (secondary cardiac tumors) are more common than primary cardiac tumors, and most commonly spread via the lymphatic route. Although metastases may involve the pericardium, epicardium, myocardium, or endocardium, pericardial involvement is the most common, followed by the epicardium. Tumors with high rates of cardiac metastases include pleural mesothelioma, melanoma, lung adenocarcinoma and squamous cell carcinoma, and breast carcinoma. Symptoms from cardiac metastases range from silent (only found on autopsy) to various nonspecific symptoms, which largely depend on the location and size (leading to presentations such as intracardiac obstruction, extracardiac embolization, coronary artery compression, and arrhythmias).

References:
1. Fox JF, Smith MM, Nuttall GA, et al. Chapter 20: Uncommon Cardiac Diseases. In: Kaplan JA, Augoustides JGT, Manecke GR, et al., eds. Kaplan's Cardiac Anesthesia. 7th ed. Elsevier; 2017:883-973.
2. Capdeville M, Hearn C, Rice TW, Starr NJ. Left atrial metastasis of a large cell carcinoma of the lung in an asymptomatic patient: transesophageal echocardiographic evaluation. J Cardiothorac Vasc Anesth, 1997; 11: 492-494.

4. A 50-year-old female patient presents with dyspnea on exertion. What would be consistent with a cardiac myxoma as the cause?
A. Mass in the left ventricle
B. A strong family history of cardiac myxoma
C. Concomitant melanoma
D. Slow progression of symptoms

Correct Answer: D

Explanation: Myxoma is the most common primary benign cardiac tumor. It is typically a large solitary pedunculated mass in the left atrium (75% of the time) or the right atrium (20%) with an attachment to the interatrial septum. Microscopically, it often resembles an organized thrombus, which may obscure its identity as a primary cardiac tumor. Myxoma usually presents around 30 to 60 years of age and is three times more common in women. Most cases occur sporadically, while 7% to 10% of atrial myxomas will occur in a familial pattern with an autosomal dominant transmission pattern known as the Carney complex. Myxoma typically proliferates slowly and may not produce symptoms until the mass is large enough. The typical signs and symptoms include dyspnea, embolism, intracardiac obstruction, and constitutional symptoms. The obstruction of blood flow may also cause hemolysis, hypotension, syncope, or sudden death. Other symptoms of mitral obstruction, similar to mitral stenosis, may occur, including hemoptysis, systemic embolization, fever, and weight loss. The risk of embolization to the central nervous system can be up to 40%. Surgical resection is the best treatment and has low mortality (between 0% and 7%).

References:

1. Fox JF, Smith MM, Nuttall GA, et al. Chapter 20: Uncommon Cardiac Diseases. In: Kaplan JA, Augoustides JGT, Manecke GR, et al., eds. Kaplan's Cardiac Anesthesia. 7th ed. Elsevier; 2017:883-973.
2. Waikar HD, et al. Left atrial myxoma presenting as cerebral embolism. J Cardiothorac Vasc Anesth, 2020; 34: 3452-3461.

5. A 60-year-old male patient with a recent stroke is undergoing an echocardiographic evaluation. What finding is consistent with a papillary fibroelastoma?
  A. Multiple cardiac lesions
  B. Valvular involvement
  C. 8 cm in size
  D. Concomitant atrial septal defect

Correct Answer: B

Explanation: Papillary fibroelastomas are rare, benign tumors that tend to affect the cardiac valves. Most papillary fibroelastomas are singular (90%), small, highly papillary, pedunculated, and avascular. They originate most commonly from valvular endocardium, usually involving the ventricular surface of the aortic valve or the atrial surface of the mitral valve, but they only infrequently render the involved valve incompetent. Many patients are asymptomatic with most papillary fibroelastoma found incidentally. When present, clinical symptoms may include myocardial ischemia and stroke from occlusion or embolization. On echo, fibroelastomas are usually small (mean size 12 × 9 mm), and their motion is independent of that of the attached valve leaflet. They may appear similar to a vegetation seen in endocarditis or they may be confused with Lambl excrescences, which tend to be more nodular in appearance. Surgical resection is curative but may require valvular repair or replacement in one-third of cases. Recurrence is very rare.

References:

1. Fox JF, Smith MM, Nuttall GA, et al. Chapter 20: Uncommon Cardiac Diseases. In: Kaplan JA, Augoustides JGT, Manecke GR, et al., eds. Kaplan's Cardiac Anesthesia. 7th ed. Elsevier; 2017:883-973.
2. Giambruno V, Karangelis D, Cucchietti C. Aortic valve papillary fibroelastoma: an insidious and unusual cause of angina. J Cardiothorac Vasc Anesth, 2015; 29: e61-e63.

6. Of the following primary malignant cardiac tumors in adults, the most common is:
  A. Lymphoma
  B. Angiosarcoma
  C. Histiocytoma
  D. Leiomyosarcoma

Correct Answer: B

Explanation: Nearly 25% of primary cardiac tumors are malignant, with 95% of these being sarcomas. Sarcomas may involve any cardiac chambers but typically infiltrate the right atrium (RA) and cause cavitary obstruction. Angiosarcomas, the most common sarcoma, are rapidly spreading vascular tumors that arise most often from the RA and appear near the inferior vena cava with extension to the mediastinum. Angiosarcoma can grow rapidly and undetected early on because of its nonspecific symptoms. Presenting symptoms include chest pain and dyspnea, progressive heart failure, and bloody pericardial effusion. Treatment is palliative because the response to chemotherapy and radiation is poor. Resection may be possible, but survival is typically less than 2 years. Rhabdomyosarcomas are the second most common sarcomas and are aggressive tumors that have cellular elements that resemble striated muscle. Other primary malignant tumors of the heart include malignant fibrous histiocytoma, fibrosarcomas, osteosarcoma, leiomyosarcoma (the rarest malignant cardiac tumor), undifferentiated sarcoma, neurogenic sarcoma, and lymphoma. All of these malignant tumors carry a poor prognosis with a median survival of approximately 1 year with treatment.

References:

1. Fox JF, Smith MM, Nuttall GA, et al. Chapter 20: Uncommon Cardiac Diseases. In: Kaplan JA, Augoustides JGT, Manecke GR, et al., eds. Kaplan's Cardiac Anesthesia. 7th ed. Elsevier; 2017:883-973.
2. Berry MF, Williams M, Welsby I, et al. Cardiac angiosarcoma presenting with right coronary artery pseudoaneurysm. J Cardiothorac Vasc Anesth, 2010; 24: 633-635.

7. Of the following disease primary malignancies, which is associated with the most with cardiac metastasis?
  A. Melanoma
  B. Glioblastoma
  C. Leukemia
  D. Hepatocellular carcinoma

Correct Answer: A

Explanation: Although rare overall, secondary or metastatic cardiac tumors are far more common than primary tumors. Metastatic tumors may involve the heart by direct extension, venous extension, or hematogenous or lymphatic spread. These tumors may affect primarily the pericardium (most common), the epicardium, the myocardium, or the endocardium. The site of metastasis frequently provides clues to the means of metastasis. Pericardial involvement, for example, often occurs via the direct extension from surrounding intrathoracic structures or from lymphatic spread, whereas endocardial lesions typically reflect hematogenous spread, and epicardial and myocardial lesions tend to arise from lymphatic extension. Tumors exhibiting high rates of cardiac metastases include mesothelioma (most common), melanoma (second most common), pulmonary adenocarcinoma, undifferentiated lung carcinoma, pulmonary squamous cell carcinoma, breast carcinoma, and esophageal carcinoma. Management for cardiac metastasis typically involves a combination of radiation, chemotherapy, and surgical resection.

References:

1. Fox JF, Smith MM, Nuttall GA, et al. Chapter 20: Uncommon Cardiac Diseases. In: Kaplan JA, Augoustides JGT, Manecke GR, et al., eds. Kaplan's Cardiac Anesthesia. 7th ed. Elsevier; 2017:883-973.
2. Yanagawa B, Chan EY, Cusimano RJ, et al. Approach to surgery for cardiac tumors: primary simple, primary complex, and secondary. Cardiol Clin, 2019; 37: 525-531.

8. What is a good indication to place a femoral (as opposed to internal jugular) central venous access for an open cardiac tumor resection?

A. Renal cell carcinoma extending to the right atrium

B. Large myxoma occluding the mitral valve

C. Metastatic pulmonary adenocarcinoma with facial edema

D. Angiosarcoma involving the inferior vena cava

Correct Answer: C

Explanation: In general, anesthetic management of patients with cardiac tumors is likely guided first by the patient's comorbidities and second by tumor location. Some factors that may require further considerations include depressed cardiac function (consider backup circulatory support), extensive right-sided involvement (possible right ventricular failure and pulmonary artery catheter avoidance), superior vena cava (SVC) compromise (place femoral central lines rather than in the neck), valvular involvement (e.g., myxoma occluding the mitral valve will act like mitral stenosis), and malignant tumors with significant myocardial invasion (may require deep hypothermic circulatory arrest). SVC syndrome may be caused by mediastinal or lung mass that compresses the SVC. It can significantly decrease venous return from the upper extremity and cause neck vein distention, facial and upper extremity edema, and occasionally cerebral edema.

References:

1. Fox JF, Smith MM, Nuttall GA, et al. Chapter 20: Uncommon Cardiac Diseases. In: Kaplan JA, Augoustides JGT, Manecke GR, et al., eds. Kaplan's Cardiac Anesthesia. 7th ed. Elsevier; 2017:883-973.
2. Potere B, Boulos R, Awad H, et al. The role of extracorporeal membrane oxygenation in the anesthetic management of superior vena cava syndrome: is it time to use a scoring system? J Cardiothorac Vasc Anesth, 2022; 36: 1777-1787.

9. Which valvular abnormality is most likely seen in carcinoid heart disease?

A. Aortic stenosis from calcification

B. Mitral regurgitation from prolapse

C. Tricuspid regurgitation from perforation

D. Pulmonary stenosis from restriction

Correct Answer: D

Explanation: Carcinoid tumors are metastasizing neuroendocrine tumors that arise primarily from the small bowel. Upon diagnosis, 20% to 30% of individuals with carcinoid tumors exhibit the symptoms of carcinoid syndrome, characterized by episodic vasomotor symptoms, bronchospasm, hypotension, diarrhea, and right-sided heart disease attributed to the release of serotonin, histamine, bradykinins, and prostaglandins, often in response to manipulation or pharmacologic stimulation. Carcinoid heart disease may occur in 20% to 50% of patients with carcinoid syndrome and still causes considerable morbidity and mortality. The median life expectancy is 5.9 years without carcinoid heart disease but falls to 2.6 years if it is present. A large majority (90%) of carcinoid heart disease mainly involves the right side of the heart. Carcinoid plaques composed of myofibroblasts, collagen, and myxoid matrix are deposited primarily on the tricuspid and pulmonary valves, bringing about immobility and thickening of the valve leaflets, causing restriction and a large coaptation defect. At the time of surgery, 80% of tricuspid valves are observed to be incompetent (significant tricuspid regurgitation) with only 20% with tricuspid stenosis, whereas the affected pulmonary valves tend to be equally divided between insufficiency and stenosis.

References:

1. Fox JF, Smith MM, Nuttall GA, et al. Chapter 20: Uncommon Cardiac Diseases. In: Kaplan JA, Augoustides JGT, Manecke GR, et al., eds. Kaplan's Cardiac Anesthesia. 7th ed. Elsevier; 2017:883-973.
2. Castillo J, Silvay G, Weiner M. Anesthetic management of patients with carcinoid syndrome and carcinoid heart disease: the Mount Sinai algorithm. J Cardiothorac Vasc Anesth, 2018; 32: 1023-1031.

10. Aortic valve involvement in carcinoid heart disease may indicate the presence of:

A. Left-to-right intracardiac shunt

B. Bronchial carcinoid

C. Low levels of circulating vasoactive substances

D. Bicuspid aortic valve

Correct Answer: B

Explanation: Fewer than 10% of those with carcinoid heart disease have left-sided heart involvement, possibly attributable to the inactivation of serotonin in the lungs. Nevertheless, the mitral or aortic valve may be affected in the presence of a bronchial carcinoid, a right-to-left intracardiac shunt, or a poorly controlled disease with high levels of circulating vasoactive substances. Aortic valve carcinoid disease includes cusp thickening with restricted motion and varying degrees of doming during diastole. With respect to the mitral valve, the subvalvular apparatus is most typically affected, resulting in chordal thickening that limits the leaflet mobility.

References:

1. Fox JF, Smith MM, Nuttall GA, et al. Chapter 20: Uncommon Cardiac Diseases. In: Kaplan JA, Augoustides JGT, Manecke GR, et al., eds. Kaplan's Cardiac Anesthesia. 7th ed. Elsevier; 2017:883-973.
2. Castillo J, Silvay G, Weiner M. Anesthetic management of patients with carcinoid syndrome and carcinoid heart disease: the Mount Sinai algorithm. J Cardiothorac Vasc Anesth, 2018; 32: 1023-1031.

11. A newly diagnosed carcinoid heart disease patient is being prepared for surgical management. Which management is considered a mainstay therapy?

A. Proton pump inhibitor
B. Heparin
C. Octreotide
D. Beta blocker

Correct Answer: C

Explanation: The mainstays of carcinoid disease treatment are symptom management (including somatostatin analogs), medical management of right-sided heart failure, chemotherapy, vascular embolization, surgical debulking, and valve replacements. Somatostatin analogs (e.g., octreotide, lanreotide) bind somatostatin receptors on carcinoid cells and prevent the release of the vasoactive mediators responsible for carcinoid syndrome. To maximize efficacy, octreotide infusion is typically started preoperatively with additional bolus given intraoperatively when carcinoid crisis occurs. Of note, severe hyperglycemia may occur with octreotide because of its inhibition of insulin secretion, especially in combination with steroids.

References:

1. Fox JF, Smith MM, Nuttall GA, et al. Chapter 20: Uncommon Cardiac Diseases. In: Kaplan JA, Augoustides JGT, Manecke GR, et al., eds. Kaplan's Cardiac Anesthesia. 7th ed. Elsevier; 2017:883-973.
2. Castillo J, Silvay G, Weiner M. Anesthetic management of patients with carcinoid syndrome and carcinoid heart disease: the Mount Sinai algorithm. J Cardiothorac Vasc Anesth, 2018; 32: 1023-1031.

12. A 50-year-old female with carcinoid heart disease is presenting for a scheduled tricuspid valve replacement. Which medication should be avoided during induction?

A. Midazolam
B. Fentanyl
C. Succinylcholine
D. Dexmedetomidine

Correct Answer: C

Explanation: Carcinoid tumor releases vasoactive neuroendocrine substances such as serotonin, histamine, tachykinins, kallikrein, and prostaglandin. The secretion of these substances may be exacerbated by various factors including stress, physical manipulation, and medications. Anesthetic management should minimize anxiety, pain, and responses to procedural stimulation including endotracheal intubation, incision, and tumor manipulation. Medications that may induce carcinoid mediators release include thiopental, meperidine, morphine, atracurium, succinylcholine, and catecholamines.

References:

1. Fox JF, Smith MM, Nuttall GA, et al. Chapter 20: Uncommon Cardiac Diseases. In: Kaplan JA, Augoustides JGT, Manecke GR, et al., eds. Kaplan's Cardiac Anesthesia. 7th ed. Elsevier; 2017:883-973.
2. Castillo J, Silvay G, Weiner M. Anesthetic management of patients with carcinoid syndrome and carcinoid heart disease: the Mount Sinai algorithm. J Cardiothorac Vasc Anesth, 2018; 32: 1023-1031.

13. Surgical resection of a renal.cell carcinoma that involves the intrahepatic inferior vena cava and extends above the diaphragm has a very high risk of:

A. Stroke
B. Left heart failure
C. Liver failure
D. Massive blood loss

Correct Answer: D

Explanation: Renal cell carcinoma may have a significant venous extension involving the vena cava and the heart. Renal cell cancers only represent 2% to 3% of adult malignancies but may have a mortality of almost 40%. The most common subtype is clear cell carcinoma (70%–80% of all renal cell tumors), followed by papillary renal cell carcinoma (10%–15%), and chromophobe renal cell carcinoma (3%–5%). According to the Mayo classification, level I tumor thrombus is confined to the ipsilateral renal vein or extends 2 cm or less into the inferior vena cava (IVC). A level II tumor thrombus extends more than 2 cm into the IVC but remains below the hepatic veins, whereas a level III mass involves the intrahepatic IVC but remains below the diaphragm. A level IV thrombus extends above the diaphragm and may involve the right atrium and right-sided heart structures. Surgery for levels III and IV renal cell carcinoma often requires cardiopulmonary bypass, sometimes with deep hypothermic circulatory arrest. There is also a high risk of significant blood loss. The average blood loss is about 1.8 liters in level III (average 7 units packed red blood cells given), as compared to 4.5 liters (with 15 units packed red blood cells) in level IV tumors. Further blood product administration such as fresh frozen plasma and platelets is significantly more likely to be required in level IV compared to level III cases due to the greater bleeding risk.

Stage I

Stage II

Stage III

Stage IV

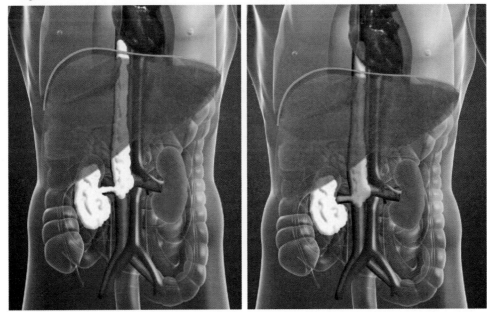

FIGURE 20.1 Renal cell carcinoma tumor thrombus staging. Stage I: Is confined to the ipsilateral renal vein or extends up to 2 cm into the inferior vena cava (IVC). Stage II: Extends more than 2 cm into the IVC but remains below the hepatic veins. Stage III: Involves the intrahepatic IVC but remains below the diaphragm. Stage IV: Extends above the diaphragm and may involve the heart structures. *IVC*, Inferior vena cava. (Reproduced with permission from Fukazawa K, Gologorsky E, Naguit K, et al. Invasive renal cell carcinoma with inferior vena cava tumor thrombus: cardiac anesthesia in liver transplant settings. J Cardiothorac Vasc Anesth, 2014; 28: 641.)

References:

1. Fox JF, Smith MM, Nuttall GA, et al. Chapter 20: Uncommon Cardiac Diseases. In: Kaplan JA, Augoustides JGT, Manecke GR, et al., eds. Kaplan's Cardiac Anesthesia. 7th ed. Elsevier; 2017:883-973.
2. Vinzant NJ, Christensen JM, Smith MM, et al. Perioperative outcomes for radical nephrectomy and level III-IV inferior vena cava tumor thrombectomy in patients with renal cell carcinoma. J Cardiothorac Vasc Anesth, 2022; 36: 3093-3100.
3. Fukazawa K, Gologorsky E, Naguit K, et al. Invasive renal cell carcinoma with inferior vena cava tumor thrombus: cardiac anesthesia in liver transplant settings. J Cardiothorac Vasc Anesth, 2014; 28: 640-646.

14. Which central venous access placement site (for large volume resuscitation) is likely ineffective in a level IV renal cell carcinoma resection?
   A. Right internal jugular vein
   B. Left internal jugular vein
   C. Either subclavian vein
   D. Either femoral vein

Correct Answer: D

Explanation: Level III and level IV renal carcinoma may have tumor extensions that occlude most of the inferior vena cava (IVC) and require interruption of IVC blood flow to resect. As such, femoral venous catheters for volume use intraoperatively may be of little use. Due to the potentially significant and rapid blood loss, adequate blood products and aggressive volume expansion should be included in the anesthetic plan. Intraoperative transesophageal echocardiography can guide central line placement (especially in patients with high tumor extension), monitor ventricular function (especially during the time of hepatic reperfusion), and assess the adequacy of surgical resection. Placement of a pulmonary artery catheter may be contraindicated in patients with cancer extending into the supradiaphragmatic IVC and right atrium.

References:

1. Fox JF, Smith MM, Nuttall GA, et al. Chapter 20: Uncommon Cardiac Diseases. In: Kaplan JA, Augoustides JGT, Manecke GR, et al., eds. Kaplan's Cardiac Anesthesia. 7th ed. Elsevier; 2017:883-973.
2. Fukazawa K, Gologorsky E, Naguit K, et al. Invasive renal cell carcinoma with inferior vena cava tumor thrombus: cardiac anesthesia in liver transplant settings. J Cardiothorac Vasc Anesth, 2014; 28: 640-646.

15. What condition may cause restrictive cardiomyopathy?
   A. Marfan syndrome
   B. Amyloidosis
   C. Amyotrophic lateral sclerosis
   D. Mycosis

Correct Answer: B

Explanation: Secondary cardiomyopathies, in which cardiac involvement occurs in the context of a systemic disorder, have multiple etiologies including infiltrative (amyloidosis, Gaucher disease) and storage (hemochromatosis, Fabry disease) diseases. Furthermore, drug toxicities (heavy metals, alcohol, cocaine), chemoradiation (doxorubicin, cyclophosphamide, adriamycin), nutritional deficiencies (beriberi, scurvy), and endocrinopathies (diabetes mellitus, hypothyroidism, hyperthyroidism, acromegaly) may also involve the heart. Inflammatory conditions (sarcoidosis, viral) and autoimmune disorders (systemic lupus erythematosus, scleroderma, rheumatoid arthritis) can also lead to secondary cardiomyopathy. Amyloidosis is a systemic disease with amyloid deposition in multiple organs including the heart, kidney, and nervous system that may lead to autonomic and sensorineural neuropathy. Cardiac amyloidosis results in stiff ventricular myocardium and a secondary restrictive cardiomyopathy. Marfan syndrome, amyotrophic lateral sclerosis, and mycosis have not been associated with restrictive myopathy.

References:

1. Fox JF, Smith MM, Nuttall GA, et al. Chapter 20: Uncommon Cardiac Diseases. In: Kaplan JA, Augoustides JGT, Manecke GR, et al., eds. Kaplan's Cardiac Anesthesia. 7th ed. Elsevier; 2017:883-973.
2. Meers JB, Townsley MM. Imaging cardiac amyloidosis: an update for the cardiothoracic anesthesiologist. J Cardiothorac Vasc Anesth, 2021; 35: 1911-1916.

16. What is TRUE regarding dilated cardiomyopathy?
   A. Second most common cardiomyopathy in adults
   B. Symptoms do not correlate with prognosis
   C. Patchy and diffuse loss of tissue with interstitial fibrosis and scarring
   D. Diastolic dysfunction occurs before systolic dysfunction

Correct Answer: C

Explanation: Dilated cardiomyopathy is the most common of the cardiomyopathies and is a leading indication for heart transplantation. It may be associated with genetic factors, toxin exposure, chemotherapy, infection, inflammatory conditions, and pregnancy. The development of symptoms has been associated with 1- and 5-year mortality rates of 25% and 50%, respectively. The myocardial histology demonstrates patchy and diffuse loss of tissue with interstitial fibrosis and scarring. The conduction system may be affected, and lead to bundle branch disease. Although systolic function typically occurs early, diastolic function is ultimately compromised. The initial management is typically medical but may later require left ventricular assist device placement and heart transplantation.

References:

1. Fox JF, Smith MM, Nuttall GA, et al. Chapter 20: Uncommon Cardiac Diseases. In: Kaplan JA, Augoustides JGT, Manecke GR, et al., eds. Kaplan's Cardiac Anesthesia. 7th ed. Elsevier; 2017:883-973.
2. Tan Z, Roscoe A, Rubino A. Transesophageal echocardiography in heart and lung transplantation. J Cardiothorac Vasc Anesth, 2019; 33: 1548-1558.

17. Typical echocardiographic findings of dilated cardiomyopathy include:
   A. Left ventricular hypertrophy
   B. Systolic anterior motion of the mitral valve
   C. Functional mitral regurgitation
   D. Thick pericardium

Correct Answer: C

Explanation: The characteristic echocardiographic findings in dilated cardiomyopathy include dilatation of all four cardiac chambers, modest thinning of the ventricular walls, and globally decreased systolic function. This pathology leads to annular dilation with consequent functional mitral and/or tricuspid regurgitation. As contractile function diminishes, stroke volume is initially maintained by augmentation of end-diastolic volume. Despite a severely decreased ejection fraction, stroke volume may remain almost normal. Increasing left atrial size may indicate worsening diastolic dysfunction in these patients, contributing significantly to functional mitral regurgitation. The onset of mitral regurgitation signals a poor prognosis because ventricular function progressively worsens without intervention. Left ventricular hypertrophy and systolic anterior motion of the mitral valve are features of hypertrophic cardiomyopathy. Thickening of the pericardium is not a typical feature of dilated cardiomyopathy.

References:

1. Fox JF, Smith MM, Nuttall GA, et al. Chapter 20: Uncommon Cardiac Diseases. In: Kaplan JA, Augoustides JGT, Manecke GR, et al., eds. Kaplan's Cardiac Anesthesia. 7th ed. Elsevier; 2017:883-973.
2. Tan Z, Roscoe A, Rubino A. Transesophageal echocardiography in heart and lung transplantation. J Cardiothorac Vasc Anesth, 2019; 33: 1548-1558.

18. Anesthetic considerations for patients with a significant dilated cardiomyopathy include:
   A. Avoiding ketamine for induction
   B. Requirement for high afterload
   C. Sensitivity to cardiac-depressant anesthetic drugs
   D. Favoring desflurane over sevoflurane for maintenance

Correct Answer: C

Explanation: The common cardiac procedures for patients with dilated cardiomyopathy include placement of a defibrillator for refractory ventricular arrhythmias, ventricular assist device placement, and heart transplantation. Anesthetic management is predicated on minimizing further myocardial depression, optimizing preload, and judiciously reducing afterload. These patients may be extremely sensitive to cardiac-depressant anesthetic drugs. Etomidate and ketamine may be safer for induction, but propofol can also be used judiciously. Of note, short-acting narcotics such as remifentanil may lead to bradycardia that may precipitate severe hypotension in this setting. Although volatile agents depress myocardial contractility, there is no clear superiority of any particular volatile agent.

References:

1. Fox JF, Smith MM, Nuttall GA, et al. Chapter 20: Uncommon Cardiac Diseases. In: Kaplan JA, Augoustides JGT, Manecke GR, et al., eds. Kaplan's Cardiac Anesthesia. 7th ed. Elsevier; 2017:883-973.
2. Ormerod JO, Yavari A. Cardiomyopathies. Medicine, 2022; 50: 492-506.

19. Sarcomeric disarray, chaotic myocytes arrangements, and beta-myosin heavy chain mutation are all associated with:
   A. Dilated cardiomyopathy
   B. Hypertrophic cardiomyopathy
   C. Restrictive cardiomyopathy
   D. Arrhythmogenic right ventricular cardiomyopathy

Correct Answer: B

Explanation: Hypertrophic cardiomyopathy is characterized by hypertrophy with diastolic dysfunction, arrhythmias, and a tendency to dynamic obstruction of the left ventricular outflow tract with associated mitral regurgitation. It is a primary myocardial abnormality with sarcomeric disarray and asymmetric left ventricular hypertrophy. The hypertrophied muscle has myocytes with bizarre shapes and multiple intercellular connections arranged in a chaotic pattern. Increased connective tissue, combined with significantly disorganized and hypertrophied myocytes, contributes to the increased chamber stiffness, impaired relaxation, and an unstable electrophysiologic substrate causing complex arrhythmias and sudden death. This cardiomyopathy is commonly inherited in an autosomal dominant fashion, with a prevalence of at least 1:200 to 1:500. Common genetic mutations in this setting include the β-myosin heavy chain and myosin-binding protein C.

References:

1. Fox JF, Smith MM, Nuttall GA, et al. Chapter 20: Uncommon Cardiac Diseases. In: Kaplan JA, Augoustides JGT, Manecke GR, et al., eds. Kaplan's Cardiac Anesthesia. 7th ed. Elsevier; 2017:883-973.
2. Addis DR, Townsley MM. Perioperative implications of the 2020 American Heart Association/American College of Cardiology guidelines for the diagnosis and treatment of patients with hypertrophic cardiomyopathy: a focused review. J Cardiothorac Vasc Anesth, 2022; 36: 2143-2153.

20. What is TRUE regarding hypertrophic cardiomyopathy?
   A. The midventricular variant is the most common type
   B. All types can be resected via the transaortic left ventricular septal myectomy approach
   C. Anomalous papillary muscle insertions can contribute to flow obstruction
   D. The basal variant is not associated with systolic anterior motion of the mitral valve

Correct Answer: C

Explanation: The most common pattern in hypertrophic cardiomyopathy involves asymmetric hypertrophy of the basal left ventricular septum with a dynamic left ventricular outflow tract obstruction and systolic anterior motion of the mitral valve (see figure). Other common morphologic types include a midventricular variant and an apical variant. Defining the location and extent of hypertrophy and the site of obstruction, if any, is important for surgical planning. Asymmetric hypertrophy of the basal septum can be treated with a standard transaortic extended left ventricular septal myectomy. On the other hand, midventricular and apical variants may require a transapical approach or a combination of transapical and transaortic approaches. Cardiac magnetic resonance imaging may characterize morphologic patterns that conventional echocardiography may miss including apical aneurysms and thrombus, as well as anomalous papillary muscle insertions that can contribute to midventricular or outflow tract obstruction.

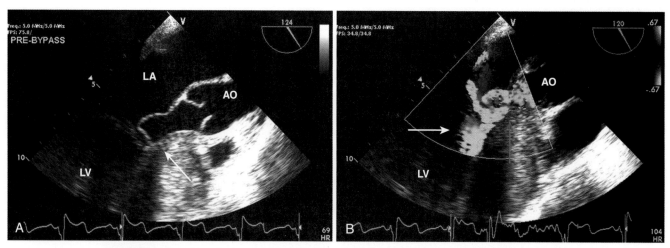

FIGURE 20.2 Transesophageal midesophageal long-axis view of the aortic valve and left ventricular outflow tract (LVOT) in a patient with hypertrophic obstructive cardiomyopathy. (A) Two-dimensional echocardiography during systole shows a thickened basal septum *(white arrow)* and systolic anterior motion (SAM) of the anterior leaflet of the mitral valve, creating dynamic LVOT obstruction. (B) Color-flow Doppler shows flow acceleration beginning at the site of the septal hypertrophy *(white arrow)* and becoming more severe in the narrowed LVOT *(pink arrow)*. Mitral regurgitation associated with SAM is typically directed posterolaterally *(red arrow)* and will typically improve if not resolved after myectomy. Jets of mitral regurgitation directed centrally or anteriorly suggest an additional cause for the regurgitation that may persist after myectomy and may need to be addressed with a separate surgical intervention on the mitral valve. *AO*, Aorta; *LA*, left atrium; *LV*, left ventricle. (Reproduced with permission from Oliver WC, Mauermann WJ, Nuttall GA. Uncommon cardiac diseases. In: Kaplan JA, Reich DL, Savino JS, eds. Kaplan's Cardiac Anesthesia: The Echo Era. 6th ed. Saunders; 2011:688.)

References:

1. Fox JF, Smith MM, Nuttall GA, et al. Chapter 20: Uncommon Cardiac Diseases. In: Kaplan JA, Augoustides JGT, Manecke GR, et al., eds. Kaplan's Cardiac Anesthesia. 7th ed. Elsevier; 2017:883-973.
2. Addis DR, Townsley MM. Perioperative implications of the 2020 American Heart Association/American College of Cardiology guidelines for the diagnosis and treatment of patients with hypertrophic cardiomyopathy: a focused review. J Cardiothorac Vasc Anesth, 2022; 36: 2143-2153.

21. What is a significant risk factor for sudden cardiac death in a patient with hypertrophic cardiomyopathy?
  A. Second-degree family history of sudden death due to hypertrophic cardiomyopathy
  B. Low resting gradient across the left ventricular outflow tract
  C. Significant late gadolinium enhancement on cardiac magnetic resonance imaging
  D. Atrial fibrillation

Correct Answer: C

Explanation: Major risk factors for sudden cardiac death in hypertrophic cardiomyopathy include a first-degree family history of sudden death, unexplained syncope, massive left ventricular hypertrophy (wall thickness ≥30 mm), repeated nonsustained ventricular tachycardia, and an inappropriate systemic systolic blood pressure response during exercise testing. The presence of significant late gadolinium enhancement (≥15% of left ventricular mass) on cardiac magnetic resonance imaging, significant obstruction of the left ventricular outflow tract at rest, apical aneurysm, systolic dysfunction, participation in strenuous competitive sports, obstructive coronary artery disease, and age above 60 years are further risk factors for cardiac death in this setting. Although atrial fibrillation is common and important, it is not an independent risk factor for sudden cardiac death in hypertrophic cardiomyopathy.

References:

1. Fox JF, Smith MM, Nuttall GA, et al. Chapter 20: Uncommon Cardiac Diseases. In: Kaplan JA, Augoustides JGT, Manecke

GR, et al., eds. Kaplan's Cardiac Anesthesia. 7th ed. Elsevier; 2017:883-973.
2. Addis DR, Townsley MM. Perioperative implications of the 2020 American Heart Association/American College of Cardiology guidelines for the diagnosis and treatment of patients with hypertrophic cardiomyopathy: a focused review. J Cardiothorac Vasc Anesth, 2022; 36: 2143-2153.

22. What is TRUE regarding the management of hypertrophic cardiomyopathy?
   A. Beta blockers are contraindicated
   B. Nondihydropyridine calcium channel blockers are second-line medications
   C. Alcohol septal ablation has a lower reintervention rate compared to surgical myectomy
   D. Surgical myectomy has a high mortality even at major centers

Correct Answer: B

Explanation: The management of hypertrophic cardiomyopathy includes avoiding factors that exacerbate the obstruction of the left ventricular outflow tract such as hypovolemia, decreased systemic vascular resistance, tachycardia, and increased contractility. Beta blockers are first-line therapy to slow the heart rate, lengthen diastolic filling, and promote stroke volume. Nondihydropyridine calcium channel blockers such as verapamil and diltiazem are second-line agents. For patients with persistent symptoms despite pharmacologic therapy, interventional therapy with either alcohol septal ablation or surgical myectomy is the next option. Alcohol septal ablation has similar survival benefits as surgical myectomy but has a higher rate of reintervention. At major centers, surgical intervention with myectomy has low mortality in the 1% range and has repeatedly been shown to offer durable freedom from outflow tract obstruction with significant clinical improvement.

References:

1. Fox JF, Smith MM, Nuttall GA, et al. Chapter 20: Uncommon Cardiac Diseases. In: Kaplan JA, Augoustides JGT, Manecke GR, et al., eds. Kaplan's Cardiac Anesthesia. 7th ed. Elsevier; 2017:883-973.
2. Addis DR, Townsley MM. Perioperative implications of the 2020 American Heart Association/American College of Cardiology guidelines for the diagnosis and treatment of patients with hypertrophic cardiomyopathy: a focused review. J Cardiothorac Vasc Anesth, 2022; 36: 2143-2153.
3. Nguyen A, Schaff HV, Hang D, et al. Surgical myectomy versus alcohol septal ablation for obstructive hypertrophic cardiomyopathy: A propensity score-matched cohort. J Thorac Cardiovasc Surg, 2019; 157: 306-315.

23. Which echocardiographic finding is likely present in a premyectomy echo in the basal septal variant of hypertrophic cardiomyopathy?
   A. High mean gradient distal to the aortic valve
   B. Respiratory variations in mitral inflow pulse wave Doppler
   C. Posteriorly directed mitral regurgitant jet
   D. Flail posterior mitral leaflet

Correct Answer: C

Explanation: Common echocardiographic findings in asymmetric basal hypertrophic cardiomyopathy include basal left ventricular hypertrophy, turbulent color flow in the left ventricular outflow tract, high gradient across the outflow tract with a unique "dagger-shaped" appearance in the Doppler signal, and systolic anterior motion of the mitral valve with posteriorly directed mitral regurgitant jet. If the jet is not directed posteriorly, or if there are multiple jets, then an additional mechanism for mitral regurgitation is likely present. This assessment is important in guiding the surgical treatment because mitral regurgitation associated with dynamic outflow tract obstruction, even when severe, rarely requires surgical intervention and will largely resolve after the basal myectomy. However, mitral regurgitation caused by organic lesions, such as mitral valve prolapse or a flail leaflet, will not. In addition to assessing postmyectomy pressure gradients, the echocardiographic evaluation should also evaluate for an iatrogenic ventricular septal defect that may complicate the myectomy procedure. Respiratory variations in mitral inflow pulse wave Doppler are not typically associated with hypertrophic cardiomyopathy.

References:

1. Fox JF, Smith MM, Nuttall GA, et al. Chapter 20: Uncommon Cardiac Diseases. In: Kaplan JA, Augoustides JGT, Manecke GR, et al., eds. Kaplan's Cardiac Anesthesia. 7th ed. Elsevier; 2017:883-973.
2. Addis DR, Townsley MM. Perioperative implications of the 2020 American Heart Association/American College of Cardiology guidelines for the diagnosis and treatment of patients with hypertrophic cardiomyopathy: a focused review. J Cardiothorac Vasc Anesth, 2022; 36: 2143-2153.

24. In the midventricular variant of hypertrophic cardiomyopathy, what echocardiographic findings is typically present?
   A. High pressure gradient in the left ventricular outflow tract
   B. Mitral stenosis
   C. Apical pouch
   D. Systolic anterior motion of the mitral valve

Correct Answer: C

Explanation: With a midventricular variant of hypertrophic cardiomyopathy, obstruction occurs at the midventricular level, attributable to the apposition of the ventricular septum and the papillary muscles. Because outflow tract obstruction is not present, systolic anterior motion of the mitral valve and associated mitral regurgitation are unlikely. Furthermore, the pressure gradient occurs not across the outflow tract but across the cavity of the ventricle, from apex to base. The elevated apical pressures, secondary to mid cavitary obstruction, may favor the formation of an apical pouch with a risk for thrombus formation due to stasis. For patients with apical variant, hypertrophy occurs predominantly at the apex, producing a small chamber size with significant impairment in diastolic filling and low stroke volumes. Typically, these do not exhibit obstruction of the outflow tract and the associated mitral regurgitation.

References:

1. Fox JF, Smith MM, Nuttall GA, et al. Chapter 20: Uncommon Cardiac Diseases. In: Kaplan JA, Augoustides JGT, Manecke GR, et al., eds. Kaplan's Cardiac Anesthesia. 7th ed. Elsevier; 2017:883-973.
2. Addis DR, Townsley MM. Perioperative implications of the 2020 American Heart Association/American College of Cardiology guidelines for the diagnosis and treatment of patients with hypertrophic cardiomyopathy: a focused review. J Cardiothorac Vasc Anesth, 2022; 36: 2143-2153.

25. Acute hypotension in a patient with hypertrophic cardiomyopathy can be treated with:
  A. Epinephrine
  B. Furosemide
  C. Phenylephrine
  D. Nitric oxide

Correct Answer: C

Explanation: Acute hypotension in a patient with hypertrophic cardiomyopathy is likely from outflow tract obstruction with systolic anterior motion of the mitral valve and subsequent significant mitral regurgitation. The treatment goals include increasing preload and afterload, while avoiding tachycardia and increased contractility. Fluid bolus and vasoconstrictors such as phenylephrine and vasopressin are the first-line treatments. Esmolol may also be used to decrease contractility and heart rate to improve preload by prolonging diastole. This syndrome should be considered in the differential diagnosis of unexpected refractory intraoperative hypotension.

References:

1. Fox JF, Smith MM, Nuttall GA, et al. Chapter 20: Uncommon Cardiac Diseases. In: Kaplan JA, Augoustides JGT, Manecke GR, et al., eds. Kaplan's Cardiac Anesthesia. 7th ed. Elsevier; 2017:883-973.
2. Addis DR, Townsley MM. Perioperative implications of the 2020 American Heart Association/American College of Cardiology guidelines for the diagnosis and treatment of patients with hypertrophic cardiomyopathy: a focused review. J Cardiothorac Vasc Anesth, 2022; 36: 2143-2153.

26. What is TRUE regarding alcohol septal ablation?
  A. Ethanol alcohol is injected directly into the hypertrophied myocardium
  B. There is almost no risk of needing a permanent pacemaker afterward
  C. Subsequent cardiac remodeling may take months
  D. It is effective even for the thickest ventricle (>30 mm)

Correct Answer: C

Explanation: For patients with severe symptoms, despite optimal medical management, and those who are not surgical candidates, alcohol septal ablation in the cardiac catheterization laboratory under fluoroscopic and echocardiographic guidance is an option. The goal is to identify a prominent anteroseptal-perforating branch of the left anterior descending coronary artery that is supplying the hypertrophied basal septum. Once the target is found, 1 to 3 mL of ethanol alcohol is infused to create a localized infarction, leading to subsequent necrosis and regression of the hypertrophied area. Although subsequent remodeling may take months, the injection can affect an immediate decrease in gradient as a result of myocardial stunning. The advantages of alcohol ablation include its minimally invasive nature and short hospital stay. It is associated, however, with a higher risk of permanent pacemaker placement, repeat procedures, and ventricular arrhythmias. Furthermore, septal ablation is often ineffective in patients with very advanced hypertrophy (≥30 mm).

References:

1. Fox JF, Smith MM, Nuttall GA, et al. Chapter 20: Uncommon Cardiac Diseases. In: Kaplan JA, Augoustides JGT, Manecke GR, et al., eds. Kaplan's Cardiac Anesthesia. 7th ed. Elsevier; 2017:883-973.
2. Addis DR, Townsley MM. Perioperative implications of the 2020 American Heart Association/American College of Cardiology guidelines for the diagnosis and treatment of patients with hypertrophic cardiomyopathy: a focused review. J Cardiothorac Vasc Anesth, 2022; 36: 2143-2153.

27. What is the hallmark of restrictive cardiomyopathy?
  A. Impaired systolic function
  B. Restricted pericardium
  C. Impaired diastolic function
  D. Dilated left ventricle

Correct Answer: C

Explanation: Restrictive cardiomyopathy is characterized by impaired myocardial relaxation and decreased ventricular compliance that leads to elevated filling pressures and severe diastolic dysfunction. The left ventricle size, thickness, and function are usually normal until late in the disease, when systolic function might deteriorate. It may be familial (autosomal dominant inheritance pattern), acquired secondary to systemic disorders (e.g., amyloidosis, hemochromatosis, Fabry disease), or idiopathic. Although its causes are varied, they may be classified as primarily myocardial or endomyocardial. Myocardial disorders are subclassified as noninfiltrative (familial, scleroderma, idiopathic), infiltrative (amyloidosis, sarcoidosis, Gaucher disease), or storage (hemochromatosis, Fabry disease). Endomyocardial disorders may be distinguished by the presence or absence of eosinophilia and include hypereosinophilic syndromes (Löffler endocarditis), endomyocardial fibrosis, and radiation-induced disorders. The echocardiographic features in this setting include biatrial enlargement, the absence of ventricular dilatation, and normal ventricular wall thickness, with grossly preserved systolic function.

References:

1. Fox JF, Smith MM, Nuttall GA, et al. Chapter 20: Uncommon Cardiac Diseases. In: Kaplan JA, Augoustides JGT, Manecke GR,

et al., eds. Kaplan's Cardiac Anesthesia. 7th ed. Elsevier; 2017:883-973.

2. Ormerod JO, Yavari A. Cardiomyopathies. Medicine, 2022; 50: 492-506.

28. A patient with severe restrictive cardiomyopathy will likely have which of the following cardiac catheterization findings?

A. Mean pulmonary artery pressure less than 15 mmHg

B. Absent A wave

C. Left ventricular end-diastolic pressure 10 mmHg greater than the right ventricular end-diastolic pressure

D. Absent Y descent

Correct Answer: C

Explanation: A classic cardiac catheterization finding in restrictive cardiomyopathy is that the left-sided filling pressures frequently exceed the right ventricular diastolic pressures by at least 5 to 10 mmHg. A rapid dip and subsequent early plateau in diastolic ventricular pressure, reflecting filling of a poorly compliant ventricle and rapid equalization of left atrial and ventricular pressures, may produce a characteristic ventricular diastolic waveform, the so-called "square root sign," although it may be absent in up to 50% of patients because it depends on both the degree of impaired ventricular relaxation and the atrial driving pressure. The atrial pressure waveform may take the appearance of an M or a W, reflecting prominent A and V waves and rapid X and Y descents. Furthermore, elevation in left-sided filling pressures produces pulmonary venous hypertension and pulmonary artery systolic pressures that may exceed 50 mmHg. Although management can be related to the etiology (e.g., enzyme-replacement therapy for Gaucher and Fabry diseases, steroids for sarcoidosis), it also should include pharmacotherapy tailored toward heart failure, including control of associated atrial fibrillation. The prognosis depends largely on the underlying cause.

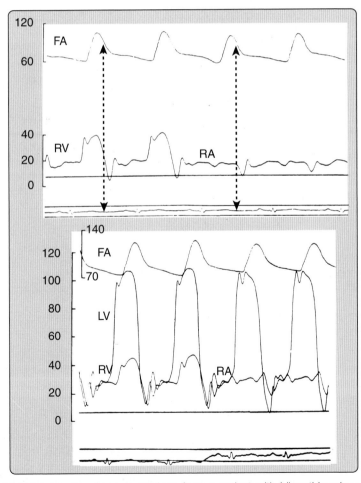

FIGURE 20.3 Intracardiac pressure tracings from a patient with idiopathic primary restrictive cardiomyopathy. (Top) Right ventricular and right atrial tracings are demonstrated with a typical diastolic square-root configuration in the right ventricular tracing and a prominent Y descent in the early diastolic period of the right atrial tracing. (Bottom) Simultaneous left ventricular–right ventricular pressures and left ventricular–right atrial pressures show a square-root configuration in the left ventricular tracing and equalization of pressures during diastole in the three chambers. *FA,* Femoral artery; *LV,* left ventricle; *RA,* right atrium; *RV,* right ventricle. (From Giuliani ER, Fuster V, Gersh BJ, et al: Cardiology: Fundamentals and Practice. St. Louis, Mosby, 1991.)

TABLE 20.1

Echocardiographic features of restrictive cardiomyopathy and constrictive pericarditis

	Restrictive Cardiomyopathy	Constrictive Pericarditis
Pericardium	Normal	Thickened
Left ventricle	Small May show systolic dysfunction No septal bounce	Small Usually intact, may be abnormal, particularly after CABG or radiation Septal bounce
Atria	Usually dilated	Usually nondilated
Mitral inflow	Increase E/A ratio, short DT No significant respiratory variation of E velocity Diastolic MR	Increase E/A ratio, short DT Expiratory increase of >25% in E velocity Diastolic MR
Tissue Doppler long velocities	Significantly reduced	Normal
Circumferential strain	Normal	Reduced
Peak radial strain class IV base	Normal	Reduced
Net twist	Normal	Reduced
Basal longitudinal strain	Reduced	Normal
Apical untwisting velocities	Normal	Reduced
Pulmonary vein inflow	Decreased (0.5) S/D ratio Prominent atrial reversal No significant respiratory change	S/D ratio = 1 Decrease in S and D[a] wave and TR velocity
Tricuspid inflow	Mild respiratory variation	Inspiratory increase of >25% in E wave and TR velocity
Inferior vena cava	Dilated	Dilated
Hepatic veins	Blunted S/D ratio	Inspiration: minimal increase in S and D velocities Expiration: decreased diastolic flow and increase in reversals Increase in atrial reversal of >25% in expiration, compared with inspiration
Peak PA pressure	>40 mm Hg	<40 mmHg
Color M-mode	Decreased Vp <45 cm/sec	Normal or increase >100 cm/sec
Mitral annular Doppler	Low velocity <8 cm/sec	High velocity >8 cm/sec

[a]One study found significantly greater decrease of D wave only with respiration in constriction.

A, Atrial transmitral filling velocity; *CABG,* coronary artery bypass graft; *D,* diastolic flow; *DT,* deceleration time; *E,* early transmitral filling velocity; *LV,* left ventricle; *MR,* mitral regurgitation. *PA,* pulmonary artery; *S,* systolic flow; *TR,* tricuspid regurgitation; *Vp,* propagation velocity.

Reproduced with permission from Naqvi TZ. Restrictive cardiomyopathy: diagnosis and prognostic implications. In: Otto CM, ed. Practice of Clinical Echocardiography. 4th ed. Saunders; 2012:557.

References:

1. Fox JF, Smith MM, Nuttall GA, et al. Chapter 20: Uncommon Cardiac Diseases. In: Kaplan JA, Augoustides JGT, Manecke GR, et al., eds. Kaplan's Cardiac Anesthesia. 7th ed. Elsevier; 2017:883-973.
2. Ormerod JO, Yavari A. Cardiomyopathies. Medicine, 2022; 50: 492-506.

29. Which finding is present in restrictive cardiomyopathy, but not constrictive pericarditis?
    A. Square root sign in the central venous pressure or right atrium waveform
    B. Minimal respiratory variation in the mitral inflow pulse wave Doppler
    C. Low right ventricular systolic pressure
    D. Mitral stenosis

Correct Answer: B

Explanation: Diagnostically, distinguishing restrictive cardiomyopathy (RCM) from constrictive pericarditis (CP) is important, considering that their treatments are quite different. In both disorders, filling pressures are high. In RCM the elevated pressures reflect a stiffened myocardium, whereas in CP, they reflect the constraint of a stiff pericardium. With cardiac catheterization, left ventricular end-diastolic pressure typically exceeds its right ventricular counterpart by 5 mmHg or more in RCM, attributable to differences in respective ventricular compliance. In CP, ventricular end-diastolic pressures are elevated and equal. Additionally, because a stiff, often thickened, pericardium constrains the total cardiac volume in CP, ventricular interdependence is exaggerated. In CP, two-dimensional echocardiography may show a thickened pericardium and may demonstrate a septal bounce consistent with ventricular interdependence and the dissociation of intracardiac and intrathoracic pressures. Mitral inflow pulsed-wave Doppler will show increased E/A ratios in both RCM and CP; however, in the latter case, there should be significant respiratory variation in the E velocity, with at least a 25% increase during expiration. Elevated natriuretic

peptides are consistent with RCM. A history of radiation, previous cardiac surgery, and thickened pericardium on cardiac imaging are consistent with CP.

References:

1. Fox JF, Smith MM, Nuttall GA, et al. Chapter 20: Uncommon Cardiac Diseases. In: Kaplan JA, Augoustides JGT, Manecke GR, et al., eds. Kaplan's Cardiac Anesthesia. 7th ed. Elsevier; 2017:883-973.
2. Ormerod JO, Yavari A. Cardiomyopathies. Medicine, 2022; 50: 492-506.

TABLE 20.2

Differentiation of pericardial constriction and myocardial restriction

Characteristic	Constrictive Pericarditis	Restrictive Cardiomyopathy
Jugular venous waveform	Elevated with less rapid Y descent	Elevated with more rapid Y descent Large A waves
LAP > RAP	Absent	Almost always
Auscultation	Early S_3 high pitched; no S_4	Late S_3 low pitched; S_4 in some cases
Mitral or tricuspid regurgitation	Frequently absent	Frequently present
Chest roentgenogram	Calcification of pericardium (20%–30%)	Pericardial calcification rare
Heart size	Normal to increased	Normal to increased
Electrocardiogram	Conduction abnormalities rare	Conduction abnormalities common
Echocardiogram	Slight enlargement of atria	Major enlargement of atria
Right ventricular pressure waveform	Square-root pattern	Square-root pattern; dip and plateau often less prominent
Right- and left-sided heart diastolic pressures	Within 5 mmHg of each other in almost all cases	Seldom within 5 mmHg of each other
Peak right ventricular systolic pressure	Almost always <60 mmHg, sometimes <40 mmHg	Usually >40 mmHg, sometimes >60 mmHg
Discordant respiratory variation of peak ventricular systolic pressures	Right and left ventricular systolic pressures are out of phase with respiration	In phase with respiration
Paradoxic pulse	Often present	Rare
CT and MRI imaging	Thickened pericardium	Rarely thickened pericardium
Endomyocardial biopsy	Normal or nonspecific changes	Nonspecific abnormalities

CT, Computed tomography; *LAP,* left atrial pressure; *MRI,* magnetic resonance imaging; *RAP,* right atrial pressure.
Reproduced with permission from Hancock EW: Cardiomyopathy: differential diagnosis of restrictive cardiomyopathy and constrictive pericarditis. Heart, 2001; 86: 343-349; and Chatterjee K, Alpert J. Constrictive pericarditis and restrictive cardiomyopathy: similarities and differences. Heart Fail Monit, 2003; 3: 118-126.

---

30. What is TRUE regarding restrictive cardiomyopathy secondary to amyloidosis?
   A. The most common type is associated with transthyretin proteins
   B. Cardiac involvement has a good prognosis
   C. Kidney is the most commonly affected organ in light chain amyloidosis
   D. Arrhythmias are rare

Correct Answer: C

Explanation: Amyloidosis is one of the more common etiologies for restrictive cardiomyopathy. There are several types

of amyloidosis that can affect the heart, with the amyloid light chain (AL) being most common (50% of cases), followed by the amyloidosis with transthyretin (ATTR) type (30% of cases). In AL amyloidosis, an increased number of plasma cells overproduce abnormal immunoglobulin light chains that form deposits in several organs. The kidney is the most commonly affected organ, followed by the heart with a prognosis of less than 6 months if not treated. In ATTR amyloidosis, there are unstable liver-derived transthyretin proteins that lead to abnormal amyloid fibrils. The clinical manifestation of cardiac amyloidosis is that of restrictive heart disease with diastolic heart failure that then progresses to systolic heart failure. With infiltration of the conduction system, a variety of arrhythmias including heart block may arise. These patients tend to be very labile during anesthetic induction, likely from a combination of severe diastolic dysfunction accompanied by a degree of systolic heart failure, and autonomic neuropathy from amyloid infiltration. Even judicious doses of drugs may have unpredictable effects. Cardiac amyloidosis may be associated with ventricular hypertrophy with a unique global longitudinal strain pattern of impaired middle and basal segments with relative apical sparing. This is different from conditions such as hypertrophic cardiomyopathy and aortic stenosis, where the reduced global longitudinal strain occurs in the most hypertrophied region.

References:

1. Fox JF, Smith MM, Nuttall GA, et al. Chapter 20: Uncommon Cardiac Diseases. In: Kaplan JA, Augoustides JGT, Manecke GR, et al., eds. Kaplan's Cardiac Anesthesia. 7th ed. Elsevier; 2017:883-973.
2. Meers JB, Townsley MM. Imaging cardiac amyloidosis: an update for the cardiothoracic anesthesiologist. J Cardiothorac Vasc Anesth, 2021; 35: 1911-1916.

31. The hallmark of arrhythmogenic right ventricular cardiomyopathy is:
   A. Severe right ventricular hypertrophy
   B. Progressive fibrofatty replacement of right ventricular myocardium
   C. Significant septal wall involvement
   D. Tricuspid stenosis

Correct Answer: B

Explanation: Arrhythmogenic right ventricular cardiomyopathy (ARVC) primarily includes progressive fibrofatty replacement of the right ventricular myocardium, which starts focally and then spreads globally to most of the right ventricle and occasionally part of the left ventricle, while relatively sparing the septum. Echocardiographic findings include right ventricular dilatation with thinning of its free wall, wall motion abnormalities, gradual systolic dysfunction, and a risk for aneurysm development. Of note, end-stage ARVC may be difficult to distinguish from dilated cardiomyopathy because the extent of left ventricular involvement has only recently been appreciated. Sudden death occurs in up to 75% of patients and, although a rare disease, accounts for 20% of sudden death in the young.

ARVC is familial in 30% to 50% of persons, with primarily autosomal dominant inheritance, variable expressivity, and reduced penetrance. The prevalence of ARVC has been estimated to be between 1:2000 and 1:5000, with men more affected than women at a ratio of 3:1. The initial presentation is often during adolescence, although it may occur in younger individuals. Its presentation most commonly begins with the onset of arrhythmias ranging from premature ventricular contractions to ventricular fibrillation originating from the right ventricle. Though challenging, ARVC patients can survive general anesthesia. A case series of 15 ARVC patients undergoing heart transplantations showed 100% intraoperative survival rate (though several did die within

months from other reasons such as donor heart failure and intracranial hemorrhage).

References:

1. Fox JF, Smith MM, Nuttall GA, et al. Chapter 20: Uncommon Cardiac Diseases. In: Kaplan JA, Augoustides JGT, Manecke GR, et al., eds. Kaplan's Cardiac Anesthesia. 7th ed. Elsevier; 2017:883-973.
2. Valchanov K, Goddard M, Ghosh S. Anesthesia for heart transplantation in patients with arrhythmogenic right ventricular dysplasia. J Cardiothorac Vasc Anesth, 2014; 28: 355-357.
3. Ormerod JO, Yavari A. Cardiomyopathies. Medicine, 2022; 50: 492-506

32. Anesthetic management of arrhythmogenic right ventricular cardiomyopathy includes which of the following?
   A. Maintaining light anesthesia
   B. Using amiodarone after treating reversible issues
   C. Avoiding general anesthesia
   D. Low threshold for placing a pulmonary artery catheter

Correct Answer: B

Explanation: In arrhythmogenic right ventricular cardiomyopathy (ARVC) there is a high risk of fatal arrhythmia due to the replacement of the myocardium with fat and fibrous tissue. In the perioperative period, anesthetic management should minimize any proarrhythmic triggers such as noxious stimuli, hypovolemia, hypercarbia, light anesthesia, and acidosis. General anesthesia alone does not appear to be arrhythmogenic. Caution should be used if inserting a pulmonary arterial catheter in patients with ARVC due to increased risks of dysrhythmias and right ventricular perforation. Management of perioperative malignant dysrhythmias in patients with ARVC targets reversible causes (e.g., light anesthesia, pain, electrolyte disturbances) followed by consideration of beta blockers and amiodarone. In the chronic setting, placement of a defibrillator or ventricular ablation is typically considered for management of ventricular arrhythmias.

References:

1. Fox JF, Smith MM, Nuttall GA, et al. Chapter 20: Uncommon Cardiac Diseases. In: Kaplan JA, Augoustides JGT, Manecke GR, et al., eds. Kaplan's Cardiac Anesthesia. 7th ed. Elsevier; 2017:883-973.
2. Ormerod JO, Yavari A. Cardiomyopathies. Medicine, 2022; 50: 492-506.

33. What is TRUE regarding mitral valve prolapse?
   A. Severe mitral regurgitation occurs in more than 30% of patients
   B. It is associated with Marfan syndrome
   C. Anterior mitral leaflet prolapse is more common than posterior leaflet prolapse
   D. Mitral valve replacement reduces mortality compared to mitral valve repair

Correct Answer: B

Explanation: Mitral valve prolapse (MVP) is a progressive degenerative mitral valve disease leading to varying degrees of mitral regurgitation. The involvement of the mitral valve ranges from a more focal fibroelastic deficiency from impaired connective tissue production to a more diffuse Barlow disease with myxomatous degeneration of the valve leaflets. MVP is likely a genetically inherited disease with an autosomal dominant pattern and with an incidence in the 1% to 2% range that has an equal distribution among men and women. Prolapse of the mitral leaflets at least 2 mm above the level of the atrioventricular ring is diagnostic for MVP. Severe mitral regurgitation develops in approximately 2% to 4% of patients with MVP, and its onset signals the need for therapeutic intervention. Left untreated, severe mitral regurgitation may lead to pulmonary hypertension, left atrial enlargement, atrial fibrillation, and heart failure. When possible, mitral valve repair is preferred over replacement due to significant morbidity and mortality improvement, although this may be challenging at times, especially with extensive bileaflet involvement.

References:

1. Fox JF, Smith MM, Nuttall GA, et al. Chapter 20: Uncommon Cardiac Diseases. In: Kaplan JA, Augoustides JGT, Manecke GR, et al., eds. Kaplan's Cardiac Anesthesia. 7th ed. Elsevier; 2017:883-973.
2. Mahmood F, Sharkey A, Maslow A, et al. Echocardiographic assessment of the mitral valve for suitability of repair: an intraoperative approach from a mitral center. J Cardiothorac Vasc Anesth, 2022; 36: 2164-2176.

34. During coronary artery bypass grafting (CABG), a patent foramen ovale (PFO) was incidentally found and the patient had no other related symptoms. What is TRUE regarding PFO?
   A. Incidence in the population is nearly 50%
   B. Prophylactic PFO closure leads to improved mortality
   C. PFO closure during a CABG does not require alteration in surgical technique
   D. Atrial septal aneurysm increases the risk of paradoxical embolus

Correct Answer: D

Explanation: Patent foramen ovale (PFO) is the most common congenital defect involving the atrial septum. PFO is relatively common, with a reported incidence of around 27% to 34% on autopsy. It is a known possible cause of embolic stroke. A paradoxical embolus is more common in the setting of an atrial septal aneurysm, a large Eustachian valve, migraines, and age above 50 years. The management includes anticoagulation, percutaneous occlusion, or surgical closure. Surgical closure requires atriotomy on cardiopulmonary bypass that may alter the surgical technique selected for coronary artery bypass grafting. When asymptomatic and found incidentally during cardiac surgery that has included atriotomy, then surgical closure is typically easily performed. Little evidence suggests that incidentally discovered PFOs in patients without any respective history increase morbidity or mortality. Certain conditions would almost mandate the

closure of the PFO, such as the insertion of a left ventricular assist device to prevent severe hypoxia from right-to-left shunting.

References:

1. Fox JF, Smith MM, Nuttall GA, et al. Chapter 20: Uncommon Cardiac Diseases. In: Kaplan JA, Augoustides JGT, Manecke GR, et al., eds. Kaplan's Cardiac Anesthesia. 7th ed. Elsevier; 2017:883-973.
2. Michel P, Villablanca PA, Ranka S, et al. Patent foramen ovale and risk of cryptogenic stroke - analysis of outcomes and perioperative implications. J Cardiothorac Vasc Anesth, 2020; 34: 819-826.

35. A patient with lung cancer is brought emergently to the operating room for significant hemoptysis. What is TRUE regarding pulmonary hemorrhage?
   A. It is relatively common and has a low mortality
   B. Refractory hypoxia is more likely to cause death than hemorrhagic shock
   C. Double-lumen endotracheal tube is contraindicated
   D. Bronchial vein embolization is a first-line therapy in refractory bleeding

Correct Answer: B

Explanation: Pulmonary hemorrhage is rare in patients with hemoptysis but has a very high mortality rate (85%). Massive hemoptysis is typically defined as more than 600 mL of expectorated blood over 24 hours or recurrent bleeding greater than 100 mL per day for several days. Four hundred milliliters of blood in the alveolar space seriously impairs oxygenation. Pulmonary hemorrhage may stabilize, only to worsen again without an obvious explanation, reflecting its unpredictable nature. Notably, death is not attributable to hemodynamic instability with hemorrhage but to excessive blood in the alveoli that causes hypoventilation and refractory hypoxia. Clot formation may lead to the occlusion of bronchial segments or even the mainstem bronchus. In the United States chronic inflammatory lung disease and bronchogenic carcinoma are the most common causes of hemoptysis. Pulmonary hemorrhage may also result from vigorous suctioning of the lungs, surgery, and improper positioning of a pulmonary arterial catheter.

Localization may be achieved by chest imaging, bronchoscopy, and/or pulmonary angiography. Medications that may be used to control bleeding include topical epinephrine, desmopressin, vasopressin, and tranexamic acid. With rapid or persistent bleeding, a double-lumen endotracheal tube may be necessary to isolate the bleeding from the unaffected lung. When this is not feasible, a bronchial blocker may be used through an existing endotracheal tube to achieve lung isolation. Continued bleeding after stabilization and conservative therapy necessitates bronchial artery embolization, which may be first-line therapy for massive hemoptysis.

References:

1. Fox JF, Smith MM, Nuttall GA, et al. Chapter 20: Uncommon Cardiac Diseases. In: Kaplan JA, Augoustides JGT, Manecke

GR, et al., eds. Kaplan's Cardiac Anesthesia. 7th ed. Elsevier; 2017:883-973.

2. Yeoh TY, Ng ES, Agasthian T, Ti LK. Lung injury from use of a suction catheter via the double-lumen tube. J Cardiothorac Vasc Anesth, 2015; 29: 1618-1620.

36. What is TRUE regarding the risks of pulmonary artery rupture with a pulmonary artery catheter?
   A. Placing the tip in the right pulmonary artery reduces the risk
   B. Deep hypothermic arrest tends to migrate the pulmonary artery catheter distally
   C. The balloon should be inflated during bypass to minimize migration
   D. Anticoagulation reduces the risk of rupture

Correct Answer: B

Explanation: Pulmonary hemorrhage is a rare but often fatal complication of pulmonary artery catheter usage. With respect to cardiac surgical patients, death may occur within minutes or up to 14 days postoperatively. A small amount of hemoptysis may herald the onset of severe pulmonary hemorrhage. Other signs of pulmonary artery rupture are hypotension, decreased arterial oxygenation, bronchospasm, pleural effusion, hemothorax, and pneumothorax. Risk factors of pulmonary artery rupture include age older than 60 years, anticoagulation, and distal migration of the catheter. Pulmonary arterial hypertension is often present and may weaken the pulmonary vasculature to increase the risk of rupture. The mechanism of pulmonary artery rupture is multifactorial, but the catheter balloon is believed to be instrumental. Catheters that reside distally will lower the inflation pressures necessary to rupture the pulmonary artery. Distal migration also occurs more easily in patients undergoing hypothermic cardiopulmonary bypass, because hypothermia stiffens the catheter. Eccentric inflation of the balloon may also contribute to pulmonary artery rupture. If the rupture occurs during cardiopulmonary bypass, then extracorporeal support should be maintained to ensure adequate oxygenation and optimal conditions for pulmonary artery repair. If pulmonary artery rupture occurs before or after cardiopulmonary bypass, then titrated positive end-expiratory pressure and maintaining catheter position with the balloon inflated may provide a temporary tamponade effect until more definitive therapies ensue. Outside the operating room, coagulopathy should be corrected, and surgical intervention considered when bleeding persists. If the patient is not intubated, one-lung isolation to separate the bleeding lung will likely help. Venoarterial extracorporeal membrane oxygenation may be required to maintain hemodynamic stability and reduce blood flow to the pulmonary vasculature. To reduce the risk of pulmonary artery rupture, the placement of a pulmonary artery catheter distally in the pulmonary artery should be avoided. Advancing the catheter more than 5 cm beyond the pulmonary valve is not advisable. The balloon should not be inflated against increased resistance, particularly if the patient has been given an anticoagulant drug or after separation from cardiopulmonary bypass. Withdrawing the catheter several centimeters prior to cardiopulmonary bypass is a common practice done by some clinicians.

References:

1. Fox JF, Smith MM, Nuttall GA, et al. Chapter 20: Uncommon Cardiac Diseases. In: Kaplan JA, Augoustides JGT, Manecke GR, et al., eds. Kaplan's Cardiac Anesthesia. 7th ed. Elsevier; 2017:883-973.

2. Addante RA, Chen J, Goswami S. Successful management of a patient with pulmonary artery rupture in a catheterization suite. J Cardiothorac Vasc Anesth, 2016; 30: 1618-1620.

37. What is TRUE regarding the pericardium?
   A. The serous or visceral pericardium is stiff and resistant to expansion
   B. It is innervated by the phrenic nerve
   C. Pericardiectomy may result in diaphragmatic paralysis
   D. The pericardial space can only accommodate 50 mL of fluid in total

Correct Answer: C

Explanation: The pericardium is a two-layer sac that encloses the heart and great vessels, with attachments to the sternum anteriorly, the parietal pleura laterally, the diaphragm inferiorly, and the mainstem bronchi, esophagus, and aorta posteriorly. The inner layer is a serous membrane (visceral pericardium) covering the surface of the heart. The outer layer is a fibrinous sac (parietal pericardium) that is attached to the great vessels, diaphragm, and sternum. The parietal pericardium is a stiff collagenous membrane that is resistant to acute expansion. The space between the inner and outer layers is called the pericardial space and normally contains 20 to 60 mL of plasma ultrafiltrate, which comes mostly from epicardial capillaries and cleared through the lymphatic system. It can gradually dilate to accept large volumes of fluid if slowly accumulated; however, rapid fluid accumulation leads to cardiac tamponade. The vagus nerve, left recurrent laryngeal nerve, and esophageal plexus innervate the pericardium, along with sympathetic contributions from the stellate ganglion, first dorsal ganglion, and other ganglia. The lateral course of the phrenic nerve on either side of the heart is an important anatomic relationship because this nerve is encapsulated in the pericardium and thus can easily be damaged during pericardiectomy. The pericardium is not essential for life, and pericardiectomy causes no apparent disability, but it has many subtle functions that are advantageous. Foremost, it acts to minimize torsion of the heart and reduces the friction from surrounding organs. In addition, the pericardium has known immunologic, vasomotor, metabolic, and fibrinolytic activities.

References:

1. Fox JF, Smith MM, Nuttall GA, et al. Chapter 20: Uncommon Cardiac Diseases. In: Kaplan JA, Augoustides JGT, Manecke GR, et al., eds. Kaplan's Cardiac Anesthesia. 7th ed. Elsevier; 2017:883-973.

2. Tuck BC, Townsley MM. Clinical update in pericardial diseases. J Cardiothorac Vasc Anesth, 2019; 33: 184-199.

38. What finding is consistent with acute pericarditis?
- **A.** ST segment abnormalities in leads II, III, and aVF
- **B.** Recent fungal infection
- **C.** Continuous pleuritic chest pain radiating to the back
- **D.** Pulsus paradoxus

Correct Answer: C

Explanation: Acute pericarditis is common, but the actual incidence is unknown because it often goes unrecognized as it is generally self-limited. The most common cause is viral (30%–50%), followed by diverse etiologies including malignancy, myocardial infarction, postcardiotomy syndrome, and uremia. Pericardial fluid analysis may suggest an infectious, neoplastic, or inflammatory cause. Acute pericarditis may present with continuous pleuritic-type chest pain, originating in the center of the chest and radiating to the back, as well as dyspnea and/or atrial arrhythmias. A pericardial friction rub is pathognomonic of pericarditis but may be heard only intermittently. Early electrocardiographic changes may include diffuse ST segment abnormalities in many leads (versus focal changes in myocardial ischemia as given in option A), followed by T wave inversions as pericarditis enters the subacute phase. Echocardiography may show normal or thickened pericardium and sometimes a noticeable pericardial effusion. Treatment of acute pericarditis consists of symptomatic relief and treating the underlying systemic illness. Symptomatic relief involves support, bed rest, and nonsteroidal anti-inflammatory agents for analgesia. A left stellate ganglion block has been used to relieve unremitting pain. Pulsus paradoxus is typically associated with chronic constrictive pericarditis. Fungal infection would typically lead to chronic pericarditis.

References:

1. Fox JF, Smith MM, Nuttall GA, et al. Chapter 20: Uncommon Cardiac Diseases. In: Kaplan JA, Augoustides JGT, Manecke GR, et al., eds. Kaplan's Cardiac Anesthesia. 7th ed. Elsevier; 2017:883-973.
2. Tuck BC, Townsley MM. Clinical update in pericardial diseases. J Cardiothorac Vasc Anesth, 2019; 33: 184-199.

39. What is most consistent with constrictive pericarditis?
- **A.** No history of cardiac surgery
- **B.** Blunted Y descent in the right atrial waveform
- **C.** Pulsus parvus et tardus
- **D.** Annulus reversus on tissue Doppler

Correct Answer: D

Explanation: Constrictive pericarditis is a dense fusion of the parietal and visceral pericardium that limits the diastolic filling of the heart, irrespective of the cause. The changes in the pericardium can be due to scarring induced by acute or chronic inflammation. Historically, tuberculosis was a major cause, but currently most cases are idiopathic. The leading identifiable causes of constrictive pericarditis are previous acute pericarditis, cardiac surgery, and mediastinal irradiation.

The clinical presentation often includes jugular venous distention, hepatomegaly, and ascites. Symptoms are nonspecific and may progress over months to years. Venous pressure waves in pericardial constriction are classically characterized by a prominent Y descent. Kussmaul sign, pulsus paradoxus, and the square-root sign may be present. Characteristic electrocardiographic changes are P mitrale (broadened P wave), low QRS voltage, T wave inversion, and atrial fibrillation (in a quarter of patients). Although pericardial calcification is very specific, it is not very sensitive for diagnosis of constrictive pericarditis. Detailed cross-sectional imaging may demonstrate the typically thickened pericardium, but it may be normal in approximately a quarter of patients that have surgically proven constrictive pericarditis. Echocardiographic findings may include a thickened pericardium, abnormal motion of the ventricular septum, dilation of the inferior vena cava, ventricular interdependence, mitral inflow respiratory variation, and annulus reversus with tissue Doppler. Annulus reversus refers to the finding that, in constrictive pericarditis, the lateral mitral annular tissue Doppler velocity is lower than the medial annular velocity due to tethering by the fibrotic constrictive pericardium. This represents a reversal of the normal scenario where the lateral annular velocity is greater than the medial annular velocity.

References:

1. Fox JF, Smith MM, Nuttall GA, et al. Chapter 20: Uncommon Cardiac Diseases. In: Kaplan JA, Augoustides JGT, Manecke GR, et al., eds. Kaplan's Cardiac Anesthesia. 7th ed. Elsevier; 2017:883-973.
2. Tuck BC, Townsley MM. Clinical update in pericardial diseases. J Cardiothorac Vasc Anesth, 2019; 33: 184-199.

40. What contributes to ventricular interdependence in patients with constrictive pericarditis?
- **A.** Decreased left ventricular filling during inspiration
- **B.** Increased intrathoracic pressure during inspiration
- **C.** Decreased right ventricular filling during inspiration
- **D.** Decreased pulmonary vascular pressure during expiration

Correct Answer: A

Explanation: Diastolic filling of the ventricles is reliant on each other, because the overall cardiac volume is fixed by the stiffened pericardium. With inspiration, intrathoracic pressure falls, as does the pressure in the pulmonary vasculature. The thickened pericardium prevents the transmission of this pressure decrease to the ventricles. Therefore, filling of the left ventricle decreases just after inspiration and is due to the fall in pressure within the pulmonary vasculature. Because the intracardiac space is fixed, a decrease in filling pressure to the left ventricle allows increased filling in the right ventricle. The result is a shift in the ventricular septum into the left ventricle during inspiration and an increase in hepatic vein diastolic flow. With expiration, intrathoracic pressure increases, the pressure in the pulmonary vasculature increases, and left ventricular filling is augmented with a shift of the ventricular septum into the right ventricle during diastole. Right ventricular filling is now decreased because of both the positive intrathoracic pressure and the flow reversals that occur during diastole in the hepatic veins. When several cardiac cycles are viewed consecutively, the ventricular septum appears to *bounce* between the left ventricle and right ventricle.

References:

1. Fox JF, Smith MM, Nuttall GA, et al. Chapter 20: Uncommon Cardiac Diseases. In: Kaplan JA, Augoustides JGT, Manecke GR, et al., eds. Kaplan's Cardiac Anesthesia. 7th ed. Elsevier; 2017:883-973.
2. Tuck BC, Townsley MM. Clinical update in pericardial diseases. J Cardiothorac Vasc Anesth, 2019; 33: 184-199.

41. The square-root sign is most likely present in:
  A. Constrictive pericarditis
  B. Dilated cardiomyopathy
  C. Aortic stenosis
  D. Tricuspid regurgitation

Correct Answer: A

Explanation: The hemodynamic changes of constrictive pericarditis are primarily related to the isolation of the cardiac chambers from respiratory effects on thoracic pressure and a fixed end-diastolic ventricular volume. The pericardium limits the filling of the left ventricle during inspiration, which leads to increased filling in the right ventricle because the pericardium is very noncompliant. With expiration, the opposite is observed as the left ventricle is overfilled and the right ventricle is limited. The limitation of right ventricular diastolic filling occurs when the cardiac volume approximates the pericardial volume, usually in mid and late diastole, and is characterized by the square root or dip-and-plateau sign of the right ventricular waveform. Filling is limited by the noncompliant pericardium. The square root sign occurs because the constricting pericardium is essentially part of the ventricular wall. When the ventricle contracts, the pericardium is deformed similar to a spring. As diastole begins, the spring is released and the ventricle fills rapidly, decreasing the ventricular pressure and creating the dip of the dip-and-plateau wave or the square root sign. As cardiac filling approaches the limit set by the fixed pericardium, the plateau of the ventricular filling curve arrives.

References:

1. Fox JF, Smith MM, Nuttall GA, et al. Chapter 20: Uncommon Cardiac Diseases. In: Kaplan JA, Augoustides JGT, Manecke GR, et al., eds. Kaplan's Cardiac Anesthesia. 7th ed. Elsevier; 2017:883-973.
2. Tuck BC, Townsley MM. Clinical update in pericardial diseases. J Cardiothorac Vasc Anesth, 2019; 33: 184-199.

42. What is a major cause of morbidity and mortality after a pericardiectomy?
  A. Cardiac tamponade
  B. Stroke
  C. Low cardiac output
  D. Massive hemorrhage

Correct Answer: C

Explanation: Pericardiectomy may be indicated for recurrent pericardial effusion and constrictive pericarditis refractory to conservative therapies. Pericardiectomy for constrictive pericarditis can be surgically challenging with an operative mortality up to 18%. After pericardial resection, significant tricuspid regurgitation and low cardiac output may develop, with a higher risk in patients with advanced disease. A low cardiac output syndrome that persists after pericardiectomy is a major cause of morbidity and mortality, with an incidence of 14% to 28% in the immediate postoperative period. Although left ventricular contractility and relaxation may be abnormal after pericardiectomy, most patients experience relief of symptoms and improvement in ventricular function over a period of weeks. The determination of myocardial function is important as an indicator for inotropic support and as a marker of patient outcome.

Good results have been reported in this setting with and without cardiopulmonary bypass. Anesthetic goals for managing patients with constrictive pericarditis for pericardiectomy include minimizing bradycardia, myocardial depression, and decreases in preload and afterload. In this scenario, cardiac output is rate-dependent due to limited and relatively fixed ventricular diastolic filling. Monitoring with a pulmonary arterial catheter is helpful, given the perioperative risk of a low cardiac output syndrome that may also complicate mediastinal dissection with hypotension and arrhythmias.

References:

1. Fox JF, Smith MM, Nuttall GA, et al. Chapter 20: Uncommon Cardiac Diseases. In: Kaplan JA, Augoustides JGT, Manecke GR, et al., eds. Kaplan's Cardiac Anesthesia. 7th ed. Elsevier; 2017:883-973.
2. Liu VC, Fritz AV, Burtoft MA, et al. Pericardiectomy for constrictive pericarditis: analysis of outcomes. J Cardiothorac Vasc Anesth, 2021; 35: 3797-3805.

43. A patient who had a mitral valve replacement 2 days ago develops acute dyspnea and hypotensive. Which finding would suggest cardiac tamponade as the etiology?
  A. Minimal respiratory variation in blood pressure measurements
  B. Right atrial pressure is nearly equal to pulmonary artery diastolic and wedge pressures
  C. Diffuse ST elevations on the electrocardiogram
  D. Tracheal deviation on chest x-ray

Correct Answer: B

Explanation: Cardiac tamponade exists when fluid accumulation in the pericardial space dramatically increases intrapericardial pressure and limits the filling of the heart. The rate of pericardial fluid accumulation, rather than the absolute volume, is the main determinant of tamponade. Some common causes of tamponade include recent cardiac surgery, malignancy, infection, and trauma. Its signs and symptoms may include dyspnea, hypotension, pulsus paradoxus, jugular venous distension, and pressure equalization in the cardiac chambers as reflected by the right atrial, as well as the pulmonary arterial, diastolic and wedge pressures. Pulsus paradoxus is not sensitive or specific for tamponade, because it may be present in obstructive pulmonary disease, right ventricular infarction, or constrictive pericarditis. Pulsus paradoxus may also be absent when left ventricular dysfunction, positive pressure breathing, atrial septal defect, and/or severe aortic regurgitation are present. The electrocardiogram may show low-voltage QRS complexes and electrical alternans with variations in the QRS amplitude due to cardiac motion in the pericardial effusion. The chest x-ray is not sensitive early in this syndrome, as the classical water bottle effect may not be evident until at least 200 cc of fluid accumulates in the pericardial space. Echocardiographic findings include diastolic collapse of the right ventricle, inversion of the right atrium during diastole, abnormal ventricular septal motion, and ventricular interdependence. Key anesthetic considerations to maintain hemodynamic stability include volume expansion, preserving sympathetic drive, minimizing bradycardia, and maintaining spontaneous ventilation when possible.

References:

1. Fox JF, Smith MM, Nuttall GA, et al. Chapter 20: Uncommon Cardiac Diseases. In: Kaplan JA, Augoustides JGT, Manecke GR, et al., eds. Kaplan's Cardiac Anesthesia. 7th ed. Elsevier; 2017:883-973.
2. Tuck BC, Townsley MM. Clinical update in pericardial diseases. J Cardiothorac Vasc Anesth, 2019; 33: 184-199.

44. A 65-year-old female patient has severe carotid artery stenosis and a triple-vessel coronary artery disease. Which of the following is TRUE?
   A. Combined carotid artery endarterectomy and coronary artery bypass grafting have high mortality
   B. Carotid artery stenting is not a feasible option in this case
   C. Carotid artery stenosis is rare in the typical candidates for coronary artery bypass grafting
   D. Carotid artery stenosis significantly increases the risk of stroke after coronary artery bypass grafting

Correct Answer: D

Explanation: Patients with concomitant symptomatic coronary and carotid disease have significantly higher perioperative risk than patients with carotid or coronary disease alone. When both carotid and coronary intervention are indicated, both procedures may be feasible in a combined or staged fashion. Carotid artery disease should be considered in ischemic heart disease, as it has an incidence of at least 10% in patients older than 60 years old who have advanced coronary artery disease. Significant carotid disease increases the risk of stroke after coronary artery bypass grafting, as do prior stroke, peripheral vascular disease, postinfarction angina, diabetes, smoking, hypertension, and advanced age. Carotid artery stenting has also gained popularity recently for carotid revascularization in this setting and may decrease the stroke risk for combined procedures. The anesthetic management for patients with both carotid and coronary artery disease should include maintenance of middle-to-upper normal blood pressure ranges and expeditious emergence to allow neurologic examination.

References:

1. Fox JF, Smith MM, Nuttall GA, et al. Chapter 20: Uncommon Cardiac Diseases. In: Kaplan JA, Augoustides JGT, Manecke GR, et al., eds. Kaplan's Cardiac Anesthesia. 7th ed. Elsevier; 2017:883-973.
2. Mehta A, Choxi R, Gleason T, et al. Carotid artery disease as a predictor of in-hospital postoperative stroke after coronary artery bypass grafting from 1999 to 2011. J Cardiothorac Vasc Anesth, 2018; 32: 1587-1596.

45. A coronary arterial fistula to the coronary sinus was incidentally found during a left heart catheterization. Which of the following is TRUE?
   A. The most common origin of the fistula is the left coronary artery
   B. The fistula should be closed or ligated before symptoms emerge
   C. Its overall incidence is less than 2%
   D. It commonly leads to a right-to-left shunt

Correct Answer: C

Explanation: Coronary arterial fistula is typically very rare, with an estimated incidence of 0.002% to 0.8%, and is usually clinically silent. It is an abnormal communication between a coronary artery and another vascular structure or cardiac chamber, bypassing the myocardial capillary network. Possible sites include the coronary sinus, cardiac vein, pulmonary artery, vena cava, pulmonary vein, or any one of the cardiac chambers. Although often congenital in origin, it may also be acquired from including inflammatory, traumatic, and/or iatrogenic etiologies. Congenital fistulas commonly occur in the right coronary artery (60%) and the left coronary artery (35%), as well as multiple locations in about 5% of cases.

These lesions may present with dyspnea, arrhythmias, infective endocarditis, myocardial ischemia, heart failure, and left-to-right shunts. The associated complications include thrombosis, embolization, pulmonary hypertension, aneurysm, hemorrhage, and sudden death. Although coronary angiography remains the gold standard in diagnosis, computed axial and/or magnetic resonance angiography can also map the relevant course and relationship with other structures. In general, significant clinical presentations are a strong indication for percutaneous closure or surgical ligation. Transesophageal echocardiography may also identify the drainage sites of a given fistula and can occasionally guide closure or ligation.

References:

1. Fox JF, Smith MM, Nuttall GA, et al. Chapter 20: Uncommon Cardiac Diseases. In: Kaplan JA, Augoustides JGT, Manecke GR, et al., eds. Kaplan's Cardiac Anesthesia. 7th ed. Elsevier; 2017:883-973.
2. Esper SA, Fink R, Rhodes JF Jr, et al. A coronary artery fistula successfully closed with the precise guidance of three-dimensional echocardiography. J Cardiothorac Vasc Anesth, 2014; 28: 194-195.

46. What is TRUE regarding cardiac surgery in pregnant patients?
- **A.** Fetal mortality is lower than maternal mortality
- **B.** Valvular disease is the most common reason for surgery
- **C.** A viable fetus should be delivered after cardiopulmonary bypass
- **D.** Nonrheumatic heart disease is the most common etiology

Correct Answer: B

Explanation: Heart disease is a major cause of maternal and fetal mortality during pregnancy. Although rheumatic heart disease has accounted for nearly 75% of maternal heart disease, congenital heart disease has become more prevalent as more women with this disease are reaching childbearing age. Significant native valve disease and prosthetic valve dysfunction explain the indications for the majority of cardiac surgical procedures in this setting. Maternal morbidity with cardiac surgery is low, but fetal mortality is high (16%–33%), and likely related to cardiopulmonary bypass, duration of the surgery, and hypothermia. In the setting of fetal viability, a cesarean section for fetal delivery is typically advised immediately before commencement of cardiopulmonary bypass. The anesthetic plan should consider the context of maternal heart disease, the influence of cardiopulmonary bypass, and the effects on the fetus. Rescue tranesophageal echocardiography should also be considered to evaluate sudden unexpected hemodynamic collapse in parturients. Amniotic fluid and other types of emboli may be demonstrated in the heart.

References:

1. Fox JF, Smith MM, Nuttall GA, et al. Chapter 20: Uncommon Cardiac Diseases. In: Kaplan JA, Augoustides JGT, Manecke GR, et al., eds. Kaplan's Cardiac Anesthesia. 7th ed. Elsevier; 2017:883-973.
2. Carlier L, Devroe S, Budts W, et al. Cardiac interventions in pregnancy and peripartum - a narrative review of the literature. J Cardiothorac Vasc Anesth, 2020; 34: 3409-3419.
3. Katz J, Shear TD, Murphy GS, et al. Cardiovascular collapse in the pregnant patient, rescue transesophageal echocardiography and open heart surgery. J Cardiothorac Vasc Anesth, 2017; 31: 203-206.

47. What is TRUE regarding cardiopulmonary bypass in a pregnant patient?
- **A.** Fetal heart rate and rate variability are rarely affected
- **B.** Hypothermia is not recommended
- **C.** Uterine contraction does not need to be monitored
- **D.** Unfractionated heparin crosses the placenta and should be avoided

Correct Answer: B

Explanation: Cardiopulmonary bypass (CPB) is associated with deleterious effects on the maternal-fetal circulation. Maternal systemic blood pressure may fall soon after initiating CPB, lowering placental perfusion secondary to factors such as hemodilution, and low systemic vascular resistance. Fetal heart rate variability is often lost, and fetal bradycardia (<80 beats per minute) may also develop. Because uterine blood flow is not autoregulated and relies on maternal perfusion pressure, decreases in maternal blood pressure cause fetal hypoxia and bradycardia. Increasing flows and/or perfusion pressure during CPB will raise maternal blood flow and usually correct the fetal hypoxia and the heart rate. If fetal bradycardia persists, other causes must be considered.

Hypothermia is not recommended for pregnant patients. Beyond the effect of hypothermia on acid-base status, coagulation, and arrhythmias, it may precipitate uterine contractions that limit placental perfusion and risk fetal ischemia and survival. A possible explanation for these contractions may be related to the severe dilution from CPB that acutely lowers progesterone levels. Accordingly, uterine monitoring is strongly recommended if CPB is required during pregnancy. If uterine contractions should begin during CPB, then stopping them is vitally important for fetal survival. Treatment includes ethanol infusion, magnesium sulfate, terbutaline, or ritodrine. Of note, many of these tocolytic agents have potential side effects and toxicities that may be detrimental to the patient with heart disease. The hematocrit should be maintained on the higher side (>28%) to optimize oxygen-carrying capacity for the mother and fetus. Arterial partial pressure of carbon dioxide ($PaCO_2$) should be slightly hypercapnic because this increases uterine blood flow. Unfractionated heparin does not cross the placenta and can be used safely.

References:

1. Fox JF, Smith MM, Nuttall GA, et al. Chapter 20: Uncommon Cardiac Diseases. In: Kaplan JA, Augoustides JGT, Manecke GR, et al., eds. Kaplan's Cardiac Anesthesia. 7th ed. Elsevier; 2017:883-973.
2. Carlier L, Devroe S, Budts W, et al. Cardiac interventions in pregnancy and peripartum - a narrative review of the literature. J Cardiothorac Vasc Anesth, 2020; 34: 3409-3419.

48. What is TRUE regarding acute kidney injury in cardiac surgery?
- **A.** Dopamine reduces kidney injury incidence
- **B.** Kidney injury increases morbidity but not mortality
- **C.** Levosimendan is contraindicated in patients with kidney injury
- **D.** Aprotinin increases risk of renal injury compared to aminocaproic acid

Correct Answer: D

Explanation: Acute kidney injury occurs frequently and is associated with increased morbidity and mortality after cardiac surgery. Patients with limited renal reserve due to chronic kidney disease are prone to acute kidney injury with complications such as fluid overload, hyponatremia, hyperkalemia, and metabolic acidosis. To date, no medication has been found to consistently be nephroprotective in cardiac surgery. Cardiopulmonary bypass may aggravate renal injury due to factors such as nonpulsatile flow, low renal perfusion, and hypothermia. Pulsatile flow and levosimendan therapy during cardiopulmonary may attenuate renal injury, although not consistently demonstrated in clinical trials. Antifibrinolytic medications may be used in renal patients to reduce bleeding, with the exception of aprotinin due to observed increases in renal injury and mortality. Tranexamic acid is considered safe but may need to be renally dosed.

References:

1. Fox JF, Smith MM, Nuttall GA, et al. Chapter 20: Uncommon Cardiac Diseases. In: Kaplan JA, Augoustides JGT, Manecke GR, et al., eds. Kaplan's Cardiac Anesthesia. 7th ed. Elsevier; 2017:883-973.
2. Zangrillo A, Alvaro G, Belletti A, et al. Effect of levosimendan on renal outcome in cardiac surgery patients with chronic kidney disease and perioperative cardiovascular dysfunction: a substudy of a multicenter randomized trial. J Cardiothorac Vasc Anesth, 2018; 32: 2152-2159.

49. A 61-year-old male with hemophilia B is scheduled to undergo coronary artery bypass grafting. His relevant factor level is 30%. Which intervention is indicated?
   A. None, the factor level is adequate
   B. Desmopressin
   C. Factor VIII concentrate
   D. Factor IX concentrate

Correct Answer: D

Explanation: Treatment of hemophilia A and B primarily depends on the replacement of factor VIII or factor IX, respectively. For hemophilia, a factor level near 50% of normal is regarded as adequate to achieve noncardiac surgical hemostasis, but in cardiac surgery the increased hemostatic demand and associated coagulation abnormalities with cardiopulmonary bypass will require a higher goal factor level of 80% to 100%. The amount of factor replacement is estimated from the priming volume of the extracorporeal circuit, the plasma volume, and the desired factor activity. To improve dosing accuracy, the factor levels should be obtained as close to the day of surgery as possible. Replacement of factor VIII or factor IX during surgery may be achieved by intermittent bolus or continuous infusions with a factor activity target of 80% to 100%, followed by no less than 70% for the first 1 to 2 days, no less than 50% for the first week, and 30% for the second week. Antifibrinolytic agents such as tranexamic acid and epsilon-aminocaproic acid are helpful to reduce blood loss and transfusion requirements. Desmopressin has been used successfully in mild-to-moderate hemophilia A to decrease intraoperative transfusion requirements. For hemophilia B, concentrated purified recombinant factor IX can be used. Of note, circulating factor IX levels will not increase as much as factor VIII after transfusion because factor IX is distributed in both intravascular and extravascular spaces. Consequently, the calculated dose may have to be doubled. Antibodies to factor VIII or factor IX ("inhibitors") may occur in patients with hemophilia who have received replacement therapy. Bleeding in the presence of factor VIII or factor IX inhibitors may be treated with prothrombin-complex concentrates that have activated forms of factors VII, IX, and X and/or recombinant factor VIIa that binds to tissue factor on the surface of activated platelets to boost coagulation.

References:

1. Fox JF, Smith MM, Nuttall GA, et al. Chapter 20: Uncommon Cardiac Diseases. In: Kaplan JA, Augoustides JGT, Manecke GR, et al., eds. Kaplan's Cardiac Anesthesia. 7th ed. Elsevier; 2017:883-973.
2. Kwak J, Mazzeffi M, Boggio LN, et al. Hemophilia: a review of perioperative management for cardiac surgery. J Cardiothorac Vasc Anesth, 2022; 36: 246-257.

50. A 55-year-old female with von Willebrand disease is scheduled to undergo a mitral valve replacement. In which type of von Willebrand disease is desmopressin the most ineffective?
   A. Type 1
   B. Type 2A
   C. Type 2N
   D. Type 3

Correct Answer: D

Explanation: Von Willebrand disease (vWD) is the most commonly inherited hemostatic abnormality. The von Willebrand factor (vWF) is both a carrier protein and stabilizer for factor VIII and is a mediator of platelet adhesion to injured sites in the vascular endothelium. Patients with vWD have an abnormality of both vWF and factor VIII. The spectrum of vWD is classified into three major types that may also have associated subtypes. Individuals with type 1 and type 2 disease make up 70% and 20% of people with vWD, respectively. Type 3 vWD represents only 10% of individuals and is autosomal recessive. Type 3 vWD individuals are severely affected and their presentation is similar to individuals with hemophilia who have a very low factor VIII activity (1%–4%). The ristocetin cofactor assay, also known as the vWF activity, is a sensitive and specific test for vWD. It measures the ability of vWF to bind to glycoprotein Ib platelet receptors. Factor VIII levels can be followed intraoperatively and then daily after surgery.

Both factor VIII and vWF levels will decrease on initiation of cardiopulmonary bypass, but vWF will subsequently increase as it is released from storage pools. Desmopressin is a synthetic analog of the natural hormone vasopressin without the vasopressor effect. Although it is the first choice for treatment in vWD, not all types of vWD will respond to this therapy. Desmopressin is effective in type 1 vWD but not in type 2B vWD because thrombocytopenia may result. It is ineffective in type 3 vWD because there are no stores of vWF to release. Antihemophilic factor/vWF complex concentrate is the current standard for replacement therapy in vWD when unresponsive to desmopressin. Antifibrinolytic agents should also be considered in patients with vWD to reduce bleeding associated with cardiac surgery.

References:

1. Fox JF, Smith MM, Nuttall GA, et al. Chapter 20: Uncommon Cardiac Diseases. In: Kaplan JA, Augoustides JGT, Manecke GR, et al., eds. Kaplan's Cardiac Anesthesia. 7th ed. Elsevier; 2017:883-973.
2. Berger J, Schwartz J, Ramachandran S, et al. Review of von Willebrand disease and acquired von Willebrand syndrome for patients undergoing cardiac surgery. J Cardiothorac Vasc Anesth, 2019; 33: 3446-3457.

CHAPTER 21

Anesthesia for Heart and Lung Transplantation

Theresa Anne Gelzinis

KEY POINTS

1. Cardiac denervation is an unavoidable consequence of heart transplantation, and reinnervation is at best partial and incomplete.
2. Drugs acting directly on the heart are the drugs of choice for altering cardiac physiology after heart transplantation.
3. Allograft coronary vasculopathy remains the greatest threat to long-term survival after heart transplantation.
4. Broadening of donor criteria has decreased time to lung transplantation.
5. Air trapping in patients with severe obstructive lung disease may impair hemodynamics and require deliberate hypoventilation.
6. Newly transplanted lungs should be ventilated with a low tidal volume and inspiratory pressure and as low an inspired oxygen concentration as can be tolerated.
7. Reperfusion injury is the most common cause of perioperative death.
8. The frequency of heart-lung transplantation has decreased as the frequency of lung transplantations has increased.

---

1. All of the following are indications for urgent heart transplantation EXCEPT:
   A. Inability to wean from inotropic medication
   B. Worsening right ventricular function with increasing pulmonary artery pressures
   C. Need for ventilatory support for intractable pulmonary edema
   D. Refractory ventricular arrhythmias

Correct Answer: B

Explanation: The four indications for urgent heart transplant include the inability to wean from inotropic medications, the need for ventilatory support for intractable pulmonary edema, refractory arrhythmias, and the need for mechanical circulatory support. Worsening right ventricular function with increasing pulmonary artery pressures is an ambulatory indication for heart transplantation. These indications are also typically assessed in real time on a frequent basis by the multidisciplinary heart transplantation team.

References:

1. Murray AW, Quinlan JJ, Blasiole B, et al. Chapter 25: Anesthesia for Heart, Lung, and Heart-Lung Transplantation. In: Kaplan JA, Augoustides JGT, Manecke GR, et al., eds. Kaplan's Cardiac Anesthesia. 7th ed. Elsevier; 2017:974-993.
2. Bhagra SK, Pettit S, Parameshwar J. Cardiac transplantation: indications, eligibility and current outcomes. Heart, 2019; 105: 252-260.

2. According to the International Society of Heart and Lung Transplantation listing criteria, all of these are criteria for listing patients for heart transplantation EXCEPT:
   A. For patients on beta blockers, a peak oxygen uptake (VO_2) of 12 mL/kg/min or less
   B. VO_2 less than 50% predicted in women candidates
   C. A minute ventilation/carbon dioxide (V_E/V_{CO2}) slope of less than 35
   D. Seattle Heart Failure Model estimated 1-year survival of less than 80%

Correct Answer: C

Explanation: Patients with persistent New York Heart Association functional class IV heart failure symptoms refractory to medical or surgical therapy are assessed by cardiopulmonary testing and by heart failure prognosis scales. With cardiopulmonary testing, a heart transplant is indicated in patients on beta blockers with a peak oxygen uptake (VO_2) of 12 mL/kg/min or less and a peak VO_2 14 mL/kg/min or less when not on beta blockers. In patients under 50 years of age or in women, a peak VO_2 under 50% predicted may also be used. Further criteria include a minute ventilation/carbon dioxide (V_E/V_{CO2}) slope greater than 35 in patients with a suboptimal cardiopulmonary test, a Seattle Heart Failure Model estimated 1-year survival of <80%, and a Heart Failure Survival Score in the high/medium risk range.

References:

1. Stone ME and Hinchey J. Chapter 28: Mechanical Assist Devices for Heart Failure. In: Kaplan JA, Augoustides JGT, Manecke GR, et al., eds. Kaplan's Cardiac Anesthesia. 7th ed. Elsevier; 2017:1042-1063.
2. Mehra MR, Canter CE, Hannan MM, et al. The 2016 International Society for Heart Lung Transplantation listing criteria for heart transplantation: a 10-year update. J Heart Lung Transplant, 2016; 35: 1-23.

3. In patients with pulmonary hypertension being considered for heart transplantation, what are the hemodynamic cutoffs for acceptance with respect to pulmonary vascular resistance (PVR) and systolic blood pressure after treatment with pulmonary vasodilators?
   A. PVR ≤3 Wood units with systolic pressure ≥85 mmHg
   B. PVR ≤3 Wood units with systolic pressure ≥80 mmHg
   C. PVR ≤3 Wood units with systolic pressure ≥75 mmHg
   D. PVR ≤3 Wood units with systolic pressure ≥70 mmHg

Correct Answer: A

Explanation: The minimum response to pulmonary vasodilators for a patient to be considered for a heart transplant is a reduction of the pulmonary vascular resistance of 3 or less Wood units with systolic blood pressure of 85 mmHg or more. These hemodynamic parameters are important to minimize the risk of right ventricular systolic failure after heart transplantation.

References:

1. Stone ME, Hinchey J. Chapter 28: Mechanical Assist Devices for Heart Failure. In: Kaplan JA, Augoustides JGT, Manecke GR, et al., eds. Kaplan's Cardiac Anesthesia. 7th ed. Elsevier; 2017:1042-1063.
2. Mehra MR, Canter CE, Hannan MM, et al. The 2016 International Society for Heart Lung Transplantation listing criteria for heart transplantation: a 10-year update. J Heart Lung Transplant, 2016; 35: 1-23.

4. Which of the following is an absolute contraindication to heart transplantation?
   A. Advanced renal disease
   B. Malignancy
   C. Active substance abuse
   D. Obesity

Correct Answer: C

Explanation: The absolute contraindications to heart transplantation include severe pulmonary hypertension with a pulmonary vascular resistance of more than 3 Wood units despite therapy with pulmonary vasodilators. Systemic illness with life expectancy less than 2 years despite heart transplantation, active substance abuse, poor compliance with medications, and multisystem disease with severe extracardiac organ dysfunction are further absolute contraindications. Relative contraindications include age greater than 70 years, a body mass index of 35 kg/m^2 (or more) or 18 kg/m^2 (or less), poorly controlled diabetes mellitus, advanced renal dysfunction, malignancy, infection, acute pulmonary embolism, tobacco or substance use within 6 months, inadequate social support, and cognitive/behavioral disability.

References:

1. Murray AW, Quinlan JJ, Blasiole B, et al. Chapter 25: Anesthesia for Heart, Lung, and Heart-Lung Transplantation. In: Kaplan JA, Augoustides JGT, Manecke GR, et al., eds. Kaplan's Cardiac Anesthesia. 7th ed. Elsevier; 2017:974-993.
2. Bhagra SK, Pettit S, Parameshwar J. Cardiac transplantation: indications, eligibility and current outcomes. Heart, 2019; 105: 252-260.

5. How long does a patient require support with veno-arterial extracorporeal membrane oxygenation before their listing status changes from status 1 to status 3?
   A. 7 days
   B. 14 days
   C. 21 days
   D. 30 days

Correct Answer: A

Explanation: According to the 2018 United Network for Organ Sharing updated heart allocation policy, patients who are supported with veno-arterial extracorporeal membrane oxygenation for up to 7 days are considered status 1, while those on this platform for more than 7 days are moved to status 3. Patients who are listed as status 1 have the highest priority for heart transplantation.

References:

1. Murray AW, Quinlan JJ, Blasiole B, et al. Chapter 25: Anesthesia for Heart, Lung, and Heart-Lung Transplantation. In: Kaplan JA, Augoustides JGT, Manecke GR, et al., eds. Kaplan's Cardiac Anesthesia. 7th ed. Elsevier; 2017:974-993.
2. Liu J, Yang BQ, Itoh A, et al. Impact of New UNOS Allocation Criteria on Heart Transplant Practices and Outcomes. Transplant Direct, 2020; 15: e642.

6. All of these indications are considered status 2 for heart transplantation EXCEPT:
   A. Circulatory support with an intra-aortic balloon pump for 7 days
   B. Circulatory support with a left ventricular assist device that requires in-hospital management

C. Circulatory support with multiple inotropes
D. Percutaneous mechanical circulatory support devices

Correct Answer: C

Explanation: The revised United Network for Organ Sharing allocation policy was developed in 2018 to simplify the allocation of hearts into three main categories. Status I patients include those supported on veno-arterial extracorporeal membrane oxygenation (VA ECMO) and nondischargeable biventricular assist devices, as well as those on mechanical support devices with life-threatening arrhythmias. Status 2 patients include those with an intra-aortic balloon pump (IABP) for less than 14 days, nondischargeable patients with a left ventricular assist device (LVAD), ventricular arrhythmias not on mechanical support, as well as those with percutaneous endovascular mechanical support devices. Status 3 patients include those with dischargeable LVADs, those requiring inotropic support, those on VA-ECMO for more than 7 days and those supported with an IABP for more than 14 days.

References:

1. Murray AW, Quinlan JJ, Blasiole B, et al. Chapter 25: Anesthesia for Heart, Lung, and Heart-Lung Transplantation. In: Kaplan JA, Augoustides JGT, Manecke GR, et al., eds. Kaplan's Cardiac Anesthesia. 7th ed. Elsevier; 2017:974-993.
2. Liu J, Yang BQ, Itoh A, et al. Impact of new UNOS allocation criteria on heart transplant practices and outcomes. transplant direct, 2020; 15: e642.

7. Which of these electrolyte abnormalities is indicative of severe systolic heart failure that may lead to hemodynamic instability during induction?
A. Hypokalemia
B. Hyperchloremia
C. Hyponatremia
D. Hypercalcemia

Correct Answer: C

Explanation: Hyponatremia, defined as a serum sodium level under 136 mEq/L, is frequently encountered in patients with advanced heart failure. This hyponatremia is due to an excess of water compared to sodium stores and increases morbidity and mortality. The etiology of this hyponatremia includes impairment in the renal excretion of water, partially due to the effect of antidiuretic hormone. The presence of preoperative hyponatremia signifies patients who are in decompensated heart failure and more likely to have hemodynamic instability during induction.

References:

1. Murray AW, Quinlan JJ, Blasiole B, et al. Chapter 25: Anesthesia for Heart, Lung, and Heart-Lung Transplantation. In: Kaplan JA, Augoustides JGT, Manecke GR, et al., eds. Kaplan's Cardiac Anesthesia. 7th ed. Elsevier; 2017:974-993.
2. Park JJ, Cho YJ, Oh IY, et al. Short and long-term prognostic value of hyponatremia in heart failure with preserved ejection fraction versus reduced ejection fraction: an analysis of the Korean Acute Heart Failure registry. Int J Cardiol, 2017; 248: 239-245.

8. What is the main indication for heterotopic heart transplantation?
A. Patients with fixed severe pulmonary hypertension
B. Pediatric patients with single ventricle physiology
C. Patients with infiltrative cardiomyopathies
D. Patients in biventricular failure

Correct Answer: A

Explanation: Heterotopic heart transplantation (HHT) is a procedure where the donor heart is grafted to the recipient heart. It used to be popular in the precyclosporin era because in cases of severe acute rejection the residual function of the native heart may be lifesaving. This was also before the advent of mechanical support devices. The two primary indications of HHT are in patients with irreversible elevated pulmonary hypertension and in donor–recipient mismatch. Orthotopic heart transplantation is indicated for all of the other indications listed above.

References:

1. Murray AW, Quinlan JJ, Blasiole B, et al. Chapter 25: Anesthesia for Heart, Lung, and Heart-Lung Transplantation. In: Kaplan JA, Augoustides JGT, Manecke GR, et al., eds. Kaplan's Cardiac Anesthesia. 7th ed. Elsevier; 2017:974-993.
2. Flècher E, Fourquet O, Ruggieri VG, et al. Heterotopic heart transplantation: where do we stand? Eur J Cardiothorac Surg, 2013; 44: 201-206.

9. From most to least common, what is the correct series for the common valvular abnormalities after orthotopic heart transplantation?
A. Tricuspid regurgitation (TR) > mitral regurgitation (MR) > pulmonic regurgitation (PR) > aortic regurgitation (AR)
B. MR > TR > AR > PR
C. TR > PR > MR > AR
D. MR > AR > TR > PR

Correct Answer: C

Explanation: The most common valvular abnormality after orthotopic heart transplant is tricuspid regurgitation (up to 84%), then pulmonic regurgitation (42%), followed by mitral regurgitation (32%), and lastly aortic regurgitation (23%). The incidence of tricuspid regurgitation after orthotopic heart transplantation is so high because of geometric annular distortion and the postbypass period, where there are significant changes in right ventricular preload, afterload, and contractility. In the majority of patients, this tricuspid regurgitation resolves over time as the donor right ventricle adapts to the new loading conditions.

References:

1. Murray AW, Quinlan JJ, Blasiole B, et al. Chapter 25: Anesthesia for Heart, Lung, and Heart-Lung Transplantation. In: Kaplan JA, Augoustides JGT, Manecke GR, et al., eds. Kaplan's Cardiac Anesthesia. 7th ed. Elsevier; 2017:974-993.
2. Nicoara A, Skubas N, Ad N, et al. Guidelines for the use of transesophageal echocardiography to assist with surgical

decision-making in the operating room: a surgery-based approach: from the American Society of Echocardiography in collaboration with the Society of Cardiovascular Anesthesiologists and the Society of Thoracic Surgeons. Am Soc Echocardiogr, 2020; 33: 692-734.

10. Which physiologic cardiovascular response is unchanged after heart transplantation?
   A. Carotid massage
   B. Baroreceptor reflex
   C. Valsalva maneuver
   D. Starling effect

Correct Answer: D

Explanation: Autonomic denervation occurs during the explantation of the native heart, resulting in the loss of cardiac autonomic nervous system function. This results in a higher resting heart rate of 90 to 130 beats per minute due to the lack of parasympathetic innervation and the increasing circulatory catecholamines. As a further consequence of this autonomic denervation, the cardiovascular responses to a Valsalva maneuver and carotid massage are all attenuated along with the baroreceptor reflexes. The Starling mechanism is, however, retained, with an increase in stroke volume and cardiac output with increased preload. Patients also have exaggerated responses to orthostatic hypotension after heart transplantation.

References:

1. Murray AW, Quinlan JJ, Blasiole B, et al. Chapter 25: Anesthesia for Heart, Lung, and Heart-Lung Transplantation. In: Kaplan JA, Augoustides JGT, Manecke GR, et al., eds. Kaplan's Cardiac Anesthesia. 7th ed. Elsevier; 2017:974-993.
2. Navas-Blanco, JR, Modak RK. Perioperative care of heart transplant recipients undergoing non-cardiac surgery. Ann Card Anaesth, 2021; 24: 140-148.

11. Which of these drugs will affect the heart rate in a transplanted heart?
   A. Epinephrine
   B. Esmolol
   C. Atropine
   D. Opioids

Correct Answer: A

Explanation: Only direct-acting agents such as epinephrine, ephedrine, isoproterenol, dopamine, and dobutamine will increase the heart rate in a transplanted heart. Of the beta blockers, esmolol and metoprolol have minimal effect on the heart. Indirect agents, such as atropine and glycopyrrolate, also have a limited effect. Opioids or muscle relaxants such as pancuronium also do not typically affect heart rate due to the disruption of the autonomic nervous system.

References:

1. Murray AW, Quinlan JJ, Blasiole B, et al. Chapter 25: Anesthesia for Heart, Lung, and Heart-Lung Transplantation. In: Kaplan JA, Augoustides JGT, Manecke GR, et al., eds. Kaplan's Cardiac Anesthesia. 7th ed. Elsevier; 2017:974-993.

2. Navas-Blanco, JR, Modak RK. Perioperative care of heart transplant recipients undergoing non-cardiac surgery. Ann Card Anaesth, 2021; 24: 140-148.

12. What is the most common indication for heart–double lung transplantation?
   A. Congenital heart disease with Eisenmenger's syndrome
   B. Idiopathic pulmonary hypertension
   C. Cystic fibrosis
   D. Idiopathic pulmonary fibrosis

Correct Answer: A

Explanation: The most common indication for heart–double lung transplantation is complex congenital heart disease with Eisenmenger's physiology, followed by idiopathic pulmonary hypertension, and cystic fibrosis. With improving treatments for pulmonary hypertension and cystic fibrosis and the discovery that performing a double lung transplant reverses the signs of isolated right ventricular dysfunction, the incidence of heart–double lung transplantation is decreasing. Further indications include acquired heart disease, idiopathic pulmonary fibrosis, and alpha-1 antitrypsin deficiency.

References:

1. Murray AW, Quinlan JJ, Blasiole B, et al. Chapter 25: Anesthesia for Heart, Lung, and Heart-Lung Transplantation. In: Kaplan JA, Augoustides JGT, Manecke GR, et al., eds. Kaplan's Cardiac Anesthesia. 7th ed. Elsevier; 2017:974-993.
2. Pasupneti S, Dhillon G, Reitz B, et al. Combined heart lung transplantation: an updated review of the current literature. Transplantation, 2017; 101: 2297-2302.

13. Compared to separate heart and double lung transplantation, heart–double lung transplant is associated with all of the following EXCEPT:
   A. Shorter survival
   B. Higher risk for cardiac allograft dysfunction
   C. Increased incidence of phrenic nerve injury
   D. More severe gastroparesis

Correct Answer: B

Explanation: Compared to isolated heart or double lung transplantation, patients receiving a heart–double lung transplant have a higher incidence of early graft failure (6.8 vs. 2.3%), defined as intrinsic graft failure resulting in death or retransplantation within the first 30 days. Patients undergoing combined heart–double lung transplantation are also at a higher risk for complications such as chylothorax, severe gastroparesis, and phrenic nerve dysfunction, leading to increased morbidity and mortality. The phrenic and vagus nerves are both near the tracheal anastomosis, where they can be easily damaged. Vagus nerve damage can result in severe gastroparesis, a risk factor for the development of chronic lung allograft dysfunction. Compared to isolated heart transplantation, these patients have less cardiac allograft dysfunction but a shorter survival. The median survival rate for combined heart-lung transplantation is 3.3 years compared to 7.1 years with double lung transplants and 10.4 years with isolated heart transplantation.

References:

1. Murray AW, Quinlan JJ, Blasiole B, et al. Chapter 25: Anesthesia for Heart, Lung, and Heart-Lung Transplantation. In: Kaplan JA, Augoustides JGT, Manecke GR, et al., eds. Kaplan's Cardiac Anesthesia. 7th ed. Elsevier; 2017:974-993.
2. Pasupneti S, Dhillon G, Reitz B, et al. Combined heart lung transplantation: an updated review of the current literature. Transplantation, 2017; 101: 2297-2302.

14. All of these are anesthetic considerations in performing a heart transplant in a patient with a total artificial heart EXCEPT:
   A. Patients typically arrive with anemia
   B. Patients have previous sternotomies
   C. Preoperative pulmonary artery catheters are easy to place
   D. These patients will arrive anticoagulated

Correct Answer: C

Explanation: The total artificial heart (TAH) is used as a bridge to transplant in patients with severe biventricular failure. The TAH is a pulsatile device that is implanted via sternotomy after the complete excision of both ventricles and preservation of the atrial posterior walls. Forward flow occurs through mechanical inflow and outflow tilting disc valves that replace the patient's native valves. These devices are placed using a sternotomy, and because the heart is replaced by the device a guidewire should only be placed in the superior vena cava, preferably under echocardiographic or fluoroscopic guidance. Pulmonary artery catheters should be placed in the new heart after separation from cardiopulmonary bypass. These patients receive anticoagulation with both warfarin and antiplatelet agents and will typically arrive anemic due to hemolysis.

References:

1. Murray AW, Quinlan JJ, Blasiole B, et al. Chapter 25: Anesthesia for Heart, Lung, and Heart-Lung Transplantation. In: Kaplan JA, Augoustides JGT, Manecke GR, et al., eds. Kaplan's Cardiac Anesthesia. 7th ed. Elsevier; 2017:974-993.
2. Yaung J, Arabia FA, Nurok M. Perioperative care of the patient with the total artificial heart. Anesth Analg, 2017; 124: 1412-1422.

15. All of the following criteria are consistent with a diagnosis of right ventricular primary graft dysfunction EXCEPT:
   A. Right atrial pressure greater than 15 mmHg
   B. Pulmonary capillary wedge pressure less than 15 mmHg
   C. Pulmonary artery systolic pressure greater than 50 mmHg
   D. Transpulmonary gradient less than 15 mmHg

Correct Answer: C

Explanation: Primary graft dysfunction (PGD) is diagnosed when dysfunction is present and a secondary cause is not identified and may involve isolated dysfunction of either the right or left ventricle or may involve both. PGD is defined as early dysfunction within 24 hours with a low cardiac index under 2.0 L/min/m^2 and/or a left ventricular ejection fraction of 40% or less. PGD of the left ventricle can be classified as mild, requiring low-dose inotropes, moderate, requiring high dose inotropes and/or an intra-aortic balloon pump, or severe, requiring further mechanical circulatory support. PGD of the right ventricle is diagnosed by a right atrial pressure over 15mmHg, a wedge pressure under 15 mmHg, a pulmonary artery systolic pressure under 50 mmHg, a transpulmonary gradient under 15 mmHg, and/or the need for right ventricular mechanical circulatory support. Right ventricular failure in this setting requires integrated aggressive management (see box for further detail).

BOX 21.1   Treatment of intraoperative right ventricular failure

- Avoid large increases in intrathoracic pressure from:
  - Positive end-expiratory pressure
  - Large tidal volumes
  - Inadequate expiratory time
- Intravascular volume
  - Increase preload if pulmonary vascular resistance is normal
  - Rely on inotropes (dobutamine) if pulmonary vascular resistance is increased
- Maintain right ventricular coronary perfusion pressure with α-adrenergic agonists
- Cautiously administer pulmonary vasodilators (avoid systemic and gas exchange effects)
  - Prostaglandin E$_1$ (0.05–0.15 µg/kg per min)
  - Inhaled nitric oxide (20–40 ppm)

References:

1. Murray AW, Quinlan JJ, Blasiole B, et al. Chapter 25: Anesthesia for Heart, Lung, and Heart-Lung Transplantation. In: Kaplan JA, Augoustides JGT, Manecke GR, et al., eds. Kaplan's Cardiac Anesthesia. 7th ed. Elsevier; 2017:974-993.
2. Kobashigawa J, Zuckermann A, Macdonald P, et al. Report from a consensus conference on primary graft dysfunction after cardiac transplantation. J Heart Lung Transplant, 2014; 33: 327-340.

16. All of these are components of the lung allocation score EXCEPT:
   A. Cardiac index
   B. Creatinine
   C. Diagnosis
   D. Hemoglobin

Correct Answer: D

Explanation: The lung allocation score (LAS) is used to stratify patients on the lung transplant waitlist in respect to waitlist urgency and post-transplant survival. It is calculated from the difference between expected 1-year post-transplant survival and waiting list urgency. The score ranges from 0 to 100, and components of the LAS include age at offer, bilirubin, body mass index, cardiac index, central venous pressure, creatinine, mechanical ventilation, diagnosis, functional capacity, forced vital capacity, oxygen requirement, and baseline carbon dioxide, as well as any changes. The hemoglobin level is not included in the calculation of the LAS.

References:

1. Murray AW, Quinlan JJ, Blasiole B, et al. Chapter 25: Anesthesia for Heart, Lung, and Heart-Lung Transplantation. In: Kaplan JA, Augoustides JGT, Manecke GR, et al., eds. Kaplan's Cardiac Anesthesia. 7th ed. Elsevier; 2017:974-993.
2. Benvenuto LJ, Arcasoy SM. The new allocation era and policy. J Thorac Dis, 2021; 13: 6504-6651.

17. All of the following are absolute contraindications to lung transplantation EXCEPT:
   A. Edible cannabis use
   B. Malignancy with high rate of recurrence
   C. Poor functional status with poor rehabilitation potential
   D. Glomerular filtration rate under 40 mL/min/1.73 m³

Correct Answer: A

Explanation: Absolute contraindications to lung transplantation include patient refusal, septic shock, extrapulmonary or disseminated infection, active tuberculosis, human immunodeficiency virus (HIV) infection with a detectable viral load, and/or malignancy with a high recurrence rate. Further contraindications include a glomerular filtration rate under 40 mL/min/1.73 m² unless being considered for multiorgan transplant, acute kidney failure with rising creatinine or on dialysis with low likelihood of recovery, and stroke within 30 days or progressive cognitive impairment. Furthermore, acute liver failure or cirrhosis unless being considered for multiorgan transplant, acute coronary syndrome or myocardial infarction within 30 days, or significant coronary heart disease not amenable to revascularization also constitute barriers to lung transplantation. Untreatable hematologic disorders, active substance use or dependence, cannabis smoking, intravenous drug use, limited functional status with poor potential for post-transplant rehabilitation, and repeated episodes of nonadherence without evidence of improvement will also prevent further consideration for lung transplantation.

References:

1. Murray AW, Quinlan JJ, Blasiole B, et al. Chapter 25: Anesthesia for Heart, Lung, and Heart-Lung Transplantation. In: Kaplan JA, Augoustides JGT, Manecke GR, et al., eds. Kaplan's Cardiac Anesthesia. 7th ed. Elsevier; 2017:974-993.
2. Benvenuto LJ, Arcasoy SM. The new allocation era and policy. J Thorac Dis, 2021; 13: 6504-6651.

BOX 21.2 Absolute contraindications for lung transplantation

- Malignancy within 2 years (preferably 5 years)
- Untreatable significant disease in another organ system
- Atherosclerotic disease not corrected
- Acute medical instability: hepatic failure
- Bleeding diathesis that is not correctable
- *Mycobacterium tuberculosis* infection
- Highly virulent or resistant microbial infections
- Chest wall deformity
- Obesity
- Medical noncompliance
- Psychiatric disease leading to noncooperation in management plan
- Absent social support system
- Substance abuse/addition
- Severely impaired functional status

BOX 21.3 Relative contraindications for lung transplantation

- Age over 65 years with limited functional reserve
- Obesity
- Malnutrition
- Severe osteoporosis
- Prior lung resection surgery
- Mechanical ventilation or extracorporeal life support
- Highly resistant bacterial colonization
- Hepatitis B and C
- HIV infection with detectable viral load
- *Burkholderia* and *Mycobacterium abscessus* infection in which good control is not expected

---

18. In patients with previous thoracic surgery, which procedure is associated with the most blood loss during lung transplantation?
   A. Video-assisted lobectomy
   B. Lung volume reduction
   C. Pneumonectomy
   D. Pleurodesis

Correct Answer: D

Explanation: Previous thoracic surgeries can affect clinical outcomes after lung transplantation including reoperation for bleeding, phrenic nerve injury, prolonged mechanical ventilation and tracheostomy rate, acute renal insufficiency, and mid-term loss of pulmonary function. Of all of the surgeries listed in the question, pleurodesis is associated with the highest incidence of protracted bleeding because it consistently causes widespread dense pleural adhesions. Predictors of early death in patients with previous thoracic surgery include age over 65 years, the presence of pulmonary hypertension, massive transfusion, and prolonged cardiopulmonary bypass. Of all of the surgeries listed in the given question, pleurodesis is associated with the highest incidence of bleeding and complications.

References:

1. Murray AW, Quinlan JJ, Blasiole B, et al. Chapter 25: Anesthesia for Heart, Lung, and Heart-Lung Transplantation. In: Kaplan JA, Augoustides JGT, Manecke GR, et al., eds. Kaplan's Cardiac Anesthesia. 7th ed. Elsevier; 2017:974-993.
2. Shigemura N, Bhama J, Gries C, et al. Lung transplantation in patients with prior cardiothoracic surgical procedures. Am J Transplant, 2012; 12: 1249-1255.

19. According to the primary graft dysfunction (PGD) scale in lung transplantation, what grade would be assigned to a lung transplant recipient if the PaO_2/FiO_2 (P/F) is 230 and there is pulmonary edema on chest radiography?
   A. PGD grade 0
   B. PGD grade 1
   C. PGD grade 2
   D. PGD grade 3

Correct Answer: C

Explanation: The International Society for Heart and Lung Transplantation developed a four-tier scoring system for primary graft dysfunction (PGD) based on the arterial to inspired oxygenation ratio (P/F) and findings on chest radiography. In this case, a P/F ratio of 230 with pulmonary edema signifies PGD grade 2.

PGD grade 0: P/F ratio over 300 and no pulmonary edema on chest radiograph

PGD grade 1: P/F ratio over 300 and pulmonary edema on chest radiograph

PGD grade 2: P/F ratio of 200 to 300 and pulmonary edema on chest radiograph

PGD grade 3: P/F ratio under 200 and pulmonary edema on chest radiograph

References:

1. Murray AW, Quinlan JJ, Blasiole B, et al. Chapter 25: Anesthesia for Heart, Lung, and Heart-Lung Transplantation. In: Kaplan JA, Augoustides JGT, Manecke GR, et al., eds. Kaplan's Cardiac Anesthesia. 7th ed. Elsevier; 2017:974-993.
2. Snell GI, Yusen RD, Weill D, et al. Report of the ISHLT Working Group on Primary Lung Graft Dysfunction, part I: definition and grading-A 2016: Consensus Group statement of the International Society for Heart and Lung Transplantation. J Heart Lung Transplant, 2017; 36: 1097-1103.

20. What is the most common cause of 30-day mortality in lung transplantation patients?
   A. Primary graft dysfunction
   B. Acute rejection
   C. Infection
   D. Renal failure

Correct Answer: A

Explanation: The two most common causes of 30-day mortality are primary graft dysfunction followed by infection. The most common infectious etiologies include bacterial bronchitis and pneumonia, but fungi, cytomegalovirus, community-acquired

BOX 21.4   Risk factors for increased mortality

- Smaller transplant center: 30 transplants per year
- Greater donor-to-recipient height mismatch
- Older recipient: older than 55 years
- Higher bilirubin
- Higher supplemental oxygen therapy
- Lower cardiac output
- Lower forced vital capacity
- Higher creatinine

respiratory viruses, and bacteria also contribute to mortality. Other causes of 30-day mortality include acute renal failure requiring dialysis, acute rejection, neurologic complications such as stroke and/or metabolic encephalopathy, and cardiac complications. Risk factors for mortality in this setting include transplant for vascular diseases, history of previous nontransplant cardiothoracic surgery, mean pulmonary pressures over 35 mmHg, disabled functional status, support with extracorporeal membrane oxygenation, high lung allocation score, and an ischemic time greater than 6 hours.

References:

1. Murray AW, Quinlan JJ, Blasiole B, et al. Chapter 25: Anesthesia for Heart, Lung, and Heart-Lung Transplantation. In: Kaplan JA, Augoustides JGT, Manecke GR, et al., eds. Kaplan's Cardiac Anesthesia. 7th ed. Elsevier; 2017:974-993.
2. Banga A, Mohanks M, Mullins J, et al. Incidence and variables associated with 30-day mortality after lung transplantation. Clin Transpl, 2019; 33: e13468.

21. After lung implantation, which pulmonary venous anastomotic diameter has been associated with increased risk for graft failure?
   A. Less than 0.15 cm
   B. Less than 0.25 cm
   C. Less than 0.5 cm
   D. Less than 0.75 cm

Correct Answer: B

Explanation: Pulmonary vein anastomoses after lung transplantation are evaluated intraoperatively using transesophageal echocardiography with color flow and pulsed wave Doppler. A normal pulmonary vein anastomosis is greater than 0.5 cm. Diameters over 0.5 cm are associated with an increased incidence of thrombosis, while diameters under 0.25 cm are associated with graft failure. Using pulsed wave Doppler, a velocity of more than 1 m/s is suggestive of an obstruction, whereas a velocity more than 1.7 m/s is suggestive of pulmonary cuff dysfunction. False positives can occur with a hyperdynamic circulation, a contralateral pulmonary artery stenosis, high cardiac output, or vasoconstriction of the donor vein. False negatives can occur with mitral valve regurgitation, diastolic dysfunction, mechanical circulatory support, or hypovolemia.

References:

1. Murray AW, Quinlan JJ, Blasiole B, et al. Chapter 25: Anesthesia for Heart, Lung, and Heart-Lung Transplantation. In: Kaplan

JA, Augoustides JGT, Manecke GR, et al., eds. Kaplan's Cardiac Anesthesia. 7th ed. Elsevier; 2017:974-993.
2. Abrams BA, Melnyk V, Allen WL, et al. TEE for lung transplantation: a case series and discussion of vascular complications. J Cardiothoracic Vasc Anesth, 2020; 34: 733-740.

22. All of these echocardiographic findings suggest pulmonary artery stenosis after lung transplantation EXCEPT:
   A. Pulmonary artery diameter under 0.8 cm
   B. Pulmonary artery anastomosis size under 75% of the native vessel
   C. Pulmonary artery velocity over 2.6 m/s
   D. Increased ipsilateral pulmonary vein flow

Correct Answer: D

Explanation: Pulmonary artery stenosis in lung transplantation is associated with graft failure, hypoxemia, prolonged mechanical ventilation, and increased mortality. Etiologies include donor–recipient size mismatch, surgical misadventure, external compression, and thrombosis. Risk factors for this complication include female gender and restrictive lung disease. Echocardiographic signs suggestive of pulmonary artery stenosis include a pulmonary artery diameter under 0.8 cm, an anastomotic diameter under 75% of the ipsilateral native pulmonary artery, a velocity over 2.6 m/s with spectral Doppler, a nonlaminar flow pattern with flow during systole, and reduced flow in the ipsilateral pulmonary veins with increased flow in the contralateral pulmonary veins.

References:

1. Murray AW, Quinlan JJ, Blasiole B, et al. Chapter 25: Anesthesia for Heart, Lung, and Heart-Lung Transplantation. In: Kaplan JA, Augoustides JGT, Manecke GR, et al., eds. Kaplan's Cardiac Anesthesia. 7th ed. Elsevier; 2017:974-993.
2. Abrams BA, Melnyk V, Allen WL, et al. TEE for lung transplantation: a case series and discussion of vascular complications. J Cardiothoracic Vasc Anesth, 2020; 34: 733-740.
3. Kumar N, Hussain N, Kumar J, et al. Evaluating the impact of pulmonary artery obstruction after lung transplant surgery: a systematic review and meta-analysis. Transplantation, 2021; 105: 711-722.

23. All of following are risk factors for postoperative anastomotic airway complications following lung transplantation EXCEPT:
   A. Donor/recipient height mismatch
   B. Glucocorticoids to treat rejection
   C. Severe primary graft dysfunction
   D. Single-lung transplantation

Correct Answer: B

Explanation: There are several risk factors associated with an increased risk of anastomotic airway complications. These include severe primary graft dysfunction, acute rejection within the first year of transplant, perioperative pulmonary infection, prolonged mechanical ventilation, single-lung transplantation, colonization with *Aspergillus fumigatus*, preoperative

Burkholderia cepacia infection, the use of sirolimus prior to complete anastomotic healing, and donor–recipient mismatch. The use of glucocorticoids to treat acute cellular rejection following lung transplantation is not associated with an increase in airway complications following lung transplantation.

References:

1. Murray AW, Quinlan JJ, Blasiole B, et al. Chapter 25: Anesthesia for Heart, Lung, and Heart-Lung Transplantation. In: Kaplan JA, Augoustides JGT, Manecke GR, et al., eds. Kaplan's Cardiac Anesthesia. 7th ed. Elsevier; 2017:974-993.
2. Crespo MM. Airway complications in lung transplantation. J Thorac Dis, 2021; 13: 6717-6724.

24. All of the following are indications for listing patients with interstitial lung disease for lung transplantation EXCEPT:
   A. Desaturation to less than 88% on 6-minute walk test
   B. Resting or exertional oxygen requirement
   C. Pulmonary hypertension
   D. Decline in forced vital capacity more than 10% in 6 months

Correct Answer: B

Explanation: Because idiopathic pulmonary fibrosis has such a rapid progression in many patients, patients with idiopathic pulmonary fibrosis are referred for lung transplantation when there is radiographic or histopathologic diagnosis of fibrosis, and when the forced vital capacity is under 80% or the diffusing capacity under 40% of predicted. Further indications for referral include a decline in pulmonary function over the past 2 years such as a decline in forced vital capacity of 10% or more with symptoms or radiographic progression, as well as a resting or exertional oxygen requirement and/or progression despite antifibrotic therapies. Patients are listed for lung transplantation with there is a hospitalization for respiratory decline, pneumothorax, or acute exacerbation, desaturation to less than 88% or more than 50-meter decline in the 6-minute walk test over 6 months, pulmonary hypertension, decline in pulmonary function over the past 6 months despite treatment as defined by measures such as decreases in forced vital capacity over 10%, and diffusion capacity over 10%.

References:

1. Murray AW, Quinlan JJ, Blasiole B, et al. Chapter 25: Anesthesia for Heart, Lung, and Heart-Lung Transplantation. In: Kaplan JA, Augoustides JGT, Manecke GR, et al., eds. Kaplan's Cardiac Anesthesia. 7th ed. Elsevier; 2017:974-993.
2. Kapnadak SG, Raghu G. Lung transplantation for interstitial lung disease. Eur Respir Rev, 2021; 30: 210017.

25. What is an acceptable delta PaO_2 following 4 to 6 hours of ex vivo lung perfusion that would be consistent with progression to lung transplantation?
   A. 250 mmHg or more
   B. 300 mmHg or more
   C. 350 mmHg or more
   D. 400 mmHg or more

Correct Answer: C

Explanation: Indications for ex vivo lung perfusion include the best arterial to inspired oxygenation ratio under 300 mmHg, pulmonary edema, poor lung compliance, high risk history, and lungs from a marginal donation in circulatory death donor. The goal of this technique is to restore lung function to allow progression to lung transplantation. After 4 to 6 hours of ex vivo lung perfusion, acceptable criteria include a delta PaO_2, defined as the difference in oxygen tension between samples from left atrium and pulmonary artery, of 350 mmHg (or more) with an inspired oxygen concentration of 100%, as well as stable or improving pulmonary artery pressures, airway pressures, and pulmonary compliance. The exclusion criteria include a delta PaO_2 under 350 mmHg, with a greater than 15% deterioration of pulmonary artery pressure, airway pressure, and pulmonary compliance.

References:

1. Murray AW, Quinlan JJ, Blasiole B, et al. Chapter 25: Anesthesia for Heart, Lung, and Heart-Lung Transplantation. In: Kaplan JA, Augoustides JGT, Manecke GR, et al., eds. Kaplan's Cardiac Anesthesia. 7th ed. Elsevier; 2017:974-993.
2. Wantanabe T, Cypel M, Keshavjee S. *Ex vivo* lung perfusion. J Thoracic Dis, 2021; 13: 6602-6617.

26. All of these patients are considered high-risk lung transplant recipients EXCEPT:
   A. Pretransplant extracorporeal membrane oxygenation
   B. Oxygen requirement greater than 5 L/min
   C. Previous tracheostomy
   D. Chronic corticosteroid use

Correct Answer: C

Explanation: Recipient characteristics that confer a higher risk during lung transplantation include preoperative extracorporeal membrane oxygenation, an oxygen requirement greater than 5 L/min, retransplantation, age over 70 years, renal or hepatic impairment, severe pulmonary hypertension, extremes of body mass index, and chronic use of corticosteroids. Previous tracheostomy does not confer a high-risk status to the patient.

References:

1. Murray AW, Quinlan JJ, Blasiole B, et al. Chapter 25: Anesthesia for Heart, Lung, and Heart-Lung Transplantation. In: Kaplan JA, Augoustides JGT, Manecke GR, et al., eds. Kaplan's Cardiac Anesthesia. 7th ed. Elsevier; 2017:974-993.
2. Buckwell E, Vickery B, Sidebotham D. Anaesthesia for lung transplantation. BJA Educ, 2020; 20: 368-376.

27. Which of these medications is not used to treat pulmonary arterial hypertension in lung transplant candidates?
   A. Pirfenidone
   B. Riociguat
   C. Bosentan
   D. Selexipag

Correct Answer: A

Explanation: The endothelin-1, nitric oxide, and prostacyclin signaling pathways are targets for the treatment of pulmonary hypertension. In pulmonary arterial hypertension, there is upregulation of the vasoconstrictor endothelin-1 and decreased production of nitric oxide and prostacyclin. The endothelin-1 pathway can be blocked by the endothelin receptor agonists bosentan, ambrisentan, and macitentan. The vasodilatory nitric oxide pathway can be enhanced by the phosphodiesterase 5 inhibitors sildenafil and tadalafil or by the stimulation of soluble guanylate cyclase with riociguat. The prostacyclin pathway can be enhanced by the prostanoid analogues epoprostenol, iloprost, and treprostinil, and by the nonprostanoid receptor agonists beraprost and selexipag. Pirfenidone is an antifibrotic used in patients with pulmonary fibrosis.

References:

1. Murray AW, Quinlan JJ, Blasiole B, et al. Chapter 25: Anesthesia for Heart, Lung, and Heart-Lung Transplantation. In: Kaplan JA, Augoustides JGT, Manecke GR, et al., eds. Kaplan's Cardiac Anesthesia. 7th ed. Elsevier; 2017:974-993.
2. Lau E, Giannoulatou E, Celermajer D, et al. Epidemiology and treatment of pulmonary arterial hypertension. Nat Rev Cardiol, 2017; 14: 603-614.

28. In patients with chronic obstructive lung disease, what BODE score would typically add a patient to the lung transplantation list?
   A. 3 or more
   B. 5 or more
   C. 7 or more
   D. 9 or more

Correct Answer: C

Discussions: The BODE scale is a scale used to predict survival in patients with chronic obstructive pulmonary disease and to refer and list patients for lung transplantation. The four components are the **B**ody mass index, airflow **O**bstruction as reflected by changes in lung function after bronchodilators, **D**yspnea, and **E**xercise capacity based on the 6-minute walk test. Each of the four categories is scored from 0 to 3. Patients are referred for transplant consideration when their BODE score is between 5 and 6, and they are listed for transplantation when their BODE score is 7 or more.

References:

1. Murray AW, Quinlan JJ, Blasiole B, et al. Chapter 25: Anesthesia for Heart, Lung, and Heart-Lung Transplantation. In: Kaplan JA, Augoustides JGT, Manecke GR, et al., eds. Kaplan's Cardiac Anesthesia. 7th ed. Elsevier; 2017:974-993.
2. Celli BR, Cote CG, Marin JM, et al The body-mass index, airflow obstruction, dyspnea, and exercise capacity index in chronic obstructive pulmonary disease. N Engl J Med, 2004; 350: 1005-1012.

29. All of these are physiologic changes following lung transplantation EXCEPT:
   A. Impaired cough
   B. Gastroesophageal reflux disease
   C. Blunted response to isocapnic hypoxia
   D. Sleep disordered breathing

Correct Answer: C

Explanation: In patients after lung transplantation, there is a reduced cough reflex due to the afferent limb of the cough reflex being interrupted during organ procurement. Mucociliary clearance is also reduced, leading to reduced airway clearance. These factors, along with oropharyngeal dysphagia, gastrointestinal reflux, and gastroparesis caused by injury to the vagus, recurrent laryngeal, and superior laryngeal nerves, can increase the risk for aspiration. There is vocal cord paresis in approximately 25% of patients. The ventilatory response to hypercapnia has been variable, and both normal and mildly blunted responses have been reported in the postoperative period. The ventilatory response to isocapnic hypoxia remains normal. Respiratory and skeletal muscle dysfunction is multifactorial, with the principal mechanisms related to deconditioning, critical care neuropathy, glucocorticoid myopathy, and diaphragmatic dysfunction from phrenic nerve injury. The incidence of diaphragmatic dysfunction following lung transplantation ranges from 3% to 30%. There is an increased incidence of sleep disordered breathing after lung transplantation due to pharyngeal muscle dysfunction, glucocorticoid-induced central fat deposition, preexisting sleep apnea, and abnormal pulmonary function.

References:
1. Murray AW, Quinlan JJ, Blasiole B, et al. Chapter 25: Anesthesia for Heart, Lung, and Heart-Lung Transplantation. In: Kaplan JA, Augoustides JGT, Manecke GR, et al., eds. Kaplan's Cardiac Anesthesia. 7th ed. Elsevier; 2017:974-993.
2. Feltracco P, Falasco G, Barbieri S, et al. Anesthetic considerations for nontransplant procedures in lung transplant patients. J Clin Anesth, 2011; 23: 508-516.

30. All of these interventions can be used to treat intraoperative right ventricular failure due to pulmonary hypertension EXCEPT:
   A. High positive end-expiratory pressures
   B. Increase preload
   C. Inotropic agents
   D. α-adrenergic agonists

Correct Answer: A

Explanation: The treatment of right ventricular dysfunction due to pulmonary hypertension is reducing pulmonary vascular tone by preventing hypoxia, hypercarbia, and acidosis, as well as avoiding increases in intrathoracic pressures from excessive positive end-expiratory pressure, large tidal volumes, and inadequate expiratory time. Further management principles include increasing preload, titrating inotropic agents with vasodilating properties when pulmonary vascular resistance is increased, and maintaining right ventricular coronary perfusion pressure with α-adrenergic agonists or vasopressin. The administration of pulmonary vasodilators such as nitric oxide or prostaglandin E₁ can unload the right ventricle due to selective pulmonary vasodilation.

The management of right ventricular failure during lung transplantation also requires meticulous attention to ventilation, as well as an understanding of the indications for rescue with cardiopulmonary bypass (see teaching boxes for further details).

References:
1. Murray AW, Quinlan JJ, Blasiole B, et al. Chapter 25: Anesthesia for Heart, Lung, and Heart-Lung Transplantation. In: Kaplan JA, Augoustides JGT, Manecke GR, et al., eds. Kaplan's Cardiac Anesthesia. 7th ed. Elsevier; 2017:974-993.
2. Buckwell E, Vickery B, Sidebotham D. Anaesthesia for lung transplantation. BJA Educ, 2020; 20: 368-376.
3. Feltracco P, Falasco G, Barbieri S, et al. Anesthetic considerations for nontransplant procedures in lung transplant patients. J Clin Anesth, 2011; 23: 508-516.

BOX 21.5 Management principles for one-lung ventilation during lung transplantation

- Tidal volume and respiratory rate
  - Maintain in patients with normal or decreased lung compliance (i.e., primary pulmonary hypertension, fibrosis)
  - Decrease both tidal volume and rate in patients with increased compliance (e.g., obstructive lung disease) to avoid hyperinflation (permissive hypercapnia)
- Maintain oxygenation by:
  - 100% inspired oxygen
  - Applying CPAP (5–10 cm H_2O) to nonventilated lung
  - Adding PEEP (5–10 cm H_2O) to ventilated lung
  - Intermittent lung reinflation if necessary
  - Surgical ligation of the pulmonary artery of the nonventilated lung
- Be alert for development of pneumothorax on nonoperative side
  - Sharp decline in oxygen saturation, end-tidal carbon dioxide
  - Sharp increase in peak airway pressures
  - Increased risk with bullous lung disease
- Therapy
  - Relieve tension
  - Resume ventilation
  - Emergency cardiopulmonary bypass

CPAP, Continuous positive airway pressure; *PEEP,* positive end-expiratory pressure.

BOX 21.6 Indications for cardiopulmonary bypass during lung transplantation

Cardiac index	<2 L/min/m²
S_vO_2	<60%
Mean arterial pressure	<50–60 mm Hg
S_aO_2	<85%–90%
pH	<7.00

CHAPTER 22

Pulmonary Thromboendarterectomy for Chronic Thromboembolic Pulmonary Hypertension

Harikesh Subramanian

KEY POINTS

1. The incidence of thromboembolic disease is difficult to estimate because of the nonspecific nature of presenting symptoms and a lack of awareness of the disorder, which makes detection difficult.

2. Chronic thromboembolic pulmonary hypertension (CTEPH) results from incomplete resolution of a pulmonary embolus (PE) or from recurrent PEs. It is an underappreciated phenomenon.

3. The cause of CTEPH after acute PE is not fully understood. Proposed mechanisms include abnormalities in fibrinolytic enzymes or resistance of the thrombus to fibrinolysis.

4. Pulmonary thromboendarterectomy (PTE) is the most effective treatment for patients with CTEPH.

5. Assessment of surgical candidacy should be performed at centers with expertise in the diagnosis and management of CTEPH. Right-sided heart catheterization defines the severity of pulmonary hypertension and the degree of cardiac dysfunction.

6. A newer surgical classification system has been developed. It describes the different levels of the resected thromboembolic specimen and corresponds to the degree of difficulty of the endarterectomy.

7. Riociguat is the first medication approved by the US Food and Drug Administration for treating certain patients with CTEPH.

8. Reperfusion pulmonary edema and airway bleeding are two of the most difficult complications of PTE to manage. Anesthesiologists should be prepared to provide diagnostic and therapeutic maneuvers for these complications.

---

1. According to the World Health Organization classification, into which group is a patient with chronic obstructive pulmonary disease classified?
   A. Group I
   B. Group II
   C. Group III
   D. Group IV

Correct Answer: C

Explanation: The classification of pulmonary hypertension by the World Health Organization is based on the etiology as outlined in the table. The first group comprises all forms of primary pulmonary artery hypertension that is primarily a disease at the arteriolar level of the pulmonary vasculature. The second group is the most common of etiologies that comprise left-sided heart diseases, including mitral stenosis, mitral regurgitation, and left ventricular failure. The third group includes respiratory diseases that may be restrictive, obstructive, or mixed in nature. The fourth group includes vascular obstructive disease due to chronic emboli and tumor. The fifth group includes pulmonary hypertensive diseases with etiologies that are unclear and/or multifactorial.

References:

1. Banks DA, Auger WR, Madani MM. Chapter 26: Pulmonary Thromboendarterectomy for Chronic Thromboembolic

TABLE 22.1
Classification of pulmonary hypertension by the World Health Organization

Group	Etiology of Pulmonary Hypertension
Group I	Pulmonary arterial hypertension (idiopathic, heritable, drug-induced, other)
Group II	Left-sided heart disease (mitral valve disease included)
Group III	Respiratory disease and hypoxemia (restrictive and obstructive etiologies)
Group IV	Chronic pulmonary thromboembolic disease/obstructive disease (also includes rare intravascular tumors)
Group V	Pulmonary hypertension with unclear etiology, idiopathic causes, and/or multifactorial mechanisms

Adapted from Galiè N, Humbert M, Vachiery JL, et al. 2015 ESC/ERS Guidelines for the diagnosis and treatment of pulmonary hypertension: The Joint Task Force for the Diagnosis and Treatment of Pulmonary Hypertension of the European Society of Cardiology (ESC) and the European Respiratory Society (ERS): Endorsed by: Association for European Paediatric and Congenital Cardiology (AEPC), International Society for Heart and Lung Transplantation (ISHLT). Eur Heart J. 2016; 37(1): 67-119.

Pulmonary Hypertension. In: Kaplan JA, Augoustides JGT, Manecke GR, et al., eds. Kaplan's Cardiac Anesthesia. 7th ed. Elsevier; 2017:994-1021.
2. Galiè N, Humbert M, Vachiery JL, et al. 2015 ESC/ERS Guidelines for the diagnosis and treatment of pulmonary hypertension: The Joint Task Force for the Diagnosis and Treatment of Pulmonary Hypertension of the European Society of Cardiology (ESC) and the European Respiratory Society (ERS): Endorsed by: Association for European Paediatric and Congenital Cardiology (AEPC), International Society for Heart and Lung Transplantation (ISHLT). Eur Heart J. 2016; 37(1): 67-119.

2. According to the World Health Organization classification, which group is defined as postcapillary pulmonary hypertension?
   A. Group I
   B. Group II
   C. Group III
   D. Group IV

Correct Answer: B

Explanation: Group II pulmonary hypertension is linked to left-sided heart disease that results in left atrial hypertension with consequent pulmonary hypertension. This disease group manifests as postcapillary pulmonary hypertension. Commonly, in this group, the transpulmonary gradient and the pulmonary vascular resistance are below 12 mmHg and 3 Wood units, respectively.

References:
1. Banks DA, Auger WR, Madani MM. Chapter 26: Pulmonary Thromboendarterectomy for Chronic Thromboembolic Pulmonary Hypertension. In: Kaplan JA, Augoustides JGT,

Manecke GR, et al., eds. Kaplan's Cardiac Anesthesia. 7th ed. Elsevier; 2017:994-1021.
2. Galiè N, Humbert M, Vachiery JL, et al. 2015 ESC/ERS Guidelines for the diagnosis and treatment of pulmonary hypertension: The Joint Task Force for the Diagnosis and Treatment of Pulmonary Hypertension of the European Society of Cardiology (ESC) and the European Respiratory Society (ERS): Endorsed by: Association for European Paediatric and Congenital Cardiology (AEPC), International Society for Heart and Lung Transplantation (ISHLT). Eur Heart J. 2016; 37(1): 67-119.
3. Gelzinis TA. Pulmonary hypertension in 2021: part 1 – definitions, classification, pathophysiology and presentation. J Cardiothorac Vasc Anesth, 2022; 36: 1552-1564.

3. Which of the following profiles is most consistent with chronic thromboembolic hypertension (mPAP = mean pulmonary artery pressure; PCWP = pulmonary capillary wedge pressure; PVR = pulmonary vascular resistance)?
   A. Mean pulmonary artery pressure (mPAP) = 18 mmHg, pulmonary capillary wedge pressure (PCWP) = 12 mmHg, pulmonary vascular resistance (PVR) = 250 dynes/s/cm^5
   B. mPAP = 27 mmHg, PCWP = 17 mmHg, PVR = 250 dynes/s/cm^5
   C. mPAP = 27 mmHg, PCWP = 10 mmHg, PVR = 400 dynes/s/cm^5
   D. mPAP = 27 mmHg, PCWP = 17 mmHg, PVR = 400 dynes/s/cm^5

Correct Answer: C

Explanation: Chronic thromboembolic pulmonary hypertension is classified as group IV pulmonary hypertension, as outlined hemodynamically by profile option C. It is associated with pulmonary hypertension with a mean pulmonary artery pressure above 25 mmHg, a pulmonary capillary wedge pressure below 15 mmHg, and an elevated pulmonary vascular resistance greater than 200 dynes/s/cm^5. Profile option A is not consistent with pulmonary hypertension since the mean pulmonary artery pressure is less than 20 mmHg. Profile option B is consistent with Group II pulmonary hypertension associated with left heart disease with postcapillary pulmonary hypertension. Profile option D is consistent with mixed disease.

References:
1. Banks DA, Auger WR, Madani MM. Chapter 26: Pulmonary Thromboendarterectomy for Chronic Thromboembolic Pulmonary Hypertension. In: Kaplan JA, Augoustides JGT, Manecke GR, et al., eds. Kaplan's Cardiac Anesthesia. 7th ed. Elsevier; 2017:994-1021.
2. Gelzinis TA. Pulmonary hypertension in 2021: part 1 – definitions, classification, pathophysiology and presentation. J Cardiothorac Vasc Anesth, 2022; 36: 1552-1564.

4. Which of the following is NOT associated with the pathology of chronic thromboembolic pulmonary hypertension?
   A. Incomplete thrombus resolution and organization
   B. Pulmonary arterial vascular remodeling
   C. Fibrin plugging of arterioles
   D. Pulmonary venous hypertension

Correct Answer: D

Explanation: Chronic thromboembolic pulmonary hypertension is defined as pulmonary hypertension that is persistent for at least 3 months in a patient with previous acute pulmonary embolism on anticoagulation. It occurs as a long-term complication in about 0.1% to 9.1% of patients with an acute pulmonary embolic event within 2 years of the event. The etiology is thought to not only include mechanical obstruction but also reorganization of the thrombus and associated vascular remodeling. Consequently, for this question, incomplete thrombus resolution and organization, pulmonary arterial vascular remodeling, and fibrin plugging of the arterioles are all correct answers. Venous hypertension is incorrect because this finding is typically associated with left heart disease rather than chronic thromboembolic hypertension.

References:

1. Banks DA, Auger WR, Madani MM. Chapter 26: Pulmonary Thromboendarterectomy for Chronic Thromboembolic Pulmonary Hypertension. In: Kaplan JA, Augoustides JGT, Manecke GR, et al., eds. Kaplan's Cardiac Anesthesia. 7th ed. Elsevier; 2017: 994-1021.
2. Gelzinis TA. Pulmonary hypertension in 2021: part 1 – definitions, classification, pathophysiology and presentation. J Cardiothorac Vasc Anesth, 2022; 36: 1552-1564.

5. Which of the following is the least valuable modality in the diagnosis and management of chronic thromboembolic pulmonary hypertension?
   A. Transesophageal echocardiography
   B. Ventilation perfusion scanning
   C. Right heart catheterization
   D. Pulmonary angiography

Correct Answer: A

Explanation: Ventilation perfusion scanning is a main imaging modality that helps to diagnose chronic thromboembolic disease. Although catheter-based pulmonary angiography has traditionally been considered the gold standard for confirming this diagnosis and for assessing the proximal extent of chronic thromboembolic disease, contrast-enhanced computed tomographic angiography with multiplanar reconstruction can also help identify the relevant pulmonary vascular abnormalities. A right heart catheterization is helpful in this setting to quantify the pulmonary hypertension and in ruling out causes related to the left heart. Of the given options, transesophageal echocardiography is least likely to be useful in diagnoses and management of this disease and may not provide additional information compared to transthoracic echocardiography.

References:

1. Banks DA, Auger WR, Madani MM. Chapter 26: Pulmonary Thromboendarterectomy for Chronic Thromboembolic Pulmonary Hypertension. In: Kaplan JA, Augoustides JGT, Manecke GR, et al., eds. Kaplan's Cardiac Anesthesia. 7th ed. Elsevier; 2017:994-1021.

2. Ranka S, Mohananey D, Agarwal N, et al. Chronic thromboembolic pulmonary hypertension – management strategies and outcomes. J Cardiothorac Vasc Anesth, 2020; 34: 2513-2523.

6. A 45-year-old woman presents for an extensive thoracic spinal fusion. In the preoperative holding area, she suddenly complains of shortness of breath and chest pain. The patient is hypotensive with advanced tachycardia and hypoxia. A point-of-care transthoracic echocardiogram demonstrates a large free clot in the right ventricle. Given that this patient has a low bleeding risk, which would be most appropriate?
   A. Unfractionated heparin bolus of 20 units/kg followed by an infusion of 18 units/kg/hour
   B. Unfractionated heparin bolus of 80 units/kg followed by an infusion of 10 units/kg/hour
   C. Unfractionated heparin bolus of 20 units/kg followed by an infusion at 10 units/kg/hour
   D. Unfractionated heparin bolus of 80 units/kg followed by an infusion of 18 units/kg/hour

Correct Answer: D

Explanation: The patient appears to have signs and symptoms suggestive of a massive or submassive pulmonary embolism. It is important to start anticoagulation early with an appropriate dose as soon as the diagnosis is made while other invasive interventions are planned. An assessment of clinical bleeding risk can guide the dosing of anticoagulation. In patients with average or low bleeding risk, the recommended goal of anticoagulation in this setting is a target partial thromboplastin time of 1.5 to 2.5 times the normal value. The contemporary approach to acute pulmonary embolism includes a multidisciplinary pulmonary embolus response team that can assist with further management options including thrombolysis, catheter-based thrombectomy, or surgical embolectomy.

References:

1. Banks DA, Auger WR, Madani MM. Chapter 26: Pulmonary Thromboendarterectomy for Chronic Thromboembolic Pulmonary Hypertension. In: Kaplan JA, Augoustides JGT, Manecke GR, et al., eds. Kaplan's Cardiac Anesthesia. 7th ed. Elsevier; 2017:994-1021.
2. Rivera-Lebron B, McDaniel M, Ahrar K, et al. Diagnosis, treatment and follow up of acute pulmonary embolism: consensus practice from the PERT consortium. Clin Appl Thromb Hemost, 2019: 25: 1076029619853037.
3. Rosovsky R, Merli G. Anticoagulation in pulmonary embolism: update in the age of direct oral anticoagulants. Tech Vasc Interv Radiol, 2017; 20: 141-151.
4. Cormican D, Morkos MS, Winter D, et al. Acute perioperative pulmonary embolism – management strategies and outcomes. J Cardiothorac Vasc Anesth, 2020; 34: 1972-1984.

7. Which of the following findings is NOT associated with pulmonary hypertension?
   A. Holosystolic murmur that increases with inspiration
   B. Right axis deviation on an electrocardiogram
   C. Enlarged hilar pulmonary arteries on chest imaging
   D. An increased pulmonary artery acceleration on transthoracic echocardiography

Correct Answer: D

Explanation: Pulmonary hypertension typically presents with a constellation of signs and symptoms. Secondary tricuspid regurgitation is common in this setting and is characterized by a holosystolic murmur that increases during inspiration. The right ventricular hypertrophy and dilation that accompany the increased afterload of pulmonary hypertrophy can progress to right axis deviation on the electrocardiogram. The associated prominent pulmonary artery vasculature associated with "pruning" or attenuation of the peripheral vasculature may also be seen on chest imaging. The echocardiographic findings include right-sided chamber enlargement, interventricular septal flattening, tricuspid regurgitation, and right ventricular systolic dysfunction, as well as a reduced pulmonary artery acceleration time (normal values are >130 msec).

References:

1. Banks DA, Auger WR, Madani MM. Chapter 26: Pulmonary Thromboendarterectomy for Chronic Thromboembolic Pulmonary Hypertension. In: Kaplan JA, Augoustides JGT, Manecke GR, et al., eds. Kaplan's Cardiac Anesthesia. 7th ed. Elsevier; 2017:994-1021.
2. Gelzinis TA. Pulmonary hypertension in 2021: part 1 – definitions, classification, pathophysiology and presentation. J Cardiothorac Vasc Anesth, 2022; 36: 1552-1564.

8. Which factor has been correlated with worse outcomes after surgical pulmonary thromboendarterectomy?
   A. Increased pulmonary capillary wedge pressure
   B. Decreased mean pulmonary artery pressure
   C. Severely increased pulmonary vascular resistance
   D. Chronic thromboembolic disease with an emphasis on the central rather than peripheral pulmonary vasculature

Correct Answer: C

Explanation: Studies have shown that patients with severe chronic thromboembolic pulmonary hypertension who display a pulmonary vascular resistance greater than 1000 dynes/s/cm^5 have increased perioperative mortality and morbidity. As a consequence, patient selection for surgical intervention in this disease is typically guided by a holistic assessment, including clinical presentation, coexisting disease, and degree of pulmonary hypertension (see teaching box). An increased wedge pressure is uncommon in this setting, given that group IV pulmonary hypertension is typically associated with low or normal wedge pressures. A significant decrease in mean pulmonary artery pressure after surgery is typically associated with significant clearance of chronic thromboembolic material, and consequently improved postoperative outcomes. Extensive thromboembolic disease in the central pulmonary arteries is readily available for surgical resection and is typically associated with improved clinical outcomes as a result (see teaching box).

References:

1. Banks DA, Auger WR, Madani MM. Chapter 26: Pulmonary Thromboendarterectomy for Chronic Thromboembolic Pulmonary Hypertension. In: Kaplan JA, Augoustides JGT,

---

> ### BOX 22.1 Patient selection criteria for pulmonary thromboendarterectomy
>
> - Presence of surgically resectable chronic thromboembolic disease
> - Symptomatic chronic thromboembolic disease, with or without pulmonary hypertension and right-sided heart dysfunction at rest
> - Absence of concurrent illnesses representing an immediate threat to life
> - Patient's desire for surgical treatment based on dissatisfaction with poor cardiorespiratory function or prognosis
> - Patient's willingness to accept the mortality risk of the pulmonary thromboendarterectomy surgical procedure

> ### BOX 22.2 University of california san diego chronic thromboemboli classification
>
> - Level I: Chronic thromboembolic disease in the main pulmonary arteries
> - Level IC: Complete occlusion of one main pulmonary artery with chronic thromboembolic disease
> - Level II: Chronic thromboembolic disease starting at the level of the lobar arteries or in the main descending pulmonary arteries
> - Level III: Chronic thromboembolic disease starting at the level of the segmental arteries
> - Level IV: Chronic thromboembolic disease starting at the level of the subsegmental arteries
> - Level 0: No evidence of chronic thromboembolic disease in either lung

From Madani MM, Jamieson SW, Pretorius V, et al. Subsegmental pulmonary endarterectomy: time for new surgical classification. Abstract presented at the International CTEPH Conference, Paris, 2014.

Manecke GR, et al., eds. Kaplan's Cardiac Anesthesia. 7th ed. Elsevier; 2017:994-1021.
2. Hartz RS, Byrne JG, Levitsky S, et al. Predictors of mortality in pulmonary thromboendarterectomy. Ann Thorac Surg, 1996; 62: 1255-1259.
3. Ranka S, Mohananey D, Agarwal N, et al. Chronic thromboembolic pulmonary hypertension – management strategies and outcomes. J Cardiothorac Vasc Anesth, 2020; 34: 2513-2523.

9. Which of the following statements is INCORRECT about a surgical endarterectomy?
   A. Pulmonary endarterectomy is usually performed without arresting the heart
   B. Most endarterectomies are performed bilaterally
   C. A complete endarterectomy extending to the segmental vessels is important to ensure therapeutic success
   D. A median sternotomy is the preferred approach for access to the pulmonary arteries

Correct Answer: A

Explanation: Pulmonary thromboendarterectomy is typically performed via median sternotomy hypothermic circulatory arrest to optimize surgical exposure. Hypothermic arrest is required because the lung receives dual blood supply from the pulmonary arteries as well as the bronchial arteries. In addition, in patients with chronic thromboembolic pulmonary hypertension, collaterals develop in the lungs from the intercostal, diaphragmatic, and pleural vessels. If circulatory arrest is not performed, the back-filling of blood from the lungs into the pulmonary arteries will interfere with surgical exposure, making it impossible to identify the dissection planes within the pulmonary arteries for the endarterectomy. Although hypothermic circulatory arrest is usually required for short periods of time, it remains essential for the procedure.

References:

1. Banks DA, Auger WR, Madani MM. Chapter 26: Pulmonary Thromboendarterectomy for Chronic Thromboembolic Pulmonary Hypertension. In: Kaplan JA, Augoustides JGT, Manecke GR, et al., eds. Kaplan's Cardiac Anesthesia. 7th ed. Elsevier; 2017:994-1021.
2. Ranka S, Mohananey D, Agarwal N, et al. Chronic thromboembolic pulmonary hypertension – management strategies and outcomes. J Cardiothorac Vasc Anesth, 2020; 34: 2513-2523.

10. Which of the following statements is true in patients with chronic thromboembolic pulmonary hypertension (CTEPH)?
    A. The majority of tricuspid valve disease in CTEPH requires surgical intervention
    B. The majority of pulmonic valve disease in CTEPH requires valve replacement
    C. A patent foramen ovale identified during a pulmonary endarterectomy requires closure
    D. Most patients with chronic thromboembolic pulmonary hypertension require a superficial endarterectomy

Correct Answer: C

Explanation: In chronic thromboembolic pulmonary hypertension, functional tricuspid and pulmonary regurgitation is common but typically improves with the significant decrease in pulmonary vascular resistance that follows pulmonary endarterectomy. On the other hand, patients who have a patent foramen ovale in this setting are likely to benefit from closure, since they are at risk of an embolic stroke from paradoxical embolism. In addition, a superficial embolectomy will be incomplete and lead to clinical relapse in chronic thromboembolic pulmonary hypertension.

References:

1. Banks DA, Auger WR, Madani MM. Chapter 26: Pulmonary Thromboendarterectomy for Chronic Thromboembolic Pulmonary Hypertension. In: Kaplan JA, Augoustides JGT, Manecke GR, et al., eds. Kaplan's Cardiac Anesthesia. 7th ed. Elsevier; 2017:994-1021.
2. Ng O, Gimenez-Mila M, Jenkins DP, et al. Perioperative management of pulmonary endarterectomy – perspective from the UK National Health Service. J Cardiothoracic Vasc Anesth, 2019; 33: 3101-3109.

11. Which is NOT a common presenting feature of chronic thromboembolic pulmonary hypertension?
    A. Syncope
    B. Hoarseness
    C. Dysphagia
    D. Palpitations

Correct Answer: C

Explanation: As chronic thromboembolic pulmonary hypertension progresses and the right heart fails, patients may develop ascites, early satiety, epigastric or right upper quadrant fullness, edema, chest pain, and/or syncope. Further presenting features may include nonproductive cough, hemoptysis, and palpitations. Left vocal cord dysfunction and hoarseness may arise from compression of the left recurrent laryngeal nerve between the aorta and an enlarged left main pulmonary artery. Dysphagia is not a typical presenting feature in chronic thromboembolic pulmonary hypertension, as the left atrium that lies over the esophagus is not progressively enlarged in this condition.

References:

1. Banks DA, Auger WR, Madani MM. Chapter 26: Pulmonary Thromboendarterectomy for Chronic Thromboembolic Pulmonary Hypertension. In: Kaplan JA, Augoustides JGT, Manecke GR, et al., eds. Kaplan's Cardiac Anesthesia. 7th ed. Elsevier; 2017:994-1021.
2. Gelzinis TA. Pulmonary hypertension in 2021: part 1 – definitions, classification, pathophysiology and presentation. J Cardiothorac Vasc Anesth, 2022; 36: 1552-1564.

12. The LEAST common cause of postoperative death among patients undergoing pulmonary thromboendarterectomy is:
    A. Residual pulmonary hypertension
    B. Reperfusion pulmonary edema
    C. Massive pulmonary hemorrhage
    D. Systemic thromboembolism

Correct Answer: D

Explanation: The common causes of postoperative mortality after pulmonary thromboendarterectomy include residual pulmonary hypertension, pulmonary edema, and massive pulmonary hemorrhage. Residual pulmonary hypertension may follow incomplete endarterectomy due to inaccessibility of the segmental branches of the pulmonary artery. Reperfusion edema is a result of reperfusion of the segments of the lung that were previously hypoperfused, resulting in relative acute hyperemia. Pulmonary hemorrhage can occur due to fistula formation between the pulmonary vasculature and the bronchiolar tree after surgical dissection. Although systemic thromboembolism is a possibility after pulmonary endarterectomy, it is relatively uncommon, as aggressive anticoagulation is a typical feature of postoperative management in this setting to reduce thrombotic complications.

References:

1. Banks DA, Auger WR, Madani MM. Chapter 26: Pulmonary Thromboendarterectomy for Chronic Thromboembolic Pulmonary Hypertension. In: Kaplan JA, Augoustides JGT, Manecke GR, et al., eds. Kaplan's Cardiac Anesthesia. 7th ed. Elsevier; 2017:994-1021.
2. Kratzert WB, Boyd EK, Saggar R, et al. Critical care of patients after pulmonary thromboendarterectomy. J Cardiothorac Vasc Anesth, 2019; 33: 3310-3326.

13. Which of the following is FALSE about airway complications after pulmonary thromboendarterectomy in patients with chronic thromboembolic pulmonary hypertension?
    A. Dark-colored bleeding from the airway is suggestive of surgical injury of the airway
    B. Pink-frothy postsurgical bleeding from the airway is most likely due to reperfusion injury
    C. A double lumen tube to isolate a bleeding source in the lungs is preferred over bronchial blocker
    D. Small bronchial bleeds resolve with isolation in 24 to 48 hours

Correct Answer: C

Explanation: After pulmonary thromboendarterectomy, dark-colored bleeding from the airway may be due to a surgical injury to the airway, including the possibility of a bronchoarteriolar fistula. Pink frothy bleeding may be due to reperfusion injury with pulmonary edema. A bronchial blocker is preferred over a double lumen tube for isolation of the bleeding lobe. Furthermore, a bronchial blocker facilitates the use of a large bronchoscope for airway hygiene and intervention as well as isolation of the bleeding segment with minimal remanipulation of the airway. Although small airway bleeds may heal spontaneously within 24 to 48 hours, the patient may require support during this period with venovenous extracorporeal membrane oxygenation.

References:

1. Banks DA, Auger WR, Madani MM. Chapter 26: Pulmonary Thromboendarterectomy for Chronic Thromboembolic Pulmonary Hypertension. In: Kaplan JA, Augoustides JGT, Manecke GR, et al., eds. Kaplan's Cardiac Anesthesia. 7th ed. Elsevier; 2017:994-1021.
2. Kratzert WB, Boyd EK, Saggar R, et al. Critical care of patients after pulmonary thromboendarterectomy. J Cardiothorac Vasc Anesth, 2019; 33: 3310-3326.

14. All of the following statements are true for the postoperative management after surgical thromboendarterectomy in chronic thromboembolic pulmonary hypertension EXCEPT:
    A. There is usually a reduction in pulmonary vascular resistance immediately after the surgery
    B. Diuresis may be required to reduce reperfusion pulmonary edema

    C. Inhaled nitric oxide therapy can improve ventilation/perfusion mismatching
    D. After surgical thomboendarterectomy for chronic thromboembolic pulmonary hypertension, patients may stop anticoagulation after 1 year

Correct Answer: D

Explanation: There is typically an immediate reduction in the mean pulmonary artery pressure and pulmonary vascular resistance after successful pulmonary thromboendarterectomy. These hemodynamic benefits can produce reperfusion injury and pulmonary edema that may require diuresis in the initial postoperative period. As an inhaled pulmonary vasodilator, nitric oxide therapy in the immediate postoperative period may improve ventilation/perfusion mismatching in select patients, but carries the risk of aggravating pulmonary hyperemia. Patients who have undergone pulmonary thromboendarterectomy for chronic thromboembolic pulmonary hypertension have an ongoing risk of recurrence that explains the recommendation for lifelong systemic anticoagulation.

References:

1. Banks DA, Auger WR, Madani MM. Chapter 26: Pulmonary Thromboendarterectomy for Chronic Thromboembolic Pulmonary Hypertension. In: Kaplan JA, Augoustides JGT, Manecke GR, et al., eds. Kaplan's Cardiac Anesthesia. 7th ed. Elsevier; 2017:994-1021.
2. Kratzert WB, Boyd EK, Saggar R, et al. Critical care of patients after pulmonary thromboendarterectomy. J Cardiothorac Vasc Anesth, 2019; 33: 3310-3326.
3. Ng O, Gimenez-Mila M, Jenkins DP, et al. Perioperative management of pulmonary endarterectomy – perspective from the UK National Health Service. J Cardiothoracic Vasc Anesth, 2019; 33: 3101-3109.

15. Which patients are at particular risk of early postoperative thrombosis in the pulmonary arteries after pulmonary endarterectomy?
    A. Patients with level I disease starting in the main pulmonary artery
    B. Patients with level IC disease with complete occlusion of one main pulmonary artery
    C. Patients with level II disease starting in the lobar arteries
    D. Patients with level III disease starting in the segmental arteries

Correct Answer: B

Explanation: The University of California San Diego surgical classification of chronic thromboembolic disease is based on the involvement of the branches of the pulmonary artery (see teaching box). Among the subgroups of this classification, patients with level IC disease (chronic thromboembolic disease with complete occlusion of one main pulmonary artery) have a relatively increased risk of early postoperative thrombosis in the pulmonary arterial vasculature that requires a therapeutic level of anticoagulation as soon as possible in the postoperative period.

References:

1. Banks DA, Auger WR, Madani MM. Chapter 26: Pulmonary Thromboendarterectomy for Chronic Thromboembolic Pulmonary Hypertension. In: Kaplan JA, Augoustides JGT, Manecke GR, et al., eds. Kaplan's Cardiac Anesthesia. 7th ed. Elsevier; 2017:994-1021.
2. Kratzert WB, Boyd EK, Saggar R, et al. Critical care of patients after pulmonary thromboendarterectomy. J Cardiothorac Vasc Anesth, 2019; 33: 3310-3326.

16. Which medical therapy for pulmonary hypertension is specifically indicated in chronic thromboembolic pulmonary hypertension?
   A. Bosentan
   B. Sildenafil
   C. Riociguat
   D. Treprostenil

Correct Answer: C

Explanation: Medical therapy for patients with chronic thromboembolic pulmonary hypertension is targeted at reducing the pulmonary vascular resistance in a multimodal fashion to improve clinical outcomes (see teaching box). The pharmacologic options in this clinical setting include the endothelin receptor agonists such as bosentan, ambrisentan, and macitentan, as well as the phosphodiesterase 5 inhibitors such as sildenafil and tadalafil. Furthermore, the guanylate cyclase stimulator riociguat has been specifically approved for patients with chronic thromboembolic pulmonary hypertension. In addition, the prostacyclin analogs such as epoprostenol, iloprost, and treprostinil, as well as the prostaglandin receptor agonists beraprost and selexipag all offer additional possibilities for pharmacologic pulmonary vasodilation. Beyond the guanylate cyclase stimulator riociguat, all the above mentioned therapeutic agents have been used in chronic thromboembolic pulmonary hypertension with varying results.

BOX 22.3   Patient groups with chronic thromboembolic pulmonary hypertension to consider for targeted medical therapy for pulmonary hypertension

- Patients with inoperable chronic thromboembolic pulmonary hypertension
- Patients with residual pulmonary hypertension after a pulmonary thromboendarterectomy surgical procedure
- Patients with chronic thromboembolic pulmonary hypertension in whom comorbidities are so significant that surgical treatment is contraindicated
- Patients who have severe pulmonary hypertension and right-sided heart failure, in whom targeted medical therapy for pulmonary hypertension may be a "clinically stabilizing bridge" to surgical treatment

---

References:

1. Banks DA, Auger WR, Madani MM. Chapter 26: Pulmonary Thromboendarterectomy for Chronic Thromboembolic Pulmonary Hypertension. In: Kaplan JA, Augoustides JGT, Manecke GR, et al., eds. Kaplan's Cardiac Anesthesia. 7th ed. Elsevier; 2017:994-1021.
2. Pepke-Zaba J, Ghofrani HA, Hoeper MM. Medical management of chronic thromboembolic pulmonary hypertension. Eur Respir Rev, 2017; 26: 160107.

17. Patients who are not candidates for a surgical thombo-embolectomy may undergo percutaneous pulmonary angioplasty. Which of the following statements is FALSE concerning balloon pulmonary angioplasty?
   A. Balloon pulmonary angioplasty may have a significant risk of reperfusion injury, especially in those with mean pulmonary artery pressure over 35 mmHg
   B. Mild to moderate hemoptysis may occur after this procedure
   C. There is usually immediate improvement in hemodynamic parameters following this procedure
   D. There is typically an improvement in functional status at 3 months

Correct Answer: C

Explanation: Transcatheter interventions such as balloon pulmonary angioplasty may be indicated in select patients with chronic pulmonary thromboembolic disease who may not be candidates for surgical pulmonary thromboendarterectomy. These percutaneous interventions also have a risk of reperfusion injury, including postprocedural hemoptysis. Although there is often improvement in functional status class at 3 months, there may not be immediate improvement in the relevant hemodynamic parameters.

References:

1. Banks DA, Auger WR, Madani MM. Chapter 26: Pulmonary Thromboendarterectomy for Chronic Thromboembolic Pulmonary Hypertension. In: Kaplan JA, Augoustides JGT, Manecke GR, et al., eds. Kaplan's Cardiac Anesthesia. 7th ed. Elsevier; 2017:994-1021.
2. Kratzert WB, Boyd EK, Saggar R, et al. Critical care of patients after pulmonary thromboendarterectomy. J Cardiothorac Vasc Anesth, 2019; 33: 3310-3326.
3. Ranka S, Mohananey D, Agarwal N, et al. Chronic thromboembolic pulmonary hypertension – management strategies and outcomes. J Cardiothorac Vasc Anesth, 2020; 34: 2513-2523.

18. All of the following are risk factors for the development of chronic thromboembolic pulmonary hypertension after an acute pulmonary embolism EXCEPT:
   A. Low pulmonary artery pressures at presentation
   B. Idiopathic thromboembolic disease
   C. Larger perfusion defects at diagnosis
   D. History of multiple pulmonary emboli

Correct Answer: A

Explanation: Risk factors for the development of chronic thromboembolic pulmonary hypertension after acute pulmonary embolism include larger perfusion defects at diagnosis, idiopathic thromboembolic disease, and high pulmonary artery pressures at the time of presentation. Furthermore, a history of multiple pulmonary emboli is also a significant risk factor because it is associated with repeated episodes of pulmonary embolic injury that can lead to chronic pulmonary hypertension.

References:

1. Banks DA, Auger WR, Madani MM. Chapter 26: Pulmonary Thromboendarterectomy for Chronic Thromboembolic Pulmonary Hypertension. In: Kaplan JA, Augoustides JGT, Manecke GR, et al., eds. Kaplan's Cardiac Anesthesia. 7th ed. Elsevier; 2017:994-1021.
2. Gelzinis TA. Pulmonary hypertension in 2021: part 1 – definitions, classification, pathophysiology and presentation. J Cardiothorac Vasc Anesth, 2022; 36: 1552-1564.

19. Which hypercoagulable state is associated with the development of chronic thromboembolic pulmonary hypertension?
   A. Protein C deficiency
   B. Antithrombin deficiency
   C. Factor V Leiden
   D. Antiphospholipid antibodies

Correct Answer: D

Explanation: In analyzing hypercoagulable syndromes and the risk of chronic thromboembolic pulmonary hypertension (CTEPH), the incidences of protein C, protein S, antithrombin deficiency, and factor V Leiden are no more frequent in patients with CTEPH than in a healthy population. There is, however, an increased risk of CTEPH in patients with antiphospholipid antibodies and lupus anticoagulant. The investigation and effective management of an underlying hypercoagulable state play an important role in achieving the best outcomes in chronic thromboembolic hypertension, including after pulmonary thromboendarterectomy.

References:

1. Banks DA, Auger WR, Madani MM. Chapter 26: Pulmonary Thromboendarterectomy for Chronic Thromboembolic Pulmonary Hypertension. In: Kaplan JA, Augoustides JGT, Manecke GR, et al., eds. Kaplan's Cardiac Anesthesia. 7th ed. Elsevier; 2017:994-1021.
2. Gelzinis TA. Pulmonary hypertension in 2021: part 1 – definitions, classification, pathophysiology and presentation. J Cardiothorac Vasc Anesth, 2022; 36: 1552-1564.
3. Simonneau G, Torbicki A, Dorfmüller P, et al. The pathophysiology of chronic thromboembolic pulmonary hypertension. Eur Respir Rev, 2017; 26: 160112.

20. Patients with which blood type are less susceptible to the development of chronic thromboembolic pulmonary hypertension?
   A. A
   B. B
   C. AB
   D. O

Correct Answer: D

Explanation: Chronic thromboembolic pulmonary hypertension is more common in patients with blood groups A, B and AB. In one study, 77% of patients with chronic thromboembolic pulmonary hypertension (CTEPH) had non-O blood group compared with 58% of patients with pulmonary arterial hypertension ($P = .003$) A European registry suggested that non-O blood group was a significant predictor for the diagnosis of CTEPH (Odds Ratio 2.09, 95% CI 1.12–3.94; $P = 0.019$). The ABO locus is a susceptibility locus for venous thromboembolism, and non-O carriers have a higher risk for venous thromboembolism than O carriers.

References:

1. Banks DA, Auger WR, Madani MM. Chapter 26: Pulmonary Thromboendarterectomy for Chronic Thromboembolic Pulmonary Hypertension. In: Kaplan JA, Augoustides JGT, Manecke GR, et al., eds. Kaplan's Cardiac Anesthesia. 7th ed. Elsevier; 2017:994-1021.
2. Simonneau G, Torbicki A, Dorfmüller P, et al. The pathophysiology of chronic thromboembolic pulmonary hypertension. Eur Respir Rev, 2017; 26: 160112.

21. Which disease is associated with chronic thromboembolic pulmonary artery hypertension?
   A. Sickle cell disease
   B. Human immunodeficiency virus infection
   C. Pulmonary capillary hemangiomatosis
   D. Schistosomiasis

Correct Answer: A

Explanation: Schistosomiasis, infection with human immunodeficiency virus, and pulmonary capillary hemangiomatosis have all been associated with group I pulmonary artery hypertension. Sickle cell disease is associated with group IV pulmonary hypertension due to chronic thromboembolic disease. Approximately 10% to 60% of patients with sickle cell disease will develop pulmonary hypertension in this fashion.

References:

1. Banks DA, Auger WR, Madani MM. Chapter 26: Pulmonary Thromboendarterectomy for Chronic Thromboembolic Pulmonary Hypertension. In: Kaplan JA, Augoustides JGT, Manecke GR, et al., eds. Kaplan's Cardiac Anesthesia. 7th ed. Elsevier; 2017:994-1021.

2. Fonseca G, Souza R. Pulmonary hypertension in sickle cell disease. Curr Opin Pulm Med, 2015; 21: 432-437.
3. Gordeuk VR, Castro OL, Machado RF. Pathophysiology and treatment of pulmonary hypertension in sickle cell disease. Blood, 2016; 127: 82.

22. According to registry data, what percentage of patients diagnosed with chronic thromboembolic pulmonary hypertension have no past history of pulmonary embolism?
   A. 5%
   B. 25%
   C. 50%
   D. 75%

Correct Answer: B

Explanation: Although the majority of patients with chronic thromboembolic pulmonary hypertension may have a history of acute pulmonary embolism, clinical registry data has indicated that approximately 25% to 30% of patients may present with this disease with no prior history of pulmonary embolism. A comprehensive evaluation including detailed chest imaging and right heart catheterization is essential to not only make the diagnosis of chronic thromboembolic pulmonary hypertension but also quantify the severity of pulmonary hypertension in a given case.

References:

1. Banks DA, Auger WR, Madani MM. Chapter 26: Pulmonary Thromboendarterectomy for Chronic Thromboembolic Pulmonary Hypertension. In: Kaplan JA, Augoustides JGT, Manecke GR, et al., eds. Kaplan's Cardiac Anesthesia. 7th ed. Elsevier; 2017:994-1021.
2. Auger WR, Channick RN, Kerr KM, et al. Evaluation of patients with suspected chronic thromboembolic pulmonary hypertension. Semin Thorac Cardiovasc Surg, 1999; 11: 179-190.
3. Bonderman D, Jakowitsch J, Adlbrecht C, et al. Medical conditions increasing the risk of chronic thromboembolic pulmonary hypertension. Thromb Haemost, 2005; 93: 512-516.
4. Gelzinis TA. Pulmonary hypertension in 2021: part 1 – definitions, classification, pathophysiology and presentation. J Cardiothorac Vasc Anesth, 2022; 36: 1552-1564.

23. Which of the following is NOT a predictor of high (>10%) mortality risk at 1 year for a patient with pulmonary arterial hypertension?
   A. World Health Organization functional class III
   B. A 6-minute walk test with a distance of 100 m
   C. Cardiac index under 2.0 L/min/m²
   D. Presence of pericardial effusion on echocardiography

Correct Answer: A

Explanation: The risk factors for a high mortality (>10%) risk at 1 year for a patient with pulmonary arterial hypertension include congestive heart failure, rapid progression of symptoms, repeated syncope, and World Health Organization functional class IV. Further predictors for high mortality in this clinical setting include a distance of less than 165 m on a 6-minute walk test, a right atrial area over 26 cm², pericardial effusion, and a

cardiac index below 2 L/min/m². It is important to identify this high-risk group in the preoperative evaluation for both cardiac and noncardiac surgery, since these patients are likely to also have the highest perioperative mortality.

References:

1. Banks DA, Auger WR, Madani MM. Chapter 26: Pulmonary Thromboendarterectomy for Chronic Thromboembolic Pulmonary Hypertension. In: Kaplan JA, Augoustides JGT, Manecke GR, et al., eds. Kaplan's Cardiac Anesthesia. 7th ed. Elsevier; 2017:994-1021.
2. Gelzinis TA. Pulmonary hypertension in 2021: part 1 – definitions, classification, pathophysiology and presentation. J Cardiothorac Vasc Anesth, 2022; 36: 1552-1564.
3. Diaz-Rodriguesz N, Nyhan SM, Koth TM, et al. How we would treat our own pulmonary hypertension if we needed to undergo cardiac surgery. J Cardiothorac Vasc Anesth, 2022; 36: 1540-1548.

24. Which are approved routes of administration of Treprostinil?
   A. Intravenous and inhaled
   B. Intravenous, inhaled, subcutaneous
   C. Intravenous, inhaled, subcutaneous, oral
   D. Intravenous only

Correct Answer: C

Explanation: It is important to note the different dosing and routes for planning clinical administration of prostanoids. Treprostinil is a versatile pulmonary vasodilator that can be administered via intravenous, inhalational, subcutaneous, and oral routes. The parenteral routes of administration can either be intermittent or continuous. In contrast, epoprostenol, another prostanoid, is only approved for continuous intravenous infusion. The inhaled use of epoprostenol, common in patients with pulmonary hypertension, constitutes off-label use.

References:

1. Banks DA, Auger WR, Madani MM. Chapter 26: Pulmonary Thromboendarterectomy for Chronic Thromboembolic Pulmonary Hypertension. In: Kaplan JA, Augoustides JGT, Manecke GR, et al., eds. Kaplan's Cardiac Anesthesia. 7th ed. Elsevier; 2017:994-1021.
2. Diaz-Rodriguesz N, Nyhan SM, Koth TM, et al. How we would treat our own pulmonary hypertension if we needed to undergo cardiac surgery. J Cardiothorac Vasc Anesth, 2022; 36: 1540-1548.

25. All of the following are risk factors for developing chronic thromboembolic pulmonary hypertension EXCEPT:
   A. Thyroid replacement therapy
   B. Nephrectomy
   C. Malignancy
   D. Ventriculoatrial shunt

Correct Answer: B

Explanation: The risk factors for developing chronic thromboembolic include thyroid replacement therapy, a history of a splenectomy, malignancy, the presence of a ventriculoatrial shunt, a prothrombotic state, and previous venous thromboembolism. A history of nephrectomy has not been associated as a risk factor for development of chronic thromboembolic pulmonary hypertension.

References:

1. Banks DA, Auger WR, Madani MM. Chapter 26: Pulmonary Thromboendarterectomy for Chronic Thromboembolic Pulmonary Hypertension. In: Kaplan JA, Augoustides JGT, Manecke GR, et al., eds. Kaplan's Cardiac Anesthesia. 7th ed. Elsevier; 2017:994-1021.
2. Marshall PS, Kerr KM, Auger WR. Chronic thromboembolic pulmonary hypertension. Clin Chest Med, 2013; 34: 779-797.

26. What is the initial screening test for the diagnosis of chronic thromboembolic pulmonary hypertension?
    A. Ventilation/perfusion scan
    B. Cardiopulmonary exercise test
    C. Echocardiography
    D. Pulmonary angiography

Correct Answer: C

Explanation: In patients with signs, symptoms, and a history suggestive of pulmonary hypertension, the current expert consensus has recommended transthoracic echocardiography as the first step. This comprehensive assessment includes an estimation of pulmonary artery systemic pressure and the detection of indirect signs of pulmonary hypertension, such as right atrial and right ventricular dilatation, impaired right ventricular contractility, and Doppler flow abnormalities in the right ventricular outflow tract. Further testing thereafter in the diagnosis and staging of chronic thromboembolic pulmonary hypertension include ventilation perfusion scanning, cardiopulmonary exercise testing, and pulmonary angiography.

References:

1. Banks DA, Auger WR, Madani MM. Chapter 26: Pulmonary Thromboendarterectomy for Chronic Thromboembolic Pulmonary Hypertension. In: Kaplan JA, Augoustides JGT, Manecke GR, et al., eds. Kaplan's Cardiac Anesthesia. 7th ed. Elsevier; 2017:994-1021.
2. Gopalan D, Delcroix M, Held M. Diagnosis of chronic thromboembolic pulmonary hypertension. Eur Respir Rev, 2017; 26: 160108.
3. Marshall PS, Kerr KM, Auger WR. Chronic thromboembolic pulmonary hypertension. Clin Chest Med, 2013; 34: 779-797.

27. Which diagnostic test can rule out the diagnosis of chronic thromboembolic pulmonary hypertension?
    A. Ventilation/perfusion scan
    B. Cardiopulmonary exercise test
    C. Pulmonary angiography
    D. Chest radiography

Correct Answer: A

Explanation: A ventilation/perfusion scan is an imaging test of choice to exclude chronic thromboembolic pulmonary hypertension. A normal ventilation/perfusion scan excludes this disease state with a high sensitivity of 90% to 100% and specificity of 94% to 100%. Cardiopulmonary exercise testing can quantify the disability burden in patients with pulmonary hypertension but does not point to the specific etiology. Pulmonary angiography is a gold standard for the diagnosis of chronic thromboembolic pulmonary hypertension but is reserved for select cases given its invasive nature. Chest radiography can detect stigmata of pulmonary hypertension at times but does not indicate the underlying etiology,

References:

1. Banks DA, Auger WR, Madani MM. Chapter 26: Pulmonary Thromboendarterectomy for Chronic Thromboembolic Pulmonary Hypertension. In: Kaplan JA, Augoustides JGT, Manecke GR, et al., eds. Kaplan's Cardiac Anesthesia. 7th ed. Elsevier; 2017:994-1021.
2 Gopalan D, Delcroix M, Held M. Diagnosis of chronic thromboembolic pulmonary hypertension. Eur Respir Rev, 2017; 26: 160108.
3. Marshall PS, Kerr KM, Auger WR. Chronic thromboembolic pulmonary hypertension. Clin Chest Med, 2013; 34: 779-797.

28. All of the following are required to be a center of excellence for the treatment of chronic thromboembolic pulmonary hypertension EXCEPT:
    A. Perform more than 50 pulmonary thromboembolectomies per year
    B. Have a surgical mortality below 5%
    C. Have a multidisciplinary pulmonary hypertension team
    D. No requirement for transcatheter therapies

Correct Answer: D

Explanation: Expert recommendations suggest that patients with suspected chronic thromboembolic pulmonary hypertension be referred to centers of excellence for further diagnosis and management. An expert center performs more than 50 pulmonary thromboembolectomy procedures per year, with a surgical mortality below 5%, and with the ability to perform segmental endarterectomies. These centers should evaluate the disease severity and related treatment modalities in a multidisciplinary team setting with an experienced surgeon, a pulmonary hypertension specialist, a pulmonary interventionist, and an expert radiologist. The treatment modalities at a center of excellence include the array of medications, transcatheter interventions, and surgical therapy to inform an integrated team-based management plan for a given patient.

References:

1. Banks DA, Auger WR, Madani MM. Chapter 26: Pulmonary Thromboendarterectomy for Chronic Thromboembolic Pulmonary Hypertension. In: Kaplan JA, Augoustides JGT, Manecke GR, et al., eds. Kaplan's Cardiac Anesthesia. 7th ed. Elsevier; 2017:994-1021.

2. Madani MM. Pulmonary endarterectomy for chronic thromboembolic pulmonary hypertension: state of the art 2020. Pulm Circ, 2021; 11: 20458940211007372.

29. According to the San Diego classification of chronic thromboembolic pulmonary hypertension, what is the classification of disease when the location of the fibrotic thromboembolic tissue starts in the subsegmental branches of the pulmonary arteries?

A. Level I
B. Level II
C. Level III
D. Level IV

Correct Answer: D

Explanation: In the San Diego classification of chronic thromboembolic pulmonary hypertension, the level of disease is classified based on the extent of pulmonary arterial involvement with respect to the central and peripheral pulmonary arteries (see teaching box for further detail). The degree of reduction in pulmonary vascular resistance has been correlated with this classification system. Patients with a predominantly central disease burden (levels I and II) can typically undergo extensive mechanical clearance of the pulmonary arterial tree, and consequently have a substantial reduction in pulmonary vascular resistance after endarterectomy, accompanied by excellent clinical outcomes.

References:

1. Banks DA, Auger WR, Madani MM. Chapter 26: Pulmonary Thromboendarterectomy for Chronic Thromboembolic Pulmonary Hypertension. In: Kaplan JA, Augoustides JGT, Manecke GR, et al., eds. Kaplan's Cardiac Anesthesia. 7th ed. Elsevier; 2017:994-1021.
2. Madani MM. Pulmonary endarterectomy for chronic thromboembolic pulmonary hypertension: state of the art 2020. Pulm Circ, 2021; 11: 20458940211007372.

30. All of these indices are signs of impending hemodynamic collapse when inducing general anesthesia in patients with chronic thromboembolic pulmonary hypertension EXCEPT:

A. Severe tricuspid regurgitation
B. Tricuspid annular plane systolic excursion of 22 mm

> **BOX 22.4   Signs of impending collapse**
> - Right ventricular end-diastolic pressure over 15 mmHg
> - Severe tricuspid regurgitation

C. Right ventricular end-diastolic pressure over 15 mmHg
D. Pulmonary vascular resistance over 1000 dynes/s/cm^5

Correct Answer: B

Explanation: During the anesthetic induction of patients with chronic thromboembolic pulmonary hypertension presenting for endarterectomy, significant right ventricular dysfunction can place the patient at risk for hemodynamic collapse under general anesthesia. The signs of impending right ventricular failure in this setting include severe tricuspid regurgitation, right ventricular end-diastolic pressure over 15 mmHg, and a pulmonary vascular resistance over 1000 dynes/s/cm^5. Whereas tricuspid annular systolic excursion can assess right ventricular systolic function, a value of 22 mm lies within the normal range, and so would not indicate a compromised right ventricle. Patients with these warning signs typically require inotropic support with epinephrine or dobutamine to prevent cardiovascular collapse associated with induction of general anesthesia.

References:

1. Banks DA, Auger WR, Madani MM. Chapter 26: Pulmonary Thromboendarterectomy for Chronic Thromboembolic Pulmonary Hypertension. In: Kaplan JA, Augoustides JGT, Manecke GR, et al., eds. Kaplan's Cardiac Anesthesia. 7th ed. Elsevier; 2017:994-1021.
2. Madani MM. Pulmonary endarterectomy for chronic thromboembolic pulmonary hypertension: state of the art 2020. Pulm Circ, 2021; 11: 20458940211007372.
3. Ranka S, Mohananey D, Agarwal N, et al. Chronic thromboembolic pulmonary hypertension – management strategies and outcomes. J Cardiothorac Vasc Anesth, 2020; 34: 2513-2523.

CHAPTER 23

Procedures in the Hybrid Operating Room

Justin Tawil

KEY POINTS

1. A hybrid operating room combines advanced imaging capabilities with a fully functioning operating suite.
2. Transcatheter aortic valve replacement (TAVR) is recommended for patients with severe symptomatic aortic stenosis who are inoperable or at high risk for needing surgical aortic valve replacement and have a predicted post-TAVR survival of more than 12 months.
3. Vascular complications are the most common complications with the transfemoral approach.
4. The concept of multimodal imaging plays an important role in preprocedural assessment.
5. The presence of a heart team is a prerequisite for establishing a TAVR program.
6. Catheter-based mitral valve repair techniques are primarily guided by transesophageal echocardiography.

---

1. Which of the following is NOT required in a hybrid operating room?
   A. High-quality fluoroscopy
   B. A control room with direct view of the surgical field
   C. Radiopaque defibrillator pads
   D. Ventilation with laminar airflow to provide smooth undisturbed air

Correct Answer: C

Explanation: Hybrid operating rooms are designed to facilitate an operating room–like environment and advanced high-quality imaging systems to facilitate both. Good quality multimodal imaging is usually present, including advanced ultrasound and fluoroscopy. A control room for technicians and supporting staff should have a good view of the ongoing procedure. The hybrid space should also have a large sterile operating room space with conventional environmental control for a sterile environment. Radiolucent defibrillator pads are required in this setting so that x-ray imaging is not blocked by traditional defibrillator pads. Foil-containing radiopaque pads can be used if strategically placed to avoid the imaging planes needed for interventional procedure, but they are not required.

References:

1. Zakhary WZA, Ender JK. Chapter 27: Procedures in the Hybrid Operating Room. In: Kaplan JA, Augoustides JGT, Manecke GR, et al., eds. Kaplan's Cardiac Anesthesia. 7th ed. Elsevier; 2017:1022-1041.
2. Tommaso CL, Bolman RM 3rd, Feldman T, et al. Multisociety (AATS, ACCF, SCAI, and STS) expert consensus statement: operator and institutional requirements for transcatheter valve repair and replacement, part 1: transcatheter aortic valve replacement. J Am Coll Cardiol, 2012; 59: 2028-2042.

2. Transcatheter aortic valve replacement procedures are required to be performed in which environment?
   A. Cardiac cath lab
   B. Operating room
   C. Hybrid room
   D. Any of the above

Correct Answer: D

Explanation: Transcatheter aortic valve replacement (TAVR) procedures can be performed in any of the above locations. The multisociety guidelines do not require any specific location. Whereas in the United States the hybrid operating room is a popular choice, the alternatives are also common options around the world. The selected space must be adequately resourced with respect to equipment and personnel to ensure procedural success and the growth of the TAVR program at a given institution.

References:

1. Zakhary WZA, Ender JK. Chapter 27: Procedures in the Hybrid Operating Room. In: Kaplan JA, Augoustides JGT, Manecke GR, et al., eds. Kaplan's Cardiac Anesthesia. 7th ed. Elsevier; 2017:1022-1041.
2. Tommaso CL, Bolman RM 3rd, Feldman T, et al. Multisociety (AATS, ACCF, SCAI, and STS) expert consensus statement: operator and institutional requirements for transcatheter valve repair and replacement, part 1: transcatheter aortic valve replacement. J Am Coll Cardiol, 2012; 59: 2028-2042.

3. How are the coronary arteries visualized prior to transcatheter aortic valve replacement deployment?
A. Intravascular ultrasound
B. Static biplane x-ray
C. Digital subtraction angiography
D. Transthoracic echocardiography

Correct Answer: C

Explanation: Digital Subtraction Angiography (DSA) is an advanced imaging technique that is able to correct images following contrast administration to maximize the fidelity of arterial structures. DSA also minimizes motion artifacts and structures not of interest. Typically, the aortic root is visualized with DSA prior to deployment by contrast injection through a pigtail in the aortic root. This allows proceduralists to ensure that they are low enough to avoid covering the coronary arteries during aortic valve deployment.

References:

1. Zakhary WZA, Ender JK. Chapter 27: Procedures in the Hybrid Operating Room. In: Kaplan JA, Augoustides JGT, Manecke GR, et al., eds. Kaplan's Cardiac Anesthesia. 7th ed. Elsevier; 2017:1022-1041.
2. Yamamoto M, Okura Y, Ishihara M, et al. Development of digital subtraction angiography for coronary artery. J Digit Imaging, 2009; 22: 319-325.

4. Which of the following is NOT associated with radiation exposure during pregnancy?
A. Organ malformation
B. Growth retardation
C. Delayed cognitive development
D. Congenital cataracts

Correct Answer: D

Explanation: Doses of radiation above 250 milligrays (mGy) are associated with organ malformation. Radiation exposure to doses above 200 mGy is associated with fetal growth retardation. More than 100 mGy of exposure during pregnancy is associated with delayed mental development. While cataracts are a known complication of occupational exposure, congenital cataracts are thought to be related to postnatal x-rays, medication exposures, and intrauterine insults, but no relationship to prenatal radiation and cataracts is known.

References:

1. Zakhary WZA, Ender JK. Chapter 27: Procedures in the Hybrid Operating Room. In: Kaplan JA, Augoustides JGT, Manecke GR, et al., eds. Kaplan's Cardiac Anesthesia. 7th ed. Elsevier; 2017:1022-1041.
2. Biso SMR, Vidovich MI. Radiation protection in the cardiac catheterization laboratory. J Thorac Dis, 2020; 12: 1648-1655.
3. Prakalapakorn SG, Rasmussen SA, Lambert SR, et al. National Birth Defects Prevention Study. Assessment of risk factors for infantile cataracts using a case-control study: National Birth Defects Prevention Study, 2000-2004. Ophthalmology, 2010; 117: 1500-1505.

5. Which of the following connotes high-risk for mortality in surgical aortic valve replacement that might then warrant consideration of transcatheter aortic valve replacement?
A. Predicted mortality of 6% with the Society of Thoracic Surgeons calculator
B. Predicted mortality of 10% with European System of Cardiac Operative Risk Evaluation
C. Two or more markers of frailty not expected to improve following surgery
D. Moderate aortic stenosis patient with metastatic cancer

Correct Answer: C

Explanation: In surgical aortic valve replacement, a mortality prediction of 8% or more with the Society of Thoracic Surgeons risk calculator is considered high. In a similar fashion, predicted mortality of 15% to 20% by the European System of Cardiac Operative Risk Evaluation is considered high risk. Two or more markers of frailty would indicate high risk of perioperative death with surgical aortic valve replacement. Patients with advanced frailty who are felt to benefit from aortic valve surgery should be evaluated for transcatheter aortic valve replacement (TAVR). Because the selection criteria for TAVR are in constant evolution, the clinical guidelines have recommended that this complex decision be reached by a multidisciplinary heart team in consultation with the patient.

References:

1. Zakhary WZA, Ender JK. Chapter 27: Procedures in the Hybrid Operating Room. In: Kaplan JA, Augoustides JGT, Manecke GR, et al., eds. Kaplan's Cardiac Anesthesia. 7th ed. Elsevier; 2017:1022-1041.
2. Nishimura RA, Otto CM, Bonow RO, et al. 2014 AHA/ACC Guideline for the Management of Patients with Valvular Heart Disease: executive summary: a report of the American College of Cardiology/ American Heart Association Task Force on Practice Guidelines. Circulation, 2014; 129: 2440-2492.

6. Which of the following criteria is consistent with severe aortic stenosis?
A. Dimensionless index = 0.48
B. Mean gradient = 50 mmHg
C. Peak velocity = 3 m/s
D. Indexed aortic valve area = 0.9 cm^2/m^2

Correct Answer: B

Explanation: Severe aortic stenosis is defined by echocardiographic criteria. The dimensionless index is the ratio of the velocity time integral (VTI) in the left ventricular outflow tract (LVOT) to that of the aortic valve jet (AV) and can be calculated as follows: LVOT VTI/AV VTI. This index is dimensionless because the units cancel out in this calculation, and a value below 0.25 is consistent with severe aortic stenosis. A transvalvular mean gradient across the aortic valve greater than 40 mm Hg also defines severe aortic stenosis. Further criteria include a peak transvalvular gradient greater than 4 m/s, an aortic valve area under 1.0 cm^2, and an indexed aortic valve area less 0.6 cm^2/m^2.

Remember that patients with reduced ejection fraction may have low-gradient aortic stenosis, as a weakened left ventricle may not be able to generate large gradients and pressures despite very high-grade aortic stenosis due to pump failure. In those patients with low-gradient aortic stenosis, the dimensionless index and dobutamine stress echocardiography can be helpful to make the diagnosis. With stress echocardiography, a rise in the aortic valve gradients will help identify those patients with a low ejection fraction who may benefit from aortic valve replacement.

References:

1. Zakhary WZA, Ender JK. Chapter 27: Procedures in the Hybrid Operating Room. In: Kaplan JA, Augoustides JGT, Manecke GR, et al., eds. Kaplan's Cardiac Anesthesia. 7th ed. Elsevier; 2017:1022-1041.
2. Nishimura RA, Otto CM, Bonow RO, et al. 2014 AHA/ACC Guideline for the Management of Patients with Valvular Heart Disease: executive summary: a report of the American College of Cardiology/American Heart Association Task Force on Practice Guidelines. Circulation, 2014; 129: 2440-2492.
3. Panayiotides IM, Nikolaides E. Transcatheter Aortic Valve Implantation (TAVI): is it time for this intervention to be applied in a lower risk population? Clin Med Insights Cardiol, 2014; 8: 93-102.

7. The risk of stroke in high-risk patients after transcatheter aortic valve replacement is approximately:
   A. Less than 1%
   B. 2%–5%
   C. 5%–10%
   D. More than 10%

Correct Answer: B

Explanation: The 30-day mortality in high-risk patients after transcatheter aortic valve replacement (TAVR) is 3% to 6%. The risk of clinically apparent major stroke after TAVR in this patient population was 3.8% at 30 days and 5.1% at 1 year. The subclinical stroke rate can be much higher, especially in the setting of detailed brain imaging to detect embolic stroke burden.

References:

1. Zakhary WZA, Ender JK. Chapter 27: Procedures in the Hybrid Operating Room. In: Kaplan JA, Augoustides JGT, Manecke GR, et al., eds. Kaplan's Cardiac Anesthesia. 7th ed. Elsevier; 2017:1022-1041.

2. Miller DC, Blackstone EH, Mack MJ, et al. Transcatheter (TAVR) versus surgical (AVR) aortic valve replacement: occurrence, hazard, risk factors, and consequences of neurologic events in the PARTNER trial. J Thorac Cardiovasc Surg, 2012; 143: 832-843 e13.

8. Which risk factor is included in common risk calculators to predict outcomes after cardiac surgery?
   A. Chronic kidney disease
   B. Calcified ascending aorta
   C. Frailty scoring
   D. Unstable aortic atheroma

Correct Answer: A

Explanation: The leading risk calculators including the model developed by the Society of Thoracic Surgeons include measures of renal function such as serum creatinine, estimated glomerular filtration rate, and renal replacement therapy. Despite these risk models, further measures of clinical significance that are not included in these scoring systems still merit consideration for patients on an individual basis. Factors that increase risk of aortic valve replacement include peripheral vascular disease, carotid stenosis, porcelain aorta, mobile aortic atheroma, and prior mediastinal radiation and may not be fully appreciated by objective scoring systems. Frailty is becoming a more recognized topic for special consideration in patient assessment. The lack of reserve that defines frailty can delay recovery from technically successful cardiac surgery. Frailty scoring may help identify patients who would particularly benefit from minimally invasive valve replacement.

References:

1. Zakhary WZA, Ender JK. Chapter 27: Procedures in the Hybrid Operating Room. In: Kaplan JA, Augoustides JGT, Manecke GR, et al., eds. Kaplan's Cardiac Anesthesia. 7th ed. Elsevier; 2017:1022-1041.
2. Sintek M, Zajarias A. Patient evaluation and selection for transcatheter aortic valve replacement: the heart team approach. Prog Cardiovasc Dis, 2014; 56: 572-582.

9. Which access route for transcatheter aortic valve replacement would be most suitable for an obese patient with a history of severe bilateral lower extremity amputations, left pleurodesis, and prior coronary artery bypass grafting with a left internal mammary graft to the left anterior descending artery?
   A. Femoral artery approach with moderate sedation
   B. Transapical approach under general anesthesia
   C. Femoral vein-transcaval approach under general anesthesia
   D. Left subclavian artery under moderate sedation

Correct Answer: C

Explanation: In the presented clinical scenario, the transcaval approach is the best choice for transcatheter aortic valve replacement. Severe peripheral arterial disease with amputations suggests diseased femoral arteries that will likely prove hostile for arterial access. The patient's history of pleurodesis will make it difficult to identify the cardiac apex via the minithoracotomy approach because of adhesions. A left subclavian artery approach may compromise the patient's left internal mammary graft.

References:

1. Zakhary WZA, Ender JK. Chapter 27: Procedures in the Hybrid Operating Room. In: Kaplan JA, Augoustides JGT, Manecke GR, et al., eds. Kaplan's Cardiac Anesthesia. 7th ed. Elsevier; 2017:1022-1041.
2. Morozowich ST, Sell-Dottin KA, Crestanello JA, et al. Transcarotid versus transaxillary/subclavian transcatheter aortic valve replacement (TAVR): analysis of outcomes. J Cardiothorac Vasc Anesth, 2022; 36: 1771-1776.

10. During transcatheter aortic valve replacement, which of these cardiac effects is caused by transvenous pacing for valve deployment?
  A. Myocardial ischemia
  B. Improved left ventricular filling
  C. Reduced oxygen consumption
  D. Increased cardiac output

Correct Answer: A

Explanation: Rapid ventricular pacing effectively induces controlled ventricular tachycardia to halt cardiac output so that the transcatheter aortic valve can be deployed with less risk of displacement. Ventricular tachycardia consumes significantly more oxygen than the resting heart. In addition to consuming more oxygen, rapid ventricular depolarization keeps the left ventricular chamber pressures high, which impairs filling. The combination of increased oxygen consumption and impaired relaxation exacerbates myocardial ischemia during pacing. Although adenosine can also induce periods of reduced cardiac output, rapid ventricular pacing is generally preferred because of its predictability and reversibility.

References:

1. Zakhary WZA, Ender JK. Chapter 27: Procedures in the Hybrid Operating Room. In: Kaplan JA, Augoustides JGT, Manecke GR, et al., eds. Kaplan's Cardiac Anesthesia. 7th ed. Elsevier; 2017:1022-1041.
2. Bokoch MP, Hiramoto JS, Lobo EP, et al. Rapid ventricular pacing for landing zone precision during thoracic endovascular aortic repair: a case series. J Cardiothorac Vasc Anesth, 2017; 31: 2141-2146.

11. During rapid pacing and deployment of a transcatheter aortic valve, the pacemaker loses capture with return of sinus rhythm and cardiac ejection. The balloon is deflated, and the patient becomes hypotensive. Intermittent ventricular tachycardia and fibrillation occur and are treated with lidocaine and electrical defibrillation, but the hypotension persists requiring high-dose vasoactive support. Prominent ST elevations are noted in lead V of the electrocardiogram. What would be the most probable finding with transesophageal echocardiography?
  A. New pericardial fluid
  B. Severe aortic insufficiency
  C. No opening of the aortic valve
  D. New regional wall motion abnormalities in the anterior and lateral left ventricle

Correct Answer: D

Explanation: This patient has suffered from an iatrogenic left coronary occlusion. The transcatheter aortic valve has been pushed away from its intended position during failed rapid ventricular pacing and is now occluding the left coronary artery ostium inducing coronary ischemia. Given this displacement of the valve with left main coronary obstruction, the echocardiogram would be expected to show normal valve function, no pericardial effusion, and hypokinesis of the anterior and lateral walls of the left ventricle. At times, mechanical circulatory support with cardiopulmonary bypass or extracorporeal membrane oxygenation may be required to achieve hemodynamic stability for further management, including percutaneous coronary stenting to restore coronary flow.

References:

1. Zakhary WZA, Ender JK. Chapter 27: Procedures in the Hybrid Operating Room. In: Kaplan JA, Augoustides JGT, Manecke GR, et al., eds. Kaplan's Cardiac Anesthesia. 7th ed. Elsevier; 2017:1022-1041.
2. Spina R, Khalique O, George I, et al. Acute left main stem coronary occlusion following transcatheter aortic valve replacement in a patient without recognized coronary obstruction risk factors: a case report. Eur Heart J Case Rep, 2018; 2: yty112.
3. Yadlapali D, Musuku SR, Pani S, et al. Rescue management of a coronary artery occlusion during a transcatheter aortic valve replacement. J Cardiothorac Vasc Anesth, 2021; 35: 1167-1171.

12. Each of the following components are part of the functional aortic annulus EXCEPT:
  A. The ring formed by the anatomic ventriculoarterial junction
  B. The ring formed by the coronary ostia
  C. The ring formed by the hinge points at the attachment of the valve leaflets to the myocardium
  D. The ring formed at the top of the valve leaflets at the sinotubular junction

Correct Answer: B

Explanation: The aortic root complex forms a functional aortic annulus with components that are important for the integrity of the aortic valve (see figure). These components include the aortic leaflets, the sinuses of Valsalva, and the ring formed by the anatomic ventriculoarterial junction. Further components include the basal virtual ring formed by the hinge points at the attachment of the valve leaflets to the heart and the superior ring at the top of the leaflets at the level of the sinotubular junction. Although the coronary artery ostia are part of the aortic root, they do not form a ring that is part of the functional aortic annulus,

References:

1. Zakhary WZA, Ender JK. Chapter 27: Procedures in the Hybrid Operating Room. In: Kaplan JA, Augoustides JGT, Manecke GR, et al., eds. Kaplan's Cardiac Anesthesia. 7th ed. Elsevier; 2017:1022-1041.

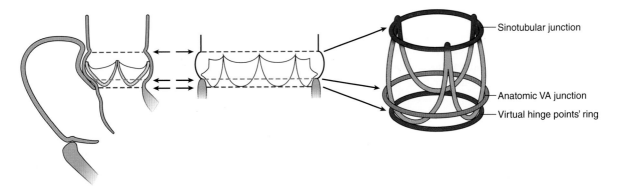

FIGURE 23.1 The various rings associated with the aortic annulus. *VA,* Ventriculoarterial. (Modified from Piazza N, de Jaegere P, Schultz C, et al. Anatomy of the aortic valvar complex and its implications for transcatheter implantation of the aortic valve. Circ Cardiovasc Interv, 2008; 1: 74–81.)

2. Patel PA, Gutsche JT, Vernick WJ, et al. The functional aortic annulus in the 3D era: focus on transcatheter aortic valve replacement for the perioperative echocardiographer. J Cardiothorac Vasc Anesth, 2015; 29: 240-245.

13. Immediately after deployment of a new transcatheter aortic valve, the patient's vital signs recover quickly with cessation of rapid pacing. The patient subsequently develops an obstructed breathing pattern associated with new-onset delirium. His airway is secured with prompt endotracheal intubation to restore ventilation. Which of the following statements is true regarding the risk of stroke in transcatheter aortic valve replacement (TAVR)?
  A. The transfemoral approach has a higher risk of stroke than the transapical approach
  B. Stroke is less common with surgical aortic valve replacement
  C. More than half of patients demonstrate evidence of cerebral ischemic injury after TAVR
  D. Strokes in TAVR exclusively arise from calcium emboli derived from the aortic valve

Correct Answer: C

Explanation: Strokes during transcatheter aortic valve replacement (TAVR) can arise during many parts of the procedure. As the device migrates retrograde through the thoracic aorta, it is possible for aortic plaques in the arch or ascending aorta to embolize. Additionally, during valvuloplasty and deployment, calcium may be dislodged from the annulus or valve leaflets. Wires and catheters may also disrupt embolic material from the aortic arch, ascending aorta, and/or the aortic valve. Prolonged hypotension during the procedure or with rapid pacing may add additional ischemic insult. Clinically evident stroke occurs in 2% to 6% of TAVR patients, which is at least equivalent to or higher than seen in surgical aortic valve replacement, depending on the level of patient risk. Furthermore, detailed neuroimaging with computed axial tomography and/or magnetic resonance imaging suggest that about 70% to 80% of patients have cerebral emboli with ischemia that may not present clinically.

References:
1. Zakhary WZA, Ender JK. Chapter 27: Procedures in the Hybrid Operating Room. In: Kaplan JA, Augoustides JGT, Manecke GR, et al., eds. Kaplan's Cardiac Anesthesia. 7th ed. Elsevier; 2017:1022-1041.
2. Parel PA, Patel S, Feinman JW, et al. Stroke after transcatheter aortic valve replacement: incidence, definitions, etiologies, and management options. J Cardiothorac Vasc Anesth, 2018; 32: 968-981.

14. The typical risks of transseptal puncture during transcatheter heart interventions include all of the following EXCEPT:
  A. Aortic injury
  B. Pericardial tamponade
  C. Stroke
  D. Ventricular tachycardia

Correct Answer: D

Explanation: The transseptal approaches for electrophysiologic and structural heart procedures carry several risks. Although the goal is to cross from the right atrium into the left atrium via the interatrial septum, it is possible for errant needles to cross too anterior and enter the aorta, the aortic annulus, or the left ventricular outflow tract. These punctures may allow blood to rapidly accumulate within the pericardium, causing tamponade. Echocardiographic guidance is useful for both preventing and detecting these events. Stroke while accessing the left heart during transseptal puncture may result from inadequate anticoagulation and thrombus formation on the device, or via iatrogenic gas embolization. These emboli can cross the newly made atrial septal defect to travel systemically and cause stroke. Ventricular arrhythmias during septal crossing and from atrial devices is uncommon.

References:
1. Zakhary WZA, Ender JK. Chapter 27: Procedures in the Hybrid Operating Room. In: Kaplan JA, Augoustides JGT, Manecke GR, et al., eds. Kaplan's Cardiac Anesthesia. 7th ed. Elsevier; 2017:1022-1041.
2. Katsiampoura A, Mufarrih SH, Sharkey A, et al. A sequential approach for echocardiographic guidance of transseptal puncture: the PITLOC protocol. J Cardiothorac Vasc Anesth, 2022; 36: 3257-3264.

15. During laser extraction of pacemaker leads in the superior vena cava, the patient becomes acutely hypotensive. Rescue echocardiography revealed hypovolemia without evidence of tamponade and normal cardiac function. A prepositioned balloon venous occluder deployed and inflated. Which venous access option would be the most effective route of resuscitation?
  A. Large-bore catheter in the left hand
  B. Large-bore catheter in right hand
  C. Introducer in the right internal jugular vein
  D. Large-bore catheter in the saphenous vein

Correct Answer: D

Explanation: Although major central venous injuries during pacemaker laser lead removal are uncommon, they can cause severe hypotension. Balloon occlusion of the injury site or a more proximal vein can prevent exsanguination but may render typical venous access ineffective. If a balloon occluder is deployed in this area, only lower extremity venous resuscitation will be effective. Large-diameter femoral central access or saphenous vein access can be used to restore circulating blood volume, although cardiopulmonary bypass may be required for hemodynamic control and venous repair.

References:

1. Zakhary WZA, Ender JK. Chapter 27: Procedures in the Hybrid Operating Room. In: Kaplan JA, Augoustides JGT, Manecke GR, et al., eds. Kaplan's Cardiac Anesthesia. 7th ed. Elsevier; 2017:1022-1041.
2. Boyle TA, Wilkoff BL, Pace J, et al. Balloon-assisted rescue of four consecutive patients with vascular lacerations inflicted during lead extraction. Heart Rhythm, 2017; 14: 757-776.
3. Sonny A, Wakefield BJ, Sale S, et al. Transvenous lead extraction: a clinical commentary for anesthesiologists. J Cardiothorac Vasc Anesth, 2018; 32: 1101-1111.

16. Implantable cardiac pacemaker laser lead removals are often performed with intraoperative echocardiographic monitoring because all the following are possible complications EXCEPT:
  A. Right ventricular avulsion
  B. Severe pulmonic regurgitation
  C. Pericardial tamponade
  D. Severe tricuspid regurgitation

Correct Answer: B

Explanation: Laser lead extraction is a high-risk procedure that is usually performed for infected leads or venous obstruction caused by the leads, or when tricuspid valve function is compromised by pacemaker leads. It is often performed under general anesthesia, with invasive monitoring, echocardiography, and cardiac surgery on standby. Bleeding from injury to major vessels like the superior vena cava, coronary sinus, subclavian vein, or ventricular perforation can be identified and treated with good preparation. Tamponade and valve injury are possible as well. Pulmonic regurgitation is not a complication of lead extraction.

References:

1. Zakhary WZA, Ender JK. Chapter 27: Procedures in the Hybrid Operating Room. In: Kaplan JA, Augoustides JGT, Manecke GR, et al., eds. Kaplan's Cardiac Anesthesia. 7th ed. Elsevier; 2017:1022-1041.
2. Okamura H. Lead extraction using a laser system: Techniques, efficacy, and limitations. J Arrhythm, 2016; 32: 279-282.
3. Sonny A, Wakefield BJ, Sale S, et al. Transvenous lead extraction: a clinical commentary for anesthesiologists. J Cardiothorac Vasc Anesth, 2018; 32: 1101-1111.

17. Which team members have the highest radiation exposure during hybrid procedures?
  A. Scrub nurses
  B. Proceduralists
  C. Catherization lab technicians
  D. Anesthesia providers

Correct Answer: D

Explanation: Anesthesia team members have the highest rate of exposure during interventional procedures. Frequent patient assessments and a location at the head of the table with fixed spaces that limit distance to the radiation source and radiation shields are all contributory. It is estimated that anesthesia team members are exposed to as much as 15 times the radiation as scrub nurses. Proceduralists also had less exposure in part due to better shielding and less scatter.

References:

1. Zakhary WZA, Ender JK. Chapter 27: Procedures in the Hybrid Operating Room. In: Kaplan JA, Augoustides JGT, Manecke GR, et al., eds. Kaplan's Cardiac Anesthesia. 7th ed. Elsevier; 2017:1022-1041.
2. Biso SMR, Vidovich MI. Radiation protection in the cardiac catheterization laboratory. J Thorac Dis, 2020; 12: 1648-1655.

18. All of the following are potential complications of transcatheter pulmonary valve replacement EXCEPT:
  A. Rupture of the right ventricular outflow tract
  B. Obstruction of the right pulmonary artery
  C. Obstruction of the right coronary artery
  D. Entrapment of the delivery device

Correct Answer: C

Explanation: All are described complications of transcatheter pulmonic valve placement except right coronary artery obstruction. The left coronary artery courses between the aorta and the right ventricular outflow tract and so may be compressed during this procedure.

References:

1. Zakhary WZA, Ender JK. Chapter 27: Procedures in the Hybrid Operating Room. In: Kaplan JA, Augoustides JGT, Manecke GR, et al., eds. Kaplan's Cardiac Anesthesia. 7th ed. Elsevier; 2017:1022-1041.
2. Gregory SH, Zoller JK, Shahanavaz S, et al. Anesthetic considerations for transcatheter pulmonary valve replacement. J Cardiothorac Vasc Anesth, 2018; 32: 402-411.

19. Following test closure of a mitral valve transcatheter edge-to-edge repair (TEER) device for severe central mitral regurgitation, the patient should be evaluated for all of the following EXCEPT:
    A. Mitral regurgitation
    B. Systolic anterior motion of the anterior mitral valve leaflet
    C. Mitral stenosis
    D. Stable motion of the mitral leaflets and TEER device

Correct Answer: B

Explanation: Mitral valve transcatheter edge-to-edge repair (TEER) is a minimally invasive transcatheter plication of the anterior and posterior mitral leaflets. Following the initial positioning of the device, a thorough evaluation of the resulting conditions should occur before it is secured in place. Changes to the mitral regurgitation should be evaluated, as should the security of the TEER device's hold on the leaflets. It is important to evaluate the mean gradient across the valve to ensure that a high degree of mitral stenosis has not been created. Systolic anterior motion of the mitral valve is not likely following TEER, because the anterior leaflet is tethered to the posterior leaflet and not free to be pulled into the left ventricular outflow tract. This mitral repair technique may be safely used in patients with predisposing anatomy for this outflow obstruction syndrome.

References:

1. Zakhary WZA, Ender JK. Chapter 27: Procedures in the Hybrid Operating Room. In: Kaplan JA, Augoustides JGT, Manecke GR, et al., eds. Kaplan's Cardiac Anesthesia. 7th ed. Elsevier; 2017:1022-1041.
2. Wu IY, Barajas MB, Hahn RT. The mitraclip procedure – a comprehensive review for the cardiac anesthesiologist. J Cardiothorac Vasc Anesth, 2018; 32: 2746-2759.

20. Which procedure is most dependent on echocardiography?
    A. Transcatheter aortic valve replacement
    B. Laser lead extraction
    C. Transcatheter mitral valve repair
    D. Thoracic endovascular aortic repair

Correct Answer: C

Explanation: Although all of these procedures benefit from real-time echocardiography for diagnosis, guidance, and evaluation of results, a successful transcatheter edge-to-edge mitral valve repair is entirely dependent on echocardiography. Transseptal puncture in this procedure is guided by echocardiography. This is followed by guided translocation of the device safely away from the atrial appendage, and away from the pulmonary veins towards the mitral valve. Echocardiographic guidance is key to guiding the device into proper orientation and to the intended grasping area. Furthermore, echocardiographic imaging also helps identify the key measures of success and any of the potential complications. This differs from the remaining procedures in this question, which can be successfully completed with fluoroscopy alone. Echocardiography in laser lead extraction can be helpful to evaluate for complications following the procedure.

References:

1. Zakhary WZA, Ender JK. Chapter 27: Procedures in the Hybrid Operating Room. In: Kaplan JA, Augoustides JGT, Manecke GR, et al., eds. Kaplan's Cardiac Anesthesia. 7th ed. Elsevier; 2017:1022-1041.
2. Wu IY, Barajas MB, Hahn RT. The mitraclip procedure – a comprehensive review for the cardiac anesthesiologist. J Cardiothorac Vasc Anesth, 2018; 32: 2746-2759.
3. Sonny A, Wakefield BJ, Sale S, et al. Transvenous lead extraction: a clinical commentary for anesthesiologists. J Cardiothorac Vasc Anesth, 2018; 32: 1101-1111.

21. Which echocardiographic finding identifies a good candidate for transcatheter edge-to-edge mitral valve repair?
    A. High-grade calcific restriction of the posterior leaflet
    B. Preprocedural transmitral mean gradient of 9 mmHg
    C. Multiple jets of equal significance
    D. Flail P2 segment

Correct Answer: D

Explanation: A flail P2 segment with severe mitral regurgitation resulting from a single lesion is a strong indication for transcatheter edge-to-edge repair (TEER) in patients who are high risk or not otherwise candidates for surgical mitral valve repair. Dense calcification or marked restriction of the posterior leaflet are relative contraindications to TEER. TEER device placement produces some degree of added stenosis in exchange for treating regurgitation. On average, the mitral valve gradient increases from 1.5 to 4.5 mmHg, secondary to the creation of a double inlet mitral orifice. A patient with moderate to severe mitral stenosis (mean gradient = 9) will be left with severe mitral stenosis and is not likely to benefit from TEER. Patients may require multiple device placements for treatment of a single regurgitant lesion, but this intervention is less ideal for treating patients with multiple jets of similar severity at different locations or those with valve clefts or perforations.

References:

1. Zakhary WZA, Ender JK. Chapter 27: Procedures in the Hybrid Operating Room. In: Kaplan JA, Augoustides JGT, Manecke GR, et al., eds. Kaplan's Cardiac Anesthesia. 7th ed. Elsevier; 2017:1022-1041.
2. Patzelt, J, Zhang W, Sauter R, et al. Elevated mitral valve pressure gradient is predictive of long-term outcome after percutaneous edge-to-edge mitral valve repair in patients with degenerative mitral regurgitation (MR), but not in functional MR. JAMA, 2019; 8: e011366.
3. Wu IY, Barajas MB, Hahn RT. The mitraclip procedure – a comprehensive review for the cardiac anesthesiologist. J Cardiothorac Vasc Anesth, 2018; 32: 2746-2759.

22. Which is not a risk factor for complications during laser lead extraction?
- **A.** Admission for heart failure
- **B.** Infection
- **C.** Pediatric patients
- **D.** Operator experience

Correct Answer: D

Explanation: Risk factors for complications during laser lead extraction include female sex, admission for heart failure, extremes of age, infection as the indication, warfarin use, number of leads extracted, and longer duration of implantation. In recent studies, operator experience has not been shown to affect the incidence of complications.

References:

1. Zakhary WZA, Ender JK. Chapter 27: Procedures in the Hybrid Operating Room. In: Kaplan JA, Augoustides JGT, Manecke GR, et al., eds. Kaplan's Cardiac Anesthesia. 7th ed. Elsevier; 2017:1022-1041.
2. Sood N, Martin DT, Lampert R, et al. Incidence and predictors of perioperative complications with transvenous lead extractions: real-world experience with national cardiovascular data registry. Circ Arrhythm Electrophysiol, 2018; 11: e004768.
3. Sonny A, Wakefield BJ, Sale S, et al. Transvenous lead extraction: a clinical commentary for anesthesiologists. J Cardiothorac Vasc Anesth, 2018; 32: 1101-1111.

23. Which patient would be considered a candidate for transcatheter pulmonic valve placement?
- **A.** Right ventricular systolic pressure one-third that of systemic systolic pressure
- **B.** Mild pulmonic stenosis
- **C.** Severe right ventricular dilation
- **D.** No prior sternotomy

Correct Answer: C

Explanation: Transcatheter valve replacement of right-sided valves is primarily for those patients with prior open cardiac surgery with high-grade stenosis and/or regurgitation. Significant pulmonic stenosis would be in the severe range with significant elevation of right ventricular systolic pressure greater than one-third of the systemic blood pressure. Significant pulmonic valve disease would be associated with advanced right ventricular hypertrophy and/or dilation, depending on the valve lesion and ventricular reserve.

References:

1. Zakhary WZA, Ender JK. Chapter 27: Procedures in the Hybrid Operating Room. In: Kaplan JA, Augoustides JGT, Manecke GR, et al., eds. Kaplan's Cardiac Anesthesia. 7th ed. Elsevier; 2017:1022-1041.
2. Gregory SH, Zoller JK, Shahanavaz S, et al. Anesthetic considerations for transcatheter pulmonary valve replacement. J Cardiothorac Vasc Anesth, 2018; 32: 402-411.

24. Which statement is TRUE concerning the intraoperative management of patients undergoing transcatheter pulmonary valve replacement?
- **A.** There is a higher risk for ostial obstruction
- **B.** Patients are usually otherwise healthy
- **C.** Echocardiographic guidance is essential
- **D.** Rapid pacing is not required

Correct Answer: D

Explanation: Patients undergoing right-sided valve replacement are usually chronically ill with extensive cardiac history and comorbidity. Valve positioning with transcatheter pulmonary valve replacement does not require rapid pacing for a number of reasons. The right ventricular pressures are lower than left ventricular pressures, making the device less likely to move due to right ventricular stroke work. Additionally, the absence of coronary ostial considerations often offers a larger safe landing zone than with transcatheter aortic valve replacement, but left-sided coronary artery obstruction is still possible. Fluoroscopy is usually sufficient for image guidance. Given the potential for a long procedure duration, general anesthesia is usually selected.

References:

1. Zakhary WZA, Ender JK. Chapter 27: Procedures in the Hybrid Operating Room. In: Kaplan JA, Augoustides JGT, Manecke GR, et al., eds. Kaplan's Cardiac Anesthesia. 7th ed. Elsevier; 2017:1022-1041.
2. Aldoss O, Carr K, Shahanavaz S, et al. Acute and mid-term outcomes of transcatheter pulmonary valve implantation in patients older than 40 years. Int J Cardiol Congen Heart Dis, 2021; 3: 100084.

25. If the temporary venous pacer loses capture at a threshold of 0.4 mA, what output should the pacemaker be set at for rapid ventricular pacing?
- **A.** Less than 0.4 mA
- **B.** 0.4 mA
- **C.** 4 mA
- **D.** 10 mA

Correct Answer: C

Explanation: The temporary venous pacer stimulation threshold is the output needed to ensure 1:1 conduction via the pacemaker. Any lower energy output will have intermittent or complete failure to stimulate depolarization of the left ventricular muscle. Loss of capture during deployment could cause left ventricular ejection that can displace the valve during deployment. The selected output should be about two- to tenfold the threshold current to ensure capture. In this case, 1 to 4 mA would be appropriate, given the threshold of 0.4 mA. Although many practitioners choose an output of 10 mA for rapid pacing to ensure capture even when the tip is repositioned during cardiac contraction, excessive current may damage cardiac muscle. It may not be appropriate to default to the maximum pacer output if a lower setting provides reliable pacing. Changes in the stimulation threshold may indicate catheter malpositioning that can be corrected prior to valve deployment.

References:

1. Zakhary WZA, Ender JK. Chapter 27: Procedures in the Hybrid Operating Room. In: Kaplan JA, Augoustides JGT, Manecke GR, et al., eds. Kaplan's Cardiac Anesthesia. 7th ed. Elsevier; 2017:1022-1041.
2. Liu M, Wu P. Myocardial injury after temporary transvenous cardiac pacing. Ther Clin Risk Manag, 2021; 18: 415-421.

26. Several minutes after a difficult femoral transvenous pacer placement and testing during transcatheter aortic valve replacement, significant hypotension develops. The arterial pulse pressure is reduced, and a significant respiratory variation is noted on the arterial waveform. The patient complains of new shortness of breath. Jugular venous distention is also noted. What would best diagnose the patient's new problem?
  A. Chest x-ray
  B. Femoral angiogram
  C. Transthoracic echocardiogram
  D. Lung ultrasound

Correct Answer: C

Explanation: This patient is experiencing obstructive shock consistent with cardiac tamponade. Pericardial tamponade reportedly occurs anywhere from 0.6% to 4.5% with transcatheter aortic valve replacement and less commonly with other transcatheter procedures (0.2%–2% for ablations). Initially patients may present with transient and then sustained hypotension. Like all obstructive shock syndromes, there is limited stroke volume and thus a narrow pulse pressure. The respiratory variation (pulsus paradoxus) results from cyclic respiratory increases and decreases in preload. Jugular venous distention results as pericardial pressures prevent normal central venous drainage, a key feature for distinguishing between retroperitoneal bleeding and obstructive shock. Chest x-ray may be helpful to rule out pneumothorax, but supine patients on fluoroscopy tables may not demonstrate the expected absence of peripheral lung markings until very late. Lung ultrasound would be more sensitive to anterior pneumothorax than supine x-ray but would not help identify tamponade. Pericardial effusion and tamponade would be best diagnosed by echocardiography.

References:

1. Zakhary WZA, Ender JK. Chapter 27: Procedures in the Hybrid Operating Room. In: Kaplan JA, Augoustides JGT, Manecke GR, et al., eds. Kaplan's Cardiac Anesthesia. 7th ed. Elsevier; 2017:1022-1041.
2. Adamczyk M, Wasilewski J, Niedziela J, et al. Pericardial tamponade as a complication of invasive cardiac procedures: a review of the literature. Postepy Kardiol Interwencyjnej, 2019; 15: 394-403.

27. Which series of personal protective equipment provides radiation reduction from most to least?
  A. Lead gloves > thyroid collars > leaded glasses > radiosorbent surgical caps
  B. Radiosorbent caps > lead gloves > thyroid collars > leaded glasses
  C. Thyroid collars > leaded glasses > leaded gloves > radiosorbent surgical caps
  D. Leaded glasses > thyroid collars > radiosorbent surgical caps > lead gloves

Correct Answer: C

Explanation: Gowns and thyroid collars reduce radiation by more than 95%, and leaded glasses reduce radiation by 35% to 90%. Leaded gloves decrease radiation by 20% to 50%, and radiosorbent surgical caps reduce radiation by 3%.

References:

1. Zakhary WZA, Ender JK. Chapter 27: Procedures in the Hybrid Operating Room. In: Kaplan JA, Augoustides JGT, Manecke GR, et al., eds. Kaplan's Cardiac Anesthesia. 7th ed. Elsevier; 2017:1022-1041.
2. Biso SMR, Vidovich MI. Radiation protection in the cardiac catheterization laboratory. J Thorac Dis, 2020; 12: 1648-1655.

28. Which treatment strategy is effective in reducing spinal cord ischemia after thoracic endovascular aortic repair?
  A. Controlled hypotension
  B. Spinal fluid drainage
  C. Large graft size
  D. Phlebotomy

Correct Answer: B

Explanation: Spinal cord ischemia following aorta grafting is a feared complication resulting from disruption of the intercostal/spinal arteries that feed the anterior spinal cord. Larger grafts cover more segments and increase the risk of spinal cord ischemia. Induced hypertension will enhance collateral blood flow to these areas, as will reducing spinal fluid pressures. Reducing the oxygen-carrying capacity via phlebotomy would not be helpful for reducing ischemia to the spinal cord.

References:

1. Zakhary WZA, Ender JK. Chapter 27: Procedures in the Hybrid Operating Room. In: Kaplan JA, Augoustides JGT, Manecke GR, et al., eds. Kaplan's Cardiac Anesthesia. 7th ed. Elsevier; 2017:1022-1041.
2. Xue L, Luo S, Ding H, et al. Risk of spinal cord ischemia after thoracic endovascular aortic repair. J Thorac Dis, 2018; 10: 6088-6096.
3. Chan CH, Desai SR, Hwang NC. Cerebrospinal fluid drains: risks in contemporary clinical practice. J Cardiothorac Vasc Anesth, 2022; 36: 2685-2699.

29. Each of the following is a risk factor for a permanent pacemaker following transcatheter aortic valve replacement EXCEPT:

A. Valve oversizing

B. Atrial flutter

C. Right bundle branch block

D. Second-degree heart block

Correct Answer: B

Explanation: Atrial arrhythmias carry no increased risk for patients requiring permanent pacemakers after transcatheter aortic valve replacement (TAVR). Valve oversizing leads to increased pressure on the conduction fibers passing through the left ventricular outflow tract and disrupts normal electrical pathways below the atrioventricular node. Similarly, preexisting infranodal electrical conduction defects such as bundle branch and second-degree heart blocks increase the risk of conduction failure after TAVR. Usually, these abnormalities present immediately following deployment but can be delayed, so postoperative telemetry is important. The rates of permanent pacemaker placement following TAVR range from 9% to 26%. The CoreValve prosthesis has been associated with higher rates of postoperative pacemaker placement compared to the Sapien valve family.

References:

1. Zakhary WZA, Ender JK. Chapter 27: Procedures in the Hybrid Operating Room. In: Kaplan JA, Augoustides JGT, Manecke GR, et al., eds. Kaplan's Cardiac Anesthesia. 7th ed. Elsevier; 2017:1022-1041.

2. Rück A, Saleh N, Glaser N, et al. Outcomes following permanent pacemaker implantation after transcatheter aortic valve replacement. JACC Cardiol Intv, 2021; 14: 2173-2181.

30. Which is TRUE with regard to transapical transcatheter aortic valve replacement (TAVR)?

A. Less painful than transfemoral TAVR

B. The valve is crimped in the usual orientation

C. Is performed under general anesthesia

D. Postinsertion blood pressure control is less important

Correct Answer: C

Explanation: Transapical transcatheter aortic valve replacement (TAVR) represents some unique challenges with regard to access and patient care. Because the left chest is opened with some rib spreading, there is more pain, and general anesthesia is required. Because of the incision into the left ventricular apex, left ventricular rupture and pseudoaneurysm are possible, especially if blood pressure is not well controlled perioperatively. Although left ventricular injury and rupture from stiff guidewires have been reported in transfemoral TAVR, the large device access through the apex in transapical TAVR carries additional risk for left ventricular injury. When the valve is inserted via the transapical approach, the valve must be inversely oriented on the delivery sheath as compared to the standard femoral approach so that leaflets open to allow flow in the correct direction.

References:

1. Zakhary WZA, Ender JK. Chapter 27: Procedures in the Hybrid Operating Room. In: Kaplan JA, Augoustides JGT, Manecke GR, et al., eds. Kaplan's Cardiac Anesthesia. 7th ed. Elsevier; 2017:1022-1041.

2. Pasic M, Buz S, Dreysse S, et al. Transapical aortic valve implantation in 194 patients: problems, complications, and solutions. Ann Thorac Surg, 2010: 90: 1463-1469.

3. Cobey FC, Ferreira R, Naseem T, et al. Anesthetic and perioperative considerations for transapical transcatheter aortic valve replacement. J Cardiothorac Vasc Anesth, 2014; 28: 1075-1087.

CHAPTER 24

Mechanical Assist Devices for Heart Failure

Theresa Anne Gelzinis

KEY POINTS

1. Mechanical circulatory support (MCS) for the failing heart has become a mainstay of the modern management of patients with both acute and chronic heart failure refractory to pharmacologic and other usual interventions.

2. Outcomes with MCS have improved so dramatically that the main focus of this arena has now shifted away from simple survival and toward mitigation of risk and minimization of adverse events.

3. Data taken from experience gained with the first generation of pulsatile devices may no longer be applicable in the current era of nonpulsatile support, but the valuable lessons learned continue to help shape management and clinical decision making.

4. In addition to the traditional indications for MCS (e.g., short-term bridge to recovery and long-term bridge to transplantation), MCS is currently employed for a variety of both short- and long-term modern indications, including acute rescue of patients from acute low cardiac output situations (bridge to immediate survival), prevention of further myocardial damage following an ischemic event, prevention of deterioration in multisystem organ function, as a temporizing measure to buy time for recovery, as a bridge to the next step of management (bridge to next decision), as a bridge to improved candidacy (for transplantation), and, increasingly, as a final management strategy for end-stage heart failure (destination therapy).

5. Patient status at the time of implementation of rescue MCS is a key factor determining outcome. Deterioration from delayed implementation is associated with worse outcome.

6. The timing of implantation of a durable left ventricular assist device (LVAD) (e.g., as a bridge to transplantation and/or as destination therapy) and perioperative optimization of the patient's nutritional status are key factors determining outcome.

7. Nonpulsatile support devices have supplanted the first generation of pulsatile ventricular assist devices worldwide, and outcomes have improved dramatically with the technology now available.

8. Extracorporeal membrane oxygenation is being incorporated more and more often into modern extracorporeal life support algorithms.

9. The implantable total artificial heart has undergone a resurgence of interest as a bridge to transplantation for patients with biventricular failure and in other scenarios where an LVAD alone would not be ideal.

10. A number of new MCS devices are in various stages of development and clinical trials.

---

1. Which Interagency Registry for Mechanical Assisted Circulatory Support profile is defined as having resting symptoms on oral home therapy?
   A. Profile 2
   B. Profile 3
   C. Profile 4
   D. Profile 5

Correct Answer: C

Explanation: There are seven Interagency Registry for Mechanical Assisted Circulatory Support profiles that are defined as follows:

Profile 1 is cardiogenic shock (crash and burn). Profile 2 is heart failure with progressive decline, with worsening end-organ damage despite therapy (sliding fast on inotropes). Profile 3 is heart failure that is clinically stable on continuous intravenous inotropes. Profile 4 is heart failure with resting symptoms on oral therapy at home. Profile 5 is heart failure with intolerance of minimal effort. Profile 6 is heart failure with exertion limited to the first few minutes of mild physical activity. Profile 7 is heart failure with New York Heart Association class III symptoms and with limitation to mild physical activity, including activities of daily living.

References:

1. Stone ME, Hinchey J. Chapter 28: Mechanical Assist Devices for Heart Failure. In: Kaplan JA, Augoustides JGT, Manecke GR, et al., eds. Kaplan's Cardiac Anesthesia. 7th ed. Elsevier; 2017:1042-1063.
2. Stevenson LW, Pagani FD, Young JB, et al. INTERMACS profiles of advanced heart failure. J Heart Lung Transplant, 2009; 6: 535-541.

2. At which Interagency Registry for Mechanical Assisted Circulatory Support profile are patients with heart failure electively implanted with a left ventricular assist device?
   A. Profile 3
   B. Profile 4
   C. Profile 5
   D. Profile 6

Correct Answer: A

Explanation: The timing of left ventricular assist device implantation (LVAD) is optimal when the patient is in end-stage class D heart failure on inotropic support to optimize end-organ function. With Interagency Registry for Mechanical Assisted Circulatory Support (INTERMACS) profiles 1 and 2, the patients are hemodynamically unstable with increasing end-organ damage, increasing the incidence of poorer outcomes. The majority of patients undergo LVAD implantation when they are at INTERMACS profile 3 heart failure.

References:

1. Stone ME, Hinchey J. Chapter 28: Mechanical Assist Devices for Heart Failure. In: Kaplan JA, Augoustides JGT, Manecke GR, et al., eds. Kaplan's Cardiac Anesthesia. 7th ed. Elsevier; 2017:1042-1063.
2. Heidenreich P, Bozkurt B, Aguilar D, et al. 2022 AHA/ACC/HFSA Guideline for the Management of Heart Failure. J Am Coll Cardiol, 2022; 79: e263-e421.

3. For maximum augmentation with an intra-aortic balloon pump, what percentage of the aorta has to be obstructed during balloon inflation?
   A. 85%
   B. 90%
   C. 95%
   D. 100%

Correct Answer: B

Explanation: For optimal augmentation while reducing the incidence of aortic trauma, maximal intra-aortic balloon pump inflation should be at 90% of the aortic diameter.

References:

1. Stone ME, Hinchey J. Chapter 28: Mechanical Assist Devices for Heart Failure. In: Kaplan JA, Augoustides JGT, Manecke GR,

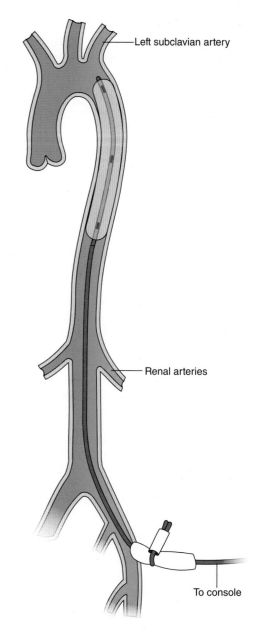

FIGURE 24.1 The intra-aortic balloon pump.

et al., eds. Kaplan's Cardiac Anesthesia. 7th ed. Elsevier; 2017:1042-1063.
2. González LS, Chaney MA. Intraaortic balloon pump counterpulsation, part I: history, technical aspects, physiologic effects, contraindications, medical applications/outcomes. Anesth Analg, 2020; 131: 776-791.

4. The electrocardiographic trigger for intra-aortic balloon pump inflation occurs during the:
   A. TP interval
   B. PR interval
   C. QRS interval
   D. ST interval

Correct Answer: A

Explanation: Optimal balloon inflation during intra-aortic balloon counterpulsation occurs immediately following aortic valve closure. The most common trigger for function of the intra-aortic balloon pump is the electrocardiogram. Inflation is triggered during the intervals between the T and P waves during ventricular diastole when the aortic valve is closed.

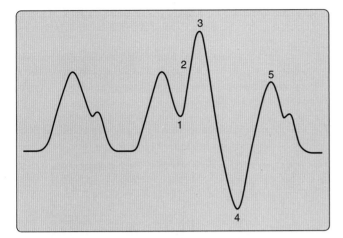

FIGURE 24.2 A well-timed intra-aortic balloon pump (IABP) inflation. The figure demonstrates an arterial pressure tracing taken from a patient with an IABP. The first pulse seen on the left is the familiar waveform of an arterial pulse. An IABP is triggered to inflate during the second pulse, generating a typical sinusoidal balloon inflation-deflation waveform. The third pulse represents an assisted ejection due to the action of the IABP. Characteristics of the typical balloon waveform include the following: (1) The balloon inflation point coinciding with the location of the patient's dicrotic notch (representing aortic valve closure at the end of systole). (2) A steep slope of increasing pressure indicating rapid balloon inflation. This creates a rapid rise in aortic root pressure to reach. (3) The assisted diastolic peak pressure perfusing the coronary arteries while the IABP is inflated. This increase in coronary perfusion pressure creates the increased myocardial oxygen supply associated with IABP action. (4) A steep slope of pressure decline indicates a rapid balloon deflation, resulting in a decrease in end-diastolic aortic root pressure. This localized decreased afterload decreases impedance to opening of the aortic valve at the beginning of systole and creates the decreased myocardial oxygen demand associated with IABP action. (5) The assisted systolic peak pressure of the next beat perfusing the body. The systolic pressure attained by this ejection was accomplished with less myocardial work thanks to the IABP. Depending on the level of assistance required, the balloon can be triggered with each cardiac cycle (so-called 1:1 assistance), every other cycle (1:2), every third cycle (1:3), and so forth.

References:

1. Stone ME, Hinchey J. Chapter 28: Mechanical Assist Devices for Heart Failure. In: Kaplan JA, Augoustides JGT, Manecke GR, et al., eds. Kaplan's Cardiac Anesthesia. 7th ed. Elsevier; 2017:1042-1063.
2. González LS, Chaney MA. Intraaortic balloon pump counterpulsation, part I: history, technical aspects, physiologic effects, contraindications, medical applications/outcomes. Anesth Analg, 2020; 131: 776-791.

5. Which timing error during intra-aortic balloon therapy produces this waveform seen in the figure below?

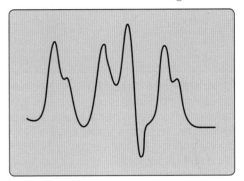

A. Early deflation
B. Late deflation
C. Early inflation
D. Late inflation

Correct Answer: A

Explanation: Early deflation allows time for aortic root pressure to return to baseline before systolic ejection and therefore fails to decrease impedance to opening the aortic valve. This fails to decrease myocardial oxygen demand.

References:

1. Stone ME, Hinchey J. Chapter 28: Mechanical Assist Devices for Heart Failure. In: Kaplan JA, Augoustides JGT, Manecke GR, et al., eds. Kaplan's Cardiac Anesthesia. 7th ed. Elsevier; 2017:1042-1063.
2. González LS, Chaney MA. Intraaortic balloon pump counterpulsation, part I: history, technical aspects, physiologic effects, contraindications, medical applications/outcomes. Anesth Analg, 2020; 131: 776-791.

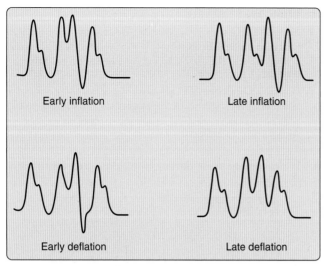

FIGURE 24.3 Intra-aortic balloon pump (IABP) timing errors. Early inflation, before the dicrotic notch (i.e., before systolic ejection is completed) immediately forces the aortic valve closed, resulting in prematurely terminated systolic ejection. This results in decreased stroke volume for that cardiac cycle and increased preload for the next cardiac cycle. Not only does this reduce an already impaired cardiac output, but acutely increased end-diastolic volumes stress the failing ventricle by increasing wall tension, which can increase myocardial oxygen demand, impair perfusion, and lead to ischemia. Thus early inflation must be corrected because it increases myocardial oxygen demand and decreases myocardial oxygen supply. Late inflation, after the dicrotic notch, fails to augment coronary perfusion pressure optimally. Therefore myocardial oxygen supply is not maximally enhanced. Early deflation allows time for aortic root pressure to return to baseline before systolic ejection and therefore fails to decrease impedance to opening the aortic valve. Thus myocardial oxygen demand is not decreased. Recall that it is the decrease in myocardial oxygen demand that most benefits the failing ventricle and allows for increased stroke volume with less myocardial work. Late deflation can be identified by a failure of the pressure to fall back to baseline or, ideally, below baseline, before the next systolic ejection. Late deflation impedes systolic ejection like an aortic cross clamp. The ventricle is forced to develop such a high pressure to open the aortic valve that ventricular wall tension is significantly increased, which increases myocardial oxygen demand, impairs perfusion, and can lead to ischemia.

6. Which timing error during intra-aortic balloon counterpulsation is associated with reduced systolic ejection, reduced stroke volume and increased left ventricular preload?
   A. Late inflation
   B. Early inflation
   C. Late deflation
   D. Early deflation

Correct Answer: B

Explanation: Early inflation, occurring before the dicrotic notch, immediately forces the aortic valve to close, prematurely terminating systolic ejection (see figure). This results in decreased stroke volume for that cardiac cycle and increased preload for the next cardiac cycle. This reduces cardiac output and acutely increases end-diastolic volumes, wall tension, and myocardial

oxygen demand, resulting in impairing perfusion and possibly ischemia. The net result is an increase in myocardial oxygen demand and a reduction in myocardial oxygen supply.

References:
1. Stone ME, Hinchey J. Chapter 28: Mechanical Assist Devices for Heart Failure. In: Kaplan JA, Augoustides JGT, Manecke GR, et al., eds. Kaplan's Cardiac Anesthesia. 7th ed. Elsevier; 2017:1042-1063.
2. González LS, Chaney MA. Intraaortic balloon pump counterpulsation, part I: history, technical aspects, physiologic effects, contraindications, medical applications/outcomes. Anesth Analg, 2020; 131: 776-791.

7. The timing abnormality during intra-aortic balloon therapy as depicted in the figure below is due to:

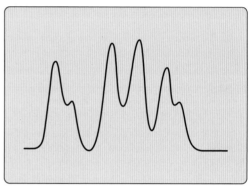

   A. Early deflation
   B. Early inflation
   C. Late deflation
   D. Late inflation

Correct Answer: C

Explanation: Late deflation can be identified by a failure of the pressure to fall back to or below the baseline before the next systolic ejection. Late deflation impedes systolic ejection forcing the ventricle to develop high pressure that opens the aortic valve, increasing left ventricular wall tension and myocardial oxygen demand, impairing perfusion, and leading to ischemia.

References:
1. Stone ME, Hinchey J. Chapter 28: Mechanical Assist Devices for Heart Failure. In: Kaplan JA, Augoustides JGT, Manecke GR, et al., eds. Kaplan's Cardiac Anesthesia. 7th ed. Elsevier; 2017:1042-1063.
2. González LS, Chaney MA. Intraaortic balloon pump counterpulsation, part I: history, technical aspects, physiologic effects, contraindications, medical applications/outcomes. Anesth Analg, 2020; 131: 776-791.

8. Which triggering event during intra-aortic balloon counterpulsation is associated with suboptimal coronary perfusion and afterload reduction with potential retrograde coronary and carotid blood flow?
   A. Early deflation
   B. Early inflation
   C. Late deflation
   D. Late inflation

Correct Answer: A

Explanation: Early deflation is associated with suboptimal diastolic augmentation, a decreased reduction in aortic end-diastolic pressure, and an increase in systolic pressure. Physiological effects include suboptimal coronary perfusion, a potential for retrograde coronary and carotid blood flow, suboptimal afterload reduction, and an increase in myocardial oxygen demand.

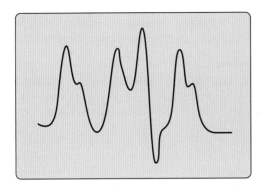

References:

1. Stone ME, Hinchey J. Chapter 28: Mechanical Assist Devices for Heart Failure. In: Kaplan JA, Augoustides JGT, Manecke GR, et al., eds. Kaplan's Cardiac Anesthesia. 7th ed. Elsevier; 2017:1042-1063.
2. Krishna M, Zacharowski K. Principles of intra-aortic balloon pump counterpulsation. Contin Educ Anaesth Crit Care Pain, 2009; 9: 24-28.

9. All of these statements are true concerning the normal function of an intraortic balloon pump EXCEPT:
   A. Peak assisted systolic blood pressure is lower than peak of unassisted systolic blood pressure
   B. Augmented diastolic blood pressure is lower than the unassisted systolic blood pressure
   C. Assisted end-diastolic blood pressure is lower than unassisted end diastolic pressure
   D. Augmented diastolic blood pressure is greater than assisted systolic blood pressure

Correct Answer: B

Explanation: With optimal timing, the blood pressure waveform reveals an augmented diastolic blood pressure greater than the unassisted systolic blood pressure, reductions in assisted end-diastolic and assisted systolic blood pressures, and an assisted systolic blood pressure less than unassisted systolic blood pressure.

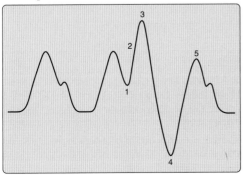

References:

1. Stone ME, Hinchey J. Chapter 28: Mechanical Assist Devices for Heart Failure. In: Kaplan JA, Augoustides JGT, Manecke GR, et al., eds. Kaplan's Cardiac Anesthesia. 7th ed. Elsevier; 2017:1042-1063.
2. González LS, Chaney MA. Intraaortic balloon pump counterpulsation, part I: history, technical aspects, physiologic effects, contraindications, medical applications/outcomes. Anesth Analg, 2020; 131: 776-791.

10. Which of these effects is due to balloon inflation during intra-aortic balloon counterpulsation?
    A. Increased stroke volume
    B. Decreased left ventricular end-diastolic volume
    C. Decreased left ventricular end-diastolic pressure
    D. Increased left ventricular compliance

Correct Answer: C

Explanation: The effects of balloon inflation include increased diastolic and mean blood pressure; increased coronary perfusion pressure, coronary blood flow, and myocardial oxygen supply; and decreased left ventricular end-diastolic pressure. The effects of balloon deflation include increased stroke volume, left ventricular ejection fraction, and left ventricular compliance; a shorter isovolumic ejection time; and decreased systolic blood pressure, left ventricular end-systolic and end-diastolic volumes, afterload, left ventricular wall tension, and myocardial oxygen demand.

References:

1. Stone ME, Hinchey J. Chapter 28: Mechanical Assist Devices for Heart Failure. In: Kaplan JA, Augoustides JGT, Manecke GR, et al., eds. Kaplan's Cardiac Anesthesia. 7th ed. Elsevier; 2017:1042-1063.
2. González LS, Chaney MA. Intraaortic balloon pump counterpulsation, part I: history, technical aspects, physiologic effects, contraindications, medical applications/outcomes. Anesth Analg, 2020; 131: 776-791.

11. By what percentage does an intra-aortic balloon pump increase cardiac output?
    A. 10%
    B. 20%
    C. 30%
    D. 40%

Correct Answer: B

Explanation: Intra-aortic balloon counterpulsation can increase cardiac output by 20%. This is possible only if the left ventricle has intrinsic contractile function that can increase cardiac output in response to the beneficial systolic and diastolic effects of this mechanical therapy.

References:

1. Stone ME, Hinchey J. Chapter 28: Mechanical Assist Devices for Heart Failure. In: Kaplan JA, Augoustides JGT, Manecke GR, et al., eds. Kaplan's Cardiac Anesthesia. 7th ed. Elsevier; 2017:1042-1063.
2. González LS, Chaney MA. Intraaortic balloon pump counterpulsation, part I: history, technical aspects, physiologic effects, contraindications, medical applications/outcomes. Anesth Analg, 2020; 131: 776-791.

12. All of the following can reduce intra-aortic balloon pump augmentation EXCEPT:

   A. Bradycardia

   B. Reduced systemic vascular resistance

   C. Elevated stroke volumes

   D. Early inflation

Correct Answer: A

Explanation: Augmentation by an intra-aortic balloon pump is reduced by tachycardia, reduced systemic vascular resistance due to increased aortic capacitance, stroke volumes higher or lower than balloon volumes, and the timing errors such as early and late inflation. The maximal augmentation occurs when the balloon volume is equal to the stroke volume.

References:

1. Stone ME, Hinchey J. Chapter 28: Mechanical Assist Devices for Heart Failure. In: Kaplan JA, Augoustides JGT, Manecke GR, et al., eds. Kaplan's Cardiac Anesthesia. 7th ed. Elsevier; 2017:1042-1063.
2. Krishna M, Zacharowski K. Principles of intra-aortic balloon pump counterpulsation. Contin Educ Anaesth Crit Care Pain, 2009; 9: 24-28.

13. All of the following are absolute contraindications to left ventricular assist device placement EXCEPT:

   A. Irreversible hepatic disease

   B. Irreversible renal disease

   C. Severe psychological limitations

   D. Untreated malignancy

Correct Answer: D

Explanation: According to the 2022 AHA/ACC/HFSA heart failure guidelines, absolute contraindications include irreversible hepatic, renal, and neurological disease, medical nonadherence, and severe psychological limitations. Relative contraindications include over 80 years of age for destination therapy, obesity and malnutrition, musculoskeletal disease that impairs rehabilitation, active systemic infection, prolonged intubation, untreated malignancy, severe peripheral vascular disease, active substance abuse, impaired cognitive function, unmanaged psychiatric disorder, and lack of social support.

References:

1. Stone ME, Hinchey J. Chapter 28: Mechanical Assist Devices for Heart Failure. In: Kaplan JA, Augoustides JGT, Manecke GR, et al., eds. Kaplan's Cardiac Anesthesia. 7th ed. Elsevier; 2017:1042-1063.
2. Heidenreich P, Bozkurt B, Aguilar D, et al. 2022 AHA/ACC/HFSA guidelines for the management of heart failure. J Am Coll Cardiol, 2022; 79: e263-e421.

14. According to the European Association of Cardiothoracic Surgery, which left ventricular ejection fraction (EF) is required before assessing a patient for a left ventricular assist device?

   A. EF of 35% or less

   B. EF of 30% or less

   C. EF of 25% or less

   D. EF of 20% or less

Correct Answer: C

Explanation: The criteria for consideration of left ventricular assist device placement according to the 2019 European Association of Cardiothoracic Surgery Expert consensus on long-term mechanical support include patients with New York Heart Association functional class IIIB to IV, a left ventricular ejection fraction of 25% or less, and at least one of the following criteria: Interagency Registry for Mechanical Assisted Circulatory Support profile 2 to 4, inotrope dependence, progressive end-organ dysfunction, and/or temporary mechanical support dependence.

References:

1. Stone ME, Hinchey J. Chapter 28: Mechanical Assist Devices for Heart Failure. In: Kaplan JA, Augoustides JGT, Manecke GR, et al., eds. Kaplan's Cardiac Anesthesia. 7th ed. Elsevier; 2017:1042-1063.
2. Potapov EV, Antonides C, Crespo-Leiro MG, et al. 2019 EACTS Expert Consensus on long-term mechanical circulatory support. Eur J Cardiothor Surg, 2019; 56: 230-270.

15. Compared to axial pumps for left ventricular assist devices, all of the following are characteristics of centrifugal pumps EXCEPT:

   A. Higher pump pulsatility

   B. Has a rotor in parallel with the pump

   C. Operates at lower speeds

   D. Is more sensitive to preload and afterload

Correct Answer: B

Explanation: The two types of pumps in contemporary left ventricular assist devices are axial and centrifugal. In an axial pump, the rotor is in parallel to the pump, which causes the blood to flow from the inlet to the outlet in a pushing fashion and requires more pressure to move blood. This requires higher speeds, causing more damage to the red blood cells and von Willebrand factor. Axial pumps also have lower sensitivity to preload and afterload, making suction events more common. Centrifugal pumps have a rotor that is parallel to the pump, moving blood from the inlet to the outlet with a throwing motion that reduces the amount of force required to move blood. Centrifugal pumps require less speed, which reduces trauma to red blood cells and von Willebrand factor, and are programmed to have a higher preload and afterload sensitivity, and can reduce the speed before a suction event occurs. During native ventricular contraction, because of their high-pressure sensitivity, centrifugal pumps have a larger change in flow compared to axial devices during native ventricular contraction, but this does not translate into clinically significant pulsatility.

References:

1. Stone ME, Hinchey J. Chapter 28: Mechanical Assist Devices for Heart Failure. In: Kaplan JA, Augoustides JGT, Manecke GR, et al., eds. Kaplan's Cardiac Anesthesia. 7th ed. Elsevier; 2017:1042-1063.
2. Giridharan GA, Koenig SC, Slaughter MS. Do Axial-Flow LVADs unload better than centrifugal-flow LVADs? ASAIO J, 2014; 60: 137-139.

16. Which of these ventricular assist devices is pulsatile and can support biventricular failure?
A. Berlin Heart Excor
B. Centrimag
C. Heartmate 3
D. Impella

Correct Answer: A

Explanation: The Berlin Heart Excor is a paracorporeal, pulsatile ventricular assist device that is used in the pediatric population. It consists of a polyurethane sac surrounded by a pneumatic pump that, when inflated, moves blood by ejecting it from the sac. It can be used as a right, left, or biventricular assist device. The Centrimag, Heartmate 3, and Impella are continuous flow devices.

References:

1. Stone ME, Hinchey J. Chapter 28: Mechanical Assist Devices for Heart Failure. In: Kaplan JA, Augoustides JGT, Manecke GR, et al., eds. Kaplan's Cardiac Anesthesia. 7th ed. Elsevier; 2017:1042-1063.
2. Almond CS, Morales DL, Blackstone EH, et al. Berlin Heart EXCOR Pediatric Ventricular Assist Device for Bridge to Heart Transplantation in US Children. Circulation, 2013; 127: 1702-711.

17. Which left ventricular assist device requires a transseptal puncture to implant?
A. Centrimag
B. Heartmate 3
C. Impella
D. TandemHeart

Correct Answer: D

Explanation: The TandemHeart left ventricular assist device is a percutaneously placed centrifugal pump that can support the left or right ventricle as a bridge to immediate survival or recovery. A percutaneously inserted femoral venous inflow cannula is advanced to the right atrium and then trans-septally inserted into the right atrium with the outflow directed into a femoral artery cannula. It can provide up to 5 liters per minute of flow. The other devices do not cross the interatrial septum.

References:

1. Stone ME, Hinchey J. Chapter 28: Mechanical Assist Devices for Heart Failure. In: Kaplan JA, Augoustides JGT, Manecke GR, et al., eds. Kaplan's Cardiac Anesthesia. 7th ed. Elsevier; 2017:1042-1063.
2. Cole SP, Martinez-Acero N, Peterson A, et al. Imaging for temporary mechanical circulatory support devices. J Cardiothorac Vasc Anesth, 2022; 36: 2114-2131.

18. In a patient who has right ventricular failure and hypoxia, an oxygenator can be placed on all of these devices EXCEPT:
A. Centrimag
B. Extracorporeal membrane oxygenation
C. Impella
D. TandemHeart

Correct Answer: C

Explanation: The only ventricular assist device that an oxygenator cannot be added to is the Impella. The full details of these devices are covered in the provided references. Extracorporeal membrane oxygenation by definition includes an oxygenator. The Centrimag and TandemHeart devices can accommodate an oxygenator in the circuit if needed.

References:

1. Stone ME, Hinchey J. Chapter 28: Mechanical Assist Devices for Heart Failure. In: Kaplan JA, Augoustides JGT, Manecke GR, et al., eds. Kaplan's Cardiac Anesthesia. 7th ed. Elsevier; 2017:1042-1063.
2. Abdelshafy M, Caliskan K, Guven G, et al. Temporary right-ventricular assist device: a systemic review. J Clin Med, 2022; 11: 613.
3. Cole SP, Martinez-Acero N, Peterson A, et al. Imaging for temporary mechanical circulatory support devices. J Cardiothorac Vasc Anesth, 2022; 36: 2114-2131.

19. When performing the prebypass transesophageal echocardiogram for placement of a left ventricular assist device, which pathology requires surgical intervention?
A. Intact mechanical aortic valve
B. Severe mitral regurgitation
C. Mild aortic insufficiency
D. Moderate pulmonic insufficiency

Correct Answer: A

Explanation: The prebypass transesophageal echocardiography exam evaluates any impediment to left ventricular assist device (LVAD) function. This includes determinants that would affect LVAD filling including right ventricular function, tricuspid regurgitation, and mitral stenosis. The aortic valve is evaluated for the presence of stenosis, regurgitation, and valve replacement. Aortic insufficiency will cause recirculation into the pump, reducing forward cardiac flow. A mechanical aortic valve predisposes the patient to thrombus formation. The rest of the exam consists of evaluating for intracardiac shunts, thrombi in the left heart, and any plaques at the aortic outflow cannula site. The surgeon should be notified about severe tricuspid regurgitation, reduced right ventricular dysfunction, mitral stenosis, aortic stenosis, aortic insufficiency greater than mild, or the presence of a mechanical aortic valve, which predisposes patients to thrombi. Other pathologies include an intracardiac shunt, which can lead to postoperative right to left shunting causing hypoxia, and any intracardiac thrombi or mobile aortic plaque, which can lead to a stroke.

References:

1. Stone ME, Hinchey J. Chapter 28: Mechanical Assist Devices for Heart Failure. In: Kaplan JA, Augoustides JGT, Manecke GR, et al., eds. Kaplan's Cardiac Anesthesia. 7th ed. Elsevier; 2017:1042-1063.
2. Sciaccaluga C, Soliman-Aboumarie H, Sisti N, et al. Echocardiography for left ventricular assist device implantation and evaluation: an indispensable tool. Heart Fail Review, 2022; 27: 891-902.

20. Which of these structures should be examined with transesophageal echocardiography after the initiation of cardiopulmonary bypass in patients with systolic heart failure?
- **A.** Aortic valve
- **B.** Hepatic veins
- **C.** Left atrial appendage
- **D.** Tricuspid valve

Correct Answer: A

Explanation: The aortic valve and intra-atrial septum should be evaluated with transesophageal echocardiography after the initiation of bypass. Prebypass aortic insufficiency can be underestimated, because patients with systolic heart failure have elevated left ventricular diastolic pressure and reduced aortic diastolic pressure. On cardiopulmonary bypass, the left ventricular diastolic pressure is reduced and any aortic insufficiency is unmasked. The intra-atrial septum should be re-evaluated once cardiopulmonary bypass is initiated, because the presence of high left atrial pressure may prevent the detection of a patent foramen ovale. After the initiation of bypass, left atrial pressure is reduced, increasing the gradient between the right and left atria, allowing the detection of a patent foramen.

References:
1. Stone ME, Hinchey J. Chapter 28: Mechanical Assist Devices for Heart Failure. In: Kaplan JA, Augoustides JGT, Manecke GR, et al., eds. Kaplan's Cardiac Anesthesia. 7th ed. Elsevier; 2017:1042-1063.
2. Flores AS, Essandoh M, Yerington GC, et al. Echocardiographic assessment for ventricular assist device placement. J Thor Dis, 2015; 12: 2139-2150.

21. Which of these echocardiographic parameters are the most sensitive for detecting right ventricular dysfunction after insertion of a left ventricular assist device?
- **A.** Tricuspid annular plane systolic excursion and right ventricle (RV) sphericity index
- **B.** RV fractional area change and RV index of myocardial performance
- **C.** Tricuspid annular systolic velocity by tissue Doppler and RV sphericity index
- **D.** RV fractional area change and RV global strain

Correct Answer: D

Explanation: Standard echocardiographic parameters of right ventricular longitudinal function, such as tricuspid annular plane systolic excursion and tricuspid annular systolic velocity by tissue Doppler, do not significantly predict for right ventricular failure after implantation of a left ventricular assist device. Free-wall longitudinal strain derived by speckle tracking echocardiography has good correlation with the right ventricular stroke work index, and it is the best predictor of right ventricular failure in this setting. According to recent studies, a fractional area change under 35% and global strain 12.5% or less are the best predictors of right ventricular failure in the early postoperative period.

References:
1. Stone ME, Hinchey J. Chapter 28: Mechanical Assist Devices for Heart Failure. In: Kaplan JA, Augoustides JGT, Manecke GR, et al., eds. Kaplan's Cardiac Anesthesia. 7th ed. Elsevier; 2017:1042-1063.
2. Sciaccaluga C, Soliman-Aboumarie H, Sisti N, et al. Echocardiography for left ventricular assist device implantation and evaluation: an indispensable tool. Heart Fail Review, 2022; 27: 891-902.
3. Raina A, Seetha Rammohan HR, Gertz ZM, et al. Postoperative right ventricular failure after left ventricular assist device placement is predicted by preoperative echocardiographic structural, hemodynamic, and functional parameters. J Card Fail, 2013; 19: 16-24.

22. Which of these variables is NOT used to calculate flow in left ventricular assist devices?
- **A.** Pulsatility
- **B.** Hematocrit
- **C.** Power
- **D.** Speed

Correct Answer: A

Explanation: The three variables that are used to calculate flow are the power, speed, and hematocrit. Pulsatility is not required in the flow calculations.

References:
1. Stone ME, Hinchey J. Chapter 28: Mechanical Assist Devices for Heart Failure. In: Kaplan JA, Augoustides JGT, Manecke GR, et al., eds. Kaplan's Cardiac Anesthesia. 7th ed. Elsevier; 2017:1042-1063.
2. Tchoukina I, Smallfield MC, Shah KS. Device management and flow optimization on left ventricular assist device support. Crit Care Clin, 2018; 34: 453-463.

23. Which of these variables is NOT associated with a risk of increased in right ventricular dysfunction following placement of a left ventricular assist device?
- **A.** Female sex
- **B.** Nonischemic cardiomyopathy
- **C.** Increased pulmonary arterial pulsatility index
- **D.** Central venous pressure/pulmonary capillary wedge pressure ratio of more than 0.63

Correct Answer: C

Explanation: Factors that predispose a patient to right ventricular dysfunction after placement of a left ventricular assist device include female sex, nonischemic cardiomyopathy, temporary support, and the severity of tricuspid regurgitation. Biochemical markers include elevated blood urea nitrogen, creatinine, bilirubin, and aspartate aminotransferase. Hemodynamic variables include an increase in right atrial pressure, reduced stroke work index, increased pulmonary vascular resistance and diastolic pulmonary gradient, and reduced pulmonary arterial pulsatility index and tricuspid annular plane systolic excursion, as well as a central venous pressure/pulmonary capillary wedge pressure ratio of more than 0.63.

References:
1. Stone ME, Hinchey J. Chapter 28: Mechanical Assist Devices for Heart Failure. In: Kaplan JA, Augoustides JGT, Manecke GR, et al., eds. Kaplan's Cardiac Anesthesia. 7th ed. Elsevier; 2017:1042-1063.
2. Cogswell R, John R, Shaffer A. Right ventricular failure after left ventricular assist device. Cardiol Clin, 2020; 38: 219-225.

24. In patients with left ventricular assist devices, which of these conditions causes hypotension with decreased flow and an elevated pulsatility index?
    A. Hypovolemia
    B. Aortic insufficiency
    C. Reduced speed
    D. Partial inflow obstruction

Correct Answer: C

Explanation: The pulsatility index is a measure of the flow pulse through the left ventricular assist device that reflects circulating blood volume and native left ventricular ejection. Of all of the choices listed, only reduced speed will reduce flow while increasing the pulsatility index. Hypovolemia, aortic insufficiency, and partial inflow obstruction will reduce flow and lower the pulsatility index. Furthermore, aortic insufficiency will lead to a blind circulatory loop where a portion of the device output will circle back into the left ventricle due to the incompetent aortic valve.

References:
1. Stone ME, Hinchey J. Chapter 28: Mechanical Assist Devices for Heart Failure. In: Kaplan JA, Augoustides JGT, Manecke GR, et al., eds. Kaplan's Cardiac Anesthesia. 7th ed. Elsevier; 2017:1042-1063.
2. Tchoukina I, Smallfield MC, Shah KS. Device management and flow optimization on left ventricular assist device support. Crit Care Clin, 2018; 34: 453-463.

25. Of these conditions listed, which one is responsible for hypotension due to increased flow and decreased pulsatility index in a patient with a left ventricular assist device?
    A. Hypertension
    B. Hypovolemia
    C. Partial inflow obstruction
    D. Vasodilation

Correct Answer: D

Explanation: Of the choices listed, only vasodilation is responsible for increased flow with a reduced pulsatility index. The pulsatility index is a measure of the flow pulse through the left ventricular assist device that reflects circulating blood volume and native left ventricular ejection. Vasodilation will increase the flow and native left ventricular ejection due to decreases in afterload, with a consequent rise in the pulsatility index. Hypovolemia and partial inflow obstruction will decrease flow, as well as the pulsatility index, due to an effective decrease in circulating volume available to the device. Systemic hypertension will decrease native left ventricular ejection due to increases in systemic vascular resistance that will consequently decrease the pulsatility index.

References:
1. Stone ME, Hinchey J. Chapter 28: Mechanical Assist Devices for Heart Failure. In: Kaplan JA, Augoustides JGT, Manecke GR, et al., eds. Kaplan's Cardiac Anesthesia. 7th ed. Elsevier; 2017:1042-1063.
2. Tchoukina I, Smallfield MC, Shah KS. Device management and flow optimization on left ventricular assist device support. Crit Care Clin, 2018; 34: 453-463.

26. All of these conditions can cause decreased flow with a decreased pulsatility index in a patient with a left ventricular assist device EXCEPT:
    A. Hypovolemia
    B. Hypertension
    C. Right ventricular failure
    D. Tamponade

Correct Answer: B

Explanation: Hypovolemia, right ventricular failure, and tamponade all decrease preload for the left ventricular assist device, which reduces both the flow and the pulsatility index. The pulsatility index is a measure of the flow pulse through the left ventricular assist device that reflects circulating blood volume and native left ventricular ejection. Systemic hypertension can decrease the pulsatility index due to decreases in native ventricular ejection that accompany elevations in systemic vascular resistance, but it typically does not decrease flow.

References:
1. Stone ME, Hinchey J. Chapter 28: Mechanical Assist Devices for Heart Failure. In: Kaplan JA, Augoustides JGT, Manecke GR, et al., eds. Kaplan's Cardiac Anesthesia. 7th ed. Elsevier; 2017:1042-1063.
2. Tchoukina I, Smallfield MC, Shah KS. Device management and flow optimization on left ventricular assist device support. Crit Care Clin, 2018; 34: 453-463.

27. Which medication should be considered in patients with left ventricular assist devices who have both high flows and a high pulsatility index?
    A. Diuretics
    B. Antihypertensives
    C. Inotropic agents
    D. Antiarrhythmic agents

Correct Answer: A

Explanation: The pulsatility index is a measure of the flow pulse through the left ventricular assist device that reflects circulating blood volume and native left ventricular ejection. The differential diagnosis for increased flow and pulsatility includes hypervolemia and myocardial recovery, so in the absence of myocardial recovery, hypervolemia is treated with diuretics. Antihypertensives would be indicated to correct systemic hypertension associated with a low pulsatility index due to high systemic vascular resistance. In the setting of high flows and a high pulsatility index, there is no clinical indication for inotropic or antiarrhythmic therapy.

References:

1. Stone ME, Hinchey J. Chapter 28: Mechanical Assist Devices for Heart Failure. In: Kaplan JA, Augoustides JGT, Manecke GR, et al., eds. Kaplan's Cardiac Anesthesia. 7th ed. Elsevier; 2017:1042-1063.
2. Tchoukina I, Smallfield MC, Shah KS. Device management and flow optimization on left ventricular assist device support. Crit Care Clin, 2018; 34: 453-463.

28. To fill a total artificial heart pump, all of these steps must be undertaken EXCEPT:

A. Administer volume
B. Increase pump rate
C. Reduce percentage systole
D. Start vacuum

Correct Answer: B

Explanation: With a total artificial heart pump, an abrupt drop to zero flow during diastole represents complete filling. If the flow does not drop to zero during diastole, then filling of the ventricles is incomplete, and augmentation of intravascular volume is indicated. Alternatively, next steps are to decrease the pump rate and/or slightly decrease the percentage systole. Once the chest is closed, the amount of vacuum can be increased to assist filling without the entrainment of air with an open chest.

References:

1. Stone ME, Hinchey J. Chapter 28: Mechanical Assist Devices for Heart Failure. In: Kaplan JA, Augoustides JGT, Manecke GR, et al., eds. Kaplan's Cardiac Anesthesia. 7th ed. Elsevier; 2017:1042-1063.
2. Rangwala Z, Banks DA, Copeland JG. Pro: The total artificial heart: is it an appropriate replacement for existing biventricular assist devices? J Cardiothorac Vasc Anesth, 2014; 28: 836-839.

29. After implantation of a left ventricular assist device, normal transesophageal echocardiographic findings include all of the following EXCEPT:

A. Midline interventricular septum
B. Pulsed wave Doppler of the inflow cannula under 1.5 m/s
C. Inflow cannula pointing to the middle scallop of the posterior mitral leaflet
D. Pulsed wave Doppler of the outflow cannula over 2 m/s

Correct Answer: D

Explanation: The transesophageal echocardiographic examination after implantation of a left ventricular assist device includes the evaluation of right ventricular function and valvular function, as well as a comprehensive evaluation for septal defects and cannula function. The ventricular loading is optimized when the interventricular septum is in the midline. Rightward shift of the septum indicates suboptimal mechanical support, while a leftward shift indicates excessive unloading. The inflow cannula should be aligned perpendicular to the mitral valve annulus and toward the middle scallop of the posterior mitral leaflet. Pulsed wave Doppler flow should demonstrate unidirectional laminar flow from the left ventricle to the inflow cannula with variable systolic augmentation and velocities under 1.5 m/s. The distal ascending aorta of the aorta can be visualized by transesophageal echocardiography in most patients. Flow from the outflow graft should be laminar and unidirectional with variable systolic augmentation. The sample volume should be positioned 1 cm proximal to the aortic anastomosis, and the normal peak velocity ranges from 1 to 2 m/s with unidirectional and slightly pulsatile flow. High flow velocities and nonlaminar flow patterns are suggestive of obstructed cannula flow.

References:

1. Stone ME, Hinchey J. Chapter 28: Mechanical Assist Devices for Heart Failure. In: Kaplan JA, Augoustides JGT, Manecke GR, et al., eds. Kaplan's Cardiac Anesthesia. 7th ed. Elsevier; 2017:1042-1063.
2. Sciaccaluga C, Soliman-Aboumarie H, Sisti N, et al. Echocardiography for left ventricular assist device implantation and evaluation: an indispensable tool. Heart Fail Review, 2022; 27: 891-902.

30. According to the International Society of Heart and Lung Transplantation guidelines, what is the maximum recommended mean arterial pressure for patients with left ventricular assist devices?

A. 60 mmHg
B. 70 mmHg
C. 80 mmHg
D. 90 mmHg

Correct Answer: C

Explanation: According to the International Society of Heart and Lung Transplantation guidelines, the recommended maximum mean arterial pressure is 80 mmHg to avoid complications such as right ventricular failure, stroke, aortic insufficiency, subendocardial ischemia, and arrhythmias.

References:

1. Stone ME, Hinchey J. Chapter 28: Mechanical Assist Devices for Heart Failure. In: Kaplan JA, Augoustides JGT, Manecke GR, et al., eds. Kaplan's Cardiac Anesthesia. 7th ed. Elsevier; 2017:1042-1063.
2. Eisen HJ, Flack JM, Atluri P, et al. Management of hypertension in patients with ventricular assist devices: a scientific statement from the American Heart Association. Circ Heart Fail, 2022; 15: e000074.

CHAPTER 25

Reoperative Cardiac Surgery

Chris Cassara

KEY POINTS

1. Reoperative cardiac surgery presents greater risk than first-time surgery because patients are usually older, have more comorbidities, and have more advanced cardiovascular disease. Also, resternotomy can be hazardous due to adhesions of cardiac structures to the sternum. Bypass conduits may not be available due to prior use, and the frequency of valve replacement versus valve repair is higher.

2. A thorough history, clinical evaluation, and review of imaging must be performed—with particular thought to weighing the risk of surgery against the possibility of medical management with multidisciplinary expertise—before making the decision to proceed.

3. Preinduction anesthetic preparations include placement of defibrillator pads, pacemaker or defibrillator adjustments, and placement of invasive monitoring in the setting of the possibility of peripheral cannulation strategies and alternative cardiopulmonary bypass techniques such as cooling before sternotomy.

4. Coagulopathy can be strategically managed using point-of-care testing to guide blood and blood product transfusion.

5. Emergency reexploration is a high-risk situation in which expeditious surgical intervention is required, usually in the setting of bleeding with pericardial tamponade. Transfusion should be anticipated, hemodynamics supported, and heparin ready to administer in anticipation of possible cardiopulmonary bypass.

---

1. A 35-year-old female with history of a previous aortic valve replacement for congenital aortic stenosis presents with increasing fatigue. Transthoracic echocardiography demonstrates severe stenosis of the bioprosthetic valve. Balloon aortic valvuloplasty is attempted but results in acute severe aortic insufficiency. What should be performed prior to going to the operating room?
   A. Transesophageal echocardiography
   B. Exercise stress test
   C. Noncontrast computed tomography of the chest
   D. Right heart catheterization

Correct Answer: C

Explanation: Patients with acute severe aortic insufficiency should be expeditiously taken to the operating room. However, plain chest computed tomography of the chest will better delineate the relationship of anatomic structures to the sternum. This imaging information can help risk stratify the sternal entry in this case and inform the design of the anesthetic plan accordingly (see table).

References:

1. Rhee AJ, Chikwe J. Chapter 29: Reoperative Cardiac Surgery. In: Kaplan JA, Augoustides JGT, Manecke GR, et al., eds. Kaplan's Cardiac Anesthesia. 7th ed. Elsevier; 2017:1064-1071.
2. Roselli EE, Pettersson GB, Blackstone EH, et al. Adverse events during reoperative cardiac surgery: frequency, characterization, and rescue. J Thorac Cardiovasc Surg, 2008; 135: 316-323.

2. A 65-year-old man with history of a three-vessel coronary artery bypass procedure presents for mitral valve replacement via right thoracotomy. Which of the following preoperative tests should be strongly considered?
   A. Pulmonary function testing
   B. Right heart catheterization
   C. Computed tomographic angiography of the coronary arteries
   D. Upper extremity ultrasound

Correct Answer: A

Explanation: To perform this procedure, one-lung ventilation must be used prior to and after cardiopulmonary bypass.

Pulmonary function testing will give the anesthesiologist insight into how well the patient will tolerate this selective lung ventilation. Generally, an anterolateral thoracotomy is used, and the patient is not fully placed in the lateral decubitus position. The patient's degree of pulmonary shunting may be aggravated by this position, and selective right lung collapse may not be well tolerated if there is significant lung disease. Upper extremity ultrasound will help demonstrate an internal jugular thrombus if present but is not strongly indicated preoperatively. The patient will have coronary angiography prior to the procedure to delineate the coronary anatomy and graft patency. Right heart catheterization might be indicated if there was presence of pulmonary hypertension or right heart dysfunction on the preoperative echocardiogram.

References:

1. Rhee AJ, Chikwe J. Chapter 29: Reoperative Cardiac Surgery. In: Kaplan JA, Augoustides JGT, Manecke GR, et al., eds. Kaplan's Cardiac Anesthesia. 7th ed. Elsevier; 2017:1064-1071.
2. Roselli EE, Pettersson GB, Blackstone EH, et al. Adverse events during reoperative cardiac surgery: frequency, characterization, and rescue. J Thorac Cardiovasc Surg, 2008; 135: 316-323.

3. A 65-year-old man with history of a three-vessel coronary artery bypass procedure presents for mitral valve replacement via right thoracotomy approach using hypothermic fibrillatory arrest. Transesophageal echocardiographic assessment of which of the following valves would be helpful prior to incision?
   A. Aortic valve
   B. Mitral valve
   C. Tricuspid valve
   D. Pulmonic valve

Correct Answer: A

Explanation: Performing the procedure under hypothermic fibrillatory arrest requires that the patient have a competent aortic valve. If there is greater than moderate aortic insufficiency, the ventricle will become distended, increasing myocardial oxygen demand. The presence of significant aortic regurgitation could result in a modified surgical plan as a result. While the other valves should be inspected as part of a complete exam, their routine assessment will not typically hinder the operation. A significant degree of tricuspid regurgitation is commonly found in this setting and can be readily addressed with annuloplasty in most cases.

References:

1. Rhee AJ, Chikwe J. Chapter 29: Reoperative Cardiac Surgery. In: Kaplan JA, Augoustides JGT, Manecke GR, et al., eds. Kaplan's Cardiac Anesthesia. 7th ed. Elsevier; 2017:1064-1071.
2. Antunes PE, Ferrão de Oliveira J, Prieto D, et al. Coronary artery bypass surgery without cardioplegia: hospital results in 8515 patients. Eur J Cardiothorac Surg, 2016; 49: 918-925.

4. A 72-year-old man with prior coronary artery bypass presents for mitral valve repair via right thoracotomy approach. During initial dissection with incomplete cardiac exposure, the patient develops ventricular fibrillation. What is the next best step in management?
   A. External defibrillation at 200 J
   B. Internal defibrillation at 20 J
   C. Reinflation of the right lung
   D. Amiodarone infusion

Correct Answer: C

Explanation: During dissection via the thoracotomy approach, the right lung must be deflated. If an arrhythmia occurs at this time, internal defibrillation will not be able to be performed, given that the entire heart is not exposed. Improved current transmission will occur through the reinflated lung and should ideally occur prior to external defibrillation.

References:

1. Rhee AJ, Chikwe J. Chapter 29: Reoperative Cardiac Surgery. In: Kaplan JA, Augoustides JGT, Manecke GR, et al., eds. Kaplan's Cardiac Anesthesia. 7th ed. Elsevier; 2017:1064-1071.
2. Pahwa S, Stephens EH, Dearani JA. High-risk reoperative sternotomy-how we do it, how we teach it. World J Pediatr Congenit Heart Surg, 2020; 11: 459-465.

5. Prior to induction of anesthesia for reoperative cardiac surgery, which of the following should be placed?
   A. External defibrillator pads
   B. Arterial pressure monitoring catheter
   C. Central venous catheter
   D. Near infrared spectroscopy

Correct Answer: A

Explanation: The rate of arrhythmia increases during redo cardiac surgery. Although certain monitoring lines may be placed prior to induction of anesthesia, external defibrillator pads should be considered for all patients undergoing reoperative cardiac surgery prior to anesthetic induction. Near infrared spectroscopy pads could also be placed prior to induction, but that is to obtain a baseline before any sedative medication is administered.

References:

1. Rhee AJ, Chikwe J. Chapter 29: Reoperative Cardiac Surgery. In: Kaplan JA, Augoustides JGT, Manecke GR, et al., eds. Kaplan's Cardiac Anesthesia. 7th ed. Elsevier; 2017:1064-1071.
2. Pahwa S, Stephens EH, Dearani JA. High-risk reoperative sternotomy-how we do it, how we teach it. World J Pediatr Congenit Heart Surg, 2020; 11: 459-465.

6. Which of the following arrhythmias is most common during the dissection phase after resternotomy?
   A. Ventricular fibrillation
   B. Ventricular tachycardia
   C. Atrial fibrillation
   D. Atrial flutter

Correct Answer: A

Explanation: External defibrillator pads should be attached to the patient prior to induction for reoperative cardiac surgery. These pads remain on the patient for the entire case because electrocautery of the adhesions may directly induce ventricular fibrillation, the most common arrhythmia in resternotomy, and internal paddles cannot be applied effectively until the heart is dissected out. Ventricular fibrillation can also be induced if there is damage to the patent bypass grafts during mediastinal dissection, causing severe myocardial ischemia. Arrhythmias can be minimized by using short bursts of cautery when in close proximity to the ventricle.

References:

1. Rhee AJ, Chikwe J. Chapter 29: Reoperative Cardiac Surgery. In: Kaplan JA, Augoustides JGT, Manecke GR, et al., eds. Kaplan's Cardiac Anesthesia. 7th ed. Elsevier; 2017:1064-1071.
2. Pahwa S, Stephens EH, Dearani JA. High-risk reoperative sternotomy-how we do it, how we teach it. World J Pediatr Congenit Heart Surg, 2020; 11: 459-465.
3. Whang B, Filsoufi F, Fischer GW, et al. The left thoracotomy approach for reoperative cardiac surgery: considerations for the anesthesiologist. J Cardiothorac Vasc Anesth, 2011; 25: 134-139.

7. During axillary artery cannulation, what is the most common complication?
   A. Cerebrovascular embolus
   B. Brachial plexus injury
   C. Upper extremity ischemia
   D. Axillary artery dissection

Correct Answer: B

Explanation: Cannulation of the axillary artery may be preferred when central aortic cannulation is hazardous in the setting of severe atheroma and/or proximity to the sternum in the reoperative setting. The rate of atherosclerotic disease of the axillary is low and therefore has favorably low rates of atheroembolism. Complications of limb ischemia and arterial dissection are reduced when a vascular graft that permits cannulation for cardiopulmonary bypass is sewn to the side of the axillary artery. Given the artery's proximity to the brachial plexus in the infraclavicular position, there is an increased rate of injury due to stretching of the nerves during the cannulation process.

References:

1. Rhee AJ, Chikwe J. Chapter 29: Reoperative Cardiac Surgery. In: Kaplan JA, Augoustides JGT, Manecke GR, et al., eds. Kaplan's Cardiac Anesthesia. 7th ed. Elsevier; 2017:1064-1071.
2. Choudhary SK, Reddy PR. Cannulation strategies in aortic surgery: techniques and decision making. Indian J Thorac Cardiovasc Surg, 2022; 38: 132-145.

8. During femoral artery cannulation in the elderly, which of the following complications is greatly increased compared to other sites?
   A. Cerebrovascular embolus
   B. Limb ischemia
   C. Arterial dissection
   D. Neurovascular injury

Correct Answer: A

Explanation: Elderly patients tend to have more atherosclerotic disease of the descending aorta when compared to younger individuals. When choosing to cannulate the femoral artery, the risk of cerebrovascular embolus is increased when retrograde flow is established during cardiopulmonary bypass. This risk is greater than other cannulation sites where they utilize antegrade flow. The degree of aortic atheroma in the descending thoracic aorta can be accurately assessed with transesophageal echocardiography. The detection of severe atheroma in this setting should prompt consideration for alternative arterial access in an effort to reduce the overall stroke risk.

References:

1. Rhee AJ, Chikwe J. Chapter 29: Reoperative Cardiac Surgery. In: Kaplan JA, Augoustides JGT, Manecke GR, et al., eds. Kaplan's Cardiac Anesthesia. 7th ed. Elsevier; 2017:1064-1071.
2. Choudhary SK, Reddy PR. Cannulation strategies in aortic surgery: techniques and decision making. Indian J Thorac Cardiovasc Surg, 2022; 38: 132-145.
3. Orihashi K, Suedra T, Okada K, et al. Detection and monitoring of complications associated with femoral or axillary arterial cannulation for repair of aortic dissection. J Cardiothorac Vasc Anesth, 2006; 20: 20-25.

9. A 70-year-old man presents for aortic valve replacement due to severe stenosis of a prosthetic aortic valve. Cardiopulmonary bypass is initiated via the femoral artery and vein prior to sternotomy due to the proximity of the ascending aorta to the sternum. There is a high-pressure alarm on cardiopulmonary bypass and low flows when attempting to increase the pump speed. Which of the following complications has most likely occurred?
   A. Femoral artery thrombus
   B. Retrograde aortic dissection
   C. Cardiopulmonary bypass "air lock"
   D. Low reservoir volume

Correct Answer: B

Explanation: High-pressure alarms on cardiopulmonary bypass are seen with impediments to flow in the arterial cannula. Femoral artery thrombosis generally occurs distal to the cannula and causes low extremity ischemia. Retrograde dissection is a complication of femoral artery cannulation and will present with higher pressures and low flows when the false lumen is pressurized. Air lock results when air enters the venous system, causing low pressure and flow.

References:

1. Rhee AJ, Chikwe J. Chapter 29: Reoperative Cardiac Surgery. In: Kaplan JA, Augoustides JGT, Manecke GR, et al., eds. Kaplan's Cardiac Anesthesia. 7th ed. Elsevier; 2017:1064-1071.
2. Choudhary SK, Reddy PR. Cannulation strategies in aortic surgery: techniques and decision making. Indian J Thorac Cardiovasc Surg, 2022; 38: 132-145.
3. Orihashi K, Suedra T, Okada K, et al. Detection and monitoring of complications associated with femoral or axillary arterial cannulation for repair of aortic dissection. J Cardiothorac Vasc Anesth, 2006; 20: 20-25.

10. A 70-year-old man presents for mitral valve replacement due to severe stenosis of the prosthetic valve. He is found to have severe pulmonary hypertension on his preoperative workup. Which technique will likely reduce the risk of injury to right-sided structures?

A. Institution of cardiopulmonary bypass prior to sternotomy

B. Axillary artery cannulation

C. Nitric oxide utilization

D. Induced systemic hypotension

Correct Answer: A

Explanation: This patient will likely have a distended right ventricle due to his pulmonary hypertension, and this will be in close proximity to the sternum. By initializing cardiopulmonary bypass prior to sternotomy, the right ventricle will be decompressed and reduce the risk of laceration on re-entry. Axillary artery cannulation, while useful in reoperation, will not decompress the right ventricle. Nitric oxide is a potent pulmonary artery vasodilator and may decompress the right ventricle, but not likely to the extent required to prevent injury. Furthermore, in this setting, it should be utilized with caution as it may precipitate pulmonary edema, since the increased transpulmonary flow will acutely increase left atrial pressure in the setting of severe prosthetic mitral stenosis.

References:

1. Rhee AJ, Chikwe J. Chapter 29: Reoperative Cardiac Surgery. In: Kaplan JA, Augoustides JGT, Manecke GR, et al., eds. Kaplan's Cardiac Anesthesia. 7th ed. Elsevier; 2017:1064-1071.
2. Breglio A, Anyanwu A, Itagaki S, et al. Does prior coronary bypass surgery present a unique risk for reoperative valve surgery? Ann Thorac Surg, 2013; 95: 1603-1608.

11. A 65-year-old man with history of a three-vessel coronary bypass procedure presents for mitral valve replacement via right thoracotomy approach. Which of the following temperature ranges should be achieved while on cardiopulmonary bypass with a hypothermic fibrillatory arrest technique?

A. 28°C to 34°C

B. 25°C to 27°C

C. 14°C to 27°C

D. Below 14°C

Correct Answer: B

Explanation: The right thoracotomy approach for cardiac surgery lessens the complications associated with sternal re-entry. However, access to the ascending aorta can prove difficult and may not allow a cross clamp to be applied. In a patient with patent bypass grafts, myocardial protection will be insufficient due to the washout from the grafts. Therefore, the surgeon may decide to perform the procedure under fibrillatory arrest. To provide adequate myocardial protection, the heart will need to be decompressed and cooled to approximately 26°C.

References:

1. Rhee AJ, Chikwe J. Chapter 29: Reoperative Cardiac Surgery. In: Kaplan JA, Augoustides JGT, Manecke GR, et al., eds. Kaplan's Cardiac Anesthesia. 7th ed. Elsevier; 2017:1064-1071.
2. Arcidi JM Jr, Rodriguez E, Elbeery JR, et al. Fifteen-year experience with minimally invasive approach for reoperations involving the mitral valve. J Thorac Cardiovasc Surg, 2012; 143: 1062-1068.

12. In patients with patent internal mammary artery grafts, all of these strategies will improve myocardial protection during aortic cross clamping for reoperative cardiac surgery EXCEPT:

A. Clamping the internal mammary artery graft

B. Using off-pump techniques

C. Cooling to 25°C to 27°C

D. Retrograde cardioplegia

Correct Answer: D

Explanation: Patients undergoing reoperative cardiac surgery usually have worse myocardial function with more advanced coronary and valvular disease than those undergoing primary surgery. Reoperation includes technical challenges that will increase the cross clamp time. Any patent internal mammary artery grafts will perfuse the coronary circulation with systemic blood flow after cross clamping of the aorta, washing out the cardioplegia, reducing the potassium concentration, and increasing the temperature of blood, causing the areas of myocardium not perfused by the mammary graft to become ischemic. Approaches to prevent this phenomenon include clamping the mammary graft, cooling the patient to 25°C to 27°C to supply the heart with cold blood, or avoiding arrest by using off-pump or beating heart techniques. Retrograde cardioplegia does not protect the heart well in this setting due to washout of cardioplegia.

References:

1. Rhee AJ, Chikwe J. Chapter 29: Reoperative Cardiac Surgery. In: Kaplan JA, Augoustides JGT, Manecke GR, et al., eds. Kaplan's Cardiac Anesthesia. 7th ed. Elsevier; 2017:1064-1071.
2. Breglio A, Anyanwu A, Itagaki S, et al. Does prior coronary bypass surgery present a unique risk for reoperative valve surgery? Ann Thorac Surg, 2013; 95: 1603-1608.

13. A 30-year-old man with a history of a tetralogy of Fallot repair presents with severe pulmonic insufficiency requiring pulmonic valve replacement. Initially, the axillary artery is cannulated. However, during sternal re-entry, massive hemorrhage is encountered. What is the next best step in management?

A. Initialization of "sucker bypass"

B. Insertion of a femoral venous cannula

C. Institution of massive transfusion protocol

D. Administration of inotropes

Correct Answer: A

Explanation: After injury to a great vessel or the right ventricle, the first measure should be to initiate cardiopulmonary bypass and decompress the heart. If a venous cannula is not in place, suction catheters should be placed in the field to return blood to the circuit and temporize the situation. Massive transfusion and administration of inotropes/pressors should occur as well to facilitate hemodynamic stability, but this will not typically keep up with the rate of bleeding from a large vessel injury.

References:
1. Rhee AJ, Chikwe J. Chapter 29: Reoperative Cardiac Surgery. In: Kaplan JA, Augoustides JGT, Manecke GR, et al., eds. Kaplan's Cardiac Anesthesia. 7th ed. Elsevier; 2017:1064-1071.
2. Gerstein NS, Panikkath PV, Mirrakhimov AE, et al. Cardiopulmonary bypass emergencies and intraoperative issues. J Cardiothorac Vasc Anesth, 2022; 6: 4505-4522.

14. A 61-year-old woman with history of prior mitral valve repair now presents with severe mitral stenosis and is undergoing a redo sternotomy for mitral valve replacement. During sternotomy, the right ventricle is lacerated, and cardiopulmonary bypass is emergently instituted. What is the dose of intravenous heparin that is required?
  A. 200 to 300 units/kg
  B. 300 to 400 units/kg
  C. 300 to 400 mg/kg
  D. 400 to 500 mg/kg

Correct Answer: B

Explanation: Heparin doses of 300 to 400 units/kg will reliably achieve activated clotting times over 350 seconds and heparin levels over 2.0 units/mL, which is required prior to the initialization of cardiopulmonary bypass. Although activated clotting times between 180 and 300 seconds have been described as safe, activated clotting time below 180 seconds will typically not protect against catastrophic thrombus formation in the cardiopulmonary bypass circuit.

References:
1. Rhee AJ, Chikwe J. Chapter 29: Reoperative Cardiac Surgery. In: Kaplan JA, Augoustides JGT, Manecke GR, et al., eds. Kaplan's Cardiac Anesthesia. 7th ed. Elsevier; 2017:1064-1071.
2. Finley A, Greenberg C. Review article: heparin sensitivity and resistance: management during cardiopulmonary bypass. Anesth Analg, 2013; 116: 1210-1222.
3. Gerstein NS, Panikkath PV, Mirrakhimov AE, et al. Cardiopulmonary bypass emergencies and intraoperative issues. J Cardiothorac Vasc Anesth, 2022; 6: 4505-4522.

15. Indications for re-exploration for bleeding after cardiac surgery include all EXCEPT:
  A. More than 400 mL of blood loss in one hour
  B. More than 1 L of blood loss in 24 hours
  C. More than 200 mL/hour for more than 2 hours
  D. Bleeding associated with hypotension

Correct Answer: B

Explanation: In general, indications that the patient may require re-exploration for bleeding include (1) greater than 400 mL bleeding in 1 hour; (2) greater than 200 mL/hour for more than 2 hours; (3) greater than 2 L of blood loss in 24 hours; (4) increasing rate of bleeding, particularly in the absence of coagulopathy; and (5) bleeding associated with hypotension, low cardiac output, or tamponade. These criteria require frequent reassessment in real time to minimize complications and facilitate prompt further investigation and clinical rescue as needed.

References:
1. Rhee AJ, Chikwe J. Chapter 29: Reoperative Cardiac Surgery. In: Kaplan JA, Augoustides JGT, Manecke GR, et al., eds. Kaplan's Cardiac Anesthesia. 7th ed. Elsevier; 2017:1064-1071.
2. Raphael J, Mazer CD, Subramani S, et al. Society of Cardiovascular Anesthesiologists clinical practice improvement advisory for management of perioperative bleeding and hemostasis in cardiac surgery patients. J Cardiothorac Vasc Anesth, 2019; 33: 2887-2899.

16. During a resternotomy, which is the structure that is most frequently damaged?
  A. Right ventricle
  B. Aorta
  C. Bypass grafts
  D. Innominate artery

Correct Answer: C

Explanation: Potentially life-threatening injuries related to resternotomy include trauma to patent bypass grafts, which are the most frequently injured structures, especially when they are in close proximity to the sternum. Further critical structures that can be injured during resternotomy include the aorta, right atrium, right ventricle, and innominate vein. Given these risks, the anesthetic plan should be adapted according to the risk of resternotomy (see Table 25.1).

References:
1. Rhee AJ, Chikwe J. Chapter 29: Reoperative Cardiac Surgery. In: Kaplan JA, Augoustides JGT, Manecke GR, et al., eds. Kaplan's Cardiac Anesthesia. 7th ed. Elsevier; 2017:1064-1071.
2. Breglio A, Anyanwu A, Itagaki S, et al. Does prior coronary bypass surgery present a unique risk for reoperative valve surgery? Ann Thorac Surg, 2013; 95: 1603-1608.

17. An aortic valve replacement has just been completed on a 70-year-old man for severe aortic stenosis. On moving the patient to the transport bed, he develops ventricular fibrillation. What is the next best step in the patient's management?
  A. External defibrillation
  B. Intravenous lidocaine
  C. Cardiopulmonary resuscitation including chest compressions
  D. Emergent re-exploration

Correct Answer: A

Explanation: Traditional advanced cardiac life support calls for immediately starting chest compressions when the patient develops a hemodynamically significant arrhythmia. After cardiac surgery, the incidence of ventricular

TABLE 25.1

Risk stratification of low, medium, high, and very high risk sternotomies, with a summary of operative strategy tailored to address risks

Preoperative Assessment of Risk		Intraoperative Strategy
Increasing risk of major injury	Low-risk resternotomy: • Prior cardiac surgery without patent coronary bypass grafts • Aorta and mediastinal structures a safe distance from the sternum (Fig. 25.1A)	• Resternotomy, dissection of adhesions, standard aortocaval cannulation; initiate bypass; proceed with residual adhesiolysis and cardiac surgical procedure • Optional: Expose peripheral cannulation sites before sternotomy
	Moderate-risk resternotomy: • Patent coronary bypass grafts that lie >1 cm from the sternum, including patent left internal mammary artery (IMA) to left anterior descending coronary artery routed lateral to the sternum (*arrow* in Fig. 25.1B)	• As previous • Optional: peripheral arterial cannulation, with 5000 units of heparin given and arterial line flushed intermittently by perfusion; resternotomy and division of adhesions as above • If major vascular injury occurs, venous cannulation can be performed peripherally, and centrally and after full heparinization cardiopulmonary bypass (CPB) is commenced.
	High-risk resternotomy: • Patent left IMA graft crossing midline close to sternum, right ventricle adherent to sternum (Fig. 25.1C), normal aorta in close proximity to sternum • Third- or fourth-time resternotomy	• Peripheral and arterial cannulation with full heparinization before resternotomy • Optional: institute CPB, stop ventilation, and drain venous return into pump reservoir to decompress right side of heart
	Very high-risk resternotomy: • Patent left IMA graft crossing midline adherent to sternum (Fig. 25.1D) and large area of myocardium at risk, aortic tube graft or aneurysm adherent to sternum	• Peripheral and arterial cannulation with full heparinization, institution of CPB, cooling before resternotomy • Optional: circulatory arrest under moderate hypothermia during sternotomy

Risk stratification and risk mitigation approaches for sternotomies. Sternotomy risk is categorized as low, medium... and very high. A review of operative approaches to minimize associated risk is provided.

Modified from Akujuo A, Fischer GW, Chikwe J. Current concepts in reoperative cardiac surgery. Semin Cardiothorac Vasc Anesth, 2009; 13: 206-214.

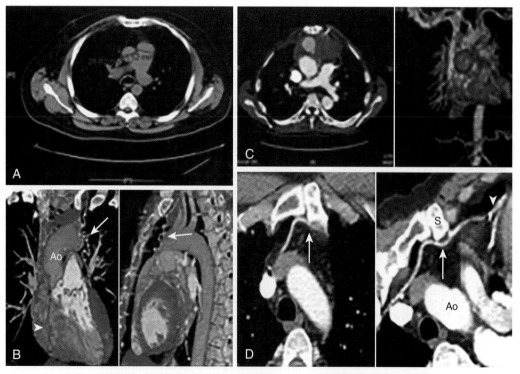

FIGURE 25.1 Cross-sectional imaging of reoperative cardiac surgery patients illustrating anatomy that poses a risk during resternotomy. (A) Low-risk resternotomy: Aorta and pulmonary artery are of normal caliber and well away from the sternum. (B) Moderate-risk resternotomy: Left internal mammary artery graft *(arrow)* is lateral to the sternum. (C) High-risk resternotomy: Right ventricle is adherent to the sternum. (D) Left internal mammary graft crosses the midline posterior to the sternum *(arrow)*. (From Akujuo A, Fischer GW, Chikwe J. Current concepts in reoperative cardiac surgery. Semin Cardiothorac Vasc Anesth. 2009;13:206–214.)

tachycardia/fibrillation is elevated, and it is recommended that the first course of action is defibrillation up to three times. If defibrillation fails, external chest compressions should be performed until the chest is prepped and resternotomy is performed. Open cardiac massage is preferred after the chest is opened.

References:

1. Rhee AJ, Chikwe J. Chapter 29: Reoperative Cardiac Surgery. In: Kaplan JA, Augoustides JGT, Manecke GR, et al., eds. Kaplan's Cardiac Anesthesia. 7th ed. Elsevier; 2017:1064-1071.
2. Society of Thoracic Surgeons Task Force on Resuscitation After Cardiac Surgery. The Society of Thoracic Surgeons Expert Consensus for the Resuscitation of Patients Who Arrest After Cardiac Surgery. Ann Thorac Surg, 2017; 103: 1005-1020.

18. A tricuspid valve replacement for infective endocarditis has been completed on a 35-year-old woman. While waiting in the operating room for a bed in the intensive care unit, the patient's systolic blood pressure decreases to 60 mmHg with a central venous pressure increase to 30 mmHg and a concomitant fall in the cardiac index to 1.1 L/min/m^2. Transesophageal echocardiogram demonstrates a circumferential effusion. Which of the following is the next best step in management?
   A. Initiate epinephrine infusion
   B. Emergent resternotomy
   C. Begin chest compressions
   D. Administer inhaled nitric oxide

Correct Answer: B

Explanation: The patient is in cardiac tamponade and should be emergently re-explored. The epinephrine infusion may temporize the situation, but definitive treatment will be release of the tamponade and identification of the bleeding source. Nitric oxide would be useful in isolated right heart failure. Chest compressions should not be the first step in management, because after resternotomy and pericardial release the hemodynamics should be restored.

References:

1. Rhee AJ, Chikwe J. Chapter 29: Reoperative Cardiac Surgery. In: Kaplan JA, Augoustides JGT, Manecke GR, et al., eds. Kaplan's Cardiac Anesthesia. 7th ed. Elsevier; 2017:1064-1071.
2. Society of Thoracic Surgeons Task Force on Resuscitation After Cardiac Surgery. The Society of Thoracic Surgeons Expert Consensus for the Resuscitation of Patients Who Arrest After Cardiac Surgery. Ann Thorac Surg, 2017; 103: 1005-1020.

19. A tricuspid valve replacement for infective endocarditis has been completed on a 45-year-old man. While waiting in the operating room for an intensive care unit (ICU) bed, the patient becomes tachycardic, and the arterial blood pressure waveform becomes flat. Transesophageal echocardiogram does not demonstrate an effusion. Which of the following is the next best step in management?
   A. Initiate epinephrine infusion
   B. Emergent resternotomy

   C. Begin formal cardiopulmonary resuscitation including chest compressions
   D. External defibrillation

Correct Answer: C

Explanation: The patient likely has pulseless electrical activity. Although he is immediately post–cardiac surgery, his management should progress down the typical cardiac arrest algorithm, and chest compressions should be initiated while a cause for this syndrome is elucidated. The differential diagnosis for pulseless electrical activity includes hypoxia, hypothermia, hypo/hyperkalemia, acidosis, hypoglycemia, tamponade, tension pneumothorax, myocardial ischemia, and pulmonary embolus. External defibrillation is the first step when the rhythm is ventricular fibrillation.

References:

1. Rhee AJ, Chikwe J. Chapter 29: Reoperative Cardiac Surgery. In: Kaplan JA, Augoustides JGT, Manecke GR, et al., eds. Kaplan's Cardiac Anesthesia. 7th ed. Elsevier; 2017:1064-1071.
2. Society of Thoracic Surgeons Task Force on Resuscitation After Cardiac Surgery. The Society of Thoracic Surgeons Expert Consensus for the Resuscitation of Patients Who Arrest After Cardiac Surgery. Ann Thorac Surg, 2017; 103: 1005-1020.

20. A tricuspid valve replacement for tricuspid regurgitation has been completed on a 69-year-old woman. On arrival at the intensive care unit, the patient's systolic blood pressure decreases to 60 mmHg with an acute increase in the central venous pressure to 25 mmHg associated with a dilated hypokinetic right ventricle on point-of-care ultrasound. Which of the following is the next best step in management?
   A. Initiate an epinephrine infusion
   B. Return to the operating room
   C. Emergent resternotomy
   D. Begin chest compressions

Correct Answer: A

Explanation: The patient developed severe acute right ventricular systolic dysfunction. Treatment involves the administration of epinephrine, and if the patient remains hypotensive the chest should be emergently opened in the intensive care unit to reduce the intrathoracic pressure, and/or the patient should be cannulated for venoarterial extracorporeal membrane oxygenation. The time to transport to the operating room will be detrimental to the patient's care and likely interfere with clinical stabilization of clinical hemodynamics.

References:

1. Rhee AJ, Chikwe J. Chapter 29: Reoperative Cardiac Surgery. In: Kaplan JA, Augoustides JGT, Manecke GR, et al., eds. Kaplan's Cardiac Anesthesia. 7th ed. Elsevier; 2017:1064-1071.
2. Society of Thoracic Surgeons Task Force on Resuscitation After Cardiac Surgery. The Society of Thoracic Surgeons Expert Consensus for the Resuscitation of Patients Who Arrest After Cardiac Surgery. Ann Thorac Surg, 2017; 103: 1005-1020.
3. Kalagara H, Coker B, Gerstein NS, et al. Point-of-care ultrasound (POCUS) for the cardiothoracic anesthesiologist. J Cardiothorac Vasc Anesth, 2022; 36: 1132-1147.

21. A patient for a redo sternotomy for a mitral valve replacement is found to have patent coronary bypass grafts that lie more than 1 cm from the sternum with a patent left internal mammary graft to the left anterior descending coronary artery lateral to the sternum. What is his risk of injury during resternotomy?
  A. Low risk
  B. Moderate risk
  C. High risk
  D. Very high risk

Correct Answer: B

Explanation: A low-risk resternotomy is defined as prior cardiac surgery without patent coronary bypass grafts with the aorta and mediastinal structures at a safe distance to the sternum. A moderate-risk resternotomy is defined as having patent coronary bypass grafts that lie more than 1 cm from the sternum, including a patent left internal mammary artery (LIMA) graft routed lateral to the sternum. A high-risk resternotomy is defined as having a patent LIMA graft crossing midline close to sternum, right ventricle adherent to sternum, or a normal aorta in close proximity to the sternum. A very high-risk resternotomy is defined as a patent LIMA graft crossing midline adherent to sternum, as well as an aortic tube graft or aneurysm adherent to sternum.

References:

  1. Rhee AJ, Chikwe J. Chapter 29: Reoperative Cardiac Surgery. In: Kaplan JA, Augoustides JGT, Manecke GR, et al., eds. Kaplan's Cardiac Anesthesia. 7th ed. Elsevier; 2017:1064-1071.
  2. Pahwa S, Stephens EH, Dearani JA. High-risk reoperative sternotomy-how we do it, how we teach it. World J Pediatr Congenit Heart Surg, 2020; 11: 459-465.
  3. Whang B, Filsoufi F, Fischer GW, et al. The left thoracotomy approach for reoperative cardiac surgery: considerations for the anesthesiologist. J Cardiothorac Vasc Anesth, 2011; 25: 134-139.

22. A 68-year-old woman is admitted to the intensive care unit after a two-vessel coronary artery bypass graft. Her rhythm deteriorates to ventricular fibrillation, and she is externally defibrillated three times without improvement. Although chest compressions, resternotomy, and internal cardiac massage fail to improve her hemodynamics, what is the next best step in management?
  A. Insertion of an intra-aortic balloon pump
  B. Return to the operating room
  C. Perform coronary angiography
  D. Initiation of venoarterial extracorporeal membrane oxygenation

Correct Answer: D

Explanation: At this point, the patient should be stabilized on venoarterial extracorporeal membrane oxygenation. Although she likely has a problem with one of her grafts that could be evaluated with coronary angiography with the possibility of graft revision in the operating room, she should first be clinically stabilized. An intra-aortic balloon pump may help augment diastolic pressure with cardiac arrest, if it is in place prior to the arrest.

References:

  1. Rhee AJ, Chikwe J. Chapter 29: Reoperative Cardiac Surgery. In: Kaplan JA, Augoustides JGT, Manecke GR, et al., eds. Kaplan's Cardiac Anesthesia. 7th ed. Elsevier; 2017:1064-1071.
  2. Society of Thoracic Surgeons Task Force on Resuscitation After Cardiac Surgery. The Society of Thoracic Surgeons Expert Consensus for the Resuscitation of Patients Who Arrest After Cardiac Surgery. Ann Thorac Surg, 2017; 103: 1005-1020.

23. Which of the following laboratory tests may significantly reduce the rate of red blood cell transfusion during redo cardiac surgery?
  A. International normalized ratio
  B. Partial thromboplastin time
  C. Thromboelastography
  D. Platelet count

Correct Answer: C

Explanation: Redo cardiac surgery predisposes the patient to requiring perioperative blood transfusion. By utilizing point-of-care thromboelastography (TEG) to direct blood product administration, the rate of transfusion can be substantially reduced and possibly affect short term clinical outcomes. The indices from TEG allow for a more targeted administration of blood products and reduce coagulopathic bleeding. Standard tests for coagulation such as the international normalized ratio, partial thromboplastin time, and platelet count may be relatively slow to result and not accurately reflect the patient's coagulation status in real time.

References:

  1. Rhee AJ, Chikwe J. Chapter 29: Reoperative Cardiac Surgery. In: Kaplan JA, Augoustides JGT, Manecke GR, et al., eds. Kaplan's Cardiac Anesthesia. 7th ed. Elsevier; 2017:1064-1071.
  2. Redfern RE, Fleming K, March RL, et al. Thrombelastography-directed transfusion in cardiac surgery: impact on postoperative outcomes. Ann Thorac Surg, 2019; 107: 1313-1318.
  3. Raphael J, Mazer CD, Subramani S, et al. Society of Cardiovascular Anesthesiologists clinical practice improvement advisory for management of perioperative bleeding and hemostasis in cardiac surgery patients. J Cardiothorac Vasc Anesth, 2019; 33: 2887-2899.

24. In patients transfused with large volumes of salvaged blood, which of the following factors is most likely responsible for continued coagulopathy?
  A. Low fibrinogen
  B. Low serum calcium
  C. Residual heparin
  D. Low platelet count

Correct Answer: C

Explanation: Despite the salvaged blood being washed, there may be a small amount of heparin in the blood that is being transfused. When the volumes of salvaged blood transfusion become large, a significant elevation in activated clotting time may be seen. The other coagulation factors will likely decrease if there is increased surgical bleeding; however, heparin reversal should be considered along with transfusion of coagulation factors. The presence of heparin can be assessed with point-of-care heparinase thromboelastography before additional protamine is administered.

References:

1. Rhee AJ, Chikwe J. Chapter 29: Reoperative Cardiac Surgery. In: Kaplan JA, Augoustides JGT, Manecke GR, et al., eds. Kaplan's Cardiac Anesthesia. 7th ed. Elsevier; 2017:1064-1071.
2. Son K, Yamada T, Tarao K, et al. Effects of cardiac surgery and salvaged blood transfusion on coagulation function assessed by thromboelastometry. J Cardiothorac Vasc Anesth, 2020; 34: 2375-2382.

25. A 65-year-old man undergoes mitral valve replacement due to bioprosthetic valve endocarditis. At the end of the procedure, there appears to be coagulopathic bleeding despite normal coagulation parameters. Which of the following may be considered to improve bleeding?
   A. Prothrombin complex concentrate
   B. Tranexamic acid
   C. Protamine
   D. Fibrinogen concentrate

Correct Answer: A

Explanation: In patients where surgical bleeding has been ruled out, point-of-care testing can be performed to determine any coagulation defects. If bleeding persists after the administration of blood products, both recombinant activated factor VIIa or prothrombin complex concentrates have been used successfully to treat bleeding after cardiac surgery. The incidences of bleeding and thrombotic complications after cardiac surgery are likely equivalent with either agent, as reflected by chest tube output, re-exploration rates, thromboembolic complications, and length of stay in the intensive care unit. Tranexamic acid, protamine, and fibrinogen may assist in restoring coagulation balance, especially when strongly indicated by relevant point-of-care coagulation indices.

References:

1. Rhee AJ, Chikwe J. Chapter 29: Reoperative Cardiac Surgery. In: Kaplan JA, Augoustides JGT, Manecke GR, et al., eds. Kaplan's Cardiac Anesthesia. 7th ed. Elsevier; 2017:1064-1071.
2. Katz A, Ahuja T, Arnouk, et al. A comparison of prothrombin complex concentrate and recombinant activated factor VII for the management of bleeding with cardiac surgery. J Intensive Care Med, 2022; 37: 231-239.
3. Raphael J, Mazer CD, Subramani S, et al. Society of Cardiovascular Anesthesiologists clinical practice improvement advisory for management of perioperative bleeding and hemostasis in cardiac surgery patients. J Cardiothorac Vasc Anesth, 2019; 33: 2887-2899.

26. A 26-year-old male with a history of congenital heart disease presents for a pulmonic valve replacement. This will be his fourth sternotomy. What is his anticipated risk for complications during sternotomy?
   A. Low
   B. Moderate
   C. High
   D. Very high

Correct Answer: C

Explanation: A third or fourth resternotomy is considered a high-risk procedure. Consequently, the preoperative chest imaging should be reviewed and the specific risks discussed with the surgical team to inform the anesthetic plan (see Table 25.1).

References:

1. Rhee AJ, Chikwe J. Chapter 29: Reoperative Cardiac Surgery. In: Kaplan JA, Augoustides JGT, Manecke GR, et al., eds. Kaplan's Cardiac Anesthesia. 7th ed. Elsevier; 2017:1064-1071.
2. Pahwa S, Stephens EH, Dearani JA. High-risk reoperative sternotomy-how we do it, how we teach it. World J Pediatr Congenit Heart Surg, 2020; 11: 459-465.

27. A 70-year-old man presents for aortic valve replacement due to severe stenosis of the prosthetic valve. Cardiopulmonary bypass is initiated via the femoral artery and vein prior to sternotomy due to the proximity of the ascending aorta to the sternum. The procedure progresses uneventfully; however, after decannulation, the patient becomes hemodynamically unstable with a decreasing hematocrit and progressive hypovolemia. Which of the following complications has most likely occurred?
   A. Femoral artery thrombus
   B. Retrograde aortic dissection
   C. Retroperitoneal hematoma
   D. Coagulopathic bleeding

Correct Answer: C

Explanation: Retrograde dissection is a complication of femoral artery cannulation and will present with higher pressures and low flows when the false lumen is pressurized. A retroperitoneal hematoma may present after a misplaced cannula; however, adequate flow on cardiopulmonary bypass would not be able to be achieved. Generally, an injury to the femoral artery is made during placement of the arterial cannula, and it is discovered after decannulation when the tamponade has been released.

References:

1. Rhee AJ, Chikwe J. Chapter 29: Reoperative Cardiac Surgery. In: Kaplan JA, Augoustides JGT, Manecke GR, et al., eds. Kaplan's Cardiac Anesthesia. 7th ed. Elsevier; 2017:1064-1071.
2. Choudhary SK, Reddy PR. Cannulation strategies in aortic surgery: techniques and decision making. Indian J Thorac Cardiovasc Surg, 2022; 38: 132-145.
3. Ghadimi K, Vernick WJ, Horak J, et al. Case 12 – 2014 Inferior vena cava compression by retroperitoneal hematoma during cardiopulmonary bypass. J Cardiothorac Vasc Anesth, 2014; 28: 1403-1409.

28. A 47-year-old man undergoes a redo mitral valve replacement for infective endocarditis. Throughout the procedure, the patient requires several units of packed red blood cells, cryoprecipitate, and platelets. The surgical field is hemostatic; however, after chest closure the mediastinal drainage tubes have increased their output to 500 mL per hour. What is the next best step in management?

A. Perform chest re-exploration
B. Administer recombinant factor VIIa
C. Administer prothrombin complex concentrate
D. Transfuse packed red blood cells

Correct Answer: A

Explanation: Significant increases in chest tube output constitute an indication for re-exploration. Indications for return to the operating room for bleeding include chest tube output over 500 mL in the first hour, 1000 mL in the first 4 hours, and/or excessive bleeding that results in hemodynamic instability, including tamponade. Patients require intensive monitoring and real-time collaborative decision-making to maintain clinical stability and prompt mediastinal exploration when indicated.

References:

1. Rhee AJ, Chikwe J. Chapter 29: Reoperative Cardiac Surgery. In: Kaplan JA, Augoustides JGT, Manecke GR, et al., eds. Kaplan's Cardiac Anesthesia. 7th ed. Elsevier; 2017:1064-1071.
2. Čanádyová J, Zmeko D, Mokráček A. Re-exploration for bleeding or tamponade after cardiac operation. Interact Cardiovasc Thorac Surg, 2012: 14, 704-707.
3. Raphael J, Mazer CD, Subramani S, et al. Society of Cardiovascular Anesthesiologists clinical practice improvement advisory for management of perioperative bleeding and hemostasis in cardiac surgery patients. J Cardiothorac Vasc Anesth, 2019; 33: 2887-2899.

29. A 64-year-old man with history of two-vessel coronary artery bypass grafting presents for aortic valve replacement. During sternotomy, the patient develops hypotension and recurrent events of ventricular fibrillation requiring aggressive vasoactive support and external defibrillation. Which complication has likely occurred?

A. Laceration of the internal mammary artery
B. Injury to the right ventricle
C. Electrocautery-induced arrhythmia
D. Electrolyte abnormality

Correct Answer: A

Explanation: Re-sternotomy after prior coronary artery bypass grafting may present unique problems for the surgeon. The internal mammary artery graft may adhere to the sternum and be injured on re-entry. This injury may present with severe hypotension, acute anterior wall motion abnormalities, and recurrent ventricular arrhythmias. Although right ventricular injury is also a possibility, it is less likely to present with recurrent ventricular fibrillation.

References:

1. Rhee AJ, Chikwe J. Chapter 29: Reoperative Cardiac Surgery. In: Kaplan JA, Augoustides JGT, Manecke GR, et al., eds. Kaplan's Cardiac Anesthesia. 7th ed. Elsevier; 2017:1064-1071.
2. Breglio A, Anyanwu A, Itagaki S, et al. Does prior coronary bypass surgery present a unique risk for reoperative valve surgery? Ann Thorac Surg, 2013; 95: 1603-1608.

30. A 65-year-old man with history of a four-vessel coronary artery grafting procedure presents for mitral valve replacement via a right thoracotomy approach. Which of the following is important when performing fibrillatory arrest while on cardiopulmonary bypass for this planned procedure?

A. Temperature 28 to 34°C
B. Correct placement of the left ventricular vent
C. Administration of amiodarone
D. Absence of a patent foramen ovale

Correct Answer: B

Explanation: In a patient with patent bypass grafts, myocardial protection will be insufficient due to the washout from the grafts. Therefore, the surgeon may decide to perform the procedure under hypothermic fibrillatory arrest. The heart is constantly perfused and provides the surgeon with a somewhat motionless field. To provide adequate myocardial protection, the left ventricle must be both decompressed to minimize wall tension and also cooled to 26°C to minimize oxygen demand.

References:

1. Rhee AJ, Chikwe J. Chapter 29: Reoperative Cardiac Surgery. In: Kaplan JA, Augoustides JGT, Manecke GR, et al., eds. Kaplan's Cardiac Anesthesia. 7th ed. Elsevier; 2017:1064-1071.
2. Arcidi JM Jr, Rodriguez E, Elbeery JR, et al. Fifteen-year experience with minimally invasive approach for reoperations involving the mitral valve. J Thorac Cardiovasc Surg, 2012; 143: 1062-1068.

CHAPTER 26

Patient Safety in the Cardiac Operating Room

Michael L. Boisen

KEY POINTS

1. Cardiac surgical patients are at significant risk from preventable adverse events. These events occur through human error, by either faulty decision making (diagnosis, decision for treatment) or faulty actions (failure to implement the plan correctly).

2. Human error is ubiquitous and cannot be prevented or eliminated by trying harder or by eliminating the one who errs. Reduction in human error requires system changes that prevent errors from occurring (forcing functions) or prevent errors from reaching the patient.

3. Sleep deprivation and fatigue can render a person more likely to make an error. Although residents' hours are limited, those of other physicians in the United States are not, unlike in other countries.

4. Nontechnical skills such as leadership, communication, cooperation, and situational awareness are critical to patient safety, but they are rarely taught. Distractions, disruptions, noise, and alarms contribute to technical errors and increase mortality rates in cardiac surgery.

5. Communication is the leading root cause of sentinel events, whether through missing information or through misunderstanding. Use of structured communication protocols reduces errors. Handoffs performed without protocol involve significant numbers of omitted items.

6. Team training reduces surgical mortality rates, but it must be done with careful preparation and with regular retraining.

7. Surgical briefings that use a checklist significantly reduce surgical mortality rates (World Health Organization Safe Surgery Saves Lives). Debriefings allow teams to identify hazards and formulate improvements.

8. Simulation is an effective means to teach both technical and nontechnical skills and to allow teams to train for rare but dangerous events.

9. Cognitive aids should be available in every operating room to provide direction during rare crisis events (e.g., malignant hyperthermia, pulseless electrical activity).

10. Medication errors occur in approximately 1 in every 150 to 200 anesthetic cases. The Anesthesia Patient Safety Foundation published a set of recommendations to reduce medication errors, including standardization, using technology such as bar codes and smart infusion pumps, having pharmacy involvement in every step of the medication process, and building a culture of safety.

11. Awareness during anesthesia occurs approximately 1 to 2 times per 1000 anesthetic cases, and it occurs more often in cardiac surgical procedures. Use of a processed electroencephalogram or achieving an end-tidal concentration of 0.7 minimum alveolar concentration is effective in reducing the incidence of awareness.

12. The culture of an organization or a unit contributes significantly to patient safety or danger. Strict hierarchical cultures typically harbor a culture of blame and shame, which inhibits identification and correction of hazards. A "just culture" acknowledges that human error occurs and seeks to redesign the system to prevent future errors, but also holds individual persons accountable for willful violations.

1. All of the following can be considered preventable adverse events EXCEPT:
   A. Syringe swap error
   B. Retained guidewire during central venous catheterization
   C. Allergic reaction in a patient with no known allergies
   D. Wrong-site surgery

Correct Answer: C

Explanation: Adverse events refer to injuries resulting from medical care rather than an underlying disease. Adverse events are considered preventable if avoidable by any means currently available, unless those means are not considered standard care. Syringe swaps are considered preventable by using best labeling practices and/or barcode scanners and smart pumps. Unintentionally retained foreign objects are considered "never events" and can affect hospital reimbursement. Wrong-site or wrong-patient surgeries are preventable using redundant systems to identify the correct site and patient. Allergic reactions are only preventable if a medication administration is inappropriate based on known allergies (negligence).

References:

1. Wahr JA, Bowdle TA, Nussmeier NA. Chapter 30: Patient Safety in the Cardiac Operating Room. In: Kaplan JA, Augoustides JGT, Manecke GR, et al., eds. Kaplan's Cardiac Anesthesia. 7th ed. Elsevier; 2017:1072-1108.
2. Merry AF, Weller J, Mitchell SJ. Improving the quality and safety of patient care in cardiac anesthesia. J Cardiothorac Vasc Anesth, 2014; 28: 1341-1351.

2. Recommended strategies for preventing human errors include all of the following EXCEPT:
   A. Implementing checklists/decision support tools
   B. Identifying and eliminating error-prone individuals
   C. Restricting duty hours to prevent fatigue
   D. Encouraging team members to express safety concerns without fear of reprisal

Correct Answer: B

Explanation: Human error cannot be eliminated, but systems can be designed to reduce the occurrence and mitigate the consequences of errors. Adverse clinical events, though often incited by human errors, usually involve multiple failures that line up to result in a clinical event, as explained by Reason's Swiss cheese model. Therefore, system changes are usually necessary, including using checklists/cognitive aids, implementing measures to prevent and recognize fatigue, and promoting open communication around safety issues in the development of a safety culture.

References:

1. Wahr JA, Bowdle TA, Nussmeier NA. Chapter 30: Patient Safety in the Cardiac Operating Room. In: Kaplan JA, Augoustides JGT, Manecke GR, et al., eds. Kaplan's Cardiac Anesthesia. 7th ed. Elsevier; 2017:1072-1108.
2. Merry AF, Weller J, Mitchell SJ. Improving the quality and safety of patient care in cardiac anesthesia. J Cardiothorac Vasc Anesth, 2014; 28: 1341-1351.

3. Which of the following is/are examples of system failures that may influence human errors?
   A. Orientation/training failures
   B. Inadequate staffing levels
   C. Poor equipment design
   D. All of the above are examples of system failures

Correct Answer: D

Explanation: System failures in the health system organization are remote from the control of individual clinicians and are usually the distal cause of structure and process failures. Decisions made at higher levels within the organization create latent conditions upstream from human failures in the accident causal chain, as outlined in the Swiss cheese model of safety events. System-based or organizational factors have been commonly implicated in anesthetic safety incidents. These failures include training and supervision problems, inadequate manpower or assistance, and equipment problems.

BOX 26.1 **Factors contributing to safety violations in healthcare**

Individual Traits
- Experience (knows a better way to get it done, which may be correct)
- Attitude toward compliance (worker's beliefs about likely outcomes)
- Previous accident (no previous incident leads to belief that violation is safe)
- Previous injury
- Laziness (reported only as a contributing factor in others)

Information, Education, Training
- Level of knowledge (knowledge of rules, policies, and regulations)
- Conflict or confusion among staff members
- Level of training (lack of familiarity with regulations)
- Level of training (may increase or decrease likelihood of violation)
- Unfamiliarity with design

Design Flaws
- Poor design requiring violation (design of tool or environment makes compliance impossible)
- Changes to approved design (rules apply to previous design and do not fit the newer design)
- Required equipment not available
- Complicated design

Safety Climate
- Poor management (lack of supervision, senior workers giving advice to violate)
- Management tolerating or approving violations (management ignores or encourages violation to meet other goals)

BOX 26.1   Factors contributing to safety violations in healthcare—cont'd

- Subjective norm to comply (normalization of deviance)
- Perceived expectations by doctors (nurse perceives expectation is to violate)

Competing Goals

- Time pressure (quicker way of working to save time)
- Work pressure (unable to complete task unless rule is violated)
- Perceived risk (if low or no risk, more likely to violate)

- Conflicting demands (cannot achieve one goal without violating another goal)
- Physical fatigue or exhaustion

Problems with Rules

- Impossible rule to work within
- Complex rule (no one understands the rule)
- Outdated rule (violation may result in greater safety)
- Difficult rule to comply with (technically difficult to comply)

Modified from Alper SJ, Karsh BT. A systematic review of safety violations in industry. Accid Anal Prev, 2009; 41: 739-754.

References:

1. Wahr JA, Bowdle TA, Nussmeier NA. Chapter 30: Patient Safety in the Cardiac Operating Room. In: Kaplan JA, Augoustides JGT, Manecke GR, et al., eds. Kaplan's Cardiac Anesthesia. 7th ed. Elsevier; 2017:1072-1108.
2. Reason J. Safety in the operating theatre – Part 2: Human error and organizational failure. Qual Saf Health Care, 2005; 14: 56-61.
3. Runciman WB, Webb RK, Lee R, et al. System failure: an analysis of 2000 incident reports. Anaesth Intens Care, 1993; 21: 684-695.
4. Nin OC, Looper JN, Summer SS, et al. Are you emotionally intelligent? Improving patient safety and quality through better communication. J Cardiothorac Vasc Anesth, 2022; 36: 936-939.

4. Which term describes an event that can result in death, permanent harm, and/or severe temporary harm?
  A. Adverse event
  B. Close call
  C. Sentinel event
  D. Never event

Correct Answer: C

Explanation: Sentinel events have been defined as "unexpected occurrences involving death or serious physiological or psychological injury, or the risk thereof." Such events are called sentinel because they signal the need for immediate investigation and response by the health system organization. Sentinel event reporting has been recommended, with state-level reporting required in many states. Adverse events are serious, undesirable, and usually unanticipated events that result in harm to the patient. A close call event is a patient safety event that could produce harm but was caught before it could do so. Similar to sentinel events, "never events" are serious adverse events that are considered preventable (such as wrong-site surgery), as defined by the National Quality Forum.

References:

1. Wahr JA, Bowdle TA, Nussmeier NA. Chapter 30: Patient Safety in the Cardiac Operating Room. In: Kaplan JA, Augoustides JGT, Manecke GR, et al., eds. Kaplan's Cardiac Anesthesia. 7th ed. Elsevier; 2017:1072-1108.
2. Merry AF, Weller J, Mitchell SJ. Improving the quality and safety of patient care in cardiac anesthesia. J Cardiothorac Vasc Anesth, 2014; 28: 1341-1351.

5. Recommended best practices for prevention of medication errors in the operating room include all of the following EXCEPT:
  A. Pre-preparation of high-alert drugs by the pharmacy in a ready-to-use form
  B. Prelabeling of empty syringes in batches
  C. Use of standardized, route-specific tubing connections
  D. Use of standardized drug libraries within infusion pumps

Correct Answer: B

Explanation: Recommendations for improving medication safety in the operating room include preparation of high-alert drugs (e.g., epinephrine) by the pharmacy, adoption of standardized route-specific connectors for tubing (e.g., intravenous, arterial, epidural platforms), and delivery of infusions with electronically controlled devices containing a drug library. The prelabeling of empty syringes in batches has not been recommended. This labeling should occur at the time a medication is transferred from the original packaging into a syringe or other container. The recommendations for medication safety are summarized in a teaching box.

References:

1. Wahr JA, Bowdle TA, Nussmeier NA. Chapter 30: Patient Safety in the Cardiac Operating Room. In: Kaplan JA, Augoustides JGT, Manecke GR, et al., eds. Kaplan's Cardiac Anesthesia. 7th ed. Elsevier; 2017:1072-1108.
2. Neira VM, Scheffler M, Wong D, et al. Survey of the preparation of cardiovascular emergency medications for adult cardiovascular anesthesia. J Cardiothorac Vasc Anesth, 2021; 35: 1813-1820.

6. Types of human errors include all of the following EXCEPT:
  A. Slips and lapses
  B. Mistakes
  C. Violations
  D. Latent

Correct Answer: D

Explanation: Human errors can be considered as unintentional failures (slips and lapses) or failures of intention (mistakes). Slips and lapses are failures to execute a plan because of attention and memory failures, respectively. Mistakes are actions that are executed as planned, but the plan is

BOX 26.2   Consensus recommendations for improving medication safety in the operating room

Standardization

1. High-alert drugs (e.g., phenylephrine and epinephrine) should be available in standardized concentrations or diluents prepared by the pharmacy in a ready-to-use (bolus or infusion) form that is appropriate for both adult and pediatric patients. Infusions should be delivered by an electronically controlled smart device containing a drug library.
2. Ready-to-use syringes and infusions should have standardized, fully compliant, machine-readable labels.
3. *Additional ideas*
   a. Interdisciplinary and uniform curriculum for medication administration safety to be available to all training programs and facilities
   b. No concentrated versions of any potentially lethal agents in the operating room
   c. Required read-back in an environment for extremely high-alert drugs such as heparin
   d. Standardized placement of drugs within all anesthesia workstations in an institution
   e. Convenient required method to save all used syringes and drug containers until the case is concluded
   f. Standardized infusion libraries and protocols throughout an institution
   g. Standardized route-specific connectors for tubing (intravenous, arterial, epidural, enteral)

Technology

1. Every anesthetizing location should have a mechanism to identify medications before drawing up or administering them (bar code reader) and a mechanism to provide feedback, decision support, and documentation (automated information system).
2. *Additional ideas*
   a. Technology training and device education for all users, possibly requiring formal certification

b. Improved and standardized user interfaces on infusion pumps
c. Mandatory safety checklists incorporated into all operating room systems

Pharmacy/Prefilled/Premixed

1. Routine provider-prepared medications should be discontinued whenever possible.
2. Clinical pharmacists should be part of the perioperative and operating room team.
3. Standardized pre-prepared medication kits by case type should be used whenever possible.
4. *Additional ideas*
   a. Interdisciplinary and uniform curriculum for medication administration safety for all anesthesia professionals and pharmacists
   b. Enhanced training of operating room pharmacists specifically as perioperative consultants
   c. Deployment of ubiquitous automated dispensing machines in the operating room suite (with communication to central pharmacy and its information management system)

Culture

1. Establish a "just culture" for reporting errors (including near misses) and discussion of lessons learned.
2. Establish a culture of education, understanding, and accountability through a required curriculum and continuing medical education and through dissemination of dramatic stories in the *APSF Newsletter* and educational videos.
3. Establish a culture of cooperation and recognition of the benefits of the STPC (standardization, technology, pharmacy/prefilled/premixed, and culture) paradigm within and among institutions, professional organizations, and accreditation agencies.

Reprinted from Eichhorn JH. APSF hosts medication safety conference: consensus group defines challenges and opportunities for improved practice. APSF Newslett, 2010; 25: 1-8.

BOX 26.3   Description of human factor levels

Organizational Influences

1. Climate: vision within the organization including policy, command structure, and culture
2. Process: means by which the vision of an organization is carried out, including operations, procedures, and oversight
3. Resource management: how human, monetary, and other resources necessary to carry out the organizational vision are managed

Unsafe Supervision

4. Inadequate supervision: oversight, management of personnel, and resources, including training, guidance, and leadership
5. Problem correction: instances when deficiencies among individual persons, equipment, training, or

other safety areas are "known" to the supervisor yet allowed to continue
6. Inappropriate operations: management of work, including aspects of risk management, crew pairing, and operational tempo

Preconditions to Unsafe Acts

7. Environmental factors
   a. Technologic environment: design of equipment and controls, display-interface characteristics, checklist layouts, task factors, and automation
   b. Physical environment: operational setting and environment (heat, lighting)
8. Adverse mental states: psychological and/or mental conditions, such as fatigue, pernicious attitudes, and misplaced motivation that negatively affect performance

BOX 26.3 Description of human factor levels—cont'd

9. Adverse physiologic states: medical and/or physiologic conditions such as illness, intoxication, and abnormalities known to affect performance

10. Physical or mental limitations: physical or mental disabilities, such as poor vision; lack of skill, aptitude, or knowledge; and other mental illnesses that affect performance

11. Teamwork: communication, coordination, and other teamwork issues that affect performance

12. Personal readiness: off-duty activities, such as adhering to rest requirements, alcohol restrictions, and other mandates required to perform optimally on the job

Unsafe Acts

13. Decision errors: "thinking" errors representing intended behavior that proceeds as designed, yet the plan proves inadequate for the situation. Errors manifest as poorly executed procedures,

improper choices, or simply misinterpretation of relevant information.

14. Skill-based errors: highly practiced behavior that occurs with little thought. These errors frequently appear as breakdown in visual patterns, forgotten intentions, and omitted items during procedures. The technique with which one performs a task is included.

15. Perceptual errors: errors arising when sensory input is degraded. Faced with acting on imperfect or incomplete information, operating room staff members run the risk of misjudging procedures as well as responding incorrectly to a variety of visual-vestibular illusions.

16. Routine violations: "bending the rules," a type of violation that is habitual and often enabled by management that tolerates departures from the rules.

17. Exceptional violations: departures from authority, neither typical of the individual nor condoned by management.

From ElBardissi AW, Wiegmann DA, Dearani JA, et al. Application of the human factors analysis and classification system methodology to the cardiovascular surgery operating room. Ann Thorac Surg, 2007; 83: 1412-1418; discussion 8-9.

inadequate to achieve the desired outcome. Violations are deviations from safe operating practices, whether deliberate or erroneous. Latent errors tend to be removed from the direct control of the human and include things such as design flaws, incorrect installation, faulty maintenance, low-quality management decisions, and poor organizational structures.

References:

1. Wahr JA, Bowdle TA, Nussmeier NA. Chapter 30: Patient Safety in the Cardiac Operating Room. In: Kaplan JA, Augoustides JGT, Manecke GR, et al., eds. Kaplan's Cardiac Anesthesia. 7th ed. Elsevier; 2017:1072-1108.
2. Reason J. Safety in the operating theatre – Part 2: Human error and organizational failure. Qual Saf Health Care, 2005; 14: 56-61.

7. Technology-related hazards in the cardiac operating rooms can result from all of these issues EXCEPT:
   A. Limited maintenance of malfunctioning equipment
   B. Flaws in equipment design
   C. Training protocols for new equipment
   D. Adverse impact of technology on human cognitive processes

Correct Answer: C

Explanation: Technology plays a key role in safety-critical systems including the cardiac operating room environment. Technology-related hazards are not limited to malfunctioning equipment, but also commonly arise due to suboptimal human–technology interactions. In an observational study of safety hazards in cardiovascular operating rooms, technology-related safety hazards were found to negatively impact provider cognition and behavior. Consideration of human factors in design of technologies and layout of physical spaces is required in order for technology to mitigate rather than amplify latent risks to patient safety. Training protocols have been

recommended to enhance patient safety during the introduction of new technology into the perioperative environment.

References:

1. Wahr JA, Bowdle TA, Nussmeier NA. Chapter 30: Patient Safety in the Cardiac Operating Room. In: Kaplan JA, Augoustides JGT, Manecke GR, et al., eds. Kaplan's Cardiac Anesthesia. 7th ed. Elsevier; 2017:1072-1108.
2. Martinez EA, Thompson DA, Errett NA, et al. Review article: high stakes and high risk: a focused qualitative review of hazards during cardiac surgery. Anesth Analg, 2011; 112: 1061-1074.
3. Pennathur PR, Thompson D, Abernathy JH 3rd, et al. Technologies in the wild (TiW): human factors implications for patient safety in the cardiovascular operating room. Ergonomics, 2013; 56: 205-219.

8. Successful intraoperative focused event management may be compromised by which aspect?
   A. High level of technical knowledge
   B. Late detection of problems
   C. Effective communication
   D. Efficient resource management

Correct Answer: B

Explanation: Reducing the latent factors throughout the healthcare organization that predispose to safety lapses is an effective strategy to improve patient safety and healthcare quality, as it interrupts the interaction of multiple errors that can result in a sentinel event. Once a problem occurs, early detection and corrective action can prevent the problem from evolving or interacting with other problems to create a crisis. Technical/medical knowledge, while necessary to correctly diagnose and treat problems, is not sufficient for successful crisis management in anesthesia. Effective management of all available resources, as well as teamwork with high-quality

BOX 26.4 **Teamwork assessment tools**

OTAS (Observational Teamwork Assessment for Surgery)	Procedural task checklist centered on patient, equipment, and communications tasks ratings • Communication • Cooperation • Coordination • Shared leadership • Shared monitoring
NOTECHS (Oxford Non-technical Skills)	Adapted from the aviation NOTECHS scale used in Europe • Cooperation and teamwork • Leadership and management • Situational awareness • Problem solving and decision making • ± Communication and interaction
ANTS (Anaesthetists' Non-technical Skills)	Based on aviation crew resource management principles, developed by industrial psychologists and anesthesiologists • Task management • Teamworking • Situation awareness • Decision making
SPLINTS (Scrub Practitioners' List of Non-technical Skills)	Psychologist-facilitated focus groups identified key nontechnical skills for scrub practitioners • Situation awareness • Communication and teamwork • Task management

Reprinted with permission. Circulation. 2013;128:1139-1169. © 2013 American Heart Association, Inc.

communication, is also necessary for optimal outcomes in the intraoperative environment.

References:

1. Wahr JA, Bowdle TA, Nussmeier NA. Chapter 30: Patient Safety in the Cardiac Operating Room. In: Kaplan JA, Augoustides JGT, Manecke GR, et al., eds. Kaplan's Cardiac Anesthesia. 7th ed. Elsevier; 2017:1072-1108.
2. Gerstein NS, Pannikkath PV, Mirrakhimov AE, et al. Cardiopulmonary bypass emergencies and intraoperative issues. J Cardiothorac Vasc Anesth, 2022; 36: 4505-4522.

9. Simulation-based training is an effective method for improving all of these competencies EXCEPT:
   A. Medical expertise
   B. Professionalism
   C. Communication
   D. Collaboration

Correct Answer: B

Explanation: Many studies of simulation-based training in anesthesiology show enhanced learning compared to conventional instruction and improvement in the acquisition of both technical and nontechnical skills. High-fidelity simulation of critical events in anesthesia crisis management training improves clinical performance and has become an established part of the maintenance of certification requirements in anesthesiology. Simulation education can considerably improve intraoperative management approaches to clinical crises, including emergencies in cardiopulmonary bypass.

With respect to targeted competencies, simulation can promote the competencies of medical expertise, communication, and collaboration. Further interventions are required for adequate and effective education in professionalism, management, and health advocacy.

References:

1. Wahr JA, Bowdle TA, Nussmeier NA. Chapter 30: Patient Safety in the Cardiac Operating Room. In: Kaplan JA, Augoustides JGT, Manecke GR, et al., eds. Kaplan's Cardiac Anesthesia. 7th ed. Elsevier; 2017:1072-1108.
2. Sanchez Novas D, Domenech G, Belitzky NG, et al. Simulation-based training for early procedural skills acquisition in new anesthesia trainees: a prospective observational study. Adv Simul, 2020; 5: 19.
3. Bruppacher HR, Alam SK, LeBlanc VR, et al. Simulation-based training improves physicians' performance in patient care in high-stakes clinical setting of cardiac surgery. Anesthesiology, 2010; 112: 985-992.
4. Aggarwal R, Mytton OT, Derbrew M, et al. Training and simulation for patient safety. BMJ Qual Safety, 2010; 19: i34-i43.

10. Cognitive aids such as checklists may provide the following benefits EXCEPT:
   A. Improved management of simulated crises
   B. Reductions in miscommunication
   C. Reductions in mortality
   D. Prevention of complications

Correct Answer: B

BOX 26.5 **Recommendations for prevention of intraoperative awareness**

- Check all equipment drugs and doses; ensure that the anesthetic agent is reaching the patient.
- Consider amnestic premedication.
- Use a peripheral nerve stimulator to titrate neuromuscular blockade; minimize it as much as possible.
- If intense paralysis is required, consider using a tourniquet on the forearm to allow movement of that hand if the patient is aware.
- Administer at least 0.5–0.7 minimum alveolar concentrations of an inhaled agent; set the alarm for an end-tidal concentration lower than this level.
- Monitor the inhaled anesthetic concentration on cardiopulmonary bypass.
- Consider vasoactive agents to manage hypotension rather than lowering the anesthetic concentration.
- If the anesthetic level cannot be maintained because of hemodynamic compromise, consider hypnotic or amnestic agents.

- Supplement hypnotic agents with analgesic agents such as opioids to decrease the experience of pain in the event of awareness.
- Consider use of a processed electroencephalogram such as a bispectral index monitor, particularly if using total intravenous anesthesia; do not seek to lower the anesthetic concentration based solely on a bispectral index number.
- Evaluate known risk factors for awareness; explicitly ask about previous episodes of awareness. In patients with a previous history, consider increasing anesthetic concentrations and using sufficient opioids.
- Redose intravenous anesthetic agents during periods when inhaled anesthesia cannot be used (during long intubation attempt or during rigid bronchoscopy).
- When planning for sedation, explicitly discuss with the patient expectations for recall.

Modified from Mashour GA, Orser BA, Avidan MS. Intraoperative awareness: from neurobiology to clinical practice. Anesthesiology, 2011; 114: 1218-1233.

Explanation: Cognitive aids include checklists, briefing tools, and crisis manuals. Crisis manuals containing key evidence-based steps for responding to common operating room crises have resulted in significant improvement in clinical team performance, as observed during simulated crises. The implementation of surgical safety checklists has reduced perioperative mortality and morbidity. Checklists and cognitive aids may not improve communication themselves, unless they are well designed and implemented with socio-cultural factors in mind.

References:

1. Wahr JA, Bowdle TA, Nussmeier NA. Chapter 30: Patient Safety in the Cardiac Operating Room. In: Kaplan JA, Augoustides JGT, Manecke GR, et al., eds. Kaplan's Cardiac Anesthesia. 7th ed. Elsevier; 2017:1072-1108.
2. Harrison TK, Manser T, Howard SK, et al. Use of cognitive aids in a simulated anesthetic crisis. Anesth Analg, 2006; 103: 551-556.
3. Ziewacz JE, Arriaga AF, Bader AM, et al. Crisis checklists for the operating room: development and pilot testing. J Am Coll Surg, 2011; 213: e10-217.
4. van Klei WA, Hoff RG, van Aarnhem EE, et al. Effects of the introduction of the WHO "Surgical Safety Checklist" on in-hospital mortality: a cohort study. Ann Surg, 2012; 255: 44-49.
5. Catchpole K, Russ S. The problem with checklists. BMJ Qual Safety, 2015; 24: 545-549.

11. Which of the following statements is TRUE concerning teamwork?
A. Leadership deficiencies are among the top contributors to sentinel events and malpractice litigation
B. Physicians are accurate at assessing their own teamwork and communication skills
C. Individual factors are more important than teamwork in analyses of adverse events
D. Nontechnical skills such as teamwork are acquired automatically with increasing clinical experience

Correct Answer: A

Explanation: In complex systems like cardiac surgery, teamwork and communication failures are common features of preventable adverse events. Although individual factors such as fatigue or stress play a role in medical errors, problems with teamwork represent equal or even greater latent risks than do individual factors. Individuals (especially physicians) generally rate their own teamwork and communication skills much more highly compared to evaluations by team members. Nontechnical skills such as communication and teamwork must be explicitly taught and monitored and are not necessarily acquired by clinical practice alone. Leadership deficiencies and communication failures factor prominently in sentinel event reviews, as well as in malpractice litigation.

References:

1. Wahr JA, Bowdle TA, Nussmeier NA. Chapter 30: Patient Safety in the Cardiac Operating Room. In: Kaplan JA, Augoustides JGT, Manecke GR, et al., eds. Kaplan's Cardiac Anesthesia. 7th ed. Elsevier; 2017:1072-1108.
2. ElBardissi AW, Wiegmann DA, Dearani JA, et al. Application of the human factors analysis and classification system methodology to the cardiovascular surgery operating room. Ann Thorac Surg, 2007; 83: 1412-1418.
3. Frankel AS, Leonard MW, Denham CR. Fair and just culture, team behavior, and leadership engagement: the tools to achieve high reliability. Health Serv Res, 2006; 41: 1690-1709.
4. Morris JA Jr, Carrillo Y, Jenkins JM, et al. Surgical adverse events, risk management, and malpractice outcome: morbidity and mortality review is not enough. Ann Surg, 2003; 237: 844-851.

12. Neglecting to turn on the ventilator after the termination of cardiopulmonary bypass is an example of what type of error?
   A. Reasoning
   B. Decision
   C. Action
   D. Cognitive

Correct Answer: C

Explanation: Errors include action errors, which can include syringe swaps or failure to complete a planned sequence, such as turning on the ventilator after bypass. Decision errors occur when the plan or diagnosis is in error from either inappropriate pattern recognition or faulty reasoning. Reasoning errors occur in the absence of a schema or rule that applies in this situation. Cognitive errors are often due to incorrect assumptions.

References:

1. Wahr JA, Bowdle TA, Nussmeier NA. Chapter 30: Patient Safety in the Cardiac Operating Room. In: Kaplan JA, Augoustides JGT, Manecke GR, et al., eds. Kaplan's Cardiac Anesthesia. 7th ed. Elsevier; 2017:1072-1108.
2. Gerstein NS, Pannikkath PV, Mirrakhimov AE, et al. Cardiopulmonary bypass emergencies and intraoperative issues. J Cardiothorac Vasc Anesth, 2022; 36: 4505-4522.

13. Which of the following is FALSE regarding perioperative checklists and team briefings?
   A. Preoperative checklist briefings are associated with reduced mortality
   B. Postoperative surgical debriefings are not as valuable as preoperative briefings
   C. A checklist review prior to central line insertion decreases line-associated bloodstream infections
   D. Simply mandating checklist use may result in substantial degrees of noncompliance

Correct Answer: B

Explanation: Proper implementation of surgical briefings as the process and use of checklists for the content has significantly improved patient safety. Use of safety checklists has led to significant reductions in postoperative mortality and complications, including bloodstream infections. Postoperative debriefings have also been associated with similar outcome improvements. Healthcare teams will lapse in compliance with safety checklists over time, highlighting the priority for periodic interventions to boost stakeholder engagement with ongoing monitoring and reinforcement.

References:

1. Wahr JA, Bowdle TA, Nussmeier NA. Chapter 30: Patient Safety in the Cardiac Operating Room. In: Kaplan JA, Augoustides JGT, Manecke GR, et al., eds. Kaplan's Cardiac Anesthesia. 7th ed. Elsevier; 2017:1072-1108.
2. Haynes AB, Weiser TG, Berry WR, et al. Safe Surgery Saves Lives Study Group. A surgical safety checklist to reduce morbidity and mortality in a global population. N Engl J Med, 2009; 360: 491-499.
3. Rose MR, Rose KM. Use of a surgical debriefing checklist to achieve higher value health care. Am J Med Qual, 2018; 33: 514-522.
4. van Klei WA, Hoff RG, van Aarnhem EE, et al. Effects of the introduction of the WHO "Surgical Safety Checklist" on in-hospital mortality: a cohort study. Ann Surg, 2012; 255: 44-49.
5. Pronovost P, Needham D, Berenholtz S, et al. An intervention to decrease catheter-related bloodstream infections in the ICU. N Engl J Med, 2006; 355: 2725-2732.

14. Which of the following is not an element of a "just culture" in healthcare?
   A. Safety errors result from multiple causes
   B. Emphasis on system redesign to minimize the risk of errors
   C. Encouraging the reporting of safety issues
   D. No accountability of individuals who willfully violate established procedures

Correct Answer: D

Explanation: Organizational culture plays a critical role in patient safety. A just and fair culture is one that learns and improves by openly identifying its own vulnerabilities and correcting them, and in which individuals feel safe and protected when voicing concerns about safety. Human error is not viewed as the cause of adverse events, but rather as a symptom of underlying issues in an imperfect system. Essential to a just culture is a commitment-based management strategy in which individual members are held accountable only when they knowingly and unnecessarily increase risk.

References:

1. Wahr JA, Bowdle TA, Nussmeier NA. Chapter 30: Patient Safety in the Cardiac Operating Room. In: Kaplan JA, Augoustides JGT, Manecke GR, et al., eds. Kaplan's Cardiac Anesthesia. 7th ed. Elsevier; 2017:1072-1108.
2. Frankel AS, Leonard MW, Denham CR. Fair and just culture, team behavior, and leadership engagement: the tools to achieve high reliability. Health Serv Res, 2006; 41: 1690-1709.
3. Khatri N, Brown GD, Hicks LL. From a blame culture to a just culture in health care. Health Care Manage Rev, 2009; 34: 312-322.

15. Which of the following statements is inaccurate concerning drug errors in anesthesiology?
   A. Drug errors are possible only with route and dose
   B. The risk of litigation does not influence the reporting of drug errors
   C. Self-reported incidence of anesthetic drug errors is approximately 0.5 to 1 in 100 cases
   D. Providers perceive themselves as being more likely to make errors than they are in reality

Correct Answer: C

Explanation: Based on reporting trends, anesthetic drug errors are estimated to occur at a rate in the range of 1 in 100 to 1 in 200 cases. There are many types of drug errors, including substitution, incorrect dose, incorrect route, or omission. It is likely medicolegal concerns lead to underreporting of errors. Whereas most anesthesiologists acknowledge making drug errors, most also believe they are LESS likely to make an error than their colleagues. Drug errors in

TABLE 26.1

Definitions of types of communication failure with illustrative examples and notes

Failure	Definition	Illustrative Example
Occasion failures	Problem in the situation or context of the communication event	The staff surgeon asks the anesthesiologist whether the antibiotics have been administered. At the point of this question, the procedure has been underway for more than an hour. Because antibiotics are optimally given within 30 minutes of incision, the timing of this inquiry is ineffective both as a prompt and as a safety redundancy measure.
Content failures	Insufficiency or inaccuracy apparent in the information being transferred	As the case is set up, the anesthesia fellow asks the staff surgeon whether the patient has an ICU bed. The staff surgeon replies that the "bed is probably not needed, and there isn't likely one available anyway, so we'll just go ahead." Relevant information is missing, and questions are left unresolved: has an ICU bed been requested, and what will the plan be if the patient does need critical care and an ICU bed is not available?
Audience failures	Gaps in the composition of the group engaged in the communication	The nurses and anesthesiologist discuss how the patient should be positioned for operation without the participation of a surgical representative. Surgeons have particular positioning needs, so they should be participants in this discussion. Decisions made in their absence occasionally lead to renewed discussions and repositioning of the patient on their arrival.
Purpose failures	Communication events in which the purpose is unclear, not achieved, or inappropriate	During a living donor liver resection, the nurses discuss whether ice is needed in the basin they are preparing for the liver. Neither knows. No further discussion ensues. The purpose of this communication—to find out whether ice is required—is not achieved.

ICU, Intensive care unit.

From Lingard L, Espin S, Whyte S, et al. Communication failures in the operating room: an observational classification of recurrent types and effects. Qual Saf Health Care, 2004; 13: 330-334.

anesthesiology commonly have involved high-alert medications such as insulin, succinylcholine, and epinephrine.

References:

1. Wahr JA, Bowdle TA, Nussmeier NA. Chapter 30: Patient Safety in the Cardiac Operating Room. In: Kaplan JA, Augoustides JGT, Manecke GR, et al., eds. Kaplan's Cardiac Anesthesia. 7th ed. Elsevier; 2017:1072-1108.
2. Neira VM, Scheffler M, Wong D, et al. Survey of the preparation of cardiovascular emergency medications for adult cardiovascular anesthesia. J Cardiothorac Vasc Anesth, 2021; 35: 1813-1820.

16. Which of the following factors are NOT associated with increased risk of awareness during anesthesia?
   A. Cardiac surgical procedures
   B. Neuromuscular blockade
   C. American Society of Anesthesiologists physical status III or IV
   D. Monitoring of end-tidal volatile agent level

Correct Answer: D

Explanation: Cardiac surgical procedures are associated with significantly increased incidence of awareness during anesthesia, a finding that has been reproduced in multiple studies. Further risk factors for this outcome include significant comorbidity, defined by the American Society of Anesthesiologists as physical status classification equal to III or IV, as well as exposure to muscle relaxants. Monitoring end-tidal

volatile agent concentrations can reduce the risk of intraoperative awareness.

References:

1. Wahr JA, Bowdle TA, Nussmeier NA. Chapter 30: Patient Safety in the Cardiac Operating Room. In: Kaplan JA, Augoustides JGT, Manecke GR, et al., eds. Kaplan's Cardiac Anesthesia. 7th ed. Elsevier; 2017:1072-1108.
2. Sebel PS, Bowdle TA, Ghoneim MM, et al. The incidence of awareness during anesthesia: a multicenter United States study. Anesth Analg, 2004; 99: 833-839.
3. Gerstein NS, Panikkath PV, Mirrakhimov AE, et al. Cardiopulmonary bypass emergencies and intraoperative issues. J Cardiothorac Vasc Anesth, 2022; 36(12): 4505-4522. doi: 10.1053/j.jvca.2022.07.011.

17. Key components in the development of evidence-based guidelines include all of the following EXCEPT:
   A. Systematic review
   B. Regular updating
   C. Inclusion of high profile authors with significant industry relationships
   D. Grading level of evidence and strength of recommendations

Correct Answer: C

Explanation: Owing to the rapid expansion of medical knowledge, access to critically appraised and synthesized evidence has become fundamental to the practice of evidence-based medicine. Published recommendations for clinical practice guideline development include the following quality indicators: a transparent process for disclosing and managing conflicts of interest; a prespecified and systematic literature review; and application of validated instruments to assess for bias and grade the evidence. These quality indicators enhance the impact of a given guideline in the perioperative environment.

References:
1. Wahr JA, Bowdle TA, Nussmeier NA. Chapter 30: Patient Safety in the Cardiac Operating Room. In: Kaplan JA, Augoustides JGT, Manecke GR, et al., eds. Kaplan's Cardiac Anesthesia. 7th ed. Elsevier; 2017:1072-1108.
2. Huang J, Firestone S, Moffatt-Bruce S, et al. 2021 Clinical practice guidelines for anesthesiologists on patient blood management in cardiac surgery. J Cardiothorac Vasc Anesth, 2021; 35: 3493-3495.

18. What is FALSE regarding sleep deprivation and fatigue?
   A. Fatigue has been implicated as a contributing factor in adverse events
   B. Psychomotor vigilance is degraded by sleep deprivation
   C. Reaction time is increased by sleep deprivation
   D. Performance is unaffected by fatigue until after 24 hours of continuous duty

Correct Answer: D

Explanation: Fatigue has been implicated as a contributor to impaired performance. The deficits in performance include lapses in vigilance, increases in reaction time, and enhanced risk of errors and critical incidents in anesthesia. It has been noted that 24-hour shifts are associated with 36% more serious medical errors than 16-hour shifts.

References:
1. Wahr JA, Bowdle TA, Nussmeier NA. Chapter 30: Patient Safety in the Cardiac Operating Room. In: Kaplan JA, Augoustides JGT, Manecke GR, et al., eds. Kaplan's Cardiac Anesthesia. 7th ed. Elsevier; 2017:1072-1108.
2. Landrigan CP, Czeisler CA, Barger LK, et al. Effective implementation of work-hour limits and systemic improvements. Jt Comm J Qual Patient Saf, 2007; 33: 19-29.

19. Distractions in cardiac surgery can result from:
   A. Communication failures
   B. Presurgical briefings
   C. Equipment problems
   D. Both A and C

Correct Answer: D

Explanation: Distractions that inhibit team performance occur frequently in the complex and dynamic cardiac operating room and are linked to major adverse events. Effective presurgical briefings should not be considered distractions, as they occur prior to surgery and are critical to optimal team performance.

References:
1. Wahr JA, Bowdle TA, Nussmeier NA. Chapter 30: Patient Safety in the Cardiac Operating Room. In: Kaplan JA, Augoustides JGT, Manecke GR, et al., eds. Kaplan's Cardiac Anesthesia. 7th ed. Elsevier; 2017:1072-1108.
2. Merry AF, Weller J, Mitchell SJ. Improving the quality and safety of patient care in cardiac anesthesia. J Cardiothorac Vasc Anesth, 2014; 28: 1341-1351.

20. All of the following are important principles to manage noise in the operating room EXCEPT:
   A. Installing video recording equipment
   B. Limiting ancillary conversations
   C. Managing alarms
   D. Avoiding loud music

Correct Answer: A

Explanation: Noise levels are often excessive in cardiac operating rooms, presenting hazards to personnel and patient safety. Human auditory processing and concentration are adversely affected by excessive noise levels. Recommended measures to manage noise include "sterile cockpit" procedures, in which conversation during critical periods is limited to the task at hand, and alarm management to reduce the number of false positive alarms that lead to appropriate alarms being disabled or silenced. Limiting loud music would also assist in reducing the overall noise level in the operating room environment and limit distractions. Installing video recording equipment would not directly manage noise in the operating room, especially if no audio is available.

References:
1. Wahr JA, Bowdle TA, Nussmeier NA. Chapter 30: Patient Safety in the Cardiac Operating Room. In: Kaplan JA, Augoustides JGT, Manecke GR, et al., eds. Kaplan's Cardiac Anesthesia. 7th ed. Elsevier; 2017:1072-1108.
2. Merry AF, Weller J, Mitchell SJ. Improving the quality and safety of patient care in cardiac anesthesia. J Cardiothorac Vasc Anesth, 2014; 28: 1341-1351.
3. Ginsberg SH, Pantin E, Kraidin J, et al. Noise levels in modern operating rooms during surgery. J Cardiothorac Vasc Anesth, 2013; 27: 528-530.
4. Way TJ, Long A, Weihing J, et al. Effect of noise on auditory processing in the operating room. J Am Coll Surg, 2013; 216: 933-938.

21. All of the following forms of structured communication are recommended in perioperative cardiothoracic practice EXCEPT:
   A. Closed-loop communication
   B. Handoff tools
   C. Briefing/debriefing tools
   D. Use of nonverbal cues

Correct Answer: D

Explanation: Structured communication is intended to improve reliability of information transfer. Closed-loop communication is a method of structured communication in which the person receiving information repeats it back to make sure the message is understood correctly, and the sender confirms to "close the loop." Closed-loop communication is a key component of crew resource management and is recommended for resuscitation teams in American Heart Association guidelines. Handoff and briefing/debriefing tools, like checklists, provide structure to critical communications and have been shown to improve reliability of information transfer and prevent adverse events. The use of nonverbal cues has been recommended when speaking with patients but is difficult to implement in an operating room setting.

References:

1. Wahr JA, Bowdle TA, Nussmeier NA. Chapter 30: Patient Safety in the Cardiac Operating Room. In: Kaplan JA, Augoustides JGT, Manecke GR, et al., eds. Kaplan's Cardiac Anesthesia. 7th ed. Elsevier; 2017:1072-1108.
2. Santos R, Bakero L, Franco P, et al. Characterization of non-technical skills in pediatric cardiac surgery: communication patterns. Eur J Cardiothorac Surg, 2012; 41: 1005-1012.
3. Lane-Fall MB, Pascual JL, Peifer HG, et al. A partially structured postoperative handoff protocol improves communication in 2 mixed surgical intensive care units: findings from the Handoffs and Transitions in Critical Care (HATRICC) prospective cohort study. Ann Surg, 2020; 271: 484-493.
4. de Vries EN, Prins HA, Crolla RM, et al. Effect of a comprehensive surgical safety system on patient outcomes. N Engl J Med, 2010; 363: 1928-1937.

22. What relatively minor intraoperative events may have significant adverse effects on patient safety?
   A. Communication problems
   B. Flow disruptions
   C. Excessive noise
   D. All of the above

Correct Answer: D

Explanation: Observational studies in cardiac surgery have shown that even minor events that, in isolation, would not contribute to patient safety have serious consequences when associated with the decreased ability to respond to major intraoperative events, leading to increased morbidity and mortality. Communication problems factor prominently in analyses of preventable adverse events. Surgical flow disruptions with deviations from the desired progression of an operation can result from equipment factors and teamwork or communication failures, and such flow disruptions strongly predict adverse events. Ambient noise adversely affects information processing in the operating room, especially with nonroutine or unexpected communications that may signal incipient problems.

References:

1. Wahr JA, Bowdle TA, Nussmeier NA. Chapter 30: Patient Safety in the Cardiac Operating Room. In: Kaplan JA, Augoustides JGT, Manecke GR, et al., eds. Kaplan's Cardiac Anesthesia. 7th ed. Elsevier; 2017:1072-1108.
2. Wiegmann DA, El Bardissi AW, Dearani JA, et al. Disruptions in surgical flow and their relationship to surgical errors: an exploratory investigation. Surgery, 2007; 142: 658-665.
3. Martinez EA, Thompson DA, Errett NA, et al. Review article: high stakes and high risk: a focused qualitative review of hazards during cardiac surgery, Anesth Analg. 2011; 112: 1061-1074.
4. Way TJ, Long A, Weihing J, et al. Effect of noise on auditory processing in the operating room. J Am Coll Surg, 2013; 216: 933-938.

23. Which statement is FALSE concerning teamwork?
   A. Simulation is an effective method of improving teamwork and communication
   B. Team training has been shown to reduce surgical mortality
   C. Self-assessment of teamwork skills is accurate
   D. Measurement tools exist for assessment of teamwork in the perioperative environment

Correct Answer: C

Explanation: Structured training of perioperative teams can improve patient safety and outcomes. Simulation training including crew resource management not only improves teamwork but was also shown in a prospective study to significantly reduce mortality. Marked discrepancies exist between individuals' self-assessed communication and teamwork skills and assessments by team members. Objective instruments for this assessment should be selected to enhance quality and accuracy. The tools for teamwork assessment include the Oxford nontechnical skills instrument and the anesthesia nontechnical skills instrument (see box 26.4 for full details).

References:

1. Wahr JA, Bowdle TA, Nussmeier NA. Chapter 30: Patient Safety in the Cardiac Operating Room. In: Kaplan JA, Augoustides JGT, Manecke GR, et al., eds. Kaplan's Cardiac Anesthesia. 7th ed. Elsevier; 2017:1072-1108.
2. Stevens LM, Cooper JB, Raemer DB, et al. Educational programs in crisis management for cardiac surgery teams including high realism simulation. J Thorac Cardiovasc Surg, 2012; 144: 17-24.
3. Powers KA, Rehrig ST, Irias N, et al. Simulated laparoscopic operating room crisis: an approach to enhance the surgical team performance. Surg Endosc, 2008; 22: 885-900.
4. Wahr JA, Prager RL, Abernathy JH 3rd, et al. Patient safety in the cardiac operating room: human factors and teamwork: a scientific statement from the American Heart Association. Circulation, 2013; 128: 1139-1169.
5. Neily J, Mills PD, Young-Xu Y, et al. Association between implementation of a medical team training program and surgical mortality. JAMA, 2010; 304: 1693-1700.

24. Which statement is FALSE regarding failure to rescue?
   A. Failure to rescue can be defined as failure or delay in recognizing and responding to a complication
   B. Rapid response systems are recommended to prevent avoidable mortality in hospitals
   C. Failure to rescue may be a better indicator of hospital quality than complications rates
   D. None of the above

Correct Answer: D

Explanation: Delay or failure in responding to complications is termed failure to rescue. Rapid response systems aim to detect clinical deterioration and intervene before the point of cardiac arrest and are the focus in perioperative patient safety. Failure to rescue may reflect hospital quality more accurately than complication rates. In a landmark multicenter study in coronary artery bypass graft surgery, failure to rescue, defined as mortality following a complication, was better correlated with in-hospital mortality than were complication rates.

References:

1. Wahr JA, Bowdle TA, Nussmeier NA. Chapter 30: Patient Safety in the Cardiac Operating Room. In: Kaplan JA, Augoustides JGT, Manecke GR, et al., eds. Kaplan's Cardiac Anesthesia. 7th ed. Elsevier; 2017:1072-1108.
2. Carthey J, de Leval MR, Reason JT. The human factor in cardiac surgery: errors and near misses in a high technology medical domain. Ann Thorac Surg, 2001; 72: 300-305.
3. Silber JH, Rosenbaum PR, Schwartz JS, et al. Evaluation of the complication rate as a measure of quality of care in coronary artery bypass graft surgery. JAMA, 1995; 274: 317-323.
4. Mpody C, Cui J, Awad H, et al. Primary stroke and failure-to-rescue following thoracic endovascular aortic aneurysm repair. J Cardiothorac Vasc Anesth, 2021; 35: 2338-2344.

25. Implementation of handover protocols in patient care has demonstrated all of the following effects EXCEPT:
   A. Decreased errors and omission
   B. Decreased adverse clinical events
   C. Improved provider satisfaction
   D. Increased handover duration

Correct Answer: D

Explanation: Drawing from other high-risk industries such as aviation, implementation of a standardized approach to handoff communication is a priority in patient safety. The implementation of structured protocols can improve all aspects of the handover without significantly increasing duration. Multiple trials have demonstrated that structured implementation of a handoff bundle reduces medical errors and adverse clinical events, and improves provider satisfaction.

References:

1. Wahr JA, Bowdle TA, Nussmeier NA. Chapter 30: Patient Safety in the Cardiac Operating Room. In: Kaplan JA, Augoustides JGT, Manecke GR, et al., eds. Kaplan's Cardiac Anesthesia. 7th ed. Elsevier; 2017:1072-1108.
2. Chatterjee S, Shake JG, Arora RC, et al. Handoffs from the operating room to the intensive care unit after cardiothoracic surgery: from the Society of Thoracic Surgeons Workforce on Critical Care. Ann Thorac Surg, 2019; 107: 619-630.
3. Catchpole KR, de Leval MR, McEwan A, et al. Patient handover from surgery to intensive care: using Formula 1 pit-stop and aviation models to improve safety and quality. Paediatr Anaesth, 2007; 17: 470-478.
4. Starmer AJ, Spector ND, Srivastava R, et al. I-PASS Study Group. Changes in medical errors after implementation of a handoff program. N Engl J Med, 2014; 371: 1803-1812.
5. Lane-Fall MB, Pascual JL, Peifer HG, et al. A partially structured postoperative handoff protocol improves communication in 2 mixed surgical intensive care units: findings from the Handoffs and Transitions in Critical Care (HATRICC) prospective cohort study. Ann Surg, 2020; 271: 484-493.

26. Root cause analysis of adverse events in healthcare seeks to:
   A. Identify persons responsible
   B. Identify system vulnerabilities
   C. Eliminate system vulnerabilities
   D. B and C

Correct Answer: D

Explanation: Root cause analysis is a structured process for the analysis of adverse events and near misses. The root cause analysis process seeks to identify underlying problems and system vulnerabilities that increase the likelihood of errors, rather than focusing on individual performance. The findings from root cause analysis typically can assist in reducing system vulnerabilities and can be a basis for system improvements to prevent future patient harm from occurring.

References:

1. Wahr JA, Bowdle TA, Nussmeier NA. Chapter 30: Patient Safety in the Cardiac Operating Room. In: Kaplan JA, Augoustides JGT, Manecke GR, et al., eds. Kaplan's Cardiac Anesthesia. 7th ed. Elsevier; 2017:1072-1108.
2. Pronovost PJ, Holzmueller CG, Martinez E, et al. A practical tool to learn from defects in patient care. Jt Comm J Qual Patient Saf, 2006; 32: 102-108.
3. Wahr JA, Prager RL, Abernathy JH 3rd, et al. Patient safety in the cardiac operating room: human factors and teamwork: a scientific statement from the American Heart Association. Circulation, 2013; 128: 1139-1169.

27. In the taxonomy hierarchy of human errors, all of the following are considered errors due to the condition of the operator, EXCEPT:
   A. Lapses in communication
   B. Adverse mental status
   C. Chronic performance limitation
   D. Adverse physiologic state

Correct Answer: A

Explanation: In the taxonomy of errors, preconditions for unsafe acts include environmental factors, personnel factors, and operator condition. The environmental factors may be physical and/or technological. The personnel factors include communication, coordination, planning, and fitness for duty. The condition of the operator includes adverse mental and physiologic states as well as chronic performance limitations.

References:

1. Wahr JA, Bowdle TA, Nussmeier NA. Chapter 30: Patient Safety in the Cardiac Operating Room. In: Kaplan JA, Augoustides JGT, Manecke GR, et al., eds. Kaplan's Cardiac Anesthesia. 7th ed. Elsevier; 2017:1072-1108.
2. Wahr JA, Prager RL, Abernathy JH 3rd, et al. Patient safety in the cardiac operating room: human factors and teamwork: a

scientific statement from the American Heart Association. Circulation, 2013; 128: 1139-1169.

28. In the operating room environment, which noise level has been associated with an increase in surgical technical errors?
  A. 20 dB
  B. 40 dB
  C. 60 dB
  D. 80 dB

Correct Answer: D

Explanation: The noise in the operating room environment can be much higher than the recommended level of 45 to 50 dB. In combination with other distractors, excessive noise levels can increase the risk of technical and communication errors in the conduct of a surgical procedure. Operating room noise levels reaching 80 dB in combination with other distractors have been associated with a significant increase in surgical technical errors. An 80-dB level of noise is equivalent to the sound of an alarm clock.

References:

1. Wahr JA, Bowdle TA, Nussmeier NA. Chapter 30: Patient Safety in the Cardiac Operating Room. In: Kaplan JA, Augoustides JGT, Manecke GR, et al., eds. Kaplan's Cardiac Anesthesia. 7th ed. Elsevier; 2017:1072-1108.
2. Wahr JA, Prager RL, Abernathy JH 3rd, et al. Patient safety in the cardiac operating room: human factors and teamwork: a scientific statement from the American Heart Association. Circulation, 2013; 128: 1139-1169.
3. Moorthy K, Munz Y, Dossis A, et al. The effect of stress-inducing conditions on the performance of a laparoscopic task. Surg Endosc, 2003; 17: 1481-1484.
4. Way TJ, Long A, Weihing J, et al. Effect of noise on auditory processing in the operating room. J Am Coll Surg, 2013; 216: 933-938.

29. The following statements are true regarding preventable adverse events in cardiac surgical patients, EXCEPT:
  A. Cardiac surgical patients are at increased risk for adverse events
  B. Infection is an uncommon adverse event
  C. Surgical adverse events are often preventable
  D. Studies likely underestimate the true incidence of adverse events

Correct Answer: B

Explanation: The adverse event rate in cardiothoracic surgery has been measured at 10.8%, a rate that is higher than that observed in many other surgical subspecialties. In a study reviewing 15,000 inpatient discharge records from Utah and Colorado, Gawande et al. found that a small number of surgical operations accounted for the majority of preventable surgical adverse events, including a rate of 4.7% for coronary artery and/or cardiac valve procedures. Although these observations may be due in large part to the inherent riskiness of cardiac surgical procedures and the severity of patient illness, the majority (54%) of all surgical adverse events were deemed preventable. These retrospective studies likely underestimate the true incidence of surgical adverse events, in part due to concerns about litigation affecting documentation. The most common types of identified adverse events included surgical technical complications, infection, and perioperative bleeding.

References:

1. Wahr JA, Bowdle TA, Nussmeier NA. Chapter 30: Patient Safety in the Cardiac Operating Room. In: Kaplan JA, Augoustides JGT, Manecke GR, et al., eds. Kaplan's Cardiac Anesthesia. 7th ed. Elsevier; 2017:1072-1108.
2. Brennan TA, Leape LL, Laird NM, et al. Incidence of adverse events and negligence in hospitalized patients: results of the Harvard Medical Practice Study I. N Engl J Med, 1991; 324: 370-376.
3. Gawande AA, Thomas EJ, Zinner MJ, et al. The incidence and nature of surgical adverse events in Colorado and Utah in 1992. Surgery, 1999; 126: 66-75.

30. Medication safety in the operating room is enhanced by which of the following?
  A. Availability of multiple concentrations of drugs for infusion
  B. Hand-written drug labels
  C. Provider-prepared drug infusions
  D. Point-of-care bar code readers

Correct Answer: D

Explanation: According to estimates, effective point-of-care medication bar codes can significantly reduce medication errors in the operating room environment. Furthermore, medication safety can be enhanced with infusions available in a single, standardized concentration and with programmed delivery by infusion devices with drug libraries. Further strategies for optimizing medication safety include minimizing the availability of concentrated versions of potentially lethal medications in the operating room; using standardized, machine-readable labels for all medications; and ensuring availability of pre-prepared medications, with high-alert drugs prepared by the pharmacy rather than the providers.

References:

1. Wahr JA, Bowdle TA, Nussmeier NA. Chapter 30: Patient Safety in the Cardiac Operating Room. In: Kaplan JA, Augoustides JGT, Manecke GR, et al., eds. Kaplan's Cardiac Anesthesia. 7th ed. Elsevier; 2017:1072-1108.
2. Wahr JA, Prager RL, Abernathy JH 3rd, et al. Patient safety in the cardiac operating room: human factors and teamwork: a scientific statement from the American Heart Association. Circulation, 2013; 128: 1139-1169.
3. Merry AF, Weller J, Mitchell SJ. Improving the quality and safety of patient care in cardiac anesthesia. J Cardiothorac Vasc Anesth, 2014; 28: 1341-1351.

CHAPTER 27

Cardiopulmonary Bypass

John G.T. Augoustides

KEY POINTS

1. Cardiopulmonary bypass (CPB) provides the extracorporeal maintenance of respiration and circulation and permits the surgeon to operate on a quiet, nonbeating heart.

2. CPB is associated with a number of profound physiologic perturbations. The central nervous system, kidneys, gut, and heart are especially vulnerable to ischemic events associated with extracorporeal circulation.

3. Advanced age is the most important risk factor for stroke and neurocognitive dysfunction after CPB.

4. Acute renal injury from CPB can contribute directly to poor outcomes.

5. Drugs such as dopamine and diuretics do not prevent renal failure after CPB.

6. Myocardial stunning represents injury caused by short periods of myocardial ischemia that can occur during CPB.

7. Blood cardioplegia has the potential advantage of delivering oxygen to ischemic myocardium, whereas crystalloid cardioplegia does not carry much oxygen.

8. Gastrointestinal complications after CPB include pancreatitis, gastrointestinal bleeding, bowel infarction, and cholecystitis.

9. Pulmonary complications such as atelectasis and pleural effusions are common after cardiac surgery with CPB.

10. Embolization, hypoperfusion, and inflammatory processes are central common pathophysiologic mechanisms responsible for organ dysfunction after CPB.

11. Controversy regarding the optimal management of blood flow, pressure, and temperature during CPB remains. Perfusion should be adequate to support ongoing oxygen requirements; mean arterial pressures of more than 70 mmHg may benefit patients with cerebral and/or diffuse arthrosclerosis. Arterial blood temperatures should never exceed 37.5°C.

12. The initiation and termination of CPB are key phases of a cardiac surgery procedure, but the anesthesiologist must remain vigilant throughout the entire bypass period.

13. Total CPB can be tailored to allow deep hypothermic circulatory arrest or partial bypass. These special techniques require sophisticated monitoring and care.

14. Organ dysfunction cannot definitively be prevented during cardiac surgery with off-pump techniques.

---

1. The most accurate assessment of atherosclerosis in the ascending aorta is possible with:
   A. Digital palpation
   B. Transesophageal echocardiography
   C. Epiaortic ultrasound
   D. Transthoracic echocardiography

Correct Answer: C

Explanation: Although digital palpation, transthoracic echocardiography, and transesophageal echocardiography can all detect ascending aortic atheroma, epiaortic imaging has the best accuracy due to its proximity and unobstructed acoustic window for all imaging zones in the ascending aorta. Transesophageal echocardiography typically has a "blind spot" in the distal ascending aorta due to the interposition of the tracheobronchial tree between the esophagus and the ascending aorta at this level. Digital palpation of the ascending aorta can detect severe atherosclerosis or a porcelain aorta, but is unreliable to assess disease severity across all zones of the ascending aorta. Transthoracic echocardiography can image the ascending aorta but does not typically have the resolution to assess atheroma accurately throughout the ascending aorta.

References:

1. Zakhary WZA, Ender JK. Chapter 31: Procedures in the Hybrid Operating Room. In: Kaplan JA, Augoustides JGT, Manecke GR, et al., eds. Kaplan's Cardiac Anesthesia. 7th ed. Elsevier; 2017:1022-1041.
2. Macknight BM, Maldonado Y, Augoustides JG, et al. Advances in imaging for management of acute aortic syndromes: focus on transesophageal echocardiography and type A aortic dissection for the perioperative echocardiographer. J Cardiothorac Vasc Anesth, 2016; 30: 1129-1141.

2. The definition by expert consensus for moderate hypothermia during cardiopulmonary bypass is:
   A. 20.1 to 28°C
   B. 28.1 to 34°C
   C. 14.1 to 20°C
   D. 10 to 14°C

Correct Answer: A

Explanation: Expert consensus has defined a classification of hypothermia levels during cardiopulmonary bypass based on nasopharyngeal temperature as follows:

LEVEL OF HYPOTHERMIA	NASOPHARYNGEAL TEMPERATURE
Profound hypothermia	Below 14°C
Deep hypothermia	14.1 to 20°C
Moderate hypothermia	20.1 to 28°C
Mild hypothermia	28.1 to 34°C

References:

1. Zakhary WZA, Ender JK. Chapter 31: Procedures in the Hybrid Operating Room. In: Kaplan JA, Augoustides JGT, Manecke GR, et al., eds. Kaplan's Cardiac Anesthesia. 7th ed. Elsevier; 2017:1022-1041.
2. Gutsche JT, Ghadmimi K, Patel PA, et al. New frontiers in aortic therapy: focus on deep hypothermic circulatory arrest. J Cardiothorac Vasc Anesth, 2014; 28: 1159-1163.

3. The most effective neuroprotective strategy during cardiopulmonary bypass is:
   A. Pulsatile perfusion
   B. Embolic reduction
   C. Mild hyperthermia
   D. Pharmacologic adjuncts

Correct Answer: B

Explanation: Although pulsatile perfusion may be neuroprotective, the current evidence is not convincing to suggest that routine pulsatile perfusion during cardiopulmonary bypass is warranted. Because cerebral emboli play a prominent role in perioperative brain injury, a multimodal approach to manage and reduce cerebral emboli during cardiopulmonary bypass has been encouraged. Although mild hypothermia may be

neuroprotective, mild cerebral hyperthermia has been associated with adverse neurocognitive outcomes and so has been discouraged in contemporary practice. Multiple drugs including propofol, ketamine, lidocaine, and steroids have been investigated for possible neuroprotection during cardiopulmonary bypass. The evidence to support these agents for routine administration in this setting is weak.

References:

1. Zakhary WZA, Ender JK. Chapter 31: Procedures in the Hybrid Operating Room. In: Kaplan JA, Augoustides JGT, Manecke GR, et al., eds. Kaplan's Cardiac Anesthesia. 7th ed. Elsevier; 2017:1022-1041.
2. Hessel E. What's new in cardiopulmonary bypass? J Cardiothorac Vasc Anesth, 2019; 33: 2296-2326.

4. The strongest contributor to the development of cognitive dysfunction after cardiopulmonary bypass is:
   A. Cerebral microemboli
   B. Cerebral hyperperfusion
   C. Systemic inflammatory response
   D. Blood-brain barrier dysfunction

Correct Answer: A

Explanation: The gaseous and particulate microemboli that arise during cardiopulmonary bypass have been linked in multiple studies to the development of cognitive dysfunction after cardiac surgery. Cerebral hypoperfusion rather than hyperperfusion has been associated with the development of stroke and cognitive dysfunction, especially in combination with cerebral emboli. Although exposure to cardiopulmonary bypass leads to a systemic inflammatory response, there is minimal evidence to link this inflammation with cognitive injury after cardiopulmonary bypass. Furthermore, recent trials have demonstrated that steroid therapy does not reduce the risk of delirium after cardiopulmonary bypass. Although the function of the blood-brain barrier is to preserve the homeostasis of the extracellular cerebral milieu, it is still not clear whether disruption of this protective barrier leads directly to cognitive injury after cardiopulmonary bypass. Furthermore, this association is further confounded by the fact that injury to the blood-brain is often secondary to a primary process such as ischemia from cerebral embolization.

References:

1. Zakhary WZA, Ender JK. Chapter 31: Procedures in the Hybrid Operating Room. In: Kaplan JA, Augoustides JGT, Manecke GR, et al., eds. Kaplan's Cardiac Anesthesia. 7th ed. Elsevier; 2017:1022-1041.
2. Crawford JH, Townsley MM. Steroids for adult and pediatric cardiac surgery: a clinical update. J Cardiothorac Vasc Anesth, 2019; 33: 2039-2045.

5. The strongest risk factor for gastrointestinal complications after cardiopulmonary bypass is:
   A. Young age
   B. Elective cardiac surgery
   C. Systemic hypertension
   D. Duration of cardiopulmonary bypass

Correct Answer: D

Explanation: Gastrointestinal complications after cardiopulmonary bypass include liver injury, pancreatitis, bleeding, bowel ischemia, and perforation. Although these complications are relatively uncommon, their occurrence significantly increases the risk of adverse clinical outcomes. Preoperative risk factors for these complications include age over 75 years, congestive heart failure, and hyperbilirubinemia. Procedural risk factors include emergency surgery, reoperation, combined procedures, and cardiac transplantation, as well as the duration of cardiopulmonary bypass and aortic clamping. Postoperative risk factors include low cardiac output, systemic hypotension, exposures to inotropes and vasopressors, renal failure, infection, and prolonged stay in the intensive care unit.

References:

1. Zakhary WZA, Ender JK. Chapter 31: Procedures in the Hybrid Operating Room. In: Kaplan JA, Augoustides JGT, Manecke GR, et al., eds. Kaplan's Cardiac Anesthesia. 7th ed. Elsevier; 2017:1022-1041.
2. Chaudry R, Zaki J, Wegner R, et al. Gastrointestinal complications after cardiac surgery: a nationwide population-based analysis of morbidity and mortality predictors. J Cardiothorac Vasc Anesth, 2017; 31: 1268-1274.

6. The protection of the gastrointestinal tract during cardiopulmonary bypass is best achieved with:
   A. Anti-inflammatory therapy
   B. Maintenance of high flow
   C. Titration of vasopressin therapy
   D. Selective gastrointestinal decontamination

Correct Answer: B

Explanation: Gastrointestinal complications after cardiopulmonary bypass often result from a multimodal injury including splanchnic hypoperfusion, mesenteric emboli, translocation of endotoxin, and the systemic inflammatory response. A major intervention to minimize the risk of these complications is to preserve splanchnic flow including the avoidance of high doses of vasopressors. Although vasopressin may enhance systemic mean arterial pressure, it is also a powerful splanchnic vasoconstrictor that may compromise splanchnic perfusion in high doses. There is little evidence to guide the selection and dosing of anti-inflammatory therapies such as steroids or complement inhibitors for visceral protection. Although selective bacterial decontamination of the gastrointestinal tract with preoperative oral antibiotics such as polymyxin and tobramycin can reduce endotoxemia after cardiopulmonary bypass, this approach has not been strongly shown to improve clinical outcomes after cardiopulmonary bypass.

References:

1. Zakhary WZA, Ender JK. Chapter 31: Procedures in the Hybrid Operating Room. In: Kaplan JA, Augoustides JGT, Manecke GR, et al., eds. Kaplan's Cardiac Anesthesia. 7th ed. Elsevier; 2017:1022-1041.
2. Chan MXF, Buitinck S, Stooker M, et al. Clinical effects of perioperative selective decontamination of the digestive tract (SDD) in cardiac surgery: a propensity score matched analysis. J Cardiothorac Vasc Anesth, 2019; 33: 3001-3009.

7. Risk factors for respiratory failure after cardiac surgery with cardiopulmonary bypass include:
   A. Infective endocarditis
   B. Cardiopulmonary bypass time over 60 minutes
   C. Ejection fraction over 40%
   D. Male gender

Correct Answer: A

Explanation: Pulmonary complications after cardiopulmonary bypass include acute lung injury, atelectasis, pneumonia, pulmonary embolism, and pleural effusions. Risk factors for pulmonary dysfunction in this setting include age over 70 years, female gender, systemic hypertension, active smoking, chronic obstructive pulmonary disease, ejection fraction less than 40%, endocarditis, and renal failure. Procedural risk factors for postoperative pulmonary complications in this setting include double valve procedures, emergency surgery, reoperative surgery, emergency surgery, and prolonged procedures with a duration of cardiopulmonary bypass greater than 180 minutes. Active endocarditis can lead to lung injury through multiple mechanisms including septic emboli, increased hydrostatic pressure from acute valvular disease, endotoxemia, upregulated systemic inflammatory responses, and complex surgical management.

References:

1. Zakhary WZA, Ender JK. Chapter 31: Procedures in the Hybrid Operating Room. In: Kaplan JA, Augoustides JGT, Manecke GR, et al., eds. Kaplan's Cardiac Anesthesia. 7th ed. Elsevier; 2017:1022-1041.
2. Fischer MO, Brotons F, Briant AR, et al. Postoperative pulmonary complications after cardiac surgery: The Venice International Cohort Study. J Cardiothorac Vasc Anesth, 2022; 36: 2344-2351.

8. Perioperative maneuvers that can reduce pulmonary complications after cardiac surgery with cardiopulmonary bypass include:
   A. Inhaled nitric oxide
   B. Ventilation bundle strategy
   C. Avoidance of neuromuscular blockade
   D. Steroid therapy

Correct Answer: B

Explanation: Pulmonary complications after cardiopulmonary bypass can be limited by a perioperative bundle strategy for lung ventilation that includes low tidal volumes, reduced fraction of inspired oxygen, and recruitment maneuvers. Inhaled pulmonary vasodilators such as nitric oxide can reduce the elevated pulmonary vascular resistance that is common in postoperative pulmonary dysfunction to reduce the workload of the right ventricle. Despite these beneficial effects, the current evidence base does not suggest that this therapy reduces pulmonary complications after cardiac surgery with cardiopulmonary bypass. Exposure to nondepolarizing neuromuscular blockade may be associated with pulmonary complications after noncardiac surgery. Their effects in cardiac surgery are still under investigation. A recent prospective randomized trial demonstrated that avoidance of nondepolarizing neuromuscular blockers was feasible but did not reduce the risk of postoperative pulmonary complications and worsened operating conditions. Although the inflammatory response to cardiopulmonary bypass may have a role in postoperative acute lung injury, steroid therapy has not been conclusively shown to reduce pulmonary complications in this setting.

References:

1. Zakhary WZA, Ender JK. Chapter 31: Procedures in the Hybrid Operating Room. In: Kaplan JA, Augoustides JGT, Manecke GR, et al., eds. Kaplan's Cardiac Anesthesia. 7th ed. Elsevier; 2017:1022-1041.
2. Gerlach RM, Shahul S, Wroblewski KE, et al. Intraoperative use of nondepolarizing neuromuscular blockade agents during cardiac surgery and postoperative pulmonary complications after cardiac surgery: a prospective randomized trial. J Cardiothorac Vasc Anesth, 2019; 33: 1673-1681.

9. The adverse effects of cold cardioplegia include:
   A. Enhancement of myocardial metabolism
   B. Decreased plasma viscosity
   C. Increased red blood cell deformability
   D. Myocardial edema

Correct Answer: D

Explanation: Cardioplegia can be classified according to temperature range as follows: cold (10–12°C) tepid (27–30°C), and warm (36–38°C). The benefits of cold cardioplegia include suppression of cardiac metabolism and consequent reduction of myocardial oxygen demand. Despite these beneficial effects, tepid and warm cardioplegia were developed to offset the disadvantages of cold cardioplegia such as increases in plasma viscosity, decreased deformability of red blood cells, and myocardial edema. The mechanism of myocardial edema with cold cardioplegia is related to inhibition of membrane ion pumps and further clusters of membrane receptors. Cold cardioplegia may include crystalloid and blood components in various ratios.

References:

1. Zakhary WZA, Ender JK. Chapter 31: Procedures in the Hybrid Operating Room. In: Kaplan JA, Augoustides JGT, Manecke GR, et al., eds. Kaplan's Cardiac Anesthesia. 7th ed. Elsevier; 2017:1022-1041.
2. Zeng J, He W, Qu Z, et al. Cold blood versus crystalloid cardioplegia for myocardial protection in adult cardiac surgery: a meta-analysis of randomized controlled studies. J Cardiothorac Vasc Anesth, 2014; 28; 674-681.

10. The advantages of blood cardioplegia as compared to crystalloid cardioplegia include:
   A. Enhanced outcomes in low-risk patients
   B. Supraphysiologic concentrations of potassium
   C. Oxygen delivery
   D. Delivery temperature

Correct Answer: C

Explanation: The composition of cardioplegia can be classified as blood-containing or non-blood-containing, often termed blood or crystalloid cardioplegia. A typical ingredient of all cardioplegia solutions is higher than physiologic concentrations of potassium to facilitate rapid cardiac arrest for prompt reduction of myocardial oxygen demand. The benefits of blood cardioplegia include enhanced oxygen delivery to ischemic myocardium, augmentation of high-energy phosphate stores, and free radical scavenging. Despite these advantages, clinical outcomes in low-risk cardiac surgical patients appear to be equivalent with either blood or crystalloid cardioplegia for myocardial protection. A meta-analysis of randomized controlled trials demonstrated that cold blood cardioplegia as compared to cold crystalloid cardioplegia may reduce perioperative myocardial infarction with no differences in perioperative atrial fibrillation, stroke, and mortality. The delivery temperature of blood or crystalloid cardioplegia can be cold, tepid, or warm, and so is not a distinguishing characteristic of blood cardioplegia.

References:

1. Zakhary WZA, Ender JK. Chapter 31: Procedures in the Hybrid Operating Room. In: Kaplan JA, Augoustides JGT, Manecke GR, et al., eds. Kaplan's Cardiac Anesthesia. 7th ed. Elsevier; 2017:1022-1041.
2. Zeng J, He W, Qu Z, et al. Cold blood versus crystalloid cardioplegia for myocardial protection in adult cardiac surgery: a meta-analysis of randomized controlled studies. J Cardiothorac Vasc Anesth, 2014; 28; 674-681.

11. The advantages of retrograde cardioplegia as compared to antegrade cardioplegia include:
   A. Reliable delivery to the right ventricle
   B. Prompt cardiac arrest
   C. Enhanced surgical conditions during aortic valve and aortic root surgery
   D. Decreased efficacy in aortic regurgitation

Correct Answer: C

Explanation: Retrograde cardioplegia is typically delivered by a cannula positioned in the coronary sinus. Although the delivery of cardioplegia by this route is reliable for the left ventricle, the delivery to the right ventricle and ventricular septum can be less reliable due to factors such as cannula position and variations in cardiac venous anatomy. Since retrograde cardioplegia is often inefficient to achieve prompt cardiac arrest, administration of antegrade cardioplegia is often selected to achieve asystole prior to initiation of retrograde cardioplegia. The administration of retrograde cardioplegia can simultaneously enhance myocardial protection and also facilitate the conduct of aortic valve and aortic root procedures. The presence of significant aortic insufficiency can interfere with the delivery of anterograde rather than retrograde cardioplegia, as the delivered cardioplegia in the aortic root will partially leak into the left ventricle rather than completely course down the coronary arteries. Severe proximal coronary artery disease can also limit the delivery of antegrade cardioplegia and is often an indication for retrograde cardioplegia administration.

References:

1. Zakhary WZA, Ender JK. Chapter 31: Procedures in the Hybrid Operating Room. In: Kaplan JA, Augoustides JGT,

Manecke GR, et al., eds. Kaplan's Cardiac Anesthesia. 7th ed. Elsevier; 2017:1022-1041.

2. Lebon JS, Couture P, Colizza M, et al. Myocardial protection fin minimally invasive mitral valve surgery: retrograde cardioplegia alone using endovascular coronary sinus catheter compared with combined antegrade and retrograde cardioplegia. J Cardiothorac Vasc Anesth, 2019; 33; 1197-1204.

12. Ischemic preconditioning of the heart:
- **A.** Can provide myocardial protection against ischemia
- **B.** Cannot be induced remotely
- **C.** May not be induced pharmacologically
- **D.** Consistently improves outcomes after cardiac surgery

Correct Answer: A

Explanation: Direct ischemic myocardial preconditioning refers to the protective effect against an ischemic insult that is developed by prior exposure of the heart to a brief ischemic episode. This direct ischemic preconditioning can be induced by intermittent coronary occlusion and has been associated with significant subsequent protection from myocardial ischemia, particularly in animal models. These protective effects can also be induced remotely with brief ischemia in another tissue bed followed by reperfusion such as occurs with intermittent limb occlusion with a pressure cuff device such as sphygmomanometer. The beneficial effects of ischemic preconditioning can also be pharmacologically replicated by exposure to volatile anesthetics. Despite these myocardial protective effects of direct and remote ischemic preconditioning, the extensive evidence to data has not consistently demonstrated an effective myocardial strategy that can be clinically implemented.

References:

1. Zakhary WZA, Ender JK. Chapter 31: Procedures in the Hybrid Operating Room. In: Kaplan JA, Augoustides JGT, Manecke GR, et al., eds. Kaplan's Cardiac Anesthesia. 7th ed. Elsevier; 2017:1022-1041.

2. Maldonado Y, Weiner MM, Ramakrishna H. Remote ischemic preconditioning in cardiac surgery: is there a proven clinical benefit? J Cardiothorac Vasc Anesth, 2017; 33; 1910-1915.

13. After aortic cross clamping on cardiopulmonary bypass, the surgical team proceeded with antegrade cardioplegia via a cannula in the proximal ascending aorta prior to planned aortic valve replacement. During the administration of the cardioplegia, there was significant elevation of the pulmonary artery pressure. The most appropriate next step would be to:
- **A.** Continue with this administration until cardiac arrest has been obtained
- **B.** Deliver antegrade cardioplegia directly via the coronary ostia with a handheld cannula
- **C.** Switch to delivery of retrograde cardioplegia
- **D.** Track left ventricular diameter with transesophageal echocardiography

Correct Answer: B

Explanation: The delivery of antegrade cardioplegia can be impaired in the setting of significant aortic valve insufficiency,

as the cardioplegic solution will leak into the left ventricle and cause left heart distension that may be accompanied by elevation of the pulmonary artery pressure. This left ventricular distention will increase wall stress and myocardial oxygen demand and aggravate ventricular ischemia during aortic cross clamping. Transesophageal echocardiography can often assess the degree of aortic regurgitation and left ventricular distention in this setting. A vena contracta of 0.3 cm for aortic regurgitation has been correlated with the risk for significant left ventricular distention that may prompt cessation of antegrade cardioplegia. Given the elevation in pulmonary artery pressure in this setting, it is likely that there is significant left ventricular distention that can be quantified by point-of-care transesophageal echocardiography. The solution to this problem is to open the aorta and proceed with direct delivery of anterograde cardioplegia to the coronary ostia with a handheld cannula to achieve prompt cardiac arrest. This solution is compatible with the planned aortic valve replacement that would require aortic valve exposure. Continuing with delivery until cardiac arrest is less ideal, as it risks worsening ventricular distention and consequent ischemia. Switching to retrograde cardioplegia allows ongoing delivery of cardioplegia but may not result in rapid cardiac asystole. Tracking of left ventricular diameter with transesophageal echocardiography does quantify the problem but does not address the cause or solve the dilemma.

References:

1. Zakhary WZA, Ender JK. Chapter 31: Procedures in the Hybrid Operating Room. In: Kaplan JA, Augoustides JGT, Manecke GR, et al., eds. Kaplan's Cardiac Anesthesia. 7th ed. Elsevier; 2017:1022-1041.

2. Canty DJ, Joshi P, Royse C, et al. Transesophageal echocardiography guidance of antegrade cardioplegia delivery for cardiac surgery. J Cardiothorac Vasc Anesth, 2015; 29; 1498-1503.

14. Recommended maneuvers to consider in the immediate management of massive arterial gas embolism during cardiopulmonary bypass include:
- **A.** Reverse Trendelenburg position
- **B.** Immediate continuation of cardiopulmonary bypass
- **C.** Retrograde cerebral perfusion
- **D.** Hyperbaric therapy 72 to 96 hours after the event

Correct Answer: C

Explanation: Massive arterial air embolism during cardiopulmonary bypass is a rare but life-threatening perfusion emergency. The recommendations for management of this scenario include steep Trendelenburg position rather than reverse Trendelenburg to discourage cerebral air embolism. Furthermore, immediate discontinuation of cardiopulmonary bypass has been advised with aspiration of air from the heart and aorta as well as clearance of air from the arterial line. Retrograde cerebral perfusion can also promote washout of gas emboli from the brain with a flow rate of about 500 cc per minute at 20°C for 1 to 2 minutes. After these deairing maneuvers, cardiopulmonary bypass may be continued if necessary to complete the cardiac surgical procedure with deepening of systemic hypothermia for neuroprotection.

Since postoperative seizures are common in this setting, prophylaxis with anticonvulsant therapy may also be reasonable to improve neurologic outcome. If available, hyperbaric therapy can promote dissolution of cerebral gas emboli and neurological recovery in the immediate postoperative period, even if delayed up to 48 hours after the event. After 48 to 72 hours, the efficacy of this intervention may be compromised, although there are reports of good neurological outcome with this intervention beyond this time point. A coordinated and rapid team response to this perfusion complication also plays an important role in the quality and success of the subsequent management.

References:

1. Zakhary WZA, Ender JK. Chapter 31: Procedures in the Hybrid Operating Room. In: Kaplan JA, Augoustides JGT, Manecke GR, et al., eds. Kaplan's Cardiac Anesthesia. 7th ed. Elsevier; 2017:1022-1041.
2. Weiner MM, Wicker J, Fischer GW, et al. Case 5-2015: Early detection and treatment of an air embolism during cardiac surgery. J Cardiothorac Vasc Anesth, 2015; 29; 791-796.

15. Acute iatrogenic aortic dissection associated with cardiopulmonary bypass:
  A. Is less commonly associated with femoral cannulation
  B. Rarely has a site of origin related to the arterial inflow cannula
  C. May not cause hypotension during cardiopulmonary bypass
  D. Is uncommonly associated with coronary artery bypass surgery

Correct Answer: C

Explanation: Acute iatrogenic aortic dissection is an uncommon but life-threatening complication associated with cardiac surgery that has an estimated mortality of 30%. This complication is less commonly associated with ascending aortic cannulation, with an 0.06% incidence, as compared to femoral arterial cannulation, which has an estimated incidence of 0.6% (tenfold higher risk). The site of origin for aortic dissection in this setting is most commonly the arterial inflow cannula in up to 30% to 35% of cases. Further common sites of origin include aortic clamp sites, whether full or partial clamping, as well as the proximal saphenous vein anastomotic locations. Although systemic hypotension may be due to an intraoperative dissection, this clinical sign may be absent in focal aortic dissection that has not yet propagated extensively. Iatrogenic aortic dissection is commonly associated with coronary artery bypass grafting (up to 60% of cases) and aortic valve surgery (up to 17% of cases). A high index of suspicion and a coordinated team response to this complication can significantly reduce mortality from this aortic emergency.

References:

1. Zakhary WZA, Ender JK. Chapter 31: Procedures in the Hybrid Operating Room. In: Kaplan JA, Augoustides JGT, Manecke GR, et al., eds. Kaplan's Cardiac Anesthesia. 7th ed. Elsevier; 2017:1022-1041.
2. Ram H, Dwarakanath S, Green AE, et al. Iatrogenic aortic dissection associated with cardiac surgery: a narrative review. J Cardiothorac Vasc Anesth, 2021; 35; 3050-3066.

16. Cardiac surgery with cardiopulmonary bypass during pregnancy:
  A. May be deleterious to the fetus, especially in the third trimester
  B. Requires pulsatile perfusion to optimize placental perfusion
  C. Is best undertaken with moderate hypothermia at a range of 20 to 28°C
  D. Should be conducted with high flow rates during cardiopulmonary bypass

Correct Answer: D

Explanation: Cardiac surgery with cardiopulmonary bypass is commonly avoided during pregnancy unless it is strongly indicated due to maternal and fetal risks. Although fetal risk is present, this risk is higher with early gestational age such as the first trimester rather than the third trimester. Further risk factors for increased fetal risk include emergency surgery and maternal comorbidities. Although pulsatile perfusion has been proposed as a way to enhance placental perfusion, there is inconclusive evidence to make this a strong recommendation. The recommended temperature range for cardiopulmonary bypass during pregnancy is in the normothermic to mild hypothermic range (32–34°C). The advantages of mild hypothermia in this setting include reduced fetal oxygen demand and a low risk of fetal arrhythmias. Further degrees of hypothermia, including moderate hypothermia and beyond, have been associated with increased fetal risk and fetal loss. The flow rate for cardiopulmonary bypass in the pregnant patient has been recommended to be in the high range (>2.5 L/min/m²) at a systemic mean arterial pressure of 60 to 70 mmHg to optimize placental perfusion.

References:

1. Zakhary WZA, Ender JK. Chapter 31: Procedures in the Hybrid Operating Room. In: Kaplan JA, Augoustides JGT, Manecke GR, et al., eds. Kaplan's Cardiac Anesthesia. 7th ed. Elsevier; 2017:1022-1041.
2. Carlier L, Devrore S, Budts W, et al. Cardiac interventions in pregnancy and peripartum – a narrative review of the literature. J Cardiothorac Vasc Anesth, 2020; 34; 3409-3419.

17. A 34-year-old woman presents to the emergency room with acute type A aortic dissection in her third trimester of a singleton pregnancy. The management approach should include:
  A. Delayed surgical intervention due to the excessive maternal and fetal risks
  B. Prompt delivery of the fetus before surgical aortic repair
  C. Compliance with the recommendations for cardiopulmonary bypass during pregnancy
  D. Central aortic repair with aortic valve preservation and total arch replacement

Correct Answer: B

Explanation: Acute Stanford type A aortic dissection is an emergency that threatens the lives of both the mother and the fetus. As such, it is also a surgical emergency that has good maternal outcome but may have a fetal mortality as high as 30%, in spite of skilled multidisciplinary management. Cardiac surgery with cardiopulmonary bypass is urgently indicated for central aortic repair after prompt delivery of the fetus. A recommended management approach is to proceed with induction of general endotracheal anesthesia and placement of invasive maternal monitoring, followed by cesarean section to deliver the viable fetus and limit further fetal risk from the acute aortic syndrome. After completion of the cesarean section, central aortic repair can then proceed with cardiopulmonary bypass in the standard fashion for the given institution. Since the fetus has already been delivered, it is not necessary for cardiopulmonary bypass to follow the recommendations for perfusion in pregnancy. Aortic repair should be guided by the extent of proximal dissection, surgical experience, and institutional preferences. While aortic valve preservation and total arch replacement may be possible in aortic centers of excellence, the focus should be on central aortic repair that is realistic and effective to secure maternal survival and limit complications.

References:

1. Zakhary WZA, Ender JK. Chapter 31: Procedures in the Hybrid Operating Room. In: Kaplan JA, Augoustides JGT, Manecke GR, et al., eds. Kaplan's Cardiac Anesthesia. 7th ed. Elsevier; 2017:1022-1041.
2. Patel PA, Fernando RJ, Mackay EJ, et al. Acute type A aortic dissection in pregnancy and peripartum - diagnostic and therapeutic challenges in a multidisciplinary setting. J Cardiothorac Vasc Anesth, 2018; 32; 1991-1997.

18. A 45-year-old woman presents to the emergency room with severe accidental hypothermia complicated by 6 hours of cardiac arrest. The management approach should consider:
- **A.** Resuscitation with protocol-driven extracorporeal life support
- **B.** Aggressive rewarming with tolerance of mild hyperthermia
- **C.** No further management given the prolonged cardiac arrest time
- **D.** No sedative and/or analgesic administration to permit assessment of neurological function

Correct Answer: A

Explanation: Accidental hypothermia can present in severe cases with core temperatures below 32°C and with no perfusing cardiac rhythm that may persist for more than 6 hours. These cases often respond to resuscitation with protocol-driven extracorporeal life support that may include exposure to cardiopulmonary bypass. The rate of rewarming should be gradual with avoidance of hyperthermia to optimize neurological recovery. Despite prolonged cardiac arrest times beyond 6 hours, this multidisciplinary management approach can result in excellent survival with no neurological sequelae. Although sedation and/or analgesia should be minimized to permit serial assessment of neurological function, these modalities may be required for patient comfort, especially if there are concomitant surgical procedures during the recovery process.

References:

1. Zakhary WZA, Ender JK. Chapter 31: Procedures in the Hybrid Operating Room. In: Kaplan JA, Augoustides JGT, Manecke GR, et al., eds. Kaplan's Cardiac Anesthesia. 7th ed. Elsevier; 2017:1022-1041.
2. Mwaura L, Rubino A, Vulsteke A. No cold death – extracorporeal life support for all victims of accidental hypothermia. J Cardiothorac Vasc Anesth, 2020; 34; 372-373.

19. A 75-year-old woman develops acute kidney injury (AKI) after undergoing aortic and mitral valve replacement with cardiopulmonary bypass. Which statement is most correct about this complication?
- **A.** AKI has little effect on long-term outcomes after cardiac surgery
- **B.** Advanced age is a described risk factor for the development of AKI
- **C.** Serum creatinine is an early and sensitive biomarker for AKI
- **D.** There is a lack of classification systems for this complication of cardiopulmonary bypass

Correct Answer: B

Explanation: Acute kidney injury (AKI) associated with cardiac surgery remains a common and important perioperative complication. Although there is a spectrum of severity in AKI, it has been demonstrated to affect morbidity and mortality in the short and long term after cardiac surgery. Advanced age is a well-described risk factor for AKI in this setting that may be partially due to the decreased renal reserve observed with aging. Although serum creatinine is commonly tracked for the diagnosis of AKI, it is a relatively late biomarker for this complication, analogous to Q waves in the evolution of myocardial infarction. The degree of AKI can be classified according to grading systems such as the RIFLE (Risk/Injury/Failure/Loss of kidney function/End-stage kidney disease) criteria, AKIN (Acute Kidney Injury Network) criteria, and the KDIGO (Kidney Disease Improving Global Outcomes) criteria.

References:

1. Zakhary WZA, Ender JK. Chapter 31: Procedures in the Hybrid Operating Room. In: Kaplan JA, Augoustides JGT, Manecke GR, et al., eds. Kaplan's Cardiac Anesthesia. 7th ed. Elsevier; 2017:1022-1041.
2. Just IA, Alborzi F, Godde M, et al. Cardiac surgery-related acute kidney injury – risk factors, clinical course, and management suggestions. J Cardiothorac Vasc Anesth, 2022; 36; 444-451.

20. A 45-year-old woman develops acute kidney injury (AKI) after undergoing aortic root replacement. Which statement is most correct about this complication?
- **A.** Thoracic aortic procedures are among the risk factors for AKI after cardiac surgery
- **B.** Genetic risk factors for AKI have not been described
- **C.** Embolic load has little role in the pathogenesis of AKI in this setting
- **D.** Hydroxyethyl starches are not nephrotoxic

Correct Answer: A

Explanation: Acute kidney injury (AKI) associated with cardiac surgery has multiple risk factors that are related to the procedure, the patient, and the perioperative setting. Procedural risk factors include emergent and reoperative surgeries, valvular interventions, and prolonged cardiopulmonary times, including thoracic aortic procedures that may require hypothermic circulatory arrest (option A). Besides advanced age, patient risk factors include systemic hypertension, diabetes, atherosclerotic vascular disease, and left ventricular dysfunction. Genetic risk factors including polymorphisms related to inflammation and vasoconstriction have been described that may explain the variability in and vulnerability to AKI across the patient spectrum. The rate of rewarming should be gradual, with avoidance of hyperthermia to optimize neurological recovery. Renal emboli including atheroemboli have been associated with AKI after cardiac surgery and may result from plaque disruption from aortic clamping and intra-aortic balloon counterpulsation (see box). Significant evidence from randomized trials and meta-analyses has suggested that hydroxyethyl starch solutions are associated with AKI after cardiac surgery. This body of evidence has led to the recommendation that these solutions be avoided in the cardiac surgery setting.

> BOX 27.1 **Contributors to renal injury during cardiopulmonary bypass**
>
> - Emboli
> - Renal ischemia
> - Reperfusion injury
> - Pigments
> - Contrast agents
> - Hydroxyethyl starches

References:
1. Zakhary WZA, Ender JK. Chapter 31: Procedures in the Hybrid Operating Room. In: Kaplan JA, Augoustides JGT, Manecke GR, et al., eds. Kaplan's Cardiac Anesthesia. 7th ed. Elsevier; 2017:1022-1041.
2. Just IA, Alborzi F, Godde M, et al. Cardiac surgery-related acute kidney injury – risk factors, clinical course, and management suggestions. J Cardiothorac Vasc Anesth, 2022; 36; 444-451.

21. A 62-year-old woman develops acute kidney injury (AKI) after undergoing orthotopic heart transplantation. Which statement is most correct about early biomarkers for this complication?
- **A.** Cystatin c reflects AKI due to accumulation from decreased glomerular clearance
- **B.** Proximal renal tubular epithelial antigen is a marker of glomerular damage in AKI
- **C.** Beta-microglobulin levels are not affected by lysine analog antifibrinolytic agents
- **D.** Neutrophil gelatinase-associated lipocalin does not reflect acute renal stress

Correct Answer: **A**

Explanation: Acute kidney injury (AKI) associated with cardiac surgery may be detected with biomarkers that rise earlier in AKI than serum creatinine (see box). Markers such as cystatin c and tryptophan glycoconjugate are categorized as serum accumulation markers since they mimic creatinine in its accumulation from decreased clearance that occurs with a drop in the glomerular filtration rate. Markers such as alpha-glutathione

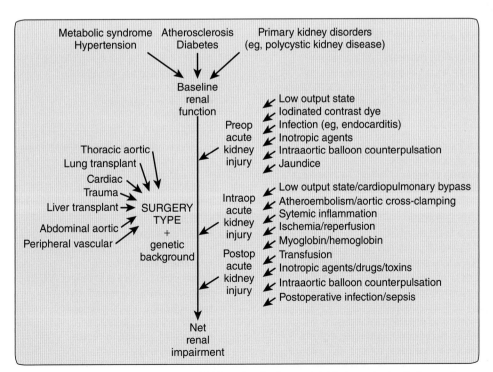

FIGURE 27.1 Numerous sources of kidney insult play a variably important role for each patient during the perioperative period. (Used with permission and modified from Stafford-Smith M, Patel UD, Phillips-Bute BG, et al. Acute kidney injury and chronic kidney disease after cardiac surgery. Adv Chronic Kidney Dis, 2008; 15: 257–277.)

s-transferase and proximal renal tubular epithelial antigen reflect AKI due to tubular cell damage with leakage of cell contents into the urine. Markers such as beta-globulin and renal tubular epithelial antigen-1 reflect AKI due to tubular cell dysfunction that results in proteinuria through impaired protein reabsorption. Lysine analog antifibrinolytic agents such as tranexamic acid and aminocaproic acid blocks these tubular receptors to cause a benign tubular proteinuria. Markers such as neutrophil gelatinase-associated lipocalin and kidney injury molecule-1 reflect AKI from renal insults that triggers an acute stress response.

References:

1. Zakhary WZA, Ender JK. Chapter 31: Procedures in the Hybrid Operating Room. In: Kaplan JA, Augoustides JGT, Manecke GR, et al., eds. Kaplan's Cardiac Anesthesia. 7th ed. Elsevier; 2017:1022-1041.
2. Siverton NA, Hall IE, Melendez NP, et al. Intraoperative urinary biomarkers and acute kidney injury after cardiac surgery J Cardiothorac Vasc Anesth, 2022; 35; 1691-1700.

22. A 62-year-old man develops acute kidney injury (AKI) after undergoing aortic valve replacement for aortic valve disease. Which statement is most correct about this complication?
    A. Mild hypothermia during cardiopulmonary bypass is strongly protective against AKI
    B. The degree of hemodilution during cardiopulmonary bypass is a risk factor for AKI
    C. Fenoldopam prevents acute renal failure requiring dialysis in this clinical setting
    D. N-acetylcysteine is an effective intervention for reduction of AKI after cardiac surgery

Correct Answer: B

Explanation: Due to its outcome importance, considerable research has evaluated strategies to reduce the risk of acute kidney injury (AKI) associated with cardiac surgery. Although hypothermia is a well-established protective strategy in renal transplantation, mild hypothermia during cardiopulmonary bypass has not been conclusively demonstrated to confer the same renal benefits. Significant hemodilution, on the other hand, has been shown to be a significant risk factor for AKI, especially when the hematocrit falls by more than 50% from baseline or when it falls below 20%. Fenoldopam is a selective agonist of dopamine D1 receptors that causes systemic vasodilation with enhanced renal perfusion, natriuresis, and diuresis. Despite these beneficial effects, randomized trials have suggested possible mild nephroprotective properties with no effect on the risk for acute renal failure requiring renal replacement therapy. Despite its attenuating effects in contrast nephropathy, perioperative N-acetylcysteine does not appear to be nephroprotective for cardiac surgical patients.

References:

1. Zakhary WZA, Ender JK. Chapter 31: Procedures in the Hybrid Operating Room. In: Kaplan JA, Augoustides JGT, Manecke GR, et al., eds. Kaplan's Cardiac Anesthesia. 7th ed. Elsevier; 2017:1022-1041.
2. Zangrillo A, Biondi-Zoccai GGL, Frati E, et al. Fenoldopam and acute renal failure in cardiac surgery - a meta-analysis of randomized placebo-controlled trials. J Cardiothorac Vasc Anesth, 2012; 26; 407-413.

BOX 27.2   Early acute kidney injury biomarkers

- **Serum accumulation markers:** reflect acute kidney injury (AKI) much like creatinine, serum accumulation, and decreased clearance with drop in glomerular filtration (Note: also useful to monitor renal recovery)
  - Cystatin C
  - Proatrial natriuretic peptide (1–98)
  - Tryptophan glycoconjugate
- **Tubular enzymuria markers:** reflect AKI through leakage of cell contents into urine after tubular cell damage
  - α-Glutathione S-transferase
  - π-Glutathione S-transferase
  - β-N-acetyl-β-d-glucosaminidase
  - γ-Glutamyl transpeptidase
  - Alkaline phosphatase
  - Lactate dehydrogenase
  - Ala-(leu-gly)-aminopeptidase
  - Proximal renal tubular epithelial antigen
  - Urinary sodium hydrogen exchanger isoform 3
- **Tubular proteinuria markers:** reflect AKI through appearance of small proteins in urine that would normally be taken up by tubular cells, reflecting

tubular cell dysfunction (Note: not useful if using lysine analog antifibrinolytic agents)
  - α_1-Microglobulin
  - β_2-Microglobulin
  - Albumin
  - Adenosine deaminase binding protein
  - Renal tubular epithelial antigen-1
  - Retinol binding protein
  - Lysozyme
  - Ribonuclease
  - Immunoglobulin G
  - Transferrin
  - Ceruloplasmin
  - Lambda and kappa light chains
  - Urinary total protein
- **Renal stress markers:** reflect AKI through various pathophysiologies reflecting or triggered by acute stress
  - Neutrophil gelatinase-associated lipocalin
  - Urinary interleukin-18
  - Platelet activating factor
  - Kidney injury molecule-1
  - Cysteine rich protein 61
  - Urinary P_{O_2}

23. A 68-year-old man develops acute kidney injury (AKI) after undergoing mitral valve replacement for mitral valve disease. Which statement is most correct about this complication?

A. Atrial natriuretic peptide infusion is strongly protective against AKI

B. Dopamine therapy prevents renal failure after cardiopulmonary bypass

C. Perioperative statin therapy does not prevent AKI in this setting

D. Insulin-like growth factor is effective for reduction of perioperative AKI after cardiac surgery

Correct Answer: C

Explanation: Due to its outcome importance, there has been a vigorous search for prevention strategies to reduce the risk of acute kidney injury (AKI) after cardiac surgery. Although a meta-analysis has suggested that atrial natriuretic peptide may be nephroprotective in cardiac surgery, these benefits have not been conclusively demonstrated in large randomized clinical trials. Despite the observations that dopamine therapy can enhance renal perfusion and diuresis, large clinical trials have highlighted that it does not reduce the risk of AKI and may have some risk, including impaired hepatosplanchnic metabolism and increased postoperative arrhythmias. Although statins have beneficial pleiotropic effects, recent meta-analysis of randomized trials has found no favorable effect on AKI in cardiac surgery. Despite its favorable effects in patients with chronic kidney disease such as improved renal function and delayed requirement for dialysis, insulin-like growth factor appears to have no beneficial renal effects in AKI (option D).

References:

1. Zakhary WZA, Ender JK. Chapter 31: Procedures in the Hybrid Operating Room. In: Kaplan JA, Augoustides JGT, Manecke GR, et al., eds. Kaplan's Cardiac Anesthesia. 7th ed. Elsevier; 2017:1022-1041.
2. Zhao BC, Shen P, Liu KX, et al. Perioperative statins do not prevent acute kidney injury after cardiac surgery: a meta-analysis of randomized controlled trials. J Cardiothorac Vasc Anesth, 2017; 361: 2086-2092.

24. The initiation of cardiopulmonary bypass in a 58-year-old man undergoing mitral valve replacement is complicated by systemic hypotension. Which statement is most correct about this phenomenon?

A. Prompt vasopressor therapy should be initiated to restore systemic perfusion

B. It may be due to changes in blood viscosity

C. It should be corrected with prompt induction of hypothermia

D. It is likely due to decreased levels of nitric oxide

Correct Answer: B

Explanation: The initiation of cardiopulmonary bypass is commonly accompanied by transitory systemic hypotension that typically does not require vasopressor therapy for correction. This phenomenon is likely due to the acute reduction in blood viscosity that accompanies the rapid hemodilution during the commencement of cardiopulmonary bypass. Because blood pressure is the product of blood viscosity and systemic vascular resistance, an acute fall in blood viscosity will be associated with a corresponding fall in the blood pressure. Although hypothermia will induce systemic vasoconstriction to improve systemic hypotension during cardiopulmonary bypass, this effect is relatively delayed, since systemic cooling takes time. A second mechanism that may explain the common transitory hypotension that accompanies the onset of cardiopulmonary bypass is the decreased binding of nitric oxide by hemoglobin due to the significant hemodilution. This decreased binding of nitric oxide will lead to increased levels of nitric oxide that cause systemic vasodilation and consequent systemic hypotension. This hypotension at the onset of cardiopulmonary bypass is typically transitory and requires little intervention. If the hypotension persists, then it should prompt a review of the checklist for cardiopulmonary bypass, and subsequent appropriate intervention (see box).

BOX 27.3	**Bypass procedure checklist**

1. Assess arterial inflow.
   a. Arterial perfusate oxygenated?
   b. Direction of arterial inflow appropriate?
   c. Evidence of arterial dissection?
   d. Patient's arterial pressure persistently low?
   e. Inflow line pressure high?
   f. Pump/oxygenator reservoir level falling?
   g. Evidence of atrial cannula malposition?
   h. Patient's arterial pressure persistently high or low?
   i. Unilateral facial swelling, discoloration?
   j. Symmetrical cerebral oximetry?
2. Assess venous outflow.
   a. Is blood draining to the pump/oxygenator's venous reservoir?
   b. Evidence of SVC obstruction?
   c. Facial venous engorgement or congestion, CVP elevated?
3. Is bypass complete?
   a. High CVP/low PA pressure?
   b. Impaired venous drainage?
   c. Low CVP/high PA pressure?
   d. Large bronchial venous blood flow?
   e. Aortic insufficiency?
   f. Arterial and PA pressure nonpulsatile?
   g. Desired pump flow established?
4. Discontinue drug and fluid administration.
5. Discontinue ventilation and inhalation drugs to patient's lungs.

CVP, Central venous pressure; *PA,* pulmonary artery; *SVC,* superior vena cava.

References:

1. Zakhary WZA, Ender JK. Chapter 31: Procedures in the Hybrid Operating Room. In: Kaplan JA, Augoustides JGT, Manecke GR, et al., eds. Kaplan's Cardiac Anesthesia. 7th ed. Elsevier; 2017:1022-1041.
2. Hwang NC. Preventive strategies for minimizing hemodilution in the cardiac surgery patient during cardiopulmonary bypass. J Cardiothorac Vasc Anesth, 2015; 29: 1663-1671.

25. During systemic rewarming and preparation for separation from cardiopulmonary bypass after completion of aortic valve replacement in a 41-year-old woman, systemic hypertension develops. Which statement is most correct about this phenomenon?
    A. The depth of anesthesia may be inappropriate
    B. It should be corrected with prompt induction of hypothermia
    C. Pump flow should be reduced to correct the hypertension
    D. It is likely transitory and therefore does not require further management

Correct Answer: A

Explanation: The preparation for separation from cardiopulmonary bypass should be a systematic sequence of events that includes completion of rewarming. With the return of normothermia, there is an increased risk of patient awareness that is likely accompanied by significant neuromuscular blockade. This scenario can trigger significant endogenous catecholamine release that can result in significant systemic hypertension. The depth of anesthesia should be promptly deepened to correct this scenario. The induction of hypothermia is not appropriate at this point because the surgical procedure has been completed and hypothermia will exacerbate the hypertension due to vasoconstriction. Although a transitory reduction in pump flow will correct the systemic hypertension, it does not address the cause of the systemic hypertension and will exacerbate tissue hypoperfusion.

Systemic vasodilation rather than systemic hypertension typically accompanies systemic rewarming due to the consequent vasodilation. Systemic hypertension should prompt a review of the checklist for preparation to separate from cardiopulmonary bypass, and lead to subsequent appropriate management (see box).

References:

1. Zakhary WZA, Ender JK. Chapter 31: Procedures in the Hybrid Operating Room. In: Kaplan JA, Augoustides JGT, Manecke GR, et al., eds. Kaplan's Cardiac Anesthesia. 7th ed. Elsevier; 2017:1022-1041.
2. Monaco F, Di Prima AL, Kim JH, et al. Management of challenging cardiopulmonary bypass separation. J Cardiothorac Vasc Anesth, 2020; 34: 1622-1635.

26. During minimally invasive mitral valve repair in a 34-year-old woman with port-access cardiopulmonary bypass, there is an acute decrease in the right-sided cerebral oximetry signal to 60% below the baseline. Which the most likely explanation for this monitoring change?
    A. The patient has suffered an embolic stroke
    B. The endoaortic clamp has migrated
    C. The oximetry pad has failed and should be replaced
    D. The retrograde cardioplegia cannula has dislodged

Correct Answer: B

Explanation: The endoaortic clamp is one of the specialty cannulas that may be selected in the conduct of port-access cardiopulmonary bypass. This cannula has an occlusion balloon that functions as an aortic clamp and a lumen that allows infusion of antegrade cardioplegia into the aortic root and coronary arteries. This cannula is typically positioned in the proximal ascending aorta about 2 to 4 cm above the aortic valve. Since this cannula can migrate distally to occlude the brachiocephalic arteries, its position is typically monitored carefully in a number of ways, including cerebral oximetry (see table). Although an embolic

---

BOX 27.4   Preparation for separation from bypass checklist

1. Air clearance maneuvers completed
2. Rewarming completed
   a. Nasopharyngeal temperature 36–37°C
   b. Rectal/bladder temperature ≥35°C, but ≤37°C
3. Address issue of adequacy of anesthesia and muscle relaxation
4. Obtain stable cardiac rate and rhythm (use pacing if necessary)
5. Pump flow and systemic arterial pressure
   a. Pump flow to maintain mixed venous saturation ≥70%
   b. Systemic pressure restored to normothermic levels
6. Metabolic parameters
   a. Arterial pH, Po_2, Pco_2 within normal limits
   b. Hct: 20%–25%

   c. K^+: 4.0–5.0 mEq/L
   d. Possibly ionized calcium
7. Ensuring all monitoring/access catheters are functional
   a. Transducers rezeroed
   b. TEE (if used) out of freeze mode
8. Respiratory management
   a. Atelectasis cleared/lungs reexpanded
   b. Evidence of pneumothorax?
   c. Residual fluid in thoracic cavities drained
   d. Ventilation reinstituted
9. Intravenous fluids restarted
10. Inotropes/vasopressors/vasodilators prepared

Hct, Hematocrit; *TEE*, transesophageal echocardiography.

stroke can cause a unilateral fall in cerebral oximetry, this would be unusual in a young adult, given the lack of aortic atheroma. The likely explanation is this setting is that the endoaortic clamp has migrated in a cephalad direction to occlude the innominate artery with a consequent fall in right-sided cerebral perfusion. This migration can also be detected through dampening of a right radial arterial line and through serial imaging of the ascending aorta with transesophageal echocardiography (see table). Although failure of the oximetry pad can result in a reduced signal, this is unusual and should be considered after exclusion of more serious etiologies such as migration of the endoaortic clamp. Although the coronary sinus cannula may dislodge and migrate into the right atrium, this event would interfere with delivery of retrograde cardioplegia and not affect cerebral perfusion.

References:

1. Zakhary WZA, Ender JK. Chapter 31: Procedures in the Hybrid Operating Room. In: Kaplan JA, Augoustides JGT, Manecke GR, et al., eds. Kaplan's Cardiac Anesthesia. 7th ed. Elsevier; 2017:1022-1041.
2. Ali J, Cody J, Maldonado Y, et al. Near-infrared spectroscopy (NIRS) for cerebral and tissue oximetry: analysis of evolving applications. J Cardiothorac Vasc Anesth, 2022; 36: 2758-2776.

27. During minimally invasive mitral and tricuspid valve repair in a 64-year-old woman with port-access cardiopulmonary bypass, there is an acute decrease in the left-sided cerebral oximetry signal to 80% below the baseline. What is the most likely explanation for this monitoring change?
    A. The hematocrit has dropped below 20%
    B. The endoaortic clamp has migrated proximally
    C. There is an intraoperative aortic dissection
    D. The endopulmonary vent has migrated distally

Correct Answer: C

Explanation: Although a fall in the hematocrit may cause a drop in cerebral oxygen delivery and a fall in cerebral oximetry, this fall should be bilateral rather than unilateral, as both cerebral hemispheres will experience this compromised oxygenation. The endoaortic clamp has an occlusion balloon that functions as an aortic clamp and a lumen that allows delivery of antegrade cardioplegia. This cannula is typically positioned in the proximal ascending aorta about 2 to 4 cm above the aortic valve. Since this cannula can migrate distally to occlude the brachiocephalic arteries, its position is typically monitored in a multimodal fashion, including cerebral oximetry. The proximal migration of this cannula would mean that it has slipped into the aortic root, and so it would not cause cerebral malperfusion. This proximal migration

TABLE 27.1
Potential strategies to monitor cerebral blood flow during port-access bypass

Monitor	Limitations	Observation With Cephalad Migration of Endoaortic Clamp[a]
Fluoroscopy	1. Must interrupt surgery to use monitor	EAC occluding great vessels
Transesophageal echocardiography	1. May be difficult to visualize EAC position during cardiopulmonary bypass	EAC in area of great vessels
Carotid ultrasound	1. Difficult to monitor signal continuously—depends on index of suspicion 2. Difficult to obtain signal with nonpulsatile blood flow	Sudden loss of blood flow signal
Transcranial Doppler	1. Difficult to monitor MCA blood flow continuously—depends on index of suspicion 2. Difficult to insonate MCA during nonpulsatile blood flow 3. Poor sensitivity/specificity	1. Loss of MCA blood flow velocity signal 2. Change in ratio of RMCA vs. LMCA blood flow velocity 3. Change in RMCA or LMCA blood flow direction
Cerebral oximetry (R vs. L signal)	1. Sensitivity/specificity?	Decrease in cerebral venous blood oxygen saturation; change in R vs. L signal[b]
Electroencephalography	1. Hypothermia, anesthetics, and roller pump artifacts limit interpretation of EEG signals	EEG slowing/change in right vs. left EEG signal
Right and left radial arterial pressures	1. Requires cannulation of both radial arteries; increased risk for hand ischemia 2. Left radial arterial free graft conduit not possible	Change in the ratio of right and left radial arteries measured MAP

[a]Hypothetical observation; the sensitivity and specificity of these monitors in this clinical setting have not been evaluated.
[b]The rate and magnitude of change depend on many factors, including the patient's cerebral temperature, magnitude of obstruction, and collateral blood flow.
EAC, Endoaortic clamp; *EEG*, electroencephalographic; *L*, left; *MAP*, mean arterial pressure; *MCA*, middle cerebral artery; *R*, right.

can be readily imaged with transesophageal echocardiography to allow subsequent correct repositioning of the endo-aortic clamp. An acute intraoperative dissection could cause left cerebral ischemia through interference with left carotid perfusion due to an intimal flap in the aortic arch. This complication can develop in the setting of femoral arterial cannulation and/or endoaortic clamping during the conduct of port-access cardiopulmonary bypass. The dissection process can be characterized with transesophageal echocardiography. Although the endopulmonary vent in the pulmonary artery may migrate distally in the pulmonary artery, this event might interfere with venting of the left ventricle and not affect cerebral perfusion.

References:

1. Zakhary WZA, Ender JK. Chapter 31: Procedures in the Hybrid Operating Room. In: Kaplan JA, Augoustides JGT, Manecke GR, et al., eds. Kaplan's Cardiac Anesthesia. 7th ed. Elsevier; 2017:1022-1041.
2. Ram H, Dwarakanath S, Green AE, et al. Iatrogenic aortic dissection associated with cardiac surgery: a narrative review. J Cardiothorac Vasc Anesth, 2021; 35: 3050-3066.

28. During preparation for minimally invasive mitral valve repair with port-access cardiopulmonary bypass, percutaneous coronary sinus catheter is placed for delivery of retrograde cardioplegia during the procedure. Which statement is most correct about this catheter?
    A. Fluoroscopy has a minimal role in its placement
    B. It does not dislodge from the coronary sinus when positioned correctly
    C. Ventricularization of the pressure tracing is typically associated with unsuccessful placement
    D. Successful placement is characterized by appropriate pressure and flow criteria

Correct Answer: D

Explanation: The placement of the percutaneous coronary sinus catheter in port-access cardiopulmonary bypass requires imaging guidance, typically with transesophageal echocardiography to engage the sinus and with fluoroscopy to advance the catheter in the sinus. Even if correctly positioned, it may dislodge from the coronary sinus during surgical manipulation of the heart. Ventricularization of the coronary sinus pressure tracing is frequently observed and is significantly associated with appropriate placement. Successful placement of this cannula is characterized by pressures greater than 30 mmHg at a flow rate of about 150 to 200 mL/minute.

References:

1. Zakhary WZA, Ender JK. Chapter 31: Procedures in the Hybrid Operating Room. In: Kaplan JA, Augoustides JGT, Manecke GR, et al., eds. Kaplan's Cardiac Anesthesia. 7th ed. Elsevier; 2017:1022-1041.
2. Lebon JS, Couture P, Rochon AG, et al. The endovascular coronary sinus catheter in minimally invasive mitral and tricuspid valve surgery: a case series. J Cardiothorac Vasc Anesth, 2010; 24: 746-751.

29. During preparation for minimally invasive mitral valve repair with port-access cardiopulmonary bypass, cardioplegia was commenced after application of the endoaortic clamp. Which statement is most correct about management of cardioplegia in this setting?
    A. Anterograde cardioplegia requires direct cannulation of the ascending aorta
    B. Retrograde cardioplegia is not an option in port-access cardiopulmonary bypass
    C. Myocardial protection is compromised with this minimally invasive approach
    D. The endoaortic clamp can serve as a left ventricular vent

Correct Answer: D

Explanation: Anterograde cardioplegia can be effectively administered via the tip of the endoaortic clamp after correct positioning in the proximal ascending aorta and after inflation of the endoaortic balloon. This delivery option obviates the need to cannulate the ascending aorta directly through a chest incision. Retrograde cardioplegia can be administered via the coronary sinus, either with direct cannulation by the surgeon or via the percutaneous coronary sinus catheter that is positioned with imaging guidance. These techniques permit effective delivery of both antegrade and retrograde cardioplegia in port-access cardiopulmonary bypass for optimal myocardial protection during the procedure. Furthermore, the lumen of the endoaortic clamp catheter that permits delivery of anterograde cardioplegia can also serve as a drainage outlet for venting of the left ventricle across the aortic valve.

References:

1. Zakhary WZA, Ender JK. Chapter 31: Procedures in the Hybrid Operating Room. In: Kaplan JA, Augoustides JGT, Manecke GR, et al., eds. Kaplan's Cardiac Anesthesia. 7th ed. Elsevier; 2017:1022-1041.
2. Lebon JS, Couture P, Rochon AG, et al. The endovascular coronary sinus catheter in minimally invasive mitral and tricuspid valve surgery: a case series. J Cardiothorac Vasc Anesth, 2010; 24: 746-751.

30. During the echocardiographic examination for minimally invasive mitral valve repair and left atrial appendage ligation with port-access cardiopulmonary bypass, a persistent left superior vena cava was diagnosed. Which statement is most correct about this venous anomaly in this setting?
    A. It does not affect the delivery of anterograde cardioplegia
    B. The diagnosis can be confirmed by intravenous administration of agitated saline in the right upper extremity
    C. It is not at risk for injury in this procedure
    D. It does not affect the placement of a pulmonary arterial catheter

Correct Answer: A

Explanation: Although uncommon, a persistent left superior vena cava can affect the delivery of retrograde cardioplegia as it drains into the coronary sinus. This venous anomaly does not affect the delivery of antegrade cardioplegia in the proximal thoracic aorta. The diagnosis can be confirmed with intravenous injection of agitated saline in the left upper extremity, as saline contrast will be imaged by transesophageal echocardiography to be entering the right atrium from the coronary sinus above the septal leaflet of the tricuspid valve. Intravenous injection of contrast injected in the right upper extremity will not travel to the right atrium via a persistent left superior vena cava. Given the proximity of the coronary sinus and persistent left superior vena cava to the mitral valve annulus and the left atrial appendage, these structures are at risk for injury during mitral valve and left atrial appendage procedures. A persistent left superior vena cava can complicate placement of a pulmonary arterial catheter if floated from the left internal or left subclavian vein, since the catheter may traverse the coronary sinus to reach the pulmonary artery.

References:

1. Zakhary WZA, Ender JK. Chapter 31: Procedures in the Hybrid Operating Room. In: Kaplan JA, Augoustides JGT, Manecke GR, et al., eds. Kaplan's Cardiac Anesthesia. 7th ed. Elsevier; 2017:1022-1041.
2. Nwana-Nzewunwa OC, Lennon Paul, Gebhardt BR, et al. Facial plethora and markedly elevated central venous pressure after mitral valve repair, maze, and left atrial appendage occlusion procedures. J Cardiothorac Vasc Anesth, 2022; 36: 1804-1806.

CHAPTER 28

Extracorporeal Devices and Related Technologies

Daniel Bainbridge and John G.T. Augoustides

KEY POINTS

1. Mechanical circulatory support (MCS) for the failing heart has become a mainstay of the modern management of patients with both acute and chronic heart failure refractory to pharmacologic and other usual interventions.

2. Outcomes with MCS have improved so dramatically that the main focus of this arena has now shifted away from simple survival and toward mitigation of risk and minimization of adverse events.

3. Data taken from experience gained with the first generation of pulsatile devices may no longer be applicable in the current era of nonpulsatile support, but the valuable lessons learned continue to help shape management and clinical decision making.

4. In addition to the traditional indications for MCS (e.g., short-term bridge to recovery and long-term bridge to transplantation), MCS is currently employed for a variety of both short- and long-term modern indications, including acute rescue of patients from acute low cardiac output situations (bridge to immediate survival), prevention of further myocardial damage following an ischemic event, prevention of deterioration in multisystem organ function, as a temporizing measure to buy time for recovery, as a bridge to the next step of management (bridge to next decision), as a bridge to improved candidacy (for transplantation), and, increasingly, as a final management strategy for end-stage heart failure (destination therapy).

5. Patient status at the time of implementation of rescue MCS is a key factor determining outcome. Deterioration from delayed implementation is associated with worse outcome.

6. The timing of implantation of a durable left ventricular assist device (LVAD) (e.g., as a bridge to transplantation and/or as destination therapy) and perioperative optimization of the patient's nutritional status are key factors determining outcome.

7. Nonpulsatile support devices have supplanted the first generation of pulsatile ventricular assist devices worldwide, and outcomes have improved dramatically with the technology now available.

8. Extracorporeal membrane oxygenation is being incorporated more and more often into modern extracorporeal life support algorithms.

9. The implantable total artificial heart has undergone a resurgence of interest as a bridge to transplantation for patients with biventricular failure and in other scenarios where an LVAD alone would not be ideal.

10. A number of new MCS devices are in various stages of development and clinical trials.

---

1. Overocclusive operation of a roller pump may result in:
   A. Spallation of the tube
   B. Roller pumps have a raceway that prevents over-occlusion
   C. Retrograde flow
   D. High arterial line pressure

Correct Answer: A

Explanation: Spallation (the generation of particulate fragmentation from the inner wall of the tubing) and hemolysis of red blood cells occurs when the occlusion of the roller pump is set too high (overocclusive operation) (see teaching box). Ideally, occlusion should be set to allow a static column of water at 30 cm above the venous reservoir to fall at 1 cm/min to prevent over-occlusion. Retrograde flow may occur when the tubing is under occluded and typically results in higher revolutions per minute for delivered flow than was calculated.

BOX 28.1 Roller pumps

- Composed of twin rollers
- Deliver flow using positive displacement of the fluid in the tubing
- Blood flow is calculated using tubing stroke volume and pump revolutions per minute
- An underocclusive roller pump may result in retrograde flow in the patient and in the cardiopulmonary bypass circuit
- An overocclusive roller pump may increase hemolysis and produce spallation of the perfusion tubing

References:

1. Groom RC, Fitzgerald D. Chapter 32: Extracorporeal Devices and Related Technologies. In: Kaplan JA, Augoustides JGT, Manecke GR, et al., eds. Kaplan's Cardiac Anesthesia. 7th ed. Elsevier; 2017:1162-1213.
2. Allison J, Spiwak B, Norbal A, et al. Extracorporeal tubing in the roller pump raceway: physical changes and particulate generation. J Extra Corpor Technol, 2008; 40: 188-192.

2. All the following are true regarding centrifugal pumps EXCEPT:
   A. They do not generate forces sufficient to cause arterial line splitting/delamination
   B. Blood flow is directly proportional to downstream resistance
   C. Hemolysis may be caused by heat generation
   D. If the pump stops, retrograde flow may result

Correct Answer: B

Explanation: As resistance increases, flow decreases, making this relationship inverse not direct (see box). The pump is unable to generate the forces required to delaminate/split the arterial line, even if clamped suddenly. However, if the line is suddenly clamped it may generate a lot of heat, which may cause blood hemolysis. If the pump stops, because it is nonocclusive, retrograde flow may occur.

References:

1. Groom RC, Fitzgerald D. Chapter 32: Extracorporeal Devices and Related Technologies. In: Kaplan JA, Augoustides JGT, Manecke GR, et al., eds. Kaplan's Cardiac Anesthesia. 7th ed. Elsevier; 2017:1162-1213.
2. Asante-Slaw J, Tyrell J, Hoschtizky A, et al. Does the use of a centrifugal pump offer any additional benefit for patients having open heart surgery? Interact Cardiovasc Thorac Surg, 2006; 5: 128-134.

BOX 28.2 Centrifugal pumps

- Operate on the constrained vortex principle
- Blood flow is inversely related to downstream resistance
- Flow rate is determined using an ultrasonic flow meter
- Increase in centrifugal pump revolutions per minute may result in heat generation and hemolysis
- If the centrifugal pump is stopped, the line must be clamped to prevent retrograde flow

3. Comparing centrifugal pumps to roller pumps, the following is TRUE for centrifugal pumps:
   A. Lower mortality
   B. Improved neurological outcomes
   C. Reduced postoperative blood loss
   D. No clinical benefit compared to roller pumps

Correct Answer: D

Explanation: Although centrifugal pumps may offer some benefits such as fewer microemboli, less platelet activation, and reduced hemolysis, these advantages have not translated into durable clinical benefits (see teaching boxes). Although the utilization of centrifugal pumps may provide safety advantages, its clinical advantages are not apparent.

References:

1. Groom RC, Fitzgerald D. Chapter 32: Extracorporeal Devices and Related Technologies. In: Kaplan JA, Augoustides JGT, Manecke GR, et al., eds. Kaplan's Cardiac Anesthesia. 7th ed. Elsevier; 2017:1162-1213.
2. Ferraris VA, Brown JR, Despotis GJ, et al. Perioperative blood transfusion and blood conservation in cardiac surgery: The Society of Thoracic Surgeons and The Society of Cardiovascular Anesthesiologists clinical practice guideline. Ann Thorac Surg, 2011; 91: 944-982.
3. Asante-Slaw J, Tyrell J, Hoschtizky A, et al. Does the use of a centrifugal pump offer any additional benefit for patients having open heart surgery? Interact Cardiovasc Thorac Surg, 2006; 5: 128-134.

4. Regarding resistance to blood flow during cardiopulmonary bypass, which is TRUE?
   A. Venous reservoir provides the least resistance
   B. The patient's systemic vascular resistance does not play a role
   C. The arterial cannula provides the greatest resistance
   D. The venous cannula provides the least resistance

Correct Answer: C

Explanation: The aortic cannula has the smallest cross-sectional area in the system and so, according to Poiseuille's law, contributes to the greatest resistance (see teaching box). Neither the venous cannula nor the venous reservoir contributes to the resistance experienced by the pump during cardiopulmonary bypass. The patient's systemic vascular resistance is a factor in the calculation of resistance during cardiopulmonary bypass as is tubing length, the oxygenator, heat exchanger, arterial line filter, and viscosity of the perfusate.

BOX 28.3 Arterial cannulae

- The arterial cannula tip is the point of highest blood flow velocity in the cardiopulmonary bypass circuit
- Some arterial cannulae have flow-dispersing tips to reduce exit velocity and reduce the risk for atheroma dislodgement from the wall of the aorta
- Cannula placement should be assessed by a test infusion from the pump and observation of a pulsatile pressure excursion

References:

1. Groom RC, Fitzgerald D. Chapter 32: Extracorporeal Devices and Related Technologies. In: Kaplan JA, Augoustides JGT, Manecke GR, et al., eds. Kaplan's Cardiac Anesthesia. 7th ed. Elsevier; 2017:1162-1213.
2. Sarkar M, Prabhu V. Basics of cardiopulmonary bypass. Indian J Anaesth, 2017; 61: 760-767.

5. Which of the following is TRUE regarding air embolism during cardiopulmonary bypass?
   A. Massive air embolism is most frequently caused by the venous reservoir
   B. The use of a level-sensing device makes air bubble detectors unnecessary
   C. Air bubble detectors are sensitive to small amounts of air
   D. Photoelectric detectors are more sensitive to air than are ultrasound detectors

Correct Answer: C

Explanation: Air bubble detectors are sensitive to small amounts of air. The latest detectors typically use ultrasound, as it is a more sensitive method than photoelectric detection. Level-sensing devices ensure that the venous reservoir does not cause air embolism due to low blood levels in the reservoir but do not detect entrained air in the circuit. Massive air embolism is usually caused by air entrainment in the surgical field, as most modern circuits use the level sensor to shut off the pumps when a low blood level is detected.

References:

1. Groom RC, Fitzgerald D. Chapter 32: Extracorporeal Devices and Related Technologies. In: Kaplan JA, Augoustides JGT, Manecke GR, et al., eds. Kaplan's Cardiac Anesthesia. 7th ed. Elsevier; 2017:1162-1213.
2. Gerstein NS, Panikkath P, Mirrakhimov AE, et al. Cardiopulmonary bypass emergencies and intraoperative issues. J Cardiothorac Vasc Anesth, 2022; 36: 4505-4522.

6. Regarding membrane oxygenators, which is TRUE?
   A. Silicone oxygenators have no blood–gas interface
   B. Microporous propylene oxygenators degrade rapidly, limiting their use for long-term extracorporeal circulation
   C. Polymethyl pentene oxygenators have reduced diffusion but less plasma leak than propylene membranes
   D. Bubble oxygenators caused less contact activation but more gaseous microemboli

Correct Answer: A

Explanation: The three materials commonly used in membrane oxygenators include silicone, propylene, and polymethyl pentene. Silicone is rarely used but allows diffusion of gases through the membrane, and thus no blood–gas interface. Propylene oxygenators (hollow fiber) have a blood–gas interface but in general are robust and can be used for long cases because they are unlikely to fracture and admit plasma (see teaching box). Polymethyl pentene oxygenators

have the best diffusion characteristics for gas, but have a tendency to fracture, and so are not used for long cases. Bubble oxygenators, of historical interest only, had both more contact activation and more gaseous microemboli.

BOX 28.4   Membrane oxygenators

- Hollow-fiber membrane oxygenators are commonly used for cardiopulmonary bypass
- An oxygen gas mixture flows through microporous polypropylene hollow fibers
- Blood flow is directed over the microporous hollow fibers
- Recently nonporous polymethylpentene (PMP) hollow fibers have been developed
- PMP fibers provided a more durable surface for prolonged oxygenation such as extracorporeal membrane oxygenation
- PMP fibers do not permit the passage of volatile anesthetics such as isoflurane

---

References:

1. Groom RC, Fitzgerald D. Chapter 32: Extracorporeal Devices and Related Technologies. In: Kaplan JA, Augoustides JGT, Manecke GR, et al., eds. Kaplan's Cardiac Anesthesia. 7th ed. Elsevier; 2017:1162-1213.
2. Sarkar M, Prabhu V. Basics of cardiopulmonary bypass. Indian J Anaesth, 2017; 61: 760-767.

7. Gas transfer in a membrane oxygenator is affected by:
   A. Oxygenator volume, partial pressure of venous gases, blood flow, and ventilation flow (sweep gas)
   B. Oxygenator surface area, partial pressure of venous gases, blood flow, and ventilation flow (sweep gas)
   C. Oxygenator volume, partial pressure of arterial gases, blood pressure, and ventilation pressure (sweep gas)
   D. Oxygenator surface area, partial pressure of arterial gases, blood pressure, and ventilation pressure (sweep gas)

Correct Answer: B

Explanation: Similar to normal physiology, the gas exchange across a membrane oxygenator is affected by its surface area, partial pressure of venous gases, blood flow, and ventilation flow (sweep gas). These factors mirror the physiologic variables in the lung, namely diffusion capacity, partial pressure of venous gases, perfusion, and ventilation. Ventilation pressure and blood pressure do not primarily affect gas transfer across a membrane oxygenator.

References:

1. Groom RC, Fitzgerald D. Chapter 32: Extracorporeal Devices and Related Technologies. In: Kaplan JA, Augoustides JGT, Manecke GR, et al., eds. Kaplan's Cardiac Anesthesia. 7th ed. Elsevier; 2017:1162-1213.
2. Sarkar M, Prabhu V. Basics of cardiopulmonary bypass. Indian J Anaesth, 2017; 61: 760-767.

8. Which of the following is FALSE regarding open venous reservoirs?

   A. They consist of a hard polycarbonate shell
   B. They have integrated venous and cardiotomy reservoirs
   C. Vacuum-assist venous return is not possible
   D. Air bubbles escape to atmosphere at the top of the reservoir

Correct Answer: C

Explanation: Vacuum-assist venous drainage is frequently employed to assist the venous drainage during cardiopulmonary bypass. Open venous reservoir systems have polycarbonate shells that are typically open to atmosphere and with both the venous and cardiotomy reservoirs integrated into one (see teaching box). In these types of reservoir systems, air bubbles reach the atmosphere at the top of the reservoir.

BOX 28.5   Venous reservoirs

Open Systems

• Open systems have polycarbonate hard-shell reservoirs and are usually equipped with an integral cardiotomy reservoir
• With open systems, venous return may be improved by applying regulated suction to the reservoir (vacuum-assisted venous drainage)
• With open systems, buoyant air bubbles escape to the atmosphere at the top of the reservoir

Closed Systems

• Closed systems consist of collapsible polyvinylchloride bags
• Closed systems require a separate cardiotomy reservoir
• Buoyant air from the venous line accumulates in the bag and must be actively aspirated
• Closed systems have a reduced contact surface of the blood with air or plastic
• A separate centrifugal pump may be used to increase venous return (kinetic-assisted venous drainage)

References:

1. Groom RC, Fitzgerald D. Chapter 32: Extracorporeal Devices and Related Technologies. In: Kaplan JA, Augoustides JGT, Manecke GR, et al., eds. Kaplan's Cardiac Anesthesia. 7th ed. Elsevier; 2017:1162-1213.
2. Sarkar M, Prabhu V. Basics of cardiopulmonary bypass. Indian J Anaesth, 2017; 61: 760-767.

9. What is FALSE regarding closed venous reservoirs?

   A. They consist of a collapsible polyvinylchloride bag
   B. Air in the venous line must be aspirated from the reservoir
   C. A separate centrifugal pump may be used to increase venous return
   D. They have integrated venous and cardiotomy reservoirs

Correct Answer: D

Explanation: As the name suggests, closed reservoirs have a collapsible bag that limits the air–blood interface, and therefore any air entrained must be aspirated separately (see teaching box).

As such, a cardiotomy reservoir, with the associated large amount of air that is aspirated, would not work in a closed system, so a separate reservoir is necessary. Furthermore, these systems may require a separate centrifugal pump to increase venous return.

References:

1. Groom RC, Fitzgerald D. Chapter 32: Extracorporeal Devices and Related Technologies. In: Kaplan JA, Augoustides JGT, Manecke GR, et al., eds. Kaplan's Cardiac Anesthesia. 7th ed. Elsevier; 2017:1162-1213.
2. Sarkar M, Prabhu V. Basics of cardiopulmonary bypass. Indian J Anaesth, 2017; 61: 760-767.
3. Zangrillo A, Garozzo FA, Biondi-Zoccai G, et al. Miniaturized cardiopulmonary bypass improves short-term outcome in cardiac surgery: A meta-analysis of randomized controlled studies. J Thorac Cardiovasc Surg, 2010; 139: 1162-1169.

10. The advantages of miniaturized over conventional cardiopulmonary bypass circuits include:

   A. Enhanced air management
   B. Enhanced management of shed blood
   C. Reduced patient transfusions
   D. Decreased mortality

Correct Answer: C

Explanation: Miniature cardiopulmonary bypass (CPB) systems are designed to limit the blood contact with foreign surfaces, including air and circuit tubing. As such, most systems are designed as closed systems with centrifugal pumps placed close to the patient to minimize the tubing length of the extracorporeal circuit. Given these goals and constraints, these closed systems are not optimized for the presence of air or shed mediastinal blood. Meta-analysis of trials looking at miniature CPB circuits suggests the main advantage is reductions in transfusions and not mortality.

References:

1. Groom RC, Fitzgerald D. Chapter 32: Extracorporeal Devices and Related Technologies. In: Kaplan JA, Augoustides JGT, Manecke GR, et al., eds. Kaplan's Cardiac Anesthesia. 7th ed. Elsevier; 2017:1162-1213.
2. Harling L, Warren OJ, Martin A, et al. Do miniaturized extracorporeal circuits confer significant clinical benefit without compromising safety? A meta-analysis of randomized controlled trials. ASAIO J, 2011; 57: 141-151.
3. Zangrillo A, Garozzo FA, Biondi-Zoccai G, et al. Miniaturized cardiopulmonary bypass improves short-term outcome in cardiac surgery: A meta-analysis of randomized controlled studies. J Thorac Cardiovasc Surg, 2010; 139: 1162-1169.

11. Regarding heat exchangers in extracorporeal circulation, which of the following statements is FALSE?

   A. They are usually designed with countercurrent flow
   B. They are frequently made of aluminum, which during prolonged use in pediatrics may lead to aluminum toxicity
   C. They are usually placed on the proximal or venous side to reduce gas emboli
   D. They are placed proximal to the oxygenator and so have low-pressure blood flow

Correct Answer: D

Explanation: The heat exchanger is typically placed proximal to the oxygenator, but distal to the pump. In this manner it has high-pressure blood flow in the system, but any gaseous microemboli that may form during rewarming then typically dissipate in the oxygenator. The device is designed for countercurrent flow to improve the heating/cooling efficiency. Although stainless steel and propylene may be used in construction, aluminum is also frequently used and may cause toxicity in pediatric patients.

References:

1. Groom RC, Fitzgerald D. Chapter 32: Extracorporeal Devices and Related Technologies. In: Kaplan JA, Augoustides JGT, Manecke GR, et al., eds. Kaplan's Cardiac Anesthesia. 7th ed. Elsevier; 2017:1162-1213.
2. Sarkar M, Prabhu V. Basics of cardiopulmonary bypass. Indian J Anaesth, 2017; 61: 760-767.

12. Arterial line filters:
   A. Can provide protection against neurocognitive dysfunction
   B. Have a filter size of 120–140 μm
   C. Must be a stand-alone filter placed as close to the arterial cannula as possible
   D. Remove only particulate microemboli, and not gaseous microemboli

Correct Answer: A

Explanation: The arterial line filter has been shown to provide protection against neurocognitive dysfunction with high-level evidence (see box). The pore size is usually 20 to 40 μm. It is used to remove both particulate and gaseous microemboli. There is a trend towards incorporation of the filters into oxygenators, which may reduce prime volumes and assist in miniaturizing of the extracorporeal circuit.

BOX 28.6 Arterial line filters

- Have been shown to reduce the rate of neurocognitive dysfunction
- Reduce the load of gaseous and particulate microemboli to the patient
- Typical pore size ranges between 20 and 40 μm
- There is a trend towards integration of the arterial filter into the oxygenator

---

References:

1. Groom RC, Fitzgerald D. Chapter 32: Extracorporeal Devices and Related Technologies. In: Kaplan JA, Augoustides JGT, Manecke GR, et al., eds. Kaplan's Cardiac Anesthesia. 7th ed. Elsevier; 2017:1162-1213.
2. Sarkar M, Prabhu V. Basics of cardiopulmonary bypass. Indian J Anaesth, 2017; 61: 760-767.
3. Wahta A, Milojevic M, De Somer FMJJ, et al. 2019 EACTS/ EACTA/EBCP guidelines on cardiopulmonary bypass in adult cardiac surgery. Eur J Cardiothorac Surg, 2020; 57: 210-251.

13. Regarding cardioplegia, which of the following is TRUE?
   A. All current solutions work to arrest the heart in a depolarized state
   B. Retrograde cardioplegia is typically delivered at pressures of 100–150 mmHg
   C. Simultaneous antegrade and retrograde cardioplegia may be used
   D. Antegrade cardioplegia is typically associated with poor perfusion of the right ventricle owing to the location of the right coronary artery

Correct Answer: C

Explanation: Simultaneous antegrade and retrograde delivery of cardioplegia is possible with venous drainage occurring through the thebesian and arteriosinusoidal veins. Solutions used to arrest the heart include potassium-containing solutions and magnesium/lidocaine-containing solutions. The former arrest the heart in a depolarized state, while the latter arrest the heart in a polarized state. Antegrade cardioplegia is typically delivered at pressures of 100 to 150 mmHg, while retrograde cardioplegia typically uses pressures of 40 to 60 mmHg. Complications of retrograde cardioplegia include: rupture of the coronary sinus, poor perfusion of the right ventricle, and nonhomogenous flow patterns.

References:

1. Groom RC, Fitzgerald D. Chapter 32: Extracorporeal Devices and Related Technologies. In: Kaplan JA, Augoustides JGT, Manecke GR, et al., eds. Kaplan's Cardiac Anesthesia. 7th ed. Elsevier; 2017:1162-1213.
2. Sarkar M, Prabhu V. Basics of cardiopulmonary bypass. Indian J Anaesth, 2017; 61: 760-767.
3. Wahta A, Milojevic M, De Somer FMJJ, et al. 2019 EACTS/ EACTA/EBCP guidelines on cardiopulmonary bypass in adult cardiac surgery. Eur J Cardiothorac Surg, 2020; 57: 210-251.

14. Regarding priming solutions for extracorporeal circulation, which of the following is FALSE?
   A. Albumin may be used to coat the surface of the cardiopulmonary bypass machine and reduce contact activation
   B. Hydroxyethyl starch reduces blood product utilization
   C. Balanced salt solutions make up the majority of the prime
   D. Heparin is frequently added, especially if the priming balanced salt solution contains calcium

Correct Answer: B

Explanation: Clinical exposure to hydroxyethyl starch has been associated with increased postoperative blood loss, reoperation for bleeding, and transfusion. As such, it has been recommended to avoid these agents during cardiopulmonary bypass. The theoretical benefit of albumin is that the protein coats the surface of the tubing and thus reduces contact activation, although the benefit of this may be reduced with bonded circuits. Heparin is frequently added to the cardiopulmonary bypass prime, and additional amounts may be added if the balanced solution contains calcium.

References:

1. Groom RC, Fitzgerald D. Chapter 32: Extracorporeal Devices and Related Technologies. In: Kaplan JA, Augoustides JGT, Manecke GR, et al., eds. Kaplan's Cardiac Anesthesia. 7th ed. Elsevier; 2017:1162-1213.
2. Navickis RJ, Haynes GR, Wilkes MM. Effect of hydroxyethyl starch on bleeding after cardiopulmonary bypass; a meta-analysis of randomized controlled trials. J Thorac Cardiovasc Surg, 2012; 144: 223-230.

15. Regarding autologous preoperative donation as a method for red blood cell conservation during cardiopulmonary bypass, which of the following is FALSE?
   A. Predonated blood is immunogenic
   B. Predonation still poses the risk of clerical error (wrong unit to wrong patient)
   C. Predonation is less commonly used owing to the many contraindications
   D. Predonation may result in the patient being anemic at the time of surgery

Correct Answer: A

Explanation: Predonated autotransfusion blood is nonimmunologic. It does still carry the risk of the wrong unit being delivered to the wrong patient, or of the patient being anemic at the time of surgery owing to removal of red blood cell mass. Cardiac patients frequently have numerous contraindications for preoperative autodonation, and some studies suggest that only 10% of patients may be candidates.

References:

1. Groom RC, Fitzgerald D. Chapter 32: Extracorporeal Devices and Related Technologies. In: Kaplan JA, Augoustides JGT, Manecke GR, et al., eds. Kaplan's Cardiac Anesthesia. 7th ed. Elsevier; 2017:1162-1213.
2. Bolliger D, Erb JM, Buser A. Controversies in the clinical practice of blood management. J Cardiothorac Vasc Anesth, 2021; 35: 3933-3941.

16. Regarding intraoperative plasmapheresis of autologous blood, which of the following is FALSE?
   A. It can sequester the various blood components from autologous blood
   B. A high centrifuge speed results in platelet-poor plasma
   C. It can be performed using the same process employed by cell saver machines
   D. It is used to remove circulating antibodies and thus reduce the immune response

Correct Answer: D

Explanation: Intraoperative plasmapheresis is used on autologous blood to separate the blood into various components, including platelet-rich plasma, platelet-poor plasma, and red blood cells. It can usually be performed using the cell saver device. Platelet-poor plasma is collected at high centrifuge rates (5200–5600 rpm), while platelet-rich plasma is collected at lower speeds (2400–3600 rpm). It is not used to remove circulating antibodies.

References:

1. Groom RC, Fitzgerald D. Chapter 32: Extracorporeal Devices and Related Technologies. In: Kaplan JA, Augoustides JGT, Manecke GR, et al., eds. Kaplan's Cardiac Anesthesia. 7th ed. Elsevier; 2017:1162-1213.
2. Bai SJ, Zeng B, Zhang L, et al. Autologous platelet-rich plasmapheresis in cardiovascular surgery: a narrative review. J Cardiothorac Vasc Anesth, 2020; 34: 1614-1621.

17. Regarding the use of cell salvage autotransfusion devices, which of the following is FALSE?
   A. Device washes shed blood to remove fat, bone, and particulate contamination
   B. Size of the collection bowl affects the minimum amount of shed blood that can be processed
   C. Reinfused product contains both red blood cells and plasma
   D. Final products for reinfusion typically have a hematocrit of 45%–60%

Correct Answer: C

Explanation: Autotransfusion cell salvage machines typically process shed blood through centrifuging and washing the shed blood with saline (see box). This results in the removal of fat, bone, and particulate contamination, as well as most of the plasma. The product for final reinfusion is thus red blood cells suspended in normal saline with a final hematocrit of 45% to 60%.

BOX 28.7 Basic components of a typical autotransfusion device

- Centrifuge
- Centrifugal bowl
- Aspiration set
- Anticoagulant cardiotomy reservoir
- Wash fluid
- Waste bag
- Reinfusion bag

References:

1. Groom RC, Fitzgerald D. Chapter 32: Extracorporeal Devices and Related Technologies. In: Kaplan JA, Augoustides JGT, Manecke GR, et al., eds. Kaplan's Cardiac Anesthesia. 7th ed. Elsevier; 2017:1162-1213.
2. Baker RA, Merry AF. Cell salvage is beneficial for all cardiac surgical patients: arguments for and against. J Extr Corpor Technol, 2012; 44: 38-41.

18. Regarding ultrafiltration during cardiopulmonary bypass, which of the following is TRUE?
   A. It removes plasma and other solutes like albumin, resulting in hemoconcentration
   B. It increases colloid oncotic pressure and therefore decreases extravascular fluid
   C. It has no effect on blood urea nitrogen
   D. The sieving coefficients are based primarily on the charge of the particle

Correct Answer: B

Explanation: Ultrafiltration is a process to remove particles and fluid based on a hydrostatic pressure through a membrane. The size of the particle is the principle determinate of what is removed, with sizes less than 50,000 Daltons being removed. Albumin is not removed, owing to its large size (65,000 Daltons), which allows the colloid oncotic pressure to increase. Blood urea nitrogen and other uremic toxins are also ultrafiltrated.

References:

1. Groom RC, Fitzgerald D. Chapter 32: Extracorporeal Devices and Related Technologies. In: Kaplan JA, Augoustides JGT, Manecke GR, et al., eds. Kaplan's Cardiac Anesthesia. 7th ed. Elsevier; 2017:1162-1213.
2. Sarkar M, Prabhu V. Basics of cardiopulmonary bypass. Indian J Anaesth, 2017; 61: 760-767.
3. Wahta A, Milojevic M, De Somer FMJJ, et al. 2019 EACTS/EACTA/EBCP guidelines on cardiopulmonary bypass in adult cardiac surgery. Eur J Cardiothorac Surg, 2020; 57: 210-251.

19. With respect to modified ultrafiltration associated with cardiopulmonary bypass, which of the following is incorrect?
- **A.** It refers to ultrafiltration of the patient after cardiopulmonary bypass
- **B.** It reduces complement, cytokines, and pyrogens
- **C.** It increases systemic vascular resistance as a result of hemoconcentration
- **D.** It does not result in reductions in blood transfusion

Correct Answer: D

Explanation: The use of modified ultrafiltration is associated with reductions in blood transfusion and is indicated in blood conservation. It is a technique that employs the arterial line and a pump for inflow and the venous cannula for outflow and is performed after cardiopulmonary bypass but before decannulation. It is primarily used to reduce fluid and raises systemic mean arterial pressure due to increases in blood viscosity and systemic vascular resistance. As an additional benefit, it filters out complement, cytokines, and pyrogens.

References:

1. Groom RC, Fitzgerald D. Chapter 32: Extracorporeal Devices and Related Technologies. In: Kaplan JA, Augoustides JGT, Manecke GR, et al., eds. Kaplan's Cardiac Anesthesia. 7th ed. Elsevier; 2017:1162-1213.
2. Sarkar M, Prabhu V. Basics of cardiopulmonary bypass. Indian J Anaesth, 2017; 61: 760-767.
3. Wahta A, Milojevic M, De Somer FMJJ, et al. 2019 EACTS/EACTA/EBCP guidelines on cardiopulmonary bypass in adult cardiac surgery. Eur J Cardiothorac Surg, 2020; 57: 210-251.
4. Aubrey-Annes W. Pro: The value of modified ultrafiltration in children after cardiopulmonary bypass. J Cardiothorac Vasc Anesth, 2019; 33: 866-869.

20. Regarding heparin-bonded extracorporeal circuits, which of the following is FALSE?
- **A.** They allow the use of lower doses of heparin (100 IU/kg)
- **B.** They reduce platelet activation
- **C.** They reduce granulocyte activation
- **D.** They minimize the binding of factor Xa to the circuit

Correct Answer: A

Explanation: While the initial expectation of heparin-bonded circuits was to reduce heparin dosing, low-dose heparin in these circuits has resulted in increased thrombus formation and so is not recommended. However, bonded circuits have shown reductions in factor activation, platelet activation, and granulocyte activation.

References:

1. Groom RC, Fitzgerald D. Chapter 32: Extracorporeal Devices and Related Technologies. In: Kaplan JA, Augoustides JGT, Manecke GR, et al., eds. Kaplan's Cardiac Anesthesia. 7th ed. Elsevier; 2017:1162-1213.
2. Mahmood S, Bilal H, Zaman M, et al. Is a fully heparin-bonded cardiopulmonary bypass circuit superior to a standard cardiopulmonary bypass circuit? Interact Cardiovasc Thorac Surg, 2012; 14: 406-414.

21. Oxygenator gas exchange failure may occur in all the following EXCEPT:
- **A.** Gas supply leak
- **B.** High patient metabolic rate
- **C.** Clotted blood deposition on the membrane
- **D.** Oversized oxygenator

Correct Answer: D

Explanation: Undersizing an oxygenator in addition to gas supply leak, high metabolic rate, and deposition of blood on the membrane will all cause poor gas exchange resulting in real or apparent oxygenator failure.

References:

1. Groom RC, Fitzgerald D. Chapter 32: Extracorporeal Devices and Related Technologies. In: Kaplan JA, Augoustides JGT, Manecke GR, et al., eds. Kaplan's Cardiac Anesthesia. 7th ed. Elsevier; 2017:1162-1213.
2. Gerstein NS, Panikkath P, Mirrakhimov AE, et al. Cardiopulmonary bypass emergencies and intraoperative issues. J Cardiothorac Vasc Anesth, 2022; 3: 4505-4522.

22. Regarding pulsatile perfusion during cardiopulmonary bypass, which of the following statements is FALSE?
- **A.** It may be done using nonpulsatile perfusion and an intra-aortic balloon pump
- **B.** It has demonstrated improvements in renal function
- **C.** Centrifugal pumps are better than roller pumps in producing pulsatile flow
- **D.** Roller pumps generate a pulse by accelerating during the systolic phase and decelerating during the diastolic phase

Correct Answer: C

Explanation: Roller pumps, as compared to centrifugal pumps, typically result in better pulsatile perfusion. The pulse in roller pumps is generated by accelerating the pump during the systolic phase and decelerating it during the diastolic phase. Intra-aortic balloon counterpulsation may also be used to generate the pulse in nonpulsatile cardiopulmonary bypass systems. A meta-analysis of randomized trials has suggested that pulsatile perfusion may improve renal function.

References:

1. Groom RC, Fitzgerald D. Chapter 32: Extracorporeal Devices and Related Technologies. In: Kaplan JA, Augoustides JGT, Manecke GR, et al., eds. Kaplan's Cardiac Anesthesia. 7th ed. Elsevier; 2017:1162-1213.
2. Sievert A, Sistino J. A meta-analysis of renal benefits to pulsatile perfusion in cardiac surgery. J Extra Corpor Technol, 2012; 44: 10-14.

23. Regarding the conduct of left heart bypass, which of the following statements is FALSE?
   A. The inflow may be from the left atrium, right atrium, pulmonary veins, or ascending aorta
   B. The outflow is into the femoral artery or thoracic aorta
   C. It does not contain an oxygenator
   D. Because of the reduced surface area and continuous flow, it does not require as much anticoagulation as routine cardiopulmonary bypass

Correct Answer: A

Explanation: Inflow to a left heart bypass device may be from the left atrium, descending aorta, or ascending aorta. Because the circuit does not typically contain an oxygenator, right atrial blood would not be suitable. It is a closed system and does not contain a venous reservoir or ability to return suctioned blood. As such it requires less heparinization than a standard cardiopulmonary bypass circuit. Blood is typically returned to the femoral artery or thoracic aorta.

References:

1. Groom RC, Fitzgerald D. Chapter 32: Extracorporeal Devices and Related Technologies. In: Kaplan JA, Augoustides JGT, Manecke GR, et al., eds. Kaplan's Cardiac Anesthesia. 7th ed. Elsevier; 2017:1162-1213.
2. Wahlgren CM, Blohme L, Gunther A, et al. Outcomes of left heart bypass versus circulatory arrest in elective open surgical descending and thoracoabdominal aortic repair. Eur J Vasc Endovasc Surg, 2017; 53: 672-678.

24. Regarding the conduct of deep hypothermic circulatory arrest for aortic arch repair, which of the following statements is TRUE?
   A. It may be safely achieved at temperatures below 23°C
   B. A safe circulatory arrest period will last for 90 to 100 minutes
   C. Systemic rewarming should be stopped when nasopharyngeal temperature is between 35 and 36°C
   D. A 15°C difference between core and perfusate temperature is ideal for rewarming

Correct Answer: C

Explanation: For deep hypothermic circulatory arrest, the patient should be cooled and subsequently rewarmed with a perfusate temperature that is no more than 10°C different from the core body temperature. Circulatory arrest may be initiated when the core temperature is below 20°C to permit a safe arrest period of 40 to 50 minutes. Systemic rewarming should cease when the nasopharyngeal temperature reaches 35°C to 36°C. This avoids cerebral hyperthermia (overshoot), which is detrimental to cerebral function.

References:

1. Groom RC, Fitzgerald D. Chapter 32: Extracorporeal Devices and Related Technologies. In: Kaplan JA, Augoustides JGT, Manecke GR, et al., eds. Kaplan's Cardiac Anesthesia. 7th ed. Elsevier; 2017:1162-1213.
2. STS/SCA/AmSECT clinical practice guidelines for cardiopulmonary bypass - temperature management during cardiopulmonary bypass. J Cardiothorac Vasc Anesth, 2015; 29: 1104-1113.

25. Which of the following statements regarding antegrade cerebral perfusion during aortic arch repair is FALSE?
   A. It involves cannulation of the brachiocephalic vessels
   B. The perfusate should be kept at 20 to 28°C (cold)
   C. Alpha stat is the preferred acid-base management technique
   D. The flows are kept between 20 and 30 mL/kg/min

Correct Answer: D

Explanation: Antegrade cerebral perfusion involves the cannulation of the brachiocephalic arteries. Blood is drawn distal to the oxygenator, cooled to 20 to 28°C, and then perfused to the brain in an antegrade fashion. The line pressures are typically maintained below 150 mmHg with flows in the 5- to 10-mL/kg/min range. Acid-base management is usually as per alpha stat.

References:

1. Groom RC, Fitzgerald D. Chapter 32: Extracorporeal Devices and Related Technologies. In: Kaplan JA, Augoustides JGT, Manecke GR, et al., eds. Kaplan's Cardiac Anesthesia. 7th ed. Elsevier; 2017:1162-1213.
2. Qu JZ, Kao LW, Smith JE, et al. Brain protection in aortic arch surgery: an evolving field. J Cardiothorac Vasc Anesth, 2022; 35: 1176-1188.

26. Regarding roller pumps during cardiopulmonary bypass, which of the following statements is FALSE?
   A. They may cause air cavitation
   B. Smaller tube size results in lower pump speed
   C. Pump speed is directly related to the magnitude of hemolysis caused by the pump
   D. The use of shims allows multiple tubing sizes to work in the same pump

Correct Answer: B

Explanation: Roller pumps are designed with the use of shims to accommodate multiple tubing sizes in the same pump (see teaching box). Smaller tubing size necessitates higher speeds for the same pump flow, which may result in an increase in hemolysis. The decompression phase of the roller, as it moves past the tubing, may result in rapid pressure drops and air cavitation.

References:

1. Groom RC, Fitzgerald D. Chapter 32: Extracorporeal Devices and Related Technologies. In: Kaplan JA, Augoustides JGT,

Manecke GR, et al., eds. Kaplan's Cardiac Anesthesia. 7th ed. Elsevier; 2017:1162-1213.

2. Sarkar M, Prabhu V. Basics of cardiopulmonary bypass. Indian J Anaesth, 2017; 61: 760-767.

3. Wahta A, Milojevic M, De Somer FMJJ, et al. 2019 EACTS/EACTA/EBCP guidelines on cardiopulmonary bypass in adult cardiac surgery. Eur J Cardiothorac Surg, 2020; 57: 210-251.

27. The largest nonendothelialized surface in a cardiopulmonary bypass machine is:

A. Oxygenator

B. Venous reservoir

C. Venous line filter

D. Arterial line filter, if separate from the oxygenator

Correct Answer: A

Explanation: The oxygenator is the largest nonendothelialized surface in the cardiopulmonary bypass circuit. The purpose of this large surface area is to facilitate effective gas exchange.

References:

1. Groom RC, Fitzgerald D. Chapter 32: Extracorporeal Devices and Related Technologies. In: Kaplan JA, Augoustides JGT, Manecke GR, et al., eds. Kaplan's Cardiac Anesthesia. 7th ed. Elsevier; 2017:1162-1213.

2. Sarkar M, Prabhu V. Basics of cardiopulmonary bypass. Indian J Anaesth, 2017; 61: 760-767.

3. Wahta A, Milojevic M, De Somer FMJJ, et al. 2019 EACTS/EACTA/EBCP guidelines on cardiopulmonary bypass in adult cardiac surgery. Eur J Cardiothorac Surg, 2020; 57: 210-251.

28. Regarding heater-cooler units during cardiopulmonary bypass, which of the following statements is FALSE?

A. Water pressure is greater than blood pressure to allow flow into the heater cooler

B. They have been associated with mycobacterium contamination

C. Blood-to-water leak should be suspected if the water becomes discolored

D. A water-to-blood leak will cause hemolysis

Correct Answer: A

Explanation: Water pressure in the heater cooler ideally is below the pressure of the blood pumped through the heater cooler. If a leak does occur, blood-to-water flow will result in discoloration of the water. If pressure in the heater cooler is greater than the blood pressure, then the possibility exists that contaminated (nonsterile) water will leak into the circulation and cause hemolysis. The heater-cooler units have also been associated with mycobacterial contamination.

References:

1. Groom RC, Fitzgerald D. Chapter 32: Extracorporeal Devices and Related Technologies. In: Kaplan JA, Augoustides JGT, Manecke GR, et al., eds. Kaplan's Cardiac Anesthesia. 7th ed. Elsevier; 2017:1162-1213.

2. Sarkar M, Prabhu V. Basics of cardiopulmonary bypass. Indian J Anaesth, 2017; 61: 760-767.

3. Wahta A, Milojevic M, De Somer FMJJ, et al. 2019 EACTS/EACTA/EBCP guidelines on cardiopulmonary bypass in adult cardiac surgery. Eur J Cardiothorac Surg, 2020; 57: 210-251.

29. Regarding aortic root cardioplegia cannulas, which of the following statements is FALSE?

A. They are designed to produce a large pressure drop across the tip to prevent air entrainment

B. They should be able to handle flows of 200 to 300 mL/min

C. Typical pressures inside the root are 60 to 100 mmHg

D. They may also function as a vent to allow removal of debris within the root

Correct Answer: A

Explanation: Aortic root cardioplegia cannulas are designed to provide a minimal drop across the cannula tip. Pressures of 60 to 100 mmHg and flows of 200 to 300 mL/min are typical. The cannula can function as a vent to allow removal of air and small debris.

References:

1. Groom RC, Fitzgerald D. Chapter 32: Extracorporeal Devices and Related Technologies. In: Kaplan JA, Augoustides JGT, Manecke GR, et al., eds. Kaplan's Cardiac Anesthesia. 7th ed. Elsevier; 2017:1162-1213.

2. Sarkar M, Prabhu V. Basics of cardiopulmonary bypass. Indian J Anaesth, 2017; 61: 760-767.

3. Wahta A, Milojevic M, De Somer FMJJ, et al. 2019 EACTS/EACTA/EBCP guidelines on cardiopulmonary bypass in adult cardiac surgery. Eur J Cardiothorac Surg, 2020; 57: 210-251.

30. Regarding vacuum-assisted venous drainage during cardiopulmonary bypass, which of the following statements is FALSE?

A. It is used in open circuits to assist in venous drainage

B. It may result in higher rates of gaseous microemboli

C. It permits the use of smaller venous cannulae

D. It reduces the risk of massive air embolism as the venous reservoir is under negative pressure

Correct Answer: D

Explanation: Vacuum-assisted venous drainage may be used to augment the venous drainage in open systems, and as such may permit the use of smaller-bore venous lines (commonly used in minimally invasive procedures). However, concern has been raised about the reported increase in gaseous microemboli caused by the negative pressure secondary to air entrainment in the venous line. There have also been reports about an increased risk for massive air embolism.

References:

1. Groom RC, Fitzgerald D. Chapter 32: Extracorporeal Devices and Related Technologies. In: Kaplan JA, Augoustides JGT, Manecke GR, et al., eds. Kaplan's Cardiac Anesthesia. 7th ed. Elsevier; 2017:1162-1213.

2. Davila RM, Rawles T, Mack MJ. Venoarterial air embolus: A complication of vacuum-assisted venous drainage. Ann Thorac Surg, 2001; 71: 1369-1371.

3. Wahta A, Milojevic M, De Somer FMJJ, et al. 2019 EACTS/EACTA/EBCP guidelines on cardiopulmonary bypass in adult cardiac surgery. Eur J Cardiothorac Surg, 2020; 57: 210-251.

CHAPTER 29

Extracorporeal Membrane Oxygenation

Daniel Bainbridge

KEY POINTS

1. Extracorporeal membrane oxygenation (ECMO) has had a profound resurgence as therapy for acute cardiopulmonary failure.
2. Advancements in equipment and improvements in techniques and management have led to better outcomes for patients undergoing ECMO.
3. Venoarterial (VA) ECMO should be considered for patients with acute cardiac or combined cardiac and respiratory failure.
4. Venovenous (VV) ECMO is indicated for patients with adequate cardiac function in the setting of severe acute respiratory failure refractory to standard management.
5. Cerebral hypoxia can complicate the management of patients on VA ECMO who have pulmonary failure and recovery of cardiac function.
6. Complete cardiac rest for patients on VA ECMO may require placement of ventricular drains or assist devices to prevent ventricular distention.
7. Bleeding and thrombosis remain the two most common complications associated with ECMO.
8. Careful titration of anticoagulation may require multiple laboratory modalities, including a heparin assay to guide anticoagulation management.
9. ECMO can produce changes in drug pharmacokinetics that may affect systemic concentrations of lipophilic or highly protein-bound medications.
10. ECMO is increasingly used for newer indications such as acute pulmonary hypertension and accidental hypothermia and to facilitate surgery in patients with compromised pulmonary or cardiac function.
11. Walking ECMO (i.e., awake ECMO) can provide a bridge to transplantation for patients with end-stage lung disease.

---

1. The following is TRUE when comparing the use of extracorporeal membrane oxygenation (ECMO) for acute respiratory failure to routine medical care:
   A. Similar mortality with increased disability in the ECMO group
   B. Decreased mortality in the ECMO group
   C. Increased mortality in the ECMO group
   D. Similar mortality with reduced disability in the ECMO group

Correct Answer: B

Explanation: Based on trials that have randomized patients with acute respiratory failure to routine medical care versus extracorporeal membrane oxygenation (ECMO), the rates of death and disability were lower in patients managed with ECMO. Ongoing trials have supported reduced rates, with mortality in the conventional medical therapy cohort as high as 50%, while the ECMO-treated cohort had mortality rates of 35% to 40%.

References:
1. Gutsche JT, Ramakrishna H. Chapter 33: Extracorporeal Membrane Oxygenation. In: Kaplan JA, Augoustides JGT, Manecke GR, et al., eds. Kaplan's Cardiac Anesthesia. 7th ed. Elsevier; 2017:1214-1228.
2. Mazzeffi MA, Rao VK, Dodd-O J, et al. Intraoperative management of adult patients on extracorporeal membrane

oxygenation: an expert consensus statement from the Society of Cardiovascular Anesthesiologists-Part I: technical aspects of extracorporeal membrane oxygenation. J Cardiothorac Vasc Anesth, 2021; 35: 3496-3512.

3. Mazzeffi MA, Rao VK, Dodd-O J, et al. Intraoperative management of adult patients on extracorporeal membrane oxygenation: an expert consensus statement from the Society of Cardiovascular Anesthesiologists-Part II: intraoperative management and troubleshooting. J Cardiothorac Vasc Anesth, 2021; 35: 3513-3527.

2. In the United States, the prevalence of extracorporeal membrane oxygenation has increased steadily between 2006 and 2011 by approximately what percentage?
   A. 5%
   B. 25%
   C. 150%
   D. 400%

Correct Answer: D

Explanation: The widespread dissemination of extracorporeal membrane oxygenation (ECMO) for the management of acute respiratory illness and specifically the outbreak of H1N1 influenza in 2009 led to a dramatic increase in the use of ECMO throughout the United States. This increase has been estimated to be in the range of 400% to 450%. Prior to this surge, the prevalence of ECMO was rather static in the United States from 1999 to 2006. The profound dissemination of this advanced technology thereafter may reflect both the evolving indications for both venovenous and venoarterial ECMO, as well as improvements in ECMO design.

BOX 29.1   Indications for venoarterial extracorporeal membrane oxygenation

- Pulmonary embolism
- Myocardial infarction
- Myocarditis
- Postcardiotomy cardiac failure
- Heart transplantation
- Acute-on-chronic heart failure
- Cardiac arrest
- Acute respiratory distress syndrome with severe cardiac dysfunction
- Refractory ventricular arrhythmia
- Cardiac trauma
- Acute anaphylaxis
- Cardiac support for percutaneous cardiac procedures

References:

1. Gutsche JT, Ramakrishna H. Chapter 33: Extracorporeal Membrane Oxygenation. In: Kaplan JA, Augoustides JGT, Manecke GR, et al., eds. Kaplan's Cardiac Anesthesia. 7th ed. Elsevier; 2017:1214-1228.
2. Sauer CM, Yuh DD, Bonde P. Extracorporeal membrane oxygenation use has increased by 433% in adults in the United States from 2006 to 2011. ASAIO J, 2015; 61: 31-36.

3. What is the expected survival following cardiac arrest in patients that are managed with extracorporeal membrane oxygenation as part of their resuscitation and subsequent care?
   A. 5%
   B. 15%
   C. 30%
   D. 60%

Correct Answer: D

Explanation: Based on a meta-analysis by Cardarelli et al. the survival in patients placed on extracorporeal membrane oxygenation (ECMO) increased from 30% in 1990 to 59% in 2007. This degree of survival will also depend on local expertise and indications for ECMO. Furthermore, ongoing refinements in ECMO expertise and hardware will likely continue to improve the prognosis in this acute care setting.

References:

1. Gutsche JT, Ramakrishna H. Chapter 33: Extracorporeal Membrane Oxygenation. In: Kaplan JA, Augoustides JGT, Manecke GR, et al., eds. Kaplan's Cardiac Anesthesia. 7th ed. Elsevier; 2017:1214-1228.
2. Cardarelli MG, Young AJ, Griffith B. Use of extracorporeal membrane oxygenation for adults in cardiac arrest (E-CPR): a meta-analysis of observational studies. ASAIO J, 2009; 55: 581-586.
3. Mazzeffi MA, Rao VK, Dodd-O J, et al. Intraoperative management of adult patients on extracorporeal membrane oxygenation: an expert consensus statement from the Society of Cardiovascular Anesthesiologists-Part I: technical aspects of extracorporeal membrane oxygenation. J Cardiothorac Vasc Anesth, 2021; 35: 3496-3512.

4. All the following are true about extracorporeal membrane oxygenation (ECMO) EXCEPT:
   A. An ECMO circuit consists of inflow and outflow tubing, a pump, and an oxygenator
   B. Blood carbon dioxide levels are controlled by adjusting the FIO_2 and pump flows
   C. The oxygenator typically has a hollow fiber membrane design
   D. A heat exchanger may be used in the circuit

Correct Answer: B

Explanation: A typical extracorporeal membrane oxygenation (ECMO) circuit consists of inflow and outflow cannulae, a pump, a membrane oxygenator, and a heat exchanger. The ECMO oxygenator typically has a hollow-fiber membrane design. The oxygenation is controlled by altering the oxygen concentration of the sweep gas passing through the oxygenator. Carbon dioxide is controlled by altering the sweep speed (flow) of the gas and is not impacted by the oxygen concentration of the sweep gas. Increasing the sweep speed consequently decreases carbon dioxide. Decreasing ECMO flow rates force more blood flow through the patient's lungs, and the effect on gas exchange is therefore dependent on the patient's ventilation.

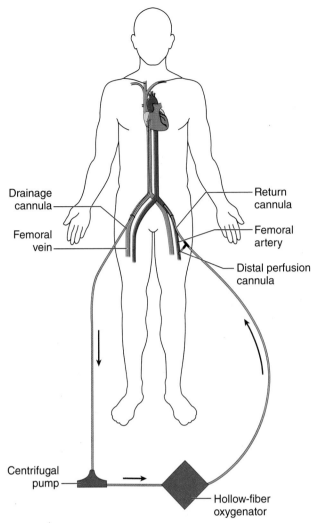

FIGURE 29.1 Standard extracorporeal membrane oxygenation circuit. (From Sidebotham D, McGeorge A, McGuinness S, et al. Extracorporeal membrane oxygenation for treating severe cardiac and respiratory failure in adults. Part 2: technical considerations. J Cardiothorac Vasc Anesth, 2010; 24: 164–172.)

Drainage cannula

Return cannula

Femoral vein

Femoral artery

Distal perfusion cannula

Centrifugal pump

Hollow-fiber oxygenator

References:

1. Gutsche JT, Ramakrishna H. Chapter 33: Extracorporeal Membrane Oxygenation. In: Kaplan JA, Augoustides JGT, Manecke GR, et al., eds. Kaplan's Cardiac Anesthesia. 7th ed. Elsevier; 2017:1214-1228.

2. Mazzeffi MA, Rao VK, Dodd-O J, et al. Intraoperative management of adult patients on extracorporeal membrane oxygenation: an expert consensus statement from the Society of Cardiovascular Anesthesiologists-Part I: technical aspects of extracorporeal membrane oxygenation. J Cardiothorac Vasc Anesth, 2021; 35: 3496-3512.

5. The following statements are true regarding oxygenators in extracorporeal membrane oxygenation EXCEPT:

  A. They typically have a hollow-fiber membrane design

  B. They have small priming volumes and offer gas exchange at flow rates from 1 to 7 L/min

  C. They may fail secondary to deposits of fibrin and platelets on the surface of the membrane

  D. Their failure usually results in gaseous microemboli, which may impact patients' cognitive function

Correct Answer: D

Explanation: Modern oxygenators in extracorporeal membrane oxygenation (ECMO) consist of hollow-fiber membranes. They have the advantage of small prime volumes, allow a wide variety of flows (1–7 L/min), have a relatively large surface area (1.5–2 m²), and reduce platelet consumption and plasma leakage. When they do fail, however, it is usually secondary to fibrin and platelet deposition, which results in high pressure and poor gas exchange in the oxygenator. Gaseous microemboli are not a typical sign of oxygenator failure in ECMO.

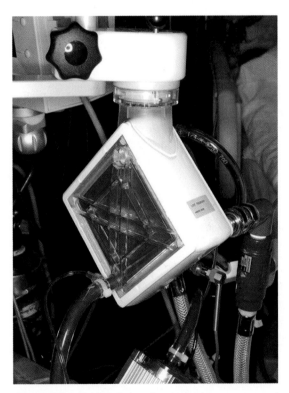

FIGURE 29.2 Polymethylpentene membrane oxygenator.

References:

1. Gutsche JT, Ramakrishna H. Chapter 33: Extracorporeal Membrane Oxygenation. In: Kaplan JA, Augoustides JGT, Manecke GR, et al., eds. Kaplan's Cardiac Anesthesia. 7th ed. Elsevier; 2017:1214-1228.

2. Mazzeffi MA, Rao VK, Dodd-O J, et al. Intraoperative management of adult patients on extracorporeal membrane oxygenation: an expert consensus statement from the Society of Cardiovascular Anesthesiologists-Part I: technical aspects of extracorporeal membrane oxygenation. J Cardiothorac Vasc Anesth, 2021; 35: 3496-3512.

6. Regarding pumps in extracorporeal membrane oxygenation (ECMO), all of the following statements are true EXCEPT:
  A. The pumps in ECMO have a centrifugal design
  B. Venous drainage relies on gravity, and so ECMO pumps are placed below the patient
  C. The pumps in ECMO have small priming volumes
  D. The pumps in ECMO have a central opening in the rotor, which improves longevity

Correct Answer: B

Explanation: The circuits in extracorporeal membrane oxygenation (ECMO) typically use centrifugal pumps, as they have small priming volumes. Their novel design includes a central opening in the rotor to improve pump longevity. Newer pumps used in ECMO have magnetically suspended, frictionless designs to reduce hemolysis through reductions in heat generation. Since the ECMO pump creates a negative downstream pressure and a positive upstream pressure as a direct result of the its centrifugal design, it does not rely on gravity drainage like the more traditional roller pump.

BOX 29.2　Initial settings and goals after implementation of venoarterial extracorporeal membrane oxygenation

Circuit flow	≥ 2 L/min/m^2
Sweep gas flow	Equal to blood flow
Fraction of inspired oxygen (sweep gas)	100%
Inlet pressure (centrifugal pump)	≥ 100 mm Hg
Oxygen saturation (outflow cannula)	100%
Oxygen saturation (inflow cannula)	>65%
Arterial oxygen saturation	>95%
Mixed venous oxygen saturation	>65%
Arterial carbon dioxide tension	35–45 mmHg
pH	7.35–7.45
Mean arterial pressure	60–90 mmHg
Hematocrit	30%–40%
Activated partial thromboplastin time	1.5–2.0 times normal
Platelet count	>100,000/mm^3

Modified from Sidebotham D, McGeorge A, McGuinness S, et al. Extracorporeal membrane oxygenation for treating severe cardiac and respiratory failure in adults. Part 2: technical considerations. J Cardiothorac Vasc Anesth, 2010; 24: 164-172.

References:

1. Gutsche JT, Ramakrishna H. Chapter 33: Extracorporeal Membrane Oxygenation. In: Kaplan JA, Augoustides JGT, Manecke GR, et al., eds. Kaplan's Cardiac Anesthesia. 7th ed. Elsevier; 2017:1214-1228.
2. Mazzeffi MA, Rao VK, Dodd-O J, et al. Intraoperative management of adult patients on extracorporeal membrane oxygenation: an expert consensus statement from the Society of Cardiovascular Anesthesiologists-Part I: technical aspects of extracorporeal membrane oxygenation. J Cardiothorac Vasc Anesth, 2021; 35: 3496-3512.

7. In patients suffering from cardiogenic shock in the intensive care unit, all the following are indications for venoarterial extracorporeal membrane oxygenation EXCEPT:
  A. Chemotherapy-induced heart failure following treatment for malignancy
  B. Autoimmune myocarditis
  C. Persistent ventricular arrhythmia
  D. Drug-induced anaphylaxis

Correct Answer: A

Explanation: Venoarterial extracorporeal membrane oxygenation has many indications, including management of anaphylaxis, management of persistent ventricular arrhythmia, and management of myocarditis. There are, however, a few contraindications, including disseminated malignancy, advanced age, severe brain injury, and unwitnessed arrest.

References:

1. Gutsche JT, Ramakrishna H. Chapter 33: Extracorporeal Membrane Oxygenation. In: Kaplan JA, Augoustides JGT, Manecke GR, et al., eds. Kaplan's Cardiac Anesthesia. 7th ed. Elsevier; 2017:1214-1228.
2. Mazzeffi MA, Rao VK, Dodd-O J, et al. Intraoperative management of adult patients on extracorporeal membrane oxygenation: an expert consensus statement from the Society of Cardiovascular Anesthesiologists-Part I: technical aspects of extracorporeal membrane oxygenation. J Cardiothorac Vasc Anesth, 2021; 35: 3496-3512.

8. A 65-year-old female suffering from cardiogenic shock in the intensive care unit is considered for treatment with venoarterial extracorporeal membrane oxygenation (VA ECMO). What condition would result in additional challenges to establishing VA ECMO in this setting?
  A. Aortic stenosis
  B. Mitral insufficency
  C. Aortic insufficency
  D. Pulmonary stenosis

Correct Answer: C

Explanation: Aortic insufficiency may cause challenges to the successful use of venoarterial extracorporeal membrane oxygenation (VA ECMO) to support the failing heart. Without a method of left ventricular drainage, and/or allowing intermittent left ventricular ejection, the left heart will significantly distend due to the aortic regurgitation, resulting in increased end-diastolic pressure that could aggravate pulmonary edema. Furthermore, the significant left ventricular distention will increase wall tension, increase oxygen consumption, and risk ventricular ischemia. Mitral insufficiency, aortic stenosis, and pulmonary stenosis do not themselves prevent the initiation of VA ECMO and/or the need to use additional special techniques.

References:

1. Gutsche JT, Ramakrishna H. Chapter 33: Extracorporeal Membrane Oxygenation. In: Kaplan JA, Augoustides JGT, Manecke GR, et al., eds. Kaplan's Cardiac Anesthesia. 7th ed. Elsevier; 2017:1214-1228.
2. Hoyler MM, Flynn B, Iannacone EM, et al. Clinical management of venoarterial extracorporeal membrane oxygenation. J Cardiothorac Vasc Anesth, 2020; 34: 2776-2792.
3. Mazzeffi MA, Rao VK, Dodd-O J, et al. Intraoperative management of adult patients on extracorporeal membrane oxygenation: an expert consensus statement from the Society of Cardiovascular Anesthesiologists-Part I: technical aspects of extracorporeal membrane oxygenation. J Cardiothorac Vasc Anesth, 2021; 35: 3496-3512.

9. A 51-year-old patient has a ventricular septal repair performed emergently following a myocardial infarction. After the surgical procedure the surgeon elects to place the patient on venoarterial extracorporeal membrane oxygenation (VA ECMO) to unload the left ventricle in the postoperative period. Which statement about this strategy is FALSE?
   A. A left ventricular assist device would provide better ventricular unloading
   B. Blood flow through the thebesian and bronchial circulation will increase left ventricular loading
   C. A left ventricular vent or Impella device may aid in unloading the ventricle
   D. VA ECMO is the best way to unload the left ventricle because it drains all blood flow to the heart

Correct Answer: D

Explanation: Although it seems intuitive that using extracorporeal membrane oxygenation (ECMO) to drain the heart would unload the left ventricle, flow through the thebesian and bronchial circulation drains directly into the left heart. This flow results in preload to the left side that must then be ejected. Left ventricular assist devices result in improved drainage by pumping this blood through the device and not the left ventricle, which occurs with ECMO. To further unload the left ventricle with ECMO in place, an Impella device or a ventricular drain may be employed.

References:

1. Gutsche JT, Ramakrishna H. Chapter 33: Extracorporeal Membrane Oxygenation. In: Kaplan JA, Augoustides JGT, Manecke GR, et al., eds. Kaplan's Cardiac Anesthesia. 7th ed. Elsevier; 2017:1214-1228.
2. Mazzeffi MA, Rao VK, Dodd-O J, et al. Intraoperative management of adult patients on extracorporeal membrane oxygenation: an expert consensus statement from the Society of Cardiovascular Anesthesiologists-Part I: technical aspects of

extracorporeal membrane oxygenation. J Cardiothorac Vasc Anesth, 2021; 35: 3496-3512.

10. Methods to vent the left ventricle during extracorporeal circulation include all the following strategies EXCEPT:
    A. Placement of a vent catheter in the aortic root
    B. Atrial septostomy
    C. Percutaneous drainage through the pulmonary artery
    D. Placement of a vent catheter in the left ventricle

Correct Answer: A

Explanation: The placement of a vent catheter in the aortic root would simply result in the shunting of blood from the outflow cannula back to the pump and would not remove blood in the left heart. Both atrial septostomy and percutaneous drainage of the pulmonary artery will result in blood being diverted away from the left ventricle. Placement of a vent in the left ventricle will result in a reduction of left ventricular filling pressure by providing a low-pressure outlet for accumulated blood.

References:

1. Gutsche JT, Ramakrishna H. Chapter 33: Extracorporeal Membrane Oxygenation. In: Kaplan JA, Augoustides JGT, Manecke GR, et al., eds. Kaplan's Cardiac Anesthesia. 7th ed. Elsevier; 2017:1214-1228.
2. Hoyler MM, Flynn B, Iannacone EM et al. Clinical management of venoarterial extracorporeal membrane oxygenation. J Cardiothorac Vasc Anesth, 2020; 34: 2776-2792.

11. Proximal-distal syndrome in venoarterial extracorporeal membrane oxygenation refers to which of the following possibilities?
    A. Lack of flow to the limb distal to the femoral arterial cannula
    B. Ejection of poorly oxygenated blood to the cardiac and arch circulation
    C. The pressure gradient in the inflow cannula that may occur from the distal cannula to the proximal pump
    D. The oxygen gradient that occurs in the arterial circulation from the proximal location of the arterial cannula to the distal circulation

Correct Answer: B

Explanation: Proximal-distal syndrome, also called the north-south syndrome, occurs when blood passing through poorly ventilated or diseased lungs is then ejected by the left ventricle, causing a watershed in which this poorly oxygenated blood is ejected into the coronary arteries and proximal arch vessels (typically right innominate artery). The watershed occurs when the arterial inflow during extracorporeal membrane oxygenation is in a peripheral vessel, usually the femoral artery, preventing blood admixture in the ascending aorta and creating two distinct blood pools. Evidence of proximal-distal syndrome may be seen from a low saturation reading on the right hand despite normal saturations in the arterial blood taken distal to the oxygenator.

References:

1. Gutsche JT, Ramakrishna H. Chapter 33: Extracorporeal Membrane Oxygenation. In: Kaplan JA, Augoustides JGT, Manecke GR, et al., eds. Kaplan's Cardiac Anesthesia. 7th ed. Elsevier; 2017:1214-1228.
2. Mazzeffi MA, Rao VK, Dodd-O J, et al. Intraoperative management of adult patients on extracorporeal membrane oxygenation: an expert consensus statement from the Society of Cardiovascular Anesthesiologists-Part I: technical aspects of extracorporeal membrane oxygenation. J Cardiothorac Vasc Anesth, 2021; 35: 3496-3512.
3. Mazzeffi MA, Rao VK, Dodd-O J, et al. Intraoperative management of adult patients on extracorporeal membrane oxygenation: an expert consensus statement from the Society of Cardiovascular Anesthesiologists-Part II: intraoperative management and troubleshooting. J Cardiothorac Vasc Anesth, 2021; 35: 3513-3527.

12. Management strategies for the proximal-distal syndrome during venoarterial extracorporeal membrane oxygenation include all the following EXCEPT:
    A. Increase the inspired oxygen concentration of the ventilator
    B. Increase the oxygen concentration supplied to the oxygenator
    C. Place a left ventricle vent
    D. Place an outflow cannula in the ascending aorta

Correct Answer: B

Explanation: Increasing the inspired concentration of the oxygenator will have no effect on the oxygen concentration in the left ventricle, as this blood passes through the lungs. Increasing the inspired concentration of the ventilator will increase the oxygen concentration in the blood bypassing the extracorporeal membrane oxygenator circuit and entering the left ventricle. Placing a left ventricular vent will remove the shunted blood before it is ejected. Placing an outflow cannula in the ascending aorta will allow oxygenated blood to mix with the deoxygenated blood and will decrease the degree of poorly oxygenated blood being delivered to the heart and proximal arch vessels.

References:

1. Gutsche JT, Ramakrishna H. Chapter 33: Extracorporeal Membrane Oxygenation. In: Kaplan JA, Augoustides JGT, Manecke GR, et al., eds. Kaplan's Cardiac Anesthesia. 7th ed. Elsevier; 2017:1214-1228.
2. Alexis-Ruiz A, Ghadimi K, Raiten J, et al. Hypoxia and complications of oxygenation in extracorporeal membrane oxygenation. J Cardiothorac Vasc Anesth, 2019; 33: 1375-1381.

13. A patient is placed on venoarterial extracorporeal membrane oxygenation, and the pump flow is increased to 5.4 L/min. The venous line develops chatter, and the blood pressure is noted to be only 40 mmHg mean. The BEST method to increase blood pressure at this point is to:
    A. Add vasopressors
    B. Turn down pump flow to reduce inflow line chatter
    C. Add milrinone to increase the patient's own cardiac function
    D. Increase oxygenator FIO_2 to improve oxygen delivery and systemic vascular tone

Correct Answer: A

Explanation: In this scenario we can assume that flows of 5.4 L/min during extracorporeal membrane oxygenation (ECMO) are adequate. Therefore, adding vasopressors would be the next step to increase the measured blood pressure. Turning down pump flows may decrease line chatter, an indication of hypovolemia during ECMO, but given that the patient has a low blood pressure this may lower it further, and therefore a better option would be to infuse volume. Milrinone will cause peripheral vasodilation and, given the use of ECMO, would not be expected to increase the patient's own endogenous cardiac output. If the patient is hypoxic then increasing oxygen delivery may be beneficial and may increase systemic vascular resistance over several hours but would not be as rapid as adding vasopressors.

References:

1. Gutsche JT, Ramakrishna H. Chapter 33: Extracorporeal Membrane Oxygenation. In: Kaplan JA, Augoustides JGT, Manecke GR, et al., eds. Kaplan's Cardiac Anesthesia. 7th ed. Elsevier; 2017:1214-1228.
2. Hoyler MM, Flynn B, Iannacone EM, et al. Clinical management of venoarterial extracorporeal membrane oxygenation. J Cardiothorac Vasc Anesth, 2020; 34: 2776-2792.

14. Regarding weaning from venoarterial extracorporeal membrane oxygenation (VA ECMO), all of the following statements are true EXCEPT:
    A. Low-flow VA ECMO is well-tolerated, and the risks of thrombosis are minimal owing to the coated circuit
    B. Metabolic derangements should be corrected, and evidence of cardiac ejection confirmed before starting to wean
    C. If VA ECMO fails because of pulmonary issues, then conversion to venovenous extracorporeal membrane oxygenation (VV ECMO) could be considered
    D. Titration of vasopressors and inotropes should be started prior to weaning to improve successful weaning from the circuit

Correct Answer: A

Explanation: The initial range of settings in venoarterial extracorporeal membrane oxygenation (VA ECMO) are summarized in the teaching box. When weaning from VA ECMO, the patient should be metabolically stable, ideally with reasonable lung function and evidence of cardiac ejection (some pulsatility in the arterial waveform). Inotropes and vasopressors are typically started prior to weaning to improve the success in separation from ECMO. While lower flows on ECMO are possible and desirable to monitor the function of the heart, patients need supplemental heparin, as low-flow states (<1 L/min) predispose the circuit to form thrombus. If VA ECMO weaning fails because of pulmonary issues, then consideration can be given to venovenous ECMO.

References:

1. Gutsche JT, Ramakrishna H. Chapter 33: Extracorporeal Membrane Oxygenation. In: Kaplan JA, Augoustides JGT, Manecke GR, et al., eds. Kaplan's Cardiac Anesthesia. 7th ed. Elsevier; 2017:1214-1228.
2. Mazzeffi MA, Rao VK, Dodd-O J, et al. Intraoperative management of adult patients on extracorporeal membrane oxygenation: an expert consensus statement from the society of cardiovascular anesthesiologists-Part I: technical aspects of extracorporeal membrane oxygenation. J Cardiothorac Vasc Anesth, 2021; 35: 3496-3512.
3. Mazzeffi MA, Rao VK, Dodd-O J, et al. Intraoperative management of adult patients on extracorporeal membrane oxygenation: an expert consensus statement from the Society of Cardiovascular Anesthesiologists-Part II: intraoperative management and troubleshooting. J Cardiothorac Vasc Anesth, 2021; 35: 3513-3527.

15. The following are conditions where venovenous extracorporeal membrane oxygenation may be considered EXCEPT:
   A. Patients with acute respiratory distress syndrome requiring high ventilatory support
   B. Patients with severe pulmonary edema secondary to cardiogenic shock
   C. Patients with isolated retention of carbon dioxide despite high ventilatory support
   D. Patients with severe air leak syndrome

Correct Answer: B

Explanation: The role of venovenous extracorporeal membrane oxygenation (VV ECMO) is to supplement pulmonary function. It is therefore indicated in patients with severe acute respiratory distress syndrome and those with advanced retention of carbon dioxide despite high ventilatory support. In patients with severe air leaks, VV ECMO may permit pulmonary rest with low ventilatory pressures to minimize air leak and to facilitate pulmonary healing. In patients with severe pulmonary edema secondary to

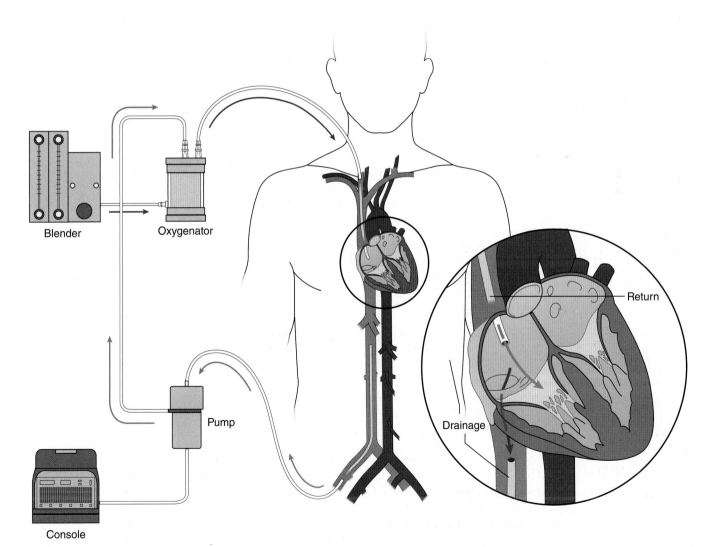

FIGURE 29.3 Central venoarterial extracorporeal membrane oxygenation cannulation and circuit.

cardiogenic shock, VV ECMO would not treat the underlying issue (heart failure), and this may be better supported by venoarterial extracorporeal membrane oxygenation until cardiac function has recovered.

References:

1. Gutsche JT, Ramakrishna H. Chapter 33: Extracorporeal Membrane Oxygenation. In: Kaplan JA, Augoustides JGT, Manecke GR, et al., eds. Kaplan's Cardiac Anesthesia. 7th ed. Elsevier; 2017:1214-1228.
2. Mazzeffi MA, Rao VK, Dodd-O J, et al. Intraoperative management of adult patients on extracorporeal membrane oxygenation: an expert consensus statement from the Society of Cardiovascular Anesthesiologists-Part I: technical aspects of extracorporeal membrane oxygenation. J Cardiothorac Vasc Anesth, 2021; 35: 3496-3512.

16. Recirculation of flow during venovenous extracorporeal membrane oxygenation can be best minimized by:
   A. Turning pump flow down
   B. Turning pump flow up
   C. Directing the inflow cannula toward the tricuspid valve
   D. Directing the inflow cannula toward the inferior vena cava

Correct Answer: C

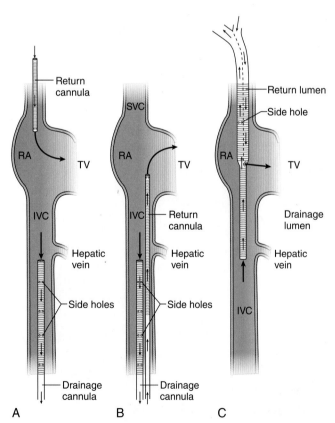

FIGURE 29.4 Common venovenous extracorporeal membrane oxygenation cannulation options. (A) Bicaval cannulation. (B) Bilateral femoral cannulation. (C) Single dual-lumen catheter. *IVC,* Inferior vena cava; *RA,* right atrium; *SVC,* superior vena cava; *TV,* tricuspid valve.

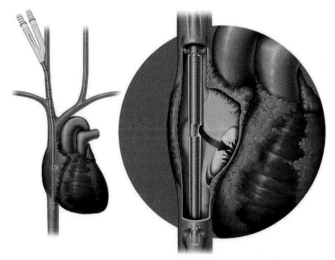

FIGURE 29.5 Peripheral bicaval cannulation venovenous extracorporeal membrane oxygenation standard cannulation and circuit.

Explanation: Recirculation during venovenous extracorporeal membrane oxygenation refers to blood leaving the outflow cannula and being pulled into the inflow cannula without first passing through the systemic circulation. It is caused by having the inflow and outflow cannulae within the venous system, often near each other. Therefore, the best method to reduce recirculation is to provide the maximum distance between the cannulas and try to ensure that blood flow from the outflow cannula is directed away from the inflow cannula, usually toward the tricuspid valve and right ventricle.

References:

1. Gutsche JT, Ramakrishna H. Chapter 33: Extracorporeal Membrane Oxygenation. In: Kaplan JA, Augoustides JGT, Manecke GR, et al., eds. Kaplan's Cardiac Anesthesia.7th ed. Elsevier; 2017:1214-1228.
2. Mazzeffi MA, Rao VK, Dodd-O J, et al. Intraoperative management of adult patients on extracorporeal membrane oxygenation: an expert consensus statement from the Society of Cardiovascular Anesthesiologists-Part I: technical aspects of extracorporeal membrane oxygenation. J Cardiothorac Vasc Anesth, 2021; 35: 3496-3512.
3. Mazzeffi MA, Rao VK, Dodd-O J, et al. Intraoperative management of adult patients on extracorporeal membrane oxygenation: an expert consensus statement from the Society of Cardiovascular Anesthesiologists-Part II: intraoperative management and troubleshooting. J Cardiothorac Vasc Anesth, 2021; 35: 3513-3527.

17. Venovenous extracorporeal membrane oxygenation is better than venoarterial extracorporeal membrane oxygenation in which of the following aspects?
   A. Superior ability to oxygenate blood
   B. Superior ability to support arterial flow
   C. Does not use an in-line oxygenator
   D. Lower risk of arterial and lower extremity injury

Correct Answer: D

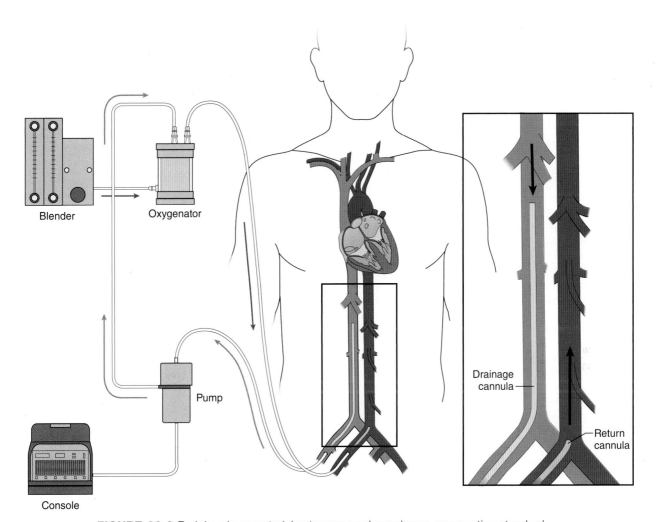

FIGURE 29.6 Peripheral venoarterial extracorporeal membrane oxygenation standard cannulation and circuit.

Explanation: Venovenous extracorporeal membrane oxygenation (VV ECMO) does not directly support arterial circulation. It also results in the venous admixture of blood, which may make support of oxygenation more difficult in patients with significant lung disease. Venoarterial extracorporeal membrane oxygenation (VA ECMO) does support blood pressure, and completely bypasses the patient's own lungs. Both VV ECMO and VA ECMO utilize in-line oxygenators. Because the cannulas in VV ECMO are restricted to the venous circulation, it is associated with lower rates of arterial and lower extremity injury as compared to VA ECMO.

References:

1. Gutsche JT, Ramakrishna H. Chapter 33: Extracorporeal Membrane Oxygenation. In: Kaplan JA, Augoustides JGT, Manecke GR, et al., eds. Kaplan's Cardiac Anesthesia. 7th ed. Elsevier; 2017:1214-1228.
2. Hoyler MM, Flynn B, Iannacone EM et al. Clinical management of venoarterial extracorporeal membrane oxygenation. J Cardiothorac Vasc Anesth, 2020; 34: 2776-2792.

18. Following the institution of venovenous extracorporeal membrane oxygenation (VV ECMO), which of the following statements is CORRECT?
    A. Inotropes and vasopressors should be turned off to rest the heart
    B. Ventilation settings should result in lowest possible inspired oxygen concentration and the avoidance of plateau pressures greater than 25 mmHg
    C. The ventilator should be switched to room air and peak pressures limited to 25 mmHg
    D. The goal should be to extubate all patients from mechanical ventilation within 24 hours of starting VV ECMO

Correct Answer: B

Explanation: Following the institution of venovenous extracorporeal membrane oxygenation (VV ECMO), ventilator settings should be reduced to achieve the lowest possible inspired oxygen concentration and to avoid plateau pressure greater than 25 mmHg. This is essentially a lung-protective strategy. As VV ECMO does not provide circulatory support (all blood flow returns to the venous side), inotropes and vasopressors should be continued. VV ECMO is unable to fully support; therefore, the ventilator should not be switched to room air but rather the lowest possible inspired oxygen concentration. Although tracheal extubation may be possible, it is typically not considered in the acute phase of initiation of VV ECMO because patients are usually quite sick. After clinical stabilization, however, the management goal is typically tracheal extubation after 48 to 72 hours if feasible.

References:

1. Gutsche JT, Ramakrishna H. Chapter 33: Extracorporeal Membrane Oxygenation. In: Kaplan JA, Augoustides JGT, Manecke GR, et al., eds. Kaplan's Cardiac Anesthesia. 7th ed. Elsevier; 2017:1214-1228.
2. Mazzeffi MA, Rao VK, Dodd-O J, et al. Intraoperative management of adult patients on extracorporeal membrane oxygenation: an expert consensus statement from the society of cardiovascular anesthesiologists-Part I: technical aspects of extracorporeal membrane oxygenation. J Cardiothorac Vasc Anesth, 2021; 35: 3496-3512.
3. Mazzeffi MA, Rao VK, Dodd-O J, et al. Intraoperative management of adult patients on extracorporeal membrane oxygenation: an expert consensus statement from the Society of Cardiovascular Anesthesiologists-Part II: intraoperative management and troubleshooting. J Cardiothorac Vasc Anesth, 2021; 35: 3513-3527.

19. All the following are signs of left ventricular distention during venoarterial extracorporeal membrane oxygenation EXCEPT:
   A. Pulmonary edema
   B. Distended left ventricle on echocardiography
   C. Ventricular arrhythmia
   D. Increased pulsatility of arterial waveform

Correct Answer: D

Explanation: Distention of the left ventricle during venoarterial extracorporeal membrane oxygenation (VA ECMO) should be avoided, as it increases oxygen consumption and will impair myocardial recovery. Signs of left ventricular distention during VA ECMO include increases in pulmonary artery pressures, pulmonary edema and ventricular arrhythmias, and a decrease in the pulsatility of the arterial waveform.

References:

1. Gutsche JT, Ramakrishna H. Chapter 33: Extracorporeal Membrane Oxygenation. In: Kaplan JA, Augoustides JGT, Manecke GR, et al., eds. Kaplan's Cardiac Anesthesia. 7th ed. Elsevier; 2017:1214-1228.
2. Hoyler MM, Flynn B, Iannacone EM et al. Clinical management of venoarterial extracorporeal membrane oxygenation. J Cardiothorac Vasc Anesth, 2020; 34: 2776-2792.

20. The continuation of venovenous extracorporeal membrane oxygenation may be futile in all the following EXCEPT:
   A. Signs of severe brain injury
   B. Lung function testing parameters less than 30% predicted

   C. Worsening pulmonary hypertension despite aggressive measures
   D. Worsening volume overload refractory to aggressive diuresis

Correct Answer: B

Explanation: Poor lung function is usually part of the indication to initiate therapy with venovenous extracorporeal membrane oxygenation (VV ECMO). Severe brain injury, severe pulmonary hypertension, and an inability to have a negative fluid balance despite aggressive measures are all signs of likely futility during management with VV ECMO.

References:

1. Gutsche JT, Ramakrishna H. Chapter 33: Extracorporeal Membrane Oxygenation. In: Kaplan JA, Augoustides JGT, Manecke GR, et al., eds. Kaplan's Cardiac Anesthesia. 7th ed. Elsevier; 2017:1214-1228.
2. Mazzeffi MA, Rao VK, Dodd-O J, et al. Intraoperative management of adult patients on extracorporeal membrane oxygenation: an expert consensus statement from the Society of Cardiovascular Anesthesiologists-Part I: technical aspects of extracorporeal membrane oxygenation. J Cardiothorac Vasc Anesth, 2021; 35: 3496-3512.
3. Mazzeffi MA, Rao VK, Dodd-O J, et al. Intraoperative management of adult patients on extracorporeal membrane oxygenation: an expert consensus statement from the Society of Cardiovascular Anesthesiologists-Part II: intraoperative management and troubleshooting. J Cardiothorac Vasc Anesth, 2021; 35: 3513-3527.

21. The following are potential non-cardiac surgical applications for venovenous extracorporeal membrane oxygenation EXCEPT:
   A. Tracheal resection
   B. Pulmonary decortication
   C. Abdominal aortic aneurysm repair
   D. Evacuation of advanced hemothorax

Correct Answer: C

Explanation: The introduction of venovenous extracorporeal membrane oxygenation (VV ECMO) would not be expected to be helpful during repair of an abdominal aortic aneurysm, as this procedure does not primarily involve the lungs. Tracheal resections, pulmonary decortication, and hemothorax evacuation all impact the pulmonary system to some degree and as such have shown benefit from the use of VV ECMO.

References:

1. Gutsche JT, Ramakrishna H. Chapter 33: Extracorporeal Membrane Oxygenation. In: Kaplan JA, Augoustides JGT, Manecke GR, et al., eds. Kaplan's Cardiac Anesthesia. 7th ed. Elsevier; 2017:1214-1228.
2. Mazzeffi MA, Rao VK, Dodd-O J, et al. Intraoperative management of adult patients on extracorporeal membrane oxygenation: an expert consensus statement from the Society of Cardiovascular Anesthesiologists-Part I: technical aspects of extracorporeal membrane oxygenation. J Cardiothorac Vasc Anesth, 2021; 35: 3496-3512.

3. Mazzeffi MA, Rao VK, Dodd-O J, et al. Intraoperative management of adult patients on extracorporeal membrane oxygenation: an expert consensus statement from the Society of Cardiovascular Anesthesiologists-Part II: intraoperative management and troubleshooting. J Cardiothorac Vasc Anesth, 2021; 35: 3513-3527.

22. When considering venovenous extracorporeal membrane oxygenation (VV ECMO) as a bridge to lung transplantation, all of the following settings are considered contraindications to VV ECMO EXCEPT:
    A. Hypercarbia causing acidosis
    B. Uncontrolled infection
    C. Uncontrolled bleeding
    D. Severe nutritional debility

Correct Answer: A

Explanation: Severe hypercarbia is an indication to initiate venovenous extracorporeal membrane oxygenation (VV ECMO) as a bridge to lung transplantation. Uncontrolled infection, severe bleeding, and/or nutritional debility are all considered relative contraindications to VV ECMO as a bridge to lung transplantation.

References:

1. Gutsche JT, Ramakrishna H. Chapter 33: Extracorporeal Membrane Oxygenation. In: Kaplan JA, Augoustides JGT, Manecke GR, et al., eds. Kaplan's Cardiac Anesthesia. 7th ed. Elsevier; 2017:1214-1228.
2. Moreno Garijo J, Cypel M, McRae K, et al. The evolving role of extracorporeal membrane oxygenation in lung transplantation: implications for anesthetic management. J Cardiothorac Vasc Anesth, 2019; 33: 1995-2006.

23. Regarding awake venovenous extracorporeal membrane oxygenation (VV ECMO), which of the following statements is CORRECT?
    A. This type of ECMO refers to patients who can follow commands despite being on mechanical ventilatory support and VV ECMO support
    B. It is not possible in patients with cystic fibrosis, due to their young age and high sedation requirements
    C. It is not suitable in patients awaiting lung transplantation
    D. It allows ambulation and improves rehabilitation

Correct Answer: D

Explanation: Awake venovenous extracorporeal membrane oxygenation (VV ECMO) describes a patient on VV ECMO who no longer requires mechanical ventilation, and who is thus able to ambulate to enhance physical rehabilitation as part of recovery and/or in preparation for lung transplantation. This strategy in VV ECMO is not only helpful in patients awaiting lung transplantation but is also indicated in select patients with cystic fibrosis or idiopathic pulmonary fibrosis when avoidance of mechanical ventilation may be desired.

References:

1. Gutsche JT, Ramakrishna H. Chapter 33: Extracorporeal Membrane Oxygenation. In: Kaplan JA, Augoustides JGT, Manecke GR, et al., eds. Kaplan's Cardiac Anesthesia. 7th ed. Elsevier; 2017:1214-1228.
2. Mazzeffi MA, Rao VK, Dodd-O J, et al. Intraoperative management of adult patients on extracorporeal membrane oxygenation: an expert consensus statement from the Society of Cardiovascular Anesthesiologists-Part I: technical aspects of extracorporeal membrane oxygenation. J Cardiothorac Vasc Anesth, 2021; 35: 3496-3512.
3. Mazzeffi MA, Rao VK, Dodd-O J, et al. Intraoperative management of adult patients on extracorporeal membrane oxygenation: an expert consensus statement from the Society of Cardiovascular Anesthesiologists-Part II: intraoperative management and troubleshooting. J Cardiothorac Vasc Anesth, 2021; 35: 3513-3527.

24. Which of the following statements is CORRECT about anticoagulation strategies for extracorporeal membrane oxygenation?
    A. The partial thromboplastin time (PTT) is not affected by thrombocytopenia
    B. The activated clotting time (ACT) is not affected by hypothermia
    C. Anticoagulation monitoring with the ACT rather than the PTT results in less bleeding
    D. The ACT uses glass beads as an activator

Correct Answer: A

Explanation: The two test that are most frequently employed to measure the degree of anticoagulation during extracorporeal membrane oxygenation (ECMO) are the activated clotting time (ACT) and the partial thromboplastin time (PTT). The ACT provides a good indication of the degree of anticoagulation. Despite its familiarity and reliability, it is affected by multiple factors including platelet function and hypothermia. The ACT is activated by either celite or kaolin and not glass beads. The PTT is most commonly used outside the operating room environment to measure anticoagulant activity, and has the advantage of not being affected by platelet counts. The monitoring of anticoagulation intensity with ACT or the PTT during ECMO does not result in a difference in major bleeding.

References:

1. Gutsche JT, Ramakrishna H. Chapter 33: Extracorporeal Membrane Oxygenation. In: Kaplan JA, Augoustides JGT, Manecke GR, et al., eds. Kaplan's Cardiac Anesthesia. 7th ed. Elsevier; 2017:1214-1228.
2. Mazzeffi MA, Rao VK, Dodd-O J, et al. Intraoperative management of adult patients on extracorporeal membrane oxygenation: an expert consensus statement from the Society of Cardiovascular Anesthesiologists-Part I: technical aspects of extracorporeal membrane oxygenation. J Cardiothorac Vasc Anesth, 2021; 35: 3496-3512.
3. Hoyler MM, Flynn B, Iannacone EM et al. Clinical management of venoarterial extracorporeal membrane oxygenation. J Cardiothorac Vasc Anesth, 2020; 34: 2776-2792.

TABLE 29.1

Factors affecting anticoagulation levels needed to prevent thrombosis

Factor	Effect
Circuit flow rate	Lower flow rates should trigger higher levels of anticoagulation.
Platelet count	Platelet counts less than 100 may increase the risk for bleeding.
Bleeding	Active hemorrhage may require anticoagulation discontinuation.
Hypothermia	Reduced platelet function may increase the risk of bleeding.
Antiplatelet agents	Reduced platelet function may increase the risk of bleeding.
Thrombophilic conditions (e.g., cancer)	May increase the levels of anticoagulation required
Heparin-induced thrombocytopenia	Requires novel anticoagulants and increased risk of pump thrombosis

25. All the following are suggestive of pump head thrombosis during extracorporeal membrane oxygenation EXCEPT:
    A. Decreasing levels of oxygen in the blood
    B. Change in pump sound
    C. Hemolysis
    D. Thrombocytopenia

Correct Answer: A

Explanation: A decreasing partial pressure of oxygen in the arterial blood during extracorporeal membrane oxygenation (ECMO) is usually seen in the setting of a failing oxygenator, likely secondary to thrombosis. Pump head thrombosis during ECMO is usually suspected when there is a change in the sound of the pump, an increase in hemolysis, or worsening thrombocytopenia.

References:

1. Gutsche JT, Ramakrishna H. Chapter 33: Extracorporeal Membrane Oxygenation. In: Kaplan JA, Augoustides JGT, Manecke GR, et al., eds. Kaplan's Cardiac Anesthesia. 7th ed. Elsevier; 2017:1214-1228.
2. Mazzeffi MA, Rao VK, Dodd-O J, et al. Intraoperative management of adult patients on extracorporeal membrane oxygenation: an expert consensus statement from the Society of Cardiovascular Anesthesiologists-Part I: technical aspects of extracorporeal membrane oxygenation. J Cardiothorac Vasc Anesth, 2021; 35: 3496-3512.
3. Mazzeffi MA, Rao VK, Dodd-O J, et al. Intraoperative management of adult patients on extracorporeal membrane oxygenation: an expert consensus statement from the Society of Cardiovascular Anesthesiologists-Part II: intraoperative management and troubleshooting. J Cardiothorac Vasc Anesth, 2021; 35: 3513-3527.

26. Which statement is CORRECT regarding mechanical failure of the circuit during venovenous extracorporeal membrane oxygenation (VV ECMO)?
    A. It is an uncommon event, occurring in only 5% of cases
    B. The negative pressure generated normally by the pump prevents cavitation in the inflow cannula
    C. Pump failure is the most common reason to change the VV ECMO circuit
    D. Thrombosis of the circuit occurs in up to 35% of cases in VV ECMO

Correct Answer: D

Explanation: Thrombosis of the circuit during venovenous extracorporeal membrane oxygenation (VV ECMO) is reported in up to 35% of cases and is the most frequent reason to change the circuit. Pump failure alone accounts for only 10% of indications to change the VV ECMO circuit. Negative pressure generated by the pump in VV ECMO may cause cavitation in the venous side secondary to inflow obstruction.

References:

1. Gutsche JT, Ramakrishna H. Chapter 33: Extracorporeal Membrane Oxygenation. In: Kaplan JA, Augoustides JGT, Manecke GR, et al., eds. Kaplan's Cardiac Anesthesia. 7th ed. Elsevier; 2017:1214-1228.
2. Mazzeffi MA, Rao VK, Dodd-O J, et al. Intraoperative management of adult patients on extracorporeal membrane oxygenation: an expert consensus statement from the Society of Cardiovascular Anesthesiologists-Part I: technical aspects of extracorporeal membrane oxygenation. J Cardiothorac Vasc Anesth, 2021; 35: 3496-3512.
3. Mazzeffi MA, Rao VK, Dodd-O J, et al. Intraoperative management of adult patients on extracorporeal membrane oxygenation: an expert consensus statement from the Society of Cardiovascular Anesthesiologists-Part II: intraoperative management and troubleshooting. J Cardiothorac Vasc Anesth, 2021; 35: 3513-3527.

27. Regarding the use of a hemoconcentration or continuous renal replacement therapy (CRRT) devices within the extracorporeal membrane oxygenation circuit, which statement is TRUE?
    A. The hemoconcentrator inflow line is positioned prepump, and the outflow line postpump
    B. The CRRT inflow line is positioned prepump, and the outflow line postoxygenator
    C. The CRRT inflow and outflow lines are positioned postpump and preoxygenator
    D. The CRRT inflow line is postoxygenator, and the inflow line prepump

Correct Answer: C

Explanation: The hemoconcentrator device during extracorporeal membrane oxygenation (ECMO) works best with a pressure gradient across the circuit, and so the inflow position should be on the postpump side and the outflow position on the prepump side. The continuous renal replacement therapy device during ECMO has the inflow and outflow cannulae postpump but preoxygenator, to utilize the high postpump driving pressure and to reduce the possibility of air embolization.

References:

1. Gutsche JT, Ramakrishna H. Chapter 33: Extracorporeal Membrane Oxygenation. In: Kaplan JA, Augoustides JGT, Manecke GR, et al., eds. Kaplan's Cardiac Anesthesia. 7th ed. Elsevier; 2017:1214-1228.

2. Mazzeffi MA, Rao VK, Dodd-O J, et al. Intraoperative management of adult patients on extracorporeal membrane oxygenation: an expert consensus statement from the Society of Cardiovascular Anesthesiologists-Part I: technical aspects of extracorporeal membrane oxygenation. J Cardiothorac Vasc Anesth, 2021; 35: 3496-3512.

28. A 56-year-old patient with a history of peripheral vascular disease develops cardiogenic shock after cardiac surgery. The surgeon decides to institute venoarterial extracorporeal membrane oxygenation (VA ECMO). Which statement regarding central versus peripheral VA ECMO is CORRECT?

A. Central cannulation allows higher cerebral flow rates

B. Central cannulation is associated with higher rates of limb ischemia

C. Peripheral cannulation avoids proximal-distal syndrome

D. Peripheral cannulation is associated with higher rates of spinal ischemia

Correct Answer: D

Explanation: Peripheral cannulation in venoarterial extracorporeal membrane oxygenation allows similar cerebral flow rates compared with central cannulation. Peripheral cannulation does increase the risk of limb ischemia, differential

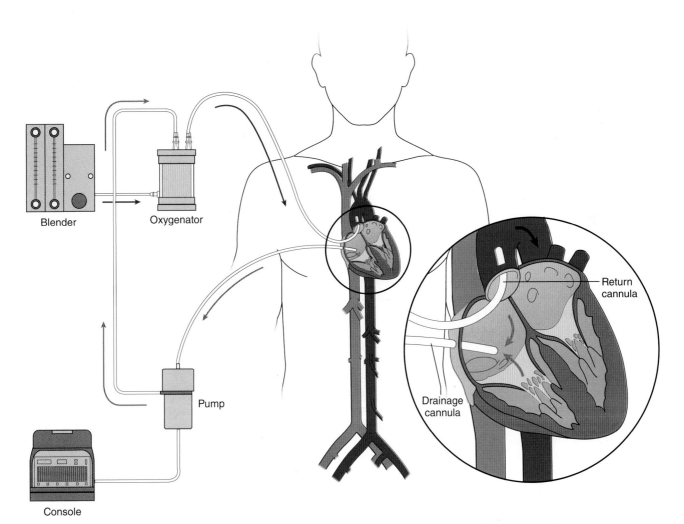

FIGURE 29.7 Single-cannula, dual-lumen venovenous extracorporeal membrane oxygenation.

hypoxia in the proximal-distal syndrome, and, for reasons not entirely clear, spinal cord ischemia.

References:

1. Gutsche JT, Ramakrishna H. Chapter 33: Extracorporeal Membrane Oxygenation. In: Kaplan JA, Augoustides JGT, Manecke GR, et al., eds. Kaplan's Cardiac Anesthesia. 7th ed. Elsevier; 2017:1214-1228.
2. Mazzeffi MA, Rao VK, Dodd-O J, et al. Intraoperative management of adult patients on extracorporeal membrane oxygenation: an expert consensus statement from the Society of Cardiovascular Anesthesiologists-Part I: technical aspects of extracorporeal membrane oxygenation. J Cardiothorac Vasc Anesth, 2021; 35: 3496-3512.
3. Mazzeffi MA, Rao VK, Dodd-O J, et al. Intraoperative management of adult patients on extracorporeal membrane oxygenation: an expert consensus statement from the Society of Cardiovascular Anesthesiologists-Part II: intraoperative management and troubleshooting. J Cardiothorac Vasc Anesth, 2021; 35: 3513-3527.

29. Which statement is FALSE regarding the extracorporeal membrane oxygenation (ECMO) and cardiopulmonary bypass (CPB) during lung transplantation?
    A. CPB is frequently instituted in the preoperative setting, allowing continuation of the support in the operating room environment
    B. ECMO decreases the risk of graft dysfunction compared to CPB
    C. The degree of heparinization is typically lower with ECMO compared to CPB
    D. ECMO has the flexibility to be used as a venovenous or venoarterial platform during surgery for lung transplantation, depending on the degree of circulatory support or pulmonary support required

Correct Answer: A

Explanation: In lung transplantation, the use of extracorporeal membrane support (ECMO) to support the patient in the preoperative, intraoperative, and postoperative settings is becoming more frequent. Venovenous ECMO is preferred in the preoperative setting, as it requires less anticoagulation and is designed to support the patient's lungs. This may be maintained during the intraoperative period if hemodynamic support is not required. It can be converted to venoarterial ECMO if the patient has hemodynamic issues. Compared to cardiopulmonary bypass, ECMO decreases the degree of graft dysfunction in lung transplantation. This mechanical support may also be slowly weaned in the postoperative phase. As compared to ECMO, the intraoperative advantages of cardiopulmonary bypass during lung transplantation include better

drainage of the right heart as well as the use of pump suction in the surgical field.

References:

1. Gutsche JT, Ramakrishna H. Chapter 33: Extracorporeal Membrane Oxygenation. In: Kaplan JA, Augoustides JGT, Manecke GR, et al., eds. Kaplan's Cardiac Anesthesia. 7th ed. Elsevier; 2017:1214-1228.
2. Moreno Garijo J, Cypel M et al. The evolving role of extracorporeal membrane oxygenation in lung transplantation: implications for anesthetic management. J Cardiothorac Vasc Anesth, 2019; 33: 1995-2006.

30. Which statement is FALSE with respect to the development of thrombocytopenia during support with extracorporeal membrane oxygenation (ECMO)?
    A. It may result in thrombosis
    B. It may result in bleeding
    C. It may be caused by the ECMO circuit
    D. Platelet transfusions should be mainly guided by the platelet count

Correct Answer: D

Explanation: Low platelet levels during extracorporeal membrane oxygenation may be due to multiple etiologies, including impaired production, enhanced sequestration, and excessive destruction. The extracorporeal membrane oxygenation circuit itself may sequestrate platelets and/or cause platelet destruction. Severe thrombocytopenia may result in bleeding due to a critical quantitative deficiency. It may be associated with thrombosis in the presence of heparin-induced thrombocytopenia. Transfusion of platelets should be considered not only on the basis of a given platelet count, but also on the risk, presence, and severity of bleeding events.

References:

1. Gutsche JT, Ramakrishna H. Chapter 33: Extracorporeal Membrane Oxygenation. In: Kaplan JA, Augoustides JGT, Manecke GR, et al., eds. Kaplan's Cardiac Anesthesia. 7th ed. Elsevier; 2017:1214-1228.
2. Mazzeffi MA, Rao VK, Dodd-O J, et al. Intraoperative management of adult patients on extracorporeal membrane oxygenation: an expert consensus statement from the Society of Cardiovascular Anesthesiologists-Part I: technical aspects of extracorporeal membrane oxygenation. J Cardiothorac Vasc Anesth, 2021; 35: 3496-3512.
3. Mazzeffi MA, Rao VK, Dodd-O J, et al. Intraoperative management of adult patients on extracorporeal membrane oxygenation: an expert consensus statement from the Society of Cardiovascular Anesthesiologists-Part II: intraoperative management and troubleshooting. J Cardiothorac Vasc Anesth, 2021; 35: 3513-3527.

CHAPTER 30

Blood and Fluid Management During Cardiac Surgery

Matthew W. Vanneman and John G.T. Augoustides

KEY POINTS

1. Practice guidelines are useful tools to guide patient management in the setting of wide practice variations or costly therapies.
2. Practice guidelines often are not effective in changing clinical practice for a variety of reasons.
3. Effective guidelines require effective implementation and the tools to follow the guidelines.
4. ABO and Rh blood groups are defined by the presence or absence of surface antigens on the red blood cell membrane.
5. The purpose of crossmatching is to reduce the mixing of patient and donor antigens and antibodies that elicit immune reactions.
6. Transfusion-related complications can be immune-mediated (e.g., graft-versus-host disease, transfusion-related acute lung injury) or non–immune-mediated (e.g., infectious transmission, transfusion-associated circulatory overload).
7. Genetic variations affect circulating levels of coagulation factors and platelet numbers.
8. It is likely that genetic variation influences the risk for perioperative hemorrhage.
9. Reoperation for bleeding is associated with increased postoperative morbidity and mortality.
10. Implementation of a massive transfusion protocol and consideration of a higher fresh frozen plasma–to–red blood cell ratio may improve hemorrhage and patient outcomes.
11. Factor replacement with recombinant factor VIIa is effective for the treatment of refractory bleeding in the perioperative setting, but it may be associated with an increased risk of thrombotic complications.
12. Human fibrinogen concentrates are approved for use in patients with dysfibrinogenemias. Use in patients with low–normal levels of fibrinogen undergoing surgery is uncertain and may place the patient at risk for thrombotic complications.
13. Prothrombin complex concentrates are prepared from pooled plasma and contain four vitamin K–dependent clotting factors: II, VII, IX, and X.
14. Appropriate volume replacement to avoid tissue hypoperfusion is more important than the choice of colloid or crystalloid.
15. Despite decades of research, there are no blood substitutes approved for clinical use in the United States.
16. Anemia while on cardiopulmonary bypass has been associated with increased perioperative renal injury and patient morbidity. However, the results of observational studies are not entirely consistent, and a specific cutoff value for a safe hematocrit while on cardiopulmonary bypass has not been determined.

1. A child with blood type B, Rhesus factor–negative is most likely to have which circulating antibodies?
   A. Anti-A antigen
   B. Anti-H antigen
   C. Anti-O antigen
   D. Anti-Rhesus factor

Correct Answer: A

Explanation: Antibodies against major blood group antigens (A and B antigens) develop early in infancy in people who lack that antigen. For example, people with a blood type B (group B antigen present, group A antigen absent) develop anti-A antibodies. People with blood type O develop anti-A and anti-B antibodies, while those with blood type AB develop neither set of antibodies. These antibodies develop very early in life, and are thought to be from cross-reactive exposure to either viral or bacterial proteins. Anti-Rhesus factor (Rh) antibodies most commonly occur in multiparous women who are themselves Rh-negative and have previously been pregnant with an Rh-positive fetus. Rh-positive fetal red blood cells enter the maternal circulation, resulting in alloimmunization against Rh-factor. This may be prevented using appropriate immunoglobulin during pregnancy. The H antigen serves as a protein base that is modified to create the A and B antigens. Antibodies to the H antigen are uncommon.

References:

1. Koch CG, Karkouti K, Body SC. Chapter 34: Blood and Fluid Management During Cardiac Surgery. In: Kaplan JA, Augoustides JGT, Manecke GR, et al., eds. Kaplan's Cardiac Anesthesia. 7th ed. Elsevier; 2017:1229-1247.
2. Faraoni D, Meier J, New HV, et al. Patient blood management for neonates and children undergoing cardiac surgery: 2019 NATA Guidelines. J Cardiothorac Vasc Anesth, 2019; 33: 3249-3263.

2. Which of the following transfusions is most likely to result in an acute hemolytic transfusion reaction?
   A. Transfusing type A, Rhesus factor (Rh)– blood into a patient who is blood type AB, Rh–
   B. Transfusing type B, Rh+ blood into a patient who is blood type B, Rh–
   C. Transfusing type AB, Rh+ blood into a patient who is blood type A, Rh+
   D. Transfusing type O, Rh+ blood into a patient who is blood type A, Rh+

Correct Answer: C

Explanation: Acute hemolytic transfusion reactions may occur when there is an ABO group mismatch between the transfused blood and the recipient's blood type. Pre-existing serum IgM antibodies in the recipient's blood stream against the A or B antigen may result in rapid complement-mediated red blood cell destruction when transfused blood contains antigens not present in the recipient. Red blood cells in type AB blood contain both group A and B antigens, and thus may trigger an acute hemolytic transfusion reaction in patients with blood type A (through anti-B antibodies), blood type B (through anti-A antibodies), or blood type O (through anti-A and anti-B antibodies). Patients with blood type AB do not have any anti-A or anti-B antibodies, as both antigens are present in the native blood stream. Type O blood has neither A nor B antigens, and is thus unlikely to result in an acute hemolytic transfusion reaction. Antibodies against Rhesus factor are associated with hemolytic disease of the newborn, not acute hemolytic transfusion reactions.

References:

1. Koch CG, Karkouti K, Body SC. Chapter 34: Blood and Fluid Management During Cardiac Surgery. In: Kaplan JA, Augoustides JGT, Manecke GR, et al., eds. Kaplan's Cardiac Anesthesia. 7th ed. Elsevier; 2017:1229-1247.
2. Faraoni D, Meier J, New HV, et al. Patient blood management for neonates and children undergoing cardiac surgery: 2019 NATA Guidelines. J Cardiothorac Vasc Anesth, 2019; 33: 3249-3263.

3. Which patient would be most likely to safely receive a red blood cell transfusion using an electronic crossmatch strategy instead of a serologic crossmatch?
   A. A patient with group A blood and anti-Duffy antibodies
   B. A patient with group B blood and anti-Kell antibodies
   C. A patient with group AB blood and anti-Kidd antibodies
   D. A patient with group O blood and anti–Rhesus factor antibodies

Correct Answer: D

Explanation: Previously, all blood crossmatching was performed serologically, testing the patient serum for antibodies against possible donor erythrocytes using an agglutination test. With the widespread availability of defined commercial red blood cells with the common major A, B, and Rhesus factor (Rh) antigens, as well as numerous clinically significant minor antigens (such as the Duffy, Kell, and Kidd minor antigens), patient serum can now be rapidly screened for the presence of antibodies against any of these antigens. The "type and screen" test determines the patient's blood type and Rh type and detects the presence of antibodies against many common minor antigens.

For patients with a negative antibody screen against minor red blood cell antigens, an electronic crossmatch can be safely performed, matching the patient's blood group and Rh type with the known blood group and Rh type of packed red blood cells (PRBC) units available in the facility. For patients with a positive antibody screen, indicating the presence of antibodies against one or more minor RBC antigens, a serologic crossmatch is recommended to identify specific units without these minor antigens that are most compatible for transfusion.

References:

1. Koch CG, Karkouti K, Body SC. Chapter 34: Blood and Fluid Management During Cardiac Surgery. In: Kaplan JA, Augoustides JGT, Manecke GR, et al., eds. Kaplan's Cardiac Anesthesia. 7th ed. Elsevier; 2017:1229-1247.
2. Boer C, Meesters MI, Milojevic M, et al. 2017 EACTS/EACTA guidelines on patient blood management for adult cardiac surgery. J Cardiothorac Vasc Anesth, 2018; 32: 88-120.

4. Which accounts for the MOST transfusion-associated deaths in the United States?
  A. Acute hemolytic transfusion reactions
  B. Anaphylactic/anaphylactoid reactions
  C. Transfusion-associated circulatory overload
  D. Transfusion-related acute lung injury

Correct Answer: C

Explanation: While prior data had indicated transfusion related acute lung injury (TRALI) was the most likely cause of transfusion-associated mortality, contemporary data from 2016-2020 now suggest that transfusion associated circulatory overload (TACO) is now a more common cause of death after transfusion. The reduction of TRALI related mortality may be due to improved donor screening and changes to donor eligibility for fresh frozen plasma utilization. TRALI remains the second most common cause of transfusion-related mortality. Acute hemolytic transfusion reactions are thankfully rare due to advancing technology and meticulous blood transfusion preparation and administration. While clinically dangerous, anaphylactic and anaphylactoid reactions from blood transfusion are also quite rare.

References:

1. Koch CG, Karkouti K, Body SC. Chapter 34: Blood and Fluid Management During Cardiac Surgery. In: Kaplan JA, Augoustides JGT, Manecke GR, et al., eds. Kaplan's Cardiac Anesthesia. 7th ed. Elsevier; 2017:1229-1247.
2. Augoustides JG, Patel P. Recent advances in perioperative medicine: highlights from the literature for the cardiothoracic and vascular anesthesiologist. J Cardiothorac Vasc Anesth, 2009; 23: 430-436.
3. Food and Drug Administration Fatalities Reported to FDA Following Blood Collection and Transfusion Annual Summary for FY2020. [(accessed on April 5 2023)]; Available online: https://www.fda.gov/media/160859/download

5. According to recent data, patients undergoing cardiac surgery who received red blood cells stored for greater than 21 days (compared to red blood cells stored for ≤10 days) are MOST likely to experience which of the following?
  A. Higher rates of mortality at day 7
  B. No differences in the multiple organ dysfunction score at day 7
  C. Shorter length of stay in the intensive care unit
  D. Longer duration of hospital length of stay

Correct Answer: B

Explanation: The Red-Cell Storage Duration Study (RE-CESS) trial randomized patients to receive red blood cell units fewer than 10 days old or greater than 21 days old and found no significant difference in the primary outcome of changes in the multiple organ dysfunction score between the two groups. Furthermore, the investigators found no significant difference in the rates of mortality, as well as length of stay in the intensive care unit or hospital. Notably, the trial was not powered for mortality as a primary end point, so further larger trials are still required. Nonetheless, despite *in vitro* studies associating storage with impaired red blood cell indices, clinical trial data suggest that the age of the transfused red blood cells may not be related to these aforementioned clinical outcomes.

References:

1. Koch CG, Karkouti K, Body SC. Chapter 34: Blood and Fluid Management During Cardiac Surgery. In: Kaplan JA, Augoustides JGT, Manecke GR, et al., eds. Kaplan's Cardiac Anesthesia. 7th ed. Elsevier; 2017:1229-1247.
2. Steiner ME, Ness PM, Assmann SF, et al. Effects of red-cell storage duration on patients undergoing cardiac surgery. N Engl J Med, 2015; 372: 1419-1429.
3. Ichikawa J, Koshino I, Arashiki N, et al. Storage-related changes in autologous whole blood and irradiated allogeneic red blood cells and their ex vivo effects on deformability, indices, and density of circulating erythrocytes in patients undergoing cardiac surgery with cardiopulmonary bypass. J Cardiothorac Vasc Anesth, 2022; 36: 855-861.

6. In a patient presenting for cardiac surgery with suspected hemophilia, which initial assay would be most useful in establishing this diagnosis?
  A. Sequencing the factor VIII gene
  B. Quantifying factor VIII mRNA levels
  C. Measuring factor VIII plasma concentration
  D. Assessing factor VIII protein activity

Correct Answer: D

Explanation: Hemophilia A and B are X-linked recessive disorders, typically presenting in males. Hemophilia A, resulting from factor VIII deficiency, is more common (1 in 5000 male births) than hemophilia B, resulting from factor IX deficiency (1 in 34,000 male births). There are hundreds of known genetic variations in the factor VIII gene, some of which alter protein production while others reduce protein effectiveness in the clotting cascade. The initial study of choice in the workup for hemophilia A is assessing plasma factor VIII activity levels, as this study will identify patients with reduced activity (due to either low amounts of protein or defective protein). The extensive genetic variability makes genetic testing a poor choice for the initial assay. Factor VIII mRNA levels and factor VIII plasma concentration may be normal in some variants of hemophilia A, as the protein may have low activity levels despite normal concentrations.

References:

1. Koch CG, Karkouti K, Body SC. Chapter 34: Blood and Fluid Management During Cardiac Surgery. In: Kaplan JA, Augoustides JGT, Manecke GR, et al., eds. Kaplan's Cardiac Anesthesia. 7th ed. Elsevier; 2017:1229-1247.
2. Lin PS, Yao YT. Perioperative management of hemophilia A patients undergoing cardiac surgery: a literature review of published cases. J Cardiothorac Vasc Anesth, 2021; 35: 1341-1350.

7. A patient with known hemophilia A is presenting for coronary artery bypass grafting. Which recommendation is MOST consistent with optimizing the patient's coagulation status during the perioperative period?
   A. Correcting plasma factor VIII levels to at least 150% of normal activity prior to surgery
   B. Maintaining plasma factor VIII activity at least greater than 50% throughout the perioperative period
   C. Administering 0.3 mcg/kg of desmopressin in the post–cardiopulmonary bypass period
   D. Monitoring and supplementing von Willebrand factor to 100% activity after intensive care unit admission

Correct Answer: B

Explanation: Hemophilia A results from factor VIII deficiency or low factor VIII activity levels. Patients presenting for cardiac surgery are at increased risk of hemorrhage; hematology consultation is strongly recommended. To minimize bleeding, factor VIII levels should be corrected to 100% of activity levels prior to surgery. During and after surgery, factor VIII levels should be monitored, and factor VIII concentrate should be administered to maintain activity levels greater than 50% throughout the perioperative period. Desmopressin may be helpful in mild or moderate hemophilia A by boosting factor VIII levels; however, this relies on some functional factor VIII already being present. Supplementation with von Willebrand factor is not the first-line therapy for patients with hemophilia A.

References:

1. Koch CG, Karkouti K, Body SC. Chapter 34: Blood and Fluid Management During Cardiac Surgery. In: Kaplan JA, Augoustides JGT, Manecke GR, et al., eds. Kaplan's Cardiac Anesthesia. 7th ed. Elsevier; 2017:1229-1247.
2. Lin PS, Yao YT. Perioperative management of hemophilia A patients undergoing cardiac surgery: a literature review of published cases. J Cardiothorac Vasc Anesth, 2021; 35: 1341-1350.

8. What is the most common type of von Willebrand disease?
   A. Type 1
   B. Type 2
   C. Type 3
   D. Type 4

Correct Answer: A

Explanation: Type 1 von Willebrand disease is a quantitative reduction of circulating von Willebrand factor (vWF) and represents 60% to 80% of cases. Most patients with type 1 disease have 10% to 50% of normal amounts of circulating vWF. The vWF in these patients is functionally normal. Type 2 disease is a mutation resulting in either loss or gain of function of the vWF protein. Type 3 disease is a rare autosomal recessive mutation resulting in no detectable vWF and low factor VIII levels. There is currently no type 4 von Willebrand disease.

References:

1. Koch CG, Karkouti K, Body SC. Chapter 34: Blood and Fluid Management During Cardiac Surgery. In: Kaplan JA, Augoustides JGT, Manecke GR, et al., eds. Kaplan's Cardiac Anesthesia. 7th ed. Elsevier; 2017:1229-1247.
2. Berger J, Schwartz J, Ramachandran S, et al. Review of von Willebrand disease and acquired von Willebrand syndrome for patients undergoing cardiac surgery. J Cardiothorac Vasc Anesth, 2019; 33: 3446-3457.

9. Desmopressin is contraindicated in which type of von Willebrand disease?
   A. Type 1
   B. Type 2A
   C. Type 2B
   D. Type 2M

Correct Answer: C

Explanation: Von Willebrand disease type 2B is caused by a gain-of-function mutation resulting in increased binding of von Willebrand factor (vWF) to platelets. The administration of desmopressin to these patients may cause additional defective vWF release that leads to platelet depletion and thrombocytopenia. Desmopressin is a known therapy for type 1 disease through its stimulation of additional vWF release. It may also be clinically indicated in types 2A, 2M, and 2N to enhance platelet aggregation. Desmopressin is not effective in type 3 disease, as in this subtype there is no detectable vWF present.

References:

1. Koch CG, Karkouti K, Body SC. Chapter 34: Blood and Fluid Management During Cardiac Surgery. In: Kaplan JA, Augoustides JGT, Manecke GR, et al., eds. Kaplan's Cardiac Anesthesia. 7th ed. Elsevier; 2017:1229-1247.
2. Berger J, Schwartz J, Ramachandran S, et al. Review of von Willebrand disease and acquired von Willebrand syndrome for patients undergoing cardiac surgery. J Cardiothorac Vasc Anesth, 2019; 33: 3446-3457.

10. Acquired von Willebrand disease may result from which pathophysiologic change?
   A. Autoantibodies against von Willebrand factor (vWF)
   B. Macrophage vWF receptor–mediated consumption
   C. Neutrophil–vWF complex activation
   D. Platelet–vWF binding, activation, and vWF consumption

Correct Answer: A

Explanation: Acquired von Willebrand disease may occur for numerous reasons. One etiology of acquired von Willebrand disease is the formation of autoantibodies against von Willebrand factor (vWF), which may be seen in hematologic malignancies. These antibodies bind the circulating vWF protein, resulting in its clearance from the circulation. As vWF levels fall, the patient develops a coagulopathy similar to inherited type 1 disease. Platelets play an important role in type 2B disease, as the vWF in this subtype has a gain-of-function mutation resulting in platelet aggregation and depletion. Platelets do not play a significant role in acquired von Willebrand disease. Neutrophils and macrophages are both phagocytic cell types in the immune system that have not been directly implicated in acquired disease.

References:

1. Koch CG, Karkouti K, Body SC. Chapter 34: Blood and Fluid Management During Cardiac Surgery. In: Kaplan JA, Augoustides JGT, Manecke GR, et al., eds. Kaplan's Cardiac Anesthesia. 7th ed. Elsevier; 2017:1229-1247.
2. Berger J, Schwartz J, Ramachandran S, et al. Review of von Willebrand disease and acquired von Willebrand syndrome for patients undergoing cardiac surgery. J Cardiothorac Vasc Anesth, 2019; 33: 3446-3457.

11. Which preoperative medication is most associated with chest re-exploration for bleeding after cardiac surgery?
   A. Aspirin
   B. Clopidogrel
   C. Heparin
   D. Warfarin

Correct Answer: B

Explanation: Clopidogrel is a thienopyridine antiplatelet agent used to block platelet aggregation by irreversibly antagonizing the P2Y12 platelet receptor. Clopidogrel is commonly used after percutaneous coronary intervention to maintain stent patency. Clopidogrel has been associated with bleeding requiring chest re-exploration after cardiac surgery in multiple studies. Ideally, a complete elimination period of approximately 5 days would be helpful to mitigate clopidogrel-associated bleeding. Unfortunately, because many patients undergo cardiac surgery on an urgent/emergent basis, this elimination period may not be possible. There are currently no reversal agents available for clopidogrel, although some studies suggest that desmopressin and antifibrinolytics may be helpful in reducing bleeding. Aspirin is not typically associated with postoperative bleeding. In patients receiving aspirin, platelet transfusion may also help mitigate bleeding. Both heparin and warfarin have well-described reversal agents, which are protamine and prothrombin complex concentrate, respectively.

References:

1. Koch CG, Karkouti K, Body SC. Chapter 34: Blood and Fluid Management During Cardiac Surgery. In: Kaplan JA, Augoustides JGT, Manecke GR, et al., eds. Kaplan's Cardiac Anesthesia. 7th ed. Elsevier; 2017:1229-1247.
2. Dalén M, van der Linden J, Holm M, et al. Adenosine diphosphate-induced single-platelet count aggregation and bleeding in clopidogrel-treated patients undergoing coronary artery bypass grafting. J Cardiothorac Vasc Anesth, 2014; 28: 230-234.

12. Administration of which intravenous fluid during cardiac surgery is most associated with increased bleeding and likelihood of resternotomy?
   A. 0.9% sodium chloride solution
   B. 4% albumin solution
   C. 20% mannitol solution
   D. Lactated Ringer's solution

Correct Answer: B

Explanation: The use of crystalloid or colloid resuscitation in cardiac surgery has been debated for decades, with no clear evidence supporting either crystalloid or colloid strategies. The recent Albumin in Cardiac Surgery (ALBICS) trial randomized patients to receive either 4% albumin or lactated Ringer's solution for intravenous volume resuscitation. The investigators found the patients in the albumin group had higher chest tube drainage, increased needs for red blood cell and platelet transfusion, and higher risks of resternotomy for bleeding. Colloid solutions such as albumin may result in excessive intravascular volume expansion, resulting in hemodilution of red blood cells, platelets, and clotting factors, that may lead to increased bleeding. A 20% mannitol solution may be used in cardiopulmonary bypass priming solutions or for osmotic diuresis; this has not been associated with increased coagulopathy or resternotomy in cardiac surgery. Neither sodium chloride nor lactated Ringer's solutions have been strongly associated with worsening bleeding or coagulation compared to colloid solutions.

References:

1. Koch CG, Karkouti K, Body SC. Chapter 34: Blood and Fluid Management During Cardiac Surgery. In: Kaplan JA, Augoustides JGT, Manecke GR, et al., eds. Kaplan's Cardiac Anesthesia. 7th ed. Elsevier; 2017:1229-1247.
2. Lange M, Ertmer C, Van Aken H, et al. Intravascular volume therapy with colloids in cardiac surgery. J Cardiothorac Vasc Anesth, 2011; 25: 847-855.
3. Pesonen E, Vlasov H, Suojaranta R, et al. Effect of 4% albumin solution vs Ringer acetate on major adverse events in patients undergoing cardiac surgery with cardiopulmonary bypass: a randomized clinical trial. JAMA, 2022; 328: 251-258.

13. According to the 2015 Pragmatic, Randomized Optimal Platelet and Plasma Ratios (PROPPR) trial, transfusing plasma, platelets, and red blood cells in a 1:1:1 ratio (compared to a 1:1:2 ratio) during acute hemorrhage is most likely to result in:
   A. Fewer intensive care unit–free days
   B. Improved exsanguination-specific 30-day mortality
   C. Similar all-cause 30-day mortality
   D. Similar rates of hemostasis

Correct Answer: C

Explanation: The Pragmatic, Randomized Optimal Platelet and Plasma Ratios (PROPPR) trial was a randomized controlled trial assessing the effect of transfusion ratio with outcomes after severe hemorrhage. The investigators randomized patients to receive transfusion ratios of either one unit of platelets, one unit of fresh frozen plasma, and one unit of packed red blood cells (the 1:1:1 group), or one unit of platelets, one unit of fresh frozen plasma, and two units of packed red blood cells (the 1:1:2 group). Although observational studies suggested a possible benefit in the 1:1:1 transfusion group, there was no significant difference between groups in 24-hour and 30-day all-cause mortality. The only secondary outcome achieving statistical significance was achievement of hemostasis (86% in 1:1:1 group, 78% in 1:1:2 group); however, this was not associated with better clinical outcomes.

References:

1. Koch CG, Karkouti K, Body SC. Chapter 34: Blood and Fluid Management During Cardiac Surgery. In: Kaplan JA, Augoustides JGT, Manecke GR, et al., eds. Kaplan's Cardiac Anesthesia. 7th ed. Elsevier; 2017:1229-1247.
2. Holcomb JB, Tilley BC, Baraniuk S, et al. Transfusion of plasma, platelets, and red blood cells in a 1:1:1 vs a 1:1:2 ratio and mortality in patients with severe trauma: the PROPPR randomized clinical trial. JAMA, 2015; 313: 471-482.
3. Seay T, Guinn N, Maisonave Y, et al. The association of increased FFP: RBC transfusion ratio to primary graft dysfunction in bleeding lung transplantation patients. J Cardiothorac Vasc Anesth, 2020; 34: 3024-3032.

14. In a patient with factor V Leiden, what is most likely to occur?
   A. Mesenteric ischemia
   B. Myocardial infarction
   C. Pulmonary embolism
   D. Stroke

Correct Answer: C

Explanation: Factor V Leiden is a gain-of-function mutation that reduces the normal proteolytic cleavage of factor V, resulting in increased factor V activity. Factor V Leiden is inherited in an autosomal dominant fashion. Patients with factor V Leiden are at greatest risk of venous thromboembolism, including deep venous thrombosis and pulmonary embolism.

Factor V Leiden is rarely associated with arterial thrombotic events such as mesenteric ischemia, myocardial infarction, and stroke. In these settings, there likely is an additional provoking event to trigger arterial thrombosis in conjunction with the factor V Leiden mutation. Despite this risk for arterial thrombosis, it remains less common than venous thromboembolic events in patients with factor V Leiden.

References:

1. Koch CG, Karkouti K, Body SC. Chapter 34: Blood and Fluid Management During Cardiac Surgery. In: Kaplan JA, Augoustides JGT, Manecke GR, et al., eds. Kaplan's Cardiac Anesthesia. 7th ed. Elsevier; 2017:1229-1247.
2. Inangil G, Yedekci AE, Sen H. Coronary artery bypass graft surgery in a patient with concomitant factor V Leiden mutation and thromboangiitis obliterans. J Cardiothorac Vasc Anesth, 2012; 26: e42-e43.

15. What is a US Food and Drug Administration–approved indication for recombinant factor VIIa administration?
   A. Prevention of bleeding in patients who decline red blood cell transfusion
   B. Prevention of bleeding in patients with idiopathic thrombocytopenia
   C. Treatment of bleeding after conventional treatments have failed
   D. Treatment of bleeding in hemophilia patients and factor inhibitors

Correct Answer: D

Explanation: Patients with hemophilia are typically managed with factor VIII (hemophilia A) or factor IX (hemophilia B) repletion. Unfortunately, these patients may develop antibodies against synthetic factors VIII or IX, as their immune systems recognize these proteins as foreign proteins. Since the synthetic factors are immunogenic, they result in the production of antibodies that neutralize the effectiveness of the synthetic clotting factor repletion. Activated factor VII (factor VIIa) bypasses factor VIII/IX in the clotting cascade, enabling resumption of the clotting cascade and boosting clotting ability. The US Food and Drug Administration (FDA) has approved factor VIIa for treatment of bleeding in hemophiliac patients with these inhibitors. Although factor VIIa has been used for rescue in massive bleeding after cardiac surgery, it does not have a formal indication for this purpose from the FDA. Additionally, factor VIIa does not have a formal indication for the prevention of bleeding in high-risk patient populations, as it has also been associated with thrombotic complications.

References:

1. Koch CG, Karkouti K, Body SC. Chapter 34: Blood and Fluid Management During Cardiac Surgery. In: Kaplan JA, Augoustides JGT, Manecke GR, et al., eds. Kaplan's Cardiac Anesthesia. 7th ed. Elsevier; 2017:1229-1247.
2. Ponschab M, Landoni G, Biondi-Zoccai G, et al. Recombinant activated factor VII increases stroke in cardiac surgery: a meta-analysis. J Cardiothorac Vasc Anesth, 2011; 25: 804-810.

16. According to current guidelines, what fibrinogen concentration should be targeted during acute hemorrhage?
   A. 0.5 to 0.8 g/L
   B. 0.8 to 1.0 g/L
   C. 1.0 to 1.5 g/L
   D. 1.5 to 2 g/L

Correct Answer: D

Explanation: Fibrinogen is a critical element of both clot initiation and clot propagation. Low fibrinogen levels may result in delayed clot formation, as well as reduced clot strength. Fibrinogen is typically produced by the liver, and normal fibrinogen levels range from 1.5 to 4.5 g/L. During acute hemorrhage, fibrinogen is consumed, as clots often form more quickly than endogenous fibrinogen is released from the liver. This consumption results in rapid fibrinogen depletion that impairs further coagulation without replacement. Prior guidelines had recommended lower repletion targets (0.8–1.0 g/L); however, contemporary studies have found that even these levels were associated with more bleeding and higher transfusion requirements. Accordingly, current guidelines now recommend targeting a higher fibrinogen level of 1.5 to 2 g/L during resuscitation.

References:

1. Koch CG, Karkouti K, Body SC. Chapter 34: Blood and Fluid Management During Cardiac Surgery. In: Kaplan JA, Augoustides JGT, Manecke GR, et al., eds. Kaplan's Cardiac Anesthesia. 7th ed. Elsevier; 2017:1229-1247.
2. Fominskiy E, Nepomniashchikh VA, Lomivorotov VV, et al. Efficacy and safety of fibrinogen concentrate in surgical patients: a meta-analysis of randomized controlled trials. J Cardiothorac Vasc Anesth, 2016; 30: 1196-1204.

17. What is an advantage of typical four-factor prothrombin complex concentrate as compared to fresh frozen plasma?
  A. Contains higher fibrinogen levels
  B. Does not require blood group matching
  C. Includes preactivated clotting factors
  D. Thaws in 1 to 5 minutes

Correct Answer: B

Explanation: Prothrombin complex concentrate (PCC) is purified, lyophilized, concentrated vitamin K–dependent factors such as factors II, VII, IX, and X (see Table 30.1). Because PCC is purified protein, it does not contain donor antibodies and thus does not require blood group matching. Additionally, because PCC is lyophilized, it can be stored without freezing and rapidly reconstituted with water and does not require any thawing time. Furthermore, because PCC is highly concentrated, it can be administered at much lower volumes to achieve similar or better results than fresh frozen plasma with reduced risk of volume overload. PCC typically does not contain fibrinogen; this may be administered separately with a dedicated fibrinogen concentrate or cryoprecipitate. Additionally, most standard PCCs do not contain activated clotting factors. While some activated PCC concentrates are commercially available, these are more typically reserved for management of patients with hemophilia and factor inhibitors.

References:

1. Koch CG, Karkouti K, Body SC. Chapter 34: Blood and Fluid Management During Cardiac Surgery. In: Kaplan JA, Augoustides JGT, Manecke GR, et al., eds. Kaplan's Cardiac Anesthesia. 7th ed. Elsevier; 2017:1229-1247.
2. Smith MM, Ashikhmina E, Brinkman NJ, et al. Perioperative use of coagulation factor concentrates in patients undergoing cardiac surgery. J Cardiothorac Vasc Anesth, 2017; 31: 1810-1819.

18. After administering 1 L of crystalloid-based intravenous solution, approximately how much volume remains in the intravascular space after steady state is achieved?
  A. 100 mL
  B. 250 mL
  C. 400 mL
  D. 650 mL

Correct Answer: B

Explanation: Crystalloid-based intravenous solutions may transiently expand the plasma volume; however, much of the infused volume is redistributed into the extravascular compartment as free water and solutes equilibrate. After 1 L of crystalloid saline is infused, approximately 20% to 25% of it will remain in the intravascular space. In contrast, colloid solutions such as albumin remain almost entirely in the intravascular space. While numerous studies have assessed the association of either crystalloid or colloid fluid resuscitation with postoperative outcomes, no clear evidence has emerged regarding the superiority of one strategy compared to another.

References:

1. Koch CG, Karkouti K, Body SC. Chapter 34: Blood and Fluid Management During Cardiac Surgery. In: Kaplan JA, Augoustides JGT, Manecke GR, et al., eds. Kaplan's Cardiac Anesthesia. 7th ed. Elsevier; 2017:1229-1247.
2. Knotzer H, Filipovic M, Siegemund M, et al. The physiologic perspective in fluid management in vascular anesthesiology. J Cardiothorac Vasc Anesth, 2014; 28: 1604-1608.

19. Which toxicity has most limited the use of hemoglobin-based oxygen carriers in humans?
  A. Anaphylaxis
  B. Hemorrhage
  C. Liver failure
  D. Systemic vasoconstriction

Correct Answer: D

Explanation: Hemoglobin-based oxygen carriers (HBOCs) have been developed as an alternative to packed red blood cell transfusion as a method of increasing blood oxygen–carrying capacity. In theory, HBOCs would avoid many of the drawbacks of red blood cells such as crossmatching, infection, and a relatively short shelf life. Unfortunately, the potential of HBOCs has been limited by toxicity, principally due to their vasoconstricting effects (see Table 30.2). Because of their hemoglobin base, HBOCs may serve as efficient nitric oxide scavengers, resulting in systemic vasoconstriction that has been associated with hypertension, stroke, and acute kidney injury. Although ongoing studies have attempted to address these challenges with HBOCs, there are currently no commercially available HBOCs in the United States. Anaphylaxis, liver failure, and hemorrhage have not been as strongly associated with HBOCs as systemic vasoconstriction.

TABLE 30.1

Constituents of commercially available prothrombin complex concentrates[a]

Product (Manufacturer); International Availability	Factor Content[b]								Antithrombotic Content				
	II		VII		IX		X		Protein C			ATIII Label (U/mL)	Heparin Label (U/mL)
	Label (U/mL)	Ratio (%)	Label (U/mL)	Ratio (%)	Label (U/mL)	Ratio (%)	Label (U/mL)	Ratio (%)	C Label (U/mL)	S Label (U/mL)	Z Label (U/mL)		
Beriplex P/N (CSL Behring); major western European countries	20–48	133	10–25	69	20–31	100	22–60	161	15–45	13–26	Not in label	0.2–1.5	0.4–2.0
Octaplex (Octapharma); major western European countries	11–38	98	9–24	66	25	100	18–30	96	7–31	7–32	Not in label	Not in label	Not in label
Prothromplex Total/S-TIM 4 Immuno (Baxter); Sweden, Germany, Austria	30	100	25	83	30	100	30	100	20	Not in label	Not in label	0.75–1.5	15
Prothromplex TIM 3 (Baxter); Italy, Austria	25	100	Not in label	—	25	100	25	100	Not in label	Not in label	Not in label	Not in label	3.75
Cofact/PPSB SD (Sanquin/CAF); Netherlands, Belgium, Austria, Germany	15	75	5	25	20	100	15	75	Not in label	Not in label	Not in label	Present, not quantified	Not in label
Kaskadil (LFB); France	40	160	25	100	25	100	40	160	Not in label	Not in label	Not in label	Not in label	Present, not quantified
Uman Complex D.I. (Kedrion); Italy	25	100	Not in label	0	25	100	20	80	Not in label	Not in label	Not in label	Present, not quantified	Present, not quantified
PPSB-human SD/Nano (Octapharma); Germany	25–55	130	7.5–20	45	24–37.5	100	25–55	130	20–50	5–25	Not in label	0.5–3	0.5–6
Profilnine (Grifols); United States	Present	150	Present	35	Present	100	Present	100	Not in label	Not in label	Not in label	Not in label	Not present
Bebulin (Baxter); United States	Present	—	Present (low)	—	Present	100	Present	—	Not in label	Not in label	Not in label	Not in label	0.15 U per U of factor IX
FEIBA (Baxter); USA	Present, not quantified (nonactivated)	Present, not quantified (activated)	500, 1000, or 2500 U per vial (nonactivated)	Present, not quantified (nonactivated)	Not in label	Not in label	Not in label	Not in label	Not in label	Not present	—	—	—

[a]Information is based on product labeling. In Europe, ranges are usually given on the product label in accordance with the European Pharmacopoeia; single values usually are from older, national registrations.
[b]Factor content ratios are based on the content of factor IX.
ATIII, Antithrombin III.
From Levy JH, Tanaka KA, Dietrich W. Perioperative hemostatic management of patients treated with vitamin K antagonists. Anesthesiology, 2008; 109: 918-926.

TABLE 30.2

Adverse events reported in the literature or publicly available sources[a]

Cohort Characteristics	Apex		Baxter		Biopure		Enzon		Hemosol		Northfield Laboratories		Sangart		Somatogen	
	Test	Ctl	Test	Ctl	Test	Ctl	Test	Ctl	Test	Ctl	Test	Ctl	Test	Ctl	Test	Ctl
No. of subjects	Not reported		504	505	708	618	Not reported		209	192	623	457	85	45	64	26
1. Death	—	—	78	61	25	14	—	—	1	4	73	39	2	0	—	—
2. Hypertension	—	—	76	38	166	59	—	—	113	75	—	—	7	1	8	0
3. Pulmonary hypertension	—	—	1	0	3	0	—	—	—	—	—	—	—	—	—	—
4. Chest pain/chest tightness	—	—	—	—	21	16	—	—	—	—	—	—	—	—	12	0
5. Congestive heart failure	—	—	0	1	54	22	—	—	0	2	17	20	—	—	—	—
6. Cardiac arrest	—	17	6	—	—	1	1	14	9	—	—	—	—	—	—	—
7. Myocardial infarction	—	—	6	1	14	4	—	—	14	7	29	2	2	0	—	—
8. Cardiac arrhythmias/ conduction abnormalities	—	—	23	17	153	100	—	—	1	1	—	—	15	5	1	1
9. Cerebrovascular accident, cerebrovascular ischemia, TIA	—	—	—	—	16	3	—	—	2	1	3	1	—	—	—	—
10. Pneumonia	—	—	—	—	35	22	—	—	—	—	27	21	—	—	—	—
11. Respiratory distress/failure	—	—	—	—	22	12	—	—	—	—	21	17	—	—	—	—
12. Acute renal failure	—	—	1	3	10	4	—	—	2	2	—	—	—	—	—	—
13. Hypoxia, cyanosis, decreased oxygen saturation	—	—	—	—	76	35	—	1	1	1	—	—	—	—	3	1
14. Hypovolemia	—	—	—	—	19	4	—	—	—	—	—	—	—	—	—	—
15. Gastrointestinal	—	—	51	31	345	195	—	—	23	1	—	—	57	20	36	6
16. Liver, LFTs abnormal	—	—	27	8	20	5	—	—	8	0	—	—	—	—	6	3
17. Pancreatitis	—	—	11	0	5	3	—	—	1	0	—	—	—	—	—	—
18. Coagulation defect, thrombo- cytopenia, thrombosis	—	—	—	—	45	17	—	—	1	0	13	4	—	—	—	—
19. Hemorrhage/bleeding/anemia	—	—	33	22	108	55	—	—	1	1	20	17	—	—	—	—
20. Sepsis, septic shock, MOF	—	—	2	2	15	6	—	—	0	1	26	20	—	—	—	—
21. Pancreatic enzyme increase	—	—	13	4	3	0	—	—	—	—	—	—	—	—	—	—
22. Lipase increase	—	—	29	9	48	12	—	—	19	2	—	—	8	4	7	1
23. Amylase increase	—	—	48	45	—	—	—	—	35	20	—	—	7	2	4	1

[a]Not all clinical trials conducted by commercial sponsors have been published, and the published results are not synonymous with line listings that would be found in a comprehensive final study report. For each paper, editorial decisions were made about what information should be included or excluded, as well as data presentation (numbers vs. percentages), making derivation of the number of subjects experiencing an event and aggregation of information to derive a comprehensive list of adverse events difficult and potentially incomplete. Not all studies were controlled. Not all enzyme elevations were captured as adverse events, and in some instances the number of subjects experiencing enzyme elevations was not captured. Differences in reporting methods may have resulted in counting subjects more than once in each category of events (i.e., rows).

Ctl, Control; LFTs, liver function tests; MOF, multisystem organ failure; TIA, transient ischemic attack; —, no information available.

From Silverman TA, Weiskopf RB. Hemoglobin-based oxygen carriers: current status and future directions. Transfusion, 2009; 49: 2495-2515.

References:

1. Koch CG, Karkouti K, Body SC. Chapter 34: Blood and Fluid Management During Cardiac Surgery. In: Kaplan JA, Augoustides JGT, Manecke GR, et al., eds. Kaplan's Cardiac Anesthesia. 7th ed. Elsevier; 2017:1229-1247.
2. Henderson R, Chow JH, Tanaka KA. A bridge to bloodless surgery: use of hemoglobin-based oxygen carriers for anemia treatment and autologous blood preservation during redo pulmonic valve replacement. J Cardiothorac Vasc Anesth, 2019; 33: 1973-1976.

20. According to the Transfusion Requirements in Cardiac Surgery (TRICS) III randomized controlled trial, patients who were randomized to an intraoperative hemoglobin target of 7.5 g/dL as compared to 9.5 g/dL had:
    A. Significantly increased amounts of chest tube output
    B. Significantly reduced rates of renal failure
    C. No significant difference in intensive care unit length of stay
    D. No significant difference in myocardial infarction

Correct Answer: D

Explanation: The Transfusion Requirements in Cardiac Surgery (TRICS) III trial randomized patients to a hemoglobin target of 7.5 g/dL (restrictive group) or 9.5 g/dL (liberal group). Patients in the liberal transfusion group were significantly more likely to receive red blood cell transfusion. The investigators found no significant difference in the composite primary outcome of death, stroke, myocardial infarction, or new renal failure, nor did they find any significant differences in each of the separate components of this outcome. There was no significant difference in almost all secondary outcomes, except with patients from the restrictive group who had a modest but statistically significant increased length of stay in the intensive care unit and hospital.

References:

1. Koch CG, Karkouti K, Body SC. Chapter 34: Blood and Fluid Management During Cardiac Surgery. In: Kaplan JA, Augoustides JGT, Manecke GR, et al., eds. Kaplan's Cardiac Anesthesia. 7th ed. Elsevier; 2017:1229-1247.
2. Mazer CD, Whitlock RP, Fergusson DA, et al. Restrictive or liberal red-cell transfusion for cardiac surgery. N Engl J Med, 2017; 377: 2133-2144.
3. Laine A, Niemi T, Schramko A. Transfusion threshold of hemoglobin 80 g/L is comparable to 100 g/L in terms of bleeding in cardiac surgery: a prospective randomized study. J Cardiothorac Vasc Anesth, 2018; 32: 131-139.

21. A patient believed to have group A blood is suspected to be suffering from an acute hemolytic transfusion reaction to a blood transfusion. Blood transfusion services report a negative direct Coombs test *in vitro*. What occurred during this test?
    A. Patient red blood cells were mixed with anti–human immunoglobulin antibody, and the cells clumped together
    B. Patient red blood cells were mixed with anti–human immunoglobulin antibody, and the cells remained suspended
    C. Patient serum was mixed with group A red blood cells, and the cells clumped together
    D. Patient serum was mixed with group A red blood cells, and the cells remained suspended

Correct Answer: B

Explanation: The direct Coombs test assesses for possible autoimmune hemolytic anemia (see figure 30.1). One cause of autoimmune hemolytic anemia is mistransfusion of incorrectly matched packed red blood cells. The ABO-mismatched blood is rapidly bound by endogenous recipient antibodies against the A or B antigen, triggering complement activation and hemolysis. The direct Coombs test uses the patient's blood, washes the red blood cell fraction, then mixes this fraction with anti-human antibodies (Coombs reagent). If antibodies are present on the red blood cell surface (an indicator of autoimmune hemolysis), then the cells will be cross-linked by the anti–human immunoglobin antibody and "agglutinate," or clump together. This is a positive direct Coombs test. If cells remain freely suspended, then antibodies are likely not present on the red blood cell surface, and this is a negative direct Coombs test. An indirect Coombs test utilizes the patient's serum, mixes it with commercially available typed red blood cells, and assesses for agglutination against specific antigens.

References:

1. Koch CG, Karkouti K, Body SC. Chapter 34: Blood and Fluid Management During Cardiac Surgery. In: Kaplan JA, Augoustides JGT, Manecke GR, et al., eds. Kaplan's Cardiac Anesthesia. 7th ed. Elsevier; 2017:1229-1247.
2. Meybohm P, Westphal S, Ravn HB, et al. Perioperative anemia management as part of PBM in cardiac surgery – a narrative updated review. J Cardiothorac Vasc Anesth, 2020; 34: 1060-1073.

22. A patient presents for cardiac surgery. After laboratory testing, the blood transfusion services recommended red blood cell transfusion with red blood cells lacking the Kidd antigen. What testing occurred?
    A. Patient red blood cells were mixed with anti-Kidd antibody, and the cells clumped together
    B. Patient red blood cells were mixed with Kidd antigen, and the cells clumped together
    C. Patient serum was mixed with red blood cells containing the Kidd antigen, and the cells clumped together
    D. Patient serum was mixed with red blood cells lacking the Kidd antigen, and the cells clumped together

Correct Answer: C

Explanation: To detect the presence of antibodies against red blood cell antigens, an indirect Coombs test is performed by mixing patient serum with a wide panel of red blood cells with known antigens (see figure). In addition to the major red blood cell A, B, and Rhesus antigens, there are approximately

DIRECT COOMBS TEST/DIRECT ANTIGLOBULIN TEST

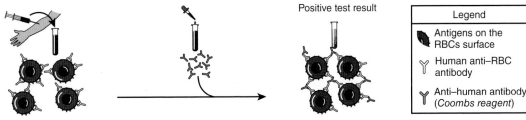

Positive test result

Legend
◣ Antigens on the RBCs surface
Y Human anti–RBC antibody
Y Anti–human antibody (*Coombs reagent*)

Blood sample from a patient with immune-mediated hemolytic anemia: antibodies are shown attached to antigens on the RBC surface.

The patient's washed RBCs are incubated with anti–human antibodies (*Coombs reagent*).

RBCs agglutinate: anti–human antibodies form links between RBCs by binding to the human antibodies on the RBCs.

INDIRECT COOMBS TEST/INDIRECT ANTIGLOBULIN TEST

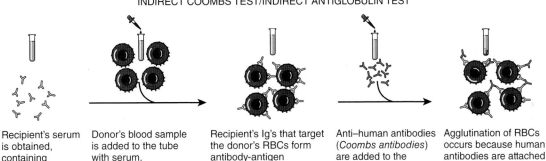

Recipient's serum is obtained, containing antibodies.

Donor's blood sample is added to the tube with serum.

Recipient's Ig's that target the donor's RBCs form antibody-antigen complexes.

Anti–human antibodies (*Coombs antibodies*) are added to the solution.

Agglutination of RBCs occurs because human antibodies are attached to RBCs.

FIGURE 30.1 Indirect and direct Coombs (antiglobulin) tests. The recipient's serum or plasma is separately mixed with three or more commercially available type O washed red blood cells (RBCs) that express about 20 of the most clinically significant RBC antigens to detect unexpected antibodies. The recipient's serum and reagent RBCs are incubated at 37°C for 30 minutes and examined. Spun cells are then washed and tested with antihuman immunoglobulin and reexamined for hemolysis or agglutination. When antibodies bind to RBC surface antigens, the cells agglutinate during incubation with an anti–human globulin (i.e., Coombs reagent), and the indirect Coombs test result is positive. (Modified from Wikipedia: Coombs test schematic. Updated March 2006. http://en.wikipedia.org/wiki/File:Coombs_test_schematic.png.)

20 known minor red blood cell surface antigens. Patients who lack certain minor antigens, such as Kell, Kidd, or Duffy (to name a few), may develop antibodies against these antigens. Red blood cells in the panel that agglutinate when mixed with patient serum indicate the presence of antibodies against that antigen. In this scenario, the patient lacks the Kidd antigen and displays anti-Kidd antibodies in the serum. These serum antibodies produce agglutination of red blood cells with the Kidd antigen, prompting the recommendation to avoid exposure to Kidd+ red blood cells. Since the patient's red blood cells lack the Kidd antigen, they will not agglutinate in the presence of anti-Kidd antibodies. Mixing the red blood cells directly with the Kidd antigen would not crosslink the cells, and so there would be no agglutination.

References:

1. Koch CG, Karkouti K, Body SC. Chapter 34: Blood and Fluid Management During Cardiac Surgery. In: Kaplan JA, Augoustides JGT, Manecke GR, et al., eds. Kaplan's Cardiac Anesthesia. 7th ed. Elsevier; 2017:1229-1247.

2. Meybohm P, Westphal S, Ravn HB, et al. Perioperative anemia management as part of PBM in cardiac surgery – a narrative updated review. J Cardiothorac Vasc Anesth, 2020; 34: 1060-1073.

23. A 25-year-old woman is brought emergently to the operating room with a Stanford type A aortic dissection. While a type and screen is pending, she requires emergency transfusion. Which blood type is the most appropriate to transfuse in this patient when using uncrossmatched packed red blood cells?

A. Blood group AB, Rhesus factor (Rh)-positive

B. Blood group AB, Rh-negative

C. Blood group O, Rh-positive

D. Blood group O, Rh-negative

Correct Answer: **D**

Explanation: Although a blood transfusion is ideally performed after completion of a type and crossmatch, emergent settings may require transfusion before this can be completed and the patient's blood type identified. In this case, uncrossmatched packed red blood cells can be administered. To minimize the risk of acute hemolytic transfusion reactions, blood group O blood is used because this blood group does not have any major antigenic surface antigens (the A or B antigen). Additionally, in women of reproductive age, Rhesus factor (Rh)-negative blood is preferred. This minimizes the risk of generating anti-Rh antibodies, which may complicate future pregnancies, as anti-Rh antibodies are associated with hemolytic anemia of the newborn. Blood group AB packed red blood cells contain both A and B major antigens and are not appropriate for transfusion into patients with an unknown blood type.

References:

1. Koch CG, Karkouti K, Body SC. Chapter 34: Blood and Fluid Management During Cardiac Surgery. In: Kaplan JA, Augoustides JGT, Manecke GR, et al., eds. Kaplan's Cardiac Anesthesia. 7th ed. Elsevier; 2017:1229-1247.
2. Boer C, Meesters MI, Milojevic M, et al. 2017 EACTS/EACTA Guidelines on patient blood management for adult cardiac surgery. J Cardiothorac Vasc Anesth, 2018; 32: 88-120.

24. Which complication is most likely associated with administration of recombinant activated factor VII in cardiac surgery?
   A. Acute kidney injury
   B. Disseminated intravascular coagulation
   C. Hyperfibrinolysis
   D. Thromboembolism

Correct Answer: D

Explanation: Recombinant activated factor VII (rVIIa) is a recombinant, activated protein that bypasses part of the clotting cascade and will directly activate factor X, resulting in thrombin generation and clot formation. Factor VIIa has been studied in cardiac surgery for refractory hemorrhage. While trials have suggested that rVIIa may be helpful in reducing bleeding, numerous trials have also found an association with excessive adverse events from thromboembolism. Accordingly, rVIIa is typically reserved for refractory, life-threatening hemorrhage after other agents, such as fresh frozen plasma, platelets, cryoprecipitate, anti-fibrinolytics, and prothrombin complex concentrates, have been ineffective. Disseminated intravascular coagulation results from excessive tissue factor release, causing microvascular thrombosis and consumption of clotting factors. Hyperfibrinolysis and acute kidney injury have not been clearly associated with rVIIa administration.

References:

1. Koch CG, Karkouti K, Body SC. Chapter 34: Blood and Fluid Management During Cardiac Surgery. In: Kaplan JA, Augoustides JGT, Manecke GR, et al., eds. Kaplan's Cardiac Anesthesia. 7th ed. Elsevier; 2017:1229-1247.
2. Ponschab M, Landoni G, Biondi-Zoccai G, et al. Recombinant activated factor VII increases stroke in cardiac surgery: a meta-analysis. J Cardiothorac Vasc Anesth, 2011; 25: 804-810.

25. Compared to four-factor prothrombin complex concentrate (PCC), three-factor PCC typically lacks which clotting agent?
   A. Factor II
   B. Factor VII
   C. Factor IX
   D. Factor X

Correct Answer: B

Explanation: Compared to four-factor prothrombin complex concentrate (PCC), three-factor PCC often has reduced or minimal levels of factor VII (see table with question 17). Although four-factor PCC is typically used for warfarin reversal or off-label treatment of hemorrhage, three-factor PCC may also be used. Despite this difference, three-factor PCC can be an effective hemostatic agent in bleeding associated with cardiac surgery.

References:

1. Koch CG, Karkouti K, Body SC. Chapter 34: Blood and Fluid Management During Cardiac Surgery. In: Kaplan JA, Augoustides JGT, Manecke GR, et al., eds. Kaplan's Cardiac Anesthesia. 7th ed. Elsevier; 2017:1229-1247.
2. Harper PC, Smith MM, Brinkman NJ, et al. Outcomes following three-factor inactive prothrombin complex concentrate versus recombinant activated factor VII administration during cardiac surgery. J Cardiothorac Vasc Anesth, 2018; 32: 151-157.

26. A patient with atrial fibrillation on therapeutic warfarin with an international normalized ratio of 2.9 is undergoing placement of a left atrial appendage occlusion device. During the procedure, the left atrium is perforated, and the patient develops cardiac tamponade. In addition to pericardial drainage, what dose of four-factor prothrombin complex concentrate is most appropriate in this situation?
   A. 25 IU/kg
   B. 35 IU/kg
   C. 50 IU/kg
   D. 75 IU/kg

Correct Answer: A

Explanation: Prothrombin complex concentrate (PCC) is a four-factor, lypophilized concentrated preparation of vitamin K–dependent proteins. PCC offers a method of rapid reversal of vitamin K antagonist anticoagulation and is approved for reversal of warfarin. PCC dosing is based upon weight and level of anticoagulation, as assessed by the patient's international normalized ratio. Current recommended dosing of PCC for this indication follows the guidelines summarized in the table:

INTERNATIONAL NORMALIZED RATIO (INR)	PCC DOSE
2.0–3.9	25 units/kg
4.0–6.0	35 units/kg
>6.0	50 units/kg

References:

1. Koch CG, Karkouti K, Body SC. Chapter 34: Blood and Fluid Management During Cardiac Surgery. In: Kaplan JA, Augoustides JGT, Manecke GR, et al., eds. Kaplan's Cardiac Anesthesia. 7th ed. Elsevier; 2017:1229-1247.
2. Smith MM, Ashikhmina E, Brinkman NJ, et al. Perioperative use of coagulation factor concentrates in patients undergoing cardiac surgery. J Cardiothorac Vasc Anesth, 2017; 31: 1810-1819.

27. Which of the following statements is most accurate regarding cold agglutinin disease?
    A. Corticosteroid therapy is recommended before cardiac surgery
    B. IgG autoantibodies are commonly present and may react with blood cell antigens at low temperatures
    C. Routine screening before cardiac surgery is not recommended
    D. Splenectomy is often beneficial in cold agglutinin disease

Correct Answer: C

Explanation: Cold agglutinin disease is a very rare (2 per 100,000 people) autoimmune disease resulting in hemolysis. Patients with cold agglutinin disease often have serum IgM antibodies (not IgG antibodies) that bind red blood cells at cold temperatures ($\sim$30°C). When the blood is rewarmed, the IgM antibodies recruit complement proteins, resulting in hemolysis. Fortunately, due to its rarity, routine screening for cold agglutinin disease is not recommended before cardiac surgery.

Neither corticosteroids nor splenectomy are clearly beneficial in cold agglutinin disease, and thus are not commonly pursued in most cases. Preoperative plasmapheresis has been utilized successfully to clear the IgM antibodies responsible for thermally triggered agglutination.

References:

1. Koch CG, Karkouti K, Body SC. Chapter 34: Blood and Fluid Management During Cardiac Surgery. In: Kaplan JA, Augoustides JGT, Manecke GR, et al., eds. Kaplan's Cardiac Anesthesia. 7th ed. Elsevier; 2017:1229-1247.
2. Yalamuri S, Heath M, McCartney S, et al. Cardiopulmonary bypass management complicated by a stenotic coronary sinus and cold agglutinins. J Cardiothorac Vasc Anesth, 2017; 31: 233-235.
3. Smith MM, Renew R, Nelson JA, et al. Reb blood cell disorders: perioperative considerations for patients undergoing cardiac surgery. J Cardiothorac Vasc Anesth, 2019; 33: 1393-1406.

28. Which strategy is most likely to result in successful implementation of clinical guidelines at an institutional level?
    A. Focusing on guidelines with level C evidence
    B. Hospital-wide email communications requesting specific guideline adherence
    C. Real-time feedback to clinicians regarding guideline implementation
    D. Widespread guideline dissemination through national societies

Correct Answer: C

Explanation: Clinical practice guidelines originate from national societies, where the latest evidence is evaluated and assimilated into recommended clinical actions. Despite widespread dissemination through national societies, most guidelines are only slowly and rarely implemented, indicating that further efforts are needed. Implementation challenges may be due to low-quality evidence (level C: very low-quality evidence), overly complex construction, and lack of clinician awareness. A successful strategy for guideline implementation has been real-time feedback to clinicians, which may facilitate behavior change and improve guideline adherence. Hospital-wide email communications are often not specific or not sufficiently targeted to achieve improved guideline adherence.

References:

1. Koch CG, Karkouti K, Body SC. Chapter 34: Blood and Fluid Management During Cardiac Surgery. In: Kaplan JA, Augoustides JGT, Manecke GR, et al., eds. Kaplan's Cardiac Anesthesia. 7th ed. Elsevier; 2017:1229-1247.
2. Gutsche JT, Kornfield ZN, Speck RM, et al. Impact of guideline implementation on transfusion practices in a surgical intensive care unit. J Cardiothorac Vasc Anesth, 2013; 27: 1189-1193.

29. What is the most common adverse transfusion reaction?
    A. Acute hemolytic transfusion reaction
    B. Delayed hemolytic transfusion reaction
    C. Febrile nonhemolytic transfusion reaction
    D. Transfusion associated circulatory overload

Correct Answer: D

Although blood transfusion is a common procedure performed in the United States, it is not without risk. The most common adverse reaction to blood transfusion is a febrile nonhemolytic transfusion reaction. The etiology of the reaction is not entirely clear, but it is hypothesized to originate from donor leukocyte degradation during blood storage, releasing inflammatory cytokines. Once transfused, these cytokines initiate a febrile reaction in the recipient. This transfusion reaction is typically treated with acetaminophen and is self-limiting. Acute and delayed hemolytic transfusion reactions are antibody-mediated processes resulting in hemolysis. These transfusion reactions are uncommon with the advent of contemporary type and screen techniques. Although transfusion associated circulatory overload is the most common cause of transfusion-associated mortality, it is fortunately less common.

References:

1. Koch CG, Karkouti K, Body SC. Chapter 34: Blood and Fluid Management During Cardiac Surgery. In: Kaplan JA, Augoustides JGT, Manecke GR, et al., eds. Kaplan's Cardiac Anesthesia. 7th ed. Elsevier; 2017:1229-1247.
2. Boer C, Meesters MI, Milojevic M, et al. 2017 EACTS/EACTA Guidelines on patient blood management for adult cardiac surgery. J Cardiothorac Vasc Anesth, 2018; 32: 88-120.

30. Which electrolyte disturbance is most likely to occur during a massive transfusion?

   A. Hypocalcemia
   B. Hypochloremia
   C. Hypokalemia
   D. Hyponatremia

Correct Answer: A

Explanation: Most blood products are collected and stored using sodium citrate, which serves to bind and chelate free divalent calcium cations. By binding calcium, a key cofactor in many coagulation proteins, citrate serves to prevent blood clotting during collection and storage. When reinfused at high levels during massive transfusion, citrate may also bind free ionic calcium in the bloodstream, resulting in profound hypocalcemia. This can be treated with administration of exogenous calcium chloride or calcium gluconate. Maintaining normal serum ionized calcium levels is important to maintain coagulation factor function and cardiovascular stability.

Massive transfusion may also be associated with hyperkalemia, which may require active management. Hyponatremia and hypochloremia are not as commonly associated with massive transfusions as hypocalcemia.

References:

1. Koch CG, Karkouti K, Body SC. Chapter 34: Blood and Fluid Management During Cardiac Surgery. In: Kaplan JA, Augoustides JGT, Manecke GR, et al., eds. Kaplan's Cardiac Anesthesia. 7th ed. Elsevier; 2017:1229-1247.
2. Dorantes RP, Boettcher BT, Woehlck HJ. Calcium chloride requirement and postreperfusion rebound during massive transfusion in liver transplantation. J Cardiothorac Vasc Anesth, 2022; 36: 2400-2405.

CHAPTER 31

Transfusion Medicine and Coagulation Disorders

Matthew W. Vanneman and John G.T. Augoustides

KEY POINTS

1. It is easiest to think of coagulation as a wave of biologic activity occurring at the site of tissue injury consisting of initiation, acceleration, control, and lysis.

2. Hemostasis is part of a larger body system: inflammation. The protein reactions in coagulation have important roles in signaling inflammation.

3. Thrombin is the most important coagulation modulator, interacting with multiple coagulation factors, platelets, tissue plasminogen activator, prostacyclin, nitric oxide, and various white blood cells.

4. The serine proteases that compose the coagulation pathway are balanced by serine protease inhibitors, termed *serpins.* Antithrombin is the most important inhibitor of blood coagulation, but others include heparin cofactor II and alpha I antitrypsin.

5. Platelets are the most complex part of the coagulation process, and antiplatelet drugs are important therapeutic agents.

6. Heparin requires antithrombin to anticoagulate blood and is not an ideal anticoagulant for cardiopulmonary bypass. Newer anticoagulants are actively being sought to replace heparin.

7. Protamine can have many adverse effects. Ideally, a new anticoagulant will not require reversal with a toxic substance such as protamine.

8. Antifibrinolytic drugs are often given during cardiac surgery; these drugs include ε-aminocaproic acid and tranexamic acid.

9. Recombinant factor VIIa is an off-label "rescue agent" to stop bleeding during cardiac surgery, but it can also be prothrombotic.

10. Every effort should be made to avoid transfusion of banked blood products during routine cardiac surgery. In fact, bloodless surgery is a reality in many cases. Patient blood management, including techniques to reduce coagulation precursors, has been shown to be cost effective and to have better outcomes than routine surgery.

11. The evolving risks of transfusion have shifted from viral transmission to transfusion-related acute lung injury and immunosuppression. Those patients who receive allogeneic blood have a measurable increased rate of perioperative serious infection (approximately 16% increase per unit transfused).

12. Cardiac centers that have adopted multidisciplinary blood management strategies have improved patient outcomes and decreased costs. The careful application of these strategies in use of coagulation drugs and products is very beneficial.

13. Whole-blood viscoelastic testing in conjunction with platelet count and fibrinogen concentration laboratory testing is of value in guiding coagulation therapy. All available testing modalities are most effective when teams have discussed and created accepted algorithms for care of the bleeding patient in their institution.

14. New purified human protein adjuncts are replacing fresh frozen plasma and cryoprecipitate with four-agent prothrombin complex concentrate and human lyophilized fibrinogen.

1. Which is most likely to initiate a clotting reaction?
  A. Coagulation factor cleavage
  B. Endothelial injury
  C. Fibrinogen binding
  D. Platelet activation

Correct Answer: B

Explanation: The clotting cascade is a dynamic process in constant equilibrium between clot formation and inhibition. Under normal circumstances this balance results in clot inhibition, as excess thrombosis may result in vessel occlusion and ischemia. Endothelial injury results in release of factors that promote clot formation and block clot inhibitors, disrupting equilibrium and initiating clot at the site of injury. This endothelial injury and protein release recruit platelets to the site of injury, promote coagulation factor cleavage, and increase fibrinogen binding and cross-linking. While all four components are important in the clotting cascade, under normal conditions the event initiating clot formation is endothelial injury.

References:

1. Spiess BD, Armour S, Horrow J, et al. Chapter 35: Transfusion Medicine and Coagulation Disorders. In: Kaplan JA, Augoustides JGT, Manecke GR, et al., eds. Kaplan's Cardiac Anesthesia. 7th ed. Elsevier; 2017: 1248-1290.
2. Furie B, Furie BC. Mechanisms of thrombus formation. N Engl J Med, 2008; 359: 938-949.
3. Kruger-Genge A, Blocki A, Franke RP, et al. Vascular endothelial cell biology: an update. Int J Mol Sci, 2019; 20: 4411.

2. Which serum cation is most important in the function of protein clotting factors?
  A. Calcium
  B. Magnesium
  C. Potassium
  D. Sodium

Correct Answer: A

Explanation: Clotting factors are serine proteases produced as zymogens, and are typically activated by upstream clotting factors as part of the clotting cascade. Once cleaved, these zymogens undergo conformation changes, resulting in clotting factor activation. Clotting factors II, VII, IX, and X require calcium as an important cation for carrying out enzymatic function, cleaving downstream targets, and propagating the clotting cascade. Many anticoagulant preservative solutions such as sodium citrate or ethylenediaminetetraacetic acid intentionally target calcium. This calcium chelation depletes free calcium in stored blood products, thus inactivating clotting factors and enabling prolonged blood storage. The effect of magnesium concentrations on clotting factor activity is not completely understood; however, it does not appear to be as critically important as calcium. Sodium and potassium are not significant cofactors for most protein clotting factors.

References:

1. Spiess BD, Armour S, Horrow J, et al. Chapter 35: Transfusion Medicine and Coagulation Disorders. In: Kaplan JA, Augoustides JGT, Manecke GR, et al., eds. Kaplan's Cardiac Anesthesia. 7th ed. Elsevier; 2017: 1248-1290.
2. Grover SP, Mackman N. Intrinsic pathway of coagulation and thrombosis. Arterioscler Thromb Vasc Biol, 2019; 39: 331-338.

3. What is the role of vitamin K in clot formation?
  A. It serves as a cofactor to enable clotting factor synthesis
  B. It serves as a cofactor to enable clotting factor protease activity
  C. It serves as a cofactor to enable clotting factor–endothelium interactions
  D. It serves as a cofactor to enable clotting factor–platelet interactions

Correct Answer: A

Explanation: Vitamin K is an important molecule in the production of the vitamin K–dependent clotting factors II, VII, IX, and X. Vitamin K is required to correctly synthesize these clotting factors by interacting with glutamate amino acid residues. This interaction enables vitamin K–dependent factors to bind calcium and assume the correct conformation for subsequent enzymatic activity. Without vitamin K, these clotting factors cannot adopt an enzymatically active conformation, and their activity levels drop precipitously. Warfarin is an anticoagulant that interferes with the vitamin K pathway. Vitamin K is not a direct cofactor enabling clotting factor activity; instead, it modifies glutamate residues to enable calcium binding. Vitamin K does not directly enable the interaction of clotting factors with either platelets or endothelial cells.

References:

1. Spiess BD, Armour S, Horrow J, et al. Chapter 35: Transfusion Medicine and Coagulation Disorders. In: Kaplan JA, Augoustides JGT, Manecke GR, et al., eds. Kaplan's Cardiac Anesthesia. 7th ed. Elsevier; 2017: 1248-1290.
2. Smith MM, Ashikhmina E, Brinkman NJ, et al. Perioperative use of coagulation factor concentrates in patients undergoing cardiac surgery. J Cardiothorac Vasc Anesth, 2017; 31: 1810-1819.

4. What is most likely to boost anti–thrombin III activity?
  A. Heparin
  B. Plasmin
  C. Protein C
  D. Thrombomodulin

Correct Answer: A

Explanation: Antithrombin III (AT III) is a critical regulator of coagulation homeostasis. To be converted to its active form, AT III requires endogenous heparan, a glycosaminoglycan present on endothelial cell surfaces. When bound to endothelial cells, the active form of AT III is responsible for inhibiting thrombin activity at sites where endothelial function is normal. At sites of endothelial damage, the endothelial cells are removed, and the heparan/AT III complex along with them. In the absence of active AT III, clot will begin to form at the site of endothelial injury. Heparin is an anticoagulant analog containing the critical sugar-based residues of endogenous heparan. Heparin, like endogenous heparan, potently increases AT III activity. Plasmin, protein C, and thrombomodulin are all critical anticoagulant proteins responsible for downregulating the clotting response. However, these proteins are not responsible for AT III activity.

References:
1. Spiess BD, Armour S, Horrow J, et al. Chapter 35: Transfusion Medicine and Coagulation Disorders. In: Kaplan JA, Augoustides JGT, Manecke GR, et al., eds. Kaplan's Cardiac Anesthesia. 7th ed. Elsevier; 2017: 1248-1290.
2. Mulloy B, Hogwood J, Gray E, et al. Pharmacology of heparin and related drugs. Pharmacol Rev, 2016; 68: 76-141.

5. Which intervention is most likely to reduce bleeding in postoperative cardiac surgery patients?
A. Administration of 0.3 ug/kg of desmopressin
B. Administration of 0.5 to 1 mg/kg of protamine
C. Forced air warming to 36.5° to 37°C core temperature
D. Mechanical ventilation with 5 to 10 cm H_2O of positive end-expiratory pressure

Correct Answer: C

Explanation: Postoperative bleeding and coagulopathy after cardiac surgery is common and multifactorial. Hypothermia, platelet dysfunction, clotting factor depletion, fibrinolysis, and anatomic bleeding all contribute to postoperative bleeding. Hypothermia (core temperature <35°C) reduces enzymatic activity of clotting factors, impeding formation and stabilization of fibrin plugs at sites of endothelial injury, resulting in bleeding (see table). Forced air warming to target core normothermia restores normal enzymatic action and may reduce bleeding in postoperative cardiac surgery and other patients. Although positive end-expiratory pressure was theorized to increase intrathoracic pressure and tamponade microvascular bleeding, this has not been demonstrated in randomized trials. Desmopressin may release von Willebrand factor; however, this does not conclusively reduce bleeding with routine

TABLE 31.1
Antihemostatic effects of hypothermia

Hemostatic Component	Effect of Hypothermia
Factors	Increased anti-factor Xa activity (by increased heparan activity?)
	Slows enzymes of the coagulation cascade
Platelets	Splanchnic sequestration
	Partial activation
Fibrinolysis	Enhanced
Endothelium	Tissue factor release

administration. Protamine may be used in the case of heparin rebound; however, the clinical association of this phenomenon with clinically significant bleeding is uncertain.

References:
1. Spiess BD, Armour S, Horrow J, et al. Chapter 35: Transfusion Medicine and Coagulation Disorders. In: Kaplan JA, Augoustides JGT, Manecke GR, et al., eds. Kaplan's Cardiac Anesthesia. 7th ed. Elsevier; 2017: 1248-1290.
2. Schöchl H, Grassetto A, Schlimp CJ. Management of hemorrhage in trauma. J Cardiothorac Vasc Anesth, 2013; 27: S35-S43.

6. Which agent is most likely to result in durable reversal of the anticoagulant effects of warfarin?
A. Fibrinogen concentrate
B. Fresh frozen plasma
C. Prothrombin complex concentrate
D. Vitamin K

Correct Answer: D

Explanation: Warfarin has a prolonged half-life (1–2 days) and inhibits the endogenous hepatic recycling of vitamin K, resulting in vitamin K depletion. Once vitamin K is depleted, hepatic synthesis of vitamin K–dependent proteins in the clotting cascade is impaired. Vitamin K repletion is crucial to provide durable reversal for warfarin-mediated anticoagulation. Importantly, however, it may take many hours for adequate factor production to restore clotting factors to levels compatible with normal hemostasis. Fresh frozen plasma (FFP) and prothrombin complex concentrate (PCC) are both effective agents to immediately reverse warfarin-induced anticoagulation. However, without administration of vitamin K, clotting factors in FFP and PCC will be depleted and not replaced, resulting in an anticoagulant state. Fibrinogen concentrate would not replace vitamin K–dependent factors, and thus is not a known reversal agent for warfarin.

References:
1. Spiess BD, Armour S, Horrow J, et al. Chapter 35: Transfusion Medicine and Coagulation Disorders. In: Kaplan JA, Augoustides JGT, Manecke GR, et al., eds. Kaplan's Cardiac Anesthesia. 7th ed. Elsevier; 2017: 1248-1290.
2. Dalia AA, Kuo A, Vanneman M, et al. Anesthesiologists guide to the 2019 AHA/ACC/HRS Focused Update for the management of patients with atrial fibrillation. J Cardiothorac Vasc Anesth, 2020; 34: 1925-1932.

7. A patient with stage V chronic kidney disease and an elevated blood urea nitrogen level is undergoing coronary artery bypass grafting. Which laboratory study is most helpful in assessing the degree of platelet inhibition from uremia?
A. Activated clotting time
B. Fibrin split products
C. Platelet count
D. Thromboelastogram

Correct Answer: D

Explanation: Measurement of the clotting cascade during cardiac surgery is important to determine what blood products may be needed to maintain hemostasis. Patients with chronic kidney disease may have significant uremia due to inadequate renal clearance. Uremia may impair platelet function, although this is typically only seen at higher levels of uremia. Viscoelastic testing such as thromboelastography and thromboelastometry may assist in detecting impaired platelet function in patients with renal failure. If platelet dysfunction is detected, desmopressin may be considered to improve clotting. In patients with chronic kidney disease, the absolute platelet count may be normal; however, platelet function may be impaired, making this study not helpful for detecting uremia-induced platelet dysfunction. Activated clotting time is a measure of anticoagulation from heparin. Fibrin split products are increased in pathologic conditions such as disseminated intravascular coagulation and are not associated with uremia-mediated platelet dysfunction.

References:

1. Spiess BD, Armour S, Horrow J, et al. Chapter 35: Transfusion Medicine and Coagulation Disorders. In: Kaplan JA, Augoustides JGT, Manecke GR, et al., eds. Kaplan's Cardiac Anesthesia. 7th ed. Elsevier; 2017: 1248-1290.
2. Meco M, Montisci A, Giustiniano E, et al. Viscoelastic blood tests use in adult cardiac surgery: meta-analysis, meta-regression, and trial sequential analysis. J Cardiothorac Vasc Anesth, 2020; 34: 119-127.

8. To which protein does tranexamic acid most strongly bind?
   A. Tissue plasminogen activator
   B. Plasminogen
   C. Plasmin
   D. Fibrin

Correct Answer: B

Explanation: Tranexamic acid is a potent antifibrinolytic important in reducing bleeding and transfusion in cardiac surgery. Normally, tissue plasminogen activator cleaves

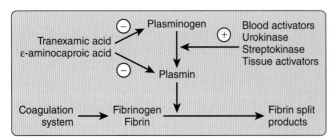

FIGURE 31.1 The fibrinolytic pathway. Antifibrinolytic drugs inhibit fibrinolysis by binding to both plasminogen and plasmin. Intrinsic blood activators (factor XIIa), extrinsic tissue activators (tissue plasminogen activator, urokinase plasminogen activator), and exogenous activators (streptokinase, acetylated streptokinase plasminogen activator complex) cleave plasminogen to form plasmin. (From Horrow JC, Hlavacek J, Strong MD, et al. Prophylactic tranexamic acid decreases bleeding after cardiac operations. J Thorac Cardiovasc Surg, 1990; 99: 70.)

inactive plasminogen to active plasmin. Once activated, plasmin breaks down cross-linked fibrin, resulting in fibrinolysis and clot dissolution. Tranexamic acid potently binds to plasminogen, blocking the conversion of plasminogen to plasmin by inhibiting the interaction between tissue plasminogen activator and plasminogen (see figure). With reduced conversion of plasminogen to plasmin and reduced plasmin levels, existing clots have prolonged life spans due to reduced fibrin destruction and fibrinolysis. Tranexamic acid does bind and inhibit plasmin but has a stronger affinity for plasminogen. It also does not directly bind tissue plasminogen activator, although it inhibits its activity by masking the cleavage site on plasminogen. Tranexamic acid also does not directly bind fibrin.

References:

1. Spiess BD, Armour S, Horrow J, et al. Chapter 35: Transfusion Medicine and Coagulation Disorders. In: Kaplan JA, Augoustides JGT, Manecke GR, et al., eds. Kaplan's Cardiac Anesthesia. 7th ed. Elsevier; 2017: 1248-1290.
2. Taam J, Yang QJ, Pang KS, et al. Current evidence and future directions of tranexamic acid use, efficacy, and dosing for major surgical procedures. J Cardiothorac Vasc Anesth, 2020; 34: 782-790.

9. A patient undergoing coronary artery bypass grafting had been receiving an intravenous infusion of unfractionated heparin prior to surgery. The patient receives 400 units/kg of heparin in preparation for cardiopulmonary bypass; however, the activated clotting time only increases from 133 seconds to 294 seconds. Which therapy is most appropriate to administer next?
   A. Antithrombin III concentrate
   B. Bivalrudin
   C. Fresh frozen plasma
   D. Heparin

Correct Answer: D

Explanation: Heparin resistance occurs when a patient does not have the anticipated anticoagulant response to heparin administration. Heparin facilitates interaction of anti–thrombin III and thrombin, resulting in thrombin inhibition. Heparin resistance is not fully understood, although one putative mechanism may be antithrombin III depletion. Because patients may require up to 800 units/kg of heparin, initial management in heparin resistance is administration of additional heparin and reassessment of the activated clotting time. Often, additional heparin administration will achieve the desired level of anticoagulation. Failing that, administration of anti–thrombin III concentrate, a recombinant preparation, may improve heparin-mediated anticoagulation as a second-line therapy. Recombinant anti–thrombin III is now recommended over fresh frozen plasma to correct anti–thrombin III deficiency to lower risks of transfusion-associated complications such as lung injury and infection. Bivalrudin, a direct thrombin inhibitor, may be used in cases of heparin-induced thrombocytopenia. It is not routinely used in heparin resistance.

References:

1. Spiess BD, Armour S, Horrow J, et al. Chapter 35: Transfusion Medicine and Coagulation Disorders. In: Kaplan JA, Augoustides JGT, Manecke GR, et al., eds. Kaplan's Cardiac Anesthesia. 7th ed. Elsevier; 2017: 1248-1290.
2. Chen Y, Phoon PY, Hwang NC. Heparin resistance during cardiopulmonary bypass in adult cardiac surgery. J Cardiothorac Vasc Anesth, 2022; 36: 4150-4160.

10. Which side effect is most likely to occur after a rapid bolus administration of 400 units/kg of heparin prior to initiating cardiopulmonary bypass?
  A. Bronchospasm
  B. Electrocardiogram changes
  C. Flushing
  D. Hypotension

Correct Answer: D

Explanation: Heparin is a critical component of cardiac surgery, enabling anticoagulation for cardiopulmonary bypass. Heparin is a large, highly negatively charged molecule. Accordingly, when administered rapidly in high doses prior to initiating cardiopulmonary bypass, heparin may complex with positively charged calcium ions. This complex may chelate calcium, depleting serum ionized calcium, resulting in reduced vascular tone and increased systemic vasodilation. Additionally, heparin may have intrinsic, calcium-independent vasodilatory properties that are less well understood. Taken together, large rapid heparin boluses such as those administered before cardiopulmonary bypass may result in hypotension. Bronchospasm may result from an allergic reaction to heparin, which is uncommon. Flushing, a skin reaction, is not typically seen with heparin bolus administration. Electrocardiographic changes are not associated with heparin.

References:

1. Spiess BD, Armour S, Horrow J, et al. Chapter 35: Transfusion Medicine and Coagulation Disorders. In: Kaplan JA, Augoustides JGT, Manecke GR, et al., eds. Kaplan's Cardiac Anesthesia. 7th ed. Elsevier; 2017: 1248-1290.
2. Dhawan R, Chaney MA. Preoperative angiotensin system inhibitor use attenuates heparin-induced hypotension in patients undergoing cardiac surgery. J Cardiothorac Vasc Anesth, 2013; 27: 828-833.

11. A positive result on which assay has the highest positive predictive value in identifying patients with heparin-induced thrombocytopenia?
  A. Luminometric platelet activation assay
  B. Platelet factor 4–heparin antibody assay
  C. Serotonin release assay
  D. Thromboxane–heparin serum activity assay

Correct Answer: C

Explanation: Heparin-induced thrombocytopenia occurs in patients who have functional antibodies against the heparin–platelet factor 4 (PF4) complex, resulting in platelet activation, aggregation, and subsequent thrombosis. Furthermore,

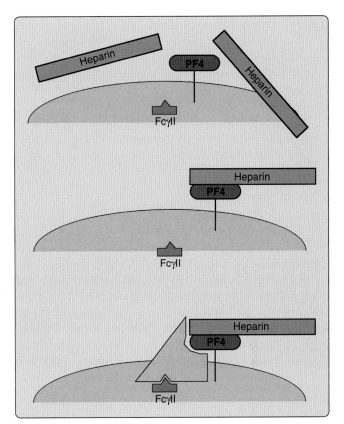

FIGURE 31.2 Presumed mechanism of the interaction among heparin, platelets, and antibody in heparin-induced thrombocytopenia. *Top,* Platelet factor 4 (*PF4*) released from platelet granules is bound to the platelet surface. *Middle,* Heparin and PF4 complexes form. *Bottom,* The antibody binds to the PF4-heparin complex and activates platelet FcγII receptors.

these antibodies may result in thrombocytopenia from platelet depletion. An important diagnostic distinction is if these PF4 antibodies are *functionally active*, and the serotonin release assay tests the functional activity of these antibodies (see figure). If positive, indicating the presence of *functional* antibodies triggering serotonin release, this assay has a very high positive predictive value for diagnosing heparin-induced thrombocytopenia.

The PF4-heparin antibody assay is a good initial diagnostic step to identify if these antibodies are present, but it does not indicate if these antibodies are functionally active. Accordingly, this antibody assay has a lower positive predictive value than the serotonin release assay. Luminometric platelet activation and thromboxane-heparin serum assays do not test for the presence of heparin-induced thrombocytopenia.

References:

1. Spiess BD, Armour S, Horrow J, et al. Chapter 35: Transfusion Medicine and Coagulation Disorders. In: Kaplan JA, Augoustides JGT, Manecke GR, et al., eds. Kaplan's Cardiac Anesthesia. 7th ed. Elsevier; 2017: 1248-1290.
2. Ivascu NS, Fitzgerald M, Ghadimi K, et al. Heparin-induced thrombocytopenia: a review for cardiac anesthesiologists and intensivists. J Cardiothorac Vasc Anesth, 2019; 33: 511-520.

12. A patient in the hospital with recently diagnosed with heparin-induced thrombocytopenia and thrombosis has now been diagnosed with an acute coronary syndrome and requires emergent coronary artery bypass graft surgery. Which agent(s) is most recommended for anticoagulation during cardiopulmonary bypass?

A. Argatroban
B. Bivalrudin
C. Heparin + cangrelor
D. Heparin + prostacyclin analog

Correct Answer: B

Explanation: Heparin-induced thrombocytopenia occurs due to functionally active platelet factor 4–heparin antibodies. For elective cardiac surgery, it is recommended to wait until complete antibody clearance (usually 2–3 months) and proceed after these antibodies are undetectable. In patients requiring urgent or emergent surgery, this delay is not possible, and avoidance of heparin is recommended. Bivalrudin, a direct thrombin inhibitor, is the recommended first-line agent for anticoagulation during cardiopulmonary bypass. Bivalrudin has a shorter half-life than argatroban, making it a better choice for shorter-term anticoagulation in cardiac surgery.

Heparin and prostacyclin infusions for anticoagulation during cardiopulmonary bypass in patients with heparin-induced thrombocytopenia has been successfully described, but is not as rigorously studied as bivalrudin, and is thus recommended as a second-line strategy. The option of cangrelor, a short-acting platelet antagonist, in conjunction with heparin does not currently have a formal recommendation in this context.

References:

1. Spiess BD, Armour S, Horrow J, et al. Chapter 35: Transfusion Medicine and Coagulation Disorders. In: Kaplan JA, Augoustides JGT, Manecke GR, et al., eds. Kaplan's Cardiac Anesthesia. 7th ed. Elsevier; 2017: 1248-1290.
2. Ivascu NS, Fitzgerald M, Ghadimi K, et al. Heparin-induced thrombocytopenia: a review for cardiac anesthesiologists and intensivists. J Cardiothorac Vasc Anesth, 2019; 33: 511-520.

13. Which adverse effect is most likely to occur in response to rapid protamine administration?

A. Arrhythmia
B. Bronchospasm
C. Right heart failure
D. Vasodilation

Correct Answer: D

Explanation: Protamine, a positively charged molecule intended to neutralize heparin, may be associated with adverse hemodynamic effects. Specifically, rapid protamine administration may result in systemic vasodilation, resulting in systemic hypotension. This effect can be mitigated by reducing the speed of protamine administration. Rapid protamine administration has also been associated with increasing pulmonary vascular resistance, although this does not frequently result in right heart failure. Protamine has also been associated with anaphylactic or anaphylactoid reactions and the associated bronchospasm; however, these reactions are thankfully rare. Protamine is not associated with the occurrence of malignant arrhythmias.

References:

1. Spiess BD, Armour S, Horrow J, et al. Chapter 35: Transfusion Medicine and Coagulation Disorders. In: Kaplan JA, Augoustides JGT, Manecke GR, et al., eds. Kaplan's Cardiac Anesthesia. 7th ed. Elsevier; 2017: 1248-1290.
2. Boer C, Meesters M, Veerhoek D, et al. Anticoagulant and side-effects of protamine in cardiac surgery: a narrative review. Br J Anesth, 2018; 120: 914-927.

14. After completion of an uneventful surgical aortic valve replacement, heparin is fully neutralized with protamine. Shortly thereafter, the patient's systemic blood pressure falls to 68/33 mmHg, pulmonary artery pressures rises to 87/45 mmHg, central venous pressure rises to 22 mmHg, and cardiac index falls to 1.2 L/min/m². The pulmonary capillary wedge pressure is 10 mmHg. Epinephrine, vasopressin, diphenhydramine, and corticosteroids are promptly administered, without significant effect. What is the next BEST step in management?

A. Administer heparin
B. Administer isoproterenol
C. Administer methylene blue
D. Administer milrinone

Correct Answer: A

Explanation: This patient is experiencing a type III protamine reaction, with profound and rapid increases in pulmonary vascular resistance with resultant acute right heart failure. Initial management involves inotropic support of the right ventricle with epinephrine, as well as empiric therapy for anaphylaxis. If these initial steps fail, returning to cardiopulmonary bypass may be necessary to restore systemic perfusion. Accordingly, heparin is the most appropriate next step, as the patient is near complete hemodynamic collapse, initial steps have failed, and anticoagulation is necessary to resume extracorporeal hemodynamic support. Although isoproterenol and milrinone may improve inotropic support of the right ventricle and reduce pulmonary vascular resistance, their systemic vasodilatory effects would worsen systemic hypotension and impair right ventricular perfusion. Methylene blue may be useful in refractory vasoplegic syndrome (hypotension and normal/elevated cardiac output), but may be contraindicated in cardiogenic shock from acute right heart failure due to its nitric oxide scavenging properties.

References:

1. Spiess BD, Armour S, Horrow J, et al. Chapter 35: Transfusion Medicine and Coagulation Disorders. In: Kaplan JA, Augoustides JGT, Manecke GR, et al., eds. Kaplan's Cardiac Anesthesia. 7th ed. Elsevier; 2017: 1248-1290.

2. Boer C, Meesters M, Veerhoek D, et al. Anticoagulant and side-effects of protamine in cardiac surgery: a narrative review. Br J Anesth, 2018; 120: 914-927.

15. Which assay has the highest predictive accuracy in estimating bleeding after cardiac surgery?
   A. Fibrin split products
   B. Platelet serotonin release assay
   C. Prothrombin time
   D. Thromboelastography

Correct Answer: D

Explanation: Hemorrhage after cardiac surgery is frequently multifactorial with derangement of multiple facets of the clotting cascade. Viscoelastic testing with thromboelastography or thromboelastometry may detect derangements in all parts of the clotting apparatus, including clotting factors, fibrinogen cross-linking, platelet function, and hyperfibrinolysis. Viscoelastic testing may predict patients at increased risk of hemorrhage and effectively guide transfusion management decisions. The platelet serotonin release assay is used for the diagnosis of heparin-induced thrombocytopenia and is not a predictor of postoperative bleeding. Prothrombin time is an *in vitro* assessment of the extrinsic clotting factors pathway and a poor predictor of hemorrhage. Fibrin split products are elevated in patients with disseminated intravascular coagulation and hyperfibrinolysis, but do not assess clot formation.

References:

1. Spiess BD, Armour S, Horrow J, et al. Chapter 35: Transfusion Medicine and Coagulation Disorders. In: Kaplan JA, Augoustides JGT, Manecke GR, et al., eds. Kaplan's Cardiac Anesthesia. 7th ed. Elsevier; 2017: 1248-1290.
2. Meco M, Montisci A, Giustiniano E, et al. Viscoelastic blood tests use in adult cardiac surgery: meta-analysis, meta-regression, and trial sequential analysis. J Cardiothorac Vasc Anesth, 2020; 34: 119-127.

16. Patients who receive excess protamine beyond what is required for heparin neutralization are at greatest risk for:
   A. Bleeding
   B. Bronchospasm
   C. Hypotension
   D. Thrombosis

Correct Answer: A

Explanation: Protamine is a positively charged ion intended for neutralization of the negatively charged heparin molecule. When administered in the appropriate ratio, protamine will bind heparin and removes its anticoagulant effect from circulation. Because of its highly positive charge, when protamine is administered in stochiometric excess of heparin, protamine may bind and inhibit negatively charged procoagulant clotting factors, thus resulting in paradoxical increases in bleeding. Although protamine has been associated with hypotension (if administered rapidly) and bronchospasm (in the context of an anaphylactoid reaction), neither of these are common after

excess protamine is administered. Protamine has not been associated with thrombotic events but may paradoxically trigger additional bleeding.

References:

1. Spiess BD, Armour S, Horrow J, et al. Chapter 35: Transfusion Medicine and Coagulation Disorders. In: Kaplan JA, Augoustides JGT, Manecke GR, et al., eds. Kaplan's Cardiac Anesthesia. 7th ed. Elsevier; 2017: 1248-1290.
2. Abuelkasem E, Mazzeffi MA, Henderson RA, et al.. Clinical impact of protamine titration-based heparin neutralization in patients undergoing coronary bypass grafting surgery. J Cardiothorac Vasc Anesth, 2019; 33: 2153-2160.

17. What is MOST likely to occur with rapid administration of desmopressin?
   A. Acidemia
   B. Diuresis
   C. Hyperkalemia
   D. Hypotension

Correct Answer: D

Explanation: Desmopressin is a vasopressin analog that also stimulates secretion of procoagulant factors such as von Willebrand factor, factor VIII, and factor XII. Desmopressin may be effective in reducing bleeding due to uremia-induced platelet dysfunction. When administered rapidly, desmopressin may induce systemic vasodilation with resultant hypotension. One putative mechanism for hypotension is rapid release of prostacyclin from endothelial cells, resulting in vasodilation. Desmopressin has anti–diuretic hormone activity, possibly resulting in clinically insignificant free water retention (not diuresis). Desmopressin may be effective in ameliorating uremia-mediated platelet dysfunction in patients with chronic kidney disease; however, it is not associated with acidemia or hyperkalemia.

References:

1. Spiess BD, Armour S, Horrow J, et al. Chapter 35: Transfusion Medicine and Coagulation Disorders. In: Kaplan JA, Augoustides JGT, Manecke GR, et al., eds. Kaplan's Cardiac Anesthesia. 7th ed. Elsevier; 2017: 1248-1290.
2. Raphael J, Mazer CD, Subramani S, et al. Society of Cardiovascular Anesthesiologists clinical practice improvement advisory for management of perioperative bleeding and hemostasis in cardiac surgery patients. J Cardiothorac Vasc Anesth, 2019; 33: 2887-2899.

18. Which medication is MOST associated with postoperative seizures in cardiac surgery?
   A. ε-Aminocaproic acid
   B. Aprotinin
   C. Prothrombin complex concentrate
   D. Tranexamic acid

Correct Answer: D

Explanation: Tranexamic acid is a potent antifibrinolytic that can stabilize clot formation and reduce bleeding associated with cardiac surgery. Tranexamic acid has been shown to reduce bleeding and improve outcomes in patients with traumatic injury and undergoing cardiac, orthopedic, or spine surgery. Tranexamic acid, particularly at higher doses, may be associated with increased risk of postoperative seizures compared to other antifibrinolytics. The clinical significance of these seizures is unknown. Aprotinin is another antifibrinolytic agent that subsequently was found to be associated with renal dysfunction and mortality. Its use in cardiac surgery has fallen substantially. ε-Aminocaproic acid is generally well tolerated even at high doses, although may be associated with rare instances of kidney dysfunction; it has not been associated with increased seizure risk. Prothrombin complex concentrate, used for reversal of warfarin-induced anticoagulation, has not been associated with seizures.

References:

1. Spiess BD, Armour S, Horrow J, et al. Chapter 35: Transfusion Medicine and Coagulation Disorders. In: Kaplan JA, Augoustides JGT, Manecke GR, et al., eds. Kaplan's Cardiac Anesthesia. 7th ed. Elsevier; 2017: 1248-1290.
2. Makhija N, Sarupria A, Kumar CS, et al. Comparison of epsilon aminocaproic acid and tranexamic acid in thoracic aortic surgery: clinical efficacy and safety. J Cardiothorac Vasc Anesth, 2013; 27: 1201-1207.
3. Kelava M, Mehta A, Sale S, et al. Effectiveness and safety of e-aminocaproic acid in overall and less-invasive cardiac surgeries. J Cardiothorac Vasc Anesth, 2022;36: 3780-3790.

19. What is MOST likely to occur after platelet transfusion?
   A. Bacterial infection
   B. Thrombosis
   C. Transfusion-associated acute lung injury
   D. Viral infection

Correct Answer: A

Explanation: Blood is collected from volunteer donors, and the platelets are separated from other blood components and stored. Platelets are stored at room temperature, whereas packed red blood cells and fresh frozen plasma are refrigerated and frozen, respectively. Because platelets are stored at room temperature, they have significantly higher risks of bacterial growth and contamination compared to other blood products. If transfused, these contaminated platelets may result in bacterial infection in the recipient. Although platelet transfusion is associated with transfusion-related acute lung injury, this complication is fortunately rare. Platelet transfusions rarely are associated with viral infection, due to extensive donor blood screening efforts. Platelet transfusion is not associated with thrombosis under normal circumstances.

References:

1. Spiess BD, Armour S, Horrow J, et al. Chapter 35: Transfusion Medicine and Coagulation Disorders. In: Kaplan JA, Augoustides JGT, Manecke GR, et al., eds. Kaplan's Cardiac Anesthesia. 7th ed. Elsevier; 2017: 1248-1290.
2. Klompas AM, Boswell MR, Plack DL, et al. Thrombocytopenia: perioperative consideratons for patients undergoing cardiac surgery. J Cardiothorac Vasc Anesth, 2022; 36: 893-905.

20. Which agent is MOST appropriate for reversal of dabigatran in a patient presenting for emergent cardiac surgery?
   A. Andexanet alfa
   B. Fresh frozen plasma
   C. Idarucizumab
   D. Prothrombin complex concentrate

Correct Answer: C

Explanation: Dabigatran is an oral direct thrombin inhibitor most commonly used for prevention of thromboembolism in patients with atrial fibrillation. Dabigatran has a specific reversal agent, an Fab antibody fragment named idarucizumab. Idarucizumab directly binds dabigatran molecules, rapidly removing them from circulating and promptly restoring thrombin function. Idarucizumab has been shown to be safe and effective in multiple clinical studies.

Andexanet alfa is a decoy factor Xa molecule that binds the factor Xa inhibitors rivaroxaban and apixaban. Andexanet alfa specifically reverses apixaban and rivaroxaban and is not effective for direct thrombin inhibitors such as dabigatran. Prothrombin complex concentrates have been described as possible reversal agents for dabigatran; however, they are less specific than the idarucizumab Fab fragment. Fresh frozen plasma has not been described as an efficient strategy for dabigatran reversal.

References:

1. Spiess BD, Armour S, Horrow J, et al. Chapter 35: Transfusion Medicine and Coagulation Disorders. In: Kaplan JA, Augoustides JGT, Manecke GR, et al., eds. Kaplan's Cardiac Anesthesia. 7th ed. Elsevier; 2017: 1248-1290.
2. Lohrmann GM, Atwal D, Augoustides JG, et al. Reversal agents for the new generation of oral anticoagulants: implications for the perioperative physician. J Cardiothorac Vasc Anesth, 2016; 30: 823-830.

21. A patient is transferred to the operating room for on-pump emergency coronary artery bypass grafting. The patient also has atrial fibrillation, and their last dose of rivaroxaban was 1 hour ago. The patient is hemodynamically stable with no signs of active bleeding. If andexanet alfa is administered, which of these periods is MOST LIKELY the best time for its administration?
   A. Before surgical incision
   B. Between incision and cardiopulmonary bypass initiation
   C. During cardiopulmonary bypass
   D. After cardiopulmonary bypass and protamine administration

Correct Answer: D

Explanation: Factor Xa inhibitors, such as rivaroxaban and apixaban, are increasingly prevalent in patients anticoagulated for atrial fibrillation who then may present for emergency cardiac surgery. Andexanet alfa is a decoy factor Xa molecule, chelating rivaroxaban and apixaban. This restores normal factor Xa clotting functions and may reduce bleeding.

In addition to anti–thrombin III, exogenous heparin also normally binds endogenous factor Xa. Unfortunately, because andexanet alfa is a decoy factor Xa molecule, andexanet alfa potently binds exogenously administered heparin, preventing its normal anticoagulant effect. This greatly complicates heparinization during cardiac surgery with or without cardiopulmonary bypass, and ideally andexanet alfa is avoided in this setting for this reason. If andexanet alfa is administered prior to cardiopulmonary bypass, extremely high doses of heparin may be required to achieve therapeutic anticoagulation, or an alternate agent such as bivalrudin may be necessary. If needed, andexanet alfa may be administered after cessation of cardiopulmonary bypass and protamine administration once the care team is confident a return to cardiopulmonary bypass is unlikely.

References:

1. Spiess BD, Armour S, Horrow J, et al. Chapter 35: Transfusion Medicine and Coagulation Disorders. In: Kaplan JA, Augoustides JGT, Manecke GR, et al., eds. Kaplan's Cardiac Anesthesia. 7th ed. Elsevier; 2017: 1248-1290.
2. Apostel HJCL, Winckers K, Bidar E, et al. Successful antithrombin administration in andexanet alfa-associated heparin resistance. J Cardiothorac Vasc Anesth, 2021; 35: 904-907.

22. A patient with heparin-induced thrombocytopenia and thrombosis presents for urgent cardiac surgery, and bivalrudin is selected as the anticoagulation strategy. What is the best method to monitor anticoagulation levels with bivalrudin while on cardiopulmonary bypass?
   A. Activated clotting time
   B. Activated partial thromboplastin time
   C. Ecarin clotting time
   D. Thrombin time

Correct Answer: A

Explanation: Bivalrudin, a direct thrombin inhibitor, has been shown in multiple studies to be a safe and effective alternative for anticoagulation in cardiac surgery in patients with heparin-induced thrombocytopenia and thrombosis. Bivalrudin increases the activated clotting time, ecarin clotting time, activated partial thromboplastin time, and thrombin time. In practice, the activated clotting time is used to monitor bivalrudin anticoagulation. This is because the activated clotting time is available as a rapidly accessible, point-of-care test that can guide real-time bivalrudin titration. Although the ecarin clotting time is a more accurate measure of bivalrudin activity than the activated clotting time, it is often not available as a point-of-care test and thus cannot reliably guide anticoagulation titration. In a similar fashion, the activated partial thromboplastin time and the thrombin time are also not available at the point of care, making them impractical for guiding anticoagulation management.

References:

1. Spiess BD, Armour S, Horrow J, et al. Chapter 35: Transfusion Medicine and Coagulation Disorders. In: Kaplan JA,

Augoustides JGT, Manecke GR, et al., eds. Kaplan's Cardiac Anesthesia. 7th ed. Elsevier; 2017: 1248-1290.
2. Erdoes G, Ortmann E, Martinez Lopez De Arroyabe BML, et al. Role of bivalirudin for anticoagulation in adult perioperative cardiothoracic practice. J Cardiothorac Vasc Anesth, 2020; 34: 2207-2214.

23. Which protein is cleaved by thrombin to support a negative feedback loop, reducing clot formation?
   A. Plasminogen
   B. Protein C
   C. Protein S
   D. Tissue plasminogen activator

Correct Answer: B

Explanation: Thrombin is the most potent and important clotting factor initiating proclotting elements of the clotting cascade. Importantly, thrombin also activates inhibitory pathways that limit clot formation and prevent excessive and deleterious clot propagation (see figure). One critical feedback step is when thrombin complexes with thrombomodulin. The thrombin-thrombomodulin complex then cleaves protein C to create activated protein C that cleaves activated factors Va and VIIa, resulting in their conversion to an inactive form and reducing clot propagation. Although thrombin also creates downstream signaling resulting in tissue plasminogen activator release from endothelial cells that creates a negative feedback loop, it does not cleave tissue plasminogen activator. Protein S is an important cofactor for activated protein C and is not cleaved by thrombin. Plasminogen is cleaved by tissue plasminogen activator, not thrombin.

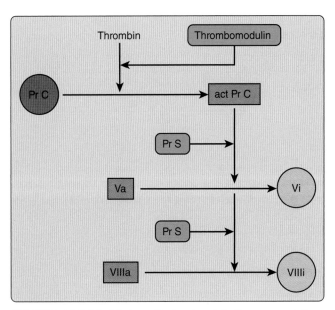

FIGURE 31.3 Modulating effects of protein C on coagulation. Thrombomodulin from endothelial cells accelerates thrombin activation of protein C (*Pr C*). In the presence of protein S (*Pr S*), activated protein C [(*act Pr C*)a] inactivates factors V and VIII. Protein C and protein S are vitamin K–dependent.

References:

1. Spiess BD, Armour S, Horrow J, et al. Chapter 35: Transfusion Medicine and Coagulation Disorders. In: Kaplan JA, Augoustides JGT, Manecke GR, et al., eds. Kaplan's Cardiac Anesthesia. 7th ed. Elsevier; 2017: 1248-1290.
2. Di Cera E. Thrombin. Mol Aspects Med, 2008; 29: 203-254.
3. Gierula M, Ahmstrom J. Anticoagulant protein S - new insights on interactions and functions. J Thromb Hemost, 2020; 18: 2801-2811.

24. What therapy is indicated for a patient with suspected heparin rebound?
   A. Anti–thrombin III factor concentrate
   B. Bivalrudin
   C. Fresh frozen plasma
   D. Protamine

Correct Answer: D

Explanation: Heparin rebound is a clinical phenomenon whereby heparin, previously neutralized by protamine, is reintroduced into the patient circulation. This may occur postoperatively due to delayed release of stored heparin in endothelial cells, more rapid endogenous degradation of protamine than heparin, or other reasons. Although multiple studies have documented the prevalence of heparin rebound, the association of heparin rebound with clinically significant bleeding is uncertain. Nonetheless, if suspected, heparin rebound may be treated with small additional doses of protamine to neutralize the free circulating heparin. Bivalirudin is a direct thrombin inhibitor used to provide anticoagulation for patients with heparin-induced thrombocytopenia; it is not indicated in heparin rebound. Anti–thrombin III factor concentrate and fresh frozen plasma may be used to supplement anti–thrombin III levels in patients with heparin resistance; they are not used for heparin rebound.

References:

1. Spiess BD, Armour S, Horrow J, et al. Chapter 35: Transfusion Medicine and Coagulation Disorders. In: Kaplan JA, Augoustides JGT, Manecke GR, et al., eds. Kaplan's Cardiac Anesthesia. 7th ed. Elsevier; 2017: 1248-1290.
2. Galeone A, Rotunno C, Guida P, et al. Monitoring incomplete heparin reversal and heparin rebound after cardiac surgery. J Cardiothorac Vasc Anesth, 2013; 27: 853-858.

25. What is most likely to occur in platelets after exposure to adenosine diphosphate?
   A. Adenosine diphosphate release
   B. Conversion of plasminogen to plasmin
   C. Glycoprotein IIb/IIIa release
   D. Protein C activation

Correct Answer: A

Explanation: Platelet activation can occur from a variety of substrates, including collagen, thrombin, and adenosine diphosphate. Adenosine diphosphate binds to the P2Y12 receptor, resulting in platelet activation. Once activated, platelets release granules containing multiple proteins including serotonin and adenosine diphosphate that aid in platelet recruitment. The release of adenosine diphosphate from platelets serves to activate nearby platelets, initiating a positive feedback loop at the site of injury to create an initial platelet plug. Platelet inhibitors such as clopidogrel, prasugrel, and ticagrelor, as well as intravenous cangrelor, all target the P2Y12 receptor and attenuate this platelet activation due to adenosine diphosphate. Although glycoprotein IIb/IIIa is an important surface receptor augmenting platelet activation that is recruited in response to adenosine diphosphate, it is not usually released from the cell surface of platelets. Conversion of plasminogen to plasmin and protein C activation both would reduce clot formation and encourage thrombolysis, but they are not triggered by platelet activation mediated by adenosine diphosphate.

References:

1. Spiess BD, Armour S, Horrow J, et al. Chapter 35: Transfusion Medicine and Coagulation Disorders. In: Kaplan JA, Augoustides JGT, Manecke GR, et al., eds. Kaplan's Cardiac Anesthesia. 7th ed. Elsevier; 2017: 1248-1290.
2. Patel PA, Lane B, Augoustides JG. Progress in platelet blockers: the target is the P2Y12 receptor. J Cardiothorac Vasc Anesth, 2013; 27: 620-624.

26. According to the 2022 randomized multicenter Outcome Impact of Different Tranexamic Acid Regimens in Cardiac Surgery with Cardiopulmonary Bypass (OPTIMAL) trial, patients who received high-dose tranexamic acid (compared to low-dose tranexamic acid) were MOST likely to experience which outcome?
   A. Higher risk of venous thromboembolism
   B. Higher risk of clinical seizures
   C. Lower amount of chest tube drainage
   D. Lower risk of red blood cell transfusion

Correct Answer: D

Explanation: The Outcome Impact of Different Tranexamic Acid Regimens in Cardiac Surgery with Cardiopulmonary Bypass (OPTIMAL) trial randomized over 3000 patients undergoing cardiac surgery across four centers to receive either high-dose (30-mg/kg bolus with a 16-mg/kg/hour infusion) or low-dose (10-mg/kg bolus with a 2-mg/kg/hour infusion) tranexamic acid therapy. This trial found that significantly fewer patients in the high-dose tranexamic acid group received red blood cell transfusions compared to the low-dose group (22% vs. 26%, $P = .004$ for superiority).

Interestingly, there was no significant difference in the amount of chest tube drainage between the high- and low-dose groups (490 mL vs. 530 mL, $P = .06$). Despite a theoretically increased risk of seizures, the OPTIMAL trial did not find a significant difference in this outcome between the high- and low-dose groups (1% vs. 0.4%, $P = .05$). It is unclear if the trial was sufficiently powered to detect a difference in this outcome. There were no significant differences in the risk of venous thromboembolism between the trial groups.

References:

1. Spiess BD, Armour S, Horrow J, et al. Chapter 35: Transfusion Medicine and Coagulation Disorders. In: Kaplan JA,

Augoustides JGT, Manecke GR, et al., eds. Kaplan's Cardiac Anesthesia. 7th ed. Elsevier; 2017: 1248-1290.

2. Shi J, Zhou C, Pan W, et al. Effect of high- vs low-dose tranexamic acid infusion on need for red blood cell transfusion and adverse events in patients undergoing cardiac surgery: the OPTIMAL randomized clinical trial. JAMA, 2022; 328: 336-347.

3. Taam J, Yang QJ, Pang KS, et al. Current evidence and future directions of tranexamic acid use, efficacy, and dosing for major surgical procedures. J Cardiothorac Vasc Anesth, 2020; 34: 782-790.

27. According to a 2011 subgroup analysis of the multicenter Blood Conservation Using Antifibrinolytics in a Randomized Trial (BART) study, patients who received tranexamic acid were most likely to experience which outcome compared to patients who received ε-aminocaproic acid?

A. Lower risk of red blood cell transfusion

B. No significant difference in the risk of massive bleeding

C. Higher risk of reoperation for bleeding

D. Higher risk of stroke

Correct Answer: B

Explanation: The multicenter Blood Conservation Using Antifibrinolytics in a Randomized Trial (BART) study was a three-armed antifibrinolytic trial randomizing patients to receive ε-aminocaproic acid, tranexamic acid, or aprotinin. In a subanalysis of this trial comparing tranexamic to ε-aminocaproic acid, the investigators found no significant differences between patients in the tranexamic and ε-aminocaproic acid groups in the primary outcome of massive postoperative bleeding, nor any differences in any of the secondary outcomes, including stroke, reoperation for bleeding, or red blood cell transfusion. Of note, seizures were not reported in the BART trial, and thus this post hoc analysis was unable to assess the end point of seizure.

References:

1. Spiess BD, Armour S, Horrow J, et al. Chapter 35: Transfusion Medicine and Coagulation Disorders. In: Kaplan JA, Augoustides JGT, Manecke GR, et al., eds. Kaplan's Cardiac Anesthesia. 7th ed. Elsevier; 2017: 1248-1290.

2. Raghunathan K, Connelly NR, Kanter GJ. Epsilon-aminocaproic acid and clinical value in cardiac anesthesia. J Cardiothorac Vasc Anesth, 2011; 25: 16-19.

28. What contains the highest concentration of fibrinogen?

A. Cryoprecipitate

B. Factor VIII inhibitor bypass agent

C. Fresh frozen plasma

D. Prothrombin complex concentrate

Correct Answer: A

Explanation: Fibrinogen is a critical element in clot formation. Fibrinogen depletion through either normal clotting or pathophysiologic states such as disseminated intravascular coagulation may result in low fibrinogen levels with associated coagulopathic bleeding. Maintaining adequate fibrinogen levels is crucial to achieving hemostasis in cardiac surgery. Cryoprecipitate contains high levels of fibrinogen in low, concentrated volumes, reducing the risk of volume overload. Commercially prepared fibrinogen concentrate also contains high amounts of fibrinogen in low volumes.

Fresh frozen plasma contains lower levels of fibrinogen in higher total volumes, making it less concentrated than cryoprecipitate. Prothrombin complex concentrate is a reversal agent for vitamin K antagonist warfarin and contains the vitamin K–dependent factors II, VII, IX, and X; it does not contain fibrinogen. Its cousin, factor VIII inhibitor bypass agent, is similar, and although it also contains small amounts of activated factor VII, it does not contain fibrinogen.

References:

1. Spiess BD, Armour S, Horrow J, et al. Chapter 35: Transfusion Medicine and Coagulation Disorders. In: Kaplan JA, Augoustides JGT, Manecke GR, et al., eds. Kaplan's Cardiac Anesthesia. 7th ed. Elsevier; 2017: 1248-1290.

2. Smith MM, Ashikhmina E, Brinkman NJ, et al. Perioperative use of coagulation factor concentrates in patients undergoing cardiac surgery. J Cardiothorac Vasc Anesth, 2017; 31: 1810-1819.

29. What outcome measures are quality indicators in blood conservation reported to the Society of Thoracic Surgeons after cardiac surgery?

A. Use of autologous normovolemic hemodilution

B. Use of hemoglobin transfusion threshold

C. Use of retrograde autologous priming

D. Use of pediatric tubes for laboratory testing

Correct Answer: C

Explanation: Patient blood management aims to reduce transfusions when possible, decreasing transfusion risks to patients and costs to hospitals. Patient blood management has many facets, and the Society of Thoracic Surgeons now tracks at least three measures of patient blood management. The tracked quality indicators in this setting include antifibrinolytic lysine analog medications such as ε-aminocaproic or tranexamic acid, retrograde autologous priming, miniature cardiopulmonary bypass circuits, and cell salvage techniques. When combined, these techniques may reduce patient red cell transfusion by minimizing bleeding, reducing hemodilution, and decreasing lost red cell mass. Although autologous normovolemic hemodilution and pediatric laboratory tubes have both been incorporated into blood management programs, they are not currently quality metrics tracked by the Society of Thoracic Surgeons. Strict hemoglobin transfusion thresholds are typically not recommended; individualized transfusion thresholds are commonly used depending on clinical context.

References:

1. Spiess BD, Armour S, Horrow J, et al. Chapter 35: Transfusion Medicine and Coagulation Disorders. In: Kaplan JA, Augoustides JGT, Manecke GR, et al., eds. Kaplan's Cardiac Anesthesia. 7th ed. Elsevier; 2017: 1248-1290.

2. Del Rio JM, Abernathy J, Taylor MA, et al. The adult cardiac anesthesiology section of STS adult cardiac surgery database: 2020 update on quality and outcomes. J Cardiothorac Vasc Anesth, 2021; 35: 22-34.

30. What is synthesized by endothelial cells under normal physiologic conditions?
   A. Streptokinase
   B. Plasmin
   C. Protein C
   D. Tissue plasminogen activator

Correct Answer: D

Explanation: Endothelial cells play a crucial role in maintaining normal clotting homeostasis and preventing clot formation in normal blood vessels. Because aberrant clotting would result in thrombosis and distal ischemia, endothelial cells release numerous agents preventing localized clot formation during normal conditions, and recanalizing formed clot after the endothelium has regenerated. Some examples of anticlotting agents released by endothelial cells are nitric oxide, prostacyclins, thrombomodulin, adenosine, and tissue plasminogen activator.

Streptokinase is a potent fibrinolytic produced by streptococcal bacteria; it is not endogenous in humans. Plasmin is converted from circulating plasminogen, which is synthesized in the liver. Protein C is produced in the liver and activated near endothelial cells by thrombin/thrombomodulin complexes.

References:

1. Spiess BD, Armour S, Horrow J, et al. Chapter 35: Transfusion Medicine and Coagulation Disorders. In: Kaplan JA, Augoustides JGT, Manecke GR, et al., eds. Kaplan's Cardiac Anesthesia. 7th ed. Elsevier; 2017: 1248-1290.
2. Kruger-Genge A, Blocki A, Franke RP. et al. Vascular endothelial cell biology: an update. Int J Mol Sci, 2019; 20: 4411.

CHAPTER 32

Discontinuing Cardiopulmonary Bypass

Matthew W. Vanneman

KEY POINTS

1. The key to successful weaning from cardiopulmonary bypass (CPB) is proper preparation.

2. After rewarming the patient, correcting any abnormal blood gases, and inflating the lungs, make sure to turn on the ventilator.

3. To prepare the heart for discontinuing CPB, optimize the cardiac rate, rhythm, preload, myocardial contractility, and afterload.

4. The worse the heart's condition, the more gradually CPB should be weaned. If hemodynamic values are not adequate, immediately return to CPB. Assess the problem, and choose an appropriate pharmacologic, surgical, or mechanical intervention before trying to terminate CPB again.

5. Perioperative ventricular dysfunction usually is caused by myocardial stunning and is a temporary state of contractile dysfunction that should respond to positive inotropic drugs.

6. In addition to left ventricular dysfunction, right ventricular failure is a possible source of morbidity and mortality after cardiac surgical procedures.

7. The presence of diastolic dysfunction during the postbypass period may contribute to impaired chamber relaxation and poor compliance, resulting in reduced ventricular filling during separation.

8. Epinephrine is frequently chosen as an inotropic drug when terminating CPB because of its mixed α- and β-adrenergic stimulation.

9. Milrinone is an excellent inodilator drug that can be used alone or combined with other drugs such as epinephrine for discontinuing CPB in patients with poor ventricular function and diastolic dysfunction.

10. In patients with high preload and/or elevated systemic vascular resistance, vasodilators such as nitroglycerin, nicardipine, clevidipine, or nitroprusside may improve ventricular function.

11. Variable gene expression and genetic polymorphism in patients presenting for cardiac surgical procedures may provide the foundation for individualized tailoring of pharmacology based on molecular genotyping in the future.

12. Intra-aortic balloon pump counterpulsation increases coronary blood flow during diastole and unloads the left ventricle during systole. These effects can help in weaning patients with poor left ventricular function and severe myocardial ischemia.

---

1. A patient has undergone an aortic arch repair requiring hypothermic circulatory arrest (minimum nasopharyngeal temperature of 25°C). The perfusionist has begun rewarming on cardiopulmonary bypass, and the patient's current nasopharyngeal temperature is 33.5°C. When providing medical direction to the perfusionist, what is the MOST appropriate blood temperature for rewarming at this time using the arterial inflow cannula?
   A. 34.5°C
   B. 36.5°C
   C. 38.5°C
   D. 40.5°C

Correct Answer: B

Explanation: Adequate patient rewarming after hypothermic circulatory arrest is crucial to prevent postoperative hypothermia and associated complications, such as infection, coagulopathy, shivering, and increased myocardial oxygen demand. Rewarming slowly but fully is important to prevent temperature loss after cardiopulmonary bypass, as thermal energy from the blood and body core redistributes to the peripheral tissues (see table). Importantly, cerebral hyperthermia (temperature >38°C) has been associated with worsened neurologic outcomes and should be avoided.

With a core temperature of 33.5°C, the most appropriate rewarming temperature at this time is 36.5°C. Current clinical practice guidelines recommend a warming gradient less than 4°C; an arterial inflow temperature of 36.5°C is within this range. Inflow temperatures of 38.5°C and 40.5°C may cause cerebral hyperthermia and would not be recommended. An inflow temperature of 34.5°C would not be adequate for the patient to arrive at normothermia prior to CPB discontinuation. Adequate temperature management is part of the general preparation for discontinuing cardiopulmonary bypass.

TABLE 32.1

General preparations for discontinuing cardiopulmonary bypass

Temperature	Laboratory Results
Adequately rewarm before weaning from CPB	Correct metabolic acidosis
Avoid overheating the brain	Optimize hematocrit
Start measures to keep patient warm after CPB	Normalize potassium
Use fluid warmer, forced air warmer	Consider giving magnesium or checking magnesium level
Warm operating room	Check calcium level and correct deficiencies

CPB, Cardiopulmonary bypass.

References:

1. Nguyen L, Roth DM, Shanewise JS, Kaplan JA. Chapter 36: Discontinuing Cardiopulmonary Bypass. In: Kaplan JA, Augoustides JGT, Manecke GR, et al., eds. Kaplan's Cardiac Anesthesia. 7th ed. Elsevier; 2017: 1291-1310.
2. Engelman R, Baker RA, Likosky DS, et al. The Society of Thoracic Surgeons, The Society of Cardiovascular Anesthesiologists, and The American Society of ExtraCorporeal Technology: clinical practice guidelines for cardiopulmonary bypass—temperature management during cardiopulmonary bypass. J Cardiothorac Vasc Anesth, 2015; 29: 1104-1113.

2. Monitoring which of the following is LEAST likely to reflect a patient's core temperature during rewarming while on cardiopulmonary bypass?

A. Arterial cannula outflow temperature

B. Bladder temperature

C. Esophageal temperature

D. Nasopharyngeal temperature

Correct Answer: B

Explanation: Temperature monitoring of both "core" and "peripheral" temperatures during rewarming on cardiopulmonary bypass (CPB) is important to prevent overly rapid

temperature correction, as well as hypothermia from heat redistribution from the core to the periphery after discontinuing CPB. The most accurate measures of "core" temperatures are the pulmonary artery, esophageal, and nasopharyngeal temperatures. Additionally, clinical practice guidelines recommend arterial cannula outflow temperatures as another reasonable surrogate of cerebral temperature. Monitoring core temperature is important to prevent cerebral hyperthermia, which has been associated with negative outcomes.

"Peripheral" temperatures such as the bladder or rectal temperatures often lag behind "core" temperatures and may not accurately reflect core temperature. Separating from CPB with a significant gradient between core and peripheral temperatures may result in core hypothermia, as heat redistributes from the core to the periphery. Accordingly, "fully" rewarming so both core and peripheral temperatures are within normothermic ranges is recommended prior to discontinuing CPB.

References:

1. Nguyen L, Roth DM, Shanewise JS, Kaplan JA. Chapter 36: Discontinuing Cardiopulmonary Bypass. In: Kaplan JA, Augoustides JGT, Manecke GR, et al., eds. Kaplan's Cardiac Anesthesia. 7th ed. Elsevier; 2017: 1291-1310.
2. Engelman R, Baker RA, Likosky DS, et al. The Society of Thoracic Surgeons, The Society of Cardiovascular Anesthesiologists, and The American Society of ExtraCorporeal Technology: clinical practice guidelines for cardiopulmonary bypass—temperature management during cardiopulmonary bypass. J Cardiothorac Vasc Anesth, 2015; 29: 1104-1113.

3. You are caring for a patient who has just completed an uncomplicated three-vessel coronary artery bypass graft surgery. While reinflating the lungs in preparation for weaning from cardiopulmonary bypass, visually inspecting the surgical field is important to avoid which potential complication of lung re-expansion?

A. Injury due to barotrauma

B. Injury due to residual pneumothorax

C. Injury from residual atelectasis

D. Injury to the left internal mammary artery

Correct Answer: D

Explanation: Adequate pulmonary re-expansion prior to weaning from cardiopulmonary bypass is important to ensure adequate lung mechanics, oxygenation, and ventilation (see teaching box). Re-expansion usually occurs with gentle manual recruitment breaths up to 30 cm H_2O. In patients who have undergone coronary artery bypass grafting, the left internal mammary artery (LIMA) may course from the left chest, through the expanding lung field. Overly aggressive expansion may damage or dislodge the LIMA graft anastomosis. Visually observing the course of the LIMA graft and carefully observing lung expansion are important to prevent this complication.

Although barotrauma may complicate pulmonary recruitment, monitoring airway pressures is a better strategy of preventing this complication than visual inspection. Transient atelectasis may be detected visually, but it is unlikely to cause significant lung injury. Residual pneumothorax is unlikely to be clinically significant while the patient is on positive pressure ventilation with an open chest. Adequate lung expansion is part of preparing the lungs for discontinuation of cardiopulmonary bypass.

BOX 32.1 Preparing the lungs for discontinuing cardiopulmonary bypass

- Suction trachea and endotracheal tube
- Inflate lungs gently by hand
- Ventilate with 100% oxygen
- Treat bronchospasm with bronchodilators
- Check for pneumothorax and pleural fluid
- Consider the need for positive end-expiratory pressure, intensive care unit ventilator, and nitric oxide

---

References:

1. Nguyen L, Roth DM, Shanewise JS, Kaplan JA. Chapter 36: Discontinuing Cardiopulmonary Bypass. In: Kaplan JA, Augoustides JGT, Manecke GR, et al., eds. Kaplan's Cardiac Anesthesia. 7th ed. Elsevier; 2017: 1291-1310.
2. Zochios V, Klein AA, Gao F. Protective invasive ventilation in cardiac surgery: a systematic review with a focus on acute lung injury in adult cardiac surgical patients. J Cardiothorac Vasc Anesth, 2018; 32: 1922-1936.

4. What is the MOST likely presentation of intracoronary air embolism during weaning cardiopulmonary bypass?
  A. Lateral wall motion abnormality
  B. Right ventricular dysfunction
  C. ST segment elevation in leads V2 to V4
  D. Ventricular fibrillation

Correct Answer: B

Explanation: Despite deairing maneuvers, intracardiac air may remain and embolize during cardiopulmonary bypass (CPB) weaning. In a supine patient, the less dense air will rise and float to the right coronary artery (RCA). Air in the RCA is most likely to present as acute ST segment elevations in the inferior leads II, III, and aVF, right ventricular dysfunction, and an inferior wall motion abnormality. Routine therapy includes returning to full CPB, increasing the mean arterial blood pressure, and waiting until restoration of normal cardiac function.

A lateral wall motion abnormality is typically indicative of circumflex artery injury, which may be seen in mitral valve procedures. ST segment elevation in leads V2 to V4 suggests left anterior descending (LAD) artery ischemia; the LAD is posterior and less likely to receive anteriorly directed intracoronary air. RCA air may uncommonly result in ventricular fibrillation, but this is not the most common presentation.

References:

1. Nguyen L, Roth DM, Shanewise JS, Kaplan JA. Chapter 36: Discontinuing Cardiopulmonary Bypass. In: Kaplan JA, Augoustides JGT, Manecke GR, et al., eds. Kaplan's Cardiac Anesthesia. 7th ed. Elsevier; 2017: 1291-1310.

2. Leyvi G, Rhew E, Crooke G, Wasnick JD. Transient right ventricular failure and transient weakness: a TEE diagnosis. J Cardiothorac Vasc Anesth, 2005; 19: 406-408.

5. Which transesophageal echocardiography view would be MOST helpful in monitoring for air embolization prior to weaning cardiopulmonary bypass?
  A. Midesophageal bicaval view (Omniplane: 90°–110°)
  B. Midesophageal long axis view (Omniplane: 120°–150°)
  C. Midesophageal right ventricular inflow/outflow view (Omniplane: 50°–70°)
  D. Transgastric mid-papillary short-axis view (Omniplane: 0°)

Correct Answer: B

Explanation: Cardiac deairing prior to weaning from cardiopulmonary bypass is important to prevent systemic air embolization (see table). Air embolization during or after cardiopulmonary bypass may be associated with neurologic injury, malignant arrhythmias, or cardiovascular collapse (in the event of intracoronary air embolism). Air can be detected during transesophageal echocardiography by mobile echobright areas with distal acoustic shadowing. The mid-esophageal long-axis view, imaging the left atrium, left ventricle (including the outflow tract), and aortic root, provides excellent imaging of multiple structures where air may accumulate. Additionally, this view provides real-time monitoring for active air egress during deairing.

The midesophageal bicaval and right ventricular inflow/outflow views predominantly image right-sided cardiac structures; air in these structures is frequently resorbed in the pulmonary tree and is rarely significant. The transgastric mid-papillary short-axis view detects segmental wall motion abnormalities due to territorial ischemia; it is less useful than the midesophageal long-axis view for detection of air accumulation.

TABLE 32.2

Final preparations for discontinuing cardiopulmonary bypass

Anesthesiologist's Preparations	Surgeon's Preparations
Level operating table	Remove macroscopic collections of air from the heart
Reset transducers to zero	Control major sites of bleeding
Activate monitors	Ensure CABG is lying nicely without kinks
Check drug infusions	Turn off or remove cardiac vents
Have resuscitation drugs and fluid volume at hand	Take clamps off the heart and great vessels
Reestablish TEE or PAC monitoring	Loosen tourniquets around caval cannulas

CABG, Coronary artery bypass graft; *PAC,* pulmonary artery catheter; *TEE,* transesophageal echocardiography.

References:

1. Nguyen L, Roth DM, Shanewise JS, Kaplan JA. Chapter 36: Discontinuing Cardiopulmonary Bypass. In: Kaplan JA, Augoustides JGT, Manecke GR, et al., eds. Kaplan's Cardiac Anesthesia. 7th ed. Elsevier; 2017: 1291-1310.
2. Reed H, Pal J, Lombaard S. Air in the left heart: a perilous situation in the presence of a left ventricular assist device. J Cardiothorac Vasc Anesth, 2016; 30: 1636-1638.

6. After completion of an uncomplicated mitral valve repair, the patient's underlying heart rhythm prior to weaning from cardiopulmonary bypass is bradycardia with first-degree atrioventricular block at 47 beats per minute. Which pacing strategy is likely to augment cardiac output the MOST?

A. AAI pacing at 90 beats per minute
B. DDD pacing at 90 beats per minute
C. DOO pacing at 90 beats per minute
D. VVI pacing at 90 beats per minute

Correct Answer: A

Explanation: Bradycardia after cardiopulmonary bypass (CPB) is common as the heart recovers from cardioplegia.

Ideally, cardiac contraction should have both atrial-ventricular synchronization and left ventricular–right ventricular synchronization. This is typically accomplished in normal sinus rhythm with native nodal conduction. This patient has underlying bradycardia, which may diminish cardiac output. AAI pacing provides electrical impulses to the atrium, which then travels down the atrioventricular node and His bundle fibers to enable native, synchronized ventricular contraction. AAI pacing thus most closely resembles normal sinus rhythm and is most likely to augment cardiac output.

DDD pacing provides pacing of both the atrium and ventricle in the event of a prolonged PR interval or first-degree atrioventricular block, which is common after CPB. DDD ventricular pacing results in right ventricular pacing with dyssynchronous right and left ventricular contraction, which likely would have a lower cardiac output compared to AAI pacing. DOO and VVI pacing similarly pace the right ventricle with associated ventricular dyssynchrony and lower cardiac output. Management of the cardiac rate and rhythm is part of preparing the heart for discontinuation of cardiopulmonary bypass (see table).

TABLE 32.3
Preparing the heart for discontinuing cardiopulmonary bypass

Hemodynamic Parameters	Preparation
Heart rate	Rate should be between 75 and 95 beats/min in most cases Treat slow rates with electrical pacing Treat underlying causes of fast heart rates Heart rate may decrease as the heart fills Control fast supraventricular rates with drugs, and then pace as needed Always have pacing immediately available during heart operations
Rhythm	Normal sinus rhythm is ideal Defibrillate if necessary when temperature >30°C Consider antiarrhythmic drugs if ventricular fibrillation persists more than a few minutes Try synchronized cardioversion for atrial fibrillation or flutter Look at the heart to diagnose atrial rhythm Try atrial pacing if atrioventricular conduction exists Try atrioventricular pacing for heart block
Preload	End-diastolic volume is the best measure of preload and can be seen with TEE Filling pressures provide a less direct measure of preload Consider baseline filling pressures Assess RV volume with direct inspection Assess LV volume with TEE Cardiac distention may cause MR and TR
Contractility	Carefully examine heart for air and employ deairing maneuvers Assess and quantify RV function with direct inspection and TEE Assess and quantify LV function with TEE Inspect for new regional wall motion abnormalities Inspect for new or worsening valvular abnormalities Quantify cardiac output by TEE or PAC Assess need for inotropic agent
Afterload	Systemic vascular resistance is a major component of afterload Keep MAP between 60 and 80 mmHg at full CPB flow Consider a vasoconstrictor if the MAP is low and a vasodilator if the MAP is high

CPB, Cardiopulmonary bypass; LV, left ventricular; MAP, mean arterial pressure; MR, mitral regurgitation; PAC, pulmonary artery catheter; RV, right ventricular; TEE, transesophageal echocardiography; TR, tricuspid regurgitation.

References:

1. Nguyen L, Roth DM, Shanewise JS, Kaplan JA. Chapter 36: Discontinuing Cardiopulmonary Bypass. In: Kaplan JA, Augoustides JGT, Manecke GR, et al., eds. Kaplan's Cardiac Anesthesia. 7th ed. Elsevier; 2017: 1291-1310.
2. Chua J, Schwarzenberger J, Mahajan A. Optimization of pacing after cardiopulmonary bypass. J Cardiothorac Vasc Anesth, 2012; 26: 291-301.

7. A patient with severe mitral regurgitation and atrial fibrillation undergoes an uncomplicated mitral valve repair, left atrial appendage amputation, and ablation procedure. While preparing to wean from cardiopulmonary bypass (CPB), the patient's native rhythm is currently atrial fibrillation at 147 beats per minute. Adequate depth of anesthesia is confirmed. Which therapy would MOST likely optimize cardiac output prior to weaning from CPB?
   A. Amiodarone bolus and infusion
   B. Esmolol bolus and infusion
   C. Repeat pulmonary vein isolation
   D. Synchronized direct current cardioversion

Correct Answer: D

Explanation: Although most ablation procedures are highly effective in reducing atrial fibrillation, they seldom immediately convert patients to normal sinus rhythm. In this case, with rapid atrial fibrillation, a synchronized direct current cardioversion is most likely to convert the patient to normal sinus rhythm to optimize cardiac contraction. If this intervention results in bradycardia, epicardial pacing wires can be used to optimize the heart rate.

Amiodarone and esmolol may reduce the heart rate and possibly result in conversion to normal sinus rhythm, but they both take longer than electrical cardioversion and may have negative inotropic properties on the recovering heart. Ablation procedures for atrial fibrillation typically require scar tissue formation over weeks to months to interrupt conduction pathways; thus, residual atrial fibrillation is common, and repeating pulmonary vein isolation is not indicated.

References:

1. Nguyen L, Roth DM, Shanewise JS, Kaplan JA. Chapter 36: Discontinuing Cardiopulmonary Bypass. In: Kaplan JA, Augoustides JGT, Manecke GR, et al., eds. Kaplan's Cardiac Anesthesia. 7th ed. Elsevier; 2017: 1291-1310.
2. Gorbaty BJ, Perelman S, Applebaum RM. Left atrial appendage thrombus formation after perioperative cardioversion in the setting of severe rheumatic mitral stenosis. J Cardiothorac Vasc Anesth, 2021; 35: 589-592.

8. Transesophageal echocardiography is MOST helpful to assess contractile function of which structure during weaning from cardiopulmonary bypass?
   A. Left atrium
   B. Left ventricle
   C. Right atrium
   D. Right ventricle

Correct Answer: B

Explanation: Transesophageal echocardiography (TEE) is a helpful tool to assess hemodynamic and filling parameters of cardiac chambers while weaning from cardiopulmonary bypass. Due to its posterior position, the left ventricle can be easily assessed with TEE, monitoring both its filling and function. TEE may be useful in assessing right ventricular function, but its utility is not as well demonstrated as assessing left ventricular function. Additionally, the right ventricle can be assessed by direct visual inspection on the surgical field, as well as with a pulmonary artery catheter. Despite being well visualized on TEE, left and right atrial contractile function are typically not as hemodynamically important when weaning from cardiopulmonary bypass.

References:

1. Nguyen L, Roth DM, Shanewise JS, Kaplan JA. Chapter 36: Discontinuing Cardiopulmonary Bypass. In: Kaplan JA, Augoustides JGT, Manecke GR, et al., eds. Kaplan's Cardiac Anesthesia. 7th ed. Elsevier; 2017: 1291-1310.
2. Monaco F, Di Prima AL, Kim JH, et al. Management of challenging cardiopulmonary bypass separation. J Cardiothorac Vasc Anesth, 2020; 34: 1622-1635.

9. Eleven minutes after aortic cross clamp removal following uncomplicated surgical mitral valve replacement, aortic valve replacement, and tricuspid valve repair, weaning from cardiopulmonary bypass is attempted. After weaning, the patient's blood pressure is 73/44 mmHg, and transesophageal echocardiography shows that the left ventricle is distended with poor contractile function, despite ongoing epinephrine and norepinephrine infusions. Which of the following is the MOST appropriate next step?
   A. Convert to central venoarterial extracorporeal membrane oxygenation
   B. Initiate cardiopulmonary bypass
   C. Place percutaneous left ventricular assist device
   D. Start milrinone infusion

Correct Answer: B

Explanation: Prolonged aortic cross clamp times and more extensive cardiac surgery are both risk factors to develop low cardiac output syndrome after cardiopulmonary bypass (CPB). In this case, attempting to wean from CPB 11 minutes after aortic cross clamp removal may not have enabled sufficient time for myocardial reperfusion and return of normal contractile function. Accordingly, a return to CPB may enable better reperfusion and restoration of contractile function, as well as possible addition of inotropic agents, if needed.

Milrinone, an inodilator, may be useful in right ventricular dysfunction, but may exacerbate hypotension in this case. A return to CPB with a trial of longer reperfusion time is more appropriate. Mechanical circulatory support such as a percutaneous left ventricular assist device or extracorporeal membrane oxygenation may be required, but only after additional weaning attempts and further pharmacologic therapy have failed.

References:

1. Nguyen L, Roth DM, Shanewise JS, Kaplan JA. Chapter 36: Discontinuing Cardiopulmonary Bypass. In: Kaplan JA, Augoustides JGT, Manecke GR, et al., eds. Kaplan's Cardiac Anesthesia. 7th ed. Elsevier; 2017: 1291-1310.
2. Monaco F, Di Prima AL, Kim JH, et al. Management of challenging cardiopulmonary bypass separation. J Cardiothorac Vasc Anesth, 2020; 34: 1622-1635.

10. Which condition MOST likely warrants a slower weaning/transition from cardiopulmonary bypass?
    A. Aortic valve replacement for severe aortic stenosis
    B. Five-vessel coronary artery bypass grafting for coronary artery disease
    C. Prebypass right ventricular fractional area of change of 37%
    D. Prebypass left ventricular ejection fraction of 21%

Correct Answer: D

Explanation: Weaning from cardiopulmonary bypass (CPB) is always challenging; however, pre-existing patient factors may portend to additional difficulties. Patients with pre-existing low left ventricular ejection fraction may poorly tolerate ischemic

TABLE 32.4

Summary of factors associated with the use of inotropic drug support or low cardiac output syndrome

Variable	Odds Ratio
Age (>60 years)	4.3
Aortic cross clamp time >90 min	2.32
Bypass time (min)	3.40
CABG + MVR	3.607
Cardiac index <2.5 L/m²/min	3.10
CHF (NYHA class >II)	1.85
CKD (stage 3–5; GFR <60 mL/1.73 m²/min	3.26
COPD	1.85
Diastolic dysfunction	4.31
Ejection fraction (%) <40	2.76
Emergency operation	9.15
Female sex	2.0
LVEDP >20 mmHg	3.58
Myocardial infarction	2.01
Moderate to severe mitral regurgitation	2.277
Regional wall motion abnormality	4.21
Repeat operation	2.38

CABG, Coronary artery bypass graft; *CHF*, congestive heart failure; *CKD*, chronic kidney disease; *COPD*, chronic obstructive pulmonary disease; *GFR*, glomerular filtration rate; *LVEDP*, left ventricular end-diastolic pressure; *MVR*, mitral valve repair or replacement; *NYHA*, New York Heart Association.

time, and therefore require additional time for reperfusion and medication titration (see table). Slowly weaning CPB enables real-time assessment of ventricular function, adjustment, and titration of intravascular volume and vasoactive medications to optimize the success of separation.

A right ventricular fractional area of change (FAC) of 37% is normal (normal FAC >35%). Patients undergoing aortic valve replacement would be predicted to have an easier time separating from CPB because the surgery removes a fixed obstruction to cardiac output. Although coronary artery disease may impair separation efforts from CPB, it is not a major significant risk factor compared to left ventricular systolic dysfunction.

References:

1. Nguyen L, Roth DM, Shanewise JS, Kaplan JA. Chapter 36: Discontinuing Cardiopulmonary Bypass. In: Kaplan JA, Augoustides JGT, Manecke GR, et al., eds. Kaplan's Cardiac Anesthesia. 7th ed. Elsevier; 2017: 1291-1310.
2. Monaco F, Di Prima AL, Kim JH, et al. Management of challenging cardiopulmonary bypass separation. J Cardiothorac Vasc Anesth, 2020; 34: 1622-1635.

11. Which action will START the process of weaning from cardiopulmonary bypass?
    A. Infusion of warm blood through the aortic root vent
    B. Occlusion of arterial outflow line
    C. Occlusion of venous drainage line
    D. Reducing cardiopulmonary bypass flows

Correct Answer: C

Explanation: Weaning from cardiopulmonary bypass (CPB) is a step-wise process. The first step is partial occlusion of the venous drainage line; this results in some blood remaining in the heart and circulating via endogenous circulation. As blood remains in the body and less blood is drained, the venous reservoir level begins to fall. Accordingly, CPB flows are reduced to prevent venous reservoir depletion. The process is repeated iteratively until the venous drainage line is fully occluded, the CPB flows are stopped, and the patient is "off" bypass.

The arterial outflow cannula is not typically occluded during CPB weaning. Infusion of warm blood through the aortic root vent may help remove residual cardioplegia if the aortic cross clamp is on; however, this process does not aid in the actual weaning process from CPB.

References:

1. Nguyen L, Roth DM, Shanewise JS, Kaplan JA. Chapter 36: Discontinuing Cardiopulmonary Bypass. In: Kaplan JA, Augoustides JGT, Manecke GR, et al., eds. Kaplan's Cardiac Anesthesia. 7th ed. Elsevier; 2017: 1291-1310.
2. Hessel EA. What's new in cardiopulmonary bypass. J Cardiothorac Vasc Anesth, 2019; 33: 2296-2326.

12. Immediately after cessation of cardiopulmonary bypass following uncomplicated ascending aorta replacement for a thoracic aortic aneurysm, the patient's blood pressure is

82/41 mmHg. Transesophageal echocardiography reveals normal biventricular function and no valvular abnormalities. The last hemoglobin was 8.9 g/dL. Which action is MOST appropriate at this time?

A. Administer epinephrine bolus

B. Infuse blood via the arterial cannula

C. Initiate norepinephrine infusion

D. Transfuse packed red blood cells via fluid warmer

Correct Answer: B

Explanation: Immediately after cessation of cardiopulmonary bypass (CPB), the venous drainage line is drained into the cardiotomy reservoir, typically resulting in 400 to 800 mL of available autologous blood for transfusion. In patients with normal biventricular function, the most reasonable initial course of action would be gradual reinfusion of this autologous blood and assessment of the patient's volume responsiveness. Typically, this autologous blood reinfusion will resolve hypotension related to volume depletion from autologous blood in the CPB reservoir.

Transfusion of packed red blood cells may be necessary, but initial management with infusion of autologous blood via the arterial cannula may resolve hypotension and anemia without allogeneic transfusion. Administration of vasoactive medication may be necessary if volume resuscitation does not resolve hypotension and vasoplegia is suspected. In a patient with normal biventricular function, autotransfusion of reservoir blood volume is a better choice to address hypovolemia than addition of inotropes such as epinephrine.

References:

1. Nguyen L, Roth DM, Shanewise JS, Kaplan JA. Chapter 36: Discontinuing Cardiopulmonary Bypass. In: Kaplan JA, Augoustides JGT, Manecke GR, et al., eds. Kaplan's Cardiac Anesthesia. 7th ed. Elsevier; 2017: 1291-1310.

2. Monaco F, Di Prima AL, Kim JH, et al. Management of challenging cardiopulmonary bypass separation. J Cardiothorac Vasc Anesth, 2020; 34: 1622-1635.

13. What is the MOST appropriate systolic blood pressure goal for aortic decannulation?

A. 70 mmHg

B. 90 mmHg

C. 110 mmHg

D. 130 mmHg

Correct Answer: B

Explanation: Blood pressure management prior to aortic decannulation is important to maintain adequate systemic perfusion while simultaneously minimizing the risk of iatrogenic aortic dissection when the aortic cannula is removed. A lower systolic blood pressure may be helpful in preventing aortic dissection on decannulation. A systolic blood pressure of 90 mmHg is likely a suitable short-term blood pressure goal to balance minimizing shear force in the aorta while also enabling systemic perfusion. A systolic blood pressure of 70 mmHg is likely insufficient for systemic

perfusion. Blood pressures of 110 or 130 mmHg have higher shear forces, and thus higher risk of aortic dissection on decannulation.

References:

1. Nguyen L, Roth DM, Shanewise JS, Kaplan JA. Chapter 36: Discontinuing Cardiopulmonary Bypass. In: Kaplan JA, Augoustides JGT, Manecke GR, et al., eds. Kaplan's Cardiac Anesthesia. 7th ed. Elsevier; 2017: 1291-1310.

2. Ram H, Dwarakanath S, Green AE, et al. Iatrogenic aortic dissection associated with cardiac surgery: a narrative review. J Cardiothorac Vasc Anesth, 2021; 35: 3050-3066.

14. After initiation of cardiopulmonary bypass (CPB), you elect to continue lung protective, positive-pressure ventilation instead of apnea. Compared to patients with apnea on CPB, patients with ongoing ventilation during CPB are MOST likely to experience which long-term outcome?

A. Longer duration of hospital length of stay

B. Lower odds of acute lung injury

C. No difference in the duration of mechanical ventilation

D. Shorter duration of intensive care unit length of stay

Correct Answer: C

Explanation: Cardiopulmonary bypass (CPB) and cardiac surgery may be associated with significant pulmonary morbidity and postoperative pulmonary complications. Consequently, efforts to reduce these complications are active areas of research. Because prolonged apnea and atelectasis were hypothesized to be one mechanism underlying pulmonary morbidity, one strategy attempting to mitigate this is continuing ventilation during CPB. Despite promise, this intervention has not been associated with any improvement in long-term pulmonary outcomes. In multiple meta-analyses of different ventilation techniques while on CPB, ventilation on CPB may be associated with small, short-term improvements in hypoxemia immediately postoperatively. However, there have been no differences in long-term clinical outcomes, such as the rates of postoperative pulmonary complications, duration of mechanical ventilation, acute lung injury, or intensive care unit or hospital lengths of stay.

References:

1. Nguyen L, Roth DM, Shanewise JS, Kaplan JA. Chapter 36: Discontinuing Cardiopulmonary Bypass. In: Kaplan JA, Augoustides JGT, Manecke GR, et al., eds. Kaplan's Cardiac Anesthesia. 7th ed. Elsevier; 2017: 1291-1310.

2. Hessel EA. What's new in cardiopulmonary bypass. J Cardiothorac Vasc Anesth, 2019; 33: 2296-2326.

15. A patient with coronary artery disease, previous stroke with no residual neurologic deficits, end-stage renal disease, and chronic systolic heart failure (left ventricular ejection fraction of 19%) undergoes a four-vessel coronary artery bypass graft and mitral valve

replacement surgery. You are preparing to initiate vasoactive medications before weaning cardiopulmonary bypass. Which medication is MOST likely to be relatively contraindicated?

A. Dobutamine
B. Epinephrine
C. Milrinone
D. Vasopressin

Correct Answer: C

Explanation: Patients with low left ventricular ejection fraction, as well as those undergoing combined coronary artery bypass grafting and mitral valve intervention, are at high risk of postoperative low cardiac output syndrome (see box). Administration of inotropes prior to weaning from cardiopulmonary bypass (CPB) is important to enable a safe transition off CPB. Milrinone, an inodilator, is almost entirely eliminated by renal excretion. In patients with end-stage kidney disease, the elimination half-life and associated systemic vasodilation of milrinone can be profoundly extended, making it less than ideal in this setting. Dobutamine, a selective β₁-agonist, has been shown to achieve similar clinical outcomes as milrinone, and is metabolized independent of renal excretion. Dobutamine, epinephrine, and vasopressin do not require dosing adjustments in patients with end-stage renal disease.

References:

1. Nguyen L, Roth DM, Shanewise JS, Kaplan JA. Chapter 36: Discontinuing Cardiopulmonary Bypass. In: Kaplan JA, Augoustides JGT, Manecke GR, et al., eds. Kaplan's Cardiac Anesthesia. 7th ed. Elsevier; 2017: 1291-1310.
2. Feneck RO, Sherry KM, Withington PS, et al. European Milrinone Multicenter Trial Group. Comparison of the hemodynamic effects of milrinone with dobutamine in patients after cardiac surgery. J Cardiothorac Vasc Anesth, 2001; 15: 306-315.

> BOX 32.2　**Risk factors for low cardiac output syndrome after cardiopulmonary bypass**
>
> - Preoperative ventricular dysfunction
> - Myocardial ischemia
> - Poor myocardial preservation
> - Reperfusion injury
> - Inadequate cardiac surgical repair or revascularization

16. In a randomized trial assigning patients in shock to receive either norepinephrine or dopamine, patients with cardiogenic shock who received dopamine (compared to norepinephrine) were MOST likely to experience:

A. Higher odds of mortality
B. Lower odds of acute kidney injury
C. Fewer days requiring vasopressors
D. Longer intensive care unit length of stay

Correct Answer: A

Explanation: In a clinical trial randomizing patients in shock to receive either norepinephrine or dopamine, the investigators found no overall differences in their composite primary outcome across the entire study cohort. However, in prespecified subgroup analysis, the investigators found a higher risk of mortality in patients with cardiogenic shock receiving a dopamine infusion compared to those receiving norepinephrine infusion. This effect was not present in patients with either septic or hypovolemic shock. Additionally, the researchers found higher rates of tachyarrhythmias in the dopamine group (see table). Patients in the dopamine and norepinephrine groups had no difference in rates of acute kidney injury, nor in the intensive care unit length of stay. Patients receiving dopamine have significantly more days receiving vasopressors compared to patients receiving norepinephrine.

References:

1. Nguyen L, Roth DM, Shanewise JS, Kaplan JA. Chapter 36: Discontinuing Cardiopulmonary Bypass. In: Kaplan JA, Augoustides JGT, Manecke GR, et al., eds. Kaplan's Cardiac Anesthesia. 7th ed. Elsevier; 2017: 1291-1310.

TABLE 32.5

Sympathomimetic agents

Drug	Dosage		Site of Action		Mechanism of Action
	Intravenous Bolus	Infusion	α	β	
Dobutamine	—	2–20 µg/kg/min	+	++++	Direct
Dopamine	—	1–10 µg/kg/min	++	+++	Direct and indirect
Epinephrine	2–16 µg	2–10 µg/min Or 0.01–0.4 µg/kg/min	+++	+++	Direct
Ephedrine	5–25 mg	—	+	++	Direct and indirect
Isoproterenol	1–4 µg	0.5–10 µg/min Or 0.01–0.10 µg/kg/min		++++	Direct
Norepinephrine	—	2–16 µg/min Or 0.01–0.3 µg/kg/min	++++	+++	Direct

2. De Backer D, Biston P, Devriendt J, et al. Comparison of dopamine and norepinephrine in the treatment of shock. N Engl J Med, 2010; 362: 779-789.
3. Guarracino F, Habicher M, Treskatsch S, et al. Vasopressor therapy in cardiac surgery-an experts' consensus statement. J Cardiothorac Vasc Anesth, 2021; 35: 1018-1029.

17. In the recent Levosimendan in Patients with Left Ventricular Systolic Dysfunction Undergoing Cardiac Surgery Requiring Cardiopulmonary Bypass (LEVO-CTS) trial, patients with a left ventricular ejection fraction less than 35% undergoing cardiac surgery were randomly assigned to receive either prophylactic levosimendan or placebo prior to skin incision. Compared to placebo, patients in the levosimendan group were MOST likely to experience which of the following?
    A. Higher rates of renal replacement therapy at 30 days
    B. Lower rates of death at 30 days
    C. No significant difference in rates of mechanical assist devices at 5 days
    D. No significant difference in rates of low cardiac output syndrome

Correct Answer: C

Explanation: Levosimendan, a calcium sensitizer, had been hypothesized to achieve superior outcomes in patients with a low ejection fraction undergoing cardiac surgery (see table). Testing this hypothesis, the recent Levosimendan in Patients with Left Ventricular Systolic Dysfunction Undergoing Cardiac Surgery Requiring Cardiopulmonary Bypass (LEVO-CTS) trial randomized patients with a left ventricular ejection fraction less than 35% undergoing cardiac surgery to receive either pre-emptive levosimendan or placebo. The investigators found no significant difference between the groups in composite outcomes including death, renal replacement therapy, myocardial infarction, and/or use of a

mechanical assist device. Furthermore, there was no significant difference between groups in any of these individual end points, nor in the vast majority of other secondary end points.

Interestingly, patients in the levosimendan group did have significantly lower risk of low cardiac output syndrome, as well as lower rates of inotropic infusion past 24 hours. Despite these findings, there were no other significant differences in clinically important end points between the groups.

References:

1. Nguyen L, Roth DM, Shanewise JS, Kaplan JA. Chapter 36: Discontinuing Cardiopulmonary Bypass. In: Kaplan JA, Augoustides JGT, Manecke GR, et al., eds. Kaplan's Cardiac Anesthesia. 7th ed. Elsevier; 2017: 1291-1310.
2. Mehta RH, Leimberger JD, van Diepen S, et al. Levosimendan in patients with left ventricular dysfunction undergoing cardiac surgery. N Engl J Med, 2017; 376: 2032-2042.
3. Faisal SA, Apatov DA, Ramakrishna H, et al. Levosimendan in cardiac surgery: evaluating the evidence. J Cardiothorac Vasc Anesth, 2019; 33: 1146-1158.

18. In a set of clinical trials randomizing patients undergoing cardiac surgery to receive intraoperative clevidipine, nitroglycerin, or sodium nitroprusside, what is MOST likely to be a true statement regarding time in goal systolic blood pressure range?
    A. Patients receiving clevidipine had significantly more time within goal ranges compared to those receiving nitroglycerin or sodium nitroprusside
    B. Patients receiving nitroglycerin had significantly more time within goal ranges compared to those receiving clevidipine or sodium nitroprusside
    C. Patients receiving sodium nitroprusside had significantly more time within goal ranges compared to those receiving clevidipine or nitroglycerin

D. Patients receiving clevidipine, nitroglycerin, or sodium nitroprusside did not have significantly different times with systolic blood pressure in goal ranges

Correct Answer: A

Explanation: Clevidipine, a short-acting calcium channel blocker, was developed for management of acute hypertension. In the set of Evaluation of Clevidipine In the Perioperative Treatment of Hypertension Assessing Safety Events (ECLIPSE) trials, patients undergoing cardiac surgery were randomized to receive intraoperative clevidipine, nitroglycerin, or sodium nitroprusside. In this evaluation, patients receiving clevidipine had significantly greater time with the systolic blood pressure in the target range compared to those receiving nitroglycerin or sodium nitroprusside. These findings were replicated in a series of subgroup and sensitivity analyses. Additionally, there were no significant differences in the occurrences of safety events between groups.

References:

1. Nguyen L, Roth DM, Shanewise JS, Kaplan JA. Chapter 36: Discontinuing Cardiopulmonary Bypass. In: Kaplan JA, Augoustides JGT, Manecke GR, et al., eds. Kaplan's Cardiac Anesthesia. 7th ed. Elsevier; 2017: 1291-1310.
2. Aronson S, Dyke CM, Stierer KA, et al. The ECLIPSE trials: comparative studies of clevidipine to nitroglycerin, sodium nitroprusside, and nicardipine for acute hypertension treatment in cardiac surgery patients. Anesth Analg, 2008; 107: 1110-1121.
3. Aronson S, Levy JH, Lumb PD, et al. Impact of perioperative blood pressure variability on health resource utilization after cardiac surgery: an analysis of the ECLIPSE trials. J Cardiothorac Vasc Anesth, 2014; 28: 579-585.

19. A patient presents for coronary artery bypass grafting; his preadmission medication list includes aspirin, atorvastatin, empagliflozin, fluoxetine, lisinopril, metoprolol succinate, and varenicline. After cardiopulmonary bypass, the patient develops hypotension with supraphysiologic cardiac output, despite norepinephrine, epinephrine, and vasopressin infusions. Vasoplegic syndrome is the presumptive diagnosis. When considering methylene blue administration, which medication represents a CONTRAINDICATION in this patient?
   A. Atorvastatin
   B. Empagliflozin
   C. Fluoxetine
   D. Lisinopril

Correct Answer: C

Explanation: The vasoplegic syndrome after cardiopulmonary bypass is a state of normal or elevated cardiac output with low systemic vascular resistance, resulting in systemic hypotension. First-line therapies for severe vasoplegia include vasoactive medications, such as norepinephrine and vasopressin. If systemic hypotension persists, methylene blue is an appropriate additional agent. Methylene blue scavenges

nitric oxide, resulting in vasoconstriction, increased systemic vascular resistance, and increased blood pressure. Methylene blue is also a potent monoamine oxidase inhibitor. When administered to patients receiving selective serotonin reuptake inhibitors such as fluoxetine, methylene blue may trigger serotonin syndrome, a serious and dangerous condition due to excessive serotonin accumulation. Methylene blue is also contraindicated in patients taking monoamine oxidase inhibitors and the antibiotic linezolid, which is also a selective serotonin reuptake inhibitor. Statins (atorvastatin), sodium-glucose transporter 2 inhibitors (empagliflozin), and angiotensin-converting enzyme inhibitors (lisinopril) do not have known interactions with methylene blue.

References:

1. Nguyen L, Roth DM, Shanewise JS, Kaplan JA. Chapter 36: Discontinuing Cardiopulmonary Bypass. In: Kaplan JA, Augoustides JGT, Manecke GR, et al., eds. Kaplan's Cardiac Anesthesia. 7th ed. Elsevier; 2017: 1291-1310.
2. Shaefi S, Mittel A, Klick J, et al. Vasoplegia after cardiovascular procedures-pathophysiology and targeted therapy. J Cardiothorac Vasc Anesth, 2018; 32: 1013-1022.

20. According to the recent double-blind, randomized controlled Vasopressin versus Norepinephrine in Patients with Vasoplegic Shock after Cardiac Surgery (VANCS) trial, patients who received vasopressin (compared to norepinephrine) as first-line therapy for treatment of distributive shock after cardiac surgery were MOST likely to experience which of the following?
   A. Lower odds of 30-day mortality
   B. Lower odds of acute renal failure
   C. Higher odds of mesenteric ischemia
   D. No significant difference in odds of atrial fibrillation

Correct Answer: B

Explanation: Vasopressin is a potent vasoconstrictor acting through a catecholamine receptor–independent mechanism. The Vasopressin versus Norepinephrine in Patients with Vasoplegic Shock after Cardiac Surgery (VANCS) trial randomized patients with vasoplegic shock after cardiac surgery to receive either vasopressin (0.01–0.06 units/min) or norepinephrine as first-line therapy. The investigators found that patients in the vasopressin group had significantly lower odds of a composite end point including 30-day mortality, mechanical ventilation >48 hours, surgical site infection, reoperation, stroke, and/or acute renal failure. This finding was entirely driven by the acute renal failure end point (10% in the vasopressin group vs. 36% in the norepinephrine group, $P < .001$). There was no significant difference in the other five primary co-end points. Furthermore, patients in the vasopressin group had significantly lower odds of atrial fibrillation, as well as shorter length of stay, both in the intensive care unit and the hospital. These results suggest that vasopressin may be a useful first-line therapy for vasoplegic syndrome after cardiac surgery.

References:

1. Nguyen L, Roth DM, Shanewise JS, Kaplan JA. Chapter 36: Discontinuing Cardiopulmonary Bypass. In: Kaplan JA, Augoustides JGT, Manecke GR, et al., eds. Kaplan's Cardiac Anesthesia. 7th ed. Elsevier; 2017: 1291-1310.
2. Hajjar LA, Vincent JL, Barbosa Gomes Galas FR, et al. Vasopressin versus Norepinephrine in Patients with Vasoplegic Shock after Cardiac Surgery: The VANCS randomized controlled trial. Anesthesiology, 2017; 126: 85-93.
3. Shaefi S, Mittel A, Klick J, et al. Vasoplegia after cardiovascular procedures-pathophysiology and targeted therapy. J Cardiothorac Vasc Anesth, 2018; 32: 1013-1022.

21. According to the Nesiritide Administered Peri-Anesthesia in Patients Undergoing Cardiac Surgery (NAPA) trial, patients with a left ventricular ejection fraction less than 40% undergoing coronary artery bypass grafting who received nesiritide (compared to placebo) were MOST likely to experience which of the following?
  A. Lower odds of 180-day mortality
  B. Higher odds of acute renal failure
  C. Higher odds of postoperative hypotension
  D. No significant difference in hospital length of stay

Correct Answer: A

Explanation: Nesiritide, a natriuretic peptide analog of human brain natriuretic peptide, may have a role in improving natriuresis and renal function in cardiac surgery. In the Nesiritide Administered Peri-Anesthesia in Patients Undergoing Cardiac Surgery (NAPA) trial, patients who received nesiritide (compared to placebo) had reduced rates of renal decline, better glomerular filtration rates, shorter hospital length of stay, and lower odds of mortality at 180 days. Furthermore, patients receiving nesiritide (compared to placebo) did not have significant differences in the number of vasoactive infusions required, nor in their postoperative systemic blood pressure. Although these findings suggest that nesiritide or other natriuretic peptide analogs may improve outcomes in cardiac surgery, further studies are needed to validate these conclusions.

References:

1. Nguyen L, Roth DM, Shanewise JS, Kaplan JA. Chapter 36: Discontinuing Cardiopulmonary Bypass. In: Kaplan JA, Augoustides JGT, Manecke GR, et al., eds. Kaplan's Cardiac Anesthesia. 7th ed. Elsevier; 2017: 1291-1310.

2. Krichevskiy LA, Kozlov IA. Natriuretic peptides in cardiac anesthesia and intensive care. J Cardiothorac Vasc Anesth, 2019; 33: 1407-1419.

22. In the recent Dobutamine Compared with Milrinone in the Treatment of Cardiogenic Shock (DOREMI) trial, patients with cardiogenic shock were randomized to receive inotropic support with milrinone or dobutamine. Patients in the milrinone group (compared to those receiving dobutamine) were MOST likely to experience:
  A. Higher odds of requiring renal replacement therapy
  B. Lower odds of nonfatal myocardial infarction
  C. Lower odds of cardiac arrest
  D. No significant difference in the odds of in-hospital mortality

Correct Answer: D

Explanation: Patients in cardiogenic shock often require inotropic support. "Inodilator agents," such as dobutamine and milrinone, may be helpful as they increase cardiac contractility while also reducing systemic vascular resistance (see table 32.5). In the Dobutamine Compared with Milrinone in the Treatment of Cardiogenic Shock (DOREMI) trial, patients in cardiogenic shock requiring inotropic support were randomly assigned to receive either milrinone or dobutamine. The primary trial outcome was a composite of in-hospital mortality, cardiac arrest, cardiac transplant, mechanical circulatory support, myocardial infarction, stroke, or new initiation of dialysis. There was no significant difference between the two groups in the composite primary end point. Furthermore, there was no significant difference in any of the individual end points between the two groups, nor in the primary composite outcome for any specific patient subgroups. While the generalizability of this specific trial to postcardiotomy shock is unknown, additional studies have also found no significant hemodynamic differences between dobutamine or milrinone in cardiac surgery.

References:

1. Nguyen L, Roth DM, Shanewise JS, Kaplan JA. Chapter 36: Discontinuing Cardiopulmonary Bypass. In: Kaplan JA, Augoustides JGT, Manecke GR, et al., eds. Kaplan's Cardiac Anesthesia. 7th ed. Elsevier; 2017: 1291-1310.

TABLE 32.6

Hemodynamic effects of inotropes

Drug	CO	dP/dt	HR	SVR	PVR	PCWP	M_{VO_2}
Dobutamine							
2–20 µg/kg per min[a]	↑↑↑	↑	↑↑	↓	↓	↓ or ↔	↑
Dopamine							
0–3 µg/kg per min	↑	↑	↑	↓	↓	↑	↑
3–10 µg/kg per min	↑↑	↑	↑	↓	↓	↑	↑
>10 µg/kg per min	↑↑	↑	↑↑	↑	(↑)	↑ or	↑↑
Isoproterenol							
0.5–10 µg/min	↑↑	↑↑	↑↑	↓↓	↓	↓	↑↑
Epinephrine							
0.01–0.4 µg/kg/min	↑↑	↑	↑	↑ (↓)	(↑)	↑ or ↔	↑↑
Norepinephrine							
0.01–0.3 µg/kg/min	↑	↑	↔ (↑↓)	↑↑	↔	↔	↑
Phosphodiesterase inhibitors[b]	↑↑	↑	↑	↓↓	↓↓	↓↓	↓
Levosimendan[c]	↑↑↑	↑↑	↑	↓↓	↓↓	↓↓	↓ or ↔

[a]The indicated dosages represent the most common dosage ranges. For the individual patient, a deviation from these recommended doses may be indicated.
[b]Phosphodiesterase inhibitors are usually given as a loading dose followed by a continuous infusion: amrinone: 0.5–1.5 mg/kg loading dose, 5–10 µg/kg per minute continuous infusion; milrinone: 50 µg/kg loading dose, 0.375–0.75 µg/kg per minute continuous infusion.
[c]Levosimendan is usually administered as a loading dose followed by an infusion for 24 hours: 8–24 µg/kg loading dose, 0.1–0.2 µg/kg per minute (Toller W, Heringlake M, Guarracino F, et al. Preoperative and perioperative use of levosimendan in cardiac surgery: European expert opinion. Int J Cardiol, 2015; 184: 323-336).
CO, Cardiac output; dP/dt, myocardial contractility; HR, heart rate; M_{VO_2}, myocardial oxygen consumption; PCWP, pulmonary capillary wedge pressure; PVR, pulmonary vascular resistance; SVR, systemic vascular resistance; ↑, mild increase; ↑↑, moderate increase; ↑↑↑, major increase; ↔, no change; ↓, mild decrease; ↓↓, moderate decrease.
Modified from Lehmann A, Boldt J. New pharmacologic approaches for the perioperative treatment of ischemic cardiogenic shock. J Cardiothorac Vasc Anesth, 2005; 19: 97-108.

2. Mathew R, Di Santo P, Jung RG, et al. Milrinone as compared with dobutamine in the treatment of cardiogenic shock. N Engl J Med, 2021; 385: 516-525.

3. Feneck RO, Sherry KM, Withington PS, et al. Comparison of the hemodynamic effects of milrinone with dobutamine in patients after cardiac surgery. J Cardiothorac Vasc Anesth, 2001; 15: 306-315.

23. Of the following outcomes, perioperative magnesium administration during cardiac surgery is MOST likely to be associated with:

   A. Higher odds of sinus bradycardia
   B. Longer duration of mechanical ventilation
   C. Lower odds of atrial fibrillation
   D. Lower odds of mortality

Correct Answer: C

Explanation: Magnesium, a divalent cation, has been associated with lower rates of postoperative atrial fibrillation after cardiac surgery when administered in the perioperative period. While individual study results have been heterogeneous, a recent systematic review and meta-analysis suggests an association of magnesium with lower rates of atrial fibrillation and ventricular arrhythmias. The optimal magnesium administration regimen—bolus, infusion, or bolus and infusion—has not been delineated.

Magnesium theoretically may be associated with hypotension due to systemic vasodilation and, at higher doses, muscle weaknesses. According to a recent systematic review, magnesium is not associated with sinus bradycardia, nor is it associated with mortality or longer duration of mechanical ventilation in cardiac surgery.

References:

1. Nguyen L, Roth DM, Shanewise JS, Kaplan JA. Chapter 36: Discontinuing Cardiopulmonary Bypass. In: Kaplan JA, Augoustides JGT, Manecke GR, et al., eds. Kaplan's Cardiac Anesthesia. 7th ed. Elsevier; 2017: 1291-1310.

2. Fairley JL, Zhang L, Glassford NJ, et al. Magnesium status and magnesium therapy in cardiac surgery: A systematic review and meta-analysis focusing on arrhythmia prevention. J Crit Care, 2017; 42: 69-77.

3. Osawa EA, Cutuli SL, Cioccari L, et al. Continuous magnesium infusion to prevent atrial fibrillation after cardiac surgery: a sequential matched case-controlled pilot study. J Cardiothorac Vasc Anesth, 2020; 34: 2940-2947.

24. Compared to milrinone, a patient receiving epinephrine is MOST likely to experience:

   A. Significantly higher cardiac output
   B. Significantly higher contractility (dP/dt)
   C. Significantly higher systemic vascular resistance
   D. Significantly higher heart rate

Correct Answer: C

Explanation: Epinephrine and milrinone are both inotropic agents aimed to increase cardiac output, and are often used in cardiogenic shock states. Epinephrine, with its mixed α- and β-adrenergic receptor activity, increases both cardiac output via β-adrenergic receptor and systemic vascular resistance via α-adrenergic receptors at higher doses. Milrinone, a phosphodiesterase inhibitor, blocks the degradation of cyclic adenosine monophosphate, in turn enhancing endogenous β-adrenergic receptor signaling. This results in increased contractility and cardiac output, as well as a significant decrease in systemic vascular resistance. Systemic hypotension is one of the known side effects of milrinone, and a key difference from epinephrine. Both milrinone and epinephrine increase cardiac output, contractility, and heart rate. Although their effects are fairly similar for each of these parameters, the crucial difference between these medications is that epinephrine will increase systemic vascular resistance via α agonism, whereas milrinone potentiates β-adrenergic signaling, with a resultant reduction in systemic vascular resistance.

References:

1. Nguyen L, Roth DM, Shanewise JS, Kaplan JA. Chapter 36: Discontinuing Cardiopulmonary Bypass. In: Kaplan JA, Augoustides JGT, Manecke GR, et al., eds. Kaplan's Cardiac Anesthesia. 7th ed. Elsevier; 2017: 1291-1310.
2. Yamada T, Takeda J, Katori N, et al. Hemodynamic effects of milrinone during weaning from cardiopulmonary bypass: comparison of patients with a low and high prebypass cardiac index. J Cardiothorac Vasc Anesth, 2000; 14: 367-373.
3. Guarracino F, Habicher M, Treskatsch S, et al. Vasopressor therapy in cardiac surgery-an experts' consensus statement. J Cardiothorac Vasc Anesth, 2021; 35: 1018-1029.

25. After completion of tricuspid valve repair and mitral valve repair, a patient is weaned from cardiopulmonary bypass. The blood pressure is 76/42 mmHg, and there is suggestion of right ventricular volume and pressure overload by transesophageal echocardiography. What would be the STRONGEST contraindication to inhaled nitric oxide therapy?
    A. Hyperdynamic left ventricular function
    B. Mitral valve mean pressure gradient of 4 mmHg
    C. Moderate residual tricuspid regurgitation
    D. Pulmonary capillary wedge pressure of 29 mmHg

Correct Answer: D

Explanation: Inhaled nitric oxide (iNO), a pulmonary vasodilator, may be useful in the setting of right ventricular failure to reduce pulmonary vascular resistance. An important contraindication for iNO therapy is if right heart failure is due to pulmonary hypertension from left heart failure. If pulmonary pressures are elevated due to high pulmonary venous and capillary pressures, inhaled pulmonary vasodilators would send additional flow to these overfilled vascular beds, resulting in pulmonary edema. Accordingly, iNO is not recommended in patients with pulmonary hypertension from left-sided heart failure, as suggested by a high pulmonary capillary wedge pressure. Hyperdynamic left ventricular function suggests a possible benefit to iNO to increase blood delivery to the left ventricle. Tricuspid regurgitation may be due to right heart failure, and thus could improve with iNO therapy; it is not a contraindication by itself. A mitral valve mean pressure gradient of 4 mmHg after repair is a normal finding (goal <5 mmHg).

References:

1. Nguyen L, Roth DM, Shanewise JS, Kaplan JA. Chapter 36: Discontinuing Cardiopulmonary Bypass. In: Kaplan JA, Augoustides JGT, Manecke GR, et al., eds. Kaplan's Cardiac Anesthesia. 7th ed. Elsevier; 2017: 1291-1310.
2. Vachiéry JL, Tedford RJ, Rosenkranz S, et al. Pulmonary hypertension due to left heart disease. Eur Respir J, 2019; 53: 1801897.

26. What MOST likely represents a contraindication to placement of an intra-aortic balloon pump?
    A. Large ventricular septal defect
    B. Patent ductus arteriosus
    C. Severe aortic regurgitation
    D. Stroke within the past 30 days

Correct Answer: C

Explanation: Intra-aortic balloon counterpulsation via a balloon pump may reduce left ventricular afterload, decrease myocardial work and oxygen demand, enhance diastolic coronary perfusion, and increase forward perfusion (see table). An important contraindication to this device is the presence of severe aortic regurgitation. In severe aortic

TABLE 32.7
Intra-aortic balloon pump counterpulsation indications and contraindications

Indications	Contraindications

1. Cardiogenic shock
  a. Myocardial infarction
  b. Myocarditis
  c. Cardiomyopathy
2. Failure to separate from CPB
3. Stabilization of preoperative patient
  a. Ventricular septal defect
  b. Mitral regurgitation
4. Stabilization of noncardiac surgical patient
5. Procedural support during coronary angiography
6. Bridge to transplantation
	1. Aortic valvular insufficiency
	2. Aortic disease
	  a. Aortic dissection
	  b. Aortic aneurysm
	3. Severe peripheral vascular disease
	4. Severe noncardiac systemic disease
	5. Massive trauma
	6. Patients with "do not resuscitate" instructions
	7. Mitral SAM with dynamic outflow tract obstruction

CPB, Cardiopulmonary bypass; *SAM,* systolic anterior motion.

regurgitation, the intra-aortic balloon pump may actually worsen myocardial work and oxygen demand by increasing the aortic regurgitant fraction in diastole, causing increased left ventricular end-diastolic volume and pressure. Another contraindication includes the presence of an aortic dissection, as this device may propagate and worsen the dissection flap. Intra-aortic balloon counterpulsation may be effective in the setting of a ventricular septal defect to reduce left ventricular afterload and improve forward perfusion. Given these benefits, a ventricular septal defect is not a contraindication to this device. A patent ductus arteriosus, if present, is usually small and not clinically significant. An intra-aortic balloon pump may slightly increase left-to-right shunt through a patent ductus arteriosus; this is unlikely to cause significant clinical changes. A recent stroke is not a contraindication to placement of this device.

References:

1. Nguyen L, Roth DM, Shanewise JS, Kaplan JA. Chapter 36: Discontinuing Cardiopulmonary Bypass. In: Kaplan JA, Augoustides JGT, Manecke GR, et al., eds. Kaplan's Cardiac Anesthesia. 7th ed. Elsevier; 2017: 1291-1310.
2. Santana JM, Dalia AA, Newton M, et al. Mechanical circulatory support options in patients with aortic valve pathology. J Cardiothorac Vasc Anesth, 2022; 36: 3318-3326.

27. According to the recent single-center Intra-aortic Balloon Counterpulsation in Patients Undergoing Cardiac Surgery (IABCS) trial, high-risk patients undergoing cardiac surgery randomized to receive preincision intra-aortic balloon pump insertion (compared to standard care) were MOST likely to experience which of the following?
   A. Increased odds of limb ischemia
   B. No significant difference in the odds of mortality or morbidity
   C. Reduced odds of cardiogenic shock
   D. Shorter intensive care unit length of stay

Correct Answer: B

Explanation: The clinical efficacy of intra-aortic balloon pump (IABP) counterpulsation remains highly controversial. Despite promising hemodynamic improvements with IABPs, these hemodynamic results have not translated into robust improvements in clinical outcomes. In a randomized controlled trial named IABP-SHOCK II, patients with cardiogenic shock from acute myocardial infarction who were randomized to receive IABP (compared to standard of care) did not demonstrate any clinical benefit.

In the Intra-Aortic Balloon Counterpulsation in Patients Undergoing Cardiac Surgery (IABCS) trial, high-risk patients undergoing cardiac surgery were randomized to prophylactic IABP insertion before surgical incision, or standard of care. There was no significant difference in the primary composite outcome of mortality, mechanical ventilation for more than 24 hours, wound infection, re-exploration, stroke, cardiogenic shock, or acute renal failure at 30 days, nor was there any

significant difference in the individual outcomes. The only significant difference between groups was that the IABP group had significantly longer use of inotropic medications and longer intensive care unit length of stay.

References:

1. Nguyen L, Roth DM, Shanewise JS, Kaplan JA. Chapter 36: Discontinuing Cardiopulmonary Bypass. In: Kaplan JA, Augoustides JGT, Manecke GR, et al., eds. Kaplan's Cardiac Anesthesia. 7th ed. Elsevier; 2017: 1291-1310.
2. Rocha Ferreira GS, de Almeida JP, Landoni G, et al. Effect of a perioperative intra-aortic balloon pump in high-risk cardiac surgery patients: a randomized clinical trial. Crit Care Med. 2018; 46: e742-e750.
3. Hessel EA 2nd. What's new in cardiopulmonary bypass. J Cardiothorac Vasc Anesth, 2019; 33: 2296-2326.

28. What is the MOST appropriate landmark for correct intra-aortic balloon pump tip position when using guidance via transesophageal echocardiography?
   A. 2 cm distal to the sinotubular junction
   B. 2 cm distal to the brachiocephalic (innominate) artery
   C. 2 cm distal to the left common carotid artery
   D. 2 cm distal to the left subclavian artery

Correct Answer: D

Explanation: Correct intra-aortic balloon pump (IABP) positioning is important not only for the desired hemodynamic effects of counter pulsation, but also to avoid possible complications. Using transesophageal echocardiography, the tip of the IABP should be positioned in the descending thoracic aorta, 1 to 2 cm distal to the left subclavian artery. This position prevents intermittent occlusion of any of the aortic arch vessels. Positions lower than this present a risk of occluding the visceral vessels such as the celiac and/or superior mesenteric arteries, which may cause mesenteric ischemia and hepatic injury. Any balloon pump positioning in the aortic arch (answer choices A, B, or C) risks occluding the cerebral vessels and/or the left subclavian artery, with possible resultant deleterious ischemia.

References:

1. Nguyen L, Roth DM, Shanewise JS, Kaplan JA. Chapter 36: Discontinuing Cardiopulmonary Bypass. In: Kaplan JA, Augoustides JGT, Manecke GR, et al., eds. Kaplan's Cardiac Anesthesia. 7th ed. Elsevier; 2017: 1291-1310.
2. Orihashi K, Hong YW, Chung G, et al. New applications of two-dimensional transesophageal echocardiography in cardiac surgery. J Cardiothorac Vasc Anesth, 1991; 5: 33-39.
3. Santana JM, Dalia AA, Newton M, et al. Mechanical circulatory support options in patients with aortic valve pathology. J Cardiothorac Vasc Anesth, 2022; 36: 3318-3326.

29. After weaning from cardiopulmonary bypass, the systemic blood pressure is 133/82 mmHg, biventricular function is excellent, and the perfusionist reports 600 mL of blood remaining in the reservoir. Which maneuver is the BEST next step to enable autotransfusion of the blood from the reservoir to the patient?

A. Administer nitroglycerin
B. Administer protamine
C. Place the patient in Trendelenburg position
D. Spin and rinse blood in cell salvage device

Correct Answer: A

Explanation: After cessation of cardiopulmonary bypass, venous decannulation, and drainage of the venous blood to the cardiotomy reservoir, it is common for there to be a residual 400 to 800 mL of blood in the reservoir. Autotransfusion of this blood back to the patient reduces anemia and returns coagulation factors and platelets. To avoid hypertension and enable aortic decannulation (especially if it is already present), nitroglycerin may be administered. Because of its venodilatory properties, nitroglycerin lowers blood pressure to permit additional autotransfusion. Additional maneuvers may include placing the patient in reverse Trendelenburg or head-up position to pool blood towards the lower extremities and lower blood pressure. Protamine administration may hasten aortic decannulation without completing autotransfusion; timing should be coordinated with the surgical team. Using a cell salvage device for blood in the venous reservoir can be done; however, it removes platelets and clotting factors, and thus is not the optimal choice.

References:

1. Nguyen L, Roth DM, Shanewise JS, Kaplan JA. Chapter 36: Discontinuing Cardiopulmonary Bypass. In: Kaplan JA, Augoustides JGT, Manecke GR, et al., eds. Kaplan's Cardiac Anesthesia. 7th ed. Elsevier; 2017: 1291-1310.
2. Kieler-Jensen N, Houltz E, Milocco I, et al. Central hemodynamics and right ventricular function after coronary artery bypass surgery. A comparison of prostacyclin, sodium nitroprusside, and nitroglycerin for treatment of postcardiac surgical hypertension. J Cardiothorac Vasc Anesth, 1993; 7: 555-559.

30. A patient with normal biventricular function undergoes an uncomplicated surgical aortic valve replacement. While weaning from cardiopulmonary bypass, the venous drainage line is clamped. What is MOST likely to occur next?

A. Bypass flows increase
B. Cardiotomy reservoir blood level rises
C. Central venous pressure rises
D. Clamping the arterial inflow line

Correct Answer: C

Explanation: The first step in weaning from cardiopulmonary bypass (CPB) is clamping the venous drainage line. With the drainage line clamped, the patient's venous blood is no longer drained into the cardiotomy reservoir and will now course through the right atrium and ventricle instead. As the blood passes through the right-sided chambers, central venous pressure will rise. After venous drainage, the cardiotomy reservoir level will fall, as it will no longer be repleted by the patient's blood via the venous drainage line. To prevent the reservoir level from falling to dangerously low levels (or depleting entirely), the perfusionist must reduce the rate of infusion from the cardiotomy reservoir to the patient; this is CPB flow rate. While clamping the arterial line and aortic decannulation is required after separating from cardiopulmonary bypass, it typically follows venous decannulation and a number of other steps after clamping the venous drainage line.

References:

1. Nguyen L, Roth DM, Shanewise JS, Kaplan JA. Chapter 36: Discontinuing Cardiopulmonary Bypass. In: Kaplan JA, Augoustides JGT, Manecke GR, et al., eds. Kaplan's Cardiac Anesthesia. 7th ed. Elsevier; 2017: 1291-1310.
2. Monaco F, Di Prima AL, Kim JH, et al. Management of challenging cardiopulmonary bypass separation. J Cardiothorac Vasc Anesth, 2020; 34: 1622-1635.

CHAPTER 33

Fast-Track Postoperative Cardiac Recovery and Outcomes

Jennette Hansen and Brigid Flynn

KEY POINTS

1. Cardiac anesthesia has fundamentally shifted from a high-dose narcotic technique to a more balanced approach using moderate-dose narcotics, shorter-acting muscle relaxants, and volatile anesthetic agents.

2. This new paradigm has also led to renewed interest in perioperative pain management involving multimodal techniques that facilitate rapid tracheal extubation, such as regional blocks, intrathecal morphine, and supplementary nonsteroidal anti-inflammatory drugs.

3. This approach has prompted a change from the classical model of recovering patients in the traditional intensive care unit manner, with weaning protocols and intensive observation, to management more in keeping with the recovery room practice of early extubation and rapid discharge, which has shifted the care of cardiac patients to more specialized post–cardiac surgery recovery units.

4. Fast-track cardiac anesthesia appears to be safe in comparison with conventional high-dose narcotic anesthesia, but if complications occur that would prevent early tracheal extubation, the management strategy should be modified accordingly.

5. The goal of a post–cardiac surgery recovery model is a postoperative unit that allows variable levels of monitoring and care based on patients' needs.

6. The initial management in the postoperative care of fast-track cardiac surgical patients consists of ensuring an efficient transfer of care from operating room staff to cardiac recovery area staff, while at the same time maintaining stable patient vital signs.

7. It is important to know the risk factors associated with cardiac surgical procedures and to review treatment options for patients with specific reference to outcomes, all within the context of cost and resource use, especially as medicine increasingly involves economic realities.

1. What has been shown to be a risk factor for delayed tracheal extubation after coronary artery bypass grafting?
   A. Male sex
   B. Atrial arrhythmias
   C. Propofol usage for sedation
   D. Diabetes

Correct Answer: B

Explanation: Although the initial definition for delayed tracheal extubation was more than 10 hours following intensive care unit arrival, the current definition has dropped this interval to 6 hours. Atrial arrhythmias can lead to hemodynamic instability and therefore delay the time to tracheal extubation. Further risk factors for delayed tracheal extubation in this setting include advanced age, female gender, postoperative intra-aortic balloon pump counterpulsation, level of inotropic support, and major bleeding. Propofol usage has been found to decrease risk of prolonged intubation. Diabetes in and of itself has not been shown to prolong time to tracheal extubation.

References:

1. Bainbri D, Cheng DCH. Chapter 37: Fast-Track Postoperative Cardiac Recovery and Outcomes. In: Kaplan JA, Augoustides JGT, Manecke GR, et al., eds. Kaplan's Cardiac Anesthesia. 7th ed. Elsevier; 2017:1313-1326.
2. Hendrikx J, Timmers M, Al Tmimi L, et al. Fast-track failure after cardiac surgery: risk factors and outcome with long-term follow-up. J Cardiothorac Vasc Anesth, 2022; 36: 2463-2472.

2. A 73-year-old female underwent mitral valve repair and coronary artery bypass surgery. Throughout the case, the ventilator settings were volume control with a set tidal volume of 525 mL, a respiratory rate of 12 breaths per minute, and 5 mmHg of positive end-expiratory pressure. During the case, 500 mL of autologous blood from the cardiopulmonary bypass circuit was directly transfused through her central vascular access. The surgical team then noticed increased blood loss following the autologous transfusion. What is the MOST likely explanation for this increase in bleeding?

A. Inadequate heparin reversal
B. Incomplete coronary anastomoses
C. Low levels of positive end-expiratory pressure
D. Deficiency of coagulation factors and platelets

Correct Answer: A

Explanation: The most common etiology of new-onset blood loss in patients who receive cardiopulmonary bypass pump blood is inadequate heparin reversal. This is due to the fact that the blood transfused directly from the pump without entering the cell salvage system will contain heparin. Returning blood from the pump is beneficial because it is whole blood; however, it also contains heparin. Because it is whole blood, it also contributes to increased inflammatory response because it contains white blood cells and inflammatory mediators. If the blood were sent through cell salvage, the heparin and white blood cells would have been removed. Cell salvage is not without consequence because transfusing greater than 1 L has been found to impair coagulation due to factors such as dilution of clotting factors and platelets.

Bleeding after cardiac surgical procedures has numerous medical causes. Platelet dysfunction is common in this setting. The cardiopulmonary bypass circuit itself leads to contact activation and degranulation of platelets, thus resulting in platelet dysfunction. It is possible that failure to achieve surgical hemostasis of a coronary anastomosis is the cause, but that is less likely than inadequate heparin reversal in this scenario. Increasing levels of positive end-expiratory pressure has not been shown to have a clinically significant effect on bleeding and transfusion burden.

References:

1. Bainbri D, Cheng DCH. Chapter 37: Fast-Track Postoperative Cardiac Recovery and Outcomes. In: Kaplan JA, Augoustides JGT, Manecke GR, et al., eds. Kaplan's Cardiac Anesthesia. 7th ed. Elsevier; 2017:1313-1326.

BOX 33.1 Management of the bleeding patient

- Review activated coagulation time, prothrombin time, international normalized ratio, and platelet count
- Administer protamine if bleeding is caused by excess heparin (reinfusion of pump blood)
- Treat the medical cause with platelets, fresh frozen plasma, and cryoprecipitate if bleeding is secondary to decreased fibrinogen
- Factor VIIa should be considered if bleeding continues despite a normal coagulation profile
- Treat the surgical cause with re-exploration

2. Boer C, Meesters MI, Vonk ABA, et al. 2017 EACTS/EACTA guidelines on patient blood management for adult cardiac surgery. J Cardiothorac Vasc Anesth, 2018; 32: 88-120.

3. A 78-year-old male with history of factor V Leiden has undergone redo coronary artery bypass grafting and aortic valve replacement. A balanced resuscitation for coagulopathy was administered, followed by recombinant factor VIIa. What complication should be closely monitored in the intensive care unit, given the factor VIIa administration?

A. Prolonged neuromuscular blockade
B. Decreased tidal volumes
C. Seizure
D. Myocardial infarction

Correct Answer: D

Explanation: A commonly cited complication associated with administration of factor VIIa is arterial thrombosis. Therefore, patients may be at increased risk for myocardial infarction and cerebral vascular accidents with administration. However, many of these early studies utilized large doses of factor VIIa. In contrast, more recent studies have utilized smaller doses of factor VIIa for cardiac surgical bleeding and have demonstrated no increased adverse events but have demonstrated benefits in terms of bleeding cessation and decreased transfusions.

Factor VIIa has been shown to reduce transfusion requirements and lead to fewer reoperations in the setting of intractable bleeding. There is no association between factor VIIa and duration of neuromuscular blockade. Patients may have prolonged ventilation related to bleeding necessitating the administration of factor VIIa, but factor VII has no direct respiratory effects. There is no evidence that factor VIIa is associated with seizures.

References:

1. Bainbri D, Cheng DCH. Chapter 37: Fast-Track Postoperative Cardiac Recovery and Outcomes. In: Kaplan JA, Augoustides JGT, Manecke GR, et al., eds. Kaplan's Cardiac Anesthesia. 7th ed. Elsevier; 2017:1313-1326.
2. Raphael J, Mazer CD, Subramani S, et al. Society of Cardiovascular Anesthesiologist clinical practice improvement advisory for management of perioperative bleeding and hemostasis in cardiac surgery patients. J Cardiothorac Vasc Anesth, 2019; 33: 2887-2889.

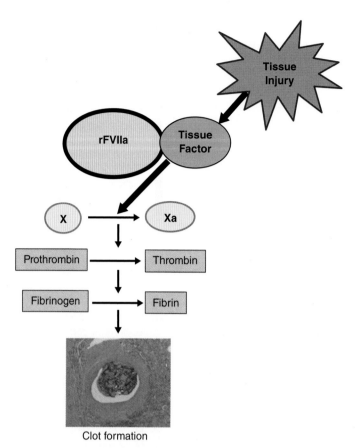

FIGURE 33.1 Simplified mechanism of action for recombinant factor VIIa when administered after injury, with subsequent tissue factor release and clot formation. (From Kidd B, Sutherland L, Jabaley CS, et al. Efficacy, safety, and strategies for recombinant-activated factor VII in cardiac surgical bleeding: a narrative review. J Cardiothorac Vasc Anesth, 2022; 36: 1157-1168.)

3. Sutherland L, Houchin A, Wang T, et al. Impact of early, low-dose factor VIIa on subsequent transfusions and length of stay in cardiac surgery. J Cardiothorac Vasc Anesth, 2022; 36: 147-154.
4. Kidd B, Sutherland L, Jabaley CS, et al. Efficacy, safety, and strategies for recombinant-activated factor VII in cardiac surgical bleeding: a narrative review. J Cardiothorac Vasc Anesth, 2022; 36: 1157-1168.

4. The majority of cardiothoracic intensive care units monitor and treat hyperglycemia following cardiac surgery in order to avoid adverse outcomes. What is an identified complication of hyperglycemia in cardiac surgical patients?
   A. Coagulopathy
   B. Hypervolemia
   C. Wound infection
   D. Increased transfusion requirement

Correct Answer: C

Explanation: Perioperative hyperglycemia has been associated with increased wound infections. Euglycemia has several definitions, but most articles target less than 180 to 200 mg/dL for cardiac surgical patients. In the past, it was believed that very tight glucose control (80–110 mg/dL) was superior, but this was later found to have increased morbidity and mortality related to hypoglycemic events. It is thought that hyperglycemia leads to glycosylation of immune cells and wound-healing proteins, thus decreasing the ability of the body to fight infection. This mechanism would inhibit collagen deposition and adequate wound healing. Hyperglycemia activates prothrombin fragments and is not associated with coagulopathy or increased transfusion requirements. Hyperglycemia can lead to relative hypovolemia due to the diuretic effect of glycosuria.

References:

1. Bainbri D, Cheng DCH. Chapter 37: Fast-Track Postoperative Cardiac Recovery and Outcomes. In: Kaplan JA, Augoustides JGT, Manecke GR, et al., eds. Kaplan's Cardiac Anesthesia. 7th ed. Elsevier; 2017:1313-1326.
2. Murray MJ, Brull SJ, Coursin DB. Strict blood glucose control in the ICU: panacea or Pandora's box? J Cardiothorac Vasc Anesth, 2004; 18: 687-689.
3. Rangasamy V, Xu X, Susheela AT, et al. Comparison of glycemic variability indices: blood glucose, risk index, and coefficient of variation in predicting adverse outcomes for patients undergoing cardiac surgery. J Cardiothorac Vasc Anesth, 2020; 34: 1794-1802.

5. What preoperative medication may reduce postoperative atrial fibrillation and decrease saphenous vein graft occlusions in patients undergoing coronary artery bypass grafting?

A. Aspirin
B. Statins
C. Clopidogrel
D. Angiotensin-converting enzyme inhibitors

Correct Answer: B

Explanation: Statins have been found to prevent neointimal formation in the saphenous vein graft, inhibiting the accelerated atherosclerosis that accompanies vein grafts. Due to inhibition of accelerated atherosclerosis, there is a significant reduction in the revascularization requirement. In some studies, statins have been found to decrease postoperative atrial fibrillation when given preoperatively. Aspirin is shown to improve mortality and to reduce myocardial infarction when given postoperatively. Clopidogrel is not given preoperatively, as it can increase bleeding. Clopidogrel is considered postoperatively in patients who cannot take aspirin or who have had an ischemic event while on aspirin. Angiotensin-converting enzyme inhibitors have not been shown to decrease atrial fibrillation or to decrease saphenous graft occlusion and have been associated with hypotension perioperatively.

> **BOX 33.2** **Medications for cardiac risk reduction after coronary artery bypass grafting**
>
> - Aspirin: all patients after bypass grafting
> - Clopidogrel: patients who have contraindication to aspirin (may have superior efficacy compared with aspirin)
> - Beta blockers: especially with perioperative myocardial infarction
> - Lipid-lowering agents: especially statin drugs

References:

1. Bainbri D, Cheng DCH. Chapter 37: Fast-Track Postoperative Cardiac Recovery and Outcomes. In: Kaplan JA, Augoustides JGT, Manecke GR, et al., eds. Kaplan's Cardiac Anesthesia. 7th ed. Elsevier; 2017:1313-1326.
2. Hinder K, Eltzschig HK, Fox AA, et al. Influence of statins on perioperative outcomes. J Cardiothorac Vasc Anesth, 2006; 20: 251-258.

6. Which of the following is a known risk factor for stroke after cardiac surgery?

A. Diabetes
B. Female sex
C. Elective surgery
D. Smoking history

Correct Answer: A

Explanation: Stroke after cardiac surgery is a serious complication because it adversely affects mortality both in the perioperative period and beyond. Identified risk factors for stroke include age, diabetes, previous history of stroke or transient ischemic attack, peripheral vascular disease, atrial fibrillation, and unstable angina. Patient gender has not been found to correlate with postoperative stroke risk. Elective surgeries have been correlated with a risk reduction for stroke after cardiac surgery. Smoking history does not have a direct correlation with postoperative stroke risk. Common sources of embolic stroke are derived from aortic manipulation during proximal anastomosis of the vein grafts, clamping, and unclamping. Hemorrhagic infarcts can occur due to perioperative anticoagulation, severe hypertension, and coexisting neurovascular abnormalities such as mycotic aneurysms in infective endocarditis. Watershed infarcts also occur secondary to cerebral hypotension during the perioperative period.

References:

1. Bainbri D, Cheng DCH. Chapter 37: Fast-Track Postoperative Cardiac Recovery and Outcomes. In: Kaplan JA, Augoustides JGT, Manecke GR, et al., eds. Kaplan's Cardiac Anesthesia. 7th ed. Elsevier; 2017:1313-1326.

TABLE 33.1
Common complications after heart operations

Complication	Incidence Rate	Risk Factors
Stroke	2%–4%	Age
		Previous stroke/TIA
		PVD
		Diabetes
		Unstable angina
Delirium	8%–15%	Age
		Previous stroke
		Duration of operation
		Duration of aortic cross clamp
Atrial fibrillation	≤35%	Age
		Male sex
		Previous atrial fibrillation
		Mitral valve operation
		Previous CHF
		Atrial fibrillation
		Blood transfusion
Renal failure	1%	Low postoperative CO
		Repeat cardiac operation
		Valve operation
		Age
		Diabetes

CHF, Congestive heart failure; *CO*, cardiac output; *PVD*, peripheral vascular disease; *TIA*, transient ischemic attack.

2. Lo EYW, Dignan R, French B. Independent predictors of post-operative stroke with cardiopulmonary bypass. J Cardiothorac Vasc Anesth, 2021; 36: 133-137.

7. A 67-year-old female who underwent aortic valve replacement has delayed awakening due to a new large parietal stroke. What is the most common cause of postoperative stroke?
- **A.** Watershed infarct
- **B.** Embolic stroke
- **C.** Intracerebral hemorrhage
- **D.** Metastatic tumors

Correct Answer: B

Explanation: Emboli are the most common cause of clinical stroke after cardiac surgery, accounting for up to two-thirds of all cases. Embolic stroke is most commonly due to manipulation of the aorta associated with cannulation and clamping events. Aortic surgery increases the risk of perioperative stroke in particular and is an independent risk factor for postoperative stroke. Cerebral hypoperfusion results in watershed strokes that may be present in up to a quarter of all strokes after cardiac surgery. Strokes due to hemorrhage and metastatic tumors are uncommon after cardiac surgery.

References:

1. Bainbri D, Cheng DCH. Chapter 37: Fast-Track Postoperative Cardiac Recovery and Outcomes. In: Kaplan JA, Augoustides JGT, Manecke GR, et al., eds. Kaplan's Cardiac Anesthesia. 7th ed. Elsevier; 2017:1313-1326.
2. Lo EYW, Dignan R, French B. Independent predictors of post-operative stroke with cardiopulmonary bypass. J Cardiothorac Vasc Anesth, 2021; 36: 133-137.

8. Which medication has been shown to be the best choice for rate control of new-onset atrial fibrillation after coronary artery bypass graft surgery?
- **A.** Beta blockers
- **B.** Calcium channel blockers
- **C.** Digoxin
- **D.** Magnesium

Correct Answer: A

Explanation: Beta blockers are a popular choice for rate control in new-onset atrial fibrillation after cardiac surgery, especially in ischemic heart disease where this medication class improves functional and symptomatic end points. Calcium channel blockers are an alternative if beta blockers are not indicated due to factors such as acute heart failure or asthma. Diltiazem is associated with less hypotension than verapamil. When beta blockers and calcium channel blockers are contraindicated, digoxin is an option, although therapeutic levels take time to achieve. Hypomagnesemia may increase the risk of postoperative atrial fibrillation and should be corrected in this setting to normal levels. However, magnesium boluses have not been shown to be effective when used for treatment of postoperative atrial fibrillation.

BOX 33.3 Treatment for complications after cardiac surgical procedures

Stroke
- Supportive treatment
- Avoidance of potential aggravating factors (e.g., hyperglycemia, hyperthermia, severe anemia)

Delirium
- Usually self-limited
- Close observation required
- Sedatives (midazolam, lorazepam) possibly required

Atrial Fibrillation
- Rate control: calcium channel blockers, beta blockers, digoxin
- Rhythm control: amiodarone, sotalol, procainamide
- Thromboembolic prophylaxis: for atrial fibrillation >48 h

Left Ventricular Dysfunction
- Volume
- Inotropes: epinephrine, milrinone, norepinephrine
- Mechanical support: intra-aortic balloon pump

Renal Failure
- Removal of the causative agent (nonsteroidal anti-inflammatory drugs, antibiotics)
- Hemodynamic support if necessary
- Supportive care

References:

1. Bainbri D, Cheng DCH. Chapter 37: Fast-Track Postoperative Cardiac Recovery and Outcomes. In: Kaplan JA, Augoustides JGT, Manecke GR, et al., eds. Kaplan's Cardiac Anesthesia. 7th ed. Elsevier; 2017:1313-1326.
2. Boons J, Van Biesen S, Fivez T, et al. Mechanisms, preventions, and treatment of atrial fibrillation after cardiac surgery: a narrative review. J Cardiothorac Vasc Anesth, 2021; 35: 3394-3403.

9. Following off-pump coronary artery bypass graft surgery, a patient's central venous pressure is 2 mmHg, pulmonary artery occlusion pressure is 8 mmHg, stroke volume is 20 mL, and cardiac index is 1.6 L/min/m². The intensive care unit team elects to administer volume. What is the recommended first-line treatment for presumed hypovolemia?
- **A.** Hydroxyethyl starch
- **B.** Albumin
- **C.** Succinylated gelatin
- **D.** Crystalloid

Correct Answer: D

Explanation: When hypovolemia is the underlying cause of low cardiac output, crystalloid can be used to optimize filling. The use of colloids in the critical care setting is controversial, given several large trials of starches that showed little efficacy in volume resuscitation end points and/or an increase in adverse events. Therefore, intravascular hypovolemia is best treated with the use of intermittent boluses of crystalloid with continuous clinical reassessment of clinical hemodynamics, including central filling pressures and cardiac output. Additionally, crystalloid is less expensive than the other options.

Hydroxyethyl starch has been associated with increased bleeding risk due to platelet dysfunction as well as risks of renal injury and mortality in critically ill patients. Albumin, although not an incorrect choice, is not recommended as first-line therapy due to lack of evidence and increased expense. Gelatin products have an increased risk of allergic reactions and are not commonly administered.

References:

1. Bainbri D, Cheng DCH. Chapter 37: Fast-Track Postoperative Cardiac Recovery and Outcomes. In: Kaplan JA, Augoustides JGT, Manecke GR, et al., eds. Kaplan's Cardiac Anesthesia. 7th ed. Elsevier; 2017:1313-1326.
2. Habicher M, Perrino A, Spies CD, et al. Contemporary fluid management in cardiac anesthesia. J Cardiothorac Vasc Anesth, 2011; 25: 1141-1153.
3. Reddy S, McGuinness S, Park R, et al. Choice of fluid therapy and bleeding risk after cardiac surgery. J Cardiothorac Vasc Anesth, 2016; 30: 1094-1103.

10. A 79-year-old male patient underwent aortic valve replacement and coronary artery bypass grafting and has been admitted to the intensive care unit, where he has developed acute kidney injury. His cardiac index is 1.2 L/min/m² with normal filling pressures and stroke volume. No regional motion abnormalities are seen on transthoracic echocardiography, and his electrocardiogram reveals no new ischemic features. The patient is on 0.1 mcg/kg/min of norepinephrine to maintain his mean arterial pressure of 65 to 70 mmHg. The urine output has been 0.5 to 0.6 cc/kg/h. What is the next best step for treatment of his renal insufficiency?
    A. Fluid bolus
    B. Increase norepinephrine
    C. Inotropic support
    D. Diuretic administration

Correct Answer: C

Explanation: This patient likely has a prerenal etiology for his acute kidney injury, suggested by hypotension and low cardiac index in the setting of normal volume status and no signs of myocardial ischemia. It is likely that inotropic therapy would improve cardiac output and hence perfusion to the kidneys to alleviate renal insufficiency. The patient is already on norepinephrine and is maintaining an adequate mean arterial pressure. Although further increasing the mean arterial pressure with additional vasopressor support might improve glomerular filtration rate, this would not be first-line therapy in the setting of low cardiac output. The patient does not have features of volume overload, so diuresis may worsen renal perfusion.

References:

1. Bainbri D, Cheng DCH. Chapter 37: Fast-Track Postoperative Cardiac Recovery and Outcomes. In: Kaplan JA, Augoustides

JGT, Manecke GR, et al., eds. Kaplan's Cardiac Anesthesia. 7th ed. Elsevier; 2017:1313-1326.
2. Just IA, Alborzi F, Godde M, et al. Cardiac surgery-related acute kidney injury risk factors, clinical course, management suggestions. J Cardiothorac Vasc Anesth, 2022; 36: 444-451.

11. A 52-year-old male had a tricuspid valve replacement for tricuspid stenosis. His left ventricular function was normal by transesophageal echocardiography prior to transfer to the intensive care unit. His hemodynamic values after admission to the intensive care unit reveal a cardiac index of 1.2 L/min/m² with central venous pressure of 18 mmHg and pulmonary artery pressures of 55/22 mmHg. His liver enzymes are mildly elevated, and his lactate is 1.9 mmol/L with a creatinine of 1.2 mg/dL. His international normalized ratio is 1.5. What is the most likely etiology of these disturbances?
    A. Right ventricular dysfunction
    B. Sepsis
    C. Bowel ischemia
    D. Fulminant liver failure

Correct Answer: A

Explanation: Right ventricular dysfunction is the most likely etiology of low cardiac index with elevations in the central venous pressure, liver function tests, international normalized ratio, and lactate. The presented laboratory profile reflects liver congestion but is not severe enough to represent fulminant liver failure. Additionally, fulminant liver failure is often associated with an increased cardiac index due to an associated low systemic vascular resistance. Pulmonary hypertension, either acute or preexisting, increases the risk for right ventricular dysfunction.

Sepsis and bowel ischemia would likely not occur during the first few hours in the intensive care unit without a history of chronic illness or prolonged preoperative hospitalization. Additionally, sepsis generally increases cardiac index. Bowel ischemia is also typically associated with higher lactate levels.

References:

1. Bainbri D, Cheng DCH. Chapter 37: Fast-Track Postoperative Cardiac Recovery and Outcomes. In: Kaplan JA, Augoustides JGT, Manecke GR, et al., eds. Kaplan's Cardiac Anesthesia. 7th ed. Elsevier; 2017:1313-1326.
2. Kim JH, Lerose CC, Landoni G, et al. Differences in biomarkers between severe isolated right and left ventricular dysfunction after cardiac surgery. J Cardiothorac Vasc Anesth, 2020; 34: 650-658.

12. A 63-year-old male with obstructive sleep apnea, tobacco abuse, obesity, hypertension, and diabetes presents with angina due to significant stenosis of his mid-left anterior descending, mid-left circumflex, and proximal posterior descending coronary arteries. What is the BEST management option for this patient?
    A. Optimal medical management
    B. Coronary artery bypass surgery
    C. Percutaneous coronary angioplasty
    D. Percutaneous coronary stents

Correct Answer: B

Explanation: Patients with multivessel disease and diabetes have better outcomes with surgical revascularization compared to multiple percutaneous interventions and/or optimal medical therapy. One trial reviewed 2600 patients and observed an absolute risk reduction in mortality rates for patients undergoing coronary artery bypass grafting of 5.6% at 5 years, 5.9% at 7 years, and 4.1% at 10 years, particularly in patients with left main, proximal left anterior descending, or three-vessel coronary disease. Surgical revascularization in diabetics with advanced coronary artery disease not only enhances survival, but also is associated with a lower risk of repeat revascularization downstream compared to percutaneous intervention and/or medical management.

TABLE 33.2

Treatment options and outcomes for coronary artery disease

Comparison	Outcome	Revascularization
Medical vs. surgical management	Absolute risk reduction in mortality	37% of medically treated patients converted to surgical treatment
	5.6% at 5 years	
	5.9% at 7 years	
	4.1% at 10 years	
	Benefit of operation greatest in LM, three-vessel disease	
Angioplasty vs. surgical management	Absolute risk reduction in mortality	50% rate of revascularization at 5 years in angioplasty group
	1.9% at 5 years	
	Rates of in-hospital MI and stroke significantly lower in angioplasty group	
	Benefit of operation greatest in diabetes, multivessel revascularization	
Stent vs. surgical management	Mortality mixed results, relative reduction ranged from a 50% reduction in favor of CABG to a 75% reduction in favor of stenting	15%–25% rate of revascularization in stent group
	MI rates at 1-year equivalent	
OPCAB vs. conventional surgical management	No difference in mortality	Most OPCAB-treated patients received fewer grafts than CCAB group (0.2 fewer grafts per patient)
	No difference in in-hospital stroke	
	No difference in in-hospital MI	

CABG, Coronary artery bypass grafting; *CCAB*, conventional coronary artery bypass; *LM*, left main coronary artery disease; *MI*, myocardial infarction; *OPCAB*, off-pump coronary artery bypass.

References:

1. Bainbri D, Cheng DCH. Chapter 37: Fast-Track Postoperative Cardiac Recovery and Outcomes. In: Kaplan JA, Augoustides JGT, Manecke GR, et al., eds. Kaplan's Cardiac Anesthesia. 7th ed. Elsevier; 2017:1313-1326.
2. Cormican D, Jayaraman Al, Sheu R, et al. Coronary artery bypass grafting versus percutaneous transcatheter coronary interventions: analysis of outcomes in myocardial revascularization. J Cardiothorac Vasc Anesth, 2019; 2569-2588.

13. Which outcome is decreased with off-pump as compared to on-pump coronary artery bypass grafting?
   A. Stroke
   B. Cognitive dysfunction
   C. Blood transfusion
   D. Transient ischemic attack

Correct Answer: C

Explanation: Meta-analysis of randomized trials has demonstrated that off-pump as compared to on-pump coronary artery bypass grafting reduces the risks of blood transfusion, atrial fibrillation, and overall resource utilization. Neuroprotective effects including freedom from stroke, transient ischemic attack, and cognitive dysfunction have not been conclusively demonstrated with off-pump coronary bypass grafting. In addition, there is ongoing concern about the quality of the vascular anastomoses with off-pump techniques, especially in low-volume centers.

References:

1. Bainbri D, Cheng DCH. Chapter 37: Fast-Track Postoperative Cardiac Recovery and Outcomes. In: Kaplan JA, Augoustides JGT, Manecke GR, et al., eds. Kaplan's Cardiac Anesthesia. 7th ed. Elsevier; 2017:1313-1326.
2. Shaefi S, Mittle A, Loberman D. Off-pump versus on-pump coronary artery bypass grafting-a systematic review and analysis of clinical outcomes. J Cardiothorac Vasc Anesth, 2019; 33: 232-244.

14. Fast-track cardiac anesthesia implies shorter times for tracheal extubation, with recent trials setting the goal for this end point within 6 hours after arrival in the intensive care. Fast-track cardiac surgical techniques have been shown to provide which of the following?
A. Decreased length of hospital stay
B. Decreased rates of renal dysfunction
C. Decreased costs
D. Decreased sternal wound infection rate

Correct Answer: C

Explanation: Tracheal extubation within 6 hours of admission to the intensive care unit is the goal of fast-track cardiac anesthesia. The multiple management techniques in this fast-track approach include decreased doses of narcotics and increased utilization of multimodal analgesia, including fascial plane blocks. Fast-track approaches have proven to be effective and safe, even in high-risk cardiac surgical patients, and significantly decrease costs, including in areas such as nursing care and laboratory testing.

> **BOX 33.4 Benefits of fast-track cardiac anesthesia**
> * Decreased duration of intubation
> * Decreased cost

Although fast-track techniques have many benefits, they have not reduced the risks of acute kidney injury and sternal wound infection after cardiac surgery. Older trials suggested shorter stays in the intensive care unit; however, recent trials have not demonstrated this benefit, perhaps due to cultural shifts in the practice of cardiac surgical intensive care. In contrast, the length of the hospital stay has not been affected by fast-track anesthesia techniques, even in older studies.

References:
1. Bainbri D, Cheng DCH. Chapter 37: Fast-Track Postoperative Cardiac Recovery and Outcomes. In: Kaplan JA, Augoustides JGT, Manecke GR, et al., eds. Kaplan's Cardiac Anesthesia. 7th ed. Elsevier; 2017:1313-1326.
2. Richey M, Mann A, He J, et al. Implementation of an early extubation protocol in cardiac surgical patients decreased ventilator time but not intensive care unit or hospital length of stay. J Cardiothorac Vasc Anesth, 2018; 32: 739-744.
3. Flynn BC, He J, Richey M, et al. Early extubation without increased adverse events in high-risk cardiac surgical patients. Ann Thorac Surg, 2019; 107: 453-459.

15. Which treatment option should be considered early in the management of a hemodynamically stable patient with nonsurgical perioperative bleeding in a cardiac surgical patient with chronic kidney disease?
A. Desmopressin
B. Recombinant factor VIIa
C. Platelet transfusion
D. Fresh frozen plasma

Correct Answer: A

Explanation: Uremia leads to a state of acquired platelet dysfunction due to both decreased platelet activation and impaired adhesion to vascular subendothelial cells. Desmopressin has been shown to promote coagulation in this setting through mechanisms that include the endothelial release of von Willebrand factor. von Willebrand factor carries factor VIII, and both are required for clot formation. These effects of desmopressin therapy can restore platelet function in the uremic patient. Factor VIIa, fresh frozen plasma, and platelet transfusion may help to decrease bleeding in a bleeding patient, but these would not be the first-line choices in a uremic patient due not only to expense, but also to lack of specificity to uremic-induced bleeding coagulopathy. Desmopressin therapy does not affect the donor pool of blood products, which should be preserved if possible.

References:
1. Bainbri D, Cheng DCH. Chapter 37: Fast-Track Postoperative Cardiac Recovery and Outcomes. In: Kaplan JA, Augoustides JGT, Manecke GR, et al., eds. Kaplan's Cardiac Anesthesia. 7th ed. Elsevier; 2017:1313-1326.
2. Rozental T, Shore-Lesserson L. Pharmacologic management of coagulopathy in cardiac surgery: an update. J Cardiothorac Vasc Anesth, 2012; 26: 669-679.

16. What has been found to be a predictor of prolonged stay in the intensive care unit?
A. Preoperative hemoglobin of 7 gm/dL
B. Preoperative statin exposure
C. Previous transient ischemic attack
D. Preoperative clopidogrel therapy

Correct Answer: D

Explanation: Preoperative potent antiplatelet medication, such as clopidogrel, increases the odds ratio of a prolonged intensive care unit stay due to increased risk of bleeding. Furthermore, if a patient undergoes cardiac surgery in the setting of a potent antiplatelet medication, it is likely that the procedure was urgent or emergent. Urgent and emergent surgeries have also been associated with increased postoperative mortality and morbidity, including a prolonged stay in the intensive care unit. Preoperative hemoglobin level and previous transient ischemic attacks have not been associated with increased length of stay. Preoperative statin therapy provides cardiovascular and other pleiotropic protective effects that often decrease the length of stay in the intensive care unit.

References:
1. Bainbri D, Cheng DCH. Chapter 37: Fast-Track Postoperative Cardiac Recovery and Outcomes. In: Kaplan JA, Augoustides JGT, Manecke GR, et al., eds. Kaplan's Cardiac Anesthesia. 7th ed. Elsevier; 2017:1313-1326.
2. Dominici C, Salsano A, Nenna A, et al. A nomogram for predicting length of stay in the intensive care unit in patients undergoing CABG: results from the multicenter E-CABG registry. J Cardiothorac Vasc Anesth, 2020; 34: 2951-2961.

17. Following an aortic valve replacement, a patient has a decreased glomerular filtration rate and increased creatinine levels. What is true regarding postoperative renal dysfunction in cardiac surgical patients?

A. Postoperative renal dysfunction after cardiac surgery occurs in more than 50% of patients

B. Postoperative renal dysfunction does not increase mortality

C. Postoperative renal dysfunction increases the length of stay in the intensive care unit

D. Glomerular filtration rate is the most common defining parameter for postoperative renal dysfunction

Correct Answer: C

Explanation: Depending on the definition, acute kidney injury in the postoperative cardiac surgical period occurs in approximately 1% to 30% of patients. Multiple definitions have been proposed for renal impairment after cardiac surgery. The RIFLE (Risk, Injury, Failure, Loss of kidney function, and End-stage kidney disease) criteria include both glomerular filtration rate and creatinine level to define the stages of renal dysfunction. The KDIGO (Kidney Disease Improving Global Outcomes) criteria utilize creatinine values to define stages of renal dysfunction. The AKIN (Acute Kidney Injury Network) criteria incorporate both creatinine and urine output values. Although the need for renal replacement therapy is a clear clinical end point, it does not consider the spectrum of patients with reductions in creatinine clearance who do not require mechanical support. Patients with varying degrees of acute kidney injury after cardiac surgery have increased mortality as well as length of stay, both in the intensive care unit and in the hospital.

References:

1. Bainbri D, Cheng DCH. Chapter 37: Fast-Track Postoperative Cardiac Recovery and Outcomes. In: Kaplan JA, Augoustides JGT, Manecke GR, et al., eds. Kaplan's Cardiac Anesthesia. 7th ed. Elsevier; 2017:1313-1326.
2. Yaqub S, Hashmi S, Kazmi MK, et al. A comparison of AKIN, KDIGO, and RIFLE definitions to diagnose acute kidney injury and predict the outcomes after cardiac surgery in a South Asian cohort. Cardiorenal Med, 2022; 12: 29-38.
3. Chew STH, Hwang NC. Acute kidney injury after cardiac surgery: a narrative review of the literature. J Cardiothorac Vasc Anesth, 2019; 33: 1122-1138.

18. Patients undergoing cardiac surgery often require blood component transfusion therapy. Which component has the greatest risk of complications?

A. Packed red blood cells

B. Fresh frozen plasma

C. Platelets

D. Cryoprecipitate

Correct Answer: C

Explanation: Platelets appear to have the highest complication rate compared to other blood products. The most common complication is sepsis from bacterial contamination because platelets are stored at 20 to 24°C. Febrile nonhemolytic reactions may also occur after platelet administration, due to recipient antibodies reacting to the human leukocyte antigen on the donor platelets. When platelets are typically pooled from multiple donors, this risk is further increased. Febrile nonhemolytic reactions can also occur as platelets near the end of their shelf life due to release of biologic mediators. Packed red blood cells, fresh frozen plasma, and cryoprecipitate are kept at cooler temperatures, and therefore have lower incidence of bacterial contamination.

References:

1. Bainbri D, Cheng DCH. Chapter 37: Fast-Track Postoperative Cardiac Recovery and Outcomes. In: Kaplan JA, Augoustides JGT, Manecke GR, et al., eds. Kaplan's Cardiac Anesthesia. 7th ed. Elsevier; 2017:1313-1326.
2. Sharma AD, Grocott HP. Platelet transfusion reactions: febrile nonhemolytic reaction or bacterial contamination? Diagnosis, detection, and current preventive modalities. J Cardiothorac Vasc Anesth, 2000; 14: 460-466.

19. A 75-year-old female is postoperative day 2 from coronary artery bypass grafting. The patient has a past medical history of tobacco abuse, atrial fibrillation, chronic obstructive pulmonary disease, peripheral vascular disease, and chronic renal disease. The patient was found to be very sleepy during the day and restless at night. The patient is oriented only to self and is being uncooperative with patient care. What is a risk factor for this scenario?

A. Chronic renal disease

B. Chronic obstructive pulmonary disease

C. Tobacco abuse

D. Atrial fibrillation

Correct Answer: D

Explanation: The description in the clinical vignette describes a typical presentation of postoperative delirium. Atrial fibrillation has been found to be linked to postoperative delirium. Further risk factors include advanced age, low albumin, perioperative stroke, ascending aortic arch replacement, long duration of the cardiac procedure, and increased C-reactive protein. Diabetes, low ejection fraction, and intraoperative blood component administration have also been associated with postoperative delirium. Chronic renal disease, chronic obstructive pulmonary disease, and tobacco abuse have not been correlated with postoperative delirium.

References:

1. Bainbri D, Cheng DCH. Chapter 37: Fast-Track Postoperative Cardiac Recovery and Outcomes. In: Kaplan JA, Augoustides JGT, Manecke GR, et al., eds. Kaplan's Cardiac Anesthesia. 7th ed. Elsevier; 2017:1313-1326.
2. Cereghetti C, Siegemund M, Schaedelin S, et al. Independent predictors of the duration of overall burden of postoperative delirium after cardiac surgery in adults: an observational cohort study. J Cardiothorac Vasc Anesth, 2017; 31: 1966-1973.
3. Stransky M, Schmidt C, Ganslmeier P, et al. Hypoactive delirium after cardiac surgery as an independent risk factor for prolonged mechanical ventilation. J Cardiothorac Vasc Anesth, 2011; 25: 968-974.

20. What is the recommended first-line treatment for post-operative delirium in the intensive care unit?
- **A.** Haloperidol
- **B.** Dexmedetomidine
- **C.** Restraints to prevent harm to self
- **D.** Reinforce orientation

Correct Answer: D

Explanation: The first-line treatment for delirium is reinforcing orientation to the patient. This can be accomplished through frequent reorientation by staff and family to person, place, time, and situation. It remains essential to ensure that a patient has the relevant sensory devices, including glasses and hearing aids. Photos of familiar people can be very useful for reorientation. The maintenance of proper sleep/wake cycle is also important. Sleep hygiene can be difficult to achieve in a critical care setting but can be ameliorated with sleep bundling of care. The best treatment for delirium in the intensive care unit is to discharge the patient from this environment as soon as clinically feasible.

Ambulating the patient has also been found to be an effective treatment for delirium. Although haloperidol and dexmedetomidine are treatments for delirium, medications should be reserved for more resistant cases. Furthermore, if medications are necessary, atypical antipsychotics, such as quetiapine, can be considered for first-line therapy. Restraints should only be used if the delirium is causing the patient to endanger themself, but are not the first-line treatment and may actually exacerbate delirium. Delirium may be associated with long-term negative outcomes, and efforts should be made to treat delirium as quickly as possible.

References:
1. Bainbri D, Cheng DCH. Chapter 37: Fast-Track Postoperative Cardiac Recovery and Outcomes. In: Kaplan JA, Augoustides JGT, Manecke GR, et al., eds. Kaplan's Cardiac Anesthesia. 7th ed. Elsevier; 2017:1313-1326.
2. Cereghetti C, Siegemund M, Schaedelin S, et al. Independent predictors of the duration of overall burden of postoperative delirium after cardiac surgery in adults: an observational cohort study. J Cardiothorac Vasc Anesth, 2017; 31: 1966-1973.

21. What is a drug of choice for preventing delirium in the cardiac surgical intensive care unit?
- **A.** Dexmedetomidine
- **B.** Fentanyl
- **C.** Ketamine
- **D.** Midazolam

Correct Answer: A

Explanation: Of the choices given, dexmedetomidine is the drug of choice for prevention of delirium. Dexmedetomidine has cardiac side effects including bradycardia and hypotension. Haloperidol is a described treatment for delirium but it is not used for prevention. Haloperidol may prolong the QT interval, requiring close monitoring after cardiac surgery, especially in patients on multiple agents that may lead to QT prolongation. Ketamine has been found in some studies to decrease delirium, but in other studies there was no difference.

Ketamine increases sympathetic tone and can lead to tachycardia that should be monitored in patients who are at risk of negative effects on the myocardium due to tachycardia. Midazolam exposure is associated with worsening delirium and should be avoided in patients at risk for delirium. Quetiapine and other atypical antipsychotics can also be used as first-line therapy in patients who can receive enteral medications.

References:
1. Bainbri D, Cheng DCH. Chapter 37: Fast-Track Postoperative Cardiac Recovery and Outcomes. In: Kaplan JA, Augoustides JGT, Manecke GR, et al., eds. Kaplan's Cardiac Anesthesia. 7th ed. Elsevier; 2017:1313-1326.
2. Pieri M, De Simone A, Rose S, et al. Trials focusing on prevention and treatment of delirium after cardiac surgery: a systematic review of randomized evidence. J Cardiothorac Vasc Anesth, 2019; 34: 1641-1654.

22. A 72-year-old male with congestive heart failure with left ventricular ejection fraction of 35% has undergone a mitral valve repair and coronary artery bypass surgery. He was transported to the intensive care unit on high doses of norepinephrine, epinephrine, and vasopressin. On the first postoperative night, his index decreased to 1.2 L/min/m² from 1.8 L/min/m², and his biventricular filling pressures increased despite increasing the inotropic support. His blood pressure was measured at 90/62 mmHg. His systemic vascular resistance was calculated to be 1875 dynes/second/cm⁻⁵. What additional measure should be considered for this patient?
- **A.** Methylene blue
- **B.** Intra-aortic balloon pump
- **C.** Increased vasoactive support
- **D.** Hydroxocobalamin

Correct Answer: B

Explanation: Intra-aortic balloon pump can be considered in a patient who is in cardiogenic shock following cardiac surgery. Intra-aortic balloon pump placement would improve coronary perfusion by increasing diastolic pressure, while augmenting ejection by deflating rapidly during systole.

This patient is at risk for postbypass cardiac dysfunction due to preexisting left-sided heart failure with an ejection fraction of 35%. Increasing the vasoactive support to supratherapeutic doses will likely only worsen side effects of these drugs. Cardiogenic shock is identified in this clinical vignette by the low cardiac index and high systemic vascular resistance. He is not in vasoplegic shock, based on a high systemic vascular resistance; thus, potent vasoconstrictors such as methylene blue and hydroxocobalamin would likely not be helpful and in fact may be harmful due to increased afterload. Methylene blue also carries risks of pulmonary vasoconstriction and serotonin syndrome.

References:
1. Bainbri D, Cheng DCH. Chapter 37: Fast-Track Postoperative Cardiac Recovery and Outcomes. In: Kaplan JA, Augoustides JGT, Manecke GR, et al., eds. Kaplan's Cardiac Anesthesia. 7th ed. Elsevier; 2017:1313-1326.

2. Saura E, Savola J, Gunn J. A 6-year single-center experience of intra-aortic balloon pump treatment—retrospective analysis of 223 patients. J Cardiothorac Vasc Anesth, 2015; 29: 1410-1414.

23. Acute kidney injury after cardiac surgery is a common and important complication. What is a cause of intrinsic renal failure?

A. Hypovolemia

B. Low cardiac output

C. Nonsteroidal anti-inflammatory drugs

D. Obstructed bladder catheter

Correct Answer: C

Explanation: Nonsteroidal anti-inflammatory drugs inhibit cyclo-oxygenase enzymes and can lead to renal ischemia by blocking prostaglandin synthesis. Prostaglandins are important for medullary oxygenation, and with prolonged hypoxia can lead to acute tubular necrosis. Both hypovolemia and low cardiac output can be prerenal etiologies for acute kidney injury. An obstructed bladder catheter can be a postrenal cause of acute kidney injury if undetected.

References:

1. Bainbri D, Cheng DCH. Chapter 37: Fast-Track Postoperative Cardiac Recovery and Outcomes. In: Kaplan JA, Augoustides JGT, Manecke GR, et al., eds. Kaplan's Cardiac Anesthesia. 7th ed. Elsevier; 2017:1313-1326.
2. Chew STH, Hwang NC. Acute kidney injury after cardiac surgery: A narrative review of the literature. J Cardiothorac Vasc Anesth, 2019; 33: 1122-1138.

24. What is a preoperative risk factor for acute renal insufficiency after cardiac surgery?

A. Congestive heart failure

B. Tobacco abuse

C. Obesity

D. Obstructive sleep apnea

Correct Answer: A

Explanation: The typical preoperative risk factors for acute renal insufficiency after cardiac surgery include advanced age, hypertension, diabetes, and heart failure. As people age, renal function declines. Heart failure is a risk factor for acute kidney injury after cardiac surgery due to low renal perfusion pressure associated with a low ejection fraction, which may be exacerbated following cardiopulmonary bypass. This is a leading mechanism of prerenal insufficiency in cardiac surgical patients. Tobacco abuse, obesity, and obstructive sleep apnea have not been found to correlate with increased risk of acute renal insufficiency after cardiac surgery. This complication after cardiac surgery remains important because it is strongly associated with increased morbidity and mortality.

References:

1. Bainbri D, Cheng DCH. Chapter 37: Fast-Track Postoperative Cardiac Recovery and Outcomes. In: Kaplan JA, Augoustides JGT, Manecke GR, et al., eds. Kaplan's Cardiac Anesthesia. 7th ed. Elsevier; 2017:1313-1326.

2. Fernando RJ, Marchant BE, Jao GT, et al. Renal function and heart failure: assessment, goals, and perioperative implications. J Cardiothorac Vasc Anesth, 2020; 34: 3175-3179.

25. A 68-year-old male underwent coronary artery bypass grafting (CABG) with saphenous vein grafts for severe multivessel disease. Which of the following is FALSE concerning aspirin therapy?

A. Preoperative aspirin use prior to CABG has no effect on graft patency

B. Initiation of aspirin within 48 hours after CABG decreases mortality

C. Beneficial effects of aspirin on saphenous vein graft patency are greatly diminished at 1 year postoperatively

D. There are currently no alternative agent recommendations for graft patency in patients with an aspirin allergy

Correct Answer: D

Explanation: Early initiation of aspirin within 48 hours after coronary artery bypass grafting has been shown to decrease the risks of both postoperative mortality and myocardial infarction. The doses of aspirin for this indication may vary and can be given orally or by suppository. No additional benefit on graft patency results from the use of aspirin preoperatively, although other cardiovascular benefits may accrue with preoperative aspirin therapy.

The beneficial effect of aspirin on saphenous vein graft patency appears to be lost after 1 year, with prolonged use of aspirin having no further benefit. Clopidogrel, prasugrel, or ticagrelor may be suitable alternatives in patients who are allergic to aspirin. Clopidogrel, through reductions in all-cause mortality, stroke, and myocardial infarction, may be superior to aspirin in patients who return with recurrent ischemic events after cardiac operations.

References:

1. Bainbri D, Cheng DCH. Chapter 37: Fast-Track Postoperative Cardiac Recovery and Outcomes. In: Kaplan JA, Augoustides JGT, Manecke GR, et al., eds. Kaplan's Cardiac Anesthesia. 7th ed. Elsevier; 2017:1313-1326.
2. Goldhammer JE, Herman CR, Sun JZ. Perioperative aspirin in cardiac and noncardiac surgery. J Cardiothorac Vasc Anesth, 2017; 31: 1060-1070.

26. A 42-year-old male underwent a mitral valve replacement with a mechanical valve. He does not have a history of atrial fibrillation, previous thromboembolic event, left ventricular dysfunction, or hypercoagulable state. What is his anticoagulation goal?

A. Daily clopidogrel

B. Warfarin with a goal international normalized ratio of 2.0 to 3.0

C. Warfarin with a goal international normalized ratio of 2.5 to 3.5

D. Aspirin alone

Correct Answer: C

TABLE 33.3

Suggested antithrombotic therapy for heart valve prophylaxis

Source	Site	Mechanical Prosthesis Target INR		Bioprosthesis		
		No Risk Factors[a]	Risk Factors[a]	Aspirin	3 Months Postoperatively	>3 Months Postoperatively
ESC/EACTS	Aortic	2.5	3.0 or 3.5[b]	Selected[c]	Aspirin or VKA	/
	Mitral	3.0 or 3.5[b]	3.0 or 3.5[b]	Selected[c]	VKA	/
AHA/ACC	Aortic	2.5	3	Systematic	Aspirin or VKA	Aspirin
	Mitral	3	3	Systematic	VKA + aspirin	Aspirin
ACCP	Aortic	2.5	2.5	If low bleeding risk	Aspirin	Aspirin
	Mitral	3	3	If low bleeding risk	VKA + aspirin	Aspirin

[a]Risk factors include atrial fibrillation, previous thromboembolic event, left ventricular dysfunction, and hypercoagulable state.
[b]According to whether prosthesis has low or intermediate thrombogenicity.
[c]Patients with concomitant atherosclerotic disease or with thromboembolism despite adequate INR.
ACC, American College of Cardiology; *ACCP,* American College of Clinical Pharmacy; *AHA,* American Heart Association; *EACTS,* European Association for Cardio-Thoracic Surgery; *ESC,* European Society of Cardiology; *INR,* international normalized ratio; *VKA,* vitamin K antagonist.
From Iung B, Rodes-Cabau J. The optimal management of anti-thrombotic therapy after valve replacement: certainties and uncertainties. Eur Heart J. 2014;35:2942–2949.

Explanation: Warfarin with an international normalized ratio of 2.5 to 3.5 for life is the current class I recommendation according to the American College of Cardiology and American Heart Association guidelines. This is true whether or not the patient has other risk factors that also require anticoagulation. A goal international normalized ratio of 2.0 to 3.0 is recommended for mechanical valves in the aortic position.

Antiplatelet therapy alone in this setting has an increased risk of valvular thrombosis. In fact, clopidogrel and aspirin combined was also found to have increased risk of thrombosis compared to warfarin. Clinical guidelines have recommended the addition of aspirin therapy to warfarin in patients who have experienced a thromboembolic event while on warfarin, those with known vascular disease, or those with a susceptibility to hypercoagulable state. The use of direct-acting oral anticoagulants, such as factor Xa inhibitors and direct thrombin inhibitors, in patients with valve replacements is not presently recommended.

References:

1. Bainbri D, Cheng DCH. Chapter 37: Fast-Track Postoperative Cardiac Recovery and Outcomes. In: Kaplan JA, Augoustides JGT, Manecke GR, et al., eds. Kaplan's Cardiac Anesthesia. 7th ed. Elsevier; 2017:1313-1326.
2. Matiasz R, Rigolin VH. 2017 focused update for management of patients with valvular heart disease: summary of new recommendations. J Am Heart Assoc, 2018; 7: e007596.
3. Patel PA, Henderson RA, Bolliger D, et al. The year in coagulation: selected highlights from 2020. J Cardiothorac Vasc Anesth, 2021; 35: 2260-2272.
4. Martin AK, Mohananey D, Ranka S, et al. The 2017 European Society of Cardiology (ESC)/European Association of Cardiothoracic Surgeons (EACTS) guidelines for management of valvular heart disease-highlights and perioperative implications. J Cardiothorac Vasc Anesth, 2018; 32: 2810-2816.

27. A 52-year-old female has undergone an aortic valve replacement with a mechanical aortic valve. She does not have a history of atrial fibrillation, previous thromboembolic event, left ventricular dysfunction, or hypercoagulable state. What is her anticoagulation goal?

A. Clopidogrel alone
B. Warfarin with a goal international normalized ratio of 2.0 to 3.0
C. Warfarin with a goal international normalized ratio of 2.5 to 3.5
D. Aspirin alone

Correct Answer: B

Explanation: Warfarin with a goal international normalized ratio of 2.0 to 3.0 for life is the current class I recommendation according to the American College of Cardiology and American Heart Association guidelines. This is true regardless of whether the patient has other risk factors that also require anticoagulation. A goal international normalized ratio of 2.5 to 3.5 is recommended for mechanical valves in the mitral position.

Antiplatelet therapy alone has been shown to have increased risk of valvular thrombosis. Clinical guidelines have recommended the addition of aspirin therapy to warfarin in patients who have experienced a thromboembolic event while on warfarin, those with known vascular disease, or those with a susceptibility to hypercoagulable state. The use of direct-acting oral anticoagulants, such as factor Xa inhibitors and direct thrombin inhibitors, in patients with valve replacements is not presently recommended.

References:

1. Bainbri D, Cheng DCH. Chapter 37: Fast-Track Postoperative Cardiac Recovery and Outcomes. In: Kaplan JA, Augoustides JGT, Manecke GR, et al., eds. Kaplan's Cardiac Anesthesia. 7th ed. Elsevier; 2017:1313-1326.
2. Matiasz R, Rigolin VH. 2017 Focused update for management of patients with valvular heart disease: summary of new recommendations. J Am Heart Assoc, 2018; 7: e007596.
3. Martin AK, Mohananey D, Ranka S, et al. The 2017 European Society of Cardiology (ESC)/European Association of Cardiothoracic Surgeons (EACTS) guidelines for management of valvular heart disease-highlights and perioperative implications. J Cardiothorac Vasc Anesth, 2018; 32: 2810-2816.
4. Patel PA, Henderson RA, Bolliger D, et al. The year in coagulation: selected highlights from 2020. J Cardiothorac Vasc Anesth, 2021; 35: 2260-2272.

28. A 72-year-old female underwent a mitral valve replacement with a bioprosthetic valve. The patient does not have a history of any thromboembolic events or atrial fibrillation. What is the anticoagulation recommendation for this patient?
    A. Aspirin and warfarin for 3 months
    B. Warfarin for life with a goal international normalized ratio of 2.5 to 3.5
    C. Clopidogrel alone
    D. Aspirin alone

Correct Answer: A

Explanation: Aspirin and warfarin for least 3 to 6 months with a goal international normalized ratio of at least 2.5 is a class IIa recommendation from the American College of Cardiology and American Heart Association after surgical bioprosthetic mitral valve replacement in patients at low risk of bleeding. Antiplatelet therapy alone has been found to have increased risk of thrombosis compared to warfarin. Warfarin therapy is not recommended past 6 months in this setting, which is one of the reasons a bioprosthetic valve is preferred in patients in whom lifelong anticoagulation is undesirable. The use of direct-acting oral anticoagulants, such as factor Xa inhibitors and direct thrombin inhibitors, in patients with valve replacements is not presently recommended.

References:

1. Bainbri D, Cheng DCH. Chapter 37: Fast-Track Postoperative Cardiac Recovery and Outcomes. In: Kaplan JA, Augoustides JGT, Manecke GR, et al., eds. Kaplan's Cardiac Anesthesia. 7th ed. Elsevier; 2017:1313-1326.
2. Patel PA, Henderson RA, Bolliger D, et al. The year in coagulation: selected highlights from 2020. J Cardiothorac Vasc Anesth, 2021; 35: 2260-2272.
3. Matiasz R, Rigolin VH. 2017 Focused update for management of patients with valvular heart disease: summary of new recommendations. J Am Heart Assoc, 2018; 7: e007596.
4. Martin AK, Mohananey D, Ranka S, et al. The 2017 European Society of Cardiology (ESC)/European Association of Cardiothoracic Surgeons (EACTS) guidelines for

29. A 73-year-old female had an aortic valve replacement with a bioprosthetic valve. She does not have a history of a thromboembolic event, reduced ejection fraction, hypercoagulable state, or atrial fibrillation. What is the recommended medical regimen for this patient after surgery?
    A. Aspirin alone
    B. Warfarin for life with a goal international normalized ratio of 2.0 to 3.0
    C. Aspirin and warfarin for 3 months
    D. Clopidogrel alone

Correct Answer: A

Explanation: The American College of Cardiology and American Heart Association recommendation for the bioprosthetic valve in the aortic position is either aspirin or warfarin. For patients with no risk factors for thromboembolism (atrial fibrillation, a history of a thromboembolic event, a hypercoagulable condition, and severely reduced left ventricular systolic function), aspirin alone can be used. For patients with a risk factor and a bioprosthetic aortic valve, aspirin plus warfarin is recommended, with warfarin discontinuing at 3 to 6 months postoperatively.

It is believed that there is lower risk of thrombosis in the aortic position and less association with atrial fibrillation immediately postoperatively compared with mitral bioprosthetic valves. For this reason, mitral bioprosthetic valves are recommended for warfarin therapy for 3 to 6 months postoperatively, even in patients without a thromboembolic risk factor. Warfarin for life is not indicated for bioprosthetic valve replacements without another reason for anticoagulation. Clopidogrel alone is not a recommendation for any valve as isolated anticoagulation. The use of direct-acting oral anticoagulants, such as factor Xa inhibitors and direct thrombin inhibitors, in patients with valve replacements is not presently recommended.

References:

1. Bainbri D, Cheng DCH. Chapter 37: Fast-Track Postoperative Cardiac Recovery and Outcomes. In: Kaplan JA, Augoustides JGT, Manecke GR, et al., eds. Kaplan's Cardiac Anesthesia. 7th ed. Elsevier; 2017:1313-1326.
2. Patel PA, Henderson RA, Bolliger D, et al. The year in coagulation: selected highlights from 2020. J Cardiothorac Vasc Anesth, 2021; 35: 2260-2272.
3. Matiasz R, Rigolin VH. 2017 Focused update for management of patients with valvular heart disease: summary of new recommendations. J Am Heart Assoc, 2018; 7: e007596.
4. Martin AK, Mohananey D, Ranka S, et al. The 2017 European Society of Cardiology (ESC)/European Association of Cardiothoracic Surgeons (EACTS) guidelines for management of valvular heart disease-highlights and perioperative implications. J Cardiothorac Vasc Anesth, 2018; 32: 2810-2816.

30. A 75-year-old male had a bioprosthetic aortic valve 6 months ago. Although he has a history of atrial fibrillation, he has no previous thromboembolic event, left ventricular dysfunction, or hypercoagulable state. What is the recommendation for his anticoagulation treatment?
   A. Aspirin and warfarin for 6 additional months for a total of 1 year of therapy
   B. Warfarin for life with a goal international normalized ratio of 2.0 to 3.0
   C. Clopidogrel alone
   D. Aspirin alone

Correct Answer: D

Explanation: It is an American Heart Association and American College of Cardiology class IIb recommendation that aspirin alone can be used for patients with a bioprosthetic aortic valve in patients without any risk factors for thrombotic events (atrial fibrillation, a history of a thromboembolic event, a hypercoagulable condition, and severely reduced left ventricular systolic function). If there is a risk factor for a thrombotic event, warfarin should be added to aspirin for 3 to 6 months. Following this, warfarin can be stopped, but aspirin should be continued for life.

The European Society of Cardiology does not recommend an antiplatelet or anticoagulation after 3 months in either mitral or aortic bioprosthetic replacements. Clopidogrel alone is not a recommendation for mechanical or bioprosthetic valves. The use of direct-acting oral anticoagulants, such as factor Xa inhibitors and direct thrombin inhibitors, in patients with valve replacements is not presently recommended.

References:

1. Bainbri D, Cheng DCH. Chapter 37: Fast-Track Postoperative Cardiac Recovery and Outcomes. In: Kaplan JA, Augoustides JGT, Manecke GR, et al., eds. Kaplan's Cardiac Anesthesia. 7th ed. Elsevier; 2017:1313-1326.
2. Patel PA, Henderson RA, Bolliger D, et al. The year in coagulation: selected highlights from 2020. J Cardiothorac Vasc Anesth, 2021; 35: 2260-2272.
3. Matiasz R, Rigolin VH. 2017 Focused update for management of patients with valvular heart disease: summary of new recommendations. J Am Heart Assoc, 2018; 7: e007596.
4. Martin AK, Mohananey D, Ranka S, et al. The 2017 European Society of Cardiology (ESC)/European Association of Cardiothoracic Surgeons (EACTS) guidelines for management of valvular heart disease-highlights and perioperative implications. J Cardiothorac Vasc Anesth, 2018; 32: 2810-2816.

CHAPTER 34

Postoperative Cardiovascular Management

Jennette Hansen and Brigid Flynn

KEY POINTS

1. Maintaining oxygen transport and oxygen delivery appropriately to meet tissue metabolic needs is the goal of postoperative circulatory control.

2. Cardiac function worsens after cardiac surgical procedures. Therapeutic approaches to reverse this dysfunction are important and often can be discontinued in the first few postoperative days.

3. Myocardial ischemia often occurs postoperatively, and it is associated with adverse cardiac outcomes. Multiple strategies have been studied to reduce this complication.

4. Postoperative biventricular dysfunction is common. It requires interventions to optimize the heart rate and rhythm, provide acceptable preload, and adjust afterload and contractility. In most patients, pharmacologic interventions can be rapidly weaned or stopped within the first 24 hours postoperatively.

5. Supraventricular tachyarrhythmias are common in the first postoperative days, with atrial fibrillation predominating. Preoperative and immediate postoperative pharmacotherapy can reduce the incidence and slow the ventricular response.

6. Postoperative hypertension has been a common complication of cardiac surgical procedures; newer vasodilator drugs are more arterial selective and allow greater circulatory stability than older, nonselective drugs.

7. Catecholamines, phosphodiesterase inhibitors, and the calcium sensitizer levosimendan have been studied for treating biventricular dysfunction.

8. Phosphodiesterase inhibitors and levosimendan are clinically effective inodilators that have important roles in patients with low cardiac output and biventricular dysfunction.

9. Long cardiopulmonary bypass times may cause a refractory vasodilated state ("vasoplegia") requiring combinations of pressors such as norepinephrine and vasopressin.

10. Positive-pressure ventilation has multiple effects on the cardiovascular system, with complex interactions that should be considered in patients after cardiac surgical procedures.

11. Critical care management of patients undergoing transcatheter aortic valve replacement who have experienced intraoperative complications includes understanding and managing the postoperative consequences of iatrogenic vascular injuries, stroke, significant paravalvular leaks, and/or cardiac conduction abnormalities.

12. Hemodynamic management after cardiothoracic operations may benefit from the use of transesophageal echocardiography to determine myocardial function and assess cardiovascular structures. Echocardiography is particularly helpful in the diagnosis of causes of obstructive shock, including pericardial effusions leading to tamponade physiology.

13. Echocardiography during the daily management of both venovenous and venoarterial extracorporeal membrane oxygenation (ECMO) may improve diagnosis of hemodynamic instability, troubleshoot common problems encountered during ECMO management, and aid in weaning the patient from mechanical support.

1. Based on the components of the oxygen delivery formula, what would be the most expedient method to improve oxygen delivery?
   A. Blood transfusion
   B. Dialysis
   C. Diuresis
   D. Intravenous iron

Correct Answer: A

Explanation: Oxygen delivery (DO_2) is determined by cardiac output (CO), arterial content of hemoglobin (Hb), and to a lesser extent oxygen saturation (SpO_2). Arterial content (CaO_2) is determined by (hemoglobin $\times$ 1.34 mL of oxygen per 1 g of hemoglobin) $\times$ (0.003 $\times$ partial pressure of oxygen [PaO_2]):

$$DO_2 = CO \times CaO_2$$
$$DO_2 = CO \times (1.34 \times Hb \times SpO_2) + (0.003 \times PaO_2)$$

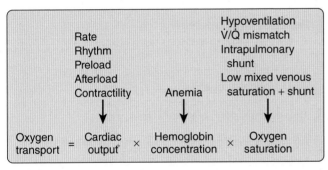

FIGURE 34.1 Important factors that contribute to abnormal oxygen transport. *V/Q*, Ventilation/perfusion.

Dialysis could be extrapolated to increase DO_2 due to beneficial effects on correction of hypervolemia leading to improved cardiac output and V/Q matching. However, blood transfusion would increase hemoglobin, which is a component of the DO_2 calculation as posed in the question. Also, volume status is unknown in this situation. Similarly, diuresis can be extrapolated to improvement of cardiac output due to optimization of filling pressures assuming a patient is fluid-overloaded. Intravenous iron may improve hemoglobin level in an iron-deficient patient, but this is not an expedient therapy to improve DO_2.

References:

1. Levy JH, Ghadimi K, Bailey JM, et al. Chapter 38: Postoperative Cardiovascular Management. In: Kaplan JA, Augoustides JGT, Manecke GR, et al., eds. Kaplan's Cardiac Anesthesia. 7th ed. Elsevier; 2017:1327-1357.
2. Burtman DTM, Stolze A, Dengelr SEKG, et al. Minimally invasive determinations of oxygen delivery and consumption in cardiac surgery: an observational study. J Cardiothorac Vasc Anesth, 2018; 32: 1266-1272.

2. A 75-year-old male has undergone a mitral valve repair and coronary artery bypass surgery. After arrival to the intensive care unit, his blood pressure is 98/62 mmHg, pulmonary artery pressure 45/22 mmHg, central venous pressure 12 mmHg, and cardiac index 1.6 L/min/m². The patient was on moderate-dose norepinephrine. His blood gases were reassuring for adequate oxygenation and ventilation, and his hemoglobin was 11.2 g/dL. What should be done to improve this patient's oxygen delivery?
   A. Blood transfusion
   B. Add epinephrine infusion
   C. Diuresis
   D. Intravenous iron

Correct Answer: B

Explanation: Oxygen delivery is determined by cardiac output multiplied by arterial oxygen content. Addition of epinephrine would improve oxygen delivery most because the patient's hemoglobin is above 10 g/dL. There is evidence that there are no benefits to transfusing patients to a hemoglobin greater than 10 g/dL. Epinephrine would improve cardiac output secondary to inotropic support increasing cardiac output.

$$DO_2 = CO \times CaO_2$$
$$DO_2 = CO \times (1.34 \times Hb \times SpO_2) + (0.003 \times PaO_2)$$

Diuresis would not be the correct answer as the patient does not appear to be volume-overloaded due to near normal central venous pressure and adequate oxygenation, but echocardiography could add to this assumption. Intravenous iron would not be indicated at this time to improve oxygen delivery, as it would take time for this therapy to increase hemoglobin levels and thus indirectly increase oxygen delivery. The patient may need an iron supplement in the future, but it would not necessarily need to be intravenous, and not enough information was provided to determine if he was iron-deficient. Although a blood transfusion may increase oxygen delivery, it may also lead to increased viscosity and decreased coronary blood flow in narrow anastomoses. Additionally, the increase in oxygen delivery when increasing hemoglobin levels from adequate levels as in this patient to supra-adequate levels is negligible and may carry risk due to increased viscosity. Finally, guidelines do not recommend blood transfusions for hemoglobin levels more than 10 g/dL in cardiac surgical patients.

References:

1. Levy JH, Ghadimi K, Bailey JM, et al. Chapter 38: Postoperative Cardiovascular Management. In: Kaplan JA, Augoustides JGT, Manecke GR, et al., eds. Kaplan's Cardiac Anesthesia. 7th ed. Elsevier; 2017:1327-1357.
2. Burtman DTM, Stolze A, Dengelr SEKG, et al. Minimally invasive determinations of oxygen delivery and consumption in cardiac surgery: an observational study. J Cardiothorac Vasc Anesth, 2018; 32: 1266-1272.

3. A 55-year-old male is admitted to the intensive care unit after coronary artery bypass grafting and mitral valve repair earlier that day. The patient has an ejection fraction of 50% and depressed right ventricular function. What is not a direct sequalae of postoperative right ventricular failure?

A. Bronchial mucous plugging
B. Tricuspid regurgitation
C. Opening of patent foreman ovale
D. Displaced septum

Correct Answer: A

Explanation: Right ventricular failure can lead to many deleterious effects following cardiac surgery.

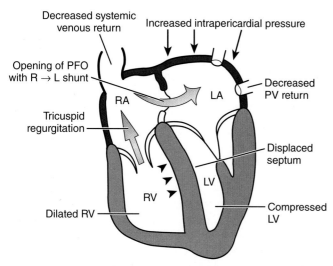

FIGURE 34.2 Mechanical changes produced by acute right ventricular failure. *LA*, Left atrium; *LV*, left ventricle; *PFO*, patent foramen ovale; *PV*, pulmonary venous; *R → L*, right-to-left; *RA*, right atrium; *RV*, right ventricle.

Increased right ventricular pressure can lead to opening of patent foreman ovale, tricuspid regurgitation, septal displacement, decreased systemic venous return, and ultimately decreased left ventricular ejection fraction and whole body oxygen deprivation. Bronchial mucous plugging should always be considered in unstable ventilated patients, but this is not directly related to right ventricular failure.

References:

1. Levy JH, Ghadimi K, Bailey JM, et al. Chapter 38: Postoperative Cardiovascular Management. In: Kaplan JA, Augoustides JGT, Manecke GR, et al., eds. Kaplan's Cardiac Anesthesia. 7th ed. Elsevier; 2017:1327-1357.
2. Patel PA, Hall A, Augoustides JG, et al. Dynamic shunting across a patent foramen ovale in adult cardiac surgery-perioperative challenges and management. J Cardiothorac Vasc Anesth, 2018; 32: 542-549.

4. Beneficial therapies aimed at directly treating postcardiotomy right ventricular failure include all of the following, EXCEPT:

A. Intravenous nitroprusside
B. Addition of inhaled nitric oxide
C. Addition of milrinone
D. Increased positive end-expiratory pressure to 12 mmHg

Correct Answer: D

Explanation: Nitroprusside is a pulmonary arterial dilator acting via the cyclic guanosine monophosphate pathway. The mechanism of nitroprusside is similar to that of inhaled nitric oxide, which relaxes the smooth muscles of the airways to dilate the pulmonary vasculature. Both of these therapies decrease pulmonary artery vascular resistance, which directly decreases right ventricular afterload and improves right ventricular cardiac output. Milrinone is an inodilator that not

---

BOX 34.1   Treatment approaches in postoperative right-sided heart failure

Preload Augmentation
- Volume, vasopressors, or leg elevation (CVP/PCWP <1)
- Decrease juxtacardiac pressures (pericardium and/or chest open)
- Establishment of atrial kick and treatment of atrial arrhythmias (sinus rhythm, atrial pacing)

Afterload Reduction (Pulmonary Vasodilation)
- Nitroglycerin, isosorbide dinitrate nesiritide
- cAMP-specific phosphodiesterase inhibitors, α_2-adrenergic agonists
- Inhaled nitric oxide
- Nebulized PGI_2
- Intravenous PGE_1 (and left atrial norepinephrine)

Inotropic Support
- cAMP-specific phosphodiesterase inhibitors, isoproterenol, dobutamine
- Norepinephrine
- Levosimendan

Ventilatory Management
- Lower intrathoracic pressures (tidal volume <7 mL/kg, low PEEP)
- Attenuation of hypoxic vasoconstriction (high FiO_2)
- Avoidance of respiratory acidosis ($PaCO_2$ 30–35 mmHg, metabolic control with meperidine or relaxants)

Mechanical Support
- Intra-aortic counterpulsation
- Pulmonary artery counterpulsation
- Right ventricular assist devices

cAMP, Cyclic adenosine monophosphate; *CVP/PCWP*, central venous pressure/pulmonary capillary wedge pressure; *FiO₂*, fraction of inspired oxygen; *PaCO₂*, partial pressure of arterial carbon dioxide; *PEEP*, positive end-expiratory pressure; *PGI₂*, prostaglandin I₂; *PGE₁*, prostaglandin E₁.

only increases right ventricular cardiac output (along with left ventricular cardiac output), but also acts as a pulmonary vasodilator by inhibiting phosphodiesterase action. Increasing the positive end-expiratory pressure (PEEP) to 12 mmHg would further increase right heart afterload by increasing intrathoracic pressure and would worsen right ventricular cardiac output. Furthermore, the increased PEEP may decrease venous return to the right heart that could lead to a further fall in right ventricular end-diastolic volume and subsequent cardiac output.

References:

1. Levy JH, Ghadimi K, Bailey JM, et al. Chapter 38: Postoperative Cardiovascular Management. In: Kaplan JA, Augoustides JGT, Manecke GR, et al., eds. Kaplan's Cardiac Anesthesia. 7th ed. Elsevier; 2017:1327-1357.
2. Patel PA, Hall A, Augoustides JGT, et al. Dynamic shunting across a patent foramen ovale in adult cardiac surgery-perioperative challenges and management. J Cardiothorac Vasc Anesth, 2018; 32: 542-549.

5. A 70-year-old male with past medical history of tobacco abuse, chronic obstructive pulmonary disease, and coronary disease arrived to the intensive care unit after coronary artery bypass surgery on moderate-dose norepinephrine. He was reported to have normal biventricular function without significant valve abnormalities. He remains on the ventilator with protocolized settings. Of the following choices, what is the best predictor of volume responsiveness in this patient?
   A. Baseline pulmonary artery systolic pressure
   B. Baseline pulmonary artery occlusion pressure
   C. Baseline central venous pressure
   D. Pulse pressure variation

Correct Answer: D

Explanation: Pulse pressure variation has been found to be a better predictor of fluid responsiveness in mechanically ventilated patients than baseline pulmonary artery occlusion pressure, pulmonary artery systolic pressure, and central venous pressure. It was found that patients with goal-directed therapy based on pulse pressure variation had less morbidity than traditional methods of measuring volume responsiveness. Pronounced pulse pressure variation with mechanical ventilation can be associated with decreased filling pressures and resultant low cardiac output. Pulse pressure is highly dependent on stroke volume and is therefore influenced by all factors that determine stroke volume (preload, afterload, and contractility). It has been shown that, in the cardiac surgical population, following the baseline values for filling pressures can be misleading and results in less improvement in stroke volume index than pulse pressure variation when relied upon for volume resuscitation.

References:

1. Levy JH, Ghadimi K, Bailey JM, et al. Chapter 38: Postoperative Cardiovascular Management. In: Kaplan JA, Augoustides JGT, Manecke GR, et al., eds. Kaplan's Cardiac Anesthesia. 7th ed. Elsevier; 2017:1327-1357.

2. Yazigi A, Khoury E, Hlais S, et al. Pulse pressure variation predicts fluid responsiveness in elderly patients after coronary artery bypass graft surgery. J Cardiothorac Vasc Anesth, 2012; 26: 387-390.

6. The following are risk factors for new-onset low cardiac output following cardiopulmonary bypass, EXCEPT:
   A. Valvular surgery
   B. Poor myocardial preservation
   C. Hypertension
   D. Long duration of aortic cross clamp

Correct Answer: C

Explanation: Low cardiac output following cardiac surgery can lead to multiple deleterious injuries and end-organ damage. Known risk factors for new-onset low cardiac output following cardiopulmonary bypass include preoperative left ventricular dysfunction, valvular surgery, long aortic cross clamp and/or total cardiopulmonary bypass time, inadequate surgical repair, ischemia/reperfusion injury, residual cardioplegia, poor myocardial preservation, and reperfusion injury with inflammatory changes. Prevention and treatment are aimed towards ensuring all elements of oxygen delivery are satisfactory. Oxygen transport is the product of cardiac output times arterial oxygen content (CaO_2). CaO_2 is composed of hemoglobin concentration $\times$ 1.34 mL of oxygen per 1 g of hemoglobin $\times$ oxygen saturation.

> **BOX 34.2   Risk factors for low cardiac output syndrome after cardiopulmonary bypass**
>
> - Preoperative left ventricular dysfunction
> - Valvular heart disease requiring repair or replacement
> - Long aortic cross clamp time and total cardiopulmonary bypass time
> - Inadequate cardiac surgical repair
> - Myocardial ischemia and reperfusion
> - Residual effects of cardioplegia solution
> - Poor myocardial preservation
> - Reperfusion injury and inflammatory changes

References:

1. Levy JH, Ghadimi K, Bailey JM, et al. Chapter 38: Postoperative Cardiovascular Management. In: Kaplan JA, Augoustides JGT, Manecke GR, et al., eds. Kaplan's Cardiac Anesthesia. 7th ed. Elsevier; 2017:1327-1357.
2. Lomivorotov VV, Efremov SM, Kirov MT, et al. Low-cardiac-output syndrome after cardiac surgery. J Cardiothorac Vasc Anesth, 2017; 31: 291-308.

7. Which drug increases cyclic guanosine monophosphate and has been studied in high-risk cardiac surgical patients to decrease afterload while increasing stroke volume, cardiac output, and natriuresis?
   A. Milrinone
   B. Nesiritide
   C. Dobutamine
   D. Epinephrine

Correct Answer: B

Explanation: Nesiritide is a medication that has been approved for patients with decompensated heart failure with dyspnea at rest or minimal activity. It was found to improve dyspnea symptoms and pulmonary capillary wedge pressure. It was also found in high-risk cardiac surgical patients with poor left ventricular function to improve renal function and 6-month mortality in one study. Caution must be used, as it is associated with hypotension due to vasodilation via cyclic guanosine monophosphate (cGMP) activation. However, this cGMP activation is also the reason for vasodilation of the systemic, pulmonary, and coronary vascular beds, which can be beneficial to high-risk patients.

Nesiritide peaks in 6 hours; therefore it may be a better medication to be used in the intensive care unit than in the operating room. Nesiritide was also found to reduce norepinephrine levels and renin release. Nesiritide improves lusitropy and induces diuresis through natriuresis.

TABLE 34.1
Novel vasodilators

Drug	Mechanism of Action	Half-Life
Nicardipine	Calcium channel blocker	Intermediate
Clevidipine	Calcium channel blocker	Ultrashort
Fenoldopam	Dopamine$_1$ agonist	Ultrashort
Nesiritide	Brain natriuretic agonist	Short
Levosimendan	K$^+$$_{ATP}$ channel modulator	Intermediate

K$^+$$_{ATP}$, Adenosine triphosphate–sensitive potassium channel.

Milrinone does share many qualities of nesiritide, but milrinone works through inhibition of breakdown of cyclic adenosine monophosphate (cAMP) via phosphodiesterase inhibition. Milrinone does cause reductions in preload and afterload. Milrinone does not directly cause natiuresis. Dobutamine can improve cardiac output and stroke volume with beta$_1$ receptor activation and increases in cAMP. Epinephrine is a potent inotropic and vasopressor medication that is accompanied by increases in cAMP.

References:

1. Levy JH, Ghadimi K, Bailey JM, et al. Chapter 38: Postoperative Cardiovascular Management. In: Kaplan JA, Augoustides JGT, Manecke GR, et al., eds. Kaplan's Cardiac Anesthesia. 7th ed. Elsevier; 2017:1327-1357.
2. Skidmore KL, Russell IA. Brain natriuretic peptide: a diagnostic and treatment hormone for perioperative congestive heart failure. J Cardiothorac Vasc Anesth, 2004; 18: 780-787.

8. A patient is found to have low blood pressure and low cardiac output. What single medication would best improve the hemodynamics of this patient?
   A. Epinephrine
   B. Milrinone
   C. Nicardipine
   D. Vasopressin

Correct Answer: A

Explanation: Epinephrine would be the most indicated in a patient with low cardiac output and low blood pressure if a single agent is desired. Epinephrine improves inotropy to improve cardiac output through beta$_1$ receptor activation, but also increases systemic vascular resistance through alpha$_1$ receptor activation. Improving both cardiac output and increasing systemic vascular resistance would increase blood pressure. Epinephrine also has adrenergic effects on beta$_2$ and alpha$_2$ receptors. Milrinone would improve cardiac output through inhibition of cyclic adenosine monophosphate breakdown but would lower systemic blood pressure secondary to vasodilation. Nicardipine is a vasodilator and would lower systemic blood pressure. Vasopressin would only increase systemic vascular resistance and is not an inotrope.

TABLE 34.2
Hemodynamic therapy guidelines

Blood Pressure	Cardiac Output	Treatment
Low	Low	Inotrope
Normal	Low	Vasodilator with or without inotrope
High	Low	Vasodilator
Low	High	Vasopressor

References:

1. Levy JH, Ghadimi K, Bailey JM, et al. Chapter 38: Postoperative Cardiovascular Management. In: Kaplan JA, Augoustides JGT, Manecke GR, et al., eds. Kaplan's Cardiac Anesthesia. 7th ed. Elsevier; 2017:1327-1357.
2. Lomivorotov VV, Efremov SM, Kirov MT, et al. Low-cardiac-output syndrome after cardiac surgery. J Cardiothorac Vasc Anesth, 2017; 31: 291-308.

9. A patient is found to have low blood pressure with normal cardiac output. What single medication would BEST increase blood pressure in this patient?
   A. Epinephrine
   B. Milrinone
   C. Nicardipine
   D. Norepinephrine

Correct Answer: D

Explanation: Of the options listed, the best answer is norepinephrine. Norepinephrine improves blood pressure by increasing systemic vascular resistance via alpha$_1$ adrenergic agonism. Norepinephrine also has beta$_1$ adrenergic receptor agonist effects, which will increase heart rate. Vasopressin acts via V$_1$ receptor to increase systemic vascular resistance and would be another good option as a first-line treatment for hypotension. In fact, vasopressin and norepinephrine act synergistically such that less of each medication is needed when used together. Epinephrine would improve the blood pressure, but would not be indicated in a patient with normal cardiac output. Milrinone would worsen the patient's blood pressure, and the patient currently does not need improvement in cardiac output. Nicardipine would lower the patient's blood pressure through vasodilation.

References:

1. Levy JH, Ghadimi K, Bailey JM, et al. Chapter 38: Postoperative Cardiovascular Management. In: Kaplan JA, Augoustides JGT, Manecke GR, et al., eds. Kaplan's Cardiac Anesthesia. 7th ed. Elsevier; 2017:1327-1357.
2. Guarracino F, Habicher M, Treskatsch S, et al. Vasopressor therapy in cardiac surgery-an experts consensus statement. J Cardiothorac Anesth, 2021; 35: 1018-1029.
3. Landry D, Oliver JA. Vasopressin in septic shock. N Engl J Med, 2008; 358: 2736-2737.

10. A patient is found to have low cardiac output with high blood pressure. What single medication would improve this patient's hemodynamics?
  A. Epinephrine
  B. Milrinone
  C. Nicardipine
  D. Norepinephrine

Correct Answer: B

Explanation: Milrinone is a phosphodiesterase III inhibitor. Phosphodiesterase breaks down cyclic adenosine monophosphate (cAMP), so inhibition of this molecule increases the amount of cAMP available. cAMP increases inotropy while causing both systemic and pulmonary vasodilation. Thus, milrinone is an ideal agent when cardiac output needs to be increased and vasodilation is desired, such as in a hypertensive patient. Like most inotropes, milrinone is associated with increased arrhythmias. Milrinone is renally cleared, and thus will have a longer half-life in patients with renal dysfunction. Epinephrine would improve cardiac output, but also increase blood pressure. Nicardipine would lower blood pressure without supplying inotropic support. Norepinephrine would increase the patient's blood pressure with minimal assistance with inotropic support.

References:

1. Levy JH, Ghadimi K, Bailey JM, et al. Chapter 38: Postoperative Cardiovascular Management. In: Kaplan JA, Augoustides JGT, Manecke GR, et al., eds. Kaplan's Cardiac Anesthesia. 7th ed. Elsevier; 2017:1327-1357.
2. Lomivorotov VV, Efremov SM, Kirov MT, et al. Low-cardiac-output syndrome after cardiac surgery. J Cardiothorac Vasc Anesth, 2017; 31: 291-308.

11. The following drugs have vasodilatory properties, EXCEPT:
  A. Nicardipine
  B. Furosemide
  C. Diphenhydramine
  D. Lisinopril

Correct Answer: C

Explanation: Nicardipine is a dihydropyridine calcium channel blocker and as such acts as an arterial vasodilator and antihypertensive. Furosemide can cause a direct vasodilation by acting on receptors in the vascular wall. A secondary effect of loop diuretics is to increase the production of prostaglandins, which results in vasodilation and increased blood supply to the kidney. Vasodilation following furosemide administration is also seen in the pulmonary vasculature due to prostaglandin synthesis. Diphenhydramine mainly works through antagonizing the histamine 1 (H1) receptor, although it has other mechanisms of action as well. When the H1 receptor is stimulated in these tissues, it produces a wide variety of actions, including increased vascular permeability and promotion of vasodilation, which is counteracted by diphenhydramine. Lisinopril is an angiotensin-converting enzyme inhibitor that decreases blood pressure through vasodilation.

References:

1. Levy JH, Ghadimi K, Bailey JM, et al. Chapter 38: Postoperative Cardiovascular Management. In: Kaplan JA, Augoustides JGT, Manecke GR, et al., eds. Kaplan's Cardiac Anesthesia. 7th ed. Elsevier; 2017:1327-1357.
2. Mukai A, Suehiro K, Kimura A, et al. Effect of systemic vascular resistance on the reliability of noninvasive hemodynamic monitoring in cardiac surgery. J Cardiothorac Vasc Anesth, 2021; 35: 1782-1791.
3. Huang X, Mees ED, Vos P, et al. Everything we always wanted to know about furosemide but were afraid to ask. Am J Physiol Renal Physiol, 2016; 310: 958-971.

12. A 75-year-old female has just undergone a coronary artery bypass surgery with four bypasses performed, including a left internal mammary graft. Upon handoff to the intensive care unit, it was said she has no regional wall motion abnormalities, and her ejection fraction is 55%. She is on minimal-dose norepinephrine to maintain a mean arterial pressure of 65 mmHg. She does not have a pulmonary artery catheter. Eight hours later she develops ST elevation in leads V2 and V3 with an acute drop in blood pressure. Chest tubes have lost 25 mL/h the last 2 hours. What is the most likely diagnosis?
  A. Cardiac tamponade
  B. Surgical bleeding
  C. Spasm of a conduit
  D. Vasoplegia

Correct Answer: C

Explanation: Spasm of a conduit is the most correct answer and is most commonly due to the internal mammary arterial bypass conduit. She has electrocardiogram (ECG) changes in the anterior wall leads, which is the location usually bypassed with the left internal mammary to the left anterior descending artery. The patient could have cardiac tamponade, and the clinician should have a high index of suspicion. However, chest tube output has been minimal, and cardiac tamponade does not typically induce regional ST elevations. Surgical bleeding is unlikely, as she has not had a large amount of blood from her chest tubes, and also this would not induce ST elevations. Vasoplegia would present with decreased blood pressure due to decreased systemic vascular resistance and generally does not occur acutely, nor would vasoplegia cause ECG changes. In this setting, graft patency should be evaluated thoroughly, potentially with emergent cardiac catheterization to ensure a stent is not needed. The treatment for conduit vasospasm includes coronary vasodilators such as nitroglyderin and/or calcium channel blockers such as nicardipine.

References:

1. Levy JH, Ghadimi K, Bailey JM, et al. Chapter 38: Postoperative Cardiovascular Management. In: Kaplan JA, Augoustides JGT, Manecke GR, et al., eds. Kaplan's Cardiac Anesthesia. 7th ed. Elsevier; 2017:1327-1357.
2. Valle MD, Hallander K. Diffuse coronary artery spasm after coronary artery bypass graft surgery. J Cardiothorac Vasc Anesth, 2002; 36: 2575-2577.
3. Carmona P, Monge E, Canal MI, et al. Coronary vasospasm-induced malignant arrhythmias and acute coronary syndrome in aortic surgery. J Cardiothorac Vasc Anesth, 2008; 22: 864-867.

13. A 71-year-old male has just undergone a coronary artery bypass surgery with four bypasses performed, including a left internal mammary graft. No regional wall motion abnormalities were noted, and his ejection fraction is 55%. Eight hours later he develops ST-elevations in leads V2 and V3 with an acute drop in systemic blood pressure. Emergent coronary angiography is negative for graft occlusion. Based on the likely diagnosis, what is the BEST treatment?
    A. Epinephrine
    B. Packed red blood cells
    C. Nitroglycerin
    D. Vasopressin

Correct Answer: C

Explanation: Vasospasm typically occurs several hours after coronary artery bypass surgery in the intensive care unit. Vasospasm occurs when the balance of vasoconstrictors and vasodilating agents becomes skewed, with the vasoconstrictors prevailing. Nitroglycerin along with dihydropyridine calcium channel blockers such as nicardipine are first-choice treatments for vasospasm. Vasodilators are used until the vasospasm resolves. Phosphodiesterase inhibition with agents such as milrinone may have a role for relief of coronary vasospasm, although the acute systemic hypotension would be concerning.

Epinephrine will likely improve systemic blood pressure and provide inotropic support, but it is not specific for alleviating vasospasm. Vasopressin and packed red blood cell transfusion would improve the systemic blood pressure but would not aid in alleviating coronary vasospasm.

References:

1. Levy JH, Ghadimi K, Bailey JM, et al. Chapter 38: Postoperative Cardiovascular Management. In: Kaplan JA, Augoustides JGT,

Manecke GR, et al., eds. Kaplan's Cardiac Anesthesia. 7th ed. Elsevier; 2017:1327-1357.
2. Gaudino M, Antoniades C, Benedetto U, et al. Mechanisms, consequences, and prevention of coronary graft failure. Circulation, 2017; 136: 1749-1764.
3. Carmona P, Monge E, Canal MI, et al. Coronary vasospasm-induced malignant arrhythmias and acute coronary syndrome in aortic surgery. J Cardiothorac Vasc Anesth, 2008; 22: 864-867.

14. A patient underwent coronary artery bypass grafting that included a radial artery conduit. Which medication has modest evidence supporting use in prevention of radial graft vasospasm?
    A. Norepinephrine
    B. Nicardipine
    C. Fenoldopam
    D. Vasopressin

Correct Answer: B

Explanation: The radial artery is often used as a bypass conduit for coronary revascularization. This conduit is known to have a propensity to spasm. However, techniques developed in the use of the internal mammary artery have been applied to the radial artery, as well as prophylactic application of calcium channel blocker infusions. The arterial selectivity of the dihydropyridine drugs such as nicardipine offers an advantage in this setting. Norepinephrine and vasopressin are vasoconstrictors that may worsen graft vasospasm. Fenoldopam is a dopamine receptor agonist that leads to vasodilation but was not found to influence coronary conduit blood flow to a clinically significant extent.

References:

1. Levy JH, Ghadimi K, Bailey JM, et al. Chapter 38: Postoperative Cardiovascular Management. In: Kaplan JA, Augoustides JGT, Manecke GR, et al., eds. Kaplan's Cardiac Anesthesia. 7th ed. Elsevier; 2017:1327-1357.
2. Gaudino M, Antoniades C, Benedetto U, et al. Mechanisms, consequences, and prevention of coronary graft failure. Circulation, 2017; 136: 1749-1764.
3. Halpenny M, Lakshmi S, O'Donnell A, et al. The effects of fenoldopam on coronary conduit blood flow after coronary artery bypass graft surgery. J Cardiothorac Vasc Anesth, 2001; 15: 72-76.

15. Following aortic valve replacement, a patient has high chest tube output for several hours and hemodynamic instability requiring multiple blood and component transfusions. Three hours into resuscitation, chest tube output decreases, and central venous pressure increases to 22 mmHg from normal baseline. What is the MOST likely diagnosis?
    A. Sepsis
    B. Myocardial infarction
    C. Aortic suture line dehiscence
    D. Cardiac tamponade

Correct Answer: D

Explanation: The mechanism of hemodynamic deterioration during cardiac tamponade is the result of impaired filling of one or more of the cardiac chambers due to blood compression. As the external pressure on the heart increases, the distending or transmural pressure (external intracavitary pressure) is decreased. The intracavitary pressure increases leading to impaired venous return and elevation of the central venous pressure. If the external pressure is high enough to exceed the ventricular pressure during diastole, diastolic ventricular collapse occurs. As the end-diastolic volume and end-systolic volume decrease, a concomitant reduction in stroke volume occurs. In the most severe form of cardiac tamponade, ventricular filling occurs only during atrial systole. Sepsis would not be expected in the immediate postoperative period. Myocardial infarction is not common following aortic valve replacement and would likely present with electrocardiogram changes accompanying hypotension. Aortic valve dehiscence is very rare and would likely present with high chest tube output that is difficult to maintain with resuscitation and without an increase in central venous pressure, but likely a decrease.

References:

1. Levy JH, Ghadimi K, Bailey JM, et al. Chapter 38: Postoperative Cardiovascular Management. In: Kaplan JA, Augoustides JGT, Manecke GR, et al., eds. Kaplan's Cardiac Anesthesia. 7th ed. Elsevier; 2017:1327-1357.
2. Carmona P, Mateo E, Casanovas I, et al. Management of cardiac tamponade after cardiac surgery. J Cardiothorac Vasc Anesth, 2012; 26: 302-311.

16. The following medications increase heart rate, EXCEPT:
   A. Vasopressin
   B. Dobutamine
   C. Epinephrine
   D. Norepinephrine

Correct Answer: A

Explanation: Vasopressin does not increase heart rate and may lead to bradycardia due to reflex bradycardia following increase in systemic vascular resistance. Dobutamine, epinephrine, and norepinephrine all increase heart rate by direct activation of beta$_1$ adrenergic receptor. Dobutamine has been cited as inducing more tachycardia than epinephrine in healthy myocardium. Isoproterenol is another beta agonist that is known to increase heart rate to a great extent and can lead to dysrhythmias.

References:

1. Levy JH, Ghadimi K, Bailey JM, et al. Chapter 38: Postoperative Cardiovascular Management. In: Kaplan JA, Augoustides JGT, Manecke GR, et al., eds. Kaplan's Cardiac Anesthesia. 7th ed. Elsevier; 2017:1327-1357.
2. Guarracino F, Habicher M, Treskatsch S, et al. Vasopressor therapy in cardiac surgery-an experts consensus statement. J Cardiothorac Anesth, 2021; 35: 1018-1029.

17. Which medication increases cyclic adenosine monophosphate through phosphodiesterase inhibition to improve lusitropy and contractility?
   A. Epinephrine
   B. Norepinephrine
   C. Milrinone
   D. Vasopressin

Correct Answer: C

Explanation: Milrinone is a phosphodiesterase III inhibitor. Phosphodiesterase breaks down cyclic adenosine monophosphate (cAMP), so inhibition of this molecule increases the amount of cAMP available. cAMP increases inotropy while causing both systemic and pulmonary vasodilation. Thus, milrinone is an ideal agent when cardiac output needs to be increased and vasodilation is desired. Milrinone can also be a useful agent to increase cAMP in patients who have beta$_1$ receptor downregulation, due to heart failure. Milrinone has been found to improve both lusitropy and contractility. Milrinone decreases preload, afterload, and pulmonary vascular resistance. Epinephrine improves contractility but does not improve lusitropy. Norepinephrine increases cAMP through beta$_1$ receptor activation improving contractility but does not improve lusitropy. Vasopressin is a vasoconstrictor that does not improve contractility or lusitropy, but rather increases systemic vascular resistance by activating endothelial V$_1$ receptor.

References:

1. Levy JH, Ghadimi K, Bailey JM, et al. Chapter 38: Postoperative Cardiovascular Management. In: Kaplan JA, Augoustides JGT, Manecke GR, et al., eds. Kaplan's Cardiac Anesthesia. 7th ed. Elsevier; 2017:1327-1357.
2. Ushio M, Egi M, Wakabayashi J, et al. Impact of milrinone administration in adult cardiac surgery patients: updated meta-analysis. J Cardiothorac Vasc Anesth, 2016; 30: 1454-1460.

18. A 64-year-old patient who underwent a coronary artery bypass grafting procedure had a prolonged intensive care unit stay due to right ventricular failure. The patient required inhaled nitric oxide (iNO) for several days and is now undergoing attempts to wean off. What can assist in hemodynamic stability during iNO wean?
   A. Isoproterenol
   B. Sildenafil
   C. Vasopressin
   D. Lisinopril

Correct Answer: B

Explanation: Sildenafil is a phosphodiesterase-5 inhibitor that increases cyclic guanosine monophosphate (cGMP), leading to relaxation of smooth muscle in the pulmonary and coronary vascular beds. The main effect is a decrease in pulmonary vascular resistance. Inhaled nitric oxide (iNO) also activates cGMP leading to potent pulmonary vasodilation.

However, iNO eventually needs to be weaned off and in doing so can elicit deleterious rebound pulmonary vasoconstriction, especially if weaned quickly. Sildenafil administration during iNO has been shown to provide pulmonary vascular vasodilation and assistance in successful iNO wean. This is especially necessary for patients with right ventricular failure who cannot tolerate increased pulmonary vascular resistance. Sildenafil has minimal systemic vasodilatory effects but can lead to systemic hypotension. Furthermore, sildenafil increases cardiac output. None of the other choices are known for pulmonary vasodilation effects and have not been studied in the setting of iNO weaning.

References:

1. Levy JH, Ghadimi K, Bailey JM, et al. Chapter 38: Postoperative Cardiovascular Management. In: Kaplan JA, Augoustides JGT, Manecke GR, et al., eds. Kaplan's Cardiac Anesthesia. 7th ed. Elsevier; 2017:1327-1357.
2. Raja SG, Danton MD, MacArthur KJ, et al. Treatment of pulmonary hypertension with sildenafil: from pathophysiology to clinical evidence. J Cardiothorac Vasc Anesth, 2006; 20: 722-735.

19. What following statement concerning commonly used cardiac hemodynamic infusions is FALSE?
   A. Cyclic adenosine monophosphate activation leads to increases in heart rate
   B. Epinephrine increases cardiac output via adrenergic agonism along with phosphodiesterase inhibition
   C. Milrinone acts specifically on phosphodiesterase-3
   D. Dopamine acts as a dopamine agonist

Correct Answer: B

Explanation: All of the choices are true except the mechanism of action for epinephrine. Epinephrine does not act on phosphodiesterase, but acts on $beta_1$, $beta_2$, $beta_3$, $alpha_1$, and $alpha_2$ adrenergic receptors. Dopamine activates D1, D2, and D3 dopamine receptors. Milrinone is specific for inhibition of phosphodiesterase-3, which leads to increased levels of cyclic adenosine monophosphate. Although there are several phosphodiesterase subtypes, phosphodiesterase-3 has a high concentration in the lung.

References:

1. Levy JH, Ghadimi K, Bailey JM, et al. Chapter 38: Postoperative Cardiovascular Management. In: Kaplan JA, Augoustides JGT, Manecke GR, et al., eds. Kaplan's Cardiac Anesthesia. 7th ed. Elsevier; 2017:1327-1357.
2. Lobato EB, Willert JL, Looke TD, et al. Effects of milrinone versus epinephrine on left ventricular relaxation after cardiopulmonary bypass following myocardial revascularization: assessment by color m-mode and tissue Doppler. J Cardiothorac Vasc Anesth, 2005; 19: 334-339.
3. Guarracino F, Habicher M, Treskatsch S, et al. Vasopressor therapy in cardiac surgery-an experts consensus statement. J Cardiothorac Anesth, 2021; 35: 1018-1029.

20. A 68-year-old man underwent coronary artery bypass grafting procedure complicated by a prolonged intensive care unit stay due to right ventricular failure. The patient required inotropic support and inhaled nitric oxide therapy. Of the following choices, which is the MOST common cause of right ventricular failure in post–cardiac surgery patients?
   A. Right-sided myocardial infarction
   B. Pulmonary embolus
   C. Coronary graft vasospasm
   D. Left ventricular failure

Correct Answer: D

Explanation: The most common cause of postoperative right ventricular failure is left ventricular impairment, as they are in contiguous system. The incidence of acute refractory right ventricular failure in adult cardiac surgery is 0.04% to 0.1%. Right ventricular failure is most common after heart transplantation and left ventricular assist device placement. Isolated right-sided myocardial infarction is rare, and inferior myocardial infarctions have variable involvement of the right ventricle. In addition to left ventricular failure, poor preservation during cardiopulmonary bypass can lead to right ventricular failure. This is because the right heart is more likely to be warm, as it is thin-walled and more exposed to the atmosphere. Depending on the conduct of retrograde cardioplegia, the solution may not adequately reach all parts of the right ventricle. Chronic or acute pulmonary hypertension increases right ventricular afterload and can lead to right ventricular failure. Pulmonary embolus is a cause of right ventricular failure, but it is not as common as left ventricular impairment after cardiac surgery due to large heparin doses used.

References:

1. Levy JH, Ghadimi K, Bailey JM, et al. Chapter 38: Postoperative Cardiovascular Management. In: Kaplan JA, Augoustides JGT, Manecke GR, et al., eds. Kaplan's Cardiac Anesthesia. 7th ed. Elsevier; 2017:1327-1357.
2. Batia M, Jia S, Smeltz A, et al. Right heart failure management: focus on mechanical support options. J Cardiothorac Vasc Anesth Surg, 2022; 36: 3278-3288.

21. Which medication should be avoided in a patient with an acute right ventricular myocardial infarction?
   A. Dobutamine
   B. Epinephrine
   C. Nitroglycerin
   D. Milrinone

Correct Answer: C

Explanation: Nitroglycerin should be avoided in patients with an acute myocardial infarction involving the right ventricle because the patients are preload- and heart rate–dependent. It is traditionally taught that nitroglycerin is a first-line treatment for acute myocardial infarction, but this is not the case with right ventricular infarction. Treatment for patients with acute right ventricular myocardial infarction centers around maintaining preload and heart rate. Epinephrine, milrinone, and dobutamine would assist in maintaining heart rate, while also providing inotropy for the ischemic right ventricle. All of the other choices may assist in maintaining hemodynamics until revascularization can be established.

References:

1. Levy JH, Ghadimi K, Bailey JM, et al. Chapter 38: Postoperative Cardiovascular Management. In: Kaplan JA, Augoustides JGT, Manecke GR, et al., eds. Kaplan's Cardiac Anesthesia. 7th ed. Elsevier; 2017:1327-1357.
2. O'Connor RE, Ali A, Brady WJ, et al. Acute coronary syndromes: 2015 American Heart Association guidelines update for cardiopulmonary resuscitation and emergency cardiovascular care. Circulation, 2015; 132: S483-S500.

22. A 59-year-old patient underwent a mitral valve replacement complicated by low cardiac output due to right ventricular dysfunction. What is LEAST useful in the management of right ventricular dysfunction?
    A. Epoprostenol
    B. Phenylephrine
    C. Inhaled nitric oxide
    D. Dobutamine

Correct Answer: B

Explanation: Nitric oxide is an inhalational pulmonary vasodilator. It diffuses across the alveolar-capillary membrane and activates cyclic guanosine monophosphate, and this leads to smooth muscle relaxation in the pulmonary vascular bed to decrease pulmonary vascular resistance. This results in less afterload for the right ventricle. Epoprostenol is an inhalational pulmonary vasodilator and synthetic prostaglandin that increases cyclic adenosine monophosphate (cAMP), resulting in a reduction in pulmonary vascular resistance and unloading of the right heart. Inhaled agents have the benefit of quick onset with fewer systemic effects and may also decrease ventilation/perfusion mismatch in hypoxic patients. Milrinone is a phosphodiesterase III inhibitor leading to increases in cAMP. cAMP causes pulmonary and systemic vasodilation and increases right ventricular contractility. Dobutamine is a beta receptor agonist and also increases cAMP, thus acting as a pulmonary vasodilator and right ventricular inotropic agent. Although phenylephrine may support blood pressure to support right ventricular perfusion, its pulmonary vasoconstrictive effects increase right ventricular afterload.

References:

1. Levy JH, Ghadimi K, Bailey JM, et al. Chapter 38: Postoperative Cardiovascular Management. In: Kaplan JA, Augoustides JGT, Manecke GR, et al., eds. Kaplan's Cardiac Anesthesia. 7th ed. Elsevier; 2017:1327-1357.
2. Rao V, Ghadimi K, Keeyapaj W, et al. Inhaled nitric oxide and inhaled epoprostenol use in cardiothoracic surgical patients:

Is there sufficient evidence for evidence-based medicine? J Cardiothorac Vasc Anesth, 2018; 32: 1452-1457.

23. Which medication when given for right ventricular support following cardiac surgery has been associated with inhibition of platelet aggregation?
    A. Milrinone
    B. Epoprostenol
    C. Epinephrine
    D. Dobutamine

Correct Answer: B

Explanation: Inhaled epoprostenol is associated with decreased platelet aggregation. Although not a choice for this question, inhaled nitric oxide as a selective pulmonary vasodilator has also been shown to inhibit platelet adhesion aggregation and stimulate disaggregation of preformed platelet aggregates. However, because these agents are given inhalationally, these effects are often not pronounced systemically. The cardiovascular bipyridines amrinone and milrinone are inotropic agents with vasodilator properties due to phosphodiesterase inhibition. Amrinone, which is rarely used today, is associated with thrombocytopenia due to accelerated peripheral loss of platelets. However, milrinone has not displayed this adverse effect. Dobutamine and epinephrine are not associated with inhibition of platelet aggregation.

References:

1. Levy JH, Ghadimi K, Bailey JM, et al. Chapter 38: Postoperative Cardiovascular Management. In: Kaplan JA, Augoustides JGT, Manecke GR, et al., eds. Kaplan's Cardiac Anesthesia. 7th ed. Elsevier; 2017:1327-1357.
2. Rao V, Ghadimi K, Keeyapaj W, et al. Inhaled nitric oxide and inhaled epoprostenol use in cardiothoracic surgical patients: Is there sufficient evidence for evidence-based medicine? J Cardiothorac Vasc Anesth, 2018; 32: 1452-1457.
3. Groves D, Blum F, Huffmyer J, et al. Effects of early inhaled epoprostenol therapy on pulmonary artery pressure and blood loss during LVAD placement. J Cardiothorac Vasc Anesth, 2014; 28: 652-660.

24. Following placement of a left ventricular assist device, a patient is brought to the intensive care unit on inhaled nitric oxide for right ventricular support. All of the following are side effects of inhaled nitric oxide, EXCEPT:
    A. Methemoglobinemia
    B. Pulmonary edema
    C. Pulmonary microemboli
    D. Pulmonary hypertension following inhaled nitric oxide discontinuation

Correct Answer: C

Explanation: Pulmonary microemboli are not associated with inhaled nitric oxide administration. In fact, this agent has been shown to inhibit platelet adhesion and aggregation and stimulate disaggregation of preformed platelet aggregates. Further potential adverse effects include toxicity from formation of nitrogen dioxide and methemoglobinemia. Nitric oxide is associated with formation of methemoglobinemia, especially in patients with renal failure; however, its clinical significance remains unclear. Methemoglobin levels can be checked on and monitored if considered a potential adverse effect of inhaled nitric oxide. Rebound pulmonary vasoconstriction and pulmonary hypertension from abrupt disconnection or withdrawal can occur and be life-threatening to patients with severe right ventricular failure. Pulmonary vascular congestion secondary to increased pulmonary blood flow from right ventricular unloading may occur in patients with compromised left ventricular function.

References:

1. Levy JH, Ghadimi K, Bailey JM, et al. Chapter 38: Postoperative Cardiovascular Management. In: Kaplan JA, Augoustides JGT, Manecke GR, et al., eds. Kaplan's Cardiac Anesthesia. 7th ed. Elsevier; 2017:1327-1357.
2. Rao V, Ghadimi K, Keeyapaj W, et al. Inhaled nitric oxide and inhaled epoprostenol use in cardiothoracic surgical patients: Is there sufficient evidence for evidence-based medicine? J Cardiothorac Vasc Anesth, 2018; 32: 1452-1457.

25. A 75-year-old female has undergone a mitral valve repair and coronary artery bypass surgery. She has a history of ejection fraction of 35%, severe mitral regurgitation, scleroderma, and atrial fibrillation. She presents to the intensive care unit on epinephrine, norepinephrine, and vasopressin. Her pulmonary pressures have now risen to 55/28 mmHg from 27/29 mmHg immediately following surgery. Echocardiography reveals moderate right ventricular dysfunction, and inhaled nitric oxide is initiated. The following morning, her oxygen requirement on the ventilator has increased, and her chest x-ray demonstrates pulmonary edema. What most likely contributed to her respiratory findings?

A. Epinephrine
B. Norepinephrine
C. Nitric oxide
D. Vasopressin

Correct Answer: C

Explanation: Inhaled vasodilators should be used with caution in patients who have left ventricular failure as the cause of their pulmonary hypertension. The increased pulmonary blood flow can worsen pulmonary edema. Inhaled nitric oxide and prostacylins (epoprostenol and iloprost) have been associated with death in patients with pulmonary veno-occlusive disease. Epinephrine and norepinephrine will provide support to the left ventricle and could decrease pulmonary edema. Norepinephrine may be beneficial due to pulmonary vasoconstrictive effects in this scenario; however, the increase in systemic afterload may worsen left ventricular cardiac output. Vasopressin will support the systemic blood pressure, with minimal to no increase in pulmonary vascular resistance, but will not worsen pulmonary edema.

References:

1. Levy JH, Ghadimi K, Bailey JM, et al. Chapter 38: Postoperative Cardiovascular Management. In: Kaplan JA, Augoustides JGT, Manecke GR, et al., eds. Kaplan's Cardiac Anesthesia. 7th ed. Elsevier; 2017:1327-1357.
2. Rao V, Ghadimi K, Keeyapaj W, et al. Inhaled nitric oxide and inhaled epoprostenol use in cardiothoracic surgical patients: Is there sufficient evidence for evidence-based medicine? J Cardiothorac Vasc Anesth, 2018; 32:1452-1457.

26. A 68-year-old male underwent urgent coronary artery bypass surgery and required multiple packed red blood cells, fresh frozen plasma, and platelets. Once in the intensive care unit, his chest tubes continued to drain copious blood for 2 hours, at which time drainage nearly ceased. Echocardiography demonstrated clot around the right ventricle. What is TRUE concerning cardiac tamponade?

A. Cardiac tamponade usually presents with an acute decrease in blood pressure
B. Cardiac tamponade occurs in 30% to 40% of cardiac surgical patients
C. Cardiac tamponade is commonly associated with pronounced respiratory variation
D. Cardiac tamponade leads to left ventricular collapse followed by right ventricular collapse

Correct Answer: C

Explanation: Cardiac tamponade occurs in 3% to 6% of patients. Patients typically have ongoing bleeding and require multiple blood transfusions after cardiac surgery. As blood accumulates around the heart, the external pressure increases, and the ability of the heart to fill decreases. In the extreme, filling only occurs during systole, and diastolic collapse of the right ventricle can be seen echocardiographically. Echocardiography may provide strong evidence for the diagnosis of cardiac tamponade and should be utilized routinely. Cardiac tamponade is associated with pronounced respiratory variation in patients on mechanical ventilation due to high filling pressures leading to low stroke volume and cardiac output. The additional external pressure applied to the heart by positive-pressure ventilation may further impair the already compromised ventricular filling in the presence of tamponade. Cardiac tamponade commonly presents as a steady increase in pressor requirements, as resuscitation efforts can maintain stability for some time. Due to its greater myocardial thickness, left ventricular compression is rarely seen in cardiac tamponade as compared to the thin-walled right ventricle.

References:

1. Levy JH, Ghadimi K, Bailey JM, et al. Chapter 38: Postoperative Cardiovascular Management. In: Kaplan JA, Augoustides JGT, Manecke GR, et al., eds. Kaplan's Cardiac Anesthesia. 7th ed. Elsevier; 2017:1327-1357.
2. Camrona P, Mateo E, Casanovas I, et al. Management of cardiac tamponade after cardiac surgery. J Cardiothorac Vasc Anesth, 2012; 26: 302-311.

27. A patient who underwent a redo sternotomy for coronary artery bypass grafting is hemodynamically unstable on high-dose norepinephrine, epinephrine, and vasopressin. Due to ongoing mediastinal bleeding, an echocardiogram is performed and demonstrates substantial circumferential pericardial fluid. While the surgical team is setting up the operating room for take-back surgery and mediastinal washout, which medication could be added to attempt to stabilize the patient?
A. Addition of milrinone
B. Addition of phenylephrine
C. Addition of dobutamine
D. Addition of inhaled nitric oxide

Correct Answer: C

Explanation: Medical management of cardiac tamponade centers around maintaining preload, maintaining heart rate, and providing inotropic support. It is also important to maintain systemic blood pressure. The patient is already on medication to support the systemic vascular resistance, and the patient would benefit from a medication that would augment his heart rate and contractility. Dobutamine is the best choice out of the options above.

Milrinone would worsen hypotension while the patient is on high-dose vasopressor therapy. Phenylephrine would decrease the patient's heart rate when his cardiac output is reliant on heart rate because the stroke volume is fixed. Inhaled nitric oxide is a pulmonary vasodilator that is commonly used for right ventricular failure following cardiac surgery. Inhaled nitric oxide would not help with increasing blood pressure or heart rate in a patient suffering from tamponade physiology.

References:

1. Levy JH, Ghadimi K, Bailey JM, et al. Chapter 38: Postoperative Cardiovascular Management. In: Kaplan JA, Augoustides JGT, Manecke GR, et al., eds. Kaplan's Cardiac Anesthesia. 7th ed. Elsevier; 2017:1327-1357.
2. Camrona P, Mateo E, Casanovas I, et al. Management of cardiac tamponade after cardiac surgery. J Cardiothorac Vasc Anest, 2012; 26: 302-311.

28. What is a risk factor for major vascular complications after transcatheter aortic valve replacement?
A. Female sex
B. Increased age
C. Renal failure
D. History of smoking

Correct Answer: A

Explanation: Female sex has been found as an independent risk factor for major vascular complications after transcatheter aortic valve replacement and is thought to be related to the large size of earlier generations of the delivery devices placed in the femoral artery. Heavily calcified femoral arterial disease has also been found to increase the risk of vascular complications. Increased age, renal failure, and history of smoking have not been found to increase risk for major vascular complication after this procedure.

References:

1. Levy JH, Ghadimi K, Bailey JM, et al. Chapter 38: Postoperative Cardiovascular Management. In: Kaplan JA, Augoustides JGT, Manecke GR, et al., eds. Kaplan's Cardiac Anesthesia. 7th ed. Elsevier; 2017:1327-1357.
2. Reidy C, Sophocles A, Ramakrishna H, et al. Challenges after the first decade of transcatheter aortic valve replacement: focus on vascular complications, stroke, and paravalvular leak. J Cardiothorac Vasc Anesth, 2013; 27: 184-189.

29. What is a preoperative risk factor for a permanent pacemaker after transcutaneous aortic valve replacement?
A. History of smoking
B. Increased age
C. Sinus bradycardia
D. Right bundle branch block

Correct Answer: D

Explanation: The risk of pacemaker implantation after transcatheter aortic valve replacement is typically higher compared to that after surgical aortic valve replacement. Preoperative right bundle branch block increases the risk for heart block in this setting, as patients are already at risk for developing a left bundle branch block after transcatheter valve deployment. This leads to complete heart block, which is the main indication for permanent pacemaker placement after this procedure. Without a right bundle branch block, the risk of new left bundle branch block is not as serious because it resolves in over 30% of cases. Increased age, sinus bradycardia, and history of smoking were not found to be a preoperative risk factors for needing a permanent pacemaker after transcatheter aortic valve replacement.

References:

1. Levy JH, Ghadimi K, Bailey JM, et al. Chapter 38: Postoperative Cardiovascular Management. In: Kaplan JA, Augoustides JGT, Manecke GR, et al., eds. Kaplan's Cardiac Anesthesia. 7th ed. Elsevier; 2017:1327-1357.
2. Ghadimi K, Patel PA, Gutsche JT, et al. Perioperative conduction disturbances after transcatheter aortic valve replacement. J Cardiothorac Vasc Anesth, 2013; 27: 1414-1420.

30. A 30-year-old female was placed on veno-venous (VV) ECMO for hypoxia related to influenza via an duel-lumen cannula in the right internal jugular vein. Following a turn to change sheets, the patient begins to desaturate despite the VV ECMO delivered oxygen content increased to 100%. What is the most likely etiology of this acute desaturation?
A. North-south syndrome
B. Recirculation
C. Low cardiac output
D. Too low of sweep setting

Correct Answer: B

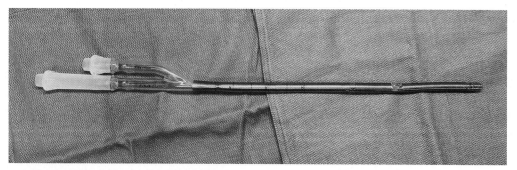

FIGURE 34.3 Example of a bi-caval dual lumen catheter able to provide deoxygenated blood removal and oxygenated blood infusion to the internal jugular vein.

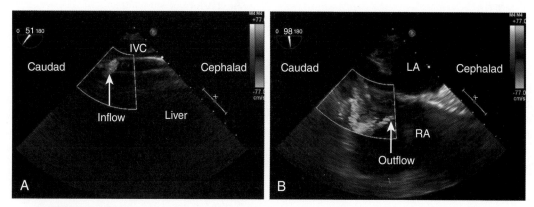

FIGURE 34.4 Transesophageal echocardiographic visualization of the Avalon Elite cannula (Maquet Cardiopulmonary, Rastatt, Germany) during venovenous extracorporeal membrane oxygenation. Caudad and cephalad directions are marked on the images for orientation. (A) The inflow lumen of Avalon Elite Bicaval Dual-Lumen Catheter and Vascular Access Kit is visible within the inferior vena cava *(IVC)* with color-flow Doppler illustrating blood flowing within the inferior intrahepatic IVC toward the inflow tip of the cannula. (B) The outflow cannula of Avalon Elite cannula is visible within the right atrium *(RA)*. Color-flow Doppler imaging illustrates blood flow from the outflow cannula directed medially toward the tricuspid valve (not seen). The color-flow Doppler box encompasses a smaller portion of the cannula outflow and shows a small amount of blood flowing away from the tricuspid valve; this finding is common but is presumably of no clinical significance (in the setting of normal flows and adequate extracorporeal gas exchange). *LA,* Left atrium. (Courtesy K. Ghadimi, MD.)

Explanation: The duel-lumen cannula is a single lumen, bidirectional cannula that allows for VV ECMO. The inflow lumen has an end hole and a side fenestrations at the tip, as well as side holes proximal to the exit site of the inflow lumen that allow drainage from the both the superior and inferior vena cavae. The outflow lumen of the single cannula opens 10 cm above the inflow cannula tip and is designed to return oxygenated blood to the right atrium.

Recirculation is seen when blood is "recirculated" directly from the oxygenated or outflow port of an duel-lumen cannula into the inflow port of the cannula that should be receiving deoxygenated blood. Thus, a fraction of oxygenated blood is not being delivered to the body. Proper placement of the duel-lumen cannula is typically aided by transesophageal echocardiography at the time of placement. Proper positioning is identified by visualizing flow within the inflow and outflow cannula lumina and the position of each limb within the inferior vena cava and the right atrium, respectively. Duel-lumen cannula positioning can be disrupted with turning of a patient, coughing or other movements.

North-south syndrome is seen in veno-arterial (VA) ECMO and is seen with upper body hypoxia due to normal or high cardiac output in the setting of poor pulmonary function. Sweep modulates carbon dioxide (CO_2), not oxygen content on ECMO.

References:

1. Levy JH, Ghadimi K, Bailey JM, et al. Chapter 38: Postoperative Cardiovascular Management. In: Kaplan JA, Augoustides JGT, Manecke GR, et al., eds. Kaplan's Cardiac Anesthesia. 7th ed. Elsevier; 2017:1327-1357.

2. Alexis-Ruiz A, Ghadimi K, Raiten J, et al. Hypoxia and complications of oxygenation in extracorporeal membrane oxygenation. J Cardiothorac Vasc Anesth, 2019; 33: 1375-1381.

31. A 52-year-old male was placed on venoarterial extracorporeal membrane oxygenation related to biventricular dysfunction and COVID infection. A right femoral arterial cannula and a left femoral venous cannula were placed, and he was initially set at 100% oxygen delivery with this platform. Echocardiography demonstrated hyperdynamic left ventricular function and an underfilled right ventricle. An arterial line was placed in his right radial artery and demonstrated an oxygen content of 80 mmHg. What is the MOST likely reason for this relative hypoxemia?

A. North-south syndrome
B. Recirculation
C. Low cardiac output
D. Low sweep setting

Correct Answer: A

Explanation: North-south syndrome is seen when a patient is cannulated bifemorally for both arterial and venous access. In patients with normal or hyperdynamic left ventricular function and poor pulmonary function, the heart continues to eject deoxygenated blood. This problem is also called proximal-distal syndrome or harlequin syndrome. The result is more deoxygenation to the upper body, especially the head and brain and hyperoxia to the lower body.

Without adequate delivery of oxygenated extracorporeal membrane oxygenation (ECMO) blood to the left ventricle for whole-body distribution, deoxygenated blood will continue to fill the left ventricle. This occurs not only to poor delivery of ECMO blood, but also ongoing shunts that continue to traverse the native circulation without being oxygenated in the lungs. This scenario commonly occurs with high cardiac output that decreases the amount of oxygenated blood from the femoral artery that reaches the upper body. This zone is termed the "mixing point." This can lead to inadequate oxygenation of the coronary and cerebral tissues. The management options include decreasing native cardiac output by decreasing inotropic support and attempting to optimize pulmonary function to aid oxygenation. Alternatively, another perfusion cannula can be added to an internal jugular vein to provide oxygenated blood to the upper body for a venoarteriovenous configuration. A further option is switching to venovenous platform, given that the cardiac output is preserved.

Recirculation occurs with venovenous ECMO due to malpositioned cannulae. Low cardiac output protects against developing the north-south syndrome. The sweep setting modulates carbon dioxide removal during extracorporeal membrane oxygenation.

References:

1. Levy JH, Ghadimi K, Bailey JM, et al. Chapter 38: Postoperative Cardiovascular Management. In: Kaplan JA, Augoustides JGT, Manecke GR, et al., eds. Kaplan's Cardiac Anesthesia. 7th ed. Elsevier; 2017:1327-1357.
2. Alexis-Ruiz A, Ghadimi K, Raiten J, et al. Hypoxia and complications of oxygenation in extracorporeal membrane oxygenation. J Cardiothorac Vasc Anesth, 2019; 33: 1375-1381.
3. Hoyler MM, Flynn BC, Iannacone E, et al. Clinical management of venoarterial extracorporeal membrane oxygenation. J Cardiothorac Vasc Anesth, 2020; 34: 2776-2792.

CHAPTER 35

Postoperative Respiratory Care

Shea Stoops and Brigid Flynn

KEY POINTS

1. Pulmonary complications following cardiopulmonary bypass are relatively common, with up to 12% of patients experiencing some degree of acute lung injury and approximately 1% requiring tracheostomy for long-term ventilation.
2. Risk factors for respiratory insufficiency include advanced age, presence of diabetes or renal failure, smoking, chronic obstructive lung disease, peripheral vascular disease, previous cardiac operations, and emergency or unstable status.
3. Impediments to weaning from mechanical ventilation and extubation include delirium, unstable hemodynamic status, respiratory muscle dysfunction, renal failure with fluid overload, and sepsis.
4. Risk factors for not being able to be wean from the ventilator include a persistent low-output state with multisystem organ failure. Echocardiography can be helpful in establishing ventricular filling, contractility, and cardiac output at baseline and during weaning trials. Long-term weaning may be best accomplished in a specialized unit rather than an acute cardiovascular recovery area.

---

1. All of the following are true concerning impaired pulmonary function following cardiac surgery, EXCEPT:
   A. General anesthesia, muscle relaxants and median sternotomy all lead to a reduction of vital capacity
   B. Intravascular lung water is decreased, leading to increased risk of development of pleural effusions
   C. Decreased functional residual capacity following cardiopulmonary bypass leads to ventilation/perfusion mismatch
   D. Increased work of breathing can increase oxygen consumption by up to 20%

Correct Answer: B

Explanation: Even in the presence of preexisting pulmonary disease, important pulmonary changes occur after cardiac operations. These include diminished functional residual capacity as a result of general anesthesia, muscle relaxants, and median sternotomy. Due to large volume fluid shifts, there is routinely increased lung water, which would likely increase, not decrease, the risk of pleural effusions. Pleural effusions and atelectasis are additional causes of pulmonary dysfunction following cardiac surgery that occur in a majority of patients. Acute functional residual capacity reduction creates arterial hypoxemia secondary to a mismatch between ventilation and perfusion and diminishes lung compliance with increased work of breathing. This additional work of breathing, which increases oxygen consumption by up to 20% in spontaneously breathing patients, also increases myocardial work at a time when myocardial reserves may be limited.

References:

1. Higgins TL, Engelman DT. Chapter 39: Postoperative Respiratory Care. In: Kaplan JA, Augoustides JGT, Manecke GR, et al., eds. Kaplan's Cardiac Anesthesia. 7th ed. Elsevier; 2017:1358-1373.
2. Fischer MO, Brotons F, Briant AR; VENICE study group, et al. Postoperative pulmonary complications after cardiac surgery: the VENICE international cohort study. J Cardiothorac Vasc Anesth, 2022; 36: 2344-2351.
3. He LL, Li XF, Jiang JL, et al. Effect of volatile anesthesia versus total intravenous anesthesia on postoperative pulmonary complications in patients undergoing cardiac surgery: a randomized clinical trial. J Cardiothorac Vasc Anesth, 2022; 36: 3758-3765.

2. A patient scheduled for coronary artery bypass grafting is concerned about postoperative respiratory complications and asks for more information during the preoperative visit. All of the following can be accurately relayed to the patient, EXCEPT:
   A. If a patient extubates <12 hours postoperatively, changes in spirometric measurements and respiratory muscle strength typically resolve upon extubation

B. Acute lung injury, sometimes progressing to acute respiratory distress syndrome, occurs in up to 12% of cardiac surgical patients

C. Approximately 6% of cardiac surgical patients require postoperative ventilation for >72 hours

D. Tracheostomy is required in approximately 1% of cardiac surgical patients due to failure to wean from ventilation in a safe time frame

Correct Answer: A

Explanation: Even in the best situations with fast-track tracheal extubation, changes in spirometric measurements and respiratory muscle strength can last up to 8 weeks postoperatively. Acute lung injury, sometimes progressing to acute respiratory distress syndrome, can occur in up to 12% of postoperative cardiac patients. Approximately 6% of cardiovascular surgical patients require more than 72 hours on the ventilator, and approximately 1% of patients undergo tracheostomy to facilitate recovery and weaning from prolonged support with mechanical ventilation.

References:

1. Higgins TL, Engelman DT. Chapter 39: Postoperative Respiratory Care. In: Kaplan JA, Augoustides JGT, Manecke GR, et al., eds. Kaplan's Cardiac Anesthesia. 7th ed. Elsevier; 2017:1358-1373.
2. Fischer MO, Brotons F, Briant AR; VENICE study group, et al. Postoperative pulmonary complications after cardiac surgery: the VENICE international cohort study. J Cardiothorac Vasc Anesth, 2022; 36: 2344-2351.
3. He LL, Li XF, Jiang JL, et al. Effect of volatile anesthesia versus total intravenous anesthesia on postoperative pulmonary complications in patients undergoing cardiac surgery: a randomized clinical trial. J Cardiothorac Vasc Anesth, 2022; 36: 3758-3765.

3. When discussing the risk of postoperative pulmonary complications with patients undergoing cardiac surgery, many risk models are available. The following factors are routinely included as risks for associated postoperative pulmonary complications, EXCEPT:

A. Increased age
B. Stage II chronic renal disease
C. Aortic valve disease
D. Diabetes

Correct Answer: C

Explanation: The Society of Thoracic Surgeons National Adult Cardiac Surgery Database is widely used in the United States, and it offers, in addition to a mortality prediction, a model customized to predict prolonged ventilation. The European System for Cardiac Operative Risk Evaluation (EuroSCORE) is commonly used in Europe. Factors common to outcome risk adjustment models include age, sex, body surface area, presence of diabetes or renal failure, chronic lung disease, peripheral vascular disease, cerebrovascular disease, previous cardiac operation, and emergency or unstable status. Chronic obstructive pulmonary disease may be a major risk for postoperative respiratory morbidity and death, and it appears as a factor in some models.

TABLE 35.1
Factors predicting postoperative respiratory outcome

	Spivack et al., 1996	Branca et al., 2001	Rady et al., 1999	Canver and Chandra, 2003
End point	Mechanical ventilation >48 h	Mechanical ventilation >72 h	Extubation failure (reintubation after initial extubation)	Mechanical ventilation >72 h
Risk factors	Reduced LVEF Preexisting CHF Angina Current smoking Diabetes	STS-predicted mortality estimate Mitral valve disease Advanced age Pressors or inotropes Renal failure Operative urgency Type of operation Preoperative ventilation Previous CABG Female sex MI within 30 days Previous stroke	Age ≥65 years Inpatient status Vascular disease COPD or asthma Pulmonary hypertension Reduced LVEF Cardiac shock Hct ≤34% BUN ≥24 mg/dL Serum albumin ≤4.0 mg/dL Do_2 ≤320 mL/L²/min >1 previous CABG Thoracic aortic operation ≥10 units of blood products Total CPB time ≥120 min	CPB time Sepsis and endocarditis GI bleeding Renal failure Deep sternal wound infection New CVA Bleeding requiring reoperation

BUN, Blood urea nitrogen, *CABG,* coronary artery bypass grafting; *CHF,* congestive heart failure; *COPD,* chronic obstructive pulmonary disease, *CPB,* cardiopulmonary bypass; *CVA,* cerebrovascular accident; *Do₂,* systemic oxygen delivery; *GI,* gastrointestinal; *Hct,* hematocrit; *LVEF,* left ventricular ejection fraction; *MI,* myocardial infarction; *STS,* The Society of Thoracic Surgeons.

References:

1. Higgins TL, Engelman DT. Chapter 39: Postoperative Respiratory Care. In: Kaplan JA, Augoustides JGT, Manecke GR, et al., eds. Kaplan's Cardiac Anesthesia. 7th ed. Elsevier; 2017:1358-1373.
2. Fischer MO, Brotons F, Briant AR; VENICE study group, et al. Postoperative pulmonary complications after cardiac surgery: the VENICE international cohort study. J Cardiothorac Vasc Anesth, 2022; 36: 2344-2351.
3. He LL, Li XF, Jiang JL, et al. Effect of volatile anesthesia versus total intravenous anesthesia on postoperative pulmonary complications in patients undergoing cardiac surgery: a randomized clinical trial. J Cardiothorac Vasc Anesth, 2022; 36: 3758-3765.

4. A 77-year-old woman with an 80-pack-year smoking history presents for her anesthesia preoperative visit prior to her coronary artery bypass surgery. She has been diagnosed with severe chronic obstructive pulmonary disease and wishes to know her postoperative pulmonary risk profile. What is TRUE regarding postoperative pulmonary complications in this patient?

A. Quantity of tobacco abuse in terms of "pack years" is the most important risk factor for postoperative pulmonary complications

B. Her risk of postoperative atrial fibrillation is the same as other women of the same age

C. Age over 75 years is a risk factor for postoperative pulmonary complications in cardiac surgical patients with chronic obstructive pulmonary disease

D. Prescribing preoperative steroids would decrease her risk of death following cardiac surgery

Correct Answer: C

Explanation: Chronic obstructive pulmonary disease (COPD) is a known risk for postoperative respiratory morbidities, with rates of pulmonary complications in approximately 12% of patients. Patients with COPD undergoing cardiac surgery also have an increased risk of death compared with patients without COPD. The risk of in-hospital mortality in patients with severe COPD is increased for patients over 75 years of age and also for patients receiving steroids for COPD. Patients with preexisting COPD appear to be at higher risk for perioperative atrial fibrillation, as well as death. Although "pack years" of tobacco abuse history is a convenient way to measure the degree of tobacco abuse, this singular data point has not been shown to predict postoperative outcomes.

References:

1. Higgins TL, Engelman DT. Chapter 39: Postoperative Respiratory Care. In: Kaplan JA, Augoustides JGT, Manecke GR, et al., eds. Kaplan's Cardiac Anesthesia. 7th ed. Elsevier; 2017:1358-1373.
2. Ball L, Volta CA, Saglietti F, et al. Associations between expiratory flow limitation and postoperative pulmonary complications in patients undergoing cardiac surgery. J Cardiothorac Vasc Anesth, 2022; 36: 815-824.

5. Prolonged tracheal intubation time following cardiac surgery has been defined as anywhere between 6 to 24 hours postoperatively. What is an intraoperative strategy that should be employed to decrease delayed tracheal extubation?

A. Decrease cardiopulmonary bypass time

B. Avoidance of morphine and use of fentanyl for analgesia

C. Administration of diuretic prior to separation from cardiopulmonary bypass decreases the risk of delayed extubation

D. Steroid administration prior to cardiopulmonary bypass decreases the risk of delayed extubation

Correct Answer: A

Explanation: Longer length of time on cardiopulmonary bypass (CPB) is repeatedly identified as a risk factor for prolonged intubation following cardiac surgery. Patients undergoing reoperation are at increased risk partly because of longer CPB times with reoperation, increased use of blood transfusion, and the additional likelihood of bleeding in this population.

Opioids and neuromuscular blocking agents with long half-lives may be expected to influence extubation time, but it is the skill of the anesthesiologist in knowing how to use these drugs well and not the specific duration of drug action that influences extubation time. Recruitment maneuvers following bypass have a variable impact on intubation time, with most studies showing these to be ineffective in reducing the need for long-term ventilatory support. No compelling data indicate that fluid management choices or the use of steroids before CPB will have substantial effects on intubation time or respiratory failure.

References:

1. Higgins TL, Engelman DT. Chapter 39: Postoperative Respiratory Care. In: Kaplan JA, Augoustides JGT, Manecke GR, et al., eds. Kaplan's Cardiac Anesthesia. 7th ed. Elsevier; 2017:1358-1373.
2. Richey M, Mann A, He J, et al. Implementation of an early extubation protocol in cardiac surgical patients decreased ventilator time but not intensive care unit or hospital length of stay. J Cardiothorac Vasc Anesth, 2018; 32: 739-744.
3. Flynn BC, He J, Richey M, et al. Early extubation without increased adverse events in high-risk cardiac surgical patients. Ann Thorac Surg, 2019; 107: 453-459.

6. Following a mitral valve repair, clinical criteria that should be met prior to tracheal extubation include all of the following EXCEPT:

A. Rapid shallow breathing index over 100

B. PaO_2/FiO_2 ratio of 200 or more

C. pH of 7.35 or higher

D. Maximal inspiratory force of 25 cm H_2O or more

Correct Answer: A

Explanation: The rapid shallow breathing index (RSBI) is an index that is both commonly applied to assess readiness for tracheal extubation and that is easy to calculate. The equation for RSBI is respiratory rate in breaths per minute divided by tidal volume in liters. A value over 100 would suggest rapid, shallow breathing and is a predictor for unsuccessful extubation. PaO_2/FiO_2 ratio is the ratio of arterial

BOX 35.1 Criteria to be met before early postoperative extubation

- *Neurologic:* Awake, neuromuscular blockade fully dissipated (head lift ≥5 s); following instructions, able to cough and protect airway
- *Cardiac:* Stable without mechanical support; cardiac index ≥2.2 L/m²/min; MAP ≥70 mmHg; no serious arrhythmias
- *Respiratory:* Acceptable CXR and ABGs (pH ≥7.35); minimal secretions, comfortable on CPAP or T-piece

- with spontaneous respiratory rate ≤20 breaths/min; MIP ≥25 cm H_2O; alternatively, a successful SBT defined as an RSBI <100 and a Pao_2/Fio_2 ≥200
- *Renal:* Undergoing diuresis well; urine output >0.8 mL/kg/h; not markedly fluid-overloaded from operative or CPB fluid administration or SIRS
- *Hematologic:* Chest tube drainage minimal
- *Temperature:* Fully rewarmed; not actively shivering

ABG, Arterial blood gas; *CPAP,* continuous positive airway pressure; *CPB,* cardiopulmonary bypass; *CXR,* chest radiograph; *MAP,* mean arterial pressure; *MIP,* maximal inspiratory pressure; Pao_2/Fio_2, ratio of arterial partial pressure of oxygen to fraction of inspired oxygen; *RSBI,* rapid shallow breathing index; *SBT,* spontaneous breathing trial; *SIRS,* systemic immune response syndrome.

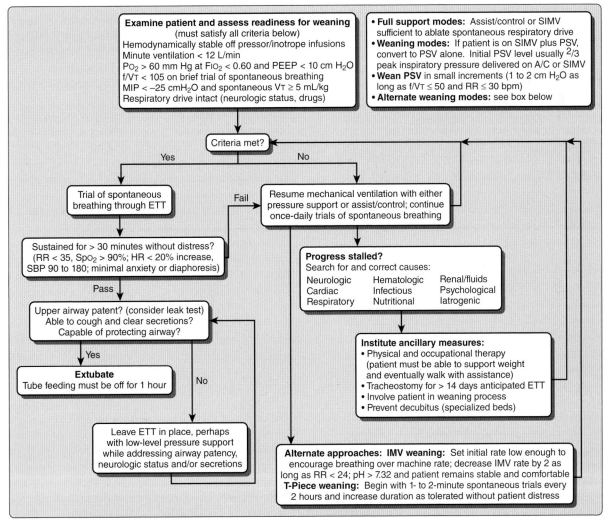

FIGURE 35.1 This flow chart addresses care of patients receiving both short-term and long-term ventilatory support in the cardiothoracic intensive care unit. All patients require periodic assessment for readiness for weaning, and if they meet criteria they are eligible for spontaneous trials leading to extubation. Patients who do not meet the criteria should have mechanical ventilation maintained until criteria are met. Pressure-support ventilation (PSV) weaning may be possible; if not, alternative approaches include intermittent mandatory ventilation (IMV) weaning and T-piece weaning. Patients who stall in their weaning process should have a comprehensive examination and an assessment of organ systems to search for correctable causes. *A/C,* Assist-control mode; *ETT,* endotracheal tube; f/V_T, frequency-to-tidal volume ratio; *MIP,* maximal inspiratory pressure; *PEEP,* positive end-expiratory pressure; PO_2, partial pressure of oxygen; *RR,* respiratory rate; *SBP,* systolic blood pressure; *SIMV,* synchronized intermittent mandatory ventilation; SpO_2, oxygen saturation measured with pulse oximetry.

oxygen partial pressure (PaO_2 in mmHg) to fractional inspired oxygen (FiO_2), in evaluation of hypoxia and is also used in extubation criteria. Prior to extubation, a PaO_2/FiO_2 ratio of more than 200 will likely not lead to hypoxia following extubation. A normal pH is important for respiratory and metabolic functions, and important for maintenance respiratory drive. A maximal inspiratory force over 25 cm H_2O demonstrates adequate airway and pulmonary strength for successful extubation.

References:

1. Higgins TL, Engelman DT. Chapter 39: Postoperative Respiratory Care. In: Kaplan JA, Augoustides JGT, Manecke GR, et al., eds. Kaplan's Cardiac Anesthesia. 7th ed. Elsevier; 2017:1358-1373.
2. Chacon M, Markin NW. Early is good, but is immediate better? considerations in fast-track extubation after cardiac surgery. J Cardiothorac Vasc Anesth, 2022; 36: 1265-1267.
3. Brovman EY, Tolis G, Hirji S, et al. Association between early extubation and postoperative reintubation after elective cardiac surgery: a bi-institutional study. J Cardiothorac Vasc Anesth, 2022; 36: 1258-1264.

7. A patient remains intubated on postoperative day 6 following an aortic and mitral valve replacement procedure. What is a strategy that has been found to help reduce ventilator-associated pneumonia?
   A. Weekly sedation titrations or interruptions
   B. Early removal of nasogastric tubes
   C. Routine changes of ventilator circuit
   D. Chest physiotherapy

Correct Answer: B

Explanation: The historical risk of ventilator-associated pneumonia (VAP) in intensive care unit patients was approximately 1% per day of ventilation. Practices that have not been considered to help prevent VAP are routine ventilator circuit changes, routine changes of in-line suction catheters, and daily replacement of heat and moisture exchangers. In a randomized controlled trial, chest physiotherapy did not change the incidence of VAP. There are multiple studies supporting early removal of nasogastric or endotracheal tubes for VAP prevention. Formal education and adherence to formal infection control programs, including hand washing, may decrease the incidence of VAP.

Further practices that help reduce the incidence of VAP include semirecumbent positioning of the patient, daily sedation interruptions, avoidance of unnecessary reintubations, adequate nutritional support, avoidance of gastric overdistention, use of the oral rather than the nasal route for intubation, scheduled drainage of condensate from ventilator circuits, and maintenance of adequate endotracheal tube cuff pressure.

References:

1. Higgins TL, Engelman DT. Chapter 39: Postoperative Respiratory Care. In: Kaplan JA, Augoustides JGT, Manecke GR, et al., eds. Kaplan's Cardiac Anesthesia. 7th ed. Elsevier; 2017:1358-1373.

2. Nam K, Park JB, Park WB, et al. Effect of perioperative subglottic secretion drainage on ventilator-associated pneumonia after cardiac surgery: a retrospective, before-and-after study. J Cardiothorac Vasc Anesth, 2021; 35: 2377-2384.
3. Mastropierro R, Bettinzoli M, Bordonali T, et al. Pneumonia in a cardiothoracic intensive care unit: incidence and risk factors. J Cardiothorac Vasc Anesth, 2009; 23: 780-788.

8. Following coronary artery bypass and mitral valve replacement surgery, a patient has continued hypoxemia while mechanically ventilated on postoperative day 3. The patient is diagnosed with acute respiratory distress syndrome (ARDS). All of the following are true concerning postcardiac surgery ARDS, EXCEPT:
   A. ARDS can be caused by blood transfusions
   B. Cardiogenic shock is a risk factor for ARDS
   C. The definition of ARDS includes cardiogenic pulmonary edema
   D. ARDS can be caused by cardiopulmonary bypass

Correct Answer: C

Explanation: Acute respiratory distress syndrome (ARDS) following cardiac surgery may develop as a sequela of blood transfusion or cardiopulmonary bypass. More commonly in the postoperative patient, ARDS is associated with cardiogenic shock, sepsis, or multisystem organ failure. Components of ARDS include diffuse alveolar damage resulting from endothelial and type I epithelial cell necrosis and noncardiogenic pulmonary edema caused by breakdown of the endothelial barrier with subsequent vascular permeability. In fact, if the pulmonary artery occlusion pressure is over 18 mmHg, pulmonary edema may have a cardiogenic etiology and is thus not considered to be ARDS.

Besides pulmonary edema being noncardiogenic in nature, the diagnosis of ARDS relies upon a low PaO_2/FIO_2 ratio of less than 300. The definition of ARDS was updated in 2012 and is called the Berlin definition. It differs from the previous American European Consensus definition by excluding the term "acute lung injury." The Berlin criteria also removed the requirement for wedge pressure less than 18 mmHg and included the requirement of positive end-expiratory pressure or continuous positive airway pressure of 5 cm H_2O or more.

References:

1. Higgins TL, Engelman DT. Chapter 39: Postoperative Respiratory Care. In: Kaplan JA, Augoustides JGT, Manecke GR, et al., eds. Kaplan's Cardiac Anesthesia. 7th ed. Elsevier; 2017:1358-1373.
2. Sanfilippo F, Palumbo GJ, Bignami E, et al. Acute respiratory distress syndrome in the perioperative period of cardiac surgery: predictors, diagnosis, prognosis, management options, and future directions. J Cardiothorac Vasc Anesth, 2022; 36: 1169-1179.
3. The ARDS Definition Task Force. Acute Respiratory Distress Syndrome: The Berlin Definition. JAMA, 2012; 307: 2526-2533.

9. Following coronary artery bypass and mitral valve replacement surgery, a patient has continued hypoxemia while mechanically ventilated on postoperative day 3. The patient is diagnosed with acute respiratory distress syndrome. Which ventilatory strategy has been shown to decrease further lung damage?
   A. Tidal volume under 6 mL/kg of ideal body weight
   B. Tidal volume under 6 mL/kg of actual body weight
   C. Peak inspiratory pressures over 35 cm H_2O to avoid atelectasis
   D. Pressure control ventilation

Correct Answer: A

Explanation: The problem in acute respiratory distress syndrome is that the lungs are no longer homogeneous, and high pressures can further damage the remaining normal lung. Direct mechanical injury may result from overdistention (volutrauma), high pressures (barotrauma), or shear injury from repetitive opening and closing. "Biotrauma" may also result from inflammatory mediator release and impaired antibacterial barriers.

Current clinical practice in patients with known or suspected lung injury is to limit inflation pressures. The maximal "safe" inflation pressure is not known, but evidence favors keeping peak inspiratory pressures lower than 35 cm H_2O and restricting tidal volumes to less than 6 mL/kg of ideal body weight in patients at risk for acute lung injury. The landmark Acute Respiratory Distress Syndrome Network (ARDSNet) trial randomized patients to 6 mL/kg versus 12 mL/kg of ideal body weight and demonstrated a significant improvement in 28-day survival rates in the group with a low tidal volume. This approach also allows for permissive hypercapnia if normal levels of $PaCO_2$ cannot be achieved with lower tidal volumes. Current data do not suggest a difference in pressure control over volume control ventilation.

References:
1. Higgins TL, Engelman DT. Chapter 39: Postoperative Respiratory Care. In: Kaplan JA, Augoustides JGT, Manecke GR, et al., eds. Kaplan's Cardiac Anesthesia. 7th ed. Elsevier; 2017:1358-1373.
2. Sanfilippo F, Palumbo GJ, Bignami E, et al. Acute respiratory distress syndrome in the perioperative period of cardiac surgery: predictors, diagnosis, prognosis, management options, and future directions. J Cardiothorac Vasc Anesth, 2022; 36: 1169-1179.
3. Brower RG, Matthay MA, Schoenfeld D, et al. Ventilation with lower tidal volumes as compared with traditional tidal volumes for acute lung injury and the acute respiratory distress syndrome. N Engl J Med, 2000; 342: 1301-1308.

10. A patient is recovering from an urgent aortic valve replacement secondary to endocarditis. The patient had preexisting sepsis prior to surgery. On postoperative day 5, the chest x-ray shows bilateral infiltrates. The PaO_2/FIO_2 ratio is 87, pH is 7.17, and $PaCO_2$ is 94 mmHg on arterial blood gas despite optimized ventilator settings. Transthoracic echocardiogram shows normal ejection fraction and appropriately functioning bioprosthetic aortic valve. What is the next BEST step in management for this patient?
    A. Lung recruitment maneuvers
    B. Venovenous extracorporeal membrane oxygenation support
    C. High-frequency oscillatory ventilation
    D. Venoarterial extracorporeal membrane oxygenation support

Correct Answer: B

Explanation: This patient has acute respiratory distress syndrome with severe hypoxemia, as well as hypercapnic respiratory failure, as seen on the arterial blood gas. Optimized ventilator settings would include low tidal volume ventilation, optimal positive end-expiratory pressure, and permissive hypercapnia. Extracorporeal membrane oxygenation (ECMO) is indicated for patients with severe refractory hypoxemia. This patient has a normal echocardiography study, suggesting the patient will likely benefit from venovenous ECMO without requiring venoarterial ECMO.

References:
1. Higgins TL, Engelman DT. Chapter 39: Postoperative Respiratory Care. In: Kaplan JA, Augoustides JGT, Manecke GR, et al., eds. Kaplan's Cardiac Anesthesia. 7th ed. Elsevier; 2017:1358-1373.
2. Sanfilippo F, Palumbo GJ, Bignami E, et al. Acute respiratory distress syndrome in the perioperative period of cardiac surgery: predictors, diagnosis, prognosis, management options, and future directions. J Cardiothorac Vasc Anesth, 2022; 36: 1169-1179.
3. Nasim R, Sukhal S, Ramakrishna H. Management strategies for severe and refractory acute respiratory distress syndrome: where do we stand in 2018? J Cardiothorac Vasc Anesth, 2019; 33: 2589-2594.

11. A 70-year-old patient undergoes a reoperative coronary artery bypass surgery with two saphenous vein grafts and one internal mammary graft. Despite a routine postoperative course, the patient is unable to be weaned from the ventilator. The arterial blood gas and chest x-ray are normal. The patient is awake and appropriately following commands with full strength. What is the most likely diagnosis?
    A. Diaphragm dysfunction
    B. Polyneuropathy
    C. Pneumonia
    D. Delirium

Correct Answer: A

Explanation: Approximately 7.6% of patients undergoing cardiac surgery have some form of diaphragmatic dysfunction. This can be permanent secondary to injury of the phrenic nerve or temporary. The phrenic nerve is at risk for injury due to location. The phrenic nerve courses bilaterally within close proximity of the internal mammary artery. It can be injured via transection or, alternatively, the blood supply to the phrenic nerve may be interrupted. Patients undergoing reoperation are more at risk because the nerve may be harder to identify given the fibrotic changes of the pericardial tissue.

References:

1. Higgins TL, Engelman DT. Chapter 39: Postoperative Respiratory Care. In: Kaplan JA, Augoustides JGT, Manecke GR, et al., eds. Kaplan's Cardiac Anesthesia. 7th ed. Elsevier; 2017:1358-1373.
2. Laghlam D, Lê MP, Srour A, et al. Diaphragm dysfunction after cardiac surgery: reappraisal. J Cardiothorac Vasc Anesth, 2021; 35: 3241-3247.

12. A 44-year old patient underwent a left ventricular assist device (LVAD) placement for nonischemic cardiomyopathy. Upon arrival to the intensive care unit, the patient has significant hypoxemia despite efforts to improve ventilation with 100% FiO_2 and positive end-expiratory pressure (PEEP) of 12 cm H_2O. Preoperative echocardiography demonstrated severe left ventricular dysfunction, mild right ventricular dysfunction and patent foramen ovale (PFO) with left to right shunt. The echocardiographic examination after LVAD implantation demonstrates a decompressed left ventricle and moderate right ventricular dysfunction. What is the MOST likely cause of this patient's refractory hypoxemia?

A. Pulmonary embolism
B. Inadequate PEEP
C. Right-to-left shunting across the PFO
D. Acute respiratory distress syndrome

Correct Answer: C

Explanation: In patients who are mechanically ventilated, shunt-induced hypoxemia should be considered if efforts to improve ventilation fail and hypoxia is not explained by pulmonary disease. Over the years there has been much discussion of what to do with the incidental finding of a patent foramen ovale (PFO). In a review of the literature, it is recommended if a PFO is found in a patient undergoing left ventricular assist device implantation, heart transplant, or other indication for arteriotomy, that the PFO be closed. The risk of a PFO converting from a left-to-right shunt to a right-to-left shunt increases with right ventricular dysfunction creating increased right ventricular and subsequently, right atrial pressures. Additionally, high levels of positive end-expiratory pressure increase right atrial pressure via transmission of pressure from the intrathoracic cavity. The patient is directly from the operating room and presumably has no known risk factors for acute pulmonary embolism and acute respiratory distress syndrome.

References:

1. Higgins TL, Engelman DT. Chapter 39: Postoperative Respiratory Care. In: Kaplan JA, Augoustides JGT, Manecke GR, et al., eds. Kaplan's Cardiac Anesthesia. 7th ed. Elsevier; 2017:1358-1373.
2. Ramakrishna H, Patel PA, Gutsche JT, et al. Incidental patent foramen ovale in adult cardiac surgery: recent evidence and management options for the perioperative echocardiographer. J Cardiothorac Vasc Anesth, 2014; 28: 1691-1695.

13. A patient who underwent a coronary artery bypass graft surgery 8 days ago has leukocytosis and fever. The sternal incision is erythematous and unstable. What is a risk for sternal dehiscence?

A. Male sex
B. Smoking
C. Use of left internal mammary graft
D. Reoperation for control of bleeding

Correct Answer: D

Explanation: Mediastinitis, sternal dehiscence, or both are complications of coronary revascularization, with an incidence of approximately 1%, a mortality rate of approximately 13%, and a tendency to prolong ventilator dependency. Predisposing factors for wound complications after cardiac operations include diabetes, low cardiac output, bilateral internal mammary artery grafts, and reoperation for control of bleeding. Keeping blood glucose lower than 200 mg/dL in the perioperative period reduces the sternal wound infection rate from 2.4% to 1.5%. Tight glucose control, however, increases the risk of hypoglycemia, and many clinicians have abandoned the very tight limits.

References:

1. Higgins TL, Engelman DT. Chapter 39: Postoperative Respiratory Care. In: Kaplan JA, Augoustides JGT, Manecke GR, et al., eds. Kaplan's Cardiac Anesthesia. 7th ed. Elsevier; 2017:1358-1373.
2. Phoon PHY, Hwang NC. Deep sternal wound infection: diagnosis, treatment and prevention. J Cardiothorac Anesth, 2020; 34: 1602-1613.

14. Which indication for intra-aortic balloon pump placement is associated with the least risk for prolonged mechanical ventilation following cardiac surgery?

A. Preoperative placement for cardiogenic shock
B. Preoperative placement for unstable angina
C. Intraoperative placement for high vasopressor requirement
D. Intraoperative placement for low cardiac output

Correct Answer: B

Explanation: Intra-aortic balloon pump (IABP) counterpulsation is associated with a higher risk of prolonged postoperative mechanical ventilation when placed for low cardiac output states, cardiac dysfunction, fluid overload, and/or associated organ injury. Additionally, patients whose IABP was placed for preoperative cardiogenic shock as an assist to separating from bypass or for low-output states in the postoperative period have a high mortality risk and frequently need prolonged ventilatory support.

When an IABP is placed preoperatively for unstable angina, the postbypass state is less likely to be associated with low cardiac output. Since the definitive surgical treatment should have corrected the reason for IABP placement, removal of the IABP and tracheal extubation need not be delayed.

References:

1. Higgins TL, Engelman DT. Chapter 39: Postoperative Respiratory Care. In: Kaplan JA, Augoustides JGT, Manecke GR, et al., eds. Kaplan's Cardiac Anesthesia. 7th ed. Elsevier; 2017:1358-1373.

B. A patient who underwent mitral valve replacement with central venous pressure of 18 mmHg

C. A patient who underwent atrial-septal defect closure with severe tricuspid regurgitation on epinephrine infusion

D. A patient who underwent aortic valve replacement with FiO_2 60% maintaining PaO_2 60 mmHg

Correct Answer: D

Explanation: Most cardiothoracic surgery patients do not benefit from excessive positive end-expiratory pressure (PEEP) settings. In fact, due to the thin wall of the right ventricle, excessive intrathoracic pressures due to ventilation settings can lead to increased right ventricular wall tension and pressure. High levels of PEEP may decrease venous return, which impedes cardiac output. Additionally, the pulmonary vasculature is also negatively affected by increased intrathoracic pressure, effectively increasing right ventricular afterload. Due to these sequalae, high levels of PEEP may lead to right ventricular dysfunction and should be avoided unless necessary in patients at risk of right ventricular dysfunction.

Maximizing oxygenation, ventilation, acid-base status, and temperature will help patients in right ventricular failure, but if hypoxemia is not present, increasing PEEP will not improve right ventricular function. Application of PEEP in the post–cardiac surgery patient usually involves balancing cardiac and pulmonary goals. The patient in scenario D of the presented question likely does not have right ventricular dysfunction and will benefit from higher PEEP to enhance alveolar recruitment and oxygenation.

References:

1. Higgins TL, Engelman DT. Chapter 39: Postoperative Respiratory Care. In: Kaplan JA, Augoustides JGT, Manecke GR, et al., eds. Kaplan's Cardiac Anesthesia. 7th ed. Elsevier; 2017:1358-1373.
2. Wang YC, Huang CH, Tu YK. Effects of positive airway pressure and mechanical ventilation of the lungs during cardiopulmonary bypass on pulmonary adverse events after cardiac surgery: a systematic review and meta-analysis. J Cardiothorac Vasc Anesth, 2018; 32: 748-759.

17. A patient with history of severe, long-standing chronic obstructive pulmonary disease and pulmonary hypertension is intubated in the intensive care unit after mitral valve repair. The patient is requiring epinephrine infusion due to right ventricular dysfunction. In order to maintain normal blood gas values, the ventilator is set at tidal volume 8 mL/kg, respiratory rate of 20 breaths per minute, and positive end-expiratory pressure (PEEP) of 8 cm H_2O. Which ventilation strategy change may improve the hemodynamics?

A. Increasing minute ventilation by increasing tidal volumes

B. Improving alveolar recruitment by increasing PEEP

C. Decreasing intrathoracic pressure by increasing the expiratory time

D. Increasing minute ventilation by increasing the respiratory rate

---

15. Which patient having a transcatheter aortic valve replacement procedure under general endotracheal anesthesia would be at highest risk for unsuccessful tracheal extubation at the end of the case?

A. A 75-year-old obese male without vasopressor requirement

B. A 64-year-old female who requires epinephrine and norepinephrine infusions after valve deployment

C. A 90-year-old female with history of chronic obstructive pulmonary disease on home oxygen

D. An 82-year-old male with history of uncontrolled diabetes having a valve-in-valve transcatheter aortic valve replacement

Correct Answer: B

Explanation: Following transcatheter aortic valve replacement (TAVR), the common risks for postoperative pulmonary complications, such as chronic obstructive pulmonary disease, diabetes, obesity, and extremes of age, should not prevent an early extubation trial if the patient meets clinical criteria. Valve-in-valve TAVR can be a more complicated procedure and require longer anesthetic and surgical times to ensure safe deployment, but this too should not prevent an early extubation trial if the patient meets respiratory and cardiovascular criteria for extubation.

However, a patient with an inotropic or large vasopressor requirement after valve deployment should not be a candidate for early extubation in case of need for additional surgical procedures or aggressive cardiogenic or pulmonary support. The TAVR-related randomized controlled studies are limited for the optimal management of these patients requiring postoperative intubation; however, extrapolating from other cardiac surgeries, hemodynamic instability would be a risk for unsuccessful extubation.

References:

1. Higgins TL, Engelman DT. Chapter 39: Postoperative Respiratory Care. In: Kaplan JA, Augoustides JGT, Manecke GR, et al., eds. Kaplan's Cardiac Anesthesia. 7th ed. Elsevier; 2017:1358-1373.
2. Raiten JM, Gutsche JT, Horak J, et al. Critical care management of patients following transcatheter aortic valve replacement. F1000Res, 2013; 2; 62.
3. Lester L, Brady MB, Brown CH 4th. Sedation versus general anesthesia for TAVR: where do we go from here? J Cardiothorac Vasc Anesth, 2017; 31: 2055-2057.

16. Which patient would most likely benefit from positive end-expiratory pressure greater than 10 mmHg?

A. A patient who underwent coronary artery bypass graft with echocardiography demonstrating right ventricular dysfunction on vasopressin infusion

---

2. Webb CA, Weyker PD, Flynn BC. Management of intra-aortic balloon pumps. Semin Cardiothorac Vasc Anesth, 2015; 19: 106-121.
3. Chacon M, Markin NW. Early is good, but is immediate better? Considerations in fast-track extubation after cardiac surgery. J Cardiothorac Vasc Anesth, 2022; 36: 1265-1267.

Correct Answer: C

Explanation: Patients with long-standing severe chronic obstructive pulmonary disease are at risk of occult positive end-expiratory pressure (PEEP) generation, known as "auto-PEEP" that may lead to air trapping and higher than anticipated intrathoracic pressures. In patients with right ventricular dysfunction, rising intrathoracic pressure decreases venous return and increases right ventricular oxygen demand due to higher afterload. Off-loading the right ventricle by decreasing the intrathoracic pressure can be accomplished by decreasing PEEP, either by increasing the expiratory time of the respiration cycle, decreasing the respiratory rate or turning off the PEEP setting on the ventilator. Auto-PEEP can be detected by respiratory waveform monitoring or by pressure monitoring with the ventilator's expiratory port held closed at end-exhalation.

References:

1. Higgins TL, Engelman DT. Chapter 39: Postoperative Respiratory Care. In: Kaplan JA, Augoustides JGT, Manecke GR, et al., eds. Kaplan's Cardiac Anesthesia. 7th ed. Elsevier; 2017:1358-1373.
2. Wang YC, Huang CH, Tu YK. Effects of positive airway pressure and mechanical ventilation of the lungs during cardiopulmonary bypass on pulmonary adverse events after cardiac surgery: a systematic review and meta-analysis. J Cardiothorac Vasc Anesth, 2018; 32: 748-759.

18. Which of the following is a benefit of increased positive end-expiratory pressure of 10 cm H_2O in cardiac surgical patients?
    A. Decreased chest tube output in bleeding patients
    B. Prevention of acute respiratory distress syndrome
    C. Improved right ventricular function
    D. Decreased atelectasis

Correct Answer: D

Explanation: Positive end-expiratory pressure (PEEP) increases the end-expiratory lung volume and counteracts airway closure by having a dominant effect in dependent lung regions. Thus, glottic levels of PEEP (5 cm H_2O for healthy lungs) seem sufficient to essentially prevent or reverse atelectasis. The negative effects of PEEP are most marked in the presence of abnormal right ventricular function, particularly if the right coronary artery is compromised. In patients with right ventricular dysfunction, increasing intrathoracic pressure decreases venous return and increases right ventricular wall tension, increasing the right ventricular oxygen demand. PEEP neither protects against the development of acute respiratory distress syndrome, nor reduces the amount of mediastinal bleeding after cardiac surgical procedures with cardiopulmonary bypass. Most clinicians routinely use 5 cm H_2O of PEEP in ventilated patients after cardiac surgery to decrease pulmonary atelectasis.

References:

1. Higgins TL, Engelman DT. Chapter 39: Postoperative Respiratory Care. In: Kaplan JA, Augoustides JGT, Manecke GR, et al., eds. Kaplan's Cardiac Anesthesia. 7th ed. Elsevier; 2017:1358-1373.

19. A patient with pulmonary hypertension is undergoing a tricuspid valve replacement. Attempts at weaning from cardiopulmonary bypass have failed due to systemic pulmonary pressures and subsequent right ventricular dysfunction. The following would be beneficial in right ventricular support when weaning from cardiopulmonary bypass in this patient, EXCEPT:
    A. Phenylephrine
    B. Inhaled iloprost
    C. Milrinone
    D. Inhaled nitric oxide

Correct Answer: A

Explanation: Elevated pulmonary artery pressure results from vasoconstriction, smooth muscle cell proliferation, and endothelial cell proliferation. Collagen vascular diseases, chronic thromboembolic obstruction of the pulmonary arteries, concomitant lung diseases, congenital heart disease, and left-sided heart failure all may be associated with pulmonary hypertension. These patients can present anesthetic and critical care challenges, especially following cardiopulmonary bypass, with complement activation, leukocyte activation, and release of inflammatory mediators. Inhaled nitric oxide, inhaled prostacyclins, such as iloprost, the endothelin-1 antagonist bosentan, and phosphodiesterase inhibitors, such as milrinone, are among the available therapies. A study of 61 high-risk adult cardiac surgical patients with pulmonary hypertension suggested that preemptive treatment using a combination of milrinone and inhaled prostacyclin before bypass reduces postbypass pulmonary pressures and the need for vasoactive support in the intensive care unit. Phenylephrine offers no right ventricular support and in fact increases right ventricular afterload by increasing pulmonary vascular resistance via alpha-receptor agonism.

References:

1. Higgins TL, Engelman DT. Chapter 39: Postoperative Respiratory Care. In: Kaplan JA, Augoustides JGT, Manecke GR, et al., eds. Kaplan's Cardiac Anesthesia. 7th ed. Elsevier; 2017:1358-1373.
2. Laflamme M, Perrault LP, Carrier M, et al. Preliminary experience with combined inhaled milrinone and prostacyclin in cardiac surgical patients with pulmonary hypertension. J Cardiothorac Vas Anesth, 2015; 29: 38-45.

20. Upon attempting to awaken a patient following mitral valve repair, the patient appears to be breathing against the ventilator and develops hemodynamic instability. These statements concerning ventilator dyssynchrony are true, EXCEPT:
    A. Ventilator dyssynchrony leads to increased intercostal and abdominal muscle tone

B. Ventilator dyssynchrony leads to increased chest cage compliance

C. Ventilator dyssynchrony is commonly due to mismatch between ventilator support and patient demand

D. Ventilator dyssynchrony may be due to insensitive systems or intrinsic positive end-expiratory pressure

Correct Answer: B

Explanation: Ventilator dyssynchrony occurs when a patient impedes inhalation or exhalation from the ventilator. Ventilator dyssynchrony leads to increased intercostal and abdominal muscle tone and pressure. This, in turn, leads to decreased chest cage compliance. During volume-cycled ventilation, a decrease in chest cage compliance results in elevated intrathoracic pressure that may reduce venous return to the right side of the heart.

The most common reason for ventilator dyssynchrony is a mismatch between ventilator support and patient demand. During the triggering phase, insensitive systems or intrinsic positive end-expiratory pressure may cause delayed or missing triggers. During flow delivery, either inadequate flow or excessive flow can be responsible. Cycling may also be mismatched if the patient's effort continues despite termination of the machine breath or if the patient is exhaling to terminate a prolonged machine breath.

References:

1. Higgins TL, Engelman DT. Chapter 39: Postoperative Respiratory Care. In: Kaplan JA, Augoustides JGT, Manecke GR, et al., eds. Kaplan's Cardiac Anesthesia. 7th ed. Elsevier; 2017:1358-1373.
2. Bignami E, Guarnieri M, Saglietti F, et al. Mechanical ventilation during cardiopulmonary bypass. J Cardiothorac Vasc Anesth, 2016; 30: 1668-1675.
3. Oto B, Annesi J, Foley RJ. Patient-ventilator dyssynchrony in the intensive care unit: A practical approach to diagnosis and management. Anaesth Intensive Care, 2021; 49: 86-97.

21. A patient had a prolonged perioperative course following an aortic and mitral valve replacement surgery. The patient was on extracorporeal membrane oxygenation for 4 days with severe ventilator dyssynchrony requiring sedative and paralytic infusions. What is TRUE concerning prolonged paralysis in the intensive care unit?

A. Critical illness polyneuropathy has only been shown to occur following steroidal paralytic agents

B. Critical illness polyneuropathy typically does not lead to delayed tracheal extubation, as the extremities are most affected

C. Accurate monitoring of the train-of-four ratio prevents critical illness neuropathy

D. Accumulation of paralytic drug metabolites is thought to lead to critical illness neuropathy

Correct Answer: D

Explanation: Critical illness polyneuropathy has been shown to occur following steroidal paralytic agents (e.g., rocuronium, vecuronium, pancuronium) and benzylisoquinolinium paralytic agents (e.g., mivacurium, atracurium, cisatracurium). Critical illness polyneuropathy is a cause of delayed tracheal extubation and delayed clinical progression as all muscle groups are affected. Even with accurate monitoring of train-of-four ratio, patients can be profoundly weak after receiving paralytic medications when critically ill. The genesis of this condition is thought to be related to the accumulation of paralytic drug metabolites.

References:

1. Higgins TL, Engelman DT. Chapter 39: Postoperative Respiratory Care. In: Kaplan JA, Augoustides JGT, Manecke GR, et al., eds. Kaplan's Cardiac Anesthesia. 7th ed. Elsevier; 2017:1358-1373.
2. Shepherd S, Batra A, Lerner DP. Review of critical illness myopathy and neuropathy. Neurohospitalist, 2017; 7: 41-48.
3. Yu PJ, Cassiere HA, Fishbein J, et al. Outcomes of patients with prolonged intensive care unit length of stay after cardiac surgery. J Cardiothorac Vasc Anesth, 2016; 30: 1550-1554.

22. A patient after aortic valve replacement has not been liberated from the ventilator after a week due to weakness and copious secretions. A tracheostomy is planned. All of the following are true in this case, EXCEPT:

A. It is uncommon to see damage to the airway epithelium or vocal cords prior to 21 days of endotracheal intubation

B. Copious secretions are an indication for tracheostomy in patients who cannot spontaneously clear their secretions

C. Pneumothorax is a known complication following tracheostomy

D. Tracheoinnominate fistulas may occur after tracheostomy

Correct Answer: A

Explanation: Prolonged endotracheal intubation results in damage to the respiratory epithelium and cilia and may lead to vocal cord damage and airway stenosis. This injury can begin as early as 10 days of endotracheal intubation. If mechanical ventilation is anticipated for longer than 14 days, consideration should be given to early tracheostomy. Other indications for tracheostomy include copious or tenacious secretions in debilitated patients who are unable to clear secretions spontaneously. Tracheostomy is relatively contraindicated in patients with ongoing mediastinitis or local infection at the tracheostomy site because of the potential for mediastinal contamination with respiratory secretions. Tracheostomy is not a risk-free procedure, and complications include pneumothorax, pneumomediastinum, subcutaneous emphysema, incisional hemorrhage, late tracheal stenosis or tracheomalacia, stomal infections, and rarely tracheoinnominate fistula.

References:

1. Higgins TL, Engelman DT. Chapter 39: Postoperative Respiratory Care. In: Kaplan JA, Augoustides JGT, Manecke GR, et al., eds. Kaplan's Cardiac Anesthesia. 7th ed. Elsevier; 2017:1358-1373.

2. Gazda AJ, Kwak MJ, Jani P, et al. Association between early tracheostomy and delirium in older adults in the United States. J Cardiothorac Vasc Anesth, 2021; 35: 1974-1980.
3. Affronti A, Casali F, Eusebi P, et al. Early versus late tracheostomy in cardiac surgical patients: a 12-year single center experience. J Cardiothorac Vasc Anesth, 2019; 33: 82-90.

23. Following an aortic valve replacement and hemiarch repair surgery, a patient has a left pleural effusion. As oxygen requirements increase, drainage of the effusion is attempted. What is TRUE regarding postoperative pleural effusions?

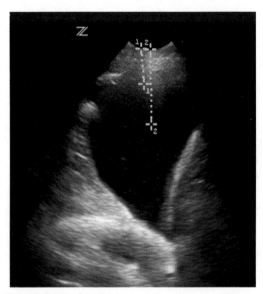

FIGURE 35.2 Pleural effusion, left hemithorax: With the patient seated erect, the transducer is oriented perpendicular to the left chest wall at the skin mark. The following measurements were obtained: depth to enter the fluid collection, 1.7 cm; depth to midfluid collection, 3.7 cm.

A. Treatment of pleural effusions always requires a thoracostomy tube to be left in place
B. Pleural effusions cause impaired gas exchange due to atelectasis
C. Since pleural effusions are in a sterile, contained environment, infection is not a risk
D. Transthoracic echocardiography is not useful in quantifying the amount of effusion present

Correct Answer: B

Explanation: Following cardiac surgery, fluid often accumulates in the pleural space. This fluid can be from bleeding or transudate and can compress lung parenchyma. This compression leads to atelectasis resulting in impaired gas exchange. An undetected pleural effusion may also act as a potential source of postoperative infection.

Transthoracic echocardiography can be used to assess the size of a pleural effusion, help mark the skin at the site that is optimal for needle insertion to drain the effusion, and verify that no lung tissue is present in the area where the operator plans to insert the needle.

Treatment of pleural effusion is with thoracentesis or placement of a tube thoracostomy. Drainage of pleural fluid can result in a significant improvement in oxygenation in acute respiratory failure patients who were refractory to treatment with mechanical ventilation and positive end-expiratory pressure.

References:

1. Higgins TL, Engelman DT. Chapter 39: Postoperative Respiratory Care. In: Kaplan JA, Augoustides JGT, Manecke GR, et al., eds. Kaplan's Cardiac Anesthesia. 7th ed. Elsevier; 2017:1358-1373.
2. Bronshteyn Y, Anderson T, Badakhsh O, et al. Diagnostic point-of-care ultrasound: recommendations from an expert panel. J Cardiothorac Vasc Anesth, 2022; 36: 22-29.

24. An 80-year-old patient is recovering from a valve replacement procedure. On postoperative day 2, she begins to perseverate and hallucinate. Her family is very concerned and voices many questions. These statements should be discussed with the family, EXCEPT:
A. Reorientation and provision of glasses and hearing aids may decrease delirium
B. Attempts to minimize narcotic administration when possible
C. Initiation of dexmedetomidine may decrease the delirium
D. Postoperative delirium is rare following cardiac surgery and only occurs in 1% to 2% of patients

Correct Answer: D

Explanation: Delirium after cardiac surgical procedures is common, with an estimated incidence of about 30% in the general cardiac surgical population that may increase to 83% in mechanically ventilated patients. Initial postoperative management of agitation consists of reassurance and orientation of the patient and control of pain. Corticosteroids increase the risk of delirium. Avoiding narcotics with a multimodal pain management technique is advised. Delirium resolves spontaneously or with pharmacologic intervention in almost all patients.

Dexmedetomidine is associated with less delirium than benzodiazepine sedation. Alcohol or benzodiazepine withdrawal should be considered in the differential diagnosis of delirium in patients with those risk factors. Newer agents such as risperidone, olanzapine, and quetiapine may also be useful. Current evidence does not support pharmacologic prophylaxis against delirium with these agents.

References:

1. Higgins TL, Engelman DT. Chapter 39: Postoperative Respiratory Care. In: Kaplan JA, Augoustides JGT, Manecke GR, et al., eds. Kaplan's Cardiac Anesthesia. 7th ed. Elsevier; 2017:1358-1373.
2. Järvelä K, Porkkala H, Karlsson S, et al. Postoperative delirium in cardiac surgery patients. J Cardiothorac Vasc Anesth, 2018; 32: 1597-1602.

3. Afonso A, Scurlock C, Reich D, et al. Predictive model for postoperative delirium in cardiac surgical patients. Semin Cardiothorac Vasc Anesth, 2010; 14: 212-217.

25. After failing to wean from mechanical ventilation, a patient who underwent a mitral valve repair is suspected of having a diaphragm injury. All of the following are true regarding diaphragmatic injury following cardiac surgery, EXCEPT:
    A. Comparing vital capacity and tidal volume in the supine and seated positions will yield the same volumes in a patient with unilateral diaphragmatic injury
    B. Diaphragmatic injury occurs in approximately 4% of patients after cardiac surgery
    C. Diaphragmatic injury appears as paradoxical movement of the diaphragm during inspiration
    D. Transient diaphragmatic paralysis can occur secondary to cold injury to the phrenic nerve

Correct Answer: A

Explanation: Diaphragmatic paralysis may complicate any cardiac procedure, but it is more common in patients undergoing reoperation, given the difficulty in identifying the phrenic nerve in fibrotic pericardial tissue. Permanent bilateral diaphragmatic paralysis is rare (<0.1% of patients after cardiac surgery), but temporary diaphragmatic weakness may occur in 4% or more of patients. The diagnosis of diaphragmatic paralysis should be suspected whenever a patient fails to be weaned from mechanical ventilation.

Patients with diaphragmatic injury will have paradoxical movement of the diaphragm during inspiration. They will also have different vital capacity and tidal volume measurements in the supine versus the seated positions. Differences in supine and seated vital capacity of more than 10% to 15% should prompt fluoroscopic examination of the diaphragm ("sniff" test). Bilateral paralysis may be missed by this test because comparison of left and right diaphragmatic excursion has lower specificity when both sides of the diaphragm are involved. Transient diaphragmatic paralysis can occur secondary to cold injury to the phrenic nerve. Less often, the phrenic nerve is injured or transected during dissection of the internal mammary arteries or during mobilization of the heart in patients undergoing reoperation due to fibrotic pericardial tissue.

References:

1. Higgins TL, Engelman DT. Chapter 39: Postoperative Respiratory Care. In: Kaplan JA, Augoustides JGT, Manecke GR, et al., eds. Kaplan's Cardiac Anesthesia. 7th ed. Elsevier; 2017:1358-1373.
2. Laghlam D, Lê MP, Srour A, et al. Diaphragm dysfunction after cardiac surgery: reappraisal. J Cardiothorac Vasc Anesth, 2021; 35: 3241-3247.

26. A homeless patient arrives to the intensive care unit following an emergent coronary artery bypass grafting procedure. The patient's albumin level was found to be 2.0 g/dL on admission labs from the emergency department. The following are associated with hypoalbuminemia prior to cardiac surgery, EXCEPT:
    A. Ventilation time
    B. Bleeding
    C. Sepsis
    D. Renal failure

Correct Answer: C

Explanation: Nutritional adequacy has a strong influence on outcomes following cardiac surgery. Hypoalbuminemia decreases a patient's ability to be weaned from ventilation. Preoperative albumin levels lower than 2.5 g/dL are associated with increased risk of reoperation for bleeding, postoperative renal failure, and prolonged ventilatory support, intensive care unit length of stay, and hospital length of stay. Weaning success occurs in approximately 93% of patients with adequate nutritional support, but in only 50% of those with inadequate nutrition. Increases in albumin and transferrin level with parenteral nutrition predict eventual ability to be weaned from ventilation. Enteral and parenteral routes appear to be similar in caloric delivery, infectious complications, and mortality rates, although hypoglycemia and vomiting are more likely with enteral delivery. Sepsis can induce hypoalbuminemia due to several pathophysiological mechanisms, but hypoalbuminemia is not a known risk factor for becoming septic.

References:

1. Higgins TL, Engelman DT. Chapter 39: Postoperative Respiratory Care. In: Kaplan JA, Augoustides JGT, Manecke GR, et al., eds. Kaplan's Cardiac Anesthesia. 7th ed. Elsevier; 2017:1358-1373.
2. Lee EH, Chin JH, Choi DK, et al. Postoperative hypoalbuminemia is associated with outcome in patients undergoing off-pump coronary artery bypass graft surgery. J Cardiothorac Vasc Anesth, 2011; 25: 462-468.
3. Karas P, Goh S, Dhital K. Is low serum albumin associated with postoperative complications in patients undergoing cardiac surgery? Interact CardioVasc Thorac Surg, 2015; 21: 777-786.

27. A patient arrives at the cardiothoracic intensive care unit following an aortic valve replacement and ascending aortic arch repair. The first arterial blood gas analysis results are as follows: 7.24/60/109/22/-1. The ventilator is set on volume control of 450 mL tidal volume, respiratory rate of 12 bpm, FiO_2 of 50%, and PEEP of 5 cm H_2O. Peak inspiratory pressure is 28 cm H_2O. What is the next BEST step in management?
    A. Administer two ampules of sodium bicarbonate
    B. Switch to pressure control ventilation mode
    C. Decrease tidal volume
    D. Increase respiratory rate

Correct Answer: D

Explanation: This patient is demonstrating an isolated respiratory acidosis due to an acidotic pH with hypercarbia in the setting of a normal serum bicarbonate level. If one wished to calculate this for acute respiratory acidosis, the expected decrease in pH = 0.08 × (measured $PaCO_2$ − 40). In this example, the pH decreases by 0.16, and the $PaCO_2$ increases by 20 mmHg (from 40 mmHg). This means that there is not a metabolic component adding to this acidosis, nor compensating the respiratory acidosis. Thus, administering sodium bicarbonate would not be recommended.

In this scenario, the minute ventilation needs to be increased. This can be accomplished by increasing the respiratory rate or the tidal volume. Because this patient's peak inspiratory pressure is already nearing upper levels, the recommendation would be to increase respiratory rate instead of tidal volume. Switching to pressure control is an option, but is not the immediate fix to the respiratory acidosis without increasing minute ventilation concomitantly.

References:

1. Higgins TL, Engelman DT. Chapter 39: Postoperative Respiratory Care. In: Kaplan JA, Augoustides JGT, Manecke GR, et al., eds. Kaplan's Cardiac Anesthesia. 7th ed. Elsevier; 2017:1358-1373.
2. Jia S, Kumar P. Con: Metabolic acidosis should not be corrected with sodium bicarbonate in cardiac surgical patients. J Cardiothorac Vasc Anesth, 2022; 36: 619-621.
3. Robba C, Siwicka-Gieroba D, Sikter A, et al. Pathophysiology and clinical consequences of arterial blood gases and pH after cardiac arrest. Intensive Care Med Exp, 2020; 8: 19.

28. A 56-year old patient arrives to the intensive care unit following cardiac surgery on volume control ventilation. What BEST describes volume control ventilation?
  A. The patient cannot initiate breaths
  B. The pressure waveform is square-shaped
  C. The inspiratory flow rate and time are set by the provider
  D. Ventilation/perfusion mismatch is less likely to occur compared with pressure control ventilation

Correct Answer: C

Explanation: With volume modes, the inspiratory flow rate, targeted volume, and inspiratory time are set by the clinician, and inspiratory peak pressure varies depending on the patient's lung compliance and synchrony with the ventilator. Volume cycling ensures consistent delivery of a set tidal volume as long as the pressure limit is not exceeded. With nonhomogeneous lung disorders, however, delivered volume tends to flow to areas of low resistance, which may result in overdistention of healthy segments of lung and underinflation of atelectatic segments with consequent ventilation/perfusion mismatching.

Volume breaths may be triggered by a timer (control mode ventilation) or by the patient's effort between the control-mode breaths. In either case, the tidal volume delivered is determined by the ventilator settings. This situation can present a problem in a patient with tachypnea as a response to neurologic injury. If the patient breathes inappropriately in response to normal arterial levels of CO_2, significant respiratory alkalosis will result. In volume control ventilation, the

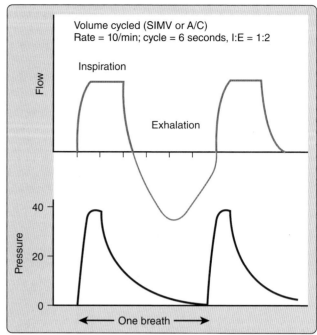

FIGURE 35.3 The top tracing shows the inspiratory flow, which is close to a square wave. Originally this flow pattern was dictated by the function of mechanical valves, but it may now be duplicated electronically. Note that the flow waveform becomes negative (opposite direction) during the exhalation phase. The typical volume cycled breath with a square waveform results in a rapid rise to peak inspiratory pressure followed by a gradual decline. If the safety pressure limit is exceeded, the peak of the pressure waveform may be truncated. *A/C,* Assist-control mode; *I:E,* inspiration-to-expiration ratio; *SIMV,* synchronized intermittent mandatory ventilation.

pressure waveform is shark-fin shaped, while the flow waveform is square shaped.

References:

1. Higgins TL, Engelman DT. Chapter 39: Postoperative Respiratory Care. In: Kaplan JA, Augoustides JGT, Manecke GR, et al., eds. Kaplan's Cardiac Anesthesia. 7th ed. Elsevier; 2017:1358-1373.
2. Morita Y, Williams B, Yamada Y, et al. Effect of anesthesia machine ventilator and ICU ventilator on intraoperative oxygenation and ventilation. J Cardiothorac Vasc Anesth, 2022; 36: 3175-3186.
3. Flynn BC, Miranda HG, Mittel AM, et al. Stepwise ventilator waveform assessment to diagnose pulmonary pathophysiology. Anesthesiology, 2022; 137: 85-92.

29. A 66-year-old patient arrives to the intensive care unit following cardiac surgery on pressure control ventilation. Which of the following BEST describes pressure control ventilation?
  A. The inspiratory flow rate is set by the provider
  B. The pressure waveform is shark-fin shaped
  C. The flow waveform is square shaped
  D. Evidence demonstrates improved oxygenation in less compliant lungs compared with volume control ventilation

Correct Answer: D

Explanation: Pressure-controlled ventilation allows the provider to specify a target inspiratory pressure. The ventilator then calculates and delivers the optimal flow rate to achieve the desired tidal volume and inspiratory-to-expiratory ratio. At a given plateau pressure (similar end-inspiratory distention), a lower tidal volume and increased positive end-expiratory pressure are associated with better recruitment and oxygenation. In pressure control ventilation, the pressure waveform is square shaped, while the flow waveform is shark-fin shaped.

References:

1. Higgins TL, Engelman DT. Chapter 39: Postoperative Respiratory Care. In: Kaplan JA, Augoustides JGT, Manecke GR, et al., eds. Kaplan's Cardiac Anesthesia. 7th ed. Elsevier; 2017:1358-1373.
2. Morita Y, Williams B, Yamada Y, et al. Effect of anesthesia machine ventilator and ICU ventilator on intraoperative oxygenation and ventilation. J Cardiothorac Vasc Anesth, 2022; 36: 3175-3186.
3. Flynn BC, Miranda HG, Mittel AM, et al. Stepwise ventilator waveform assessment to diagnose pulmonary pathophysiology. Anesthesiology, 2022; 137: 85-92.

30. A patient arrived at the intensive care unit 4 hours ago after having a mitral valve repair. The patient arrived on volume control ventilation and has been switched to pressure support ventilation. Which statement about pressure support ventilation is TRUE?

   A. Pressure support ventilation requires the provider to set a level of pressure assist

   B. Pressure support ventilation generally requires more sedation

   C. Pressure support ventilation requires the provider to set the respiratory rate

   D. Pressure support ventilation requires less patient effort

Correct Answer: A

Explanation: Pressure support augments the patient's spontaneous inspiratory effort with a clinician-selected level of pressure. Advantages include improved comfort for the patient and faster weaning. The volume delivered with each breath depends on the pressure set for inspiratory assist, as well as the patient's lung compliance. The utility of pressure support in weaning from long-term ventilation support is that it allows the patient's ventilatory muscles to assume part of the workload while augmenting tidal volume, thus preventing atelectasis, sufficiently stretching lung receptors, and keeping the patient's spontaneous respiratory rate within a reasonable physiologic range. Tidal volume varies markedly with the patient's lung compliance, so close clinical observation is needed with the initiation of pressure support.

References:

1. Higgins TL, Engelman DT. Chapter 39: Postoperative Respiratory Care. In: Kaplan JA, Augoustides JGT, Manecke GR, et al., eds. Kaplan's Cardiac Anesthesia. 7th ed. Elsevier; 2017:1358-1373.
2. Morita Y, Williams B, Yamada Y, et al. Effect of anesthesia machine ventilator and ICU ventilator on intraoperative oxygenation and ventilation. J Cardiothorac Vasc Anesth, 2022; 36: 3175-3186.
3. Flynn BC, Miranda HG, Mittel AM, et al. Stepwise ventilator waveform assessment to diagnose pulmonary pathophysiology. Anesthesiology, 2022; 137: 85-92.

CHAPTER 36

Central Nervous System Dysfunction After Cardiopulmonary Bypass

Shea Stoops and Brigid Flynn

KEY POINTS

1. Despite a progressive decrease in cardiac surgical mortality, the incidence of postoperative neurologic complications has remained relatively unchanged over the decades. During this same interval, the age, acuity, and extent of comorbidities in cardiac surgical patients have increased.

2. The risk for stroke in patients undergoing coronary artery surgery increases progressively with increasing age, ranging from 0.5% for patients younger than 55 years to 2.3% for those older than 75 years.

3. Age-associated increased risk of stroke and adverse central nervous system (CNS) outcome appear to be powered primarily by comorbidities, particularly ascending and aortic arch atherosclerosis.

4. Neurologic events in cardiac surgical patients are associated with increased postoperative mortality, prolonged intensive care unit stay, longer hospital stay, decreased quality of life, and decreased long-term survival.

5. Neurologic complications range from coma, stroke, and visual field deficits to impairments of cognitive processes (e.g., delirium, impaired memory and attention, mood alterations).

6. Mechanisms for neurologic injury in cardiac surgery include some combination of cerebral embolism, hypoperfusion, and inflammation, associated vascular disease, and altered cerebral autoregulation, rendering the brain more susceptible to injury.

7. Progression of underlying disease is a confounder in assessing late postoperative CNS complications.

8. Although occlusive carotid disease is associated with increased risk of perioperative stroke, such stroke is not infrequently contralateral, and concomitant perioperative carotid endarterectomy may increase risk of stroke and other major adverse events.

9. Perioperative risk factors for neurologic complications include renal dysfunction, diabetes mellitus, hypertension, prior cerebrovascular disease, aortic atheromatosis, manipulation of ascending aorta, complex surgical procedures, bypass time longer than 2 hours, hypothermic circulatory arrest, hemodynamic instability during and after bypass, new-onset atrial fibrillation, hyperglycemia, hyperthermia, and hypoxemia.

10. Routine epiaortic scanning before instrumentation of the ascending aorta is a sensitive and specific technique used to detect nonpalpable aortic atheromatosis.

11. In patients with significant ascending aorta atheromatosis, avoidance of aortic manipulation ("no-touch technique") is associated with decreased perioperative stroke.

12. Strategies to decrease the impact of cardiopulmonary bypass (CPB) on embolization, inflammation, and coagulation will decrease neurologic complications.

13. Cerebrovascular disease renders patients who experience wide hemodynamic perturbations during CPB at greater risk for perioperative stroke.

14. Modular minimally invasive extracorporeal circulation is a new approach to physiologically integrated CPB and is associated with a variety of improved outcomes.

15. Minimal access (minimally invasive) surgery can produce greater physiologic derangements and risk of adverse outcomes compared with conventional CPB.

KEY POINTS— cont'd

16. Cerebral near-infrared spectroscopy (cerebral oximetry) can detect cerebral ischemia and is associated with decreased incidence of stroke and improved outcomes after cardiac surgery.
17. There is a greater incidence of early postoperative cognitive dysfunction in patients exposed to conventional CPB compared with off-pump and noncardiac surgical patients.
18. The incidence of late cognitive dysfunction and stroke appears to be similar between groups undergoing conventional CPB, percutaneous coronary intervention, or medical management, implying progression of underlying disease and atrial arrhythmias as primary mechanisms of late stroke.
19. Pharmacologic management should be directed primarily toward intraoperative usage of volatile anesthetics, continuance of perioperative aspirin and statin medications, minimization of hyperglycemia, and vigilant therapy for postoperative atrial arrhythmia.

1. Patients undergoing which of the following are at the lowest risk of early stroke?
   A. Coronary artery bypass grafting
   B. Coronary artery bypass grafting and aortic valve replacement
   C. Coronary artery bypass grafting and mitral valve repair
   D. Off-pump coronary artery bypass

Correct Answer: D

Explanation: Patients undergoing off-pump versus on-pump coronary artery bypass are at significantly lower risk of early stroke. A possible reason for this significant difference is less manipulation of the aorta in the off-pump approach. The stroke risk after cardiac surgery is significantly increased in combined coronary and valve procedures, such as those described in options B and C.

References:

1. Flier S, Murkin JM. Chapter 40: Central Nervous System Dysfunction After Cardiopulmonary Bypass. In: Kaplan JA, Augoustides JGT, Manecke GR, et al., eds. Kaplan's Cardiac Anesthesia. 7th ed. Elsevier; 2017:1374-1406.
2. Nishiyama K, Horiguchi M, Shizuta S, et al. Temporal pattern of strokes after on-pump and offpump coronary artery bypass graft surgery. Ann Thorac Surg, 2009; 87: 1839-1844.
3. Ridderstolpe L, Ahlgren E, Gill H, et al. Risk factor analysis of early and delayed cerebral complications after cardiac surgery. J Cardiothorac Anesth, 2002; 16: 278-285.
4. Lo EYW, Dignan R, French B. Independent predictors of postoperative stroke with cardiopulmonary bypass. J Cardiothorac Vasc Anesth, 2022; 36: 133-137.

2. A patient who underwent coronary artery bypass grafting and aortic valve replacement demonstrated left facial droop and left facial weakness. Cerebral imaging obtained at postoperative hour 8 revealed no abnormalities. Within 12 hours, the weakness resolved, and the exam was back to baseline. What is TRUE regarding postoperative neurologic complications?
   A. A stroke is defined as any new focalized sensorimotor deficit with persistence beyond 24 hours and with confirmation by brain imaging
   B. A transient ischemic attack is defined as brief neurologic dysfunction persisting for less than 24 hours
   C. Delirium is described as a transient global impairment of cognitive function, reduced level of consciousness, and focal sensorimotor weakness
   D. Neurologic dysfunction lasting longer than 4 days, but less than 7 days, is termed a reversible ischemic neurologic deficit

Correct Answer: B

Explanation: A stroke is defined clinically as any new focal sensorimotor deficit persisting longer than 24 hours, either identified on clinical grounds only or, ideally, confirmed by brain imaging. Transient ischemic attack is defined as brief neurologic dysfunction persisting for less than 24 hours. Neurologic dysfunction lasting longer than 24 hours but less than 72 hours is termed a reversible ischemic neurologic deficit. Delirium is described as a transient global impairment of cognitive function, reduced level of consciousness, profound changes in sleep pattern, and attention abnormalities. Delirium is not usually associated with focal sensorimotor deficits or weakness, which is more indicative of transient ischemic attack, reversible ischemic neurologic deficit, or stroke.

References:

1. Flier S, Murkin JM. Chapter 40: Central Nervous System Dysfunction After Cardiopulmonary Bypass. In: Kaplan JA, Augoustides JGT, Manecke GR, et al., eds. Kaplan's Cardiac Anesthesia. 7th ed. Elsevier; 2017:1374-1406.
2. Kashani HH, Mosienko L, Grocott BB, et al. Postcardiac surgery acute stroke therapies: a systematic review. J Cardiothorac Vasc Anesth, 2020; 34: 2349-2354.
3. Ridderstolpe L, Ahlgren E, Gill H, et al. Risk factor analysis of early and delayed cerebral complications after cardiac surgery. J Cardiothorac Anesth, 2002; 16: 278-285.
4. Lo EYW, Dignan R, French B. Independent predictors of postoperative stroke with cardiopulmonary bypass. J Cardiothorac Vasc Anesth, 2022; 36: 133-137.

3. Following cardiac surgery, early strokes are defined as those occurring upon emergence from anesthesia. Delayed strokes are those that develop more than 24 hours

postoperatively, and late strokes develop more than 30 days postoperatively. Which risk factor has NOT been associated with early stroke following cardiac surgery?

A. Advanced age
B. Unstable angina
C. Duration of cardiopulmonary bypass
D. High preoperative creatinine level

Correct Answer: B

Explanation: Risk factors for early stroke following cardiac surgery include advanced age, high preoperative creatinine level, aortic atherosclerosis, and duration of cardiopulmonary bypass. Female gender, unstable angina, previous cerebrovascular disease, inotropic support requirement, and postoperative atrial fibrillation are factors that contribute to delayed stroke. Early stroke is associated with increased mortality mainly in the acute perioperative period, whereas delayed stroke was associated with increased longer-term mortality.

References:

1. Flier S, Murkin JM. Chapter 40: Central Nervous System Dysfunction After Cardiopulmonary Bypass. In: Kaplan JA, Augoustides JGT, Manecke GR, et al., eds. Kaplan's Cardiac Anesthesia. 7th ed. Elsevier; 2017:1374-1406.
2. Kashani HH, Mosienko L, Grocott BB, et al. Postcardiac surgery acute stroke therapies: a systematic review. J Cardiothorac Vasc Anesth, 2020; 34: 2349-2354.
3. Ridderstolpe L, Ahlgren E, Gill H, et al. Risk factor analysis of early and delayed cerebral complications after cardiac surgery. J Cardiothorac Anesth, 2002; 16: 278-285.
4. Lo EYW, Dignan R, French B. Independent predictors of postoperative stroke with cardiopulmonary bypass. J Cardiothorac Vasc Anesth, 2022; 36: 133-137.

4. A patient has tonic-clonic movement of his right upper extremity during emergence from anesthesia following aortic valve replacement surgery. Brain imaging was unremarkable. What risk factor has NOT been associated with seizures after cardiac surgery?

A. Open-chamber cardiac surgery
B. Poor hepatic function
C. Tranexamic acid exposure
D. Deep hypothermic circulatory arrest

Correct Answer: B

Explanation: Seizures can be diagnosed based on physical examination findings of convulsive activity or can be "silent," with only electroencephalographic findings detected. The risk factors for seizures after cardiac surgery include open-chamber cardiac surgery, deep hypothermic circulatory arrest, aortic calcification or atheroma, critical preoperative state, tranexamic acid exposure, preoperative cardiac arrest, long cardiopulmonary time, previous cardiac surgery, poor renal function, age 75 years or older, and peripheral vascular disease.

References:

1. Flier S, Murkin JM. Chapter 40: Central Nervous System Dysfunction After Cardiopulmonary Bypass. In: Kaplan JA,

Augoustides JGT, Manecke GR, et al., eds. Kaplan's Cardiac Anesthesia. 7th ed. Elsevier; 2017:1374-1406.
2. Hunter GR, Young GB. Seizures after cardiac surgery. J Cardiothorac Anesth, 2011; 25: 299-305.
3. Awad H, Essandoh M. Goal-directed oxygen delivery during cardiopulmonary bypass: can this perfusion strategy improve biochemical and clinical neurologic outcomes? J Cardiothorac Vasc Anesth, 2018; 32: 2493-2494.

5. A patient has facial twitching upon emergence from anesthesia following mitral valve replacement surgery. The patient received tranexamic acid prophylactically to decrease bleeding. A subsequent electroencephalogram demonstrates focal seizure activity. What is the mechanism of action of tranexamic acid with respect to this increased seizure risk?

A. Presynaptic blockade of γ-aminobutyric acid (GABA)
B. Presynaptic blockade of glutamate
C. Postsynaptic blockade of GABA
D. Postsynaptic blockade of glutamate

Correct Answer: C

Explanation: The association of tranexamic acid and seizures following cardiac surgery is thought to be due to direct postsynaptic receptor blockade by tranexamic acid of the inhibitory neurotransmitter γ-aminobutyric acid (GABA) in the cerebrospinal fluid. Blockade of GABA transmission creates impaired neuronal inhibition and subsequent enhanced neuronal excitation. Further risks for seizures after cardiac surgery are open-chamber procedures, stroke, prolonged cardiopulmonary bypass time, and renal failure.

References:

1. Flier S, Murkin JM. Chapter 40: Central Nervous System Dysfunction After Cardiopulmonary Bypass. In: Kaplan JA, Augoustides JGT, Manecke GR, et al., eds. Kaplan's Cardiac Anesthesia. 7th ed. Elsevier; 2017:1374-1406.
2. Taam J, Yang QJ, Pang KS, et al. Current evidence and future directions of tranexamic acid use, efficacy, and dosing for major surgical procedures. J Cardiothorac Anesth, 2020; 34: 782-790.
3. Hunter GR, Young GB. Seizures after cardiac surgery. J Cardiothorac Anesth, 2011; 25: 299-305.

6. An 85 year-old patient is assessed on the first day after coronary bypass grafting. During examination, it is noted that the patient is only oriented to self. Which statement regarding postoperative delirium is FALSE?

A. Beating heart surgery, including off-pump cardiac surgery, has a decreased risk of delirium compared with on-pump cardiac surgery
B. Increased levels of inflammatory markers are associated with delirium
C. Preoperative ventricular function is associated with delirium
D. Delirium is transient by definition and is not typically associated with long-term effects

Correct Answer: D

Explanation: Risk factors for delirium after cardiac surgery include older age, cerebrovascular disease, peripheral vascular disease, atrial fibrillation, diabetes mellitus, left ventricular ejection fraction of 30% or less, preoperative cardiogenic shock, urgent operation, intraoperative hemofiltration, operation time of 3 hours or more, and a high perioperative transfusion requirement. However, beating-heart surgery and younger patient age were identified as having a significant protective effect against postoperative stroke.

The incidence rate of delirium after cardiac surgery is typically in the 20% to 30% range and is associated with significantly increased mortality and readmission to the hospital. The mechanisms of postoperative delirium include a heightened inflammatory response as characterized by biomarkers such as interleukin-2 and tumor necrosis factor.

References:

1. Flier S, Murkin JM. Chapter 40: Central Nervous System Dysfunction After Cardiopulmonary Bypass. In: Kaplan JA, Augoustides JGT, Manecke GR, et al., eds. Kaplan's Cardiac Anesthesia. 7th ed. Elsevier; 2017:1374-1406.
2. Milne B, Gilbey T, Gautel L, et al. Neuromonitoring and neurocognitive outcomes in cardiac surgery: a narrative review. J Cardiothorac Anesth, 2022; 36: 2098-2113.
3. Afonso A, Scurlock C, Reich D, et al. Predictive model for postoperative delirium in cardiac surgical patients. Semin Cardiothorac Vasc Anesth, 2010; 14: 212-217.

7. Following uncomplicated cardiac surgery, a patient sustains hypoxic brain injury as demonstrated on magnetic resonance imaging. Which statement about brain injury after cardiac surgery is FALSE?

   A. Cerebral hypoperfusion is a rare cause of brain injury due to near-infrared spectroscopy use
   B. Microgaseous emboli can be a source of brain injury
   C. Inflammation can exacerbate brain injury following cardiopulmonary bypass
   D. Both extracranial and intracranial atherosclerotic disease are associated with postoperative brain injury

Correct Answer: A

Explanation: The primary mechanisms for brain injury after cardiac surgery are cerebral hypoperfusion and cerebral emboli. Perioperative hypoperfusion, particularly in patients with intracranial and extracranial atherosclerosis, is a common cause of postoperative brain injury. Intraoperative cerebral embolization of particulate and microgaseous elements also plays a significant role in the genesis of perioperative cerebral events in cardiac surgical patients. Additionally, the effects of inflammatory processes triggered during exposure to surgery and bypass may exacerbate brain injury. Intracranial atherosclerotic disease is a strong independent predictor of development of brain injury after cardiac surgery. Additionally, the presence of both extracranial and intracranial atherosclerotic disease was even more strongly associated with adverse perioperative neurologic outcomes than intracranial atherosclerotic disease alone.

BOX 36.1 **Factors related to cerebral injury in cardiac surgery**

- Age[8,27,28]
- Aorta atheromatosis[160,161,163,164,166,168,391–393]
- Carotid disease[30,394]
- Diabetes mellitus[6,8,21,131,174,218,395]
- Hypertension[6,8,395,396]
- Peripheral vascular disease[6,68,165,218,395,397]
- Renal dysfunction[8,398]
- Stroke or cerebrovascular disease[6,21,30,131,399]
- Recent unstable angina or acute myocardial infarction[6,218,398,400]
- Preoperative low output/low ejection fraction[397,398]
- Combined/complex procedures[15,395]
- Redo surgery[218,395]
- Prolonged cardiopulmonary bypass time[22,68,395]
- Intraoperative hemodynamic instability[15,22,149,395]
- Postoperative atrial fibrillation[149,168,398,399]

Risk factors consistently reported for perioperative cerebral injury in cardiac surgery patients.

References:

1. Flier S, Murkin JM. Chapter 40: Central Nervous System Dysfunction After Cardiopulmonary Bypass. In: Kaplan JA, Augoustides JGT, Manecke GR, et al., eds. Kaplan's Cardiac Anesthesia. 7th ed. Elsevier; 2017:1374-1406.
2. Milne B, Gilbey T, Gautel L, et al. Neuromonitoring and neurocognitive outcomes in cardiac surgery: a narrative review. J Cardiothorac Anesth, 2022; 36: 2098-2113.

8. Of the following areas of the brain, which is MOST prone to ischemia due to hypotension during cardiac surgery?

   A. Brainstem
   B. Anterior cerebral artery territory
   C. Watershed territory
   D. Hypothalamus

Correct Answer: C

Explanation: Watershed territories are border zones between the territories of two major cerebral arteries such as occurs between the middle and posterior, or the anterior and middle, cerebral arteries. In watershed territories, terminal arteriolar anastomoses exist, making the region dependent on a single vessel to deliver blood and oxygen. A profound reduction in systemic blood pressure is the most frequent cause of watershed infarcts. These areas are thought to be more susceptible to ischemia resulting from hypotension because of their critical dependence on a single blood supply. Although watershed infarcts commonly arise from profoundly hypotensive episodes, watershed lesions are not pathognomonic of a hypotensive episode, as they may also be the result of cerebral emboli. Embolization and hypoperfusion acting together play a synergistic role and either cause or magnify brain damage in cardiac surgical patients.

References:

1. Flier S, Murkin JM. Chapter 40: Central Nervous System Dysfunction After Cardiopulmonary Bypass. In: Kaplan JA, Augoustides JGT, Manecke GR, et al., eds. Kaplan's Cardiac Anesthesia. 7th ed. Elsevier; 2017:1374-1406.
2. Lo EYW, Dignan R, French B. Independent predictors of postoperative stroke with cardiopulmonary bypass. J Cardiothorac Vasc Anesth, 2022; 36: 133-137.
3. Milne B, Gilbey T, Gautel L, et al. Neuromonitoring and neurocognitive outcomes in cardiac surgery: a narrative review. J Cardiothorac Anesth, 2022; 36: 2098-2113.
4. Awad H, Essandoh M. Goal-directed oxygen delivery during cardiopulmonary bypass: can this perfusion strategy improve biochemical and clinical neurologic outcomes? J Cardiothorac Vasc Anesth, 2018; 32: 2493-2494.

9. Cerebral microemboli associated with cardiopulmonary bypass are likely to cause what clinical neurologic change in the postoperative period?
    A. Brain death
    B. Vision loss
    C. Weakness in left arm and left leg
    D. Subtle cognitive changes

Correct Answer: D

Explanation: Cerebral emboli during cardiopulmonary bypass can be arbitrarily differentiated into macroemboli (e.g., calcific or atherosclerotic debris) and microemboli (e.g., microgaseous bubbles, microparticulate matter). Overt and focal neurologic damage likely reflects the occurrence of cerebral macroemboli, generated during valve tissue removal or instrumentation of an atheromatous aorta. Microemboli are associated with less focal neurologic dysfunction than has been ascribed to cerebral macroemboli. Microemboli are typically detected by their characteristic findings on transcranial Doppler of the middle cerebral artery. Microemboli appear to have some role in diffuse, subtle neurologic and cognitive disturbances, whereas macroemboli likely produce clinically apparent catastrophic strokes.

References:

1. Flier S, Murkin JM. Chapter 40: Central Nervous System Dysfunction After Cardiopulmonary Bypass. In: Kaplan JA, Augoustides JGT, Manecke GR, et al., eds. Kaplan's Cardiac Anesthesia. 7th ed. Elsevier; 2017:1374-1406.
2. Melnyk V, Fedorko L, Djaiani G. Microemboli on cardiopulmonary bypass: should we care? J Cardiothorac Vasc Anesth 2020;34:1504-1505.

10. While undergoing an aortic valve replacement and ascending aortic arch repair, the central venous pressure acutely increases from 6 mmHg to 40 mmHg. The anesthesiologist suspects central venous hypertension and alerts the surgeon. At which part of the procedure is this MOST likely to occur?
    A. Myocardial dislocation
    B. Aortic cannulation
    C. Bicaval cannulation prior to snaring
    D. Pulmonary artery vent placement

Correct Answer: A

Explanation: During cardiopulmonary bypass, cerebral venous hypertension can result from partial obstruction of the superior vena cava, particularly in the presence of a single two-stage venous cannula. Cerebral venous hypertension may cause cerebral edema and produce a disproportionate decline in cerebral perfusion pressure relative to arterial pressure. Surgical dislocation of the heart during bypass increases proximal superior vena cava pressure and can result in significant decreases in cerebral blood flow velocity as measured with transcranial Doppler. The surgeon and perfusionist should be alerted immediately, as cerebral ischemia will result if uncorrected. Typically, repositioning of the heart or the superior vena cava cannula will fix the issue. If not, replacement of the cannula in the superior vena cava will relieve the venous obstruction.

References:

1. Flier S, Murkin JM. Chapter 40: Central Nervous System Dysfunction After Cardiopulmonary Bypass. In: Kaplan JA, Augoustides JGT, Manecke GR, et al., eds. Kaplan's Cardiac Anesthesia. 7th ed. Elsevier; 2017:1374-1406.
2. Sakamoto T, Duebener LF, Laussen PC, et al. Cerebral ischemia caused by obstructed superior vena cava cannula is detected by near-infrared spectroscopy. J Cardiothorac Vasc Anesth, 2004; 18: 293-303.
3. Niazi AK, Reese AS, Minko P, et al. Superior vena cava syndrome and otorrhagia during cardiac surgery. Cureus, 2019; 11: e4602.

11. Following cardiac surgery, early strokes are defined as those occurring upon emergence from anesthesia. Delayed strokes are those that develop more than 24 hours postoperatively, and late strokes develop more than 30 days postoperatively. What is associated with delayed stroke following cardiac surgery?
    A. Male gender
    B. Extent of aortic atherosclerosis
    C. Inotropic support requirement
    D. High preoperative creatinine

Correct Answer: C

Explanation: Factors associated with delayed stroke include female gender, unstable angina, previous cerebrovascular disease, inotropic support requirement, and postoperative atrial fibrillation. Early stroke is associated with increased mortality mainly in the acute perioperative period, whereas delayed stroke is associated with increased longer-term mortality. Risk factors for early stroke following cardiac surgery include advanced age, high preoperative creatinine level, aortic atherosclerosis, and duration of cardiopulmonary bypass. Late strokes reflect progression of comorbid disease and atrial arrhythmias for the most part, and thus are not as easily prevented through care management modifications.

References:

1. Flier S, Murkin JM. Chapter 40: Central Nervous System Dysfunction After Cardiopulmonary Bypass. In: Kaplan JA, Augoustides JGT, Manecke GR, et al., eds. Kaplan's Cardiac Anesthesia. 7th ed. Elsevier; 2017:1374-1406.
2. Kashani HH, Mosienko L, Grocott BB, et al. Postcardiac surgery acute stroke therapies: a systematic review. J Cardiothorac Vasc Anesth, 2020; 34: 2349-2354.
3. Ridderstolpe L, Ahlgren E, Gill H, et al. Risk factor analysis of early and delayed cerebral complications after cardiac surgery. J Cardiothorac Anesth, 2002; 16: 278-285.
4. Lo EYW, Dignan R, French B. Independent predictors of postoperative stroke with cardiopulmonary bypass. J Cardiothorac Vasc Anesth, 2022; 36: 133-137.

12. An 86-year-old patient suffered an acute posterior communicating artery territory stroke following mitral valve replacement. What is TRUE regarding older age and stroke risk following cardiac surgery?
   A. Preoperative anemia is associated with stroke due to increased need for blood transfusions
   B. Lower body surface area is associated with decreased risk of stroke
   C. Isolated coronary artery bypass grafting carries the highest risk for stroke
   D. Preoperative anemia is associated with stroke due to decreased oxygen delivery

Correct Answer: D

Explanation: Numerous trials have demonstrated that type I cerebral injury, defined as stroke, transient ischemic attack, or coma, is significantly increased in patients older than 80 years undergoing cardiac surgery. Factors related to intraoperative brain oxygenation, including preoperative anemia, have been shown to be the most critical determinant of stroke in the older patients. Furthermore, the stroke rate in older patients has also been shown to be inversely related to body surface area, which may again reflect a decrease in red cell mass and a greater degree of hemodilution during bypass. The stroke risk in older patients has also been shown to be directly proportional to serum creatinine concentration, as well as presence of valvular heart disease and other comorbidities. The stroke risk after cardiac surgery is typically higher in combined and thoracic aortic procedures as compared to isolated coronary artery bypass grafting.

References:

1. Flier S, Murkin JM. Chapter 40: Central Nervous System Dysfunction After Cardiopulmonary Bypass. In: Kaplan JA, Augoustides JGT, Manecke GR, et al., eds. Kaplan's Cardiac Anesthesia. 7th ed. Elsevier; 2017:1374-1406.
2. Alexander KP, Anstrom KJ, Muhlbaier LH, et al. Outcomes of cardiac surgery in patients ≥ 80 years: results from the National Cardiovascular Network. J Am Coll Cardiol, 2000; 35: 731-738.
3. Lo EYW, Dignan R, French B. Independent predictors of postoperative stroke with cardiopulmonary bypass. J Cardiothorac Vasc Anesth, 2022; 36: 133-137.

13. During cardiopulmonary bypass, alpha-stat pH management has become the standard of care for adult patients. Which of the following are attributes of alpha-stat pH management compared with pH-stat management?
   A. Only cerebral blood flow increase
   B. Cerebral blood flow decrease and cerebral metabolic rate decrease
   C. Cerebral blood flow increase and cerebral metabolic rate decrease
   D. Cerebral blood flow increase and cerebral metabolic rate increase

Correct Answer: B

Explanation: During pH-stat acid-base management, the patient's pH is maintained at a constant level by managing pH at the patient's actual temperature. In other words, it is temperature-corrected and aims for a partial pressure of carbon dioxide (pCO_2) of 40 mmHg and pH of 7.40 at the patient's actual temperature. Compared to alpha-stat, pH stat leads to higher pCO_2 levels and resultant relative respiratory acidosis. Higher pCO_2 levels increase cerebral blood flow due to vasodilation. Often CO_2 is deliberately added to maintain a pCO_2 of 40 mmHg during hypothermia.

Alpha-stat pH management is not temperature-corrected and assumes gas pressures are measured at 37°C. As the patient's temperature falls, the pCO_2 decreases due to increased solubility. A hypothermic patient with a pH of 7.40 and a pCO_2 of 40 mmHg will actually have a lower pCO_2, resulting in a relative respiratory alkalosis. The lower pCO_2 values result in decreased cerebral blood flow. Alpha-stat pH management maintains the coupling of cerebral blood flow and cerebral metabolic rate; thus cerebral metabolic rate is also decreased. Theoretically, this maintains autoregulation.

Because of the vasodilatory effects of increased carbon dioxide in patients with cerebrovascular disease, pH-stat management could theoretically induce redistribution of regional cerebral blood flow from marginally perfused to well-perfused regions, resulting in intracerebral steal. However, this has not been demonstrated in studies.

References:

1. Flier S, Murkin JM. Chapter 40: Central Nervous System Dysfunction After Cardiopulmonary Bypass. In: Kaplan JA, Augoustides JGT, Manecke GR, et al., eds. Kaplan's Cardiac Anesthesia. 7th ed. Elsevier; 2017:1374-1406.
2. Qu JZ, Kao LW, Smith JE, et al. Brain protection in aortic arch surgery: an evolving field. J Cardiothorac Vasc Anesth, 2021; 35: 1176-1188.

14. What type of oxygenator has been found to have the least amount of cerebral microemboli during cardiopulmonary bypass?
   A. Screen
   B. Rotating disc
   C. Bubble
   D. Membrane

Correct Answer: D

Explanation: The two oxygenators during cardiopulmonary bypass machines are bubble and membrane oxygenators. The early oxygenators in this setting had a bubble design that utilized oxygen bubbles added directly to the blood. This was associated with continuous cerebral emboli, as assessed by transcranial Doppler of the middle cerebral artery. However, when a membrane oxygenator was selected, there was a significant reduction in the burden of cerebral emboli.

It is apparent that emboli may be generated continuously during cardiopulmonary bypass and that equipment modifications, including arterial line microfiltration and preferential usage of membrane oxygenators, can decrease the generation of such emboli. Membrane oxygenators are currently recommended for cardiopulmonary bypass.

References:

1. Flier S, Murkin JM. Chapter 40: Central Nervous System Dysfunction After Cardiopulmonary Bypass. In: Kaplan JA, Augoustides JGT, Manecke GR, et al., eds. Kaplan's Cardiac Anesthesia. 7th ed. Elsevier; 2017:1374-1406.
2. Nigro Neto C, Arnoni R, Rida BS, et al. Randomized trial on the effect of sevoflurane on polypropylene membrane oxygenator performance. J Cardiothorac Vasc Anesth, 2013; 27: 903-907.
3. Melnyk V, Fedorko L, Djaiani G. Microemboli on cardiopulmonary bypass: should we care? J Cardiothorac Vasc Anesth, 2020; 34: 1504-1505.

15. Which modification to the cardiopulmonary circuit equipment decreases the amount of microemboli transmitted to the cerebral vasculature?
   A. Arterial line filtration
   B. Suction
   C. Centrifugal pump
   D. Roller pump

Correct Answer: A

Explanation: In a study assessing the microembolic burden during cardiopulmonary bypass with Doppler ultrasound in the middle cerebral arteries, it was found that addition of an arterial line filter significantly decreased the intensity of cerebral microemboli. The arterial line filter resulted in a 58.9% reduction of microemboli, with only 4.4% of the signals detected after the arterial filter.

It has also been shown that emboli from air within the venous line of the bypass circuit, injection of drugs into the venous line, or from cardiotomy suction can pass through the oxygenator and appear as microemboli within the arterial line, even in the presence of a venous line defoamer and a membrane oxygenator. Centrifugal pumps are known for less hemolysis than roller pumps, but neither pump is known to affect microemboli loads.

References:

1. Flier S, Murkin JM. Chapter 40: Central Nervous System Dysfunction After Cardiopulmonary Bypass. In: Kaplan JA, Augoustides JGT, Manecke GR, et al., eds. Kaplan's Cardiac Anesthesia. 7th ed. Elsevier; 2017:1374-1406.
2. Nigro Neto C, Arnoni R, Rida BS, et al. Randomized trial on the effect of sevoflurane on polypropylene membrane oxygenator performance. J Cardiothorac Vasc Anesth, 2013; 27: 903-907.
3. Melnyk V, Fedorko L, Djaiani G. Microemboli on cardiopulmonary bypass: should we care? J Cardiothorac Vasc Anesth, 2020; 34: 1504-1505.
4. Georgiadis D, Hempel A, Baumgartner RW, et al. Doppler microembolic signals during cardiac surgery: comparison between arterial line and middle cerebral artery. J Thorac Cardiovasc Surg, 2003; 126: 1638-1639.

16. A patient is found to have an early middle cerebral artery territory stroke following aortic arch repair. Which inflammatory marker is MOST associated with stroke events in the postoperative period following cardiac surgery?
   A. Erythrocyte sedimentation rate
   B. Procalcitonin
   C. Interleukin 12
   D. C-reactive protein

Correct Answer: D

Explanation: Acute ischemic stroke may trigger an inflammatory response that leads to increased levels of C-reactive protein. High levels of this biomarker may be associated with poor outcome. While all of the choices are markers of inflammation, C-reactive protein, if elevated postoperatively, has been associated with major cardiac and stroke events. A cardiac surgical study in patients with new brain infarcts after coronary artery bypass grafting found that most lesions detectable by magnetic resonance imaging were clinically silent, located in the cortical territory, small in diameter, and not related to the underlying cerebral arterial abnormality.

BOX 36.2   Clinical strategies that may decrease neurologic complications in cardiac surgery

- Early and aggressive control of hemodynamic instability
- Perioperative euglycemia between 100 and 180 mg/dL
- Routine epiaortic scanning before manipulation of ascending aorta
- Avoidance of manipulation of ascending aorta in severe atheromatosis
- Maintenance of adequate cerebral perfusion pressure (neuromonitoring/cerebral oximetry)
- Monitoring of cerebral venous pressure via a proximal central venous pressure catheter or the introducer port of a pulmonary artery catheter

- Alpha-stat pH management during moderate hypothermic cardiopulmonary bypass (CPB)
- Avoidance of arterial inflow temperature greater than 37°C
- Use of CPB circuitry incorporating membrane oxygenator and 40-mcm arterial line filter
- Use of surface-modified and reduced-area CPB circuitry
- Use of cerebral oximetry

Older age, cardiopulmonary bypass, significant aortic plaque, and high levels of high-sensitivity C-reactive protein have been demonstrated as independent predictors of new brain infarction, suggesting that a systemic inflammatory response may also contribute to the pathogenesis of new infarcts after cardiac surgery.

References:

1. Flier S, Murkin JM. Chapter 40: Central Nervous System Dysfunction After Cardiopulmonary Bypass. In: Kaplan JA, Augoustides JGT, Manecke GR, et al., eds. Kaplan's Cardiac Anesthesia. 7th ed. Elsevier; 2017:1374-1406.
2. Hall R. Identification of inflammatory mediators and their modulation by strategies for the management of the systemic inflammatory response during cardiac surgery. J Cardiothorac Vasc Anesth, 2013; 27: 983-1033.
3. Nah HW, Lee JW, Chung CH, et al. New brain infarcts on magnetic resonance imaging after coronary artery bypass graft surgery: lesion patterns, mechanism, and predictors. Ann Neurol, 2014; 76: 347-355.

17. A patient with which of the following vascular lesions is MOST at risk for perioperative stroke following cardiac surgery?
  A. A patient with right carotid stenosis of 65%
  B. A patient with left carotid stenosis of 75%
  C. A patient with right carotid stenosis of 50% and left carotid stenosis 50%
  D. A patient with right carotid stenosis of 90%

Correct Answer: C

Explanation: There have been multiple trials looking at carotid stenosis and stroke risk after cardiac surgery. The risk for postoperative stroke is 2% for patients with mild stenosis of less than 50%; 10% with moderate stenosis (>50% artery stenosis); and 11% to 19% with severe stenosis (80% stenosis or more). Although bilateral carotid disease is uncommon, it increases patient risk for stroke to approximately 20% after cardiac surgery.

It is estimated that, at most, 40% of perioperative strokes after cardiac surgery may be directly attributable to ipsilateral carotid artery disease. Carotid intervention may be indicated at times to decrease a patient's stroke risk. Concomitant carotid stenosis likely indicates a high likelihood of aortic and/or concomitant intracerebral disease that significantly affect stroke risk as well in this setting.

References:

1. Flier S, Murkin JM. Chapter 40: Central Nervous System Dysfunction After Cardiopulmonary Bypass. In: Kaplan JA, Augoustides JGT, Manecke GR, et al., eds. Kaplan's Cardiac Anesthesia. 7th ed. Elsevier; 2017:1374-1406.
2. Naylor AR, Mehta Z, Rothwell PM, et al. Carotid artery disease and stroke during coronary artery bypass: A critical review of the literature. Eur J Vasc Endovasc Surg, 2002; 23: 283-294.
3. Mehta, A. Carotid artery disease as a predictor of in-hospital postoperative stroke after coronary artery bypass grafting from 1999 to 2011. J Cardiothorac Vasc Anesth, 2018; 32: 1587-1596.

18. A patient with a history of multiple lower extremity arterial bypasses and known carotid stenosis presents for aortic and mitral valve replacements. Due to known arterial disease, there is suspicion of ascending aortic plaque. Which technique is MOST recommended for intraoperatively assessment for atherosclerotic plaque in this setting?
  A. Epiaortic scanning
  B. Fluoroscopy
  C. Transesophageal echocardiogram
  D. Manual palpation

Correct Answer: A

Explanation: Epiaortic scanning before instrumentation of the ascending aorta is a sensitive and specific technique to detect nonpalpable aortic atheroma. This should ideally occur before manipulation of the aorta. It is especially important in patients with known arterial vascular disease, and thus those at high risk for aortic vascular disease. This imaging technique allows the surgeon to look at the aorta in real time and identify where plaques are located. Therefore, aortic cannulation and cross clamp can avoid the plaques and, hopefully, subsequent cerebral emboli.

Manual palpation has a very low sensitivity. Although transesophageal echocardiography can identify aortic plaque, it has blind spots due to image limitations. The high acoustic reflectance attributable to the air-tissue interface resulting from the overlying right main bronchus and trachea limits its assessment of the upper ascending aorta, where cannulation is generally undertaken. Fluoroscopy may be specific for detection of atheroma, but it carries risks for the patient and the care team due to radiation exposure.

References:

1. Flier S, Murkin JM. Chapter 40: Central Nervous System Dysfunction After Cardiopulmonary Bypass. In: Kaplan JA, Augoustides JGT, Manecke GR, et al., eds. Kaplan's Cardiac Anesthesia. 7th ed. Elsevier; 2017:1374-1406.
2. Shapeton AD, Leissner KB, Zorca SM, et al. Epiaortic ultrasound for assessment of intraluminal atheroma; insights from the REGROUP Trial. J Cardiothorac Vasc Anesth, 2020; 34: 726-732.

19. A patient is undergoing tricuspid and mitral valve repair. Intraoperative transesophageal echocardiography demonstrates copious air within the ventricles. The following increase the efficacy of deairing, EXCEPT:
  A. Aortic root venting
  B. Carbon dioxide insufflation
  C. Administration of intravenous albumin instead of crystalloid
  D. Manual manipulation of the heart

Correct Answer: C

Explanation: A primary determinant of the number and duration of microgaseous emboli during open-chamber procedures relates to methodologies for removal of intracavitary air. Although needle aspiration and/or aortic root venting are standard techniques for air removal, carbon dioxide insufflation, either continuously or immediately before closure of ventriculotomy, has been shown to significantly increase the efficacy of deairing, resulting in decreased systemic gaseous emboli.

Although there has been a general expectation of improvements in neurologic and cognitive outcomes due to carbon dioxide insufflation, it has been surprisingly difficult to demonstrate. Even though this technique has improved survival in small studies, there is no high-quality evidence of a sustained reduction of cerebrovascular complications.

Aortic root venting and needle aspiration are standard practices and widely used techniques to reduce the burden of gaseous emboli. In combination with aortic root venting and/or needle aspiration, manual manipulation of the heart is also effective. Administration of albumin rather than crystalloid has not been associated with reductions in gaseous emboli.

References:

1. Flier S, Murkin JM. Chapter 40: Central Nervous System Dysfunction After Cardiopulmonary Bypass. In: Kaplan JA, Augoustides JGT, Manecke GR, et al., eds. Kaplan's Cardiac Anesthesia. 7th ed. Elsevier; 2017:1374-1406.
2. Persson, M. et al. What is the optimal device for carbon dioxide deairing of the cardiothoracic wound and how should it be positioned? J Cardiothorac Vasc Anesth, 2004; 18: 180-184.

20. Which cardiac surgical procedure carries the highest risk for perioperative stroke in patients younger than 80 years of age?
    A. Off-pump coronary artery bypass
    B. Coronary artery bypass grafting
    C. Coronary artery bypass and aortic valve replacement
    D. Coronary artery bypass and mitral valve repair or replacement

Correct Answer: D

Explanation: Several studies have supported the incidence of stroke to be lowest in isolated coronary artery bypass grafting in the range of 1% to 4.2%. Patients undergoing combined coronary and aortic valve procedures have a higher stroke risk in the 5% to 9.1% range. The highest risk for postoperative stroke has been associated in patients undergoing coronary artery bypass grafting and mitral valve procedures with an observed risk in the 8% to 11.2% range. Further risk factors for postoperative stroke include aortic atherosclerosis and any open-chamber procedure.

References:

1. Flier S, Murkin JM. Chapter 40: Central Nervous System Dysfunction After Cardiopulmonary Bypass. In: Kaplan JA,

Augoustides JGT, Manecke GR, et al., eds. Kaplan's Cardiac Anesthesia. 7th ed. Elsevier; 2017:1374-1406.
2. Alexander KP, Anstrom KJ, Muhlbaier LH, et al. Outcomes of cardiac surgery in patients > or = 80 years: results from the National Cardiovascular Network. J Am Coll Cardiol, 2000; 35: 731-738.
3. Kashani HH, Mosienko L, Grocott BB, et al. Postcardiac surgery acute stroke therapies: a systematic review. J Cardiothorac Vasc Anesth, 2020; 34: 2349-2354.
4. Ridderstolpe L, Ahlgren E, Gill H, et al. Risk factor analysis of early and delayed cerebral complications after cardiac surgery. J Cardiothorac Anesth, 2002; 16: 278-285.
5. Lo EYW, Dignan R, French B. Independent predictors of postoperative stroke with cardiopulmonary bypass. J Cardiothorac Vasc Anesth, 2022; 36: 133-137.

21. A 66-year-old patient is scheduled for hemiarch aortic repair with circulatory arrest. The patient is concerned about postoperative cognitive dysfunction. Which of the following should be described to the patient as the most recommended strategy for cerebral protection during this case?
    A. Retrograde cerebral perfusion
    B. Selective antegrade cerebral perfusion
    C. Normothermic circulatory arrest
    D. Hypothermic circulatory arrest

Correct Answer: D

Explanation: There is much debate about optimal cerebral protection during circulatory arrest. The most common strategy is hypothermic circulatory arrest. Hypothermic circulatory arrest can be accomplished with deep (<25°C) or moderate hypothermia (25°C–30°C). Multiple trials have analyzed patient outcomes with retrograde and antegrade perfusion in comparison with hypothermic circulatory arrest. A degree of hypothermic circulatory arrest is strongly neuroprotective and is typically combined retrograde or anterograde cerebral perfusion. Retrograde cerebral perfusion through the superior vena cava is thought to accomplish brain protection by providing metabolic substrate, removing gaseous and particulate emboli from cerebral blood vasculature, and maintaining cerebral hypothermia. However, it has been noted that not all blood returns to the aortic arch, with a potential risk for cerebral edema. Selective antegrade cerebral perfusion is typically accomplished via right axillary or subclavian cannulation. Normothermic circulatory arrest would be outside the standard of care.

References:

1. Flier S, Murkin JM. Chapter 40: Central Nervous System Dysfunction After Cardiopulmonary Bypass. In: Kaplan JA, Augoustides JGT, Manecke GR, et al., eds. Kaplan's Cardiac Anesthesia. 7th ed. Elsevier; 2017:1374-1406.
2. Qu JZ, Kao LW, Smith JE, et al. Brain protection in aortic arch surgery: an evolving field. J Cardiothorac Vasc Anesth, 2021; 35: 1176-1188.

22. A 66-year-old patient is scheduled for hemiarch aortic repair with hypothermic circulatory arrest. The patient is concerned about postoperative cognitive dysfunction and wants to learn more about hypothermic circulatory arrest. What temperature should be stated as qualifying for deep hypothermia?
  A. 33 to 35°C
  B. 28 to 32°C
  C. Below 28°C
  D. Below 20°C

Correct Answer: D

Explanation: During complex aortic arch repair, surgical access may require interruption of systemic perfusion for relatively protracted periods. Hypothermic circulatory arrest is considered an important part of the multimodal approach to neuroprotection in this setting. The definition of hypothermic levels in aortic arch surgery has progressed over time. Most recently, in 2013, expert consensus has defined deep hypothermia as a nasopharyngeal temperature range from 14.1 to 20°C. Moderate hypothermia was defined as a nasopharyngeal temperature range of 20.1 to 28°C. Mild hypothermia was defined as a nasopharyngeal temperature range of 28.1 to 34°C. This expert panel also defined profound hypothermia as a nasopharyngeal temperature below 14.1°C.

References:

1. Flier S, Murkin JM. Chapter 40: Central Nervous System Dysfunction After Cardiopulmonary Bypass. In: Kaplan JA, Augoustides JGT, Manecke GR, et al., eds. Kaplan's Cardiac Anesthesia. 7th ed. Elsevier; 2017:1374-1406.
2. Qu JZ, Kao LW, Smith JE, et al. Brain protection in aortic arch surgery: an evolving field. J Cardiothorac Vasc Anesth, 2021; 35: 1176-1188.

23. A patient is hemodynamically stable and nearing hospital discharge following left ventricular assist device placement. The patient asks about potential adverse events, specifically stroke risk. The patient should be advised that which of the following time periods carries the highest risk for stroke?
  A. 1 month postimplantation
  B. 12 months postimplantation
  C. 24 months postimplantation
  D. 36 months postimplantation

Correct Answer: D

Explanation: The reported rates of stroke after implantation of a left ventricular assist device are variable and reflect differences in follow-up and patient population. Neurologic events seem to be relatively common and are associated with adverse patient outcome. The early stroke risk after device insertion is low but increases steadily over time. The risk of stroke at 1 month is around 3%, increasing to 11% at 12 months, 17% at 24 months, and 19% at 36 months after implantation. The increasing risk is presumably due to the constant thrombogenic threat of artificial hardware in the main vasculature.

These data do not include newer data from HeartMate 3 devices, which have been shown to confer lower risk of stroke. The MOMENTUM 3 study (Multicenter Study of MagLev Technology in Patients Undergoing Mechanical Circulatory Support Therapy With HeartMate 3) has demonstrated that the HeartMate 3 pump is associated with a reduced rate of stroke compared with the HeartMate II device.

References:

1. Flier S, Murkin JM. Chapter 40: Central Nervous System Dysfunction After Cardiopulmonary Bypass. In: Kaplan JA, Augoustides JGT, Manecke GR, et al., eds. Kaplan's Cardiac Anesthesia. 7th ed. Elsevier; 2017:1374-1406.
2. Colombo PC, Mehra MR, Goldstein DJ, et al. Comprehensive analysis of stroke in the long-term cohort of the MOMENTUM 3 study. Circulation, 2019; 139: 155-168.
3. Augoustides JG, Riha H. Recent progress in heart failure treatment and heart transplantation. J Cardiothorac Vasc Anesth, 2009; 23: 738-748.

24. A patient with previous cerebrovascular events is scheduled to undergo a redo aortic valve replacement. The following could be useful in detecting inadequate cerebral perfusion during the case, EXCEPT:
  A. Transcranial Doppler
  B. Portable computed axial scanning performed pre- and postbypass
  C. Near-infrared spectroscopy
  D. Electroencephalography

Correct Answer: B

Explanation: Intraoperative neurophysiologic monitoring may be of benefit to decrease neurologic injury. Intraoperative transcranial Doppler has been demonstrated to detect embolic events in real time and allows modification of perfusion and surgical techniques. It has been shown that the numbers of emboli generated by perfusionist interventions such as drug injection and blood return, as well as episodes of entrainment of air from the surgical field, can be rapidly identified and corrected with detection of intraoperative emboli with this technology.

Brain oximetry, or near-infrared spectroscopy, has shown promising results for neuroprotection. An active treatment algorithm to minimize cerebral desaturation has been shown to be associated with decreased neurocognitive dysfunction and decreased markers of brain dysfunction. Electroencephalography patterns consistent with ischemia include increased slow wave activity and diffuse slowing of neural activity. These patterns have been reported to occur during cardiopulmonary bypass episodes thought to be associated with cerebral hypoperfusion. Notably, the electroencephalogram becomes progressively attenuated with advanced hypothermia, making cerebral oximetry a better means of monitoring and detecting onset of cerebral ischemia during deep hypothermic arrest. Portable intraoperative brain imaging with computed tomography has not been adequately evaluated for monitoring cerebral perfusion in this setting.

References:

1. Flier S, Murkin JM. Chapter 40: Central Nervous System Dysfunction After Cardiopulmonary Bypass. In: Kaplan JA, Augoustides JGT, Manecke GR, et al., eds. Kaplan's Cardiac Anesthesia. 7th ed. Elsevier; 2017:1374-1406.
2. Qu JZ, Kao LW, Smith JE, et al. Brain protection in aortic arch surgery: an evolving field. J Cardiothorac Vasc Anesth, 2021; 35: 1176-1188.

25. A patient is placed on central venoarterial extracorporeal membrane oxygenation (VA ECMO) after failing to wean from cardiopulmonary bypass. On postoperative day 2, clinical examination reveals a dilated right pupil with identification of a large stroke on brain imaging. What is TRUE regarding strokes while on VA ECMO?
    A. Estimated stroke incidence while on VA ECMO is 6%
    B. Ischemic strokes are extremely rare on ECMO due to routine use of anticoagulation
    C. Estimated stroke incidence while on VA ECMO is approximately 20%
    D. Anoxic brain injury is easily diagnosed because it leads to failure of the ECMO machine to flow

Correct Answer: A

Explanation: Venoarterial extracorporeal membrane oxygenation (VA ECMO) insertion is performed only in very high-risk patients and involves considerable risk for adverse neurologic events. The reported pooled estimate stroke rate from numerous studies is 5.9%. The overall neurological complication rate is 13.3%, with events such as hemorrhagic stroke, ischemic stroke, coma, anoxic brain injury, and brain death. Despite most patients being anticoagulated on ECMO, ischemic and embolic strokes are common, likely secondary to inflammation and extracorporeal circulation creation of microthrombi. The diagnosis of brain injury on ECMO can be difficult due to sedation requirements and lack of ECMO machine function changes with brain injury.

References:

1. Flier S, Murkin JM. Chapter 40: Central Nervous System Dysfunction After Cardiopulmonary Bypass. In: Kaplan JA, Augoustides JGT, Manecke GR, et al., eds. Kaplan's Cardiac Anesthesia. 7th ed. Elsevier; 2017:1374-1406.
2. Cormican DS, Elapavaluru S. Acute neurologic injury in VA ECMO for post-cardiotomy shock: caveat emptor. J Cardiothorac Vasc Anesth, 2021; 35: 1997-1998.
3. Hessel EA, Betz AC. The challenges of venoarterial ECMO for postcardiotomy shock. J Cardiothorac Vasc Anesth, 2021; 35: 48-50.

26. A patient with severe mitral regurgitation is being evaluated for MitraClip versus open mitral replacement procedure. All of the following are true regarding neurologic injury and mitral valve procedures, EXCEPT:
    A. The 30-day incidence of stroke following MitraClip is less than 1%
    B. The risk of stroke following open mitral replacement is 2% to 4%
    C. MitraClip procedures require cardiopulmonary bypass similarly to open mitral surgeries, thus imparting the same stroke risk
    D. Mitral valve repair has less risk of stroke compared to mitral valve replacement

Correct Answer: C

Explanation: The MitraClip procedure is used to treat patients with moderate-to-severe and severe mitral regurgitation. During this procedure, a device is advanced via the femoral vein into the right atrium and then via a transseptal route antegrade into the left atrium and further into the left ventricle with echocardiographic and fluoroscopic guidance. In most patients general anesthesia is used, but typically cardiopulmonary bypass and aortic cannulation are avoided. This may be the reason for a decreased risk of stroke following MitraClip procedures compared with open mitral valve procedures. The 30-day stroke incidence following MitraClip is 0.7%, and the 1-year stroke rate is 1.1%. The reported incidence of stroke after MitraClip is considerably lower than the stroke rate after open mitral valve surgery with cardiopulmonary bypass. For isolated surgical mitral valve replacement and repair, the incidence of stroke is 2.1% to 4.5% and 1.4%, respectively.

References:

1. Flier S, Murkin JM. Chapter 40: Central Nervous System Dysfunction After Cardiopulmonary Bypass. In: Kaplan JA, Augoustides JGT, Manecke GR, et al., eds. Kaplan's Cardiac Anesthesia. 7th ed. Elsevier; 2017:1374-1406.
2. Musuku SR, Mustafa M, Pulavarthi M, et al. Procedural, short-term, and intermediate-term outcomes in propensity-matched patients with severe mitral valve regurgitation undergoing urgent versus elective mitraclip percutaneous mitral valve repair. J Cardiothorac Vasc Anesth, 2022; 36: 1268-1275.

27. Many patients with coronary artery disease may have disease profiles amenable to percutaneous coronary intervention (PCI) or surgical coronary artery bypass grafting (CABG). Which of the following is TRUE regarding large trials comparing neurologic outcomes following PCI versus CABG?
    A. The risk of death at 5 years is higher in patients undergoing CABG
    B. The risk of delayed (>30 days) stroke is higher in patients undergoing PCI
    C. The risk of periprocedural stroke is higher in patients undergoing CABG
    D. Aortic manipulation is greater in PCI, resulting in the higher incidence of periprocedural stroke

Correct Answer: C

Explanation: Multiple large trials have compared outcomes in patients undergoing revascularization for stable multivessel coronary disease with coronary artery bypass grafting (CABG) versus percutaneous coronary intervention (PCI). These studies have demonstrated that the 5-year composite event rate of death, myocardial infarction, and stroke favored CABG, whereas the risk of stroke alone favored PCI. The difference is due to a higher 30-day stroke rate for CABG of 1.55% versus 0.37% for PCI. It is believed that the incidence of late stroke (>30 days) is similar for CABG and PCI. As such, these findings affirm that it is primarily intraoperative factors associated with CABG that give rise to the increased stroke risk. Notably, the rate of repeat revascularization is higher in patients who undergo PCI compared with CABG.

References:

1. Flier S, Murkin JM. Chapter 40: Central Nervous System Dysfunction After Cardiopulmonary Bypass. In: Kaplan JA, Augoustides JGT, Manecke GR, et al., eds. Kaplan's Cardiac Anesthesia. 7th ed. Elsevier; 2017:1374-1406.
2. Edwards FH, Shahian DM, Grau-Sepulveda MV, et al. Composite outcomes in coronary bypass surgery versus percutaneous intervention. Ann Thorac Surg, 2014; 97: 1983-1988.
3. Athappan G, Chacko P, Patvardhan E, et al. Late stroke: comparison of percutaneous coronary intervention versus coronary artery bypass grafting in patients with multivessel disease and unprotected left main disease: a meta-analysis and review of literature. Stroke, 2014; 45: 185-193.
4. Hassler KR, Schumer EM, Crestanello JA, et al. FFR-guided PCI versus CABG: analysis of new data. J Cardiothorac Vasc Anesth, 2022; 36: 3389-3391.
5. Shekhar S, Mohananey D, Villablanca P, et al. Revascularization strategies for stable left main coronary artery disease: analysis of current evidence. J Cardiothorac Vasc Anesth, 2022; 36: 3370-3378.

28. The following statements concerning pharmacologic neurologic protection for patients undergoing cardiac surgery are true, EXCEPT:
    A. Aspirin decreases risk of perioperative stroke via platelet inhibition
    B. 3-hydroxy-3-methyl-glutaryl coenzyme–A reductase inhibitors, or statins, decrease risk of stroke through anti-inflammatory and plaque-stabilizing mechanisms
    C. Calcium channel blockers have not been shown to be neuroprotective in cardiac surgery
    D. The majority of available evidence supports the use of beta blockade to reduce incidence of perioperative stroke

Correct Answer: D

Explanation: Aspirin has been shown to decrease mortality and stroke risk following cardiac surgery. The mechanism is thought to be through platelet inhibition. Recent evidence has suggested that statins not only have a lowering effect on cholesterol but also present pleiotropic and neuroprotective effects, including in stroke prevention. Statins are thought to possess antiatherosclerotic properties, increase plaque stability, and exert favorable effects on inflammation, vasomotor function, local fibrinolysis, and platelet activity. A Cochrane review on calcium antagonists in ischemic stroke in the perioperative cardiac surgical period failed to find a beneficial effect.

Beta blockade had previously been shown to lower incidences of perioperative stroke. However, some of this published data has since been retracted. Additionally, perioperative beta blocker therapy was associated with increased risk of stroke compared to placebo in the PeriOperative ISchemic Evaluation (POISE) trial. Although significantly fewer patients in the beta blocker group than in the placebo group had a myocardial infarction, there were more deaths associated with exposure to beta blockade due to fatal stroke.

References:

1. Flier S, Murkin JM. Chapter 40: Central Nervous System Dysfunction After Cardiopulmonary Bypass. In: Kaplan JA, Augoustides JGT, Manecke GR, et al., eds. Kaplan's Cardiac Anesthesia. 7th ed. Elsevier; 2017:1374-1406.
2. Devereaux PJ, Yang H, Yusuf S, et al. Effects of extended-release metoprolol succinate in patients undergoing non-cardiac surgery (POISE trial): a randomized controlled trial. Lancet, 2008; 371: 1839-1847.
3. Guay J, Ochroch EA. β-blocking agents for surgery: influence on mortality and major outcomes. A meta-analysis. J Cardiothorac Vasc Anesth, 2013; 27: 834-844.

29. All of the following are beneficial effects of statins, when taken preoperatively prior to cardiac surgical period, EXCEPT:
    A. Decreased risk of postoperative hepatic injury
    B. Decreased postoperative atrial fibrillation
    C. Enhanced vasomotor function
    D. Platelet inhibition

Correct Answer: A

Explanation: The statins not only have a lowering effect on cholesterol but also present pleiotropic and neuroprotective effects, including several studies demonstrating decreased postoperative stroke. Statins are thought to possess antiatherosclerotic properties, increase plaque stability, and exert favorable effects on inflammation, vasomotor function, local fibrinolysis, and platelet activity.

Another plausible mechanism for statin-induced neuroprotection may be the prevention of postoperative atrial fibrillation through their pleiotropic properties, leading to less postoperative stroke. Some studies have shown preoperative statin use to decrease hospital length of stay following cardiac surgery, likely due to the beneficial effects described. Statins have not been shown to be protect from hepatic injury and in fact have a small risk of causing liver injury.

References:

1. Flier S, Murkin JM. Chapter 40: Central Nervous System Dysfunction After Cardiopulmonary Bypass. In: Kaplan JA, Augoustides JGT, Manecke GR, et al., eds. Kaplan's Cardiac Anesthesia. 7th ed. Elsevier; 2017:1374-1406.
2. Elmarsafawi AG, Abbassi MM, Elkaffas S, et al. Efficacy of different perioperative statin regimens on protection against

post-coronary artery bypass grafting major adverse cardiac and cerebral events. J Cardiothorac Vasc Anesth, 2016; 30: 1461-1470.

3. Zhang C. Does statin reloading before cardiac surgery improve postoperative outcomes? J Cardiothorac Vasc Anesth, 2018; 32: e23-e24.

30. A patient undergoing aortic hemiarch repair has decreased unilateral reading of the left near-infrared spectroscopy from 86% to 45%. The surgeon and perfusionist are made aware and begin investigating cannulae and catheter positions and cardiopulmonary bypass mechanics. The following are recommended actions on the part of the anesthesiologist in management of decreased brain oximetry readings, EXCEPT:

A. Transfuse for hemoglobin goal more than 7 g/dL

B. Ensure mixed venous oxygen saturation over 60%

C. Adjust ventilation for goal end-tidal carbon dioxide of under 35 mmHg

D. Maintain mean arterial blood pressure greater than 65 mmHg

Correct Answer: C

Explanation: Brain oximetry, or near-infrared spectroscopy, has shown promising results for neuroprotection. An active treatment algorithm to minimize cerebral desaturation has been shown to be associated with decreased neurocognitive dysfunction and decreased markers of brain dysfunction.

If brain oximetry decreases during cardiac surgery, an algorithmic assessment and management is recommended. These steps include maintaining hemoglobin over 7 g/dL with transfusions as needed and maintaining mixed venous oxygen saturation greater than 60% with echocardiographic assessment and employment of inotropic agents as needed. Additionally, maintaining mean arterial blood pressure over 65 mmHg with pressors and optimizing systemic oxygen saturation is recommended. End-tidal carbon dioxide should be maintained at 35 to 40 mmHg to promote cerebral vasodilation and perfusion.

Bilateral, and perhaps especially unilateral, decrease in cerebral oximetry readings should prompt the surgeon to inspect cannulation and catheters, especially if anterograde or retrograde cerebral perfusion is being utilized. The position of the heart should be adjusted to attempt to increase blood flow if superior vena cava syndrome is suspected. The perfusionist should be prompted to assess cardiopulmonary bypass machine flows and pressures.

References:

1. Flier S, Murkin JM. Chapter 40: Central Nervous System Dysfunction After Cardiopulmonary Bypass. In: Kaplan JA, Augoustides JGT, Manecke GR, et al., eds. Kaplan's Cardiac Anesthesia. 7th ed. Elsevier; 2017:1374-1406.

2. Qu JZ, Kao LW, Smith JE, et al. Brain protection in aortic arch surgery: an evolving field. J Cardiothorac Vasc Anesth, 2021; 35: 1176-1188.

CHAPTER 37

Long-Term Complications and Management

Jennette Hansen and Brigid Flynn

KEY POINTS

1. After undergoing cardiac surgery, a small percentage of patients have complicated courses and prolonged stays in the intensive care unit (ICU).
2. These patients have an increased mortality rate, not always due to cardiac complications, but often due to multisystem organ dysfunction.
3. Infections, acute kidney injury, nutritional issues, and surgical complications are common etiologies of prolonged ICU length of stay following cardiac surgery.
4. The use of mechanical circulatory support, including ventricular assist devices and extracorporeal membrane oxygenation, leads to additional complications such as bleeding and thrombotic morbidities.
5. Palliative care teams can help with numerous aspects of prolonged ICU care.

1. A patient who received a cardiac-implanted electronic device (CIED) 5 years ago presents with fatigue. A transesophageal echocardiogram identified thickening of the right ventricular lead raising concern for infection. What is TRUE concerning CIED infections?
   A. Blood cultures in CIED infections are more sensitive than in infections caused by endocarditis
   B. The incidence of CIED infections is rare, with fewer than 0.05% of patients with CIEDs encountering infection in their lifetime
   C. Diabetes mellitus has not been shown to be a risk factor for CIED infection
   D. The most common pathogens reported for CIED infections are *Staphylococci* and other gram-positive bacteria

Correct Answer: D

Explanation: The diagnosis of cardiac-implanted electronic device (CIED) infections can be challenging. Most patients exhibit nonspecific symptoms, and fewer than 10% develop septic shock. Both blood cultures and echocardiography are less sensitive in CIED infections compared with endocarditis. The incidence of CIED infection is 0.5% to 2.2% of patients, with a two- to fivefold increase after a revision. Diabetes is a risk factor for CIED infection, along with other organ dysfunction. *Staphylococci* and other gram-positive bacteria are the most common organisms involved in CIED

infection. In fact, these bacteria account for 68% to 93% of all CIED infections.

References:

1. Birch M, Lupei MI, Wall M, et al. Chapter 41: Long-Term Complications and Management. In: Kaplan JA, Augoustides JGT, Manecke GR, et al., eds. Kaplan's Cardiac Anesthesia. 7th ed. Elsevier; 2017:1407-1424.
2. Cronin B, Essandoh M. Update on cardiovascular implantable electronic devices for anesthesiologists. J Cardiothorac Vasc Anesth, 2017; 32: 1871-1884.

2. Identified risk factors for cardiac-implanted electronic device (CIED) infections include all of the following EXCEPT:
   A. CIED device replacement due to device failure
   B. High-volume centers
   C. Young men
   D. Lack of antibiotic prophylaxis

Correct Answer: B

Explanation: In a study of more than 40,000 patients who were followed over 14 years, the incidence of cardiac-implanted electronic device (CIED) infections has been reported to be 2.45 per 1000 CIED years. This study found that risks for CIED infection included young men and patients requiring replacement of the CIED device. Other studies have shown CIED infection risks to include increased number of prior complex procedures and the lack of antibiotic prophylaxis. High-volume centers have been shown to have a lower incidence of infection rates. The management of CIED infections, including the number and sequence of blood cultures and antibiotic therapy, should be guided by the clinical severity.

TABLE 37.1

Management of cardiac-implanted electronic device–related infection with lead or endocarditis involvement

Evidence of Severe Sepsis	No Evidence of Severe Sepsis
Initial actions: 1. Conduct blood cultures testing twice within 1 hour. 2. Start empirical intravenous antimicrobial therapy within 1 hour, after blood cultures are tested. 3. Obtain an urgent echocardiographic scan within 24 hours.	*Initial actions:* 1. Perform blood culture testing three different times (>6 hours apart). 2. Obtain an echocardiographic scan. 3. Follow blood culture and echocardiographic results.
Positive blood cultures and/or echocardiographic evidence of vegetations: 1. Remove system and repeat echocardiographic scan. 2. If native cardiac structures are involved, then conduct 4 weeks of empirical antimicrobial therapy. 3. Extracardiac focus is a 6-week course of antibiotic therapy. 4. If it is a lead only infection, then consider a short course (2 weeks) of antibiotic therapy.	*No positive blood cultures and/or echocardiographic evidence of vegetations:* 1. Review diagnosis and repeat echocardiographic scan and blood cultures as clinically indicated. 2. If generator pocket infection signs are present, then consider 10–14 days of antibiotic treatment after the removal of the system.

Modified from Sandoe JA, Barlow G, Chambers JB, et al. Guidelines for the diagnosis, prevention and management of implantable cardiac electronic device infection. Report of a joint Working Party project on behalf of the British Society for Antimicrobial Chemotherapy (BSAC, hot organization), British Heart Rhythm Society (BHRS), British Cardiovascular Society (BCS), British Heart Valve Society (BHVS) and British Society for Echocardiography (BSE). J Antimicrob Chemother, 2015; 70: 325-359.

References:

1. Birch M, Lupei MI, Wall M, et al. Chapter 41: Long-Term Complications and Management. In: Kaplan JA, Augoustides JGT, Manecke GR, et al., eds. Kaplan's Cardiac Anesthesia. 7th ed. Elsevier; 2017:1407-1424.
2. Cronin B, Essandoh M. Update on cardiovascular implantable electronic devices for anesthesiologists. J Cardiothorac Vasc Anesth, 2017; 32: 1871-1884.

3. A 49-year-old male who received a HeartMate III left ventricular assist device (LVAD) 2 years ago is found to have an elevated white blood cell count and skin irritation with purulence near the driveline exit site. What is TRUE regarding LVAD drive-line infections?
   A. Gram-negative bacteria are the most common cause of LVAD drive-line infections
   B. Treatment of drive-line infections requires urgent LVAD exchange
   C. The incidence of drive-line infections is 16% to 20% in patients with an LVAD beyond 30 days
   D. Smaller body mass index is a risk factor for drive-line infection

Correct Answer: C

Explanation: Left ventricular assist device (LVAD) drive-line infections compromise the care of 16% to 20% of patients with LVADs. The majority of these infections occur more than 30 days from LVAD implantation. Patients who suffer drive-line infections require more hospitalizations and more frequent reoperations and are at increased risk for stroke. Risk factors for drive-line infections include larger body mass index and diabetes mellitus. The most common organism identified in drive-line infections is *Staphylococcus aureus*. Drive-line infections are commonly identified by examination of the drive-line exit site with red, tender, or inflamed-appearing skin prompting more evaluation. Computed tomography scans are commonly employed to evaluate the depth of the infection by looking for abscess formation or gaseous, filled pockets. Typical initial treatment of drive-line infections includes systemic antibiotics and close follow-up in patients who are stable. However, many patients will require surgical care with washouts, debridements, antibiotic bead implantation, and, ultimately, LVAD exchange if other therapies are not curative.

References:

1. Birch M, Lupei MI, Wall M, et al. Chapter 41: Long-Term Complications and Management. In: Kaplan JA, Augoustides JGT, Manecke GR, et al., eds. Kaplan's Cardiac Anesthesia. 7th ed. Elsevier; 2017:1407-1424.
2. Desai S, Hwang N. Advances in left ventricular assist devices and mechanical circulatory support. J Cardiothorac Vasc Anesth, 2018; 32: 1193-1213.

4. A patient who underwent a coronary artery bypass grafting a month ago presents to the emergency department with an elevated white blood cell count and a red, fluctuant, and tender sternotomy incision. Saphenous venous grafts were used for all bypasses. Which of the following is TRUE regarding sternal wound infections following cardiac surgery?
   A. The incidence of sternal wound infections following cardiac surgery is approximately 0.77%
   B. Fungal infections account for the majority of sternal wound infectious organisms
   C. The risk would be lower with bilateral mammary arteries as bypass grafts

D. Postoperative re-exploration decreases the risk of development of sternal wound infection

Correct Answer: A

Explanation: Although rare, sternal wound infections can have deleterious consequences on patient outcomes following cardiac surgery. Sternal wound infections have been estimated to occur at a rate of 0.47% to 0.77%. Older age, diabetes, previous stroke and transient ischemic attacks, heart failure, and use of bilateral mammary grafts for the coronary artery bypass grafting are risk factors associated with deep sternal wound infections. Patients who suffer sternal wound infections more commonly have increased duration of mechanical ventilation and hospital length of stay. *Staphylococcus aureus* and other gram-positive bacteria are the most common infective organisms. Risk factors associated with sternal wound infections include female gender, hypertension, diabetes, and re-exploration for bleeding. Some authors advocate the use of nasal mupirocin and preoperative chlorhexidine showering to reduce the incidence of sternal wound infection.

References:

1. Birch M, Lupei MI, Wall M, et al. Chapter 41: Long-Term Complications and Management. In: Kaplan JA, Augoustides JGT, Manecke GR, et al., eds. Kaplan's Cardiac Anesthesia. 7th ed. Elsevier; 2017:1407-1424.
2. Phoon P, Hwang N. Deep sternal wound infection: diagnosis, treatment and prevention. J Cardiothorac Vasc Anesth, 2019; 34: 1602-1613.

5. A patient who underwent bioprosthetic aortic valve replacement 2 years ago presents with fever, new murmur, and two positive blood cultures for *Staphylococcus aureus*. A transthoracic echocardiography study demonstrates normal valvular function but a decrease in systolic function from baseline. The patient is admitted for intravenous antibiotics due to concern for infective endocarditis. Which is the NEXT best step?

A. Transition to oral antibiotics, as aortic prostheses are less likely than mitral prostheses to lead to the development of endocarditis

B. Transition to oral antibiotics, as bioprosthetic valve endocarditis is more easily treated than mechanical bioprosthetic endocarditis

C. Discharge on intravenous antibiotics because surgical intervention for endocarditis is only indicated in patients with valve dehiscence

D. Obtain a positron emission tomography/computed tomography scan to aid diagnosis

Correct Answer: D

Explanation: The modified Duke criteria remain the gold standard for infective endocarditis diagnosis. The risk of endocarditis is considered high if two major, one major and three minor, or five minor clinical criteria are met. The risk of developing endocarditis is not different for mitral or aortic prosthesis or for mechanical versus bioprosthetic valves. *Staphylococcus aureus* is the most common organism (34%), followed by *Streptococcus* species (23%), *Enterococcus* species (19%),

TABLE 37.2
Modified duke criteria for diagnosing infective endocarditis

Major Criteria	Minor Criteria
1. Two positive blood cultures with typical microorganisms collected at least 12 hours apart (or one positive blood culture for *Coxiella burnetii*) 2. Evidence of endocardial involvement (new murmur, echocardiographic evidence of a cardiac mass, abscess, valve dehiscence)	1. Fever >38°C 2. Vascular phenomena (systemic emboli, Janeway lesions) 3. Immunologic phenomena (Osler nodes, Roth spots) 4. Predisposition to infective endocarditis (previous infective endocarditis or intravenous drug abuse) 5. Microbiologic evidence that does not meet major criteria

Adapted from J.S. Li, D.J. Sexton, N. Mick, et al. Proposed modifications to the Duke criteria for the diagnosis of infective endocarditis. Clin Infect Dis, 30 (2000), pp. 633-638.

and coagulase-negative *Staphylococcus* (18%). Although echocardiography, especially transesophageal echocardiography, may confirm diagnosis, newer evidence indicates that positron emission tomography/computed tomography scans may be superior in evaluating prosthetic valve endocarditis and cardiac-implanted electronic device–associated infections.

Uncomplicated cases of endocarditis, including those without hemodynamic instability, heart failure, valvular dysfunction, dehiscence, abscess, or fistula formation, do not require surgical intervention. However, some evidence demonstrates that surgery improves survival and is ideally performed when the patient is not in extremis. The recommendation for prophylactic antibiotics before dental and surgical procedures remains for all patients with prosthetic valves.

References:

1. Birch M, Lupei MI, Wall M, et al. Chapter 41: Long-Term Complications and Management. In: Kaplan JA, Augoustides JGT, Manecke GR, et al., eds. Kaplan's Cardiac Anesthesia. 7th ed. Elsevier; 2017:1407-1424.
2. Starakis I, Mazokopakis EE. Prosthetic valve endocarditis: diagnostic approach and treatment options. Cardiovasc Hematol Disord Drug Targets, 2009; 28: 249-260.

6. Following coronary artery bypass grating surgery, a patient's creatinine increases from a baseline of 0.8 mg/dL to 2.4 mg/dL, but there is no indication for hemodialysis. What would be TRUE for this patient with acute kidney injury after cardiac surgery (AKI-CS)?

A. Mortality risk is not increased, because hemodialysis is not required

B. Based on the Kidney Disease Improving Global Outcomes Criteria, this patient is in stage 3 renal failure

C. Aortic cross clamp time has not been shown to affect the development of AKI-CS

D. The use of prophylactic N-acetylcysteine is recommended by the American Heart Association in high-risk patients to decrease the risk of AKI-CS

Correct Answer: B

Explanation: The risk of mortality for patients who sustain acute kidney injury after cardiac surgery (AKI-CS) increases from less than 1% to 20% when moderate AKI develops. Furthermore, if dialysis is required, the risk of mortality increases to 50%. Defining AKI has been attempted by several groups, resulting in the Risk, Injury, Failure, Loss of kidney function, and End-stage kidney disease (RIFLE) criteria, followed by the Acute Kidney Injury Network (AKIN) criteria and, in 2012, the Kidney Disease Improving Global Outcomes (KDIGO) criteria. AKIN and KDIGO simplified the definitions by excluding the glomerular filtration rate criteria and use only serum creatinine and urine output to define stages 1, 2, and 3 of kidney injury.

TABLE 37.3
RIFLE criteria

	Glomerular Filtration Rate Criteria	Urine Output Criteria
Risk	1.5 × increase in baseline Cr or GFR decrease by 25%	UO <0.5 cc/kg/h × 6 hours
Injury	2 × increase in baseline Cr or GFR decrease by 50%	UO <0.5 cc/kg/h × 12 hours
Failure	3 × increase in baseline Cr or Cr >4 or GFR decrease by 75%	UO <0.3 cc/kg/h × 24 hours or anuria
Loss	Persistent ARF: Complete loss of renal function >4 weeks	
ESRD	End-stage renal disease	

RIFLE, Risk, Injury, Failure, Loss of kidney function, and End-stage kidney disease; *GFR,* glomerular filtration rate; *Cr,* creatinine; *UO,* urine output; *ARF,* acute renal failure; *ESRD,* end-stage renal disease.
Modified from Bellomo R, Ronco C, Kellum JA, et al. Acute renal failure—definition, outcome measures, animal models, fluid therapy and information technology needs: the Second International Consensus Conference of the Acute Dialysis Quality Initiative (ADQI) Group. Crit Care, 2004; 8: R204-R212.

The incidence of AKI-CS ranges from 10% to 40% of patients, depending on the definition of the AKI-CS. Risk factors for AKI-CS include advanced age, female gender, chronic obstructive pulmonary disease, diabetes, peripheral vascular disease, congestive heart failure, baseline renal insufficiency, cardiogenic shock, emergent surgery, and left main coronary disease. Longer cardiopulmonary bypass time, aortic cross clamp time, transfusion requirements, valvular surgery, and off-pump procedures have been shown to be associated with AKI-CS. Medications studied in attempts to decrease the risk of AKI-CS include fenoldopam, natriuretic peptides, sodium bicarbonate, and N-acetylcysteine. However,

TABLE 37.4
Acute Kidney Injury Network criteria

AKI Stage	Serum Creatinine Criteria	Urine Output Criteria
1	Absolute increase >0.3 mg/dL or Cr 1.5 × baseline	<0.5 cc/kg/h × 6 hours
2	Cr 2–3 × baseline	<0.5 cc/kg/h × >12 hours
3	3 × baseline Cr or value > 4 mg/dL with absolute increase >0.5 mg/dL or receiving renal replacement therapy	<0.3 cc/kg/h or anuria × 12 hours

AKI, Acute kidney injury; *Cr,* creatinine.
Modified from Mehta RL, Kellum JA, Shah SV, et al. Acute Kidney Injury Network: report of an initiative to improve outcomes in acute kidney injury. Crit Care, 2007; 11: R31.

TABLE 37.5
Kidney Disease Improving Global Outcomes criteria

Stage	Serum Creatinine (Cr)	Urine Output
1	1.5–1.9 × baseline Cr or >0.3 mg/dL increase	<0.5 cc/kg/h × 6 hours
2	2–2.9 × baseline Cr	<0.5 cc/kg/h × 12 hours
3	3 × baseline Cr or Cr > 4 mg/dL or initiation of RRT	<0.3 cc/kg/h × 24 hours or anuria >12 hours

RRT, Renal replacement therapy.
From http://kdigo.org/home/guidelines/acute-kidney-injury/

none have uniformly demonstrated benefit and thus are not recommended as prophylaxis.

References:

1. Birch M, Lupei MI, Wall M, et al. Chapter 41: Long-Term Complications and Management. In: Kaplan JA, Augoustides JGT, Manecke GR, et al., eds. Kaplan's Cardiac Anesthesia. 7th ed. Elsevier; 2017:1407-1424.
2. Just I, Alborzi F, Godde M, et al. Cardiac surgery-related acute kidney injury: risk factors, clinical course, management suggestions. J Cardiothorac Vasc Anesth, 2021; 36: 444-451.

7. The leadership of a cardiothoracic intensive care unit notice an unusually high rate of acute kidney injury after cardiac surgery (AKI-CS) and explore strategies to decrease this risk. What may prevent AKI-CS?

A. Delaying cardiac surgery, if possible, in patients with contrast-associated acute kidney injury is recommended

B. Providing early renal replacement therapy in patients who meet indications for dialysis

C. Utilizing intermittent hemodialysis instead of continuous renal replacement therapy will promote renal recovery

D. If renal replacement therapy is required, continuing challenges of intravenous diuretic therapy will aid renal recovery

Correct Answer: A

Explanation: There are no known curative treatments for acute kidney injury after cardiac surgery (AKI-CS). The best solution is to attempt to prevent this morbidity. Strategies cited in the literature include delaying surgery until contrast-associated kidney injury subsides (American College of Cardiology/American Heart Association guideline recommendation), less bleeding and fewer transfusions, shorter aortic cross clamp and cardiopulmonary bypass times, and avoidance of nephrotoxins. There is no evidence that early dialysis decreases the risk of AKI. Intermittent dialysis is not superior to continuous renal replacement therapy for renal recovery in this setting. Intermittent dialysis allows for clearance of harmful electrolytes or toxins more quickly but may not be tolerated by unstable patients. There are no recommendations regarding intravenous diuretic therapy while on dialysis and renal recovery.

References:

1. Birch M, Lupei MI, Wall M, et al. Chapter 41: Long-Term Complications and Management. In: Kaplan JA, Augoustides JGT, Manecke GR, et al., eds. Kaplan's Cardiac Anesthesia. 7th ed. Elsevier; 2017:1407-1424.
2. Liu Y, Davari-Farid S, Arora P, et al. Early versus late initiation of renal replacement therapy in critically ill patients with acute kidney injury after cardiac surgery: a systematic review and meta-analysis. J Cardiothorac Vasc Anesth, 2014; 28: 557-563.

8. Enteral nutrition may be required in patients who have prolonged and complicated cardiothoracic surgical intensive care unit courses to ensure adequate caloric intake. Known sequelae of starting enteral nutrition include:
A. Increased risk of sepsis due to increased bacterial translocation across the gut wall
B. Immune response modulation and decreased inflammatory response
C. Decreased insulin resistance
D. Ability for critically ill patients to meet metabolic demand requirements

Correct Answer: A

Explanation: The American Society of Parenteral and Enteral Nutrition (ASPEN) and the European Society for Clinical Nutrition and Metabolism (ESPEN) have recommended initiation of enteral nutrition support for all critically ill patients who cannot meet metabolic requirements on their own. However, the level of evidence for this is not strong. Enteral nutrition is favorable for maintaining gut integrity to prevent gut permeability and bacterial translocation. This likely decreases multisystem organ failure and sepsis. Further benefits of enteral nutrition include immune response modulation and decreased inflammatory response, decreased insulin resistance, and the provision of energy substrates for critically ill patients to meet metabolic demand requirements.

References:

1. Birch M, Lupei MI, Wall M, et al. Chapter 41: Long-Term Complications and Management. In: Kaplan JA, Augoustides JGT, Manecke GR, et al., eds. Kaplan's Cardiac Anesthesia. 7th ed. Elsevier; 2017:1407-1424.
2. Lopez-Delgado J, Munoz-del Rio G, Flordelis-Lasierra J, et al. Nutrition in adult cardiac surgery: preoperative evaluation, management in the postoperative period, and clinical implications for outcomes. J Cardiothorac Vasc Anesth, 2019; 33: 3143-3162.

9. A patient who is postoperative day 3 from coronary artery bypass grafting with stage 3 renal injury has failed speech and swallow evaluation due to risk of aspiration with oral food intake. When considering initiation of nutrition, what is most accurate?
A. Enteric nutrition with more protein to promote wound healing does not pose risk
B. Guidelines advise holding all nutrition and reassessing swallowing evaluation in 24 hours
C. Parenteral nutrition should be initiated
D. Enteric nutrition containing 2 kcal/mL is superior to 1 kcal/mL in this patient

Correct Answer: D

Explanation: Major society guidelines recommend initiation of enteral nutrition within 24 hours of admission to the intensive care unit. Studies have shown decreased ventilator-free days, lower infection rates, and lower mortality. However, these studies were not solely performed in cardiac surgical patients, up to 50% of whom may have delayed gastric emptying, so caution is warranted. In patients with renal injury, nutritional formulas that contain less protein, potassium, and phosphorous are advised due to inability to efficiently metabolize and clear these byproducts. Also, patients with renal injury are usually initiated on more energy-dense formulas to decrease volume because they may become fluid-overloaded due to decreased urine output. Parenteral nutrition may be associated with increased morbidity and mortality. Enteral nutrition, if available, is the preferred first-line administration route due to benefits regarding gut integrity and immune modulation.

References:

1. Birch M, Lupei MI, Wall M, et al. Chapter 41: Long-Term Complications and Management. In: Kaplan JA, Augoustides JGT, Manecke GR, et al., eds. Kaplan's Cardiac Anesthesia. 7th ed. Elsevier; 2017:1407-1424.
2. Lopez-Delgado J, Munoz-del Rio G, Flordelis-Lasierra J, et al. Nutrition in adult cardiac surgery: preoperative evaluation, management in the postoperative period, and clinical implications for outcomes. J Cardiothorac Vasc Anesth, 2019; 33: 3143-3162.

10. A 90-year-old patient presents with severe aortic stenosis, an ejection fraction of 45%, hypertension, hyperlipidemia, and acid reflux. Based on the Placement of Aortic Transcatheter Valve (PARTNER) trials, what is TRUE concerning the potential options of transcatheter aortic valve replacement (TAVR), surgical aortic valve replacement (SAVR), and nonsurgical medical management?

A. This patient's expected mortality is equal with TAVR and SAVR
B. The transfemoral approach for TAVR has a decreased periprocedural risk of death compared with the transapical approach for TAVR
C. Medical management has comparable 30-day mortality risk compared with TAVR
D. Medical management has less risk of death at 1 year, but increased risk of death at 2 years, compared to TAVR

Correct Answer: B

Explanation: Placement of Aortic Transcatheter Valve (PARTNER) A compared the outcomes of high-risk patients treated with transcatheter aortic valve replacement (TAVR) versus surgical aortic valve replacement (SAVR). PARTNER B compared the outcomes of inoperable patients treated with TAVR versus standard therapy. PARTNER A demonstrated 30-day mortality rates of 3.4% for TAVR and 6.5% for SAVR, 1-year mortality rates of 24% and 25%, respectively, and similar mortality rates at 2 years. The transfemoral approach had a decreased periprocedural mortality rate compared with both transapical TAVR and SAVR. When comparing TAVR to no surgical intervention and only medical management, described as standard therapy in the PARTNER trials, patients who underwent TAVR actually had a higher 30-day mortality rate (5% vs. 2.8%). However, mortality and other risks favored TAVR at 1- and 2-year follow-up. At 1 year, TAVR mortality was 30% compared with 50% for standard therapy, and at 2-year follow-up it was 43% compared with 68% for standard therapy.

References:

1. Birch M, Lupei MI, Wall M, et al. Chapter 41: Long-Term Complications and Management. In: Kaplan JA, Augoustides JGT, Manecke GR, et al., eds. Kaplan's Cardiac Anesthesia. 7th ed. Elsevier; 2017:1407-1424.
2. Kodali SK, Williams MR, Smith CR, et al. Two-year outcomes after transcatheter or surgical aortic-valve replacement. N Engl J Med, 2012; 366: 1686-1695.

11. Which of the following is true concerning the risks of transcatheter aortic valve replacement (TAVR) compared with surgical aortic valve replacement (SAVR)?

A. Compared with SAVR, TAVR has a decreased risk of stroke at 30 days postprocedure
B. The incidence of paravalvular leak at 1-year follow-up is greater following SAVR than TAVR
C. Moderate aortic regurgitation is more frequent after TAVR at 1- and 2-year follow-up compared with SAVR
D. Major vascular complications are similar for TAVR and SAVR

Correct Answer: C

Explanation: Although mortality is favorable with transcatheter aortic valve replacement (TAVR) compared with surgical aortic valve replacement (SAVR), there are major morbidities associated with TAVR. The risk of stroke is higher for TAVR compared to SAVR. At 30 days, the incidence of stroke after TAVR is 4.6% versus 2.4% after SAVR. Suffering a stroke increases the hazard of death. The incidence of perivalvular leak at both 1- and 2-year follow-up is higher in TAVR patients versus SAVR patients. Additionally, moderate aortic regurgitation is more frequent in TAVR patients compared with SAVR patients at both 1- and 2-year follow-up. Lastly, TAVR patients have an increased risk of major vascular complications compared to SAVR at 1 year (11% vs. 3.8%), likely due to arterial access complications.

References:

1. Birch M, Lupei MI, Wall M, et al. Chapter 41: Long-Term Complications and Management. In: Kaplan JA, Augoustides JGT, Manecke GR, et al., eds. Kaplan's Cardiac Anesthesia. 7th ed. Elsevier; 2017:1407-1424.
2. Reidy C, Sophocles A, Ramakrishna H, et al. Challenges after the first decade of transcatheter aortic valve replacement: focus on vascular complications, stroke, and paravalvular leak. J Cardiothorac Vasc Anesth, 2012; 27: 184-189.

12. A patient with multivessel coronary artery disease presents for coronary artery bypass grafting (CABG). The patient suffers from chronic back pain and has been taking oxycodone for 2 years. The patient has asked for a minimally invasive approach due to ongoing issues with chronic pain. Which of the following is evidence-based information that can help guide the decision for minimally invasive off-pump CABG (OPCAB) surgery versus standard CABG surgery?

A. Patients who receive minimally invasive OPCAB surgeries have been shown to have increased intubation times
B. Patients who receive minimally invasive OPCAB surgeries tend to have increased incidence of atrial fibrillation in the perioperative period
C. Surgeries performed with the minimally invasive OPCAB technique have shorter operative times
D. Patients who receive minimally invasive OPCAB surgeries tend to have an increased need for postoperative pain medications

Correct Answer: D

Explanation: The Sternotomy Versus Thoracotomy (STET) trial demonstrated that left anterolateral thoracotomy off-pump coronary artery bypass grafting OPCAB surgery was associated with shorter intubation times and fewer arrhythmias. However, OPCAB surgery was also associated with longer operative time, a greater need for postoperative pain relief, and worse lung function at discharge compared with standard, open OPCAB surgery.

References:

1. Birch M, Lupei MI, Wall M, et al. Chapter 41: Long-Term Complications and Management. In: Kaplan JA,

Augoustides JGT, Manecke GR, et al., eds. Kaplan's Cardiac Anesthesia. 7th ed. Elsevier; 2017:1407-1424.

2. Maj G, Regesta T, Campanella A, et al. Optimal management of patients treated with minimally invasive cardiac surgery in the era of enhanced recovery after surgery and fast-track protocols: a narrative review. J Cardiothorac Vasc Anesth, 2021; 36: 766-775.

13. An 83-year-old patient with severe coronary artery disease presents for coronary artery bypass grafting (CABG). The patient asks about the risks of on-pump versus off-pump CABG surgery. Which of the following is TRUE about on-pump versus off-pump CABG, if both are performed with median sternotomy?
    A. Mortality at 1 year is relatively increased with the off-pump approach
    B. The risk of stroke is lower with the off-pump technique
    C. Transitioning from off-pump to on-pump during the CABG procedure does not affect outcomes
    D. The number of coronary artery grafts that need to be bypassed does not influence the decision to proceed with the off-pump approach

Correct Answer: B

Explanation: Mortality at 1 year is comparable after on-pump and off-pump revascularization for coronary artery disease. The risk of stroke is decreased with an off-pump approach, especially for patients older than 80 years. Conversion to on-pump surgery during the procedure can significantly increase the risks of mortality and morbidity. Thus, conversion midprocedure is not a prudent back-up plan. Due to technical challenges such as surgical exposure, the off-pump technique may not always permit the completion of all the bypass grafts, and therefore this approach may not be optimal in patients who require four to five grafts.

References:

1. Birch M, Lupei MI, Wall M, et al. Chapter 41: Long-Term Complications and Management. In: Kaplan JA, Augoustides JGT, Manecke GR, et al., eds. Kaplan's Cardiac Anesthesia. 7th ed. Elsevier; 2017:1407-1424.
2. Shaefi S, Mittel A, Loberman D, et al. Off-pump versus on-pump coronary artery bypass grafting – a systematic review and analysis of clinical outcomes. J Cardiothorac Vasc Anesth, 2019; 33: 232-244.

14. Which statement is FALSE with respect to survival of patients with end-stage heart failure?
    A. Ventricular assist devices offer similar survival benefit and quality of life in patients with heart failure compared with optimal medical management
    B. Current left ventricular assist device (LVAD) mechanical support devices are used as destination therapy and also as bridge-to-transplant therapy
    C. At 2 years postimplant, survival of patients with LVAD support is approximately 80%
    D. Postoperative survival rates following heart transplantation compared with LVAD at 10 years favor heart transplantation

Correct Answer: A

Explanation: The Randomized Evaluation of Mechanical Assistance for the Treatment of Congestive Heart Failure (REMATCH) trial was the first large trial demonstrating that patients with heart failure have improved survival and quality of life when treated with left ventricular assist devices (LVADs) compared with medical management. LVADs may be destination therapy but can also be used as a bridge to transplant in patients awaiting a heart transplant. As technology has improved, current survival rates of patients who receive nonemergent LVAD therapy is similar at 2 years compared to patients who receive heart transplantation, at approximately 80%. However, due to adverse events associated with LVAD therapy, including bleeding and clotting, survival rates after 2 years favor heart transplantation when compared with LVAD. It is notable that this natural history may evolve with ongoing refinements in VAD design and function.

References:

1. Birch M, Lupei MI, Wall M, et al. Chapter 41: Long-Term Complications and Management. In: Kaplan JA, Augoustides JGT, Manecke GR, et al., eds. Kaplan's Cardiac Anesthesia. 7th ed. Elsevier; 2017:1407-1424.
2. Martin AK, Ripoll JG, Wilkey BJ, et al. Analysis of outcomes in heart transplantation. J Cardiothorac Vasc Anesth, 2020; 34: 551-561.

15. A patient who received a HeartMate 3 left ventricular assist device (LVAD) 2 years ago phones his physician due to a high-power LVAD alarm. With suspicion of pump thrombosis, the patient is admitted to the hospital. Which of the following is TRUE regarding LVAD pump thrombosis?
    A. Faster rates of blood flow through the pump increase the risk of thrombosis
    B. Pump thrombosis is the second leading cause of device failure following electrical issues
    C. Hemolysis labs, such as lactate dehydrogenase and haptoglobin, rarely aid the diagnosis since these do not change for several days following diagnosis of pump thrombosis
    D. High-power alarms on the LVAD may be the first sign of pump thrombosis

Correct Answer: D

Explanation: Left ventricular assist device (LVAD) pump thrombosis is associated with major morbidity and mortality. Pump thrombosis is the most common cause of device failure. Risks factors for this complication include low flow states and lack of anticoagulation. Hemolytic indicators such as lactate dehydrogenase (LDH) and haptoglobin acutely change in the setting of pump thrombosis, with elevated LDH and decreased haptoglobin levels. Further tests that aid the diagnosis include echocardiography, computed tomography scan, and the evaluation of pump parameters, especially flow and power. Commonly, power spikes are the first indication of pump thrombosis. It is likely that the risk of pump thrombosis will decrease with further advances in LVAD design and performance.

References:

1. Birch M, Lupei MI, Wall M, et al. Chapter 41: Long-Term Complications and Management. In: Kaplan JA, Augoustides JGT, Manecke GR, et al., eds. Kaplan's Cardiac Anesthesia. 7th ed. Elsevier; 2017:1407-1424.
2. Jain A, Wilhelm M, Falk V, et al. Left ventricular assist device thrombosis is associated with an increase in the systolic-to-diastolic velocity ratio measured at the inflow and outflow cannulae. J Cardiothorac Vasc Anesth, 2017; 31: 497-504.

16. Factors that predispose patients with continuous flow left ventricular devices (LVADs) to suffer gastrointestinal bleeding include:

   A. Requirement for systemic anticoagulation
   B. Increased levels of von Willebrand factor
   C. Gastrointestinal mucosa vasculature is altered in patients with LVAD support
   D. Low pulse pressure may contribute to the formation of arteriovenous malformations

Correct Answer: B

Explanation: Gastrointestinal bleeding is common in patients with left ventricular assist device (LVAD) support, with a reported prevalence of 10% to 40%. There are multiple contributing factors to the development of this complication. Patients with LVADs are usually systemically anticoagulated to decrease the risk of pump thrombosis. Aspirin is also prescribed for platelet inhibition that can further aggravate the bleeding risk. Due to shear stress on blood cells when in contact with the mechanical bearings of the LVAD, the levels of von Willebrand factor decrease, resulting in a functional deficiency that can precipitate mucosal bleeding. Furthermore, the ongoing LVAD support induces arteriovenous malformations in the vasculature of the gastrointestinal mucosa, possibly due to continuous instead of pulsatile blood flow.

References:

1. Birch M, Lupei MI, Wall M, et al. Chapter 41: Long-Term Complications and Management. In: Kaplan JA, Augoustides JGT, Manecke GR, et al., eds. Kaplan's Cardiac Anesthesia. 7th ed. Elsevier; 2017:1407-1424.
2. Gutsche JT, Atluri P, Augoustides JG. Treatment of ventricular-assist-device-associated gastrointestinal bleeding with hormonal therapy. J Cardiothorac Vasc Anesth, 2013; 27: 939-943.

17. A patient is placed on venoarterial extracorporeal membrane oxygenation (VA ECMO) due to failure to wean off cardiopulmonary bypass following aortic valve replacement and coronary artery bypass grafting. Which is TRUE regarding VA ECMO?

   A. The overall mortality rate for VA ECMO is less than the mortality rate for patients requiring venovenous extracorporeal membrane oxygenation
   B. ECMO pumps rely on pulsatile pumps in order to ensure adequate perfusion pressure
   C. Due to advances in ECMO pump technology, hemolysis is rare for patients on ECMO
   D. Systemic anticoagulation for patients on ECMO should be individualized

Correct Answer: D

Explanation: Overall, the mortality rates for venovenous extracorporeal membrane oxygenation (VV ECMO) are typically lower than those for venoarterial extracorporeal membrane oxygenation (VA ECMO). The mortality for VV ECMO ranges from 20% to 40%, as compared to VA ECMO, which may have an associated mortality in the 40% to 60% range. ECMO pumps are centrifugal pumps that deliver continuous flow blood supply to the body. Despite the numerous advances in ECMO circuitry, such as heparin-coated circuits and hollow-fiber oxygenators, there is still a risk of hemolysis due to shear stress of blood passing through the extracorporeal circuit. Hemolysis may lead to anemia, hyperbilirubinemia, and acute kidney injury. The risks of bleeding versus the risks of circuit thrombosis must be weighed on an individual basis in ECMO, depending on patient comorbidities and oxygenator microthrombi, as well as the type of ECMO and its duration.

References:

1. Birch M, Lupei MI, Wall M, et al. Chapter 41: Long-Term Complications and Management. In: Kaplan JA, Augoustides JGT, Manecke GR, et al., eds. Kaplan's Cardiac Anesthesia. 7th ed. Elsevier; 2017:1407-1424.
2. Mazzeffi M, Rao VK, Doddo J, et al. Intraoperative management of adult patients on extracorporeal membrane oxygenation: an expert consensus statement from the Society of Cardiovascular Anesthesiologists Part I: technical aspects of extracorporeal membrane oxygenation. J Cardiothorac Vasc Anesth, 2021; 35: 3496-3512.

18. A patient on venoarterial extracorporeal membrane oxygenation (ECMO) with femoral arterial and femoral venous cannulation suddenly sustains decreased ECMO flow to 1 L/min and becomes hypotensive without any forewarning. All of the following are true concerning acute decreases in ECMO flow, EXCEPT:

   A. Kinking of a vascular cannula can lead to acute decreases in ECMO flow
   B. Excessive flow rates can lead to venous collapse or "suck down" and resultant low flows
   C. Venous collapse or "suck down" is unlikely without chattering or chugging of the cannulas
   D. Hypovolemia secondary to bleeding or over-diuresis can lead to venous collapse or "suck down"

Correct Answer: C

Explanation: A common complication of peripheral venoarterial extracorporeal membrane oxygenation (ECMO) is venous collapse or "suck down." The most common reasons this occurs is due to high flow rates, especially in venoarterial ECMO. The venous cannula becomes occluded because the vein collapses around it, preventing venous drainage. This is clinically manifested as an acute drop in ECMO flows. Venous collapse is usually precipitated by the warning sign of tubing chattering or chugging, but this is not always the case. The collapse can usually be treated by transiently decreasing the revolutions per minute, administering a fluid bolus, or both. Echocardiography is useful to confirm cannula placement and volume status. Checking the cannulae for kinks that limit flow is an easily correctable issue.

References:

1. Birch M, Lupei MI, Wall M, et al. Chapter 41: Long-Term Complications and Management. In: Kaplan JA, Augoustides JGT, Manecke GR, et al., eds. Kaplan's Cardiac Anesthesia. 7th ed. Elsevier; 2017:1407-1424.
2. Mazzeffi M, Rao VK, Doddo J, et al. Intraoperative management of adult patients on extracorporeal membrane oxygenation: an expert consensus statement from the Society of Cardiovascular Anesthesiologists Part II: intraoperative management and troubleshooting. J Cardiothorac Vasc Anesth, 2021; 35: 3413-3527.

19. A patient is placed on femoral-femoral venoarterial extracorporeal membrane oxygenation (VA ECMO) following failure to separate from cardiopulmonary bypass. The following are common complications following femoral VA ECMO that providers should be vigilant for, EXCEPT:
  A. Brachial plexus neuropathy
  B. Acute kidney injury
  C. Lower extremity ischemia
  D. Infection

Correct Answer: A

Explanation: Venoarterial extracorporeal membrane oxygenation (VA ECMO) has associated comorbidities in patients who survive. The most common comorbidities are acute kidney injury (55%), renal replacement therapy (46%), major bleeding (40%), infection (30%), lower extremity ischemia (16%), compartment syndrome or fasciotomy (10%), stroke (5.9%), and lower extremity amputation (4.7%). Upper extremity neuropathy would likely be unrelated to femoral VA ECMO.

References:

1. Birch M, Lupei MI, Wall M, et al. Chapter 41: Long-Term Complications and Management. In: Kaplan JA, Augoustides JGT, Manecke GR, et al., eds. Kaplan's Cardiac Anesthesia. 7th ed. Elsevier; 2017:1407-1424.
2. Mazzeffi M, Rao VK, Doddo J, et al. Intraoperative management of adult patients on extracorporeal membrane oxygenation: an expert consensus statement from the Society of Cardiovascular Anesthesiologists Part I: technical aspects of extracorporeal membrane oxygenation. J Cardiothorac Vasc Anesth, 2021; 35: 3496-3512.

20. An 84-year-old patient who underwent high-risk cardiac surgery has failed to wean from the ventilator, inotropic support, and pressors 18 days following surgery. The course is further complicated by pneumonia and the need for renal replacement therapy. The family wishes to discuss goals of care. What is TRUE concerning end-of-life care for patients in the intensive care unit (ICU)?
  A. Some 20% of Americans who die each year do so during or shortly after a stay in the ICU
  B. Patients with advanced directives or living wills do not need family discussions, as there is little ambiguity in these documents
  C. Legally executed living wills define "reasonable chance of recovery" as ability to live at home
  D. It would be considered euthanasia to stop life-sustaining inotropic and pressor support in any circumstance

Correct Answer: A

Explanation: Unlike many countries, 20% of Americans who die each year do so during or shortly after a stay in the intensive care unit. Unfortunately, even with advance directives or living wills, created by the patient and executed by attorneys, the act of shifting medical care to end-of-life care is often fraught with ambiguity that requires extensive conversations among family members. Statements such as "heroic measures" and "reasonable hope of recovery" often have different meanings to patients, intensivists, surgeons, and family members. Euthanasia is defined as the painless killing of a patient and would not apply to stopping unwanted medical therapies.

TABLE 37.6

Complications of extracorporeal membrane oxygenation for cardiac failure

	Rate	95% Confidence Interval
Lower extremity ischemia	16.5	12.5–22.6
Compartment syndrome or fasciotomy	10.3	7.3–14.5
Lower extremity amputation	4.7	2.3–9.3
Stroke	5.9	4.2–8.3
Other neurologic injury	13.3	9.9–17.7
Acute kidney injury	55.6	35.5–74
Renal replacement therapy	46	36.7–55.5
Major bleeding	40.6	26.8–56.6
Reoperation for bleeding or tamponade	41.6	24.3–61.8
Infection	30.4	15.5–44

Modified from Cheng R, Hachamovitch R, Kittleson M, et al. Complications of extracorporeal membrane oxygenation for treatment of cardiogenic shock and cardiac arrest: a meta-analysis of 1,866 adult patients. Ann Thorac Surg, 2014; 97: 610-616.

References:

1. Birch M, Lupei MI, Wall M, et al. Chapter 41: Long-Term Complications and Management. In: Kaplan JA, Augoustides JGT, Manecke GR, et al., eds. Kaplan's Cardiac Anesthesia. 7th ed. Elsevier; 2017:1407-1424.
2. Klinedinst R, Kornfield ZN, Hadler R. Palliative care for patients with advanced heart disease. J Cardiothorac Vasc Anesth, 2018; 33: 833-843.

21. When prognosticating survival after cardiac surgery, what is accurate?

A. Patients with few comorbidities may have a 3.2% risk of 30-day mortality after elective coronary artery bypass grafting (CABG)

B. Venoarterial extracorporeal membrane oxygenation for weaning from cardiopulmonary bypass does not increase the risk of perioperative mortality

C. Decreased left ventricular ejection fraction does not increase risk of mortality following CABG surgery, since revascularization is the treatment for decreased ejection fraction

D. Age, in and of itself, without consideration for other comorbid conditions, has not been shown to impart mortality risk after cardiac surgery

Correct Answer: A

Explanation: Overall, a patient's risk of death following coronary artery bypass grafting (CABG) surgery is in the 2% to 3% range. The risk of death even for patients with few comorbid conditions never approaches zero due to the inherent risk of cardiac surgery. The risk of 30-day mortality for CABG surgery increases with decreased left ventricular ejection fraction such that a patient with an ejection fraction less than 20% has a mortality risk in the 8% to 10% range at 30 days. Age remains an important risk factor for mortality after cardiac surgery both in the short and long term. The use of venoarterial extracorporeal membrane oxygenation to wean from cardiopulmonary bypass due to cardiogenic shock increases the risk of death in adult patients undergoing cardiac surgery.

References:

1. Birch M, Lupei MI, Wall M, et al. Chapter 41: Long-Term Complications and Management. In: Kaplan JA, Augoustides JGT, Manecke GR, et al., eds. Kaplan's Cardiac Anesthesia. 7th ed. Elsevier; 2017:1407-1424.
2. McDonald, B, Walraven C, McIsaac D. Predicting 1-year mortality after cardiac surgery complicated by prolonged critical illness: derivation and validation of a population-based risk model. J Cardiothorac Vasc Anesth, 2020; 34: 2628-2637.
3. https://www.sts.org/resources/risk-calculator. Accessed June 28, 2022.

22. There are several scoring systems aimed at predicting outcomes following cardiac surgery. In the Cardiac Anesthesia Risk Evaluation (CARE) system and cardiac surgical risk scoring systems, which of the following is NOT cited as a risk for poor outcomes?

A. Emergent surgery

B. Previous uneventful cardiac surgery

C. Prostate cancer 2 years ago

D. Clinical rating of the surgeon

Correct Answer: D

Explanation: There are numerous scoring systems validated in predicting morbidity and mortality following cardiac surgery. The most often utilized is the Society of Thoracic Surgeons score (STS score) and the European System for Cardiac Operative Risk Evaluation (EuroSCORE). The Cardiac Anesthesia Risk Evaluation (CARE) system was developed as an anesthesia risk evaluation score.

BOX 37.1   Cardiac Anesthesia Risk Evaluation score

1. Patient with stable cardiac disease and no other medical problem: a noncomplex surgery is undertaken.
2. Patient with stable cardiac disease and one or more controlled medical problems[a]: a noncomplex surgery is undertaken.
3. Patient with any uncontrolled medical problem[b] or patient in whom a complex surgery is undertaken.[c]
4. Patient with any uncontrolled medical problem *and* in whom a complex surgery is undertaken.
5. Patient with chronic or advanced cardiac disease for whom cardiac surgery is undertaken as a last hope to save or improve life.
6. Emergency surgery is performed as soon as the diagnosis is made, and the surgical unit is available.

[a]Examples: Controlled hypertension, diabetes mellitus, peripheral vascular disease, chronic obstructive pulmonary disease, controlled systemic diseases, and others as judged by clinicians.

[b]Examples: Unstable angina treated with intravenous heparin or nitroglycerin, preoperative intra-aortic balloon pump, heart failure with pulmonary or peripheral edema, uncontrolled hypertension, renal insufficiency (creatinine level >140 μmol/L), debilitating systemic diseases, and others as judged by clinicians.

[c]Examples: Reoperation, combined valve and coronary artery surgery, multiple valve surgery, left ventricular aneurysmectomy, repair of ventricular septal defect after myocardial infarction, coronary artery bypass of diffuse or heavily calcified vessels, and other as judged by clinicians.

Modified from Dupuis JY, Wang F, Nathan H, et al. The cardiac anesthesia risk evaluation score: a clinically useful predictor of mortality and morbidity after cardiac surgery. Anesthesiology, 2001; 94: 194-204.

TABLE 37.7

Probabilities of mortality, morbidity, and prolonged postoperative length of stay in hospital, as predicted by the CARE score

CARE Score	Mortality (%)	Morbidity (%)	Prolonged LOS (days)
1	0.5 (0.3–0.9)	5.4 (4.3–6.8)	2.9 (2.2–3.9)
2	1.1 (0.7–1.7)	10.3 (8.9–12.1)	5.1 (4.2–6.3)
3	2.2 (1.6–3.1)	19.0 (17.2–20.9)	8.8 (7.6–10.2)
3E	4.5 (3.5–5.7)	32.1 (29.3–35.0)	14.7 (12.8–16.8)
4	8.8 (6.9–11.3)	48.8 (44.1–53.6)	23.5 (20.1–27.3)
4E	16.7 (12.4–22.1)	65.8 (59.5–71.6)	35.4 (29.3–42.0)
5	29.3 (20.8–39.6)	79.6 (73.2–84.7)	49.4 (40.4–58.5)
5E	46.2 (32.4–60.5)	88.7 (83.5–92.5)	63.6 (52.5–73.4)

Values obtained from the logistic regression analysis performed in the reference population (n = 2000). Numbers in parentheses are 95% confidence intervals.
CARE, Cardiac Anesthesia Risk Evaluation; *LOS,* length of stay.
Modified from Dupuis JY, Wang F, Nathan H, et al. The cardiac anesthesia risk evaluation score: a clinically useful predictor of mortality and morbidity after cardiac surgery. Anesthesiology, 2001; 94: 194-204.

The STS and EuroSCORE scores are more detailed than most other scoring systems and have been extensively validated. All scoring systems in this setting take into account type of surgery, complexity of surgery, and past medical history, including comorbidities. In general, emergent surgery garners the highest risk for poor outcomes following cardiac surgery. No currently validated scoring system takes into account the clinical rating of the surgeon.

References:
1. Birch M, Lupei MI, Wall M, et al. Chapter 41: Long-Term Complications and Management. In: Kaplan JA, Augoustides JGT, Manecke GR, et al., eds. Kaplan's Cardiac Anesthesia. 7th ed. Elsevier; 2017:1407-1424.
2. McDonald, B, Walraven C, McIsaac D. Predicting 1-year mortality after cardiac surgery complicated by prolonged critical illness: derivation and validation of a population-based risk model. J Cardiothorac Vasc Anesth, 2020; 34: 2628-2637.
3. https://www.sts.org/resources/risk-calculator. Accessed June 28, 2022.
4. https://www.euroscore.org/. Accessed June 29, 2022.

23. A patient with chronic systolic heart failure is admitted to the intensive care unit after cardiac surgery. The left ventricular ejection fraction is 45% with moderate diastolic dysfunction. The patient has an advanced directive stating they do not wish for heroic efforts for their care. The intensivist places a palliative care consult. What is TRUE regarding this consult?
A. The consult is not warranted; palliative care specialists do not consider chronic problems
B. This consult is warranted; palliative care specialists aim to relieve suffering and enhance disease-specific therapies as part of the practice of palliative care
C. The consult in not warranted; there are no plans to stop any therapies

D. The consult is warranted; the chance of survival in this patient is extremely low and advanced directives must be followed

Correct Answer: B
Explanation: Palliative care consults are becoming more common in cardiac surgical and cardiac medical patients. Palliative care providers do not only assist in end-of-life discussions and plans but can also assist in the entire care plan of the patient. Indeed, palliative care consultation can include curative treatment, pain relief, and improvements in quality of life when the patient is expected to survive. Most cardiac surgical patients have a comorbid condition and, depending on institutional availability of palliative care teams, may benefit from palliative care consultation.

References:
1. Birch M, Lupei MI, Wall M, et al. Chapter 41: Long-Term Complications and Management. In: Kaplan JA, Augoustides JGT, Manecke GR, et al., eds. Kaplan's Cardiac Anesthesia. 7th ed. Elsevier; 2017:1407-1424.
2. Klinedinst R, Kornfield Z, Hadler R. Palliative care for patients with advanced heart disease. J Cardiothorac Vasc Anesth, 2018; 33: 833-843.

24. A department of cardiothoracic surgery is interested in increasing the availability of palliative care consultation. Palliative care consults may result in all of the following, EXCEPT:
A. Increased patient life span
B. Increased use of extracorporeal membrane oxygenation
C. Increased patient satisfaction
D. Decreased costs

Correct Answer: B

Explanation: Palliative care consults have been shown to be beneficial in several distinct areas of patient care. Patients' life spans have been found to be increased when palliative care providers are involved in the care. Patient satisfaction is also increased, and costs are decreased when palliative care consults are obtained. There are few apparent drawbacks to obtaining palliative care consultation. If disease processes change, the goals of palliative care can change accordingly. There is no evidence that palliative care consultation changes extracorporeal membrane oxygenation utilization.

References:

1. Birch M, Lupei MI, Wall M, et al. Chapter 41: Long-Term Complications and Management. In: Kaplan JA, Augoustides JGT, Manecke GR, et al., eds. Kaplan's Cardiac Anesthesia. 7th ed. Elsevier; 2017:1407-1424.
2. Klinedinst R, Kornfield Z, Hadler R. Palliative care for patients with advanced heart disease. J Cardiothorac Vasc Anesth, 2018; 33: 833-843.

25. Many cardiac surgical patients have prolonged clinical courses in the intensive care unit. Family members often participate significantly in the care plan for these patients. Recommendations concerning family members include all of the following EXCEPT:
   A. Scheduled times for family meetings with providers
   B. "Family rounds" whereby families are invited to intensive care unit rounds
   C. No requirement for a medical decision maker, as all family member opinions are considered
   D. Encouragement of questions from family members concerning patient care

Correct Answer: C

Explanation: Care of the family is an important consideration when caring for critically ill patients. Family members have a chance to interact with and ask questions of providers concerning the care of their loved one. Scheduled times for family and provider meetings are helpful to facilitate this communication. Additionally, family members can be invited to attend critical care rounds in so-called "family rounds." An important step when involving family members in the decision-making for a patient is to identify who will be the medical decision maker, to avoid confusion and conflict.

References:

1. Birch M, Lupei MI, Wall M, et al. Chapter 41: Long-Term Complications and Management. In: Kaplan JA, Augoustides JGT, Manecke GR, et al., eds. Kaplan's Cardiac Anesthesia. 7th ed. Elsevier; 2017:1407-1424.
2. Klinedinst R, Kornfield Z, Hadler R. Palliative care for patients with advanced heart disease. J Cardiothorac Vasc Anesth, 2018; 33: 833-843.

26. An intensive care unit wishes to increase adherence to best practices and quality measures concerning patient family engagement. Palliative care bundles can be useful in this endeavor. Recommendations included in these bundles include all of the following EXCEPT:
   A. Determining advanced directive existence and content
   B. Conducting family meetings in dedicated spaces
   C. Determining resuscitation status
   D. Avoiding pain medicines and other sedatives in patients who cannot follow commands

Correct Answer: D

Explanation: Palliative care bundles are becoming an increasing adjunct to critical care in cardiac surgical patients. Adhering to best practices concerning family members of critically ill patients is a large component of this quality measure. Determination of the existence and content of advanced directives and resuscitation status needs to be carried out early in the clinical course. Additionally, it is recommended that a family member be identified as the medical decision maker and that family meetings are held in dedicated spaces. Striving for adequate pain management is a necessary component of patient care, regardless of mental status. Involving social work and spiritual support services has also been recommended.

BOX 37.2   Bundle of minimal palliative care quality measures in the intensive care unit

ICU Day 1 Goals
- Identify the medical decision maker.
- Determine whether there is an advance directive.
- Determine resuscitation (DNR/DNI) status.
- Give institutional ICU information, if applicable.
- Perform regular pain assessments, strive for optimal pain management.

ICU Day 3 Goals
- Involve social work support if not already done.
- Involve spiritual support if not already done.

ICU Day 5 Goals
- Conduct an interdisciplinary family meeting in a dedicated space.

DNI, Do not intubate; *DNR,* do not resuscitate; *ICU,* intensive care unit.
Adapted from Nelson JE, Mulkerin CM, Adams LL, Pronovost PJ. Improving comfort and communication in the ICU: a practical new tool for palliative care performance measurement and feedback. Qual Saf Health Care. 2006;15(4): 264–271.

References:

1. Birch M, Lupei MI, Wall M, et al. Chapter 41: Long-Term Complications and Management. In: Kaplan JA, Augoustides JGT, Manecke GR, et al., eds. Kaplan's Cardiac Anesthesia. 7th ed. Elsevier; 2017:1407-1424.
2. Klinedinst R, Kornfield Z, Hadler R. Palliative care for patients with advanced heart disease. J Cardiothorac Vasc Anesth, 2018; 33: 833-843.

27. A patient with a cardiac-implanted electronic device presents to the emergency department with 2 days of fever of unknown origin, leukocytosis, and systemic hypotension. A cardiology consult is placed, and there is concern for device infection with sepsis. All of the following should be completed with 24 hours of this suspected diagnosis, EXCEPT:
A. Echocardiography
B. Cardiac surgical consult
C. Two sets of blood cultures
D. Empiric antibiotic initiation

Correct Answer: B

Explanation: Patients with cardiac-implanted electronic devices (CIEDs) and signs of infection should be evaluated for device infection. This can be accomplished with history and physical examination or with more invasive modalities. Suspicion of CIED infection with sepsis should be evaluated and treated expeditiously. Within an hour of presentation, patients should have two separate sets of blood cultures drawn followed by broad spectrum antibiotic initiation. Antibiotics can be tapered pending culture results and patient response. Within 24 hours, echocardiographic assessment of the device leads and heart should be obtained. Although transthoracic echocardiography is an adequate noninvasive initial assessment, transesophageal echocardiography may be required to accurately diagnose device infection. Cardiac surgical consultation can be obtained after 24 hours, depending on the clinical assessment and test results.

References:

1. Birch M, Lupei MI, Wall M, et al. Chapter 41: Long-Term Complications and Management. In: Kaplan JA, Augoustides JGT, Manecke GR, et al., eds. Kaplan's Cardiac Anesthesia. 7th ed. Elsevier; 2017:1407-1424.
2. Cronin B, Essandoh M. Update on cardiovascular implantable electronic devices for anesthesiologists. J Cardiothorac Vasc Anesth, 2017; 32: 1871-1884.

28. Three days after a mitral valve replacement, a patient has blood cultures taken due to a high fever. Coagulase-negative *Staphylococcus* is isolated in three of four bottles. He has continued to require central venous access for vasopressor medication administration, and there is concern for infection. Which of the following is FALSE concerning central line–associated bloodstream infection (CLABSI)?
A. The incidence of CLABSI has reduced in the past 20 years
B. Diagnosis of CLABSI can be made with a positive blood culture that is not related to an infection at another site
C. CLABSI is associated with prolonged hospitalization, but not mortality
D. Diagnosis of CLABSI can be made with two positive blood cultures with a common skin contaminant associated with signs and symptoms of infection

Correct Answer: C

Explanation: Central line–associated bloodstream infection (CLABSI) is a serious complication of central venous access. Patients who sustain CLABSI have not only increased length of hospitalization, but also increased risk of mortality. The Centers for Disease Control and Prevention defines CLABSI as either a positive blood culture not related to an infection at another site or two positive blood cultures with a common skin contaminant associated with signs and symptoms of infection. Due to prevention strategies, the incidence of CLABSI has decreased in the past 2 decades by 58% in the United States with a rate of 2 per 1000 central-line days. The international rate of CLABSI is nearly fourfold that of the United States, at 7.6 per 1000 central-line days.

References:

1. Birch M, Lupei MI, Wall M, et al. Chapter 41: Long-Term Complications and Management. In: Kaplan JA, Augoustides JGT, Manecke GR, et al., eds. Kaplan's Cardiac Anesthesia. 7th ed. Elsevier; 2017:1407-1424.
2. Merry A, Weller J, Mitchell S. Improving the quality and safety of patient care in cardiac anesthesia. J Cardiothorac Vasc Anesth, 2014; 28: 1341-1351.

29. A 46-year-old male patient has been hospitalized for 2 weeks following colon resection for cancer and is found to have a non–ST-elevated myocardial infarction. The patient has a white blood cell count of $3.4 \times 10^9/L$ and has been on parenteral nutrition for 1 week. Coronary catheterization demonstrates triple vessel disease, and he is scheduled for coronary artery bypass grafting. A new central venous catheter is placed for the surgery. All of the following increase this patient's risk for central line–associated bloodstream infections, EXCEPT:
A. Male gender
B. Use of parenteral nutrition
C. Prolonged hospitalization prior to central catheter insertion
D. Neutropenia

Correct Answer: A

Explanation: Recognized risk factors for central line–associated bloodstream infections (CLABSIs) include prolonged hospitalizations before catheter insertion, femoral catheterization, prolonged catheterization, neutropenia, concomitant total parenteral nutrition, extensive catheter manipulation, and a reduced nurse-to-patient ratio. Male gender is not a described risk factor for this complication. Implementation of various preventative measures have been successful in reducing the incidence of CLABSI such that the current goal is to achieve a minimal CLABSI incidence in the United States.

References:

1. Birch M, Lupei MI, Wall M, et al. Chapter 41: Long-Term Complications and Management. In: Kaplan JA, Augoustides JGT, Manecke GR, et al., eds. Kaplan's Cardiac Anesthesia. 7th ed. Elsevier; 2017:1407-1424.

2. Merry A, Weller J, Mitchell S. Improving the quality and safety of patient care in cardiac anesthesia. J Cardiothorac Vasc Anesth, 2014; 28: 1341-1351.

30. Several organisms are known to cause central line–associated bloodstream infections (CLABSIs). Which statement is TRUE regarding infectious organisms in CLABSI?
   A. Gram-negative bacterial species rarely (<1%) cause CLABSI.
   B. Coagulase-negative *Staphylococci* is typically a contaminant and rarely (<1%) causes CLABSI.
   C. Fungal species rarely (<1%) cause CLABSI.
   D. *Enterococcus* species are more common than *Staphylococcus aureus* in CLABSI

Correct Answer: D

Explanation: The National Healthcare Safety Network states that 60% of central line–associated bloodstream infection (CLABSI) cases are caused by gram-positive organisms. Coagulase-negative *Staphylococci* is the causative agent in 34%, *Enterococcus* in 16%, and *Staphylococcus aureus* in 10% of cases. As for other species known to cause CLABSI, gram-negative bacteria are responsible for 18% and *Candida* species for 12% of cases.

References:
1. Birch M, Lupei MI, Wall M, et al. Chapter 41: Long-Term Complications and Management. In: Kaplan JA, Augoustides JGT, Manecke GR, et al., eds. Kaplan's Cardiac Anesthesia. 7th ed. Elsevier; 2017:1407-1424.
2. Merry A, Weller J, Mitchell S. Improving the quality and safety of patient care in cardiac anesthesia. J Cardiothorac Vasc Anesth, 2014; 28: 1341-1351.

CHAPTER 38

Postoperative Pain Management for the Cardiac Patient

Cheen Alkhatib

KEY POINTS

1. Inadequate postoperative analgesia or perioperative surgical stress has significant pathophysiological consequences in multiple organ systems. This includes cardiovascular, pulmonary, gastrointestinal, hematological, immunologic, and endocrine.
2. Adequate postoperative analgesia prevents patient discomfort, decreases morbidity, and decreases hospital stay and costs.
3. Analgesia should consist of a multimodal method, and the choice of medication, dose, route, and duration should be individualized.
4. Neuraxial (thoracic epidural, spinal anesthesia) and regional (paravertebral, intercostal nerve blocks, etc.) anesthesia may also be used to manage intraoperative and postoperative pain.
5. Cyclooxygenase-2 inhibitors possess analgesic benefits and lack effects on platelet function and bleeding compared to nonselective nonsteroidal anti-inflammatory drugs.

---

1. There are several pain management techniques aimed at decreasing sternal pain following cardiac surgery with sternotomy. Which nerve bundles innervate the sternum and should be targeted for this purpose?
   A. Sympathetic trunk
   B. Anterior and posterior branches of the intercostal nerves
   C. Long thoracic nerve
   D. Phrenic nerve

Correct Answer: B

Explanation: The anterior and posterior branches of the intercostal nerves innervate the sternum. Multiple investigations regarding pain management in cardiac surgeries have been conducted. Post–coronary artery bypass grafting pain has been well described and is believed to be secondary to direct mechanical trauma to the chest wall. The intercostal nerves are formed by the anterior rami of thoracic nerves 1 to 11. The first thoracic nerve provides contribution to the brachial plexus, whereas anterior branches of upper thoracic nerves 2 to 6 strictly innervate the chest wall, and posterior cutaneous branches innervate skin over the scapula and latissimus dorsi.

Sympathetic trunk are nerve fibers that run from the base of the skull to the coccyx. They are the major component of the sympathetic nervous system.

The long thoracic nerve originates from the C5 to C7 nerve roots and descends in the axilla, posterior to the brachial plexus, to innervate the serratus anterior muscle, which anchors the scapula to the chest wall. Injury to the phrenic nerve causes diaphragmatic dysfunction.

References:

1. Chaney MA. Chapter 42: Postoperative Pain Management for the Cardiac Patient. In: Kaplan JA, Augoustides JGT, Manecke GR, et al., eds. Kaplan's Cardiac Anesthesia. 7th ed. Elsevier; 2017:1425-1457.
2. Mamoun N, Wright MC, Bottiger B, et al. Pain trajectories after valve surgeries performed via midline sternotomy versus minithoracotomy. J Cardiothorac Vasc Anesth, 2022; 36: 3596-3602.

2. A 42-year-old, otherwise healthy female is scheduled for robotically assisted mitral valve repair with a thoracotomy incision. Intercostal nerve blockade is planned as an adjunct in the multimodal pain management strategy. Intercostal nerve blocks are effective by blocking what fibers to the spinal cord?
   A. Unmyelinated A-alpha fibers
   B. A-beta fibers
   C. Myelinated A-delta fibers
   D. Unmyelinated C fibers

Correct Answer: D

Explanation: Blockade of intercostal nerves interrupts C fiber afferent transmission of impulses to the spinal cord. The intercostal nerve block can be used for thoracic surgery and performed intraoperatively or postoperatively. It can provide sufficient analgesia lasting approximately 6 to 12 hours, depending on the amount and type of local anesthetic used.

Group A nerve fibers are subdivided into unmyelinated A-alpha fibers, A-beta fibers, and myelinated A-delta fibers. These subdivisions differ in amount of myelination and axon thickness. Group A fibers transmit signals at different speeds, with larger diameter axons and more myelin insulated axons having faster signal propagation. Group A nerves are found in both motor and sensory pathways.

References:

1. Chaney MA. Chapter 42: Postoperative Pain Management for the Cardiac Patient. In: Kaplan JA, Augoustides JGT, Manecke GR, et al., eds. Kaplan's Cardiac Anesthesia. 7th ed. Elsevier; 2017:1425-1457.
2. Reuben SS, Yalavarthy L. Preventing the development of chronic pain after thoracic surgery. J Cardiothorac Vasc Anesth, 2008; 22: 890-903.
3. Pai P, Hong J, Phillips A, et al. Serratus anterior plane block versus intercostal block with incision infiltration in robotic-assisted thoracoscopic surgery: a randomized controlled pilot trial. J Cardiothorac Vasc Anesth, 2022; 36: 2287-2294.
4. Zhang J, Luo F, Zhang X, et al. Ultrasound-guided continuous parasternal intercostal block relieves postoperative pain after open cardiac surgery: a case series. J Cardiothorac Vasc Anesth, 2022; 36: 2051-2054.

3. In preparation for off-pump coronary bypass graft surgery, a patient received bilateral paravertebral blocks. What is TRUE regarding paravertebral blocks?
   A. Paravertebral blocks should not be performed if cardiopulmonary bypass is planned
   B. The incidence of paralysis due to hematoma following paravertebral block is the same as that of epidural hematoma due to anatomical proximity
   C. Paravertebral blocks can be maintained with continuous local anesthetic infusion via catheter insertion
   D. Paravertebral blocks are injected in a medial manner exterior to the supraspinous process of the vertebra

Correct Answer: C

Explanation: Paravertebral blocks can be used as analgesia for abdominal, thoracic, and cardiac surgery. Longitudinal spread of local anesthetic is unpredictable with a single injection; thus, multiple injections or catheter placement for continuous infusion of local anesthetic is recommended. There are numerous reports of successful paravertebral blockade prior to and following cardiac surgery with cardiopulmonary bypass and associated large intravenous heparin doses. These analyses do not report bleeding complications due to the block. Additionally, if a paravertebral hematoma is formed, it would be less likely to compress the spinal cord because the paravertebral space, unlike the epidural space, is not surrounded by rigid bone.

Some reports describe the use of continuous-infusion catheters during cardiac surgery without complications. In contrast to intrapleural administration of local anesthetics, extrapleural administration of local anesthetic, such as paravertebral blockade, depends primarily on diffusion of the local anesthetic into the paravertebral region. Local anesthetics then affect not only the ventral nerve root, but also afferent fibers of the posterior primary ramus.

Finally, placement of a paravertebral block is often done under ultrasound guidance with a paramedian needle position. The local anesthetic is ideally placed external to the parietal pleura under the transverse process.

References:

1. Chaney MA. Chapter 42: Postoperative Pain Management for the Cardiac Patient. In: Kaplan JA, Augoustides JGT, Manecke GR, et al., eds. Kaplan's Cardiac Anesthesia. 7th ed. Elsevier; 2017:1425-1457.
2. Mazzeffi M, Khelemsky Y. Poststernotomy pain: a clinical review. J Cardiothorac Vasc Anesth, 2011; 25: 1163-1178.
3. Minami K, Yoshitani K, Inatomi Y, et al. A retrospective examination of the efficacy of paravertebral block for patients requiring intraoperative high-dose unfractionated heparin administration during thoracoabdominal aortic aneurysm repair. J Cardiothorac Vasc Anesth, 2015; 29: 937-941.

4. The mechanism of action regarding pain relief for nonsteroidal anti-inflammatory drugs is most consistent with:
   A. Activation of mu (μ), kappa (κ), and delta (δ) receptors
   B. Inhibition of cyclo-oxygenase (COX) enzyme in peripheral tissues
   C. Alpha-2 (α_2) adrenergic antagonism
   D. Inhibition of COX enzyme in central tissue

Correct Answer: B

Explanation: Nonsteroidal anti-inflammatory drugs (NSAIDs) exert their analgesic, antipyretic, and anti-inflammatory effects peripherally by interfering with prostaglandin synthesis after tissue injury. NSAIDs inhibit cyclo-oxygenase (COX), the enzyme responsible for the conversion of arachidonic acid to prostaglandin. NSAIDS have comparable efficacy in both spontaneous and moment-evoked pain.

Opioids mimic the actions of endogenous opioid peptides by interacting with mu (μ), kappa (κ), and delta (δ) opioid receptors. Dexmedetomidine activates alpha-2 (α_2) adrenoceptor, which inhibits the release of norepinephrine, terminating the propagation of pain signals. Acetaminophen acts within the central nervous system to increase the pain threshold by inhibiting central COX. Acetaminophen does not inhibit prostaglandin synthesis in peripheral tissues, which is the reason for its lack of peripheral anti-inflammatory effects.

References:

1. Chaney MA. Chapter 42: Postoperative Pain Management for the Cardiac Patient. In: Kaplan JA, Augoustides JGT, Manecke GR, et al., eds. Kaplan's Cardiac Anesthesia. 7th ed. Elsevier; 2017:1425-1457.

2. Ochroch J, Usman A, Kiefer J, et al. Reducing opioid use in patients undergoing cardiac surgery - preoperative, intraoperative, and critical care strategies. J Cardiothorac Vasc Anesth, 2021; 35: 2155-2165.

5. A 79-year-old female is admitted to the intensive care unit following aortic valve replacement. She arrives intubated and on a continuous infusion of dexmedetomidine. Which of the following is TRUE regarding dexmedetomidine?

A. Dexmedetomidine is not known to cause vasoconstriction

B. Dexmedetomidine is an alpha1 (α1)-adrenergic agonist

C. Dexmedetomidine acts on the substantia gelatinosa for analgesia

D. Dexmedetomidine has been shown to decrease opioid requirements following surgery

Correct Answer: D

Explanation: Systemic administration of α_2-adrenergic agonists, such as dexmedetomidine, has produced antinociception and sedative affects. α_2-Adrenergic agonists provide analgesia, sedation, and sympatholysis.

Dexmedetomidine exerts the sedative effect via stimulation of α_2-adrenergic agonists in the locus ceruleus and spinal cord. The locus ceruleus is a nucleus in the pons of the brainstem involved with physiological responses to stress and panic. It is a part of the reticular activating system. Opioids exert analgesic effects by acting on the substantia gelatinosa.

Typical physiologic effects of dexmedetomidine include decreased heart rate, decreased systemic vascular resistance, and possibly indirectly decreased myocardial contractility leading to decreased cardiac output and decreased blood pressure. However, at high doses dexmedetomidine causes vasoconstriction.

Existing evidence indicates that α_2-agonists enhance the analgesic effects of the opioids via an unknown mechanism of action. Several mechanisms of action have been postulated for the analgesia noted with α_2-adrenergic agonists, including supraspinal, ganglionic, spinal, and peripheral mechanisms.

References:

1. Chaney MA. Chapter 42: Postoperative Pain Management for the Cardiac Patient. In: Kaplan JA, Augoustides JGT, Manecke GR, et al., eds. Kaplan's Cardiac Anesthesia. 7th ed. Elsevier; 2017:1425-1457.

BOX 38.1 Pain and cardiac surgery

- Originates from many sources.
- Most commonly originates from the chest wall.
- Preoperative expectations influence postoperative satisfaction.
- Quality of postoperative analgesia may influence morbidity.

2. Curtis JA, Hollinger M, Jain HB. Propofol-based versus dexmedetomidine-based sedation in cardiac surgery patients. J Cardiothorac Vasc Anesth, 2013; 27: 1289-1294.

3. Chitnis S, Mullane D, Brohan J, et al. Dexmedetomidine use in intensive care unit sedation and postoperative recovery in elderly patients post-cardiac surgery (DIRECT). J Cardiothorac Vasc Anesth, 2022; 36: 880-892.

6. A 67-year-old patient on chronic methadone therapy for a history of polysubstance abuse is scheduled for elective coronary bypass graft surgery. The anesthesia team places a thoracic epidural (T3–T4 insertion) 4 hours prior to anesthetic induction for intra- and postoperative pain control. What is TRUE regarding thoracic epidural anesthesia and cardiovascular effects?

A. Thoracic epidural anesthesia (TEA) blocks cardiac sympathetic nerve activity

B. TEA increases myocardial oxygen demand

C. TEA will not cause vasodilation of stenotic coronary artery segments

D. TEA has no effect on systemic mean arterial blood pressure

Correct Answer: A

Explanation: Thoracic epidural anesthesia with local anesthetic infusion will block cardiac sympathetic nerve afferent and efferent fibers. A frequent unwanted side effect of epidural block is hypotension due to the epidurally injected local anesthetic blocking the sympathetic nerves, and thus the patient's response to hypotension, which is commonly due to hypovolemia or unopposed parasympathetic nervous system action via the vagus nerve.

Patients with sympathetic coronary artery disease can benefit from a cardiac sympathectomy due to the increase in the diameter of stenotic coronary artery segments without dilation of coronary arterioles. During myocardial ischemia, cardiac sympathectomy increases the endocardial-epicardial blood flow ratio, creating beneficial effects on collateral blood flow. This favors the determinants of myocardial oxygen demand and can improve left ventricular function.

References:

1. Chaney MA. Chapter 42: Postoperative Pain Management for the Cardiac Patient. In: Kaplan JA, Augoustides JGT, Manecke GR, et al., eds. Kaplan's Cardiac Anesthesia. 7th ed. Elsevier; 2017:1425-1457.

BOX 38.2 Epidural techniques

- Advantages
  - Reliable analgesia
  - Stress-response attenuation
  - Cardiac sympathectomy
- Disadvantages
  - Labor intensive
  - Hematoma formation risk increased
  - Side effects of epidural opioids

2. Sarica F, Erturk E, Kutanis D, et al. Comparison of thoracic epidural analgesia and traditional intravenous analgesia with respect to postoperative respiratory effects in cardiac surgery. J Cardiothorac Vasc Anesth, 2021; 35: 1800-1805.

3. Bulte CS, Boer C, Hartemink KJ, et al. Myocardial microvascular responsiveness during acute cardiac sympathectomy induced by thoracic epidural anesthesia. J Cardiothorac Vasc Anesth, 2017; 31: 134-141.

7. An immunocompromised, diabetic patient presents to the operating room for a robotically assisted mitral valve repair via thoracotomy incision. A thoracic epidural was placed 4 hours prior to administration of general anesthesia. At the completion of the procedure, the patient emerges from general anesthesia with complaints of back pain and decreased strength in their feet. How should the anesthesiologist proceed?

A. Administer narcotics for the back pain, likely due to positioning

B. Increase the systemic blood pressure

C. Order emergent magnetic resonance imaging

D. Order blood coagulation testing

Correct Answer: C

Explanation: Epidural hematoma is a rare occurrence that can lead to cord compression, cord ischemia, or myelopathy like that caused by a space-occupying tumor. Signs and symptoms of epidural hematoma may progress rapidly from mild sensory or motor deficits to devastating paraplegia and incontinence. Early signs include back pain and pressure, with motor and sensory deficits. The back pain associated with epidural hematoma may be severe and persistent. These symptoms should raise concerns and prompt emergent magnetic resonance imaging, along with consultation with a neurologist and neurosurgeon.

References:

1. Chaney MA. Chapter 42: Postoperative Pain Management for the Cardiac Patient. In: Kaplan JA, Augoustides JGT, Manecke GR, et al., eds. Kaplan's Cardiac Anesthesia. 7th ed. Elsevier; 2017:1425-1457.

2. Kupersztych-Hagege, E, Dubuisson E, Szekely B, et al. Epidural hematoma and abscess related to thoracic epidural analgesia: a single-center study of 2,907 patients who underwent lung surgery. J Cardiothorac Vasc Anesth, 2017; 31: 446-452.

8. After discussing analgesic techniques with a patient who is scheduled for minimally invasive mitral valve repair surgery, the patient desires a preoperative, single-shot spinal block. The anesthesiologist injects spinal dose bupivacaine and morphine into the intrathecal space at T3-T4. What is considered the MOST commonly reported side effect of intrathecal opioid administration?

A. Pruritus

B. Nausea and vomiting

C. Urinary retention

D. Respiratory depression

Correct Answer: A

BOX 38.3   Intrathecal techniques

- Advantages
  - Simple, reliable analgesia
  - Stress-response attenuation
  - Less hematoma risk than epidural techniques
- Disadvantages
  - No cardiac sympathectomy
  - Hematoma risk increased
  - Side effects of intrathecal opioids

Explanation: Opioids interact with specific receptors that are widely distributed within the central nervous system to produce a variety of pharmacologic effects. The most common side effect of neuraxial opioid administration is pruritus. The incidence varies widely (0%–100%) due to reporting because it is commonly only identified after directly questioning the patient. Severe pruritus is rare and only occurs in 1% of patients.

The incidence of nausea and vomiting is approximately 30%. The incidence of urinary retention also varies widely (from 0% to 80%) and occurs most frequently in young male patients. These various effects are due to the fact that the μ receptor has two subtypes: a high-affinity μ1 receptor and a low-affinity μ2 receptor. The supraspinal mechanisms of analgesia are thought to involve μ1 receptors, whereas spinal analgesia, respiratory depression, and gastrointestinal effects are associated with the μ2 receptor.

References:

1. Chaney MA. Chapter 42: Postoperative Pain Management for the Cardiac Patient. In: Kaplan JA, Augoustides JGT, Manecke GR, et al., eds. Kaplan's Cardiac Anesthesia. 7th ed. Elsevier; 2017:1425-1457.

2. Gurkan T, Goren S, Korfali G, et al. Combination of intrathecal morphine and remifentanil infusion for fast-track anesthesia in off-pump coronary artery bypass surgery. J Cardiothorac Vasc Anesth, 2005; 19: 708-713.

3. Latham P, Zarate E, White PF, et al. Fast-track cardiac anesthesia: a comparison of remifentanil plus intrathecal morphine with sufentanil in a desflurane-based anesthetic. J Cardiothorac Vasc Anesth, 2000; 14: 645-651.

4. Kiran U, Zuber K, Kakani M. Intrathecal morphine in patients undergoing minimally invasive direct coronary artery bypass surgery. J Cardiothorac Vasc Anesth, 2005; 19: 815-816.

9. After discussing analgesic techniques with a patient who is scheduled for minimally invasive atrial septal defect repair surgery, the patient desires a preoperative, single-shot spinal block. The anesthesiologist plans spinal dose bupivacaine and would like to add another nociceptive medication to the spinal. Which medication, if added to bupivacaine, will exhibit a delayed respiratory depression when administered intrathecally?

A. Fentanyl

B. Morphine

C. Sufentanil

D. Dexmedetomidine

Correct Answer: B

Explanation: The incidence of respiratory depression that requires intervention after conventional doses of intrathecal and epidural opioids is approximately 1%. Delayed respiratory depression occurs most commonly with morphine. This is due to cephalad migration of morphine in the cerebral spinal fluid, which stimulates opioid receptors in the ventral medulla due to the hydrophilicity of morphine.

Early respiratory depression occurs within minutes of fentanyl and sufentanil administration due to high lipophilicity. Factors that increase the risk for respiratory depression include large and/or repeated doses of opioids, intrathecal use, advanced age, and concomitant use of intravenous sedatives. The magnitude of postoperative respiratory depression is profoundly influenced by the dose of intrathecal or epidural morphine administered and the type and amount of intravenous analgesics and amnestics used for the intraoperative baseline anesthetic.

References:

1. Chaney MA. Chapter 42: Postoperative Pain Management for the Cardiac Patient. In: Kaplan JA, Augoustides JGT, Manecke GR, et al., eds. Kaplan's Cardiac Anesthesia. 7th ed. Elsevier; 2017:1425-1457.
2. Cohen E. Intrathecal morphine: the forgotten child. J Cardiothorac Vasc Anesth, 2013; 27: 413-416.
3. Latham P, Zarate E, White PF, et al. Fast-track cardiac anesthesia: a comparison of remifentanil plus intrathecal morphine with sufentanil in a desflurane-based anesthetic. J Cardiothorac Vasc Anesth, 2000; 14: 645-651.
4. Kiran U, Zuber K, Kakani M. Intrathecal morphine in patients undergoing minimally invasive direct coronary artery bypass surgery. J Cardiothorac Vasc Anesth, 2005; 19: 815-816.

10. A patient on chronic opioid therapy is prescribed a patient-controlled analgesia (PCA) following coronary artery bypass and mitral valve repair. What is TRUE concerning PCA for pain relief in cardiac surgical patients?

A. In general, studies demonstrate decreased additional morphine-equivalent requirements with PCA

B. In general, studies demonstrate improved respiratory function due to better pain relief with PCA

C. The majority of studies demonstrate no improvement in the immediate postoperative period in pain assessment scores with PCA

D. Atelectasis, determined by chest x-ray, is decreased with PCA

Correct Answer: C

Explanation: Although patient-controlled analgesia (PCA) is a well-established technique that has been used for more than two decades and offers the benefits of reliable analgesic effect and improved patient autonomy, whether it truly offers significant clinical advantages compared with traditional nurse-administered analgesia immediately after cardiac surgery remains to be determined. Several studies have been performed on PCA use after cardiac surgery, with most reporting no difference in the amount of adjunctive opioid requirement and respiratory status. In a study that analyzed atelectasis on chest x-ray, no differences were found in the PCA group versus the control group. Finally, the vast majority of studies find no improvement in pain assessment scores as analyzed by visual analog scale until postoperative day 3 of PCA use.

Most authors surmise that there are additional patient limitations to the effective use of PCA immediately after cardiac surgery, even though patients can obey simple commands and acknowledge discomfort. When analyzed, authors found that patients lacked the ability to understand the requirements of PCA, particularly in the early postoperative period when they were either confused or too weak to operate the demand button.

References:

1. Chaney MA. Chapter 42: Postoperative Pain Management for the Cardiac Patient. In: Kaplan JA, Augoustides JGT, Manecke GR, et al., eds. Kaplan's Cardiac Anesthesia. 7th ed. Elsevier; 2017:1425-1457.
2. Wehrfritz A, Senger AS, Just P, et al. Patient-controlled analgesia after cardiac surgery with median sternotomy: no advantages of hydromorphone when compared to morphine. J Cardiothorac Vasc Anesth, 2022; 36: 3587-3695.
3. Bignami E, Castella A, Pota V, et al. Perioperative pain management in cardiac surgery: a systematic review. Minerva Anestesiol, 2018; 84: 488-503.

11. According to The American Society of Anesthesiologists Task Force on Acute Pain Management in the Perioperative Setting, which combination would be considered a superior analgesic regimen with reduced adverse effect profile?

A. Intravenous ketamine and oral morphine

B. Intravenous ketamine and intravenous fentanyl

C. Intravenous dexmedetomidine and oral fentanyl

D. Oral acetaminophen and intravenous fentanyl

Correct Answer: B

Explanation: The American Society of Anesthesiologists Task Force on Acute Pain Management in the Perioperative Setting reports that the administration of two analgesic agents that act by different mechanisms via a single route provides superior analgesic efficacy with equivalent or reduced adverse effects. The literature is insufficient to evaluate the postoperative analgesic effects of oral opioids combined with nonsteroidal anti-inflammatory drugs, cyclooxygenase–2 inhibitors, or acetaminophen compared to oral opioid alone.

References:

1. Chaney MA. Chapter 42: Postoperative Pain Management for the Cardiac Patient. In: Kaplan JA, Augoustides JGT, Manecke GR, et al., eds. Kaplan's Cardiac Anesthesia. 7th ed. Elsevier; 2017:1425-1457.

2. The American Society of Anesthesiologists Task Force on Acute Pain Management. Practice Guidelines for Acute Pain Management in the Perioperative Setting: An Updated Report by the American Society of Anesthesiologists Task Force on Acute Pain Management. Anesthesiology, 2012; 116: 248-273.

3. Sarica F, Erturk E, Kutanis D, et al. Comparison of thoracic epidural analgesia and traditional intravenous analgesia with respect to postoperative respiratory effects in cardiac surgery. J Cardiothorac Vasc Anesth, 2021; 35: 1800-1805.

12. What is NOT considered a benefit for attaining high-quality postoperative analgesia in cardiac surgery?
  A. Increased hemodynamic instability
  B. Enhanced metabolic stability
  C. Less stress biomarker release
  D. Less hematologic alterations

Correct Answer: A

Explanation: There are numerous advantages to adequate pain relief in the perioperative period. Although there is insufficient evidence to confirm a standard of care for postoperative pain management in cardiac surgery, it is important to achieve quality postoperative analgesia. Obtaining postoperative analgesia is important because it may prevent adverse hemodynamic (tachycardia, hypertension, vasoconstriction), metabolic (increased catabolism), immunologic (impaired immune response), and hemostatic (platelet activation) alterations. Adequate postoperative pain relief is also thought to attenuate the stress response, which is likely partially responsible for the beneficial metabolic and immunologic effects. In general, it is recommended to avoid an intense, single-modality therapy for the treatment of acute postoperative pain. No single technique is clearly superior, as each possess advantages and disadvantages, and multimodal techniques have been shown to be superior.

> **BOX 38.4   Potential clinical benefits of adequate postoperative analgesia**
>
> - Hemodynamic stability
> - Metabolic stability
> - Immunologic stability
> - Hemostatic stability
> - Stress-response attenuation
> - Decreased morbidity

References:

1. Chaney MA. Chapter 42: Postoperative Pain Management for the Cardiac Patient. In: Kaplan JA, Augoustides JGT, Manecke GR, et al., eds. Kaplan's Cardiac Anesthesia. 7th ed. Elsevier; 2017:1425-1457.

2. Sarica F, Erturk E, Kutanis D, et al. Comparison of thoracic epidural analgesia and traditional intravenous analgesia with respect to postoperative respiratory effects in cardiac surgery. J Cardiothorac Vasc Anesth, 2021; 35: 1800-1805.

13. A patient scheduled for a coronary artery bypass graft procedure would like to discuss postoperative pain management options. The patient states that they would like a continuous, direct infusion of local anesthetic into the surgical wound. What is NOT a complication reported to the US Food and Drug Administration related to continuous local anesthetic infusion devices?
  A. Renal failure
  B. Tissue necrosis
  C. Surgical wound infection
  D. Catheter tip migration

Correct Answer: A

Explanation: Pain after cardiac surgery is often related to median sternotomy, peaking during the first 2 postoperative days. An alternative to traditional intravenous opioid analgesia and nonsteroidal anti-inflammatory drugs would be a continuous infusion of local anesthetic. In cardiac surgical patients with sternotomy, ropivacaine and bupivacaine have both been studied as continuous infusions at the sternal wound site. These studies demonstrated better postoperative pain control, earlier ambulation, and reduced length of hospital stay compared with standard of care. In the study that evaluated postoperative pulmonary function, no difference was observed between the groups.

Multiple clinical investigations have reported the use of local anesthetic continuous infiltration devices in a wide variety of surgeries, other than cardiac, and have found adverse events including tissue necrosis, surgical wound infection, and cellulitis. A cardiac surgical analysis of a local anesthetic infusion device observed a catheter tip migration requiring surgical re-exploration.

References:

1. Chaney MA. Chapter 42: Postoperative Pain Management for the Cardiac Patient. In: Kaplan JA, Augoustides JGT, Manecke GR, et al., eds. Kaplan's Cardiac Anesthesia. 7th ed. Elsevier; 2017:1425-1457.

2. Guay J, Kopp SL. Postoperative pain management for cardiac surgery: do we need new blocks? J Cardiothorac Vasc Anesth, 2020; 34: 2994-2995.

3. Tsui BCH, Brodt J, Pan S, et al. Alternating Side Programmed Intermittent Repeated (ASPIRe) bolus regimen for delivering local anesthetic via bilateral interfascial plane catheters. J Cardiothorac Vasc Anesth, 2021; 35: 3143-3145.

14. A patient undergoing coronary artery bypass graft surgery with sternotomy incision receives bilateral intercostal blocks by the surgeon prior to sternal wound closure. What is TRUE regarding an intercostal nerve blocks for sternotomy pain in cardiac surgical patients?
  A. The intercostal nerve block can only be performed following cessation of cardiopulmonary bypass
  B. Intercostal nerve blocks are an inferior pain control option compared to the thoracic epidural technique
  C. An indwelling continuous intercostal nerve infusion catheter is contraindicated due to a potentially high amount of local anesthesia systemic absorption
  D. Intercostal nerve blockade interrupts C-fiber afferent transmission of impulses to the spinal cord

Correct Answer: D

Explanation: Blockade of intercostal nerves interrupts C-fiber afferent transmission of impulses to the spinal cord. The intercostal nerves innervate the major parts of the skin and musculature of the chest, sternum, and abdominal wall. A block of the two dermatomes above and the two dermatomes below the level of surgical incision is required to improve respiratory parameters. Thus, numerous levels will need to be infiltrated for sternal pain following sternotomy.

The intercostal nerve block can be performed prior to cardiopulmonary bypass with sternal opening for hopes of intraoperative analgesia or with wound closure. It can provide lasting analgesia for 6 to 24 hours depending on the amount and type of local anesthetic used. Local anesthetics may be administered via multiple, single-shot injections or via an indwelling intercostal catheter. Although local anesthetic absorption varies (intercostal blocks > caudal > epidural > brachial plexus > sciatic/femoral > subcutaneous), with proper dosing and monitoring local anesthetic administration via intercostal catheters can be safely performed.

References:

1. Chaney MA. Chapter 42: Postoperative Pain Management for the Cardiac Patient. In: Kaplan JA, Augoustides JGT, Manecke GR, et al., eds. Kaplan's Cardiac Anesthesia. 7th ed. Elsevier; 2017:1425-1457.
2. Zhang J, Luo F, Zhang X, et al. Ultrasound-guided continuous parasternal intercostal block relieves postoperative pain after open cardiac surgery: a case series. J Cardiothorac Vasc Anesth, 2022; 36: 2051-2054.
3. Padala SRAN, Badhe AS, Parida S, et al. Comparison of preincisional and postincisional parasternal intercostal block on postoperative pain in cardiac surgery. J Card Surg, 2020; 35: 1525-1530.

15. A 57-year-old patient presents for a robotically assisted mitral valve repair. Medical history is concerning for chronic obstructive pulmonary disease, coronary artery disease, hypothyroidism, low back pain, and chronic pain medication use. At the completion of the procedure the patient has a pain rating of 10/10. Of the given choices, which regional anesthesia technique would be most appropriate at this time?
    A. Interscalene brachial plexus block
    B. Intercostal nerve block
    C. Supraclavicular block
    D. Rectus sheath block

Correct Answer: B

Explanation: Uncontrolled pain in the postanesthesia care unit can cause a reduction in respiratory mechanics, reduced mobility, and increased hormonal and metabolic activity. Deterioration can lead to myocardial ischemia or infarction, cerebrovascular accidents, thromboembolism, delayed wound healing, increased morbidity, and prolonged hospital stay.

The most commonly used nerve block techniques for minimally invasive cardiac surgery and nonsternotomy incisions are intercostal nerve blocks, intrapleural administration of local anesthetic, and thoracic paravertebral block.

All of these blocks can be specified to only the affected surgical side, thus decreasing local anesthetic dose compared with bilateral techniques. Intrathecal and epidural techniques are also effective for thoracotomy incisional pain. The other options would not provide pain relief to the thoracic area.

References:

1. Chaney MA. Chapter 42: Postoperative Pain Management for the Cardiac Patient. In: Kaplan JA, Augoustides JGT, Manecke GR, et al., eds. Kaplan's Cardiac Anesthesia. 7th ed. Elsevier; 2017:1425-1457.
2. Wang S, Li Y, Fei M, Zhang H, et al. Clinical analysis of the effects of different anesthesia and analgesia methods on chronic postsurgical pain in patients with uniportal video-assisted lung surgery. J Cardiothorac Vasc Anesth, 2020; 34: 987-991.
3. Zhang J, Luo F, Zhang X, et al. Ultrasound-guided continuous parasternal intercostal block relieves postoperative pain after open cardiac surgery: a case series. J Cardiothorac Vasc Anesth, 2022; 36: 2051-2054.

16. A patient with chronic pain syndrome and fibromyalgia is scheduled for minimally invasive cardiac surgery via thoracotomy to repair an atrial septal defect. The anesthesia team plans a preoperative unilateral paravertebral block. Which of the following is MOST correct concerning this block?
    A. Unilateral paravertebral blocks are associated with a similar degree of sympathectomy as with an epidural block
    B. Unilateral paravertebral blocks are often associated with a higher serum level of local anesthetic than that achieved with an intercostal nerve block, due to high vascularity of the paravertebral area
    C. Unilateral paravertebral blocks are not likely to be associated with the complication of pneumothorax
    D. Unilateral paravertebral blocks may lead to epidural spread of local anesthetic

Correct Answer: D

Explanation: Paravertebral blocks involve the injection of a local anesthetic adjacent to the thoracic vertebrae close to where the spinal nerves emerge from the intervertebral foramina. Unilateral paravertebral blocks are advantageous in obtaining post-thoracotomy analgesia because one-sided blocks can be performed, which avoids unnecessary nerve blockade of the nonaffected side. This provides the advantage of decreased risk of local anesthetic toxicity due to less local anesthetic being required for this block.

Paravertebral blocks have a reduced sympathectomy compared to epidural or spinal anesthesia. Paravertebral blocks have a reduced local anesthetic systemic absorption compared with intercostal nerve blocks. Two major concerns for potential complications are development of pneumothorax and variable degrees of local anesthetic epidural spread, especially when placing bilateral paravertebral blocks. The risk of epidural spread following a paravertebral block is increased in patients who are hypovolemic.

References:

1. Chaney MA. Chapter 42: Postoperative Pain Management for the Cardiac Patient. In: Kaplan JA, Augoustides JGT, Manecke GR, et al., eds. Kaplan's Cardiac Anesthesia. 7th ed. Elsevier; 2017:1425-1457.
2. D'Ercole, F, Arora H, Kumar PA. Paravertebral block for thoracic surgery. J Cardiothorac Vasc Anesth, 2018; 32: 915-927.
3. Minami K, Yoshitani K, Inatomi Y, et al. A retrospective examination of the efficacy of paravertebral block for patients requiring intraoperative high-dose unfractionated heparin administration during thoracoabdominal aortic aneurysm repair. J Cardiothorac Vasc Anesth, 2015; 29: 937-941.

17. A patient with a history of alcohol abuse and panic attacks presents with complex, occluded left anterior coronary artery disease not amenable to percutaneous coronary intervention. He is scheduled for minimally invasive direct coronary artery bypass grafting via left chest keyhole incisions. Paravertebral blockade is performed preoperatively. After the surgery in the postanesthesia care unit, the patient complains of a new-onset left arm paresthesia and weakness. Vital signs remain stable, along with strong and equal bilateral upper extremity pulses. The MOST likely diagnosis is:
    A. Surgery-related brachial plexus nerve injury
    B. Alcohol withdrawal
    C. Complication of the paravertebral block
    D. Residual paralysis

Correct Answer: A

Explanation: The most likely cause of unilateral brachial plexus distribution findings, such as paresthesia and weakness, is secondary to injury during surgery. The keyhole incisions and instrumentation required for the three to four small chest incisions of minimally invasive coronary artery bypass grafting should be well below the left brachial plexus avoiding direct injury. However, retraction due to the instrumentation can occur. Positioning in the lateral decubitus position can also lead to brachial plexus injuries.

The level of paravertebral blocks in the scenario was the T3 to T6 dermatomes. Therefore, the brachial plexus, which covers the C4 to T1 dermatomes, should not be affected by the paravertebrally injected local anesthetic. Thoracic paravertebral blocks involve injection of local anesthetic adjacent to the thoracic vertebrae close to the spinal nerves emerging from the intervertebral foramina. Alcohol withdrawal does not present with focal weakness, but commonly presents with confusion, anxiety, tachycardia, and hypertension. Residual paralysis would affect all muscle groups and usually presents with respiratory insufficiency.

References:

1. Chaney MA. Chapter 42: Postoperative Pain Management for the Cardiac Patient. In: Kaplan JA, Augoustides JGT, Manecke GR, et al., eds. Kaplan's Cardiac Anesthesia. 7th ed. Elsevier; 2017:1425-1457.
2. D'Ercole, F, Arora H, Kumar PA. Paravertebral block for thoracic surgery. J Cardiothorac Vasc Anesth, 2018; 32: 915-927.

3. Gianoli M, de Jong AR, Jacob KA, et al. Minimally invasive surgery or stenting for left anterior descending artery disease - meta-analysis. Int J Cardiol Heart Vasc, 2022; 40: 101046.

18. Persistent pain after cardiac surgery, defined as pain present 2 or more months after surgery, is reported in almost 30% of patients who undergo cardiac surgery. Which characteristic is not associated with persistent pain after coronary artery bypass graft surgery?
    A. Older age
    B. Postoperative sternal wound infection
    C. Injury to intercostal nerves
    D. Increased pain medication requirement in the postoperative period

Correct Answer: A

Explanation: Persistent pain after cardiac surgery can impair the quality of life of cardiac surgical patients. The cause of persistent pain after sternotomy is multifactorial, yet tissue destruction, intercostal nerve trauma, scar formation, rib fractures, sternal infection, stainless-steel wire sutures, and costochondral separation may all play roles. Such chronic pain is often localized to the arms, shoulders, or legs.

Postoperative brachial plexus neuropathies also may occur and have been attributed to rib fracture fragments, internal mammary artery dissection, suboptimal positioning of the patient during surgery, or central venous catheter placement. Postoperative neuralgia of the saphenous nerve has also been reported after harvesting of saphenous veins for coronary artery bypass grafting.

Younger patients appear to be at greater risk for the development of chronic, long-lasting pain. Some studies report increased postoperative pain medication requirement as a risk for developing persistent pain after cardiac surgery. Despite enhanced postoperative analgesia offered via epidural techniques, such analgesia does not appear to decrease the incidence of persistent pain after cardiac surgery.

References:

1. Chaney MA. Chapter 42: Postoperative Pain Management for the Cardiac Patient. In: Kaplan JA, Augoustides JGT, Manecke GR, et al., eds. Kaplan's Cardiac Anesthesia. 7th ed. Elsevier; 2017:1425-1457.
2. Yu H, Xu Z, Dai SH, et al. The effect of propofol versus volatile anesthetics on persistent pain after cardiac surgery: a randomized controlled trial. J Cardiothorac Vasc Anesth, 2021; 35: 2438-2446.

19. A 47-year-old male is scheduled for elective coronary artery bypass graft ×4 surgery with cardiopulmonary bypass. Due to high doses of preoperative narcotic requirement secondary to chronic back pain, there is concern for severe postoperative pain that will inhibit tracheal extubation and progression of care. Placement of a preoperative thoracic epidural is planned. Which statement is MOST correct concerning this practice?
    A. The patient should be admitted 2 days prior to surgery for epidural placement

B. Epidural analgesia for cardiac surgery decreases persistent pain, defined as pain lasting more than 2 months

C. Epidural analgesia for cardiac surgery decreases mortality

D. Epidural placement for cardiac surgery decreases incidence of dysrhythmia in the postoperative period

Correct Answer: D

Explanation: Although the risk of epidural hematomas is low in cardiothoracic procedures, there are certain precautions that decrease the risk. A neuraxial block should not be performed in a patient with known coagulopathy from any cause. Surgery should be delayed 24 hours in the event of a traumatic tap when placing the neuraxial block.

Systemic intravenous heparin administration can be considered safe if given 1 hour or longer after neuraxial block. Many centers do admit the patient the day prior to cardiac surgery to place the epidural, allowing more than 10 hours from placement to systemic heparinization for cardiopulmonary bypass. Time periods beyond this length are not necessary.

In a large meta-analysis, epidural techniques for cardiac surgical pain did not affect the incidences of mortality or myocardial infarction. However, epidural analgesia was associated with reduced risk for arrhythmias (atrial fibrillation and tachycardia) and pulmonary complications (pneumonia and atelectasis), reduced time to tracheal extubation, and reduced analog pain scores. Despite enhanced postoperative analgesia offered via epidural techniques, such analgesia does not appear to decrease the incidence of persistent pain after cardiac surgery.

References:

1. Chaney MA. Chapter 42: Postoperative Pain Management for the Cardiac Patient. In: Kaplan JA, Augoustides JGT, Manecke GR, et al., eds. Kaplan's Cardiac Anesthesia. 7th ed. Elsevier; 2017:1425-1457.
2. Pisano A, Torella M, Yavorovskiy A, et al. The impact of anesthetic regimen on outcomes in adult cardiac surgery: a narrative review. J Cardiothorac Vasc Anesth, 2021; 35: 711-729.
3. Sarica F, Erturk E, Kutanis D, et al. Comparison of thoracic epidural analgesia and traditional intravenous analgesia with respect to postoperative respiratory effects in cardiac surgery. J Cardiothorac Vasc Anesth, 2021; 35: 1800-1805.
4. Bulte CS, Boer C, Hartemink KJ, et al. Myocardial microvascular responsiveness during acute cardiac sympathectomy induced by thoracic epidural anesthesia. J Cardiothorac Vasc Anesth, 2017; 31: 134-141.

20. Nonsteroidal anti-inflammatory drugs (NSAIDs) are often used as part of multimodal analgesic therapy following cardiac surgery. Some of the potential advantages of adding NSAIDs to a pain regimen include all of the following, EXCEPT:

A. Decreased opioid requirements

B. Decreased postoperative pain intensity

C. Decreased constipation compared with opioid therapy

D. Improved wound healing

Correct Answer: D

Explanation: Recommendations support the administration of two analgesic agents that act by different mechanisms via a single route for providing superior analgesic efficacy with equivalent or reduced adverse effects. Nonsteroidal anti-inflammatory drugs (NSAIDs), in contrast with the opioids' central nervous system mechanism of action, primarily exert their analgesic, antipyretic, and anti-inflammatory effects peripherally by interfering with prostaglandin synthesis after tissue injury. NSAIDs inhibit cyclo-oxygenase, the enzyme responsible for the conversion of arachidonic acid to prostaglandin.

NSAID administration has been shown to decrease opioid requirements, decrease postoperative pain intensity, and indirectly decrease opioid side effects. NSAIDS have several potential side effects and risks, including gastrointestinal bleeding, renal injury, and the potential to impair wound healing. Because all of these adverse effects are common following cardiac surgery, NSAIDs are not the first-line management for pain but are used as adjuncts for patients with inadequate pain control.

References:

1. Chaney MA. Chapter 42: Postoperative Pain Management for the Cardiac Patient. In: Kaplan JA, Augoustides JGT, Manecke GR, et al., eds. Kaplan's Cardiac Anesthesia. 7th ed. Elsevier; 2017:1425-1457.
2. Ochroch J, Usman A, Kiefer J, et al. Reducing opioid use in patients undergoing cardiac surgery - preoperative, intraoperative, and critical care strategies. J Cardiothorac Vasc Anesth, 2021; 35: 2155-2165.

21. A patient is scheduled to have mitral valve repair and aortic valve replacement. Prior to the procedure, what is NOT considered a benefit of adequate postoperative analgesia following cardiothoracic procedures?

A. Hemodynamic stability

B. Stress-response attenuation

C. Normothermia

D. Hemostasis

Correct Answer: C

Explanation: Inadequate analgesia during the intraoperative and postoperative period can lead to adverse outcomes for cardiothoracic patients. Inadequate pain management can lead to hemodynamic instability consisting of tachycardia, hypertension, and vasoconstriction leading to the potential for myocardial ischemia. Pain relief attenuates the stress response during the perioperative period. This is especially important in cardiac surgery, as initiation of cardiopulmonary bypass causes a substantial increase in stress hormones, including norepinephrine and epinephrine. With pain-induced stress, patients can suffer from myocardial ischemia.

Hemostatic alterations, including platelet activation, can also occur due to inadequate analgesia. Adequate analgesia may potentially decrease morbidity in the postoperative period and enhance health-related quality of life. Regulation of body temperature is not directly affected by adequate analgesia.

References:

1. Chaney MA. Chapter 42: Postoperative Pain Management for the Cardiac Patient. In: Kaplan JA, Augoustides JGT, Manecke GR, et al., eds. Kaplan's Cardiac Anesthesia. 7th ed. Elsevier; 2017:1425-1457.
2. Wang S, Li Y, Fei M, Zhang H, et al. Clinical analysis of the effects of different anesthesia and analgesia methods on chronic postsurgical pain in patients with uniportal video-assisted lung surgery. J Cardiothorac Vasc Anesth, 2020; 34: 987-991.

22. A 64-year-old patient is in the intensive care unit after an elective aortic valve replacement. On postoperative day 2, his pain levels have increased, and intravenous fentanyl is administered multiple times. He exhibits respiratory depression, and bilevel positive airway pressure is initiated. What specific opioid receptor caused the respiratory depression in this patient?

A. $\mu 1$ (mu 1)
B. $\mu 2$ (mu 2)
C. κ (kappa)
D. δ (delta)

Correct Answer: B

Explanation: Opioids induce respiratory depression via activation of $\mu 2$-opioid receptors at specific sites in the central nervous system. Currently, three major distinct opioid-receptor types are recognized: mu (μ), kappa (κ), and delta (δ). The μ receptor has two subtypes: a high-affinity $\mu 1$ receptor and a low-affinity $\mu 2$ receptor. The supraspinal mechanisms of analgesia due to opioids are thought to involve $\mu 1$ receptors. The $\mu 2$ receptors affect respiratory depression, spinal analgesia, and gastrointestinal effects. Selective κ agonist may have therapeutic potential in analgesia. $\delta 1$ receptors appear to mediate spinal anesthesia, whereas $\delta 2$ receptors mediate supraspinal analgesia.

References:

1. Chaney MA. Chapter 42: Postoperative Pain Management for the Cardiac Patient. In: Kaplan JA, Augoustides JGT, Manecke GR, et al., eds. Kaplan's Cardiac Anesthesia. 7th ed. Elsevier; 2017:1425-1457.
2. Tempe DK. Opioid stewardship in cardiac anesthesia practice. J Cardiothorac Vasc Anesth, 2022; 36: 2262-2264.
3. Ochroch J, Usman A, Kiefer J, et al. Reducing opioid use in patients undergoing cardiac surgery - preoperative, intraoperative, and critical care strategies. J Cardiothorac Vasc Anesth, 2021; 35: 2155-2165.

23. An 84-year-old patient underwent transcutaneous aortic valve replacement. The case was complicated by femoral arterial hematoma, and the patient received fentanyl boluses during prolonged manual compression of the site. The SpO_2 decreased, and bilevel positive airway pressure ventilation was instituted. What is considered the primary mechanism for the respiratory effect following administration of opioids?

A. Reduction in the sensitivity of the respiratory center in the central nervous system to carbon dioxide

B. Reduction in the sensitivity of peripheral chemoreceptors detecting changes in oxygen tension
C. Reduction of sensory input from the pulmonary and airway mechanoreceptors within the respiratory tract
D. Reduction in sensitivity of baroreceptors located in the aortic arch and carotid sinuses to oxygen tension

Correct Answer: A

Explanation: The purpose of respiration is to maintain adequate oxygenation and remove excess carbon dioxide. Respiratory rhythm is generated in the ventrolateral medulla. Neuronal interactions with several other respiratory nuclei located in the medulla and pons shape the final pattern of rhythmic drive that coordinates the activation of the rib cage and abdominal and upper airway musculature.

The primary respiratory effect of opioids is a reduction in the sensitivity of the respiratory center to carbon dioxide, together with depression of both medullary and peripheral chemoreceptors. The primary respiratory effect of opioids is a reduction in the sensitivity of the respiratory center to carbon dioxide. Initially, respiratory rate is affected more than tidal volume, which may increase. With increasing doses, respiratory rhythmicity is disturbed, resulting in irregular gasping breathing. In addition to retention of carbon dioxide, respiratory depression may also result in hypoxia.

References:

1. Chaney MA. Chapter 42: Postoperative Pain Management for the Cardiac Patient. In: Kaplan JA, Augoustides JGT, Manecke GR, et al., eds. Kaplan's Cardiac Anesthesia. 7th ed. Elsevier; 2017:1425-1457.
2. Ochroch J, Usman A, Kiefer J, et al. Reducing opioid use in patients undergoing cardiac surgery - preoperative, intraoperative, and critical care strategies. J Cardiothorac Vasc Anesth, 2021; 35: 2155-2165.

24. What is NOT a characteristic of remifentanil?
A. Hydrolyzed by plasma and tissue esterases
B. Half-life of 60 seconds
C. Causes muscle rigidity
D. Attains steady state in approximately 3 minutes during continuous infusion

Correct Answer: B

Explanation: Remifentanil has a very fast onset and ultrashort duration of action due to its unique susceptibility to hydrolysis by nonspecific esterases in the blood and tissue. It has an elimination half-life of 10 to 20 minutes, and the time required for a 50% reduction in blood concentration after discontinuation of an infusion is 3 minutes. Caution must be taken when using remifentanil in nonintubated patients, as it is a potent respiratory depressant and can cause muscle rigidity with inability to mask-ventilate.

References:

1. Chaney MA. Chapter 42: Postoperative Pain Management for the Cardiac Patient. In: Kaplan JA, Augoustides JGT, Manecke GR, et al., eds. Kaplan's Cardiac Anesthesia. 7th ed. Elsevier; 2017:1425-1457.

2. Angst MS. Intraoperative use of remifentanil for TIVA: postoperative pain, acute tolerance, and opioid-induced hyperalgesia. J Cardiothorac Vasc Anesth, 2015; 29 Suppl 1: S16-S22.
3. Anwar S, O'Brien B. The impact of remifentanil infusion during cardiac surgery on the prevalence of persistent postsurgical pain. J Cardiothorac Vasc Anesth, 2021; 35: 467-469.

25. A patient is recovering in the intensive care unit after a three-vessel coronary artery bypass graft procedure. Sedation consists of dexmedetomidine. Which of the following physiologic changes are not expected to occur with dexmedetomidine sedation?
A. Decreased heart rate
B. Decreased cardiac output
C. Decreased tidal volume
D. Increased respiratory rate

Correct Answer: D

Explanation: Multiple cardiovascular and respiratory changes occur with alpha-adrenergic agonists, such as dexmedetomidine. The effects on the respiratory system include a decrease in tidal volume, minimal changes to respiratory rate, and a rightward shift and depression of slope of the carbon dioxide response curve. Cardiovascular changes consist of decreased heart rate and decreased systemic vascular resistance, both of which could lead to decreased cardiac output and decreased blood pressure in susceptible patients.

References:

1. Chaney MA. Chapter 42: Postoperative Pain Management for the Cardiac Patient. In: Kaplan JA, Augoustides JGT, Manecke GR, et al., eds. Kaplan's Cardiac Anesthesia. 7th ed. Elsevier; 2017:1425-1457.
2. Gallego-Ligorit L, Vives M, Vallés-Torres J, et al. Use of dexmedetomidine in cardiothoracic and vascular anesthesia. J Cardiothorac Vasc Anesth, 2018; 32: 1426-1438.

26. A patient presents for pectus excavatum surgery. A spinal anesthetic is placed prior to surgery consisting of intrathecal morphine and clonidine. The following are side effects of clonidine administration, EXCEPT:
A. Decreased cardiac contractility
B. Bradycardia
C. Hypotension
D. Decreased systemic vascular resistance

Correct Answer: A

Explanation: Intrathecal anesthesia prior to cardiac surgery can provide intraoperative and postoperative analgesia, as well as postoperative stress-response attenuation. The addition of intrathecal clonidine in various amounts (100 μg or 1 μg/kg) may potentiate intrathecal morphine-induced postoperative analgesia.

Clonidine is an alpha (α2)-adrenergic agonist. Alpha (α2)-adrenergic agonists exhibit analgesia, sedation, and sympatholytic effects, which aid in decreasing anesthetic requirements. Sympatholytic effects following α2-adrenergic agonist administration may present as hypotension, bradycardia, and decreased systemic vascular resistance. Intrathecal or enteral clonidine has negligible, if any, effects on cardiac contractility. Clonidine also produces hypotension by activation of postsynaptic α2-adrenoceptors in the brain stem and by directly inhibiting sympathetic presynaptic α2-adrenoceptor neurons in the spinal cord.

References:

1. Chaney MA. Chapter 42: Postoperative Pain Management for the Cardiac Patient. In: Kaplan JA, Augoustides JGT, Manecke GR, et al., eds. Kaplan's Cardiac Anesthesia. 7th ed. Elsevier; 2017:1425-1457.
2. Nader ND, Li CM, Dosluoglu HH, et al. Adjuvant therapy with intrathecal clonidine improves postoperative pain in patients undergoing coronary artery bypass graft. Clin J Pain, 2009; 25: 101.

27. A 56-year-old patient is scheduled for mitral and tricuspid repair. Preoperatively, the patient is administered celecoxib, a selective cyclo-oxygenase (COX)-2 inhibitor. What is the primary advantage of a COX-2 inhibitor versus a nonselective nonsteroidal anti-inflammatory drug?
A. Lack of effect on platelet function
B. Decrease in opioid requirements
C. Compromised wound healing
D. Less hypotension

Correct Answer: A

Explanation: The primary advantage of cyclo-oxygenase (COX)-2 inhibitors, compared with nonselective nonsteroidal anti-inflammatory drugs (NSAIDs), is the lack of negative effect on platelet function and resultant increased risk of bleeding. NSAIDs that nonselectively inhibit COX-1 inhibit platelet aggregation, which leads to lack of hemostasis. All NSAIDs exert their analgesic, antipyretic, and anti-inflammatory effects peripherally by interfering with prostaglandin synthesis after tissue injury. Additionally, COX-2–selective NSAIDs demonstrate less bronchoconstriction risk in patients with aspirin-induced asthma due to lack of COX-1 inhibition.

Nonselective NSAIDs are inhibitors of both COX-1 and COX-2. Some examples of nonselective NSAIDs are the "-profens" (ibuprofen, ketoprofen, flurbiprofen) and naproxen. COX-2–specific inhibitors have varying degrees of inhibition for the COX-2 isoenzymes. Some examples of COX-2 inhibitors are celecoxib, valdecoxib, and rofecoxib. Neither class of NSAIDs is associated with blood pressure effects, and both are found to decrease opioid requirements.

All NSAIDs may impede reparative inflammatory responses and increase susceptibility to sternal wound infections. Another possible implication of NSAIDs and sternal wound infections is reduced fever and tachycardia due to NSAID use. This delays detection of infection, resulting in further progression and greater consequence.

References:

1. Chaney MA. Chapter 42: Postoperative Pain Management for the Cardiac Patient. In: Kaplan JA, Augoustides JGT, Manecke GR, et al., eds. Kaplan's Cardiac Anesthesia. 7th ed. Elsevier; 2017:1425-1457.
2. Gerstein NS, Gerstein WH, Carey MC, et al. The thrombotic and arrhythmogenic risks of perioperative NSAIDs. J Cardiothorac Vasc Anesth, 2014; 28: 369-378.

28. A 36-year-old male is postoperative day 1 following a surgical aortic valve replacement. His past medical history includes bicuspid aortic valve and asthma. Despite copious opioid administration, he remains in pain. Intravenous ketorolac is given with substantial relief; thus, it is ordered every 8 hours for 2 days. The following are side effects that providers should monitor for in regards to ketorolac administration, EXCEPT:

A. Acute kidney injury
B. Postoperative delirium
C. Asthma exacerbation
D. Bleeding

Correct Answer: B

Explanation: Ketorolac is a nonsteroidal anti-inflammatory drug (NSAID) that acts as a nonselective cyclo-oxygenase (COX) inhibitor, meaning both COX-1 and COX-2 are inhibited. Inhibition of COX-1 leads to inhibition of platelet aggregation, which may lead to bleeding. All NSAIDs exert their analgesic, antipyretic, and anti-inflammatory effects peripherally by interfering with prostaglandin synthesis after tissue injury. Additionally, COX-1 inhibition can lead to asthma exacerbations. NSAIDs likely decrease the incidence of postoperative delirium through opioid sparing.

All NSAIDs have unwanted side effects, including alterations in the gastric mucosal barrier, alterations in renal tubular function, hepatocellular injury, anaphylactoid reactions, tinnitus, and urticaria. Despite these risks, clinical investigations indicate that NSAIDs provide substantial analgesia in patients after cardiac surgery without untoward effects.

References:

1. Chaney MA. Chapter 42: Postoperative Pain Management for the Cardiac Patient. In: Kaplan JA, Augoustides JGT, Manecke GR, et al., eds. Kaplan's Cardiac Anesthesia. 7th ed. Elsevier; 2017:1425-1457.
2. Engoren MC, Habib RH, Zacharias A, et al. Postoperative analgesia with ketorolac is associated with decreased mortality after isolated coronary artery bypass graft surgery in patients already receiving aspirin: a propensity-matched study. J Cardiothorac Vasc Anesth, 2007; 21: 820-826.
3. Oliveri L, Jerzewski K, Kulik A. Black box warning: is ketorolac safe for use after cardiac surgery? J Cardiothorac Vasc Anesth, 2014; 28: 274-279.

29. A 58-year-old female who had mitral valve repair is having difficulty with deep breathing due to pain. Her opioid medication causes nausea, so she is administered ketorolac as an opioid-sparing analgesic. What is TRUE regarding ketorolac?

A. Ketorolac is a selective cyclo-oxygenase–2 inhibitor
B. Ketorolac does not inhibit thromboxane A2
C. Ketorolac does not inhibit prostaglandin I2
D. Ketorolac inhibits platelet aggregation

Correct Answer: D

Explanation: Nonsteroidal anti-inflammatory drugs (NSAIDs) primarily exert their analgesic, antipyretic, and anti-inflammatory effects peripherally by interfering with prostaglandin synthesis after tissue injury. NSAIDs inhibit cyclo-oxygenase (COX) enzymes, which are involved in the conversion of arachidonic acid to prostaglandin, thromboxane, and prostacyclin. COX-1 is involved with platelet aggregation and gastric mucosal protection. COX-2 is involved with pain, inflammation, and fever. Thromboxame A2 (TXA2) has prothrombotic and vasoconstricting properties. Prostacyclin I2, or prostaglandin I2 (PGI2), has antithrombotic and vasodilating properties.

Ketorolac is a nonselective inhibitor of COX-1 and COX-2 enzymes, along with TXA2 and PGI2. Selective COX-2 drugs can be used, but these have fallen out of favor due to a potential increase in thrombotic issues.

References:

1. Chaney MA. Chapter 42: Postoperative Pain Management for the Cardiac Patient. In: Kaplan JA, Augoustides JGT, Manecke GR, et al., eds. Kaplan's Cardiac Anesthesia. 7th ed. Elsevier; 2017:1425-1457.
2. Gerstein NS, Gerstein WH, Carey MC, et al. The thrombotic and arrhythmogenic risks of perioperative NSAIDs. J Cardiothorac Vasc Anesth, 2014; 28: 369-378.
3. Oliveri L, Jerzewski K, Kulik A. Black box warning: is ketorolac safe for use after cardiac surgery? J Cardiothorac Vasc Anesth, 2014; 28: 274-279.

30. A 67-year-old patient is found to have 100% left anterior descending coronary artery occlusion. He is scheduled for urgent minimally invasive direct coronary artery bypass. An epidural is placed in the preoperative bay. Which opioid given epidurally would result in the greatest incidence of delayed respiratory depression?

A. Morphine sulfate
B. Fentanyl
C. Alfentanil
D. Hydromorphone

Correct Answer: A

Explanation: Morphine sulfate has the highest potential for inducing respiratory depression through cephalad migration in the central nervous system following epidural administration. This is due to the hydrophilicity of morphine. The increased hydrophilicity of morphine also increases the duration of action of analgesia. Lipophilic agents, such as fentanyl and sufentanil, have a more localized effect than do hydrophilic opioids, such as morphine sulfate. The major sites of action of opioids are the opiate receptors within the second and third laminae of the substantia gelatinosa in the dorsal horn of the spinal cord.

References:

1. Chaney MA. Chapter 42: Postoperative Pain Management for the Cardiac Patient. In: Kaplan JA, Augoustides JGT, Manecke GR, et al., eds. Kaplan's Cardiac Anesthesia. 7th ed. Elsevier; 2017:1425-1457.

2. Kwanten LE, O'Brien B, Anwar S. Opioid-based anesthesia and analgesia for adult cardiac surgery: history and narrative review of the literature. J Cardiothorac Vasc Anesth, 2019; 33: 808-816.

3. Sarica F, Erturk E, Kutanis D, et al. Comparison of thoracic epidural analgesia and traditional intravenous analgesia with respect to postoperative respiratory effects in cardiac surgery. J Cardiothorac Vasc Anesth, 2021; 35: 1800-1805.

INDEX